— THE —
MINERAL FIX

How to Optimize Your Mineral Intake
for Energy, Longevity, Immunity, Sleep and More

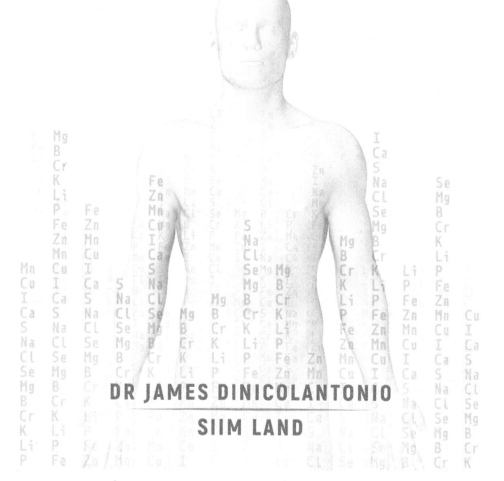

DR JAMES DINICOLANTONIO
SIIM LAND

The Mineral Fix

How to Optimize Your Mineral Intake for Energy, Longevity, Immunity, Sleep and More.

Dr. James DiNicolantonio

author of The Salt Fix

Siim Land

author of Metabolic Autophagy

DISCLAIMER

Table of Contents

About the Authors

James DiNicolantonio, PharmD
As a cardiovascular research scientist and Doctor of Pharmacy Dr. James J. DiNicolantonio has spent years researching nutrition. A well-respected and internationally known scientist and expert on health and nutrition, he has contributed extensively to health policy and medical literature.

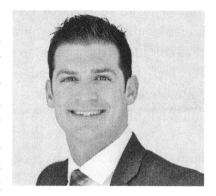

Dr. DiNicolantonio is the author of 4 best-selling health books, The Salt Fix, Superfuel, The Longevity Solution and The Immunity Fix. His website is www.drjamesdinic.com. You can follow Dr. DiNicolantonio on Twitter and Instagram at @drjamesdinic and Facebook at Dr. James DiNicolantonio.

He is the author or co-author of more than 250 medical publications, including several high-profile articles related to nutrition, including a December 2014 opinion piece about sugar addiction in *The New York Times* that was the newspaper's most emailed article during the 24 hours following its publication. Dr. DiNicolantonio has testified in front of the Canadian Senate regarding the harms of added sugars and serves as the Associate Editor of British Medical Journal's (BMJ) Open Heart, a journal published in partnership with the British Cardiovascular Society. He is also on the Editorial Advisory Board of several other medical journals, including Progress in Cardiovascular Diseases and International Journal of Clinical Pharmacology & Toxicology.

Siim Land

Siim Land is an author, speaker, content creator and renown biohacker from Estonia. Despite his young age, he is considered one of the top people in the biohacking and health optimization community with thousands of followers worldwide.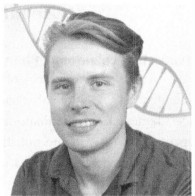

Siim Land has written books like Metabolic Autophagy, Stronger by Stress and The Immunity Fix. His website is www.siimland.com. You can follow Siim on Instagram @siimland and as Siim Land on YouTube.

Siim started researching and doing self-experiments with nutrition, exercise, and other strategies to improve his performance and health after high school when he enrolled in the military for a year. He then obtained a bachelor's degree in anthropology in Tallinn University and University of Durham in the UK. By now he has written several books about diet, creates content online, and keeps himself up to date with the latest knowledge in science.

Introduction

You might have heard the term *micro*nutrients before. These are the smaller nutrients (hence the term micro) that are found in the foods that you eat. Examples of micronutrients are vitamins and minerals. Many of them, but not all of them, are considered essential for maintaining healthy physiological functioning of the body and thus need to be consumed from the diet. For example, micronutrient deficiencies during pregnancy, such as a lack of folic acid, iodine, zinc or iron can lead to birth defects or preterm birth.[1] Maintaining adequate nutrient status, especially b-vitamins and omega-3s, may slow or reduce cognitive decline in aging[2]. Thus, getting appropriate amounts of micronutrients can prevent severe acute consequences or prevent the decline in your health. To put this differently, your nutrition directly determines how well you age.

When we think of nutrition, many debate about what percentage of calories should come from *macro*nutrients (carbs, fats and protein). Those following a ketogenic diet tend to eat a higher fat, moderate protein, lower carbohydrate diet, while a more plant-based diet is higher in carbs, moderate in protein, and lower in fat. Then there are the high protein advocates who believe in consuming more protein because they tend to be more active and have more muscle. Regardless of which macronutrient camp you fall under all of us need to consume micronutrients.

Don't let the term 'micro' fool you. Micronutrients do not have a micro effect on your health. In fact, when it comes to your health *micro*-nutrients have *macro*-effects on your healthspan and lifespan. This is because micronutrients are what your body uses to perform nearly all of its tasks such as regulating your heartbeat, allowing your body to cool off when it's too hot, synthesizing energy (ATP), DNA and protein. If you can think of a physiological function in the body, there is a good chance that micronutrients are involved. Many enzyme systems in the human body require micronutrients as cofactors[3].

Essential macronutrients include protein and fat, whereas the body can synthesize glucose making dietary carbohydrates technically non-essential [4] . However, **this book focuses on micronutrients, specifically minerals.** Just like with fats and protein, there are essential minerals that must be consumed otherwise we perish. Another example of essential micronutrients are vitamins. There are minerals that are considered non-essential and yet if we are not obtaining enough of them in the diet this can lead to worse health outcomes. Thus, both essential and non-essential minerals are extremely important for health and longevity.

The criteria for essential nutrients were established in the 1960s and 1970s[5,6,7,8]. It included the following requirements:

1. The element must be able to react with biological materials or form chelates.
2. The element must be ubiquitous in sea waters and the earth's crust. In other words, it had to be present during the evolution of many organisms and the development of their essential functions.
3. The element must be present in a significant amount in living animals.
4. The element should be toxic only at extremely high intakes compared to regular nutritional intakes.
5. The body should have homeostatic mechanisms for regulating the element's levels consistently.
6. Deficiencies in the element must have consistent and adverse effects on the body's biological functions and this change is reversible or preventable with physiological intakes of the element.

In the Western world, you would have a hard time finding someone who is deficient in macronutrients, e.g., carbs, fats or protein. However, **much of the population is deficient in micronutrients and in particular minerals.** It's not only likely that you are *deficient* in numerous minerals, but **a large percentage of the general population has a *suboptimal* level of at least one mineral in their body**[9]. For example, there is a big difference in preventing a frank nutrient deficiency, such as scurvy, which causes bleeding gums and visible bruising, versus a suboptimal intake of vitamin C, which increases your risk of cardiovascular disease. Preventing scurvy only requires around 7-10 mg of vitamin C per day, whereas to fully saturate all body tissues with vitamin C and provide *optimal* antioxidant protection, around 1,000 mg of vitamin C per day (500 mg twice daily) or more may be needed[10]. In other words, with vitamin C, there is a 100-fold difference between an intake that prevents frank deficiency (10 mg/day) and an intake that provides optimal health (1,000 mg/day).

Another example would be magnesium. You can prevent frank magnesium deficiency by only consuming around 150-180 mg per day, however, optimal intakes of magnesium sit anywhere from 450 to 1,800 mg per day or more[11]. Thus, **there can be a 10 or even a 100-fold difference in the amount of a micronutrient that prevents a frank deficiency versus one that provides optimal health and longevity. That is the key message of this book!** In the following pages, we will reveal what those optimal intakes are for each mineral based on the evidence in the medical literature.

There are two kinds of minerals: macrominerals, which you need rather large amounts of, typically more than 100 milligrams (mg) per day, **and trace minerals**, which are typically consumed in amounts less than 100 mg per day.

There are 17 *essential* **minerals**, although there is considerable debate on this number [12] . However, in general, there are **7 essential macrominerals and 10 essential trace minerals**. These essential minerals cannot be produced by the body and are considered essential to get in the diet in order for us to live. **There are at least 5 minerals that could be considered essential** but have yet to be deemed as such. Below is a list of these minerals, their food sources, and the recommended dietary allowance (RDA) or adequate intake (AI) for each in adults 19 years or older. It is important to note that **the RDA/AI is to prevent mineral deficiencies and does not represent an optimal mineral intake.**

17 Essential Minerals

7 Macrominerals (in general you need more than 100 mg of each per day)

Macromineral	Dietary Sources	RDA/AI in adults
Calcium	Spinach, nuts, dairy & mineral waters	1,000-1,200 mg
Chloride	Salt, seaweed, celery	Upper limit is typically set at 3,600 mg or 1 tsp of salt. However, intake depends on salt needs.
Magnesium	Spinach, nuts, seeds, meat, whole grains & mineral waters	400-420 mg
Phosphorus	Meat	700 mg
Potassium	Potatoes, beans, greens, tomatoes and fish	2,600-3,400 mg
Sodium	Salt	Upper limit is usually set at 2,300 mg but this will change based on salt loss.
Sulfur	Garlic, onions, eggs, Brussel sprouts & mineral water	No RDA set

10 Trace Minerals (in general you need less than 100 mg of each per day)

Trace mineral	Dietary sources	RDA/AI in adults
Chromium	Brewer's yeast, lobster, mushrooms, chicken, shrimp, black pepper & broccoli	25-35 mcg
Cobalt	Liver, fish & beef (comes from food sources of B12 or cobalamin)	No RDA but 10-20 mcg has been suggested
Copper	Liver, oysters, potatoes, mushrooms, shellfish, nuts, seeds and whole grains	0.9 mg
Fluoride	Black tea, coffee, shrimp, raisins and grapes	3-4 mg
Iodine	Seaweed or nori, oysters, milk, eggs, pink salt, iodized salt, liver, cheese, shrimp & tuna	150 mcg (220 to 290 mcg for pregnancy and lactation, respectively)
Iron	Oysters, white beans, dark chocolate, liver, lentils, red meat, sardines & spinach	8 mg for men and 18 mg for women (19-50), 8 mg for men and women 51 years and older.
Manganese	Mussels, whole grains, hazelnuts, pecans, brown rice, oysters, clams, chickpeas,	1.8-2.3 mg

	spinach, pineapple and almonds	
Molybdenum	Black-eyed peas, beef liver, lima beans, yogurt, milk, potatoes and bananas	45 mcg
Selenium	Brewer's yeast, selenium from yeast, brazil nuts, tuna, halibut, sardines, ham, shrimp & beef	55 mcg
Zinc	Oysters, beef, crab, lobster, pork, baked beans, chicken, pumpkin seeds, yogurt, cashews & cheese	8-11 mg

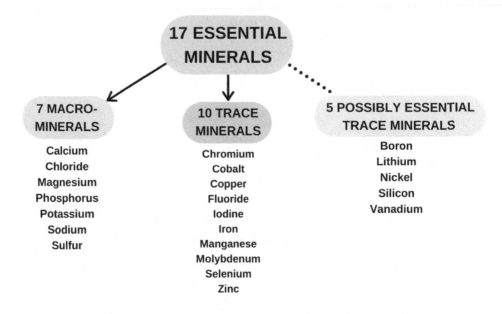

17 ESSENTIAL MINERALS

7 MACRO-MINERALS

Calcium
Chloride
Magnesium
Phosphorus
Potassium
Sodium
Sulfur

10 TRACE MINERALS

Chromium
Cobalt
Copper
Fluoride
Iodine
Iron
Manganese
Molybdenum
Selenium
Zinc

5 POSSIBLY ESSENTIAL TRACE MINERALS

Boron
Lithium
Nickel
Silicon
Vanadium

5 Possibly Essential Trace Minerals

Trace mineral	Dietary Sources	RDA/AI in adults
Boron	Prunes, raisins, almonds, peanuts, hazelnuts, dates & apples	No RDA/AI established but a diet high in boron is considered to contain 3.25 mg/2,000 calories[13]
Lithium	Mineral water, grains, vegetables, mustard, kelp, pistachios, dairy, fish and meat	No RDA/AI
Nickel	Black tea, nuts and seeds, cacao, chocolate, meat, fish and grains	No RDA/AI
Silicon	Whole grains, fruits & vegetables	No RDA/AI
Vanadium	Mushrooms, shellfish, black pepper, beer, wine, grains and certain unrefined salts	No RDA/AI

Looking at the below data we can see how dismal the situation really is when it comes to the prevalence of mineral deficiencies in the United States. **Based on 2,000 hair samples, JD Campbell noted in 2001 that:**

The 12 most common mineral deficiencies were[14]

1.Chromium (56%)

2.Magnesium (49%)

3.Zinc (47%)

4.Calcium (46%)

5.Manganese (40%)

6.Selenium (40%)

7.Potassium (37%)

8.Iron (25%)

9.Copper (25%)

10.Molybdenum (15%)

11.Phosphorus (9%)

12.Sodium (6%)

It's important to note that hair mineral analysis is a longer-term reflection of the mineral status in blood. However, we know that blood mineral levels do not necessarily reflect overall mineral status. Although to be fair, **typically when the body is deficient in a mineral, blood levels will be on the low-normal end and this would also be reflected in the hair.** However, many factors affect mineral levels in the blood and hence hair mineral analysis. In particular, high levels of **inflammation**, as found in infections, Rheumatoid arthritis and other inflammatory disorders, **can cause levels of iron, zinc and selenium to drop in the blood and hence in the hair. High amounts of inflammation can increase copper levels in the blood and in the hair even when there is copper deficiency.** Thus, hair mineral analysis has limitations considering that many things can affect the mineral status in the blood (and hence in the hair). Thus, hair mineral analysis needs to be treated with extreme caution although as it is a better tool for determining heavy metal toxicity.

In general, there isn't one test that can tell you whether you are deficient in a mineral. Indeed, it takes at least 2 or more tests to diagnose subclinical mineral deficiencies. Subclinical deficiency meaning there isn't anything apparently wrong with you on the surface but because you are ingesting a suboptimal amount of one or more minerals you may have weaker bones (osteoporosis), atherosclerosis or calcifications that are building up in your arteries (cardiovascular disease) or your brain is accumulating amyloid beta plaques (reduced cognition). On the outside, you appear fine, but on the inside, you are essentially rusting and breaking down. Later in the book, we will cover the best tests for measuring mineral status as each mineral has different tests to better determine its levels in the body.

When it comes to mineral intake in the United States, we know that the outlook is bad. Based on the National Health and Nutrition Examination Survey (NHANES) 2007-2010 (2009-2014 for potassium) and the United States Department of Agriculture 2009 data

The % of the U.S. population not meeting the RDA or AI for minerals is as follows[15,16,17]

1. Boron (no RDA established, > 75% are likely deficient based on our estimate)

2. Manganese (~75%, *our estimate*)

3. Magnesium (52.2-68%)

4. Potassium (~ 50-60%)

5. Calcium (44.1-73%)

6. Zinc (42%)

7. Iron (34%)

8. Copper (31%)

9. Selenium (15%)

Neither of the above data looked at manganese intake but considering that adult females need 1.8 mg and adult males need 2.3 mg per day it's highly likely that around 75% of U.S. adults are not hitting the RDA for manganese. This is because manganese is an extremely difficult nutrient to obtain in the diet unless you are eating mussels, oysters, certain nuts or unrefined whole grains.

Based on the above data and estimated dietary intakes, approximately:

- **1 out of every 3 people in the United States has at least 10 minerals they are deficient in**
  - Those 10 minerals being **potassium, manganese, magnesium, calcium, zinc, iron, copper, selenium, chromium, molybdenum and boron**.
  - Thus, **about a third of the U.S. population is likely deficient in the below 10 minerals** (estimated % not hitting RDA/AI or estimated % deficient)
    1. Boron (> 75%)
    2. Manganese (~ 75%)
    3. Magnesium (52.2-68%)
    4. Chromium (56%)
    5. Calcium (44.1-73%)
    6. Zinc (42-47%)
    7. Iron (25-34%)
    8. Copper (25-31%)
    9. Selenium (15-40%)
    10. Molybdenum (15%)

Why Are So Many of Us Deficient in Minerals?

Here are the main reasons for such widespread mineral and overall nutrient deficiencies:

Number 1: The Overconsumption of Highly Refined Foods

How could so many people be mineral deficient? If anything, people overeat in the United States so what's the deal? The reasons are many. For example, the foods we eat today are highly refined with many of the minerals stripped from them during their processing. This is the classic case of 'overfed but undernourished'. In fact, **being overfed and undernourished is probably the biggest reason why people are suffering from chronic disease and early death**.

At the time Campbell published his hair mineral analysis paper in 2001, the average American was consuming 134 pounds of sugar per year! Annual intakes of other refined foods included 756 doughnuts, 60 pounds of cakes and cookies, 23 gallons of ice cream, 7 pounds of potato chips, 22 pounds of candy, 365 servings of soda pop, and 90 pounds of pure fat[18]. Thus, **the most likely reason why so many of us are mineral deficient is because of the overconsumption of highly refined foods**. Not only do these foods lack minerals but they also require minerals to liberate their calories[19] and they also damage the body so that it starts to lose minerals out the stool and the urine[20,21]. The inflammation that occurs in the body when we overconsume these processed foods also increases mineral demand as more minerals get shunted towards antioxidant enzymes to handle increased oxidative stress rather than being utilized for other essential purposes. Many of these processed foods also induce high insulin levels, which cause us to lose calcium and magnesium out the urine and insulin resistance reduces the entry of magnesium and potassium into the cell[22]. Talk about a triple-whammy to your mineral status!

Essentially, **the more refined foods you eat the more micronutrient depleted you become**!

Number 2: Soil Erosion, Fertilizers, Pesticides, Herbicides and Insecticides

Plants get their nutrients from the soil and animals get their nutrients from plants. Thus, the more nutrient depleted the soil is, the fewer nutrients the vegetation growing on it will have. In just the last 70 to 80 years, the micronutrient content of food has plummeted[23]. Between 1940-1999, the amount of magnesium in vegetables has decreased by 24%, in fruit by 17%, in meat by 15%, and in cheese by 26%[24]. The reduction in magnesium in vegetables from the 1930s to the 1980s was approximately 35% in the UK[25]. In the U.K. from 1840 to 2000, the mineral reduction in wheat was, copper (-33%), magnesium (-33%), iron (-25%) and zinc (-38%)[26].

The food that we now eat is about 30% less nutritious than the same food from 1940. That means you literally need to eat 30% more food to get the same level of minerals that someone used to get who lived just 80 years ago. And who knows how less nutritious our food was back in 1940 compared to what we evolved eating tens of thousands of years ago. We could literally need to eat 2 to 3 times as much food to get the same levels of minerals we got during Paleolithic times.

The majority of the population already suffers from overfeeding. Approximately 34% of U.S. adults have metabolic syndrome[27] and approximately 42% are obese[28]. About 1.9 billion people worldwide are overweight and 650 million are obese (with a BMI above 25-30)[29]. Thus, trying to eat more could add fire to the flames of obesity and insulin resistance. **The problem lies in not getting enough calories and macronutrients but missing out on the key micronutrients, especially minerals.**

MINERAL DEPLETION OVER TIME

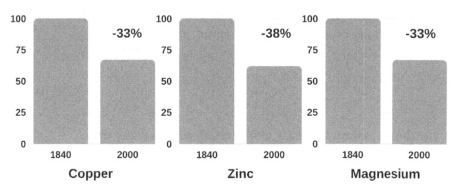

MINERAL CONTENT IN WHEAT

Data from: Mayer (1997) and Davis (2011)[30,31]

The reduction of minerals in our food is the result of using pesticides and fertilizers that kill off beneficial bacteria, earthworms, and bugs in the soil that create many of the essential nutrients in the first place and inhibit the uptake of nutrients into the plant. Fertilizing crops with nitrogen, phosphorus and potassium has led to declines in magnesium, zinc, iron and iodine[32]. For example, there has been on average about a 30% decline in the magnesium content of wheat. This is partly due to potassium being an antagonist for magnesium absorption by plants. Lower magnesium levels in soil also occur with acidic soils and around 70% of the arable land on earth is now acidic[33]. Thus, the overall characteristics of soil determines the accumulation of minerals in plants. Indeed, nowadays our soil is less healthy and so are the plants grown on them.

Even the seeds of today are lower in nutrients than before. For example, wheat seed micronutrient contents in Kansas from 1920 to 2000 showed decreases in numerous minerals including zinc (-11 to -31%), iron (-24%) and selenium (-16%)[34]. The way we grow broccoli has also led to reductions in the manganese content by around 27% compared to 1950[35].

Other issues that damage the soil's nutrient content include possible mineral binding due to the herbicide glyphosate making minerals less available to plants. Indeed, glyphosate drift has been found to reduce the concentrations of calcium, manganese, and magnesium in young leaves of non-glyphosate resistant soybean plants and the seed concentrations of calcium, magnesium, iron and manganese[36]. These results suggest that glyphosate may interfere with the uptake of several minerals by binding and forming complexes with them.

Number 3: Heavy Metals Competing with Absorption

Heavy metals like aluminum, lead, cadmium, arsenic, and mercury can accumulate in the food supply from industrial pollution. These heavy metals can compete for mineral absorption as well as mineral binding sites on enzymes. Thus, heavy metals deplete and reduce the functions of minerals in the body.

One of the best ways to prevent against heavy metal toxicity is by eating a diet high in minerals due to competition for absorption. This is why, for example, **the selenium to mercury ratio of seafood matters more than the overall mercury content** as selenium reduces mercury toxicity[37,38] and in many instances foods that are highest in mercury, such as tuna, are also very high in selenium.

Based on the same 2,000-hair sample study by Campbell it was noted that:

The 5 most common heavy metal toxins in the body are[39]

1. Aluminum (9.4%)

2. Lead (3.0%)

3. Cadmium (0.8%)

4. Arsenic (0.1%)

5. Mercury (0.1%)

Our modern environment exposes us to a lot of heavy metals and other pollutants than ever before. Besides urban areas, fossil fuels, and food, we also get heavy metals from skin care products, shampoos and medications. We will discuss more about heavy metals later in the book.

Heavy metals also increase inflammation in the body, which can increase the body's mineral requirements, as there is a greater need for antioxidant enzymes to counteract heavy metal-induced inflammation. It just so happens that some of our antioxidant enzymes, such as superoxide dismutase is made up of minerals. For example, there is copper,zinc-superoxide dismutase (Cu,ZnSOD). There is another superoxide dismutase in the mitochondria that needs manganese to function (MnSOD). Glutathione peroxidase and peroxiredoxin, both of which helps handle hydrogen peroxide, requires selenium. Selenium is needed to reduce thioredoxin, which donates an electron to peroxiredoxin to help it reduce and take care of hydrogen peroxide. Peroxiredoxin is also needed to reduce the toxic oxidant peroxynitrite, which is formed when superoxide combines with nitric oxide. Hence, selenium is needed to also handle peroxynitrite. Thioredoxin reductase and methionine sulfoxide reductase also require selenium and both are needed to protect methionine residues on proteins from oxidizing and to recycle them once they get oxidized. Thus, **our mineral status helps determine how resistant our cells are to inflammation and oxidative stress and how well they repair after damage has ensued.** Moreover, a lack of certain minerals can reduce other antioxidant levels in the body. For example, **magnesium deficiency can reduce glutathione levels and increase the susceptibility of our tissues to oxidative stress**[40]. This may be due to the requirement for magnesium for the synthesis of glutathione in red blood cells[41]. Thus, **antioxidant levels in the body are dependent on both the mineral and heavy metal status of the body.**

Why Do Mineral Deficiencies Matter? Because They Drive Most Chronic Disease!

So now that you know about minerals and how common their deficiencies are, why does any of this matter? Well, mineral deficiencies matter because they drive, or contribute to, nearly all chronic diseases. Take magnesium deficiency for example, which can cause elevated blood lipids, high blood pressure, atherosclerosis, coronary heart disease, sudden cardiac death, heart failure, kidney stones, and more[42]. That's what can happen with just one mineral deficiency!

While a death certificate might state that someone died from a heart attack, this doesn't reveal the true underlying cause of why the heart attack occurred. Both animal and human studies suggest that magnesium deficiency can cause plaque to build up in the coronary arteries as well as coronary vasospasms, both of which can actually *cause* a heart attack[43].

We need to treat the underlying causes of chronic diseases not just manage them with medications, which are typically just band-aids. There is no such a thing as an aspirin deficiency or a statin deficiency. And while these medications may provide *some* benefit, they aren't treating the underlying cause of chronic diseases like cardiovascular disease. If we start to look for the underlying causes of disease, we can start preventing them from occurring in the first place. As the saying goes, an ounce of prevention is worth a pound of cure! That is why there is a tremendous need for research into finding the best ways to diagnose subclinical mineral deficiencies and getting the health care system to pay for these tests so everyone around the world can be checked for these deficiencies.

Imagine if you could walk into a doctor's office and get screened for 22 mineral deficiencies. That could tell you a lot about your diet and overall health. Unfortunately, our healthcare system isn't built this way. However, our body is built out of minerals and there is a minimum amount that we must consume every day otherwise we slowly become depleted in them. The Mineral Fix will provide you with the information about not only the minimum amount of minerals that are needed to survive but the optimal amount of minerals to thrive!

Chapter 1
How Minerals Drive the Body's Essential Processes

The importance of minerals cannot be understated. They are necessary for virtually all bodily processes, starting with energy production and ending with hormonal balance. Chronic deficiencies in these nutrients will eventually lead to diseases and suboptimal wellbeing because there aren't enough resources to carry out essential functions for health.

In this chapter, we will go through the essential processes in the body that require minerals to function properly. By the end of it, you will realize that it's the minerals that are driving the entire show and supporting the pathways that lead to optimal health.

Minerals Driving Energy Production

Every chemical reaction involved in life, especially the assimilation of calories and nutrients from food, is collectively called metabolism. Its purpose is to convert food into energy, building blocks in the body and the removal of waste material. Our metabolism is divided into catabolism (breaking down) and anabolism (building up). There are numerous metabolic pathways wherein each step is governed by specific enzymes. Enzymes work like catalysts that initiate metabolic processes and regulate their expression. The most basic metabolic pathways are remarkably similar across species and life forms[44].

You might remember from your high school chemistry class that: **the mitochondria are the powerhouse of the cell.** That's technically correct, as the mitochondria are a type of organelle inside cells that help to convert the food we eat into smaller molecules and produce ATP or the energy currency in our body. In total, there are **up to 22 vitamins and minerals that support mitochondrial enzymes and are needed for energy production**[45]. **Minerals also help to activate**

antioxidant enzymes that protect the mitochondria from oxidative stress. Deficiencies in these minerals can lead to a reduction in ATP production, mitochondrial degradation [46] and can accelerate mitochondrial aging[47]. Organs with the highest energy requirements and the highest concentration of mitochondria, such as the heart, liver and the brain, will be affected the most by this depletion, speeding up the aging process[48].

Energy, or ATP, is one of the most essential currencies needed for all bodily processes, including maintenance of health and resilience against disease. Ventilated patients in the ICU show a compromised ability to produce ATP (about 50% less ATP synthesis in skeletal muscle mitochondria)[49]. This is called bioenergetic failure and it's associated with ICU weakness[50] and severity in septic shock[51]. The number of mitochondria and their function was reduced in the skeletal muscle of these patients. The lack of movement in these patients, and a reduction in GLUT4 translocation and/or insulin resistance, likely led to a reduction in glucose delivery into the muscle and hence a reduction in ATP production and weakness[52].

Importantly, magnesium is needed as a cofactor in several electron transport chain complex subunits, including methylenetetra-hydrofolate dehydrogenase 2 and pyruvate dehydrogenase phosphatase[53], and controls GLUT4 translocation to the cell membrane surface[54]. GLUT4 is a glucose transporter that helps bring glucose into the cell for energy production. Thus, magnesium deficiency can contribute to a lack of ATP production in the mitochondria[55]. The ability to replenish functional mitochondria is an independent predictor of survival in those who are critically ill[56]. Importantly, **minerals are extremely important for preventing mitochondrial dysfunction, growing new mitochondria (called mitochondrial biogenesis) and improving mitochondrial function, especially magnesium**[57,58].

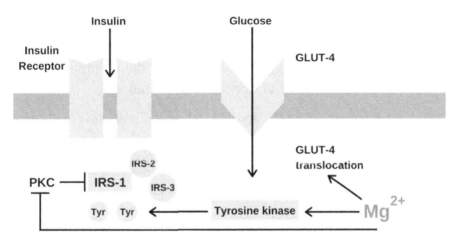

Magnesium is required for insulin action & glucose utilization

Adapted from Takaya J, Higashino H and Kobayashi Y. Intracellular magnesium and insulin resistance. Magnesium Research. 2004;17(2):126-135.

ATP and energy production are fundamentally dependent on vitamins and minerals. **Insufficient micronutrient status results in poor ATP production in the mitochondria.** The health of the mitochondria also controls the production of hormones, regulates the immune system, metabolism, fat loss, muscle growth, sleep, mood, and so much more. Thus, your micronutrient status will determine your overall health.

Almost every eukaryotic cell has mitochondria. The inner mitochondrial membrane contains the electron transport chain (ETC), which is a series of 5 complexes that transfers electrons and protons across the membrane. This drives the creation of ATP by complex V (otherwise known as ATP synthase). Energy containing cofactors like NADH and coenzymes like FADH are used to deliver electrons to the electron transport chain for ATP production[59]. The entire ETC is comprised of a series of enzymatic events wherein electrons are being passed on until they reach oxygen. This passage of electrons releases energy, which is used to transport protons into the intermembrane space[60]. During aerobic respiration, this process is called oxidative phosphorylation.

Nicotinamide adenine dinucleotide or NAD+ is a co-enzyme that's found in all living cells. It's required for carrying out many vital biological processes in the body. NAD+ helps turn nutrients into energy and controls energy homeostasis[61]. In the electron transport chain, NAD+ functions as an electron transfer molecule.

NAD has two forms: NAD+ and NADH which both govern electron transfer reactions:

- NAD+ is an oxidizing agent that picks up electrons from other molecules and thus becomes reduced.

- NADH is a reducing agent that forms from reduced NAD+ and it can then be used to donate electrons to other molecules, thus becoming NAD+ again.

Electrons of NADH can store energy that gets converted into ATP in the mitochondria during oxidative phosphorylation. A higher NAD+ to NADH ratio creates more readily available energy and makes the cells produce their own energy more efficiently. An abundance of energy from food raises NADH and lowers NAD+ levels. This type of NAD cycling helps with transporting electrons around and producing energy. It's also important for vitality and health.

There are 5 membrane-bound complexes in the mitochondrial electron transport chain – complex I, II, III, IV and V. They are all embedded inside the inner mitochondrial membrane. Here is an overview of their role and function:

- **Complex I** – In complex I, NADH gets stripped of two electrons that get transported to a lipid-soluble carrier called ubiquinone (Q). Every electron passes through an iron-sulfur cluster. As electrons become oxidized and reduced, an electron current gets formed, which powers the transport of 4 protons per 2 electrons of NADH into the intermembrane space[62,63].

- **Complex II** – In complex II, additional electrons are delivered to Q by succinate dehydrogenase (SDHA), fatty acids, glycerol 3-phosphate, and other electron donors. Complex II doesn't carry any protons into the intermembrane space, thus contributing less total energy to the electron transport chain.
- **Complex III** – In complex III, electrons are carried to cytochrome c within the intermembrane space through a proton movement system called the Q-cycle. It works by sequential oxidation and reduction of coenzyme Q10 (CoQ10).
- **Complex IV** – In complex IV, 4 electrons are removed from the 4 molecules of cytochrome c and transported to molecular oxygen (O_2). This creates 2 water molecules. Complex IV contains copper ions and multiple heme groups.
- **Complex V (ATP synthase)** – Complex V is also called ATP synthase because it generates ATP from ADP and inorganic phosphate created by the proton electrochemical gradient[64]. ATP synthase consists of two sub-units F_O and F_1, which work as a rotational motor[65]. Calcium stimulates ATP synthase[66].

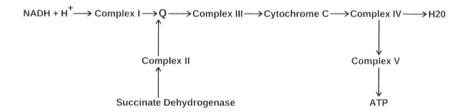

It is important to note that **oxidative stress directly reduces ATP production by inhibiting the above complexes of the respiratory chain**. Peroxynitrite is one example of an ETC complex inhibitor and as you will find out in Chapter 2, minerals are needed to make the cells resistant from oxidative stress[67].

Carbohydrates, proteins, fatty acids and ketones will ultimately be broken down into acetyl-CoA, which then delivers the acetyl group into the citric acid cycle (TCA or Krebs cycle). Acetyl-CoA created from carbohydrates happens via glycolysis and via beta-oxidation from fatty acids. **These pathways require zinc, magnesium and chromium**[68]**, which ensure the capacity for energy expenditure and muscle performance**[69]. Zinc is required to form pyruvic acid from lactic acid – the metabolic product of glucose metabolism[70]. Several reports have shown that **selenium deficiency causes defects in mitochondrial structure, integrity, and electron transport chain function** [71, 72]. Removal of extracellular magnesium ion inhibits glycolysis and limits glucose transport by red blood cells[73]. **The availability of zinc, iron and chromium are necessary for the synthesis of insulin and glucose utilization, which contributes to ATP production by the mitochondria**[74]. Mitochondrial fat oxidation, which also contributes to ATP production, is initiated by calcium[75]. Calcium is a key regulator of mitochondrial function because it is involved in many mitochondrial enzymes, such as pyruvate dehydrogenase and α-ketoglutarate dehydrogenase as a cofactor[76].

These are the minerals needed to create ATP (energy) in the body

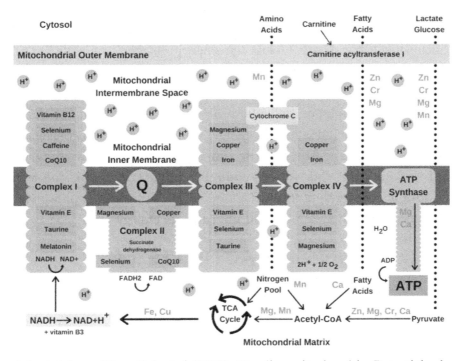

Adapted from: Wesselink et al (2019), 'Feeding mitochondria: Potential role of nutritional components to improve critical illness convalescence.' Clinical Nutrition, 38(3), 982–995.

Ca = calcium, Cr = chromium, Cu = copper, Fe = iron, Mg = magnesium, Mn = manganese and Zn = zinc.

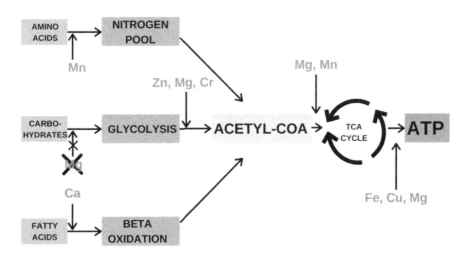

The entry of acetyl-CoA into the TCA cycle needs magnesium and manganese, which creates NADH and FADH2 to then feed into the electron transport chain (which needs iron and copper) to produce adenosine triphosphate (ATP) the energy currency of cells[77]. All reactions where ATP is involved require magnesium ions[78]. The magnesium ion is an integral part of the last enzyme in the respiratory chain, which initiates reduction of molecular oxygen[79]. As a component of membranes and nucleic acids, magnesium is present in the mitochondria[80]. **Magnesium and copper are the star minerals for making ATP and without enough ATP or energy this can lead to fatigue.** By binding to ATP and releasing the terminal phosphate, **magnesium activates ATP and liberates its energy**[81].

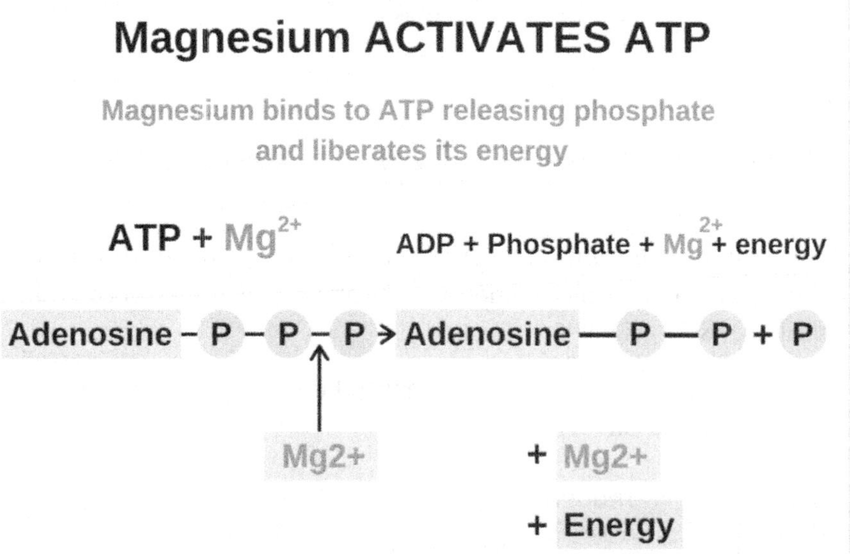

Magnesium ACTIVATES ATP

Magnesium binds to ATP releasing phosphate
and liberates its energy

$$ATP + Mg^{2+} \quad ADP + Phosphate + Mg^{2+} + energy$$

Adenosine – P – P – P > Adenosine — P — P + P

Mg2+   + Mg2+

+ Energy

Adapted From: Toto and Yucha (1994). 'Magnesium: homeostasis, imbalances, and therapeutic uses.' Critical care nursing clinics of North America, 6(4), 767–783. ATP = adenosine triphosphate, ADP = adenosine diphosphate.

A deficiency in magnesium can lead to mitochondrial damage and decreased ATP formation through potassium depletion and sodium and calcium overload[82]. Administrating magnesium can improve symptoms of chronic fatigue and these benefits are associated with increasing low magnesium levels in red blood cells in these patients[83].

Patients treated with magnesium report improved energy levels, better emotional state and less pain. Thus, it might be that people with chronic fatigue or burnout are actually deficient in magnesium or other minerals involved with energy production.

Magnesium deficiency causes mitochondrial damage and decreased ATP formation

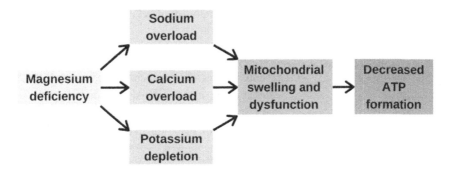

Adapted From: Aithal and Toback (1978). 'Defective mitochondrial energy production during potassium depletion nephropathy.' Laboratory investigation; a journal of technical methods and pathology, 39(3), 186–192. Na = sodium, Ca = calcium and K = potassium.

The thyroid regulates energy homeostasis and metabolic rate. The thyroid hormones thyroxine (T4) and triiodothyronine (T3) are produced by thyroid cells that take up iodine from food and combine it with the amino acid tyrosine. Once released into the bloodstream they affect body temperature, metabolic rate, breathing and heartbeat. Hypothyroidism can cause chronic fatigue, sensitivity to cold, frailty, joint pain, high cholesterol and weight loss plateaus[84,85,86,87]. Low thyroid function can make you more susceptible to other immunocompromised and immunodisordered states like diabetes, obesity, autoimmunity and inflammation[88,89,90]. **Zinc, selenium, iron, copper, manganese, magnesium and iodine are all needed for proper thyroid functioning**[91,92,93,94,95,96].

Mineral	Function in Energy Metabolism
Magnesium	• Essential for nerves and muscle function • Co-factor in over 600 enzymatic reactions • Required for ATP production and transportation
Calcium	• Essential for nerves and muscle function • Initiates fat oxidation • Carries ATP with magnesium
Phosphorus	• Structural component of ATP and creatine phosphate • Part of energy metabolism as it makes up ATP
Copper	• Essential co-factor of cytochrome c oxidase – the last part of the mitochondrial electron transport chain • Involved in iron metabolism and balance
Chromium	• Potentiates the actions of insulin and thus glucose uptake • Needed for glycolysis and ATP production
Iron	• Essential part of hemoglobin for oxygen transport • Facilitates transfer of electrons in the respiratory chain • Necessary for red blood cell function
Manganese	• Co-factor of enzymes involved in carbohydrate metabolism and gluconeogenesis
Zinc	• Essential for glycolysis and beta-oxidation • Part of over 100 enzymes involved in energy metabolism • Needed for producing thyroid hormones
Selenium	• Needed for producing thyroid hormones • Needed for glutathione and antioxidant production
Iodine	• Needed for producing thyroid hormones • Affects metabolic rate and energy metabolism

Adapted from Huskisson et al (2007) 'The Role of Vitamins and Minerals in Energy Metabolism and Well-Being', The Journal of International Medical Research, 2007; 35: 277 – 289[97].

Electrolytes and Minerals

Electrolytes are electrically charged minerals in your body. They can be found in the muscle tissue, blood, urine, sweat and other bodily fluids. Electrolyte balance usually refers to the balance of electrolytes in the body, i.e., between the intra- and extracellular fluid concentrations[98].

The main electrolytes are sodium, potassium, magnesium, phosphate, calcium, chloride and bicarbonate. There are others like zinc, copper, iron, manganese, molybdenum and chromium. You obtain these minerals from food, water and supplements.

Electrolytes, especially sodium, help your body maintain normal fluid levels in the blood, within cells and outside of cells. How much fluid each of these compartments hold depends on the amount and concentration of electrolytes in it.

- If the electrolyte concentration is too low, fluid will leave that particular compartment (blood or intra-, extracellular space)

- If the electrolyte concentration is too high, fluid will move into that particular compartment (a process called osmosis)

The body can actively adjust fluid levels by moving electrolytes in and out of cells. Fluid and electrolyte balance is determined by the right concentration of electrolytes. The kidneys help maintain electrolyte balance by filtering and reabsorbing electrolytes and water from blood. Some of it will be excreted through urine and some gets reabsorbed back into the blood.

Moving sodium and potassium across cell membranes is an active transport process that involves hydrolysis of ATP. It involves an enzyme called the Na^+/K^+-ATPase aka Sodium Potassium Pump. The Sodium-Potassium Pump moves sodium ions out and potassium ions into the cell. This is powered by magnesium and ATP. For every ATP that gets broken down, 3 sodium ions move out and 2 potassium ions move in.

Electrolyte imbalances can have many negative health consequences such as heart failure, arrythmias, oxidative stress or

even death[99,100]. It happens when you either have too low or too high levels of certain electrolytes in your blood. Fluid and electrolyte imbalances are most often caused by dehydration, excessive sweating, vomitting, diarrhea and nutrient deficiencies[101]. Certain conditions like kidney disease[102], anorexia nervosa[103] and medical burns can also cause this[104]. Symptoms of electrolyte imbalances include chronic fatigue, irregular heartbeat, high blood pressure, brain fog, sleeping problems, muscle weakness, cramping, headaches and numbness[105].

Here are the reference ranges for electrolytes measured through blood:

- Calcium: 5–5.5 mEq/L

- Chloride: 97–107 mEq/L

- Potassium: 3.5–5.3 mEq/L

- Magnesium: 1.5-2.5 mEq/L

- Sodium: 136–145 mEq/L

To avoid electrolyte imbalances you have to be obtaining enough minerals from food and liquids. You also need to avoid damage to your organs like your intestines, liver and kidneys so you don't lose the ability to absorb, reabsorb and/or utilize these minerals. The most obvious solution is to pay more attention to what kinds of foods you eat, which supplements you may need and how much salt to consume in relation to your losses.

Magnesium is what primarily regulates the sodium potassium pump[106]. However, a lack of sodium can lead to magnesium deficiency[107,108,109], as can a lack of vitamin B6 or selenium[110]. Thus, salt, vitamin B6 and selenium also control the sodium potassium pump indirectly because they control magnesium status in the body. When in a magnesium deficient state, calcium and sodium accumulate in the cell, promoting hypertension and cardiomyopathy[111]. Magnesium protects against potassium loss and muscle potassium levels won't normalize unless magnesium status is restored even when serum potassium rises[112,113,114].

Chapter 2
Minerals Needed by the Body

As you've learned from Chapter 1, minerals are intrinsically involved with almost every energetic process in the body. It's the creation and utilization of energy that allows living organisms to be alive. Thus, without minerals that help synthesize ATP, life as we know it wouldn't exist.

The body consists of various different parts that have one thing in common – they run on energy and need minerals. Just the process of growing up and physically developing requires minerals. Mineral- and water-enrichment reduces stunting in full-term, low-birth-weight infants[115]. In this chapter, we will go through the minerals needed by various organs and tissues.

Minerals Needed by the Brain

The brain's functioning and cognitive processes are governed by numerous neurotransmitters. They are chemical messengers that send messages from a nerve cell to a target cell via a synapse. Here are the most known and relevant neurotransmitters needed for sleep, health and wellbeing.

- **Serotonin or 5-hydroxytryptamine (5HT)** regulates cognition, mood, and sleep in the central nervous system[116]. Serotonin is both an inhibitory and excitatory neurotransmitter. In the enteric (intestinal) nervous system, serotonin affects digestion, motility and sensation[117]. A serotonin deficiency in the brain causes symptoms of depression and decreased social exploration[118]. Serotonin also gets converted into melatonin, which is called the main sleep hormone, but it also governs central antioxidant and repair processes during nocturnal sleep.
  - **To make serotonin and melatonin, you need magnesium, calcium, iron, copper, cobalt and zinc** [119]. About 2% of the circulating amino acid

tryptophan is converted into 5-hydroxytryptophan (5HTP) by tryptophan hydroxylase, which is an enzyme that uses 5-MTHF (the active form of folate), iron, calcium, and vitamin B3 as co-factors[120]. 5HTP is further converted into serotonin by an enzyme called dopa decarboxylase, which uses magnesium, zinc, vitamin B6 and vitamin C as co-factors.

- Melatonin is also synthesized in local tissues outside of the brain, such as the retina, bone marrow, gastrointestinal tract and the innate immune system[121], which takes place in the mitochondria[122]. Besides the retina, melatonin production outside of the pineal gland in the brain does not follow circadian rhythms and functions primarily as an antioxidant[123, 124]. Melatonin is primarily a mitochondrial-targeted antioxidant that protects the mitochondria against oxidative stress and damage[125].

o **The magnesium ion is required for activating vitamin B6, which helps the conversion of serotonin into melatonin**[126]. Dietary magnesium deficiency decreases melatonin levels in rats[127]. Supplemental magnesium improves subjective measures of insomnia such as sleep onset latency and efficiency in the elderly[128]. In patients with primary insomnia, administration of melatonin, zinc and magnesium improves the quality of sleep and quality of life[129].

o Calcium helps tryptophan to be converted into 5-HTP by tryptophan hydroxylase, thus enabling melatonin production[130]. A study found that fixing a calcium deficiency helped to regain normal REM sleep[131].

o Potassium supplementation has a positive effect on sleep quality[132] and slow-wave-sleep.

Since magnesium controls the levels of potassium in the body this further highlights the importance of both magnesium and potassium for sleep.

Magnesium, Calcium, Iron and Zinc are Needed to Make Serotonin and Melatonin in the Brain[133,134,135,136,137,138,139]

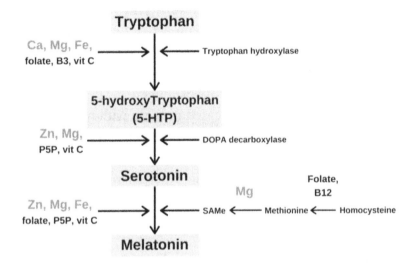

Ca = calcium, Fe = iron, Mg = magnesium

- **Dopamine** is both a hormone and a neurotransmitter that regulates mood, motivation, well-being and the feeling of reward[140]. Imbalances in dopamine affect fatigue in multiple sclerosis and other neurological disorders[141]. With aging, dopamine levels decrease, causing cognitive inflexibility and rigidity[142]. Not producing enough dopamine may cause symptoms of depression[143], anxiety, apathy and promote pleasure seeking from harmful activities like drugs or alcohol[144,145].
  - Dopamine is created from the amino acid L-tyrosine. Tyrosine hydroxylase converts L-tyrosine to L-dopa, which gets converted into dopamine. Both tyrosine hydroxylase and tryptophan hydroxylase contain iron[146]. **Iron deficiency is associated with anxiety, depression, social problems, and behavioral abnormalities**[147]. Magnesium and zinc also help with potentiating dopamine production[148]. During protein

41

turnover, the active form of vitamin B6, pyridoxal 5-phosphate, requires Mg-ATP and potassium for its reformation in the salvage pathway[149]. Thus, **both magnesium and potassium help to keep active vitamin B6 levels at sufficient levels.** Additionally, magnesium is used with active vitamin B6 to convert L-dopa to dopamine, which then requires copper to be converted into norepinephrine. Norepinephrine is the third primary neurotransmitter in the brain and its levels are typically decreased in those with major depressive disorder. Medications that treat depression block the reuptake of serotonin and norepinephrine increasing their levels in the brain, whereas minerals help to boost their levels naturally.

Magnesium, Iron and Copper Create Dopamine and Norepinephrine in the Brain[150,151,152,153,154,155]

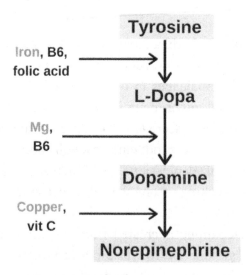

Related to cognition, creation of neurotransmitters, mental health and prevention of neurodegenerative disease:

- **Magnesium**, as noted previously, is needed for creating neurotransmitters and hormones like serotonin, dopamine, norepinephrine and melatonin. **Low magnesium intake is associated with depression in a near linear fashion**[156,157]. Magnesium supplementation of 450 mg per day was found to improve symptoms of depression and was comparable to the antidepressant drug imipramine[158]. Magnesium can also be helpful in treating anxiety symptoms[159]. Magnesium deficiency induces anxiety and HPA axis dysfunction[160]. In bipolar disorder and mania, magnesium can stabilize mood[161,162]. There is a clearly established link between the development of migraines and magnesium[163]. Oral magnesium supplementation may reduce the frequency of migraine headaches[164].

- **Iron** is an essential cofactor for the synthesis of neurotransmitters and myelin[165]. Deficient iron levels are associated with cognitive decline in the elderly[166]. In toddlers, a deficiency in iron causes poor cognitive development, which impairs brain morphology and cognition[167,168]. However, high iron levels in the brain are associated with Alzheimer's disease[169]. That is because iron is a major source of reactive oxygen species and oxidation. In reality, the loss in the ability to utilize iron, which can occur with copper deficiency for example, may be driving many of these iron 'overload' issues.

- **Zinc** is the most concentrated metal in the brain next to iron[170]. It has an important role in synaptic transmission, nucleic acid metabolism and axonal transmission[171]. There is an association between higher zinc levels during aging and healthy brain aging[172]. In the elderly, zinc concentrations are higher in those with unimpaired cognitive function compared to those with memory impairment[173]. Children with ADHD have reduced ADHD symptoms when given a zinc supplement for 12 weeks[174]. And zinc imbalances may cause neuronal death, neurological disorders, stroke, epilepsy and Alzheimer's disease[175].

In addition to the brain, there are other body parts and organs that also need minerals to carry out their vital processes. Here are the most important organs and tissues that need various minerals.

- **Heart** – related to cardiac function, cardiovascular disease risk, atherosclerosis, hypertension and stroke.
  - o **Magnesium** has a central role in protecting against cardiovascular disease and regulating the function of the heart[176]. In addition to activating ATP, magnesium also runs the sodium potassium pump, thus controlling blood pressure [177], [178], [179]. **Magnesium deficiency promotes hypertension via cellular accumulation of calcium and sodium**[180]. Magnesium is also a cofactor for the enzymes involved in cardiac mitochondria. Self-reported magnesium intake is inversely associated with arterial calcification, stroke and fatal coronary heart disease[181] and its supplementation has been found to reduce the incidence of cardiac arrhythmias[182].
  - o **Potassium** intake is inversely related to overall mortality [183], stroke, hypertension [184] and heart disease [185]. It controls the heartbeat and muscle function [186]. Potassium deficiency contributes to cardiovascular disease by promoting atherosclerosis and hypertension[187]. Because of its relationship with sodium, potassium affects intracellular fluid concentration and plasma volume[188]. The primary role of potassium is that it allows the body to effectively use and handle sodium. Hence, many people who cannot tolerate normal sodium intakes simply need more dietary potassium and/or magnesium[189].
  - o **Zinc** status affects heart health by regulating heart muscle and cardiac function[190]. Low zinc is associated with diabetic cardiomyopathy [191] and animal studies

have found that zinc supplementation protects against this[192]. There is also a link between zinc deficiency and heart failure as revealed by a 2018 meta-analysis[193]. Heart failure is also found to be connected to lower selenium and zinc and higher copper concentration[194]. In overweight type-2 diabetic subjects, zinc supplementation reduces inflammation and oxidative stress[195], which are risk factors for cardiovascular disease[196]. Zinc supplementation (40 mg plus 1 mg of copper twice daily) in those 50-80 years old significantly reduced mortality by 27% in the AREDS study.

- **Intestine** – everything related to the gut, intestines, intestinal lining and the microbiome.
    - It is estimated that 80-90% of the serotonin in the body is made in the gut with the help of microbes[197]. That process requires magnesium, zinc and iron. In magnesium-deficient mice, intestinal bifidobacteria levels (the bacteria considered to be beneficial) are associated with inflammation induced by magnesium deficiency[198]. Low magnesium signals the intestinal colonization of *Escherichia coli*, which is a pathogen responsible for hemorrhage of the intestines[199]. Magnesium deficiency alters the gut microbiota and causes depressive-like behavior[200].
    - Melatonin is also produced by the enterochromaffin (EC) cells in the gastrointestinal (GI) tract[201]. EC cells take up tryptophan from the bloodstream and converts it into 5-HTP by tryptophan-5-hydroxylase[202]. 5-HTP then gets decarboxylated into serotonin or 5-HT[203]. The melatonin synthesis rate-limiting enzyme AANAT acetylates serotonin into N-acetyl serotonin (NAS)[204], which gets further methylated by HIOMT into melatonin[205]. Zinc and magnesium enhance melatonin production by binding to AANAT, thus increasing serotonin's affinity for binding to AANAT[206,207]. There

is a direct correlation between serum zinc and melatonin levels in human patients [208]. In rodents, **omega-3 fatty acid deficiency reduces nighttime melatonin, which is normalized by DHA supplementation**[209,210].

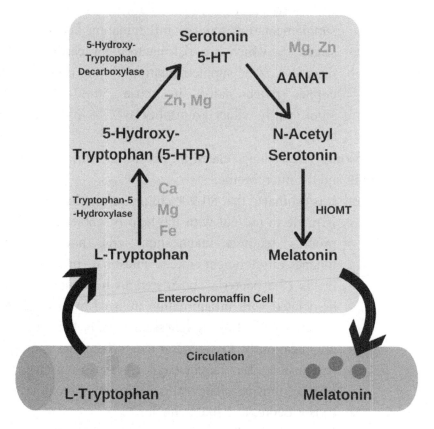

Adapted From: Pal et al (2019) 'Enterochromaffin cells as the source of melatonin: key findings and functional relevance in mammals', Melatonin Research. 2, 4 (Dec. 2019), 61-82.

- o Malabsorption, intestinal permeability and lack of digestive enzymes can cause low magnesium levels due to lack of intestinal absorption[211]. Dietary magnesium also helps to decrease the intestinal absorption of lead [212]. Zinc supplementation has been shown to improve intestinal barrier function and resolve permeability in patients with Crohn's disease[213].

- o **Daily consumption of magnesium-rich mineral water improves bowel movement frequency and stool consistency in subjects with constipation**[214]. Even magnesium oxide, which tends to have low solubility but very high elemental magnesium levels, has been shown to improve bowel movements in chronic constipation[215].

- **Liver** – everything related to liver function and energy metabolism is controlled by the liver.
  - o In both alcoholic- and non-alcoholic fatty liver disease, low magnesium levels have been found and a magnesium deficiency may be a risk factor for these conditions[216]. Higher magnesium levels are associated with a reduced risk of mortality from liver disease[217]. Excess iron can also cause liver damage because of its high oxidative capacity[218].
  - o Liver detoxification pathways require zinc, selenium, magnesium and molybdenum[219]. The liver also produces bile, which is a substance that helps to break down fat from food[220] and removing toxins from the body[221]. In rats, magnesium protects against bile duct ligation-induced liver injury[222].

- **Eyes** – everything related to vision, eye health, and preventing macular degeneration.
  - o Blurry vision might be caused by a magnesium deficiency. Oral magnesium supplementation in normotensive glaucoma patients improves visual fields and vision[223]. **Magnesium may even protect against glaucoma and retinal neuropathy**[224].
  - o Selenium has been shown to slow down the development of Graves' eye disease and orbitopathy[225]. And a selenium deficiency promotes Graves' eye disease[226].
  - o Zinc supplementation with vitamin C and E reduces the risk of developing age-related macular degeneration[227]. However, high levels of zinc are found in age-related

macular degeneration suggesting a loss in zinc utilization[228].

- **Collagen** – everything related to the skin, tendons, ligaments and soft tissue.
  - Copper is essential for collagen and elastin synthesis[229]. In young women, copper supplementation increased collagen formation[230]. Zinc deficiency slows down tissue regenerative processes and administrating zinc normalizes this[231]. Additionally, zinc may promote bone formation by stimulating cell proliferation similarly to the way it does with collagen synthesis[232].

Minerals for Managing Stress and Steroid Hormones

Dealing with chronic stress is extremely demanding on the body and it's typically not the body's first priority because short-term survival is much more important than stress management[233]. And while acute stress is not necessarily harmful and actually can have healthy effects through the phenomenon of hormesis[234], chronic stress is associated with many ailments such as cardiovascular disease and obesity[235]. Chronic stress also weakens the immune system[236]. All nutrients and minerals follow a hormetic U-shaped curve where not getting enough causes harm and getting too much is also potentially dangerous[237].

- **Magnesium** is one of the most relevant minerals for the nervous system and stress management. Stress depletes magnesium by activating the sympathetic nervous system and supplementation helps to reduce this effect[238]. Although not conclusive, studies on humans as well as animals show that **magnesium supplementation can alleviate many of the negative side-effects of stress like anxiety, depression and sleeping problems**[239].

- **Potassium** is important for cardiovascular function, nerve firing, muscles and endurance. Deficiencies in potassium can weaken muscle contraction, cause arrhythmias and impair insulin production[240,241,242].

- **Sodium** is important for energy production, digestion, and electrolyte balance. Deficiencies in sodium can cause muscle cramping, brain fog, fatigue, water retention and even insulin resistance [243]. Low-salt diets also raise triglycerides, LDL cholesterol and lower HDL[244]. Although reducing salt intake can lower blood pressure in hypertensive subjects[245], **there is no evidence that salt restriction reduces the risk of heart attacks or mortality**[246,247]. In fact, several reports show that less than 3,000 mg of sodium per day is linked to a significantly higher chance of dying overall or from heart disease[248,249,250,251]. Thus, the real problem isn't salt, which is composed of two essential minerals sodium and chloride, it's insulin resistance and metabolic syndrome that doubles the risk of cardiovascular disease and increases all-cause mortality[252].

- **Iron** is essential for hemoglobin transportation, which helps to transfer oxygen to muscles and cells. Iron deficiency anemia is one of the most common nutrient deficiencies in the world and it causes chronic fatigue and lethargy (although some of these cases may actually be due to copper deficiency). Excess iron is a risk factor for cardiovascular disease and can be toxic. Consult your doctor first before supplementation or increasing dietary iron intake[253].

- **Zinc** plays an important role as a structural agent of proteins and cell membranes preventing oxidative stress[254]. Low zinc status can cause gastrointestinal problems and increase the risk of pneumonia[255].

The body deals with stress by producing different hormones and defense systems, one of which are corticosteroids. Corticosteroids are a class of steroid hormones that are synthesized in the adrenal cortex from cholesterol. The most common steroid hormones are aldosterone, testosterone, cortisol, cortisone, pregnenolone, progesterone, DHEA and others. Steroid hormones regulate metabolism, inflammation, body composition, immunity, stress adaptation, and recovery from injuries[256]. With enough steroid hormones, the body has sufficient

49

resources to respond to stressors. Without them, damage or illness may ensue.

In order to make steroid hormones, vitamin D and DHEA, you need complex II, III, and IV[257]**, which are dependent on selenium, copper, magnesium, and iron.** You also need ferredoxin and ferredoxin reductase for producing steroid hormones[258], which are iron-sulfur proteins (thus we need iron and sulfur). Anytime iron is needed in a reaction that automatically means copper is needed because copper is needed to oxidize ferrous iron ($Fe2+$) to ferric iron ($Fe3+$) so iron can move and be transported around the body. Thus, **you need adequate levels of numerous minerals to produce sex hormones, corticosteroids and other steroid hormones**.

Steroid hormone synthesis is regulated by trophic hormones like adrenocorticotropin hormone (ACTH) and luteinizing hormone (LH) [259]. They activate G protein-coupled receptors, promoting intracellular cyclic AMP (cAMP) levels[260], which supports cAMP-dependent protein kinase (PKA), protein synthesis, and protein phosphorylation. All of these processes assist in delivering cholesterol from the outer mitochondrial membrane to the inner one, which overcomes the rate-limiting step in producing steroid hormones[261,262]. Hormones are produced by glands like the thyroid gland or adrenal glands. Those glands and hormones are also dependent on minerals like iodine, zinc, magnesium, and selenium, as discussed before. For example, **zinc deficiency is associated with lower testosterone in men and supplementation can improve testosterone levels** [263]. **Magnesium also affects free and total testosterone levels** in both sedentary people as well as athletes [264]. It has been shown that magnesium sulphate helps with the formation of cyclic AMP and governs its antiplatelet effects[265], thus affecting steroidogenesis. ATP is also required for steroid synthesis[266], which requires iron, copper, manganese and magnesium.

The immune system needs key nutrients and minerals to function properly. Malnourished individuals are more vulnerable to infections and illness because their immune system lacks the nutrients to function properly[267].

- Selenium is an essential mineral that helps increase glutathione levels[268]. It's also important for hormonal balance, antioxidant defense and balancing oxidative stress in the body.

- Magnesium is important for all bodily processes, including immunity [269]. Magnesium deficiency elevates pro-inflammatory cytokines like TNF-alpha[270] and reduces CD8+ T cells [271]. **Magnesium deficiency in immune cells can reduce their ability to kill viruses and increase Epstein-Barr activation**[272].

- Zinc is important for synthesizing hormones and for a strong immune system[273]. Studies on children show that regular use of zinc can prevent the incidence of the flu[274]. **Zinc acetate and zinc gluconate lozenges have been shown to inhibit cold viruses from latching onto cells and shorten flu duration**. Lozenges are beneficial only if used in the early stages of infection. The optimal total daily dose is above 75 mg/day divided into multiple doses taken 2–3 hours apart. The best results are achieved when starting within 24 hours of first symptoms[275].

One of the most impactful forms of oxidative stress is DNA damage that results in mutations and genomic instability. This may lead to cancer, chronic diseases and accelerated aging because the DNA replication mechanism stops working properly[276]. Unrepaired DNA damage leads to the accumulation of misfolded proteins, inflammatory cytokines, and dysfunctional cells, which can spread inflammation and lead to accelerated aging[277,278].

Cellular senescence occurs in response to DNA damage that results from exposure to reactive oxygen species (ROS) and free radicals[279,280]. Deficiencies in DNA repair mechanisms increase the frequency of mutations and leaves cells more vulnerable to malignancies[281]. Reduced DNA repair protein activity are seen in early stages of cancer and are thought to contribute to the genetic instability of cancer[282].

- **Magnesium deficiency increases the risk of oxidative damage to DNA**[283]. Importantly, magnesium is needed to activate the enzymes involved with DNA repair, DNA replication and transcription[284,285].
- **Zinc can antagonize the toxic heavy metal cadmium, an inducer of oxidative stress that plays a role in DNA damage and premature cellular aging**[286]. Zinc is important in maintaining DNA integrity and zinc deficiency increases DNA damage[287]. Moreover, a 12 week clinical study in elderly subjects with low serum zinc levels showed that supplemental zinc (20 mg/day of zinc from zinc carnosine) reduced DNA damage and improved the antioxidant profile[288]. Zinc deficiency in human cells causes the release of more oxidants, resulting in oxidative damage to DNA.[289]

DNA damage is one of the triggers for autophagy and autophagy modulates several DNA repair pathways[290]. **Autophagy** is the process of cell turnover and intracellular cleanup. Autophagy has a protective role against many metabolic and age-related diseases such as insulin resistance[291], heart disease[292,293], atherosclerosis[294], inflammation[295], Crohn's[296], bacterial infections[297], neurodegeneration[298], gut health[299], fatty liver[300] and aging in general.

- In vitro studies have shown that **zinc is critical for basal autophagy**[301,302]. In yeast, zinc depletion induces non-selective autophagy by inhibiting mTORC1, which leads to the recycling of zinc from degraded proteins[303].
- Calcium has been shown to control various stages of autophagic flux by triggering autophagy but also inhibiting it[304]. **Low potassium activates calcium signaling, which results in chronically excessive autophagy, leading to calcification**[305]. So, activating autophagy with calcium isn't a good thing.
- Magnesium is needed for calcium absorption and without enough magnesium calcium will begin to accumulate in soft tissue. Elevated levels of magnesium inhibits extracellular

matrix calcification and protects articular cartilage via Erk/autophagy pathway[306].

The body needs dozens of essential nutrients to function optimally. This includes minerals as well as vitamins. Those nutrients work synergistically with each other – sometimes requiring each other to work and at other times antagonizing each other. The chart below reveals the interactions between these nutrients. For reference, the relationships refer to high doses of these nutrients and moderate intake of these nutrients is not enough to trigger these interactions.

Nutrient	Synergistic Relationship	Varies Based on Nutrient Levels	Antagonistic Relationship
Vitamin A	Iodine, Iron, Zinc	Vitamin E	Vitamin K, Vitamin D
Vitamin B1 (Thiamine)	Magnesium		Vitamin B6
Vitamin B2 (Riboflavin)			Calcium
Vitamin B3 (Niacin)	Zinc		
Vitamin B5 (Pantothenic Acid)			Copper
Vitamin B6 (Pyridoxine)			Vitamin B1, Vitamin B9, Zinc
Vitamin B7 (Biotin)		Vitamin B5	
Vitamin B9 (Folic Acid)			Vitamin B6, Vitamin B12, Zinc
Vitamin B12 (Cobalamin)			Vitamin B9, Vitamin C

Vitamin C	Vitamin E	Copper, Iron, Selenium	Vitamin B12
Vitamin D	Vitamin K, Calcium, Magnesium, Selenium		Vitamin A, Vitamin E
Vitamin E	Vitamin C, Selenium, Zinc	Vitamin A	Vitamin D, Vitamin K
Vitamin K	Calcium	Vitamin D	Vitamin A, Vitamin E
Calcium	Vitamin D, Potassium		Magnesium, Phosphorus, Sodium, Iron, Manganese, Zinc
Magnesium	Vitamin B1, Vitamin B6, Vitamin D, Potassium		Calcium, Phosphorus, Zinc
Phosphorus			Calcium, Magnesium
Potassium	Calcium, Manganese, Sodium		
Sodium	Potassium		Calcium
Copper		Vitamin C	Iron, Molybdenum, Selenium, Zinc
Iodine	Vitamin A, Selenium		
Iron	Vitamin A, Vitamin C		Vitamin E, Calcium, Copper, Manganese, Zinc
Manganese			Calcium, Iron
Molybdenum			Copper

Selenium	Vitamin D, Vitamin E, Iodine	Vitamin C	Copper
Zinc	Vitamin A, Vitamin B3		Calcium, Magnesium, Copper, Iron
Sulfur	Molybdenum		

Data obtained from Minich (2018) 'Vitamin-Mineral Interactions', Metagenics, Inc.[307]

Low micronutrient intakes can even accelerate the so-called degenerative diseases of aging. This is known as the triage theory invented by Bruce Ames[308]. The idea is that if you are deficient in a particular micronutrient it gets triaged where it is needed most for survival while non-vital functions suffer causing insidious diseases such as cancer, metabolic disease and vascular calcifications. Although virtually impossible to prove with long-term randomized controlled trials[309], this logic is consistent with evolutionary theory, wherein natural selection favors short-term survival and reproduction over long-term health and nutritional status[310]. For example, if you are deficient in vitamin K, the vitamin K-dependent anti-calcification proteins suffer[311]. However, the vitamin-K dependent clotting factors remain intact to prevent you from bleeding out and dying if you get a cut[312]. Thus, you've traded living with functioning clotting factors for an increased risk of accumulating arterial calcifications. Sometimes life makes hard choices for you, and you don't even realize it.

Many of the leading causes of death, such as heart disease, stroke, heart failure, kidney disease, and diabetes are actually caused or contributed by mineral deficiencies. Magnesium deficiency is a perfect example of how a deficiency in one mineral can lead to cardiovascular disease[313]. **Chromium, vanadium and magnesium are some of the most common deficiencies associated with diabetes**[314]. The public needs to be informed about the importance of minerals and hopefully in the future insurance companies will actually pay for testing for mineral deficiencies. Until then, the tremendous lack of knowledge on this topic among doctors and the general public is one of the greatest health threats of our time. Hopefully, this book will help turn the tides and doctors and their patients will start to realize the importance of minerals once again.

Chapter 3
Superoxide Anions Drive Chronic Disease and Minerals Are the Antidote

Most of you have probably heard of free radicals and the importance of antioxidants in the diet to prevent those free radicals from damaging our bodies. A free radical is a molecule with a single unpaired electron in its outer layer. Most free radicals are very reactive and they can cause oxidative damage. However, **free radicals are also important for inducing hormesis, whereby a small exposure to free radicals makes our body more resilient to them in the future.** So the balance between getting some free radicals, but not too much, determines our overall health. Additionally, we have natural systems in place to help keep this balance, such as antioxidants and other reducing agents. A reducing agent is a compound that can donate an electron to a free radical to neutralize it. For example, NADPH is the universal electron donar in the body and it helps to recycle or "reduce" oxidized glutathione back to its reduced or unoxidized form.

The free radical theory of aging states that organisms get chronic disease, age and die because of the accumulation of free radical damage to the cells over time[315]. Denham Harman was one of the first to propose this idea in 1956[316]. He furthered his ideas in the 70s by describing the production of reactive oxygen species (ROS) by the mitochondria.[317] which is one of the most widely accepted theories of aging. According to the classical free radical theory of aging,
energy production by the mitochondria damages mitochondrial macromolecules, including mitochondrial DNA (mtDNA), which promotes aging[318]. After a certain threshold, this produces too much ROS, causing cell death and degradation.

In 1980, the subject shifted into implicating the mitochondria as the main targets of ROS damage, which is called the Mitochondrial Free Radical Theory of Aging[319]. It happens when electrons leak out of the electron transport chain and react with water to create a free radical called superoxide radical. These radicals damage DNA and other proteins. Age-related impairments in the mitochondrial respiratory chain decrease ATP synthesis, damage DNA, and make the cells more susceptible to oxidative stress[320].

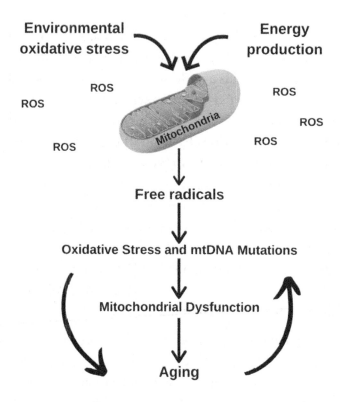

Damage to your cells and especially to your mitochondria within your cells is a consistent finding in aging. Age-related impairments in the mitochondrial respiratory chain decrease ATP synthesis, damage DNA, and make the cells more susceptible to oxidative stress. It is inevitable that our cells will become damaged or decayed from unchecked oxidative stress but how quickly this occurs is up to you. The foods and minerals that you put in your body are your weapons against this oxidative damage. It's up to you whether you want to have your shields up at full capacity, or at 50%. If your body were the U.S.S. Enterprise, would you want to go into battle with shields at 100% or 50%? That's the mentality that you want to have each day, "Are my shields at 100%?" And one way you can help bring those shields up, is by getting optimal intakes of all the minerals each day from the food that you eat, and in certain instances, beneficial supplements to help you achieve those optimal levels.

In this chapter, we will talk about how you can prevent excessive oxidative stress and mitochondrial dysfunction in order to slow the aging process. Minerals play a crucial role in regulating and expressing the body's own antioxidant defenses that help mitigate the collateral damage of reactive oxygen species in the body.

Superoxide and Peroxynitrite – Worst of the Free Radicals

Oxidative stress results from an imbalance in the proinflammatory molecules compared to the anti-inflammatory enzymes and antioxidants in the cell – more pro-oxidants than anti-oxidants means chronic inflammation and mitochondrial/tissue damage. Free radicals are implicated in serious health conditions like atherosclerosis, diabetes, cancer and neurodegeneration[321]. Inflammation is involved in many pathological processes and disease[322]. The balance between free radicals and antioxidants is vital for maintaining health and preventing disease onset[323]. Reducing exposure to free radicals and increasing the intake of antioxidant-rich foods is proposed to enhance the body's ability to deal with oxidative stress and free radicals[324]. However, it's also important to induce some oxidative stress in the body, such as exercise, sunlight, sauna and so on to induce hormesis.

Harmful free radicals include superoxide anion radical (O_2^*), reactive oxygen species (ROS), superoxide anion (O_2^*), hydrogen peroxide (H_2O_2), singlet oxygen, hydroxyl radical ($OH^•$), peroxy radical, as well as the second messenger nitric oxide ($NO^•$), which can react with O_2^* to form peroxynitrite ($ONOO^-$). They can be created from internal sources during mitochondrial energy production or through exposure to external stimuli like pollution or poor diet.

The body has an entire grid of antioxidant systems that consists of multiple lines of defense:

- The first line of defense includes antioxidant enzymes called superoxide dismutase (SOD), catalase (CAT) and glutathione peroxidase (GPX) that suppress or prevent the formation of free radicals[325]. They are quick to neutralize any molecule that has the potential to turn into a free radical.

- The second line of defense refers to antioxidants that scavenge active free radicals and thus inhibit a chain reaction of oxidative stress. Antioxidants belonging to this group include ascorbic acid, vitamin E, glutathione and ubiquinol. By donating one of their electrons to the free radical they neutralize it. In the process these antioxidants become free radicals themselves (but much less damaging ones) and will get neutralized by other antioxidants.

- The third line of defense is utilized once free radical damage has already occurred. It includes DNA damage repair proteins, enzymes, and lipids, such as the DNA repair enzyme systems (polymerases, glycosylases, and nucleases) and proteolytic enzymes (proteinases, proteases, and peptidases). They are important for repairing damage including post-insult damage as is seen in COVID-19 long haulers or radiation exposure.

- The fourth line of defense involves forming and transporting antioxidants to the site of injury for adaptation and to prevent additional free radicals from being created there[326]. They react to the signals created by free radicals.

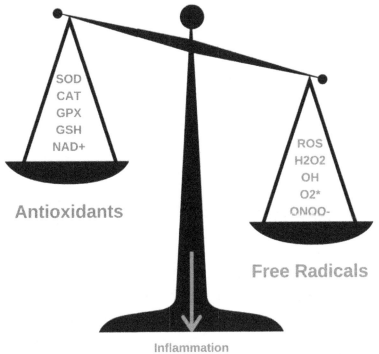

SOD
CAT
GPX
GSH
NAD+

Antioxidants

ROS
H2O2
OH
O2*
ONOO-

Free Radicals

Inflammation
Neurodegeneration
Atherosclerosis
DNA Damage

One of the most harmful forms of oxidative stress occurs with DNA damage that results in mutations and genomic instability. This may lead to certain cancers, disease and accelerated aging because the DNA replication mechanism stops working properly[327]. Your body can repair damaged DNA but sometimes it's not enough. Unrepaired DNA damage leads to the accumulation of misfolded proteins, inflammatory cytokines and dysfunctional cells, which can spread inflammation and induce accelerated aging[328,329].

To deal with environmental stress and oxidative damage, organisms have evolved systems of DNA damage response (DDR)[330]. This includes DNA repair mechanisms, damage tolerance and adaptation. The rate of DNA repair depends on many factors, such as cell type, age of cell and the surrounding environment. A cell that has accumulated too much DNA damage, or no longer repairs itself, can go into one of three states:

- **Senescence** – zombie cell in irreversible dormancy and disease. These cells can also secrete proinflammatory molecules damaging healthy surrounding tissues.

- **Apoptosis** – programmed cell death or suicide (which is a good thing).

- **Tumorigenesis** – unregulated cell division into cancer or tumors.

When DNA damage occurs, the cell can either start to repair itself or induce cell death through apoptosis. Apoptosis functions as a defence mechanism against tumorigenesis to prevent the spreading of DNA damage and potential cancerous cell formation[331]. **Having enough DHA in the cardiolipin of the mitochondria is extremely important for a cells ability to induce apoptosis and controlled cell and/or cancer cell death**[332,333,334,335]. Next to apoptosis and cell senescence, there's the process of cellular turnover also known as autophagy. It recycles damaged proteins and organelles into new ones. Studies have shown that defective autophagy increases DNA damage and the occurrence of tumors and neurodegenerative diseases[336]. During the DNA damage response, autophagy may act as a source of energy for maintaining cell cycle arrest and sustaining DNA repair activities[337]. Cells with deletion of the essential autophagy gene *Atg7* exhibit degradation and attenuated activation of checkpoint kinase 1 (Chk1) and diminished repair of DNA double-strand breaks by homologous recombination[338]. A lot of genes that seem to promote lifespan and longevity like autophagy, sirtuins and FOXO proteins are involved in DNA repair and protection[339]. SIRT7 depletion causes impaired DNA repair and genome instability[340]. **One of the best activators of sirtuins is melatonin**[341,342,343,344,345]. Thus, **maintaining good levels of melatonin production throughout the day, with things like morning light exposure, avoiding light at night and consuming an optimal amount of nutrients (so the body can synthesize melatonin) can help with sirtuin activation and DNA repair.**

There are at least 169 enzymes involved in DNA repair pathways, including superoxide dismutase, glutathione, Nrf2 and others. They all require minerals to work, such as copper, zinc, selenium and magnesium.

- **Selenium** is involved in repairing oxidized methionine residues, thus playing a role in oxidized protein repair systems[346].

  Cooking protein-rich food like meat at high temperatures creates carcinogenic compounds called heterocyclic amines and polycyclic aromatic hydrocarbons [347], which might be mitigated in the presence of adequate selenium.

- **Magnesium** is essential for base excision repair enzymes[348], which is a type of DNA damage response. In large quantities, magnesium can suppress N-Methylpurine-DNA glycosylase (MPG) that initiates base excision repair in DNA. However, magnesium is required for all the downstream actions of base excision repair proteins like apurinic/apyrimidinic endonuclease, DNA polymerase β and ligases [349]. Thus, magnesium regulates repair processes to ensure a balanced repair of damaged DNA bases.

- **Zinc** deficiency promotes oxidative stress, DNA damage and undermines antioxidant defenses in rats[350,351]. In humans, zinc deficiency causes DNA damage [352]. Zinc is involved in hundreds of proteins, including DNA-binding proteins, copper/zinc superoxide dismutase (CuZnSOD), and DNA damage repair proteins like p53[353]. Zinc is also needed for activating poly (ADP-ribose) polymerase that are involved in DNA repair at DNA damage sites[354].

- **Iron** is a cofactor to many DNA repair and replication proteins like Pol #, Rad 3/XPD and Dna2 [355]. Mutations of iron-requiring proteins are associated with diseases of DNA repair defects in mammals. Base excision repair glycosylases that remove damaged bases contain the iron-sulfur cluster protein cofactor[356]. Hence, good iron (and thus by default copper) and sulfur status are important for DNA repair.

You can't avoid all oxidative stress and DNA damage and you actually want some to induce hormesis. So it's inevitably going to happen to a certain extent. What you can do instead is alleviate excessive oxidative damage and improve the repair of damaged tissues. The presence of an optimal amount of minerals in the body is key for keeping your antioxidant defenses strong as well as repairing the damage that has already occured (think COVID-19 long haulers, stroke or heart attack victims or those with traumatic brain injury).

One free radical most relevant to our health is superoxide. Superoxide is exactly what it sounds like - a superoxide or super oxidant. It is molecular oxygen O_2 with one unpaired electron, giving the superoxide anion $O_2^{\cdot}$. This unpaired electron makes superoxide a highly reactive free radical. Superoxide can also combine with nitric oxide to form the highly reactive nitrogen species peroxynitrite $(ONOO^-)$[357]. Even though there are other oxidants that are formed in the body like hydroxyl radicals, for example, peroxynitrite has a much longer half-life, it can penetrate into multiple cells and it causes significant and relevant damage to the body. Peroxynitrite creates a burst of oxidative stress, mitochondrial dysfunction, inflammation, DNA damage, lipid peroxidation, necrosis and shuts down many enzymes[358]. It also modifies tyrosine into nitrotyrosines, which are associated with atherosclerosis, myocardial ischemia, and inflammatory bowel disease[359]. In fact, peroxynitrite is implicated in nearly every pathology, starting with hypertension, heart failure and ending with diabetes and vascular aging[360]. Thus, **the production of superoxide anions and the subsequent formation of peroxynitrite can be viewed as one of the most harmful and relevant oxidative stressors that occurs within our bodies**.

The main way your body deals with oxidative stress and DNA damage is by activating sirtuins and a group of enzymes called PARPs (poly ADP ribose polymerases). Both of them consume NAD+ and can lead to energy depletion. When that happens, you're left with chronic fatigue, getting sick easily, lackluster performance, brain fog and decelerated healing. NAD deficiency causes tissue damage in response to ionizing radiation, which also increases peroxynitrite [361] and administrating NAD protects against these effects[362]. NADPH is also essential for lowering oxidative stress and inflammation[363].

Superoxide is generated by two main pathways in the body, NADPH oxidase and in the electron transport chain of mitochondria. This is important because **in almost all chronic diseases NADPH-oxidase is activated, which increases the production of superoxide anions**[364,365]. In fact, the damage that comes from high glucose levels and free fatty acids in the body are actually due to the activation of NADPH oxidase[366]. Additionally, in the mitochondria, there is an approximate 3-4% loss of electrons that spill from the electron transport chain, leading to the formation of superoxide, which can damage and degrade our mitochondria. Thus, **chronic diseases can be thought of as a state of superoxide and peroxynitrite excess and nitric oxide deficiency**. This is primarily driven by the activation of NADPH oxidase, which is caused by many factors such as acute and chronic infections, nutrient deficiencies, heavy metals and the overconsumption of refined foods.

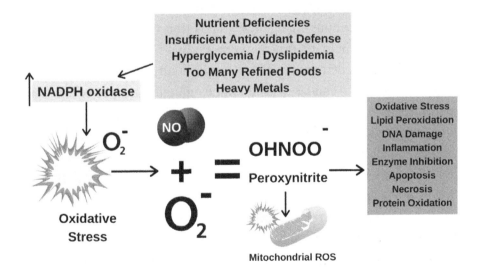

However, the body has a natural antidote to superoxide, and that is an antioxidant enzyme called superoxide dismutase (SOD). This enzyme dismutases or 'declaws' superoxide to hydrogen peroxide and oxygen, which are less damaging molecules. To be more precise, the superoxide dismutase enzymes that do this are called **copper,zinc**-superoxide dismutase (Cu,Zn-SOD) and **manganese**-superoxide dismutase (Mn-SOD). In other words, **if you want to remove superoxide anions in the body you need to have the minerals copper, zinc and manganese** as they are cofactors for superoxide dismutase enzymes in your body. If you are lacking in these minerals, then the function of your antioxidant enzyme superoxide dismutase goes down and more superoxide will bind to nitric oxide, **thereby depleting nitric oxide levels** and forming the toxic peroxynitrite. Talk about a double whammy! All of this leads to increased tissue/organ damage and a decline in overall health.

There is a total of three superoxide dismutases in humans: superoxide dismutase (SOD)-1 and superoxide dismutase (SOD)-3 contain copper and zinc and are found in the cytoplasm and extracellular space, respectively, superoxide dismutase (SOD)-2, which is found in the mitochondria, contains manganese. Thus, the minerals copper, zinc, and manganese help to protect your body from some of the most harmful oxidants that get produced. Additionally, other molecules and enzymes such as catalase, glutathione, glutathione peroxidase and peroxiredoxin help to eliminate the toxic hydrogen peroxide that gets created after superoxide dismutase does its job eliminating superoxide anions. Glutathione, glutathione peroxidase and peroxiredoxin depend on iron, selenium, magnesium and copper. Additionally, catalase levels are decreased with selenium deficiency[367] and the peroxynitrite that is formed from the combination of nitric oxide and superoxide requires peroxiredoxin and thioredoxin for its elimination, which depend on manganese, iron and selenium. **Considering that we are now exposed to an ever-increasing oxidative load from air pollution, chronic diseases, heavy metals and so on we need to ensure that our antioxidant enzymes are supported more than ever.** Thus, if we are lacking in any minerals, especially iron, copper, zinc, selenium, magnesium and manganese we are at a significant disadvantage and a higher risk for developing numerous chronic diseases.

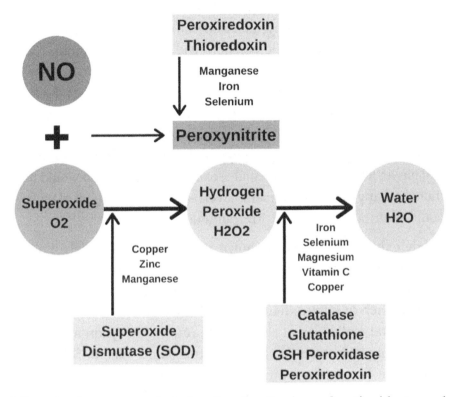

Minerals that are needed for the functioning of antioxidants and antioxidant enzymes[368,369,370,371]

Nitric Oxide (NO) is an important signaling molecule that's known for its benefits on the cardiovascular system and its antiviral effects. Nitric oxide (NO) suppresses platelet aggregation[372], lowers blood pressure[373], reduces blood clot formation[374], prevents blood vessel inflammation[375] and improves the transport of lipids and cholesterol[376]. It promotes blood flow through vasodilation and reduces the time these particles stay in your bloodstream. **Reduced availability of nitric oxide has been implicated in the pathogenesis of hypertension and atherosclerosis**[377]. In patients with hypertension, a single administration of an orally disintegrating lozenge that generates nitric oxide in the oral cavity, restores endothelial function, decreases blood pressure and improves vascular

67

compliance[378]. Increased oxidative stress and reduced nitric oxide contribute to hypertension and something called pulmonary hypertension[379]. Therapeutic applications of nitric oxide can even help with erectile dysfunction by increasing blood flow[380]. Nitric oxide is the main mediator of penile erection that activates relaxation of the smooth muscles in the penis[381]. This is why hypertension and sexual dysfunction are linked with each other[382]. Signs of sexual dysfunction and erectile dysfunction can indicate low nitric oxide levels and cardiovascular problems or even atherosclerosis. Endothelial nitric oxide synthase (eNOS) also regulates female genital tract structures and has an important role in female sexual arousal[383]. Who would have thought that your body's mineral levels, and hence nitric oxide levels, could contribute to your sex life, but it does!

Nitric oxide has even been shown to fight against certain viruses and bacterial infections [384]. Supplementation with nitric oxide boosters (such as L-arginine, but more importantly L-citrulline, as well as foods rich in nitrates like beets and leafy greens) has potential to reduce viral replication of severe acute respiratory syndrome (SARS) coronavirus and others[385]. Indeed, nitric oxide inhibits SARS-CoV replication in two ways. First, nitric oxide and its derivatives reduce the palmitoylation of nascently expressed spike (S) protein, which affects the fusion between the S protein and its cognate receptor, angiotensin converting enzyme (ACE). Secondly, nitric oxide and its derivatives reduce viral RNA production during the early stages of viral replication.[386] In fact, during the 2003 SARS outbreak in Beijing, inhalable nitric oxide was used to treat patients[387]. These individuals saw improved arterial oxygenation, reduced need for oxygen therapy and decreased spread of lung infiltrates with benefits persisting even after the inhaled nitric oxide therapy stopped.

Endogenous nitric oxide is mostly created from enzymatic pathways as well as through non-enzymatic ways. Enzymatic nitric oxide creation is initiated by nitric oxide synthase (NOS) by degrading L-arginine, L-citrulline, and nitric oxide in the presence of oxygen and NADPH[388,389]. L-arginine is an amino acid that can be derived from dietary sources or the body's own protein, is converted into citrulline and nitric oxide in the presence of NADPH and oxygen. Importantly,

exogenous intake of citrulline is better at increasing arginine and nitric oxide levels in the body compared to arginine intake because citrulline has better bioavailability and gets converted to arginine in the body[390].

Here is how nitric oxide is formed and catalyzed by NOS[391]:

2 L-arginine (citrulline is better at increasing endogenous arginine levels) + 3 NADPH + 3 H^+ + 4 O_2 ⇌ 2 citrulline + 2 **nitric oxide** + 4 H_2O + 3 $NADP^+$

Nicotinamide Adenine Dinucleotide Phosphate ($NADP+$) is a form of NAD that promotes anabolic reactions, in plants this includes things like photosynthesis or in animals nucleic acid synthesis. It's used by all forms of cellular life[392]. NADPH is the reduced (unoxidized) form of $NADP+$. The extra phosphate gets added during the de-novo or salvage pathway by the NAD+ kinase. This allows nicotinamide synthesis and conversion of NADPH back into NADH to maintain balance[393]. **NADPH protects against the oxidative stress from excessive reactive oxygen species (ROS) because it is the universal electron donor.** It also allows for the regeneration of glutathione (GSH), which is our body's master antioxidant[394]. NADPH is important because it will reduce and neutralize oxidized antioxidants and free radicals by donating electrons.

The enzymatic nitric oxide synthase (NOS) and NADPH pathways are dependent of essential co-factors that require iron and calcium to work properly[395].

Here are the nutrients needed for nitric oxide production and cardiovascular health[396]

- **Citrulline/arginine** – Arginine and citrulline are substrates needed to form nitric oxide. They are one of the main amino acids in the urea cycle. Short-term L-citrulline supplementation has been shown to improve arterial stiffness, independent of blood pressure, in middle-aged men[397]. It also increases blood flow during exercise and improves erectile dysfunction[398,399]. Supplemental arginine has been found to be unreliable in raising nitric oxide[400]. Citrulline is more readily absorbed than arginine, having shown twice the potency of arginine in relation to raising arginine levels in the blood [401]. Supplementing extra glutathione with citrulline may promote NO synthesis and stabilize it[402]. Some cells can't make NO without glutathione[403].

- **Calcium** –Endothelial NOS (eNOS) and neuronal NOS (nNOS) are controlled by intracellular calcium[404]. Increasing intracellular calcium with glutamate stimulates nNOS to promote nitric oxide[405]. Calcium also initiates the electron flow in the NOS reaction from NADPH to heme and oxygen. **The long-chain omega-3 fatty acid EPA has been shown to increase nitric oxide synthesis** by increasing intracellular calcium[406].

- **Iron** – Heme, which is an iron-containing and oxygen carrying substance, is an essential part of NOS. An iron deficiency has been shown to reduce nNOS and ileal NOS in rats[407,408].

- **Copper** –is required for the movement and utilization of iron in the body as well as the formation of ATP.

- **Zinc** – Zinc is bound to all isoforms of NOS, thereby it is necessary for NOS activity[409]. In high concentrations, zinc inhibits eNOS and nNOS[410]. Thus, a loss in the control of zinc levels may reduce nitric oxide production.

- **Manganese** – Increasing extracellular manganese stimulates nitric oxide synthesis in murine astrocytes[411]. High amounts of

70

administered manganese or lead in the brain of rats interferes with calcium-mediated nitric oxide synthesis and causes neuronal dysfunction[412]. Thus, when the body loses the ability to regulate minerals, especially copper, iron and manganese this can lead to negative consequences.

- **Magnesium** – Activates vitamin D, which increases eNOS gene expression[413]. Magnesium ions also seem to directly enhance endothelial nitric oxide production in healthy humans in a dose-dependent manner[414]. Thus, magnesium deficiency reduces nitric oxide synthesis and magnesium supplementation can restore endothelium-dependent vasorelaxation[415].

- **Carbohydrates** – Glucose metabolism is the major source of NADPH for nitric oxide synthesis[416]. Thus, nitric oxide synthesis is very much glucose-dependent and a deficiency in the utilization of glucose molecules can reduce nitric oxide synthesis. On the flip side, **hyperglycemia (elevated blood sugar) impairs nitric oxide-mediated endothelial function** [417] and causes vascular dysfunction in diabetic patients [418]. Thus, maintaining a normal blood sugar is beneficial because you don't need a high amount of carbohydrates to facilitate NADPH. We also know that **a deficiency in copper, magnesium and chromium leads to hyperglycemia,**[419,420,421] **which lowers nitric oxide** further. In rats, increasing dietary fructose also impairs vascular relaxation, causes hypertension, fatty liver and induces insulin resistance[422]; effects that are partially induced by a **fructose-induced depletion of copper and magnesium**[423,424].

Thus, to improve high blood pressure, atherosclerosis and enhance the immune system we need good levels of nitric oxide.

Having optimal levels of nitric oxide is highly dependent on various enzymatic processes in the body that all require minerals, especially copper, zinc, magnesium, iron, manganese and selenium.

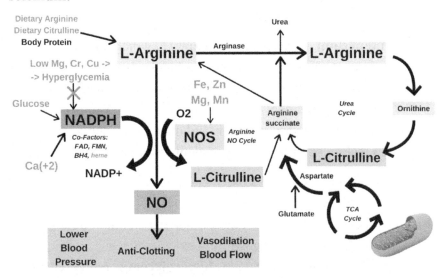

Adapted From: Luiking et al (2011) 'Regulation of Nitric Oxide Production in Health and Disease', Curr Opin Clin Nutr Metab Care. 2010 Jan; 13(1): 97–104. Ca = calcium, Cr = chromium, Cu = copper, Fe = iron, Mg = magnesium, Mn = manganese and Zn = zinc.

Glutathione (GSH) is another internal antioxidant in the body. It protects against reactive oxygen species and free radicals like peroxides, lipid peroxides and heavy metals[425]. Glutathione promotes the regulation of nitric oxide by enhancing citrulline function[426]. Without enough NADPH, your body can't recharge glutathione after it becomes oxidized. This will put breaks on all the detoxification systems. Glutathione is extremely important for protecting red blood cells from oxidative stress and its levels are highly dependent on magnesium.[427] Additionally, magnesium helps to provide the ATP required for glutathione synthesis and two ATP molecules are used for the biosynthesis of one glutathione molecule[428]. **A depletion in magnesium will deplete ATP levels and hence glutathione levels.**

Selenium is a cofactor for the antioxidant glutathione peroxidase, boosting its expression and activity, this is important for reducing inflammation during viral infections[429]. **Supplementing selenium replete humans with 200 mcg/day of selenium can improve T-lymphocyte mediated immune responses[430], increase cytotoxic lymphocyte-mediated tumor cytotoxicity and natural killer cell activity compared to baseline**[431]. Furthermore, taking 297 mcg/day vs. 13 mcg/day of selenium improves the activation and proliferation of B-lymphocytes, enhances cytotoxic T lymphocytes and improves activated T-cell function[432]. Having a low selenium status even increases the risk of influenza virus mutations[433]. Lastly, a low selenium intake has been shown to increase all-cause mortality in mice infected with virulent influenza by 3-fold[434] and in humans infected with COVID-19 by 5-fold[435]. Thus, **selenium is an extremely important mineral for helping the body fight viral infections by improving the function of immune cells and reducing inflammation.**

Another antioxidant defense mechanism against free radicals are metallothioneins (MTs), which are small, cysteine-rich, heavy metal-binding proteins[436,437]. They are mostly known for detoxifying heavy metals, in particular cadmium and maintaining metal ion homeostasis[438,439]. Human cells with excessive MTs are resistant to cadmium poisoning[440]. In mammals, MTs bind zinc[441] but if there's excess cadmium, MTs will bind cadmium instead of zinc[442]. During stress, MTs release zinc when nitric oxide and ROS levels increase[443,444]. Although zinc itself raises the zinc-binding activity of metallothionein, zinc is needed to upregulate MTs through metal regulatory transcription factor 1 (MTF-1)[445]. Thus, **the antioxidant effects of MTs are dependent on zinc**[446]. **Zinc is also needed for glutathione production**, as revealed by studies wherein zinc deficiency is accompanied by a deficiency of glutathione and increased oxidative stress[447]. Zinc also protects endothelial cells from hydrogen peroxide via Nrf2-dependent stimulation of glutathione biosynthesis[448].

There are 8 primary minerals that control our antioxidant defenses. These include calcium, chromium, copper, iron, zinc, selenium, manganese and magnesium. A deficiency in any one of these minerals will put a kink in your internal armor against oxidative stress and predispose you to chronic disease and early death.

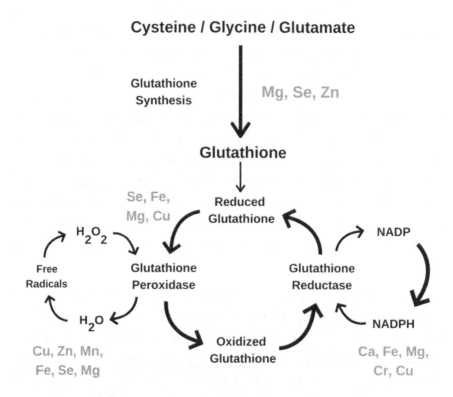

Ca = calcium, Cr = chromium, Cu = copper, Fe = iron, Mg = magnesium, Mn = manganese, Se = selenium and Zn = zinc.

Adapted from Lushchak (2012). 'Glutathione Homeostasis and Functions: Potential Targets for Medical Interventions.' Journal of Amino Acids, 2012, 1–26. doi:10.1155/2012/736837

Unchecked oxidative stress can cause damage to the proteins, fats and DNA in your body, which not only accelerate aging but may also promote cancer, atherosclerosis and other degenerative diseases such as Alzheimer's, Parkinson's and multiple sclerosis[449,450,451,452]. When oxidants and free radicals damage neurons, your brain and cognition suffer, or when they attack your myelin sheath, your ability to walk may be impaired and so on and so forth for every part of your body. Thus, **to enhance your internal antioxidant defenses you need to ensure optimal intakes of all minerals.**

Minerals for Preventing Premature Aging and Promoting Longevity

The mitochondria are always either fusing (combining together) or fissioning (breaking apart). These kinds of mitochondrial dynamics enable the repair of defective mitochondria, mitochondrial replication and selective removal of broken mitochondria via mitophagy (mitochondrial autophagy) [453]. Such mitochondrial plasticity is essential for normal functioning of the cell and protecting against age-related dysfunction [454]. Mitochondrial fission (fragmentation) is associated with metabolic disorders like hyperglycemia[455,456].

Premature aging is primarily caused by two things. Damage to tissues from numerous factors and reduced cellular repair. This leads to an accumulation of dysfunctional enzymes, proteins, and cellular membranes and if it reaches a certain threshold, it can present as disease and ultimately death. As you've just learned, the major cause of this damage in the body is from the activation of NADPH oxidase, which produces the harmful superoxide anion and the reactive nitrogen species peroxynitrite. Now that you know what the antidote is for quenching this oxidative stress (optimal mineral status) you can start to build a diet and supplement regimen to optimize your mineral intake to help you fight premature aging and get you back on a path to a healthier and longer life.

Inflammasomes Drive a Vast Range of Acute and Chronic Inflammatory Diseases

Inflammation is considered one of the main contributing factors to many chronic diseases like cardiovascular disease[457]**, cancer**[458]**, autoimmunity**[459] **and brain aging**[460]. T cell aging and chronic low grade inflammation – a term called inflammaging – are implicated in many age-related diseases [461]. Inflammasomes, which are protein complexes that assemble in response to certain pro-inflammatory signals exert pro-inflammatory and pro-apoptotic effects[462]. They have been shown to have a pathogenic role in diabetes[463], neurodegenerative diseases [464,465], autoimmune disorders like rheumatoid arthritis [466], psoriasis[467], asthma[468], allergies[469] and acne[470]. **Inflammasomes mediate acute inflammatory conditions such as gout[471] and the acute respiratory distress syndrome (ARDS) seen in COVID-19[472,473].** Inflammasomes can also trigger a type of cell death called pyroptosis, which essentially spills the cells' guts releasing its inflammatory materials driving many chronic inflammatory conditions[474].

The most known inflammasome is the NLRP3/ASC/caspase-1 complex, which is initiated by NF-kB-mediated oxidative stress[475]. NLRP3 regulates aging-associated chronic inflammation and insulin resistance[476]. NLRP3 can also be triggered by low intracellular potassium[477].

Potassium depletion is needed for NLRP3 to be bound by NEK7[478], which is an accessory protein of the NLRP3/ASC/caspase-1 complex. Not getting enough sodium or magnesium can also cause low intracellular potassium. **A lack of salt can lead to magnesium deficiency, which causes a loss of potassium in the cell.**[479,480,481,482] In many situations, cellular potassium depletion is mediated by the P2X7 receptor (P2X7R) that is enhanced by extracellular ATP. During inflammation and oxidative stress, ATP is pushed out of the cell where it can connect with P2X7R. This activation creates a pore in the plasma membrane, allowing potassium to leach out and calcium to move in.[483,484,485]

Furthermore, activated P2X7R also promotes NADPH oxidase activation and oxidative stress[486,487,488]. Fortunately, **magnesium can bind to ATP, forming Mg-ATP, releasing the terminal phosphate to release energy.** Thus, this binding with magnesium might help to prevent and reduce inflammasome activation. Additionally, **magnesium is needed to activate vitamin D into calcitriol**[489] and calcitriol, through its binding to vitamin D receptors, can inhibit NF-kB activation, which is the main driver of NLRP3 inflammasomes[490].

The assembly of inflammasomes requires NLRP3 connecting with thioredoxin interacting protein (TXNIP)[491]. When TXNIP is tied up with thioredoxin it cannot merge with and activate NLRP3[492]. However, when oxidation increases, thioredoxin is summoned to reduce oxidized proteins[493]. This can leave TXNIP open to bind to

NLRP3 and trigger inflammation. Reconverting thioredoxin back into its reduced, unoxidized form is done by thioredoxin reductase, which uses NADPH as a reductant and selenium as a cofactor[494]. Thus, oxidative damage to thioredoxin will liberate TXNIP so it can begin to interact with NLRP3, whereas adequate thioredoxin reductase helps to keep thioredoxin reduced or unoxidized so it can remain attached to TXNIP, thereby preventing inflammasome activation. Boosting NADPH and selenium intake is important for forming reduced thioredoxin through their required action on thioredoxin reductase. In other words, **if you have low NADPH or selenium levels, this will increase the activation of NLRP3 inflammasomes and increase the risk of acute or chronic inflammatory diseases**.

Several key antioxidant enzymes are needed for eliminating hydrogen peroxide and selenium is needed for keeping thioredoxin in a reduced state and for the proper functioning of glutathione peroxidase and thioredoxin reductase[495]. In mice, selenium has been shown to regulate NLRP3 inflammasomes[496]. **A selenium deficiency may increase the risk of dying from COVID-19**[497], **whereas sufficient zinc and selenium has been associated with an improved survival**[498]. In fact, in China, **those with a poor selenium status have a 3-fold higher risk of experiencing bad outcomes with COVID-19 and a 5-fold higher risk of dying**[499]. It's estimated that up to 40% of the U.S. population may be selenium deficient[500] and 15% do not meet the RDA for selenium[501].

COVID-19 patients also have significantly lower levels of zinc compared to healthy controls[502]. Among those subjects, a **zinc deficiency doubles the risk of having a poor COVID-19 outcome and lengthens hospital stay by two days**. It's estimated that about 47% of U.S. adults are deficient in zinc[503] with 42% of these individuals not getting the RDA[504]. Thus, adequate selenium and zinc status may help to prevent inflammasome activation, especially in regions where these minerals in the diet are low.

One of the primary regulators of our body's antioxidant systems is Nrf2 or Nuclear Factor Erythroid 2-Related Factor 2, which is a transcription factor that binds to DNA to express various genes. Nrf2 works by activating the antioxidant response element (ARE), which increases antioxidants like glutathione, NADPH, bilirubin, thioredoxin and cell protection[505], producing major anti-inflammatory changes[506] and lowering oxidative stress[507].

Compounds that activate NRF2/ARE include broccoli sprouts (sulforaphane), curcumin, coffee (chlorogenic/caffeic/ferulic acid and diterpenes such as cafestol)[508], red wine (quercetin and resveratrol)[509], whole grains (ferulic acid), olive oil, green tea (EGCG), garlic, onions[510], cinnamon[511], hops plant (xanthohumol), spirulina (heme-oxygenase 1, phycocyanin)[512,513,514,515] astaxanthin[516], berberine, berries (especially blueberries), nuts (pterostilbene), grapes, passion fruit, white tea, Japanese knotweed (piceatannol)[517], buckwheat and asparagus (rutin)[518].

Ferulic acid appears to have anti-inflammatory actions that suppress NF-kB activity[519], thus being able to curb the activation and formation of inflammasomes. In various cell models and rodents, ferulic acid has been shown to suppress the NLRP3 inflammasome[520,521]. Ferulic acid is bioavailable orally and a recent clinical study showed that 500 mg of ferulic acid twice a day reduced serum C-reactive protein by about one-third in hyperlipidemic patients[522]. Ferulic acid can be obtained from the ingestion of pycnogenol and many other plant anthocyanins (like black elderberry for example), coffee and unrefined whole grains. The exact mechisms surrounding the benefiits of ferulic acid are not fully understood, but ferulic acid might reduce the expression of the coupling factor MyD88, which is a key mediator in several pro-inflammatory signaling pathways that activate NF-kB and MAP kinases, which drives chronic inflammation[523].

How to Suppress NLRP3 Inflammasome Activation:

- Optimal selenium levels

- Maintain optimal NADPH levels

  o Periodic ketosis, intermittent fasting, regular exercise, improve insulin resistance (restrict refined carbohydrates, sugars and omega-6 seed oils), glycine intake, optimal mineral intake, sunlight and exercise.

- Activate Nrf2

  o Plant polyphenols, alpha lipoic acid, melatonin, ferulic acid (includes coffee and unrefined whole grains), pycnogenol, broccoli sprout powder (sulforaphane), quercetin (found in onions and leeks), EGCG (from green tea), regular exercise, intermittent fasting.

- EPA/DHA from whole food seafood and fatty fish. Avoid overcooking to prevent oxidation of the fats.

- Zinc and glucosamine

- Inhibit NF-kB

  o Turmeric, magnesium, intermittent fasting, optimal omega-6/3 balance, avoid oxidized vegetable and seed oils, sulforaphane, ketosis and quercetin.

- Increase hydrogen sulfide (H2S)

  o NAC, taurine and methyl donors (folate, B12 and betaine)

- Activate AMPK

  o Intermittent fasting, exercise, heat exposure, ketosis, berberine, curcumin, plant polyphenols, coffee, green tea, quercetin.

- Inhibit NOX (NADPH oxidase)

  o Spirulina, glycine, bilirubin, exercise, fasting and improve insulin resistance.

The active form of vitamin D, known as calcitriol, can also suppress MAP kinase, which is a major driver of inflammation during infections and sepsis but vitamin D requires magnesium for its activation[524,525]. It has been found that 15 ng/ml of vitamin D which is considered an insufficient serum vitamin D level in humans, does not supprress lipopolysaccharide(LPS)-induced inflammation[526,527].

Whereas, **inhibition of LPS (i.e., endotoxin) inflammation was significantly reduced with vitamin D levels at 30 ng/ml but maximal inhibition occurred at a vitamin D level of 50 ng/ml**[528].

NADPH oxidase or NOX is a complex of enzymes bound to the cellular membrane. It senses the presence of oxygen and nutrients to balance the body's ROS[529]. Inhibiting NOX increases NADPH and combats oxidative stress. NOX proteins are involved in the inflammation of the vasculature[530]. However, NOX also generates free radicals that destroy pathogens through a process called the respiratory burst[531]. So, some small amounts of oxidative stress are still needed for optimal cellular homeostasis.

Here are several ways to increase NADPH to promote the regeneration of antioxidant defenses in the body such as glutathione and thioredoxin:

- **Increase NAD** – NAD+ or *Nicotinamide adenine dinucleotide* is a key co-enzyme involved with virtually all cellular processes and energy production. NAD+ deficiencies are linked to aging and disease[532]. The extra phosphate group of NADP+ is added by NAD+ kinase[533].

    o   NAD can be synthesized from the amino acids tryptophan or aspartic acid and vitamin B3 or niacin[534]. **Fermented foods like sauerkraut and kimchi have B vitamins and increase NAD+.** The fermentation process produces NADH and lactate, which regenerates NAD+[535].

    o   **Fasting** and calorie restriction increase NAD+ and SIRT1 levels, which has many anti-aging benefits[536,537,538]. Fasting promotes the recycling of NAD by activating NAMPT, which governs the NAD resalvage pathway by promoting AMPK[539].

- o **Exercise** also increases NAD+ and sirtuins[540,541] as does heat exposure and **sauna sessions**[542]. They also help to recycle NAD .

- **Ketosis** - Ketone bodies lower the production of reactive oxygen species in the mitochondria by increasing NADH oxidation into NAD+ [543] . However, hyperketonemia (excessively high ketones in the blood) upregulates NOX4 and oxidative stress [544]. Such hyperketonemia or ketoacidosis usually occurs in states of insulin deficiency like type-1 diabetes, type-2 diabetes or alcohol poisoning[545].

  - o **Refined carbohydrate restriction can be an effective strategy for lowering inflammation, hyperglycemia and raising NAD+** [546] . Both inflammation and hyperglycemia deplete NAD and NADPH[547]. At the same time, glucose is a major source of NADPH[548] but you don't need high amounts of glucose to facilitate that response. Furthermore, the body can create glucose itself through endogenous means. Whether or not it's more beneficial to obtain 150 grams of carbohydrates from whole food sources to reduce the potential stress placed on the body when it's forced to endogenously make glucose is a matter of current debate.

- **Glycine** – The amino acid glycine, as well as collagen, inhibit NOX and raise NADPH[549]. This occurs by increasing chloride in cells that would generate oxidative stress. Glycine is one of the main amino acids that comprises glutathione as does glutamine and cysteine[550]. A 2019 paper by McCarty and DiNicolantonio writes: *"Supplemental glycine may be useful for the prevention and control of atherosclerosis, heart failure, angiogenesis associated with cancer or retinal disorders and a range of inflammation-driven syndromes, including metabolic syndrome."* [551].

81

- **Bilirubin** – Bilirubin is a yellow compound that gets created during heme breakdown. It's needed for clearing waste products from the death of red blood cells. Elevated levels of bilirubin might be indicative of some disease [552] but physiological intracellular levels have been shown to inhibit NOX[553,554]. Oral administration of bilirubin is not feasible because of its very low water solubility, however, biliverdin, which is a more water soluble precursor to bilirubin, can be taken orally[555].

  o **Spirulina or Blue-Green Algae** – Biliverdin's metabolite phycocyanobilin (PhyCB) can be converted by biliverdin reductase to phycocyanorubin, which is analogous to bilirubin in the body and can inhibit NOX complexes[556,557,558]. This might explain why spirulina (specifically phycocyanobilin, which is the light harvester in spirulina) has been shown to have antioxidant and anti-inflammatory effects in numerous clinical studies[559,560].

- **Improve Insulin Resistance** – NOX appears to have a role in inducing insulin resistance and cytokines in hypertrophied fat cells[561,562,563,564]. Bilirubin works in many ways to reduce obesity and its health complications, primarily by lowering NOX[565]. It's been found that plasma levels of bilirubin are inversely correlated with the risk of metabolic syndrome and diabetes[566]. In cross-sectional and prospective studies, higher bilirubin levels are associated with improved insulin sensitivity and reduced risk of metabolic syndrome and type-2 diabetes independent of BMI[567,568]. To fix insulin resistance, you need to lose weight, specifically visceral fat[569], increase physical activity[570] and avoid hyperglycemia.

- **Don't Overeat Calories** - One of the biggest consumers of NADPH is fat storage and de novo lipogenesis[571]. In essence, if your body has to store fat, it depletes NADPH and reduces its antioxidant capacity thus making you more vulnerable to oxidative stress and free radicals. When given the option to either get fat for the coming winter or preserve antioxidant defenses, the body will prioritize the storage of calories because they are scarcer.

The real way to extend lifespan and healthspan is through the consumption of a diet that optimizes the intake of minerals and provides certain phytonutrients to protect against oxidative stress. The use of the term 'balanced diet' is not unintentional it is literal. This is because consuming just one type of food will not provide optimal amounts of all minerals. Nature unfortunately didn't make one superfood to cover all your needed micronutrients. Thus, you should consume a balanced diet in order to hit your optimal nutrient and mineral intake and we will show you how to do precisely that in the coming chapters. Let *The Mineral Fix* by your key to transforming your health and putting you on the path to a longer life!

Chapter 4
Calcium, Magnesium, Hard Water and Your Heart

Heart disease is one of the leading causes of death worldwide, especially in the United States[572]. About 655,000 Americans die from heart disease every year, which is 1 out of 4 deaths[573]. Based on data from 2014-2015, this costs the U.S. $219 billion annually. The most common type of cardiovascular disease is coronary artery disease which leads to heart attacks and strokes being second[574].

Almost half of all adults have at least one of the major risk factors for heart disease: hypertension, high cholesterol or smoking[575]. Obesity and metabolic syndrome are additional contributors to cardiovascular disease development[576]. Metabolic syndrome doubles the risk of cardiovascular disease and increases all-cause mortality by 1.5 times[577].

Although it has some genetic component, cardiovascular disease is mostly a lifestyle disease that is caused by your everyday choices, such as whether or not you smoke, do you engage in regular physical activity and what foods you eat and in what amounts. Even your water quality, more specifically its mineral content, plays a major role in this.

In this chapter, we're going to talk about the connection between water, minerals and heart disease. Water is one of the most common substances we consume on a daily basis. It is one of the most essential things for life so you should get a high-quality source. Imagine what poor quality water consumption, or even harmful water consumption can do to your long-term health if you consume it every day for the rest of your life.

Hard Water vs. Soft Water

Around 20% of your daily fluid intake comes from food while the rest is provided by what you drink. The advice about how much liquid should be consumed in a day varies greatly. Let's face it, if you enjoy eating watermelons and salads, both of which consist mostly of water, you are probably going to feel less thirsty than after a meal of steak and fries. But how often do you consider the quality of that water you are drinking and cooking with on a daily basis? Taking this one step further, have you ever considered the quality of your local water supply?

In 1960, Dr. Henry Schroeder was one of the first to find a substantial correlation between average hardness of drinking water and mortality from cardiovascular disease in the US[578,579]. Water hardness simply means the mineral content of the water. Similar discoveries were noted in Japan by Jun Kobayashi in 1957 who related lower water hardness to an increased risk of sudden death[580]. These associations were negative, meaning the softer the water the higher rate of cardiovascular disease. In 1962, Morris *et al* made a direct link between human health and the composition of the local water supply[581]. The leading researcher, Margaret Crawford, was a pioneer in the field of cardiovascular disease epidemiology and in 1968 she and her colleagues saw that softness (lack of minerals) of the water supply is strongly associated with a higher risk of cardiovascular diseases[582,583].

- **Soft Water** – water low in calcium and magnesium. Calcium and magnesium concentration is less than 100 mg/L.
- **Hard Water** – water with moderate calcium and magnesium. Calcium and magnesium concentration of 100-200 mg/L.
- **Very Hard Water** – water high in calcium and magnesium. Calcium and magnesium concentration exceeding 200 mg/L.

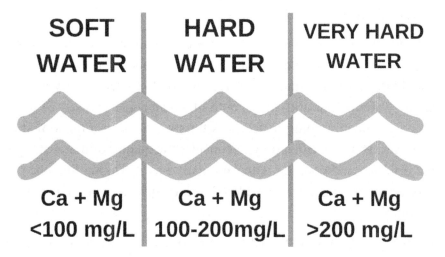

SOFT WATER	HARD WATER	VERY HARD WATER
Ca + Mg <100 mg/L	Ca + Mg 100-200mg/L	Ca + Mg >200 mg/L

Sidenote: Sodium, potassium and lithium are considered monovalent cations (or single positively charged molecules) and do not contribute to the hardness of water, only divalent cations (such as calcium or magnesium) contribute. It's important to note that drinking waters can have a similar total level of hardness but at the same time have very different concentrations of calcium and magnesium[584]. More on that topic coming up.

The association between soft water intake and cardiovascular disease was further supported in 1981 when Masironi and Shaper, citing 11 publications from different parts of the world, showed that populations consuming mineral waters with a higher mineral content enjoyed lower rates of heart attacks and deaths from arteriosclerotic disease, coronary heart disease, hypertensive heart disease as well as sudden deaths due to coronary heart disease[585]. There are 3 case-control studies that have seen that the risk of death from a heart attack is inversely related to the amount of magnesium in the drinking water[586,587,588]. In other words, **people who drink waters that are higher in magnesium are at a lower risk of dying from a heart attack.** Similar results were found by the U.S. Environmental Protection Agency who took a close look at 35 separate geographic regions in the United States. The agency noted that, "...*hardness and calcium appear to follow the normal trend of negative associations with the mortality rates for most groups of* *cardiovascular diseases"*[589]. So, what do we learn from this? ***Put simply, the higher the mineral content in drinking water, the lower the rate of death from cardiovascular disease.***

Most of the people in industrialized societies consume soft water or water that lacks minerals. The reason is because soft water is cheaper and easier to use. Soft water requires less soap, both for personal hygiene and when washing clothes or dishes and it causes less scaling of pipes and leaves fewer stains in pots and pans and enamel sinks. There is a counterpoint to that however: over time, soft water does the opposite of depositing limescale, as it is more corrosive and it can dissolve some of the metals found in the water distribution pipes, which can include copper, zinc and cadmium[590]. Masironi and Shaper noted that, ***"Soft waters could be carrying trace levels of toxic elements from pipes or soil into supply; hard waters could be protective due to their content in calcium and magnesium or in beneficial trace elements.*** *"* [591] That is illustrated by those Cornish mineworkers who suffered from lead-induced gout and traveled North to take the waters in Bath a few hundred years back. They were unknowingly moving from a soft water zone to a region that naturally provided harder spring water. Their cleansing, detoxification process, was effectively achieved by replacing their tainted soft water with calcium rich hard water. Even today, the remnants of lead piping in our water supply get encrusted with calcium in hard water areas, thus taking away much of the danger of toxicity being leached into the water.

There are undoubtedly other factors at work. Some who have written on the topic believe the harmful effect of soft water to be at least in part because of higher levels of cadmium while others believe that the protection associated with hard water is due to higher amounts of other minerals such as chromium, iodine and lithium[592]. Many researchers cite the lack of magnesium in the water supply as a significant factor. Magnesium deficiency is considered a principal driver of cardiovascular disease that increases the risk of heart disease substantially[593]. This problem is magnified by the fact that about 50-75% of the population isn't meeting the 350-420 mg RDA for magnesium[594]. Magnesium regulates vascular smooth muscle cells, affecting blood pressure[595], calcification[596], atherosclerosis[597], kidney disease[598], arrhythmias[599] and thrombosis (clots)[600].

Challenging the Food-Mineral Hypothesis

It's often said that food is sufficiently rich in minerals to provide you everything needed for general well-being. Unfortunately, **the typical whole foods we eat nowadays is severely depleted in many essential nutrients compared to just 70 to 80 years ago**.

In the introduction, we outlined the main reasons why so many people are deficient in minerals. Namely, the overconsumption of refined foods, soil depletion by fertilizers, and heavy metals competing with mineral absorption. Trying to get all your essential vitamins and minerals from just food is not a reliable option in the post-industrialized world because of these additional factors. Yet from a historical standpoint, water too has been seen as a significant source of minerals for both humans and animals, at least until the softening of water occurred.

Consuming high mineral waters provides you with an excellent way to help meet your nutrient requirements, allowing optimization of your mineral intake without overconsuming calories. Given that the majority of the population is already consuming too many calories, optimizing the water mineral content should be a matter of high priority. Just think of high mineral waters as being a more natural way to get minerals compared to how we typically get them in a multivitamin/mineral supplement.

Humans typically consume around two to three liters of water per day (perhaps more in hotter climates). Our challenge to you is not necessarily to convince you to drink more or to drink more frequently, it is to suggest that you make the most out of your everyday thirst. More specifically, just quenching your natural thirst gives you the unique opportunity to take on board important minerals. And, on average, tap water is said to contribute about 60% of the liquid balance into the body each and every day[601]. Imagine what it would do to your overall health if you allocated 60% of your hydration to an optimal source of water.

Yet when it comes to it, most of us don't even give a second thought to the quality of the water we consume on a daily basis, as long as it's safe. Tap water is essentially free in most areas and we drink it and cook with it because it is freely available, yet our health may be suffering because of what is in that tap water, or more often than not, what is missing from it. The overall long-term impact may in part be due to a decreased intake of important minerals, but it can also be because of an increased and undesirable intake of heavy metals.

A lower intake of minerals increases the absorption and the toxic effect of heavy metals, so in this way, by not consuming mineral rich water, we may increase the risk of certain diseases and enhance the harmful effects of toxic heavy metals found in the environment such as aluminum, cadmium, lead, mercury, and arsenic. We should bear in mind that, calcium, which is contained in substantially greater amounts in hard water, may help protect us against lead and cadmium absorption[602]. This can provide an additional benefit as it reduces the heavy metals from competing with the absorption of other minerals as well.

Getting precise national figures is not easy, but a 2004 survey of households in the Phoenix, Arizona area showed that a quarter used water softening equipment for their daily water intake[603], at the time, a relatively recent phenomenon. **Looking back at human history, we never used to drink artificially "*softened*" water**, even when it became available from a piped system. We used to drink the hard water, which was higher in healthy minerals, that nature provides for many of us naturally. The availability of such water is also changing. With the rise of modern agricultural systems, our soil has been steadily depleted of minerals, and so has much of the water running through it. Unsurprisingly, for most of us, the tap water we now consume contains lower levels of the healthiest minerals than it once did. This gradual change is not without its consequences. Harder water may leave deposits that cause the visible scaling of the kettles and pipes in your home but when it comes to the human body, its mineral rich nature appears to have the opposite effect, helping to dissolve the calcifications in the arteries. Quoting once more from Masironi's extensive review: *"Because of the amount taken in, as well as of the free, ionic easily absorbable form in which the chemical elements are present, water is a source of trace and major elements in human nutrition that cannot be disregarded."*[604]

It is known that socioeconomic status contributes to cardiovascular disease risk factors and outcomes[605]. In high income countries, low socioeconomic status is associated with a higher risk of cardiovascular disease and mortality[606,607,608]. This is primarily due to worse lifestyle options, such as increased consumption of cheaper processed food that has more calories, prevalence of obesity, lack of healthcare, insufficient sleep and more financial stress[609]. Less wealthy people also tend to live in areas where there are more environmental toxins and pollutants that impose an additional stressor on the body that affects nutrient status. Furthermore, it is also known that low socioeconomic status is linked with poor water quality[610]. In developing countries, it affects primarily the bacteriological component of the water, increasing the prevalence of bacterial diseases like cholera[611]. In affluent countries, tap water is mostly clean and sanitized but it is still soft water, especially in poorer regions. Morris *et al* (1961) also recognized that the regions in the UK with mostly soft water were old industrial revolution sites as well (Lancashire and South Wales)[612].

According to some authors, more than 10% of the human daily need for elements such as lithium, fluorine, calcium, copper, magnesium, iron, and zinc can be supplied by tap water if it hasn't been softened… and while you might think that 10% does not sound like much, consider this. If there were abundant supplies of minerals in the food we eat, you would be right to question water's impact, but the mineral levels of our increasingly processed food supply chain have been decreasing for years. For example, refining oils eliminates all magnesium, safflower seeds contain 680 mg of magnesium per 1000 calories, but safflower oil has no magnesium at all[613]. Refining grains, rice and wheat decreases the magnesium content by 80-90% and refining sugar decreases the magnesium content by 95-100%[614]. Many readers may be experiencing marginal mineral deficiencies, and that additional 10-20% from harder water could be providing the difference between life-long suboptimal levels and an optimal health status. And to be fair, the daily intake of certain hard waters can easily provide 50% of the RDA for calcium and magnesium, which is certainly relevant.

Bottom Line? **Given we are now at greater risk of marginal nutritional deficiencies due to refined food, poor diet and chronic diseases, drinking water with elevated levels of minerals could make the crucial difference between optimal health and long life, and illness.**

We're not just talking about drinking water. To maximize the potential benefits from water that is rich in minerals, it should be used when cooking and preparing your foods too. Boiling pasta, rice and vegetables in the right water endows those foods with a higher mineral content, the proportion of water in your food being higher than you may at first imagine. It's worth bearing in mind that dry pasta more than doubles its weight with the addition of boiling water and white rice can even triple it. Indeed, since the chemical composition of your cooking water influences the chemical composition of the food you eat, it stands to reason that if that water is poor in minerals (passing through a water-softener for example) cooked food will contain less minerals. The opposite is also true, namely that food will gain minerals after being cooked in hard water." [615]

Bottom line? **It pays to cook your food in hard water.**

The Ratio of Minerals to Toxic Heavy Metals in Water is Just as Important as Absolute Values

According to Crawford, higher calcium levels in water are important for two quite separate reasons. As we have learned, calcium is thought to inhibit the absorption of toxic elements from pipes and soil and hard water is much less corrosive than soft water. That explains why there would be less leaching of harmful metals such as lead and cadmium from water pipes, with hard waters, particularly those high in calcium, providing you this protective effect. Second, your body's absorption of toxic metals such as lead and cadmium is inversely related to the concentration of calcium. This means that high-calcium water may well have a double protective effect, containing decreased amounts of toxic heavy metals as well as reducing their degree of absorption into the body[616]. Put simply, although from a practical point of view, you may be frustrated by the calcium rich 'hard' water furring-up the pipes and kitchen equipment such as coffee makers and kettles, it is precisely that calcium lining of those water pipes which blocks any leaching effect giving you double protection.

However, just getting more calcium, especially if it's being provided in high amounts from supplements or food fortification, is not always beneficial and could even be harmful. Although this does not appear to be the case from naturally high calcium waters as the intake of calcium is slower and doesn't spike blood levels like higher amounts of calcium can do from supplements and food fortifications. Indeed, a high intake of supplemental calcium is associated with increased risk of cardiovascular disease death in both men and women[617]. Calcium supplementation without co-administered vitamin D increases the risk of having a heart attack[618]. Some evidence shows that there is an inverse relationship between calcium and blood pressure, reducing systolic blood pressure in patients with hypertension[619]. The complete mechanisms for that result are unclear[620]. It is hypothesized low calcium would result in changes in vitamin D and parathyroid hormones, which result in increasing intracellular calcium and thus causing vascular smooth muscles to increase blood pressure[621]. However, extra calcium intake through supplementation results in higher circulating calcium, leading to calcification and calcium deposition in the coronary arteries and extra-skeletal muscle tissue[622].

To promote calcium absorption and to keep calcium out of the arteries and into the bones, you need sufficient vitamin D and vitamin K2. Vitamin D regulates calcium levels in the blood and vitamin K2 directs it into the right place such as the bones and teeth[623]. Vitamin D toxicity and vitamin K deficiency are associated with soft tissue calcification[624, 625]. Low levels of vitamin K are also linked to cardiovascular disease[626]. Supplementing with vitamin K has been shown to reduce coronary artery calcification[627]. Unfortunately, the majority of people are also deficient in vitamin D and K[628], which might explain the susceptibility to calcification with calcium supplementation. On top of that, magnesium is needed to activate vitamin D and move it around the body[629]. Deficient magnesium can reduce the active form of vitamin D, also known as calcitriol, and impair the parathyroid hormonal response[630]. This can lead to magnesium-dependent vitamin-D-resistant rickets[631]. Thus, **optimizing vitamin D levels requires an optimal magnesium status**[632]. Importantly, **active vitamin D is needed to produce vitamin K-dependent proteins and helps to activate them, which requires magnesium**[633].

Dietary calcium intake is considered safe compared to supplemental calcium[634]. Among 132,823 participants over the course of 17.5 years, dietary calcium intake was not associated with all-cause mortality, but men taking ≥ 1000 mg/d of supplemental calcium had a higher risk of all-cause mortality and cardiovascular disease-specific mortality[635]. Thus, it is not recommended to be taking a calcium supplement, at least at doses above 500-1,000 mg, especially in the presence of other mineral deficiencies, and try to get it from dietary sources.

Minerals from water are easier for your body to absorb than those from food and most supplements. Most of us get our calcium from the food we eat but many of us are not getting enough calcium. According to the U.S. National Institutes of Health, nearly half of all Americans now take a regular supplement that includes calcium[636]. Yet even if you have a diet that is poor in calcium, you might be able to get a substantial amount of the calcium you need from your drinking water. According to Crawford's research, in the UK the difference in calcium intake between hard- and soft-water areas can amount to as much as 2 grams per day, which represents a significant factor. Not all of that would be absorbed by the body of course. In fact, it is estimated that less than 30% of the calcium ingested through food is absorbed, but if you consider the factors that affect your body's absorption, the importance of water as a source of calcium may be greater than most of us appreciate[637]. Consider the fact that the more calcium you take in at one time, the harder it is for your body to process it, which speaks for the steady 'supplementation' provided by your hard water supply, rather than occasionally swallowing calcium-rich pills[638].

Bottom line? **Minerals from water are more bioavailable when compared to minerals from food and supplements.**

Magnesium in Mineral Waters Provide Optimal Heart Health

There's a second mineral involved in hard water besides calcium and that's magnesium. Calcium usually plays the bigger role but even a low-calcium, magnesium-rich water source would be categorized as hard water. This is where the interaction with your health gets to be even stronger because, whereas the link between calcium and healthier hearts is mostly down to correlation, the hypothesis that magnesium is a heart-healthy mineral is more clearly persuasive.

Take for example the findings that the magnesium concentration in the hearts of subjects dying of heart disease is 24% lower than that of those subjects dying from accidents [639]. There is also a link between magnesium deficiency and sudden death, suggesting that (1) sudden death is common in areas where community water supplies are magnesium deficient, (2) Myocardial magnesium content is low in people who die of sudden death, (3) Cardiac arrhythmias and coronary artery vasospasm can be caused by magnesium deficiency and (4) Intravenous magnesium reduces the risk of arrhythmia and death immediately after a heart attack[640]. Thus, sufficient magnesium levels are strongly and negatively correlated with rates of sudden cardiac death even after adjusting for other risk factors [641]. In Taiwan, magnesium in drinking water has been shown to have a significant protective effect on the risk of cerebrovascular disease (strokes)[642].

Magnesium deficiency promotes the development of cardiovascular disease by increasing arterial calcifications, thrombosis, atherosclerosis, inflammation, and oxidative stress[643]. Masironi wrote in 1981: *"It is difficult to judge whether the apparently lower magnesium content of a damaged heart is a result or a cause of that damage."* [644] It seems to be the case that magnesium deficiency may well be damaging to those hearts which are already damaged or malfunctioning, but also that higher levels may well be protective. This is highlighted by the following quote: *"**High coronary heart disease rates in Ohio were found in areas with less than 15 mg of magnesium per liter in the drinking water, whereas low CHD rates were found in areas with 36 mg/liter. Similar findings were reported by other investigators.**"*[645]

Low serum magnesium increases the risk of thrombosis (clotting)[646,647], which does not only promote cardiovascular disease but also complications in severe COVID-19 [648, 649]. In the body, magnesium has anti-thrombotic effects and reduces mortality in pulmonary thromboembolism[650]. This suggests that magnesium has anti-coagulant properties. Magnesium deficiency has been implicated in insulin resistance, type-2 diabetes, hyperglycemia, and hyperinsulinemia[651,652], all of which are considered risk factors of heart disease[653].

Whereas levels of calcium can be quite high, even in modern processed food, which tend to be calcium-fortified, magnesium is usually present at much lower levels and the accepted daily requirement levels are seldom attained. Although this does not usually translate into a clear-cut magnesium deficiency, among those eating a modern Western diet (and that's most Americans), the recommended daily level of 350-500 mg is difficult to reach, which demonstrates yet again the important role that drinking and cooking with hard water can play. It is estimated that up to 30% of the population has a subclinical magnesium deficiency simply based on low magnesium blood levels, however, utilizing more advanced measurements for magnesium status, this can be as high as 90% in certain populations[654]. We should repeat here that just because your water is classified as hard that does not mean there is necessarily ample magnesium in it, it may simply be high in calcium.

Research from Canada shows that water areas with high magnesium concentrations can contribute as much as 20% of a person's total daily magnesium intake compared with about 1% in water areas with a low magnesium concentration[655]. The same study calculated that people in

95

Canada who consume water with a hardness above 150 mg/l as calcium carbonate obtain an additional 50 mg of magnesium than those living in soft water areas even when eating a similar diet. This amount may be important under circumstances where requirements might be raised by stressful situations[656]. This is because additional stressors, such as psychological stress, insulin resistance, and environmental toxins deplete magnesium[657].

The average concentration of magnesium in European drinking water is relatively low (about 12 mg/liter) and constitutes 10% of the daily intake[658]. However, bottled mineral water that is widely consumed in some parts of Europe might contribute an average of 40% of the total daily magnesium[659]. This observation was made long before drinking bottled water became a mainstay of U.S. drinking habits, something almost unheard of in 1976, but considered quite normal today.

Other Relevant Minerals in Your Water Supply

So far, we have expounded on two of the larger contributors to so-called 'hard' water - calcium and magnesium. These two certainly drive many of the discussions on minerals and health. Now it is time to extend our repertoire and we will take a look at a number of other important minerals commonly found in water.

- **Chromium** - Looking at the polished chrome plated fenders and pipes of a Harley Davidson motorbike, you can see the brilliant, shiny result of the hexavalent chromium plating solution, which protects the metal underneath the plating from corrosion. Trace elements of this hexavalent chromium compound can be found in polluted water and its toxicity is dangerous. However, there is another form of the element chromium, that being tri-valent and non-toxic, which is both essential and beneficial for your body.
  - **Chromium has been shown to play an important role in glucose metabolism, which influences glucose tolerance**[660]. Chromium picolinate, specifically, has been shown to reduce insulin resistance and may even

reduce the risk of cardiovascular disease and type-2 diabetes[661]. A report on four meta-analyses of human studies saw a significant reduction in fasting plasma glucose levels from chromium supplementation[662]. A 2016 review covering six meta-analyses concluded that chromium decreases fasting blood glucose and HbA1C[663]. Thus, you do not want to be deficient in chromium because that is associated with diabetes and hyperglycemia[664].

o   With an epidemic of Type-2 diabetes circling the globe, the ability to improve our glucose tolerance represents an important health factor. In the U.S. alone, an estimated 100 million adults or more now live with diabetes or pre-diabetes according to the Centers for Disease Control and Prevention[665]. Across the United States, most of the population may be in a state of marginal chromium deficiency[666].

o   A further reported benefit of chromium is that it has also been found to be protective against atherosclerotic lesions (so it protects blood vessels), but to date, this has only been observed in experimental animals[667]. In rabbits, giving chromium resulted in a 50% reduction in aortic intimal plaque area and in aortic total cholesterol content[668]. Chromium picolinate has been shown to significantly decrease triglycerides, insulin, HOMA-IR, inflammation, and insulin resistance in patients with non-alcoholic fatty liver disease[669].

o   Although a number of researchers have demonstrated this inverse association between cardiovascular disease and the chromium content of drinking water, it is important to add that the causal relationship is not proven. It remains an area worthy of further investigation, but certainly suggests that chromium can be significant as a nutritional source when it is present in your drinking water[670].

- **Lithium** is the lightest solid element in the periodic table, and it is an essential trace mineral with many recommending an intake of 1 mg/day to meet requirements[671]. You will instantly recognize the name because of its use in batteries around the world to power our electronic devices. In miniscule doses, lithium has been shown to have a number of health-related benefits. **Observational studies in Japan have noted that low-dose lithium in drinking water is associated with better longevity[672].**

  o Lithium has been associated with the low prevalence of both coronary heart disease and of gastroduodenal ulcers among the Pima Indians of Arizona, where levels in their water supplies can exceed 100 ug/l. That's over fifty times the U.S. average. Other teams of researchers found a negative correlation between lithium levels in drinking water and cardiovascular death rates in the U.S. and given that lithium has for years been prescribed as a mood stabilizer, associations with less aggressive behavior among the populations using the water could lie behind a lower incidence of mental disorders, violence and also of heart attacks[673].

  o More recently in Denmark, higher levels of lithium in the local water supply have been linked to lower levels of dementia[674]. **Higher lithium levels in drinking water have also been shown to have a protective effect on the risk of suicide in countries across the entire world[675].** Therapeutic doses of lithium (600-1800 mg/day) are commonly used to treat mania and depression in patients of bipolar disorder[676].

  o Lithium administration has been shown to protect against hyponatraemia or low sodium levels in the blood[677]. The mechanisms for that are proposed to be lithium's ability to reduce water retention in diabetes insipidius[678]. Lithium toxicity, however, can cause hypotension and cardiovascular complications, which is why its serum levels have to be monitored carefully[679]. Maternal use of lithium during the first trimester has been found to increase the risk of cardiac malformations[680].

- **Iodine** - The regular consumption of iodine is important because it allows our bodies to make the all-important thyroid hormones[681]. Low thyroid function leads to hypothyroidism, which can raise cholesterol[682], promote weight gain, and predispose you to metabolic syndrome[683]. A telltale goiter (neck swelling) is one of the most visible signs of iodine deficiency.

  o We find iodine often added to salt - in some countries it is mandatory - to ensure adequate levels are available. In Canada for example, all salt sold to consumers for table and household use must be iodized with 0.01% potassium iodide, but there are exceptions for the more specialized and exotic salts or those used for pickling vegetables[684]. If you are lucky enough to receive iodine naturally from your tap water, you may be among the best protected.

  o There is also evidence linking the iodine content in water to other health benefits: *"**Water may contribute significantly to the daily requirement of iodine, perhaps up to 20%**. The iodine content in water is negatively correlated to cardiovascular disease (CVD) rates in Finland. The susceptibility of the Finnish population to CVD apparently increases when there is less than 2-3 ug of iodine per liter of drinking water."* [685]

- **Fluoride** - The mineral fluorine presents us with a somewhat different situation, since many authorities around the world add fluoride to the water supply, usually citing studies which have shown how this measure can reduce the prevalence of tooth decay[686]. Untreated dental caries can lead to weight gain, impair growth, increase the risk of infections, affect school performance and possibly lead to death [687, 688]. Adequate fluoride intake inhibits demineralization and bacterial activity in dental plaque[689,690].

- o Fluoride is the ionic form of fluorine, which promotes bone formation and fights tooth decay[691]. Teeth and bones store 99% of the fluoride in the human body. In adults, 50% of absorbed fluoride gets retained and 50% is excreted through urine. In children the absorption rate is up to 80% because their bones and teeth are in the growth stage[692].

- o A 2015 review of 20 observational studies discovered that water fluoridation reduces the risk of tooth decay and fillings by 35% and permanent loss of adult teeth by 26% in children receiving fluoridated water compared to children receiving unfluoridated water[693]. A 2018 cross-sectional study in the U.S. found that living in a county where 75% or more of the drinking water is fluoridated with at least 0.7 mg/L of fluoride was associated with a 30% reduction in the rate of primary teeth caries and a 12% reduction in the rate of caries in primary teeth [694]. In Australian adults, exposure to fluoridated municipal water for at least 14 years associates with an 11-12% lower rate of decayed, missing or filled teeth than those whose water had negligible amounts of fluoride[695]. The average rate of decayed, missing or filled teeth in Australian Defense Force members aged 17-56 is 24% lower in those whose water that contained 0.5-1.0 mg/L of fluoride for at least half of their lifetime compared to those exposed for less than 10% of their lifetime[696]. **However, the benefit of fluoride is from its topical use, not its oral ingestion, and there are potential side effects from consuming fluoridated water.** One group of authors concluded, "Fluoride has modest benefit in terms of reduction of dental caries but significant costs in relation to cognitive impairment, hypothyroidism, dental and skeletal fluorosis, enzyme and electrolyte derangement, and uterine cancer. Given that most of the toxic effects of fluoride are due to ingestion, whereas its predominant beneficial effect is obtained via topical application, ingestion or inhalation of fluoride predominantly in any form constitutes an unacceptable risk with virtually no proven benefit."[697]

o   Within the countries of the European Union, only Ireland mandates the addition of fluoride though others are selective in its application. In the UK for example, the mineral is added to tap water only in regions where they consider natural levels are too low. In this context, the U.S. first began adding fluoride to selected water supplies in the 1940s and today, over one-third of Canadians and about two-thirds of Americans have access to fluoridated water[698]. Compounds containing the mineral fluoride have been added to many community water supplies throughout the U.S., yet some feel that nowadays, with so many toothpastes and mouthwashes containing fluoride, the potential risks may outweigh the benefits. In fact, in 2014, for the very first time, the total daily recommended levels for fluoride were reduced.

o   The daily adequate intake (AI) for fluoride in adults is 3-4 mg, 3 mg in teens aged 14-18, 1-2 mg in children aged 4-13, 0.7 mg in 1-3-year-olds, 0.5 mg in 7-12-month-olds and 0.01 mg in newborns less than 6 months of age[699]. The U.S. Public Health Service recommends a fluoride concentration of 0.7 mg/L in drinking water for prevention of dental caries. The maximum allowable concentration established by the EPA is 4.0 mg/L and maximum recommended concentration is 2.0 mg/L[700]. Average fluoride intakes in the U.S. from both foods and fluorinated drinking water is 1.2-1.6 mg for infants less than 4 years old, 2.0-2.2 mg for 4-11-year-olds, 2.4 mg for 11-14-year-olds and 2.9 mg for adults[701].

101

o Most toothpaste in the U.S. contains sodium fluoride or monofluorophosphate, usually at a concentration of 1,000-1,100 mg/L (about 1.3 mg per quarter of a teaspoon used for one brushing). How much fluoride is absorbed from toothpaste depends on the amount used and how much a person swallows it. It is estimated that adults ingest 0.1 mg/d from toothpaste, children aged 6-12 ingest 0.2-0.3 mg/d and children less than 5 years old 0.1-0.25 mg/d. Other dental products that contain fluoride are mouth washes, orthodontic bracket adhesives and cavity liners.[702] Oral antifungal medicine like voriconazole provides 65 mg/d of fluoride, which in the long-term can cause high serum fluoride levels[703,704].

o Serious systemic fluoride toxicity can be caused by doses of 5 mg/kg (about 375 mg for a 165 lb. person)[705]. That threshold is almost impossible to reach by being exposed to drinking water or dental care products. Excess fluoride intake causes gastrointestinal distress, nausea, abdominal pain and diarrhea. Ingestion of large doses of sodium fluoride (60 mg) can promote skeletal fluorosis, causing osteoporosis and bone fractures[706].

o Excess fluoride intake above the recommended intake, especially in childhood, can lead to dental fluorosis, characterized by white or brown lines or flecks on the teeth[707,708]. NHANES data has discovered that the rates of dental fluorosis have increased from 29.7% in 2001-2002 to 61.3% in 2011-2012[709]. High fluoride intake in children may also be associated with lower IQ and impaired cognition[710,711,712,713].

o **A meta-analysis of all available studies on the topic from 2018 indicated that exposure to high levels of fluoride in water were strongly associated with reduced levels of intelligence in children**[714]. This was further endorsed by research published in 2019, focused on mother-child pairs from six Canadian cities which found that **high fluoride exposure during pregnancy was correlated with lower IQ scores among young children, especially boys**. It led to the author's recommendation for pregnant mothers to reduce their fluoride intake during pregnancy, but the topic is controversial. It even led to the editor of the JAMA Pediatrics who published the findings, writing something of a disclaimer and reminding us that "scientific inquiry is an iterative process" [715]. With the benefit of hindsight however, on the topic of fluoride and its various compounds, the jump to mandatory addition to the water supply in certain areas may have been taken too hastily.

o **Brewed tea is one of the highest sources of dietary fluoride** because the tea plants absorb fluoride from the soil. Fluoride levels in tea brewed with distilled water can range from 0.3 to 6.5 mg/L (0.07 to 1.5 mg/cup)[716]. **One cup of coffee contains 0.22 mg of fluoride.** Other foods like shrimp, pork, beef and tuna have 0.02-0.17 mg of fluoride per 3 oz. serving, while a medium baked potato has 0.08 mg[717]. The amount of fluoride in breast milk and cow's milk is almost undetectable. Thus, most food sources are relatively low in fluoride and unless you are regularly drinking tea, it would be difficult to reach the adequate intake of 3-4 mg/d. Fluorinated municipal drinking water accounts for 60% of the fluoride intake in the U.S.

o Overall, drinking only tap water might be problematic for infants and children in developing years but complete avoidance may lead to fluoride deficiencies. Even supplementing fluoride 0.25-1 mg/d for 24-55 months in children living in communities without fluorinated drinking water has resulted in a 24% reduced rate of decayed, missing and filled tooth surfaces[718]. In areas where water fluoridation rates are lower than 0.6 mg/L, fluoride supplementation of 0.25-1 mg/d may reduce the rate of caries in primary teeth by 48-72% in children aged 6-10[719]. Thus, a moderate consumption of fluorinated water (1-1.5 liters a day) should be acceptable and may even be beneficial. Cooking your food and vegetables with fluorinated water may also be recommended if you have a low intake of fluoride.

- **Silicon** is best known to most of us as the base material for semiconductor manufacturing and the creation of the computer chip beginning with silica sand, which is made up of silicon dioxide. As the eighth most common element in the universe, making up more than 90% of the earth's crust, it should be no surprise that trace elements (mostly silicon dioxides) are found in our drinking water. That's probably a good thing.

  o We have already read that hard water is associated with lower death rates from coronary heart disease, but across the U.S., where the water contains above average levels of silicon - 15mg per liter vs. 8 mg per liter – that association becomes even more positive. This can be related to the silica content in natural water supplies which is commonly in the 5 to 25 mg/L range[720]. The association is further supported by the situation in Eastern Finland, where **lower silicon concentration levels in the water are associated with more heart disease than found in the west of the country**.

  o There are further benefits associated with silicon. Researchers at UK's Keele University found that **drinking around a liter of silicon-rich mineral water every day can speed up the removal of toxic aluminum from the body via the kidneys and ultimately urine**. They even recommend selecting your bottled water according to its silicon content[721]!

- **Cadmium -** *In its natural state, cadmium* is a lustrous and silver-white, malleable metal, often used together with chromium in the electro-plating of steel, but you can also find it in hard and soft drinking water, albeit in miniscule quantities.

- o Working in the late 1950s, Dr. Henry Schroeder was also among those carrying out research which indicated that soft water was linked to higher levels of heart disease. He suggested that the action of soft water increased hypertension and pointed his finger particularly at higher cadmium levels.

His four considerations were namely that:

1. Cadmium induced hypertension in rats
2. Cadmium levels were higher in humans who died of hypertension
3. The higher cadmium concentration in human subjects who died of hypertension was due to the leaching of cadmium from pipes through the corrosive action of soft water and
4. The relationship between soft water and cardiovascular mortality is linked to hypertension

- o This theory is supported by both experimental and clinical evidence[722], making cadmium something to watch out for, avoiding higher levels where you can. The wide use of cadmium in nickel-cadmium batteries, the coloration of plastics and in various discarded electronic products has led to cadmium getting into water supplies in certain areas. A potential environmental hazard to be aware of.[723]

Minerals/Metals in Water

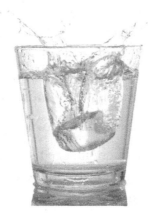

Beneficial	Harmful
Calcium	Lead
Magnesium	Aluminum
Sodium	Arsenic
Silicon	Mercury
Iodine	Cadmium
Chromium	Excess Copper
Sulfate	Excess Fluoride
Lithium	Excess Lithium
Copper	Excess Sulfate

A Geographical Advantage? Tap Water from the Western United States and from Southern Europe May Provide Greater Health Benefits

Although calcium and magnesium levels determine the hardness of water, where they are present in greater quantities, you invariably find a rich cocktail of other minerals too. Following his initial fieldwork in the early 1970s, Roberto Masironi and his colleagues went on to study how where you live is associated with water hardness, and whether that too relates to cardiovascular disease (CVD). To the north of Europe, vast and incredibly old geological substrata underlie surface rocks and topsoil meaning that the underground water flows are soft by nature. This represents a North-South direction, but a similar divisive feature can also be found in North America, albeit this time running in an East-West direction. In both continents, associations with cardiovascular disease are consistent with the softness of the water, which led the team to deduce (by elimination) that your latitude – that being how far North or South of the equator you are – plays little if any role in the matter. However, where you live in terms of your relationship to the underlying local geology consistently showed similar relationships concerning water hardness and cardiovascular disease[724]. Your fate is, at least to some extent, influenced by the very nature of the structural rock upon which the community where you live was founded.

Across the USA, there's some irony to be found in the number of water softeners now being used, each of which changes the positive heart-related qualities of hard water. Seen from the perspective of reduced build-up of deposits in kettles, water heaters and pipes, this makes all the sense in the world, but our hearts seem to 'see' and experience this differently. Masironi et al state: *"...in hard water areas of the US, it is estimated that 60-70% of residences use water softeners."* [725] In fact, one study found that half of the people living in a "hard water" area drank softened or bottled water by preference[726] (... and that figure is almost certainly higher today).

Is it time to reconsider drinking your soft tap water? There are notable cumulative benefits to sticking with hard water for drinking and cooking, and here is another to add to the list. As well as the many heart related correlations, it appears that **the rates of stones formed in the bladder or urinary tract are also higher in areas that drink soft water**[727]. Admittedly, this particular research only took place with rabbits, but it's worth also noting that when given distilled water instead of hard water, they developed more atherosclerosis[728]. Instead of the much touted idea that eating fatty food clogs your arteries, could it be that soft water is potentially more harmful?

What lies behind the water hardness theory of cardiovascular disease?

It is time to take a closer look at what is actually happening in your household water pipes. Whereas a water softener will prevent them 'furring up' with limescale (that being mostly calcium carbonate), what you might not know if you have soft water flowing through your household piping system, is that it too can affect your pipes. As we had alluded to previously, water is just slightly acidic and that's down to the carbon dioxide content. Over time, this is what gives the water a cumulative, corrosive nature which can allow the water to strip cadmium, lead and other harmful elements from your piping, depending of course on what that piping is made of. This over time leads to adverse effects on your personal cardiovascular condition and represents a biologically plausible mechanism for how soft water supplies are associated with cardiovascular disease. That is in contrast to supplies of harder water which contain calcium and importantly, other beneficial minerals for your heart and health such as magnesium. [729]

The situation is not much changed from when in 1975, researchers concluded:

> *"According to a WHO expert group, evidence from many properly designed epidemiological studies undertaken by independent investigators shows that hardness of drinking water (and particularly the calcium content) in Canada, the UK, and the US is inversely associated with cardiovascular mortality, and with adult mortality in general... This was also the conclusion of an international group of experts who met in 1975 under the auspices of the Commission of the European Communities."* [730]

That major work carried out by R. Masironi from the Cardiovascular Disease Unit of the World Health Organization (WHO) in Geneva together with A.G Shaper from the Royal Free Hospital School of Medicine in London represented the most comprehensive piece of research on the topic, and it is still relevant today. They looked at data from different countries and teams of researchers in Ontario and found that up to 10% of the variability in chronic heart disease (CHD) was associated with differences in the water hardness, particularly citing the calcium and magnesium content of the water. In soft-water areas of the U.S., cardiovascular mortality was found to be elevated by 15% compared to that in the hard-water areas. The National Academy of Sciences of the U.S. stated that "...*the body of evidence is sufficiently compelling to treat the "water story" as plausible, particularly when the number of potentially preventable deaths from cardiovascular diseases is considered*." At that time in the United States, cardiovascular diseases accounted for more than one-half of the approximate 2 million deaths occurring each year. The WHO report estimated that access to better quality drinking water would have the potential to reduce annual cardiovascular disease mortality rates by as much as 15%. Nevertheless, and as so often is the case with such associative research, they were not prescriptive with their solution. The researchers acknowledged that more definitive information would be needed in order to identify the precise nature of remedial water treatment actions that should be considered.[731]

The Vital Role Played by Magnesium

Chalkiness in the form of calcium carbonate will be what you most often identify when looking at the limescale build-up in your household water pipes, kettle or coffee machine. Yet it is the magnesium content of that scale which may be having the biggest influence on your heart and surprisingly, on your taste buds too. Even when your local Starbucks provides consistency in the quality and degree of roast used for their coffee beans, it may be the hardness of the water affecting the taste more than you might realize. That's why the same brand of coffee can taste quite different in Tampa Florida, where the water that comes out of the tap ranges in hardness from 140 to 300 parts per million (note: that's hard) compared to the coffee mecca, Portland Oregon, where water has typically 3 to 8 parts of dissolved minerals per million (that's really soft)[732]. But which coffee tastes better and why?

Christopher Hendon, a chemist at the University of Bath in England found that water composition was key to the proportions of sugars, starches, bases and acids extracted from a particular coffee roast. Whereas hard water is generally considered to be bad for better tasting cups of Java, when working with a local coffee shop, he found that it was less a matter of hard or soft but more to do with the type of hardness affecting the taste. "While high bicarbonate levels are bad," Hendon explains, "high magnesium ion levels increase the extraction of coffee into water and improve the taste."[733] His research showed that sodium rich waters produced by water softeners didn't help the taste but that using magnesium-rich water was best. And his research insights bore fruit, bringing him competitive success as well. Moving from theory to practice, in the 2014 global barista championships, which took place in Rome among more than 50 competitors, his barista partner, Maxwell Colonna-Dashwood went on to take fifth place overall[734] – using their specially selected water. If you would like to know more about the effects of water on your coffee, the pair of them even brought out a book entitled, "Water for Coffee".

The reason then that you may consider using bottled water with a higher magnesium content in your coffee machine would ostensibly be to improve the taste, but it's really your heart that could be getting the major benefit. The Chipperfields, a husband-and-wife team working from the biochemistry and chemistry departments of the University of Hull in England found that magnesium is essential for heart muscle contraction and for oxidative phosphorylation in heart mitochondria. That may sound overly complex, but it is important because oxidative phosphorylation is the process by which adenosine triphosphate (ATP) is formed, considered by biologists to be the energy currency of life itself. It is the high energy molecule which stores the energy we need to do just about everything we do, and it has been suggested that a magnesium-ATP complex is the true substrate for all reactions involving ATP.[735]

Studies have shown there is a rapid loss of magnesium from the heart when there is a lack of oxygen under experimental conditions, indicating that chronic angina (chest pain) may well lead to magnesium loss in the heart. Experiments on animals have also shown that a diet which is deficient in magnesium predisposes those animals to the development of myocardial fiber necrosis (death), but importantly, magnesium salts can reverse many of the changes that have taken place[736,737,738,739]. There is also good evidence that pretreatment with magnesium salts can protect against many of the changes in the heart caused by a lack of oxygen, representing further evidence for a diet which is high in magnesium being able to prevent the harm caused by an acute ischemic event such as a heart attack. It has even been suggested that the higher incidence of heart disease in Scotland compared to England can be attributed to a twenty-fold higher level of magnesium in English beer compared to Scottish Whisky. But I think we'll set that story aside!

Water Hardness and Magnesium – Their Role in Heart Muscle

As a broad statement, it clearly looks as if the less magnesium there is in your drinking water, the less magnesium there is in your heart and this might be what explains the greater incidence of sudden cardiac deaths in areas of low magnesium drinking water. This was certainly found to be the case in Ontario, where after examining the heart muscle from people dying after accidents in soft-water areas, they found significantly lower concentrations of magnesium. Incidentally, the magnesium/potassium ratio in their hearts was also found to be lower when it was compared with normal heart muscle from those living in hard water areas [740]. The authors concluded rather bluntly that, *"Western diets are probably often low in magnesium, so that the magnesium in hard drinking water may help to protect its consumers from ischemic heart disease."* Admittedly, it was not a large study but in all, 64 Canadian males had died as the result of accidents and thus were considered representative of the general population when compared with victims who die from "natural causes". Of those 64 men, 20 were residents of three different hard-water areas while 44 of them were residents of five soft-water areas. The mean magnesium concentrations in wet heart tissue for the hard and soft water residents were 222.3 ug/gran and 206.7 ug/gram, respectively (the difference being statistically significant at the 0.01 level). Another way of interpreting these results would suggest that although the very fact of suffering heart disease per se may lead to a reduction in magnesium levels in the heart, drinking from a soft water supply that is lower in magnesium seems also to lead to a reduction in magnesium content.[741]

Worthy of note is that after calcium, sodium and potassium, magnesium is the fourth most commonly found mineral in the human body. Of the 25 grams of magnesium present in an average 70-kilogram human (155 pounds), you will find half of it in your bones, around a quarter in your muscle tissue and the rest distributed among soft tissue and blood[742]. A lack of magnesium is to be taken seriously, as it contributes not only to heart problems but to numerous health conditions, the mineral being necessary for the efficient biochemical functioning of numerous metabolic pathways.

The human body is no one-trick pony, relying on the interplay of many interdependent factors to maintain balance and health, and magnesium is by no means the only consideration in your water supply. As well as the need to get decent levels of calcium, let us not forget that sodium also has its role to play. A study of 4200 adults from 35 geographic areas in the United States, analyzed the quality of tap water from each participant's residence. Although hardness and calcium followed the normal trend of negative associations with the mortality rates for most groups of cardiovascular diseases, they found that higher sodium levels were also (and as they noted, unexpectedly) negatively related to both the male and female cardiovascular mortality rates[743]. So just as we saw earlier with magnesium, higher sodium levels in the resident's tap water were also found to play their part in lowering the rates of cardiovascular, kidney and ischemic heart disease mortality.

What is without question true, is that individual drinking water exposure is directly related to cardiovascular health, so in the following chapters, we will examine both the good and the bad when it comes to minerals and other trace elements in your water supply. Meanwhile, if you've not done so already, now might be the time to get informed by your local water authority or supplier about just how much of which minerals are present in your daily glasses of water, your cups of tea and coffee, and your boiled vegetables and dry goods. It might provide an interesting eye opener for you and your family and provide you with a great starting point for this mineral-based journey.

Bottom line: Isn't it about time you checked out your local water content?

Chapter 5
Taking the Waters: Mineral Waters with Magnesium and Calcium

We know that nutrient deficiencies are widespread because of poor diet, soil depletion and how we grow our food. Hopefully, the previous chapter opened up a new way of thinking about this topic because water is another source of essential minerals. Drinking water is something we all do every day, and it is essential for life. However, staying hydrated does not necessarily equate to drinking water. Drinking just plain water might not do the trick if it doesn't have any minerals in it. In fact, overhydration with plain water could worsen mineral deficiency and dehydration. Unless you compensate for your mineral deficiencies with the right foods or water, you could end up excreting more minerals out the urine.

Although most tap water is safe, it doesn't have the essential minerals found in more natural sources. The most common minerals found in spring water are calcium, sodium and magnesium. Older man-made water systems used copper for plumbing. Copper is important for energy production and it has antimicrobial properties, but it can also corrode easily and contribute to excess copper.

In Ancient Rome, they used water pipes made of lead, which is now known to be poisonous and can be lethal. The Roman writer Vitruvius had documented the potential harms of lead[744]. It was said to cause abdominal pain and create a dark, ghoulish look [745]. Historians nowadays think that lead poisoning because of lead water pipes played a major role in the downfall of the Roman Empire[746,747]. Lead was readily available and cheap, which is why it was used for water pipes[748].

Water is by far a more bioavailable source of minerals because they are dissolved and charged in the liquid, rather than bound to food particles. Different foods also have ingredients and compounds, such as phytates, fiber or phytonutrients, that will decrease the amount of minerals you will absorb. At the end of the day, what matters is what you end up absorbing. With food, the absorption of minerals is never as high as what occurs from liquid because some of the nutrients are lost in the stool due to lack of digestion.

In this chapter, we will talk about the health benefits of mineral waters. First, we will go through some of the history about mineral-rich waters in the form of spa therapy or liquid consumption. Then, we will include recommendations for ensuring an adequate intake of calcium, sodium and magnesium from water.

History of Spa and Mineral Water Therapy

There are 22 different minerals that make up about 5% of our body weight. Those same minerals were present as rocks on Earth when life first formed. Life on Earth began in the oceans where there is an abundance of minerals, salt and electrolytes. They are essential for cellular functioning and energy production. The kidneys are what regulate the body's fluid and electrolyte balance.

Minerals, and mineral-infused waters, have been considered to have medicinal properties for centuries. Some of the earliest bathing descriptions originate from Ancient Greece in the 5th century BC[749]. The baths were considered sacred and were dedicated to many idols[750]. Hippocrates thought that bathing could help to re-establish a healthy balance in bodily fluids and thus treat disease[751].

The Romans began 'taking the waters' in spa towns over 2,000 years ago, and 'the right kind of water' has been reputed to cure all sorts of ailments, whether you are bathing in it or drinking copious amounts[752]. Galen, the Roman surgeon, promoted the effects of mineral water on various diseases[753]. Romans also built spas across Europe in newly conquered lands to treat wounded soldiers and recover from physical exertion.

During the Renaissance, Italian doctors began to associate the health benefits of spas with the waters high in minerals[754]. By the 17th century, many spa treatment resorts and centres were built in many regions of Europe, such as France, England, Italy, Germany, Austria and Eastern

Europe[755]. The term 'spa' comes from a small town in Belgium called Spa that had the name *Aquae Spadanae* in Roman times.

Nowhere are the benefits of mineral-rich water better demonstrated than at Epsom Springs, located just southwest of London. Epsom Springs was discovered in 1618 and legend has it that, in the midst of a dry spell of weather, a local village farmer named Henry Wicker found a trickle of water in the hollow hoofprint of a cow. He proceeded to dig up a hole around it in the hope that it would fill up overnight. The next morning it was indeed brimming over with water, but his thirsty cattle would still not drink it. He tried some himself, becoming the first person to experience the effects of Epsom salts, and he understood why. What he at the time referred to as their cleansing effect (Epsom salts are a strong laxative) led him to promote the waters as a medicine and they became increasingly well-known and successful[756]. Their reputation grew and, fast-forwarding one hundred years, a larger borehole was drilled closer to the town, leading to yet more commerce and an 18th century property and entertainment boom - but this was not to last. Epsom's water supplies were quite limited compared to other spa resorts, which were steadily increasing in popularity across Europe. Epsom's salty springs possessed highly concentrated mineral rich waters, and that intensity of taste was due to the local rocks being richly endowed in magnesium and sulfate. While supplies lasted, these, sometimes cloudy waters, were used for bathing as well as consumption, sometimes in quantities of 'several pints after another' according to anecdotal tales[757]. One can only assume, given the effect that must have had, that in view of a lack of water closets at the time, there were enough trees for patients to hide behind as the Epsom Salts demonstrated their laxative effects. Other than its famous laxative properties, a dose of Epsom salts was said to be something of a cure-all, promising relief from bodily aches and pains as well as healing colds and congestion. Yet, by the start of the 19th century, Epsom Salts had become a generic term for mixtures and lotions based on its main constituent, magnesium sulfate, most of which by then was produced as a residue from sea-salt manufacture. Time has moved on, and if you visit the suburban sprawl of Epsom today, apart from souvenir shops selling their 'original' Epsom salt, you will find just a small monument at the site where the original springs were located.

Today, the Epsom Salt Council based in the United States provides information on the many benefits and uses associated with the salty tasting compound[758], from a gardening aid to facial masks to magnesium's role in lowering stress and inflammation. Randomized controlled trials have also seen benefits of spa therapy on rheumatoid arthritis and osteoarthritis[759,760,761]. A combination of spa and exercise therapy has been shown to be effective in patients with ankylosing spondylitis, which is a type of arthritis of the spine joints[762].

Still to this day, there is much debate as to whether a soothing bath in water infused with Epsom salts provides genuine benefits – the skin after all is generally a barrier that stops for example, the salt in seawater penetrating the body. Was it perhaps just a topical effect? Or maybe it was the drinking of magnesium rich water that did the trick? Contemporary research suggests both may be true[763], but at the same time those seeking a cure for constipation were visiting Epsom, elsewhere around Europe, more and more spas were opening encouraging both the bathing-in and the drinking-of such natural waters. Although generally, these spa waters were not as rich in minerals as the magnesium infused Epsom salt waters, many of them provided an added advantage, namely, the bathing water was warm. In Germany, spa towns like Baden-Baden (literally baths, baths) and Aachen profited from their natural thermal springs, while the English city of Bath provided waters to enjoy at a constant 115 degrees Fahrenheit (46°C) – a little on the warm side for most.

The use of minerals and other chemicals in medicine was pioneered by the Renaissance Swiss physician Paracelsus (1493-1541) who is considered the 'father of toxicology' and the 'godfather of modern chemotherapy'[764]. He is also credited for giving 'zinc' its name, calling it *zincum*[765]. Paracelsus believed all diseases are the poisoning of a combustible element (sulphur), a fluid element (mercury) and a solid element (salt)[766]. According to him, these three substances are at the root of all physiological processes in the body – metabolism (sulphur), genetics (mercury) and enzymatic reactions (salt/minerals)[767]. Salt controls the body's liquids so that materials could be moved around. If there's excessive mineralization, arthritis and kidney stone formation occurs. Paracelsus figured out that some compounds that are poisonous in large amounts can be beneficial in smaller quantities, laying the foundation to future science about hormesis[768].

In 18-19th century England, many people suffering from lead intoxication, caused by the widespread use of lead in household goods, cosmetics, food and plumbing, were sent to Bath Hospital. Out of 3,377 patients sent to Bath between 1760 and 1879, 45% were cured of lead poisoning and 93% saw improvements in their symptoms[769]. The reported health benefits are attributed to the warm water promoting excretion of lead and other minerals[770].

The year 1742 saw Britain's first public hospital open in Bath, located right beside the hot springs, and in hindsight, this is seen as a first step to what would become much later, the British National Health Service. People 'took the waters' in Bath to fight rheumatic disorders, help with skin ailments and purge themselves of the palsy, caused mostly by excess exposure to lead which at the time was used extensively in water pipes, cooking and drinking utensils (they were initially unaware of this causation). Although officially, the impressive Georgian styled building was known as the Royal National Hospital for Rheumatic Diseases, locally, it was more frequently called The Min, an abbreviated form of the Royal Mineral Water Hospital. The Min is still there today, though the original building was closed a couple of years back, and a new hospital opened down the road. Apparently, plans are currently being drawn up to develop the property into a luxury hotel (with spa facilities, of course).

Across the channel in one of the hillier parts of Eastern Belgium, naturally sparkling mineral springs had been found in 1326, and the town, which grew up around them, was aptly named Spa, an acronym coming from the Latin words – Salude Per Aqua – meaning 'health or healing through water'. Agustino, the private physician to King Henry VIII 'took the waters' in 1547, helping spread knowledge about the Spa waters[771] and much later, in the 18th century, casinos and hotels were built to cope with and entertain the early health-tourists. Today it is quite easy to enjoy the pleasures of Spa water, Spa being one of the most popular brands of both flat and carbonized bottled water in the country. Of course, you can visit the thermal springs and immerse your body in the warm waters. The oldest water source at Spa is known as the Marie-Henriette spring and is still naturally carbonated to this day. The water there is eminently drinkable, though rich in both iron and manganese[772], it sometimes possesses a rather off-putting rusty color.

Returning to the long traditions and everyday word-of-mouth supporting the benefits associated with immersion in such mineral waters, you might ask whether the matter has been scientifically proven? Whereas many research papers show the strong association between drinking magnesium rich water or taking supplements and a reduction in heart disease and strokes[773], it is still questionable whether lying in magnesium rich water contributes to anything similar. Indeed, scientists in England published a paper on this very topic in 1985, albeit relating to the warm natural spring waters found in the city of Bath[774]. Eight healthy subjects were immersed in the waters for two hours and controlled for various factors including monitoring of their hearts, analysis of their blood and frequency and amount of urination – something which incidentally doubled after their efforts. The participants also exhibited something called natriuresis, which in plain English, means that their urine was also exceptionally salty. That being said, although Bath mineral water is naturally rich in sodium, potassium, magnesium and calcium, no absorption through the skin was recorded. Interestingly, when they redid the research with the same eight subjects, each relaxing for two hours in warm, plain tap water, the results were almost identical. So, in summary, **the idea of being immersed in water and potentially 'washing away disease' may be linked to this bodily cleansing process, particularly bearing in mind that an excess of lead was flushed from the body giving rise to many early health claims.** There are many, surprisingly well documented cases of the cumulative, curative effect of Bath's mineral waters dating from the early years of that original mineral hospital that most likely, the minerals acted rather like chelating agents in the water that was drunk (1 to 1 and 1/2 pints daily). That combination of drinking, together with immersion in warm water

118

worked its wonders. Records show that between 1799 and 1828, 49% of the patients seeking cures for what was often lead poisoning (mostly palsy and paralysis) were discharged as cured. Even so, can we really trust such information from the past? Funnily enough, we probably can, and we know that thanks in great part to the American NASA space program.

In the early 1970s, Americans working on the space program discovered they could simulate the effects of weightlessness by immersing potential astronauts up to their necks in water at 35°C. So, they carried out numerous physical and psychological experiments. It was found, similarly to the research conducted in Bath, that the urinary excretion of water, sodium and calcium were as a result of warm immersion, markedly increased. Because the body handles calcium and lead in a similar way, it is now thought possible that **this kind of up-to-the-neck immersion could also increase urinary lead excretion**. Separate experiments were later set up in the Immersion Laboratory in the Bristol Royal Infirmary which substantiated this. The NASA scientists also deduced that as water pressure increases with depth, the legs and abdomen are lightly compressed, expelling blood and some interstitial fluid, the thin liquid layer which surrounds the body's cells. The fluid is pushed up into blood vessels in the chest, producing a marked increase in available central blood volume, which leads to an increase of about 50% in cardiac output. There being no associated rise in blood pressure, the resistance of the rest of the body's veins and arteries has to go down – a factor that could be of great significance when treating conditions of poor blood circulation or early stages of paralysis. On balance, while the relaxing nature of bathing, the influences of water pressure on your blood circulation and the increased need to urinate after a long hot bath are worthy of note, it seems the main influence that minerals have is most closely linked to the eating and drinking of mineral rich substances.

Britain's Queen Victoria was reputed to occasionally fortify her claret wine with a drop of Scotch whisky, which could be one of the reasons she selected a remote area of the Scottish Highlands to establish her summer residence. To this day, Balmoral Castle is a preferred summer location for her direct descendant Queen Elisabeth II, and it is nearby, just a brisk walk from the castle, that you can find the Lochnagar distillery. John Begg, the gentleman who established the distillery in 1845, took advantage of the very first visit by Queen Victoria and her husband, Prince Albert, in 1848 to introduce them to the buildings, the machinery and the whisky. This proved to be a wise initiative and within days, he received a royal warrant for the premises, quickly renaming the distillery as Royal Lochnagar. What was the secret of his excellent whisky? John Begg stressed the importance of a steady supply of excellent, crystal-clear water from the Scarnock Springs, whose origins lie deep under the granite rich Cairngorm mountains beside the River Dee. The local spa waters were already well-known for their health promoting qualities, with neighboring Pannanich Wells being famous since the times of the Knights Templars. Lord Byron and Sir Walter Scott were among the many famous people who bathed there and drank the waters with Queen Victoria writing pleasurably of her visits in her 1870 diary.

When it comes to excellence in the making of whiskey (whisky is used for those made in Scotland), the quality and mineral content of water is not just important for the initial fermentation phase when the sprouted barley (known as malted) begins to ferment, but also for the later production stages. After 8 or more years in oak barrels, the whiskey is then diluted to usually hit a final level of alcohol which ranges between 40 and 45 percent. Limestone rocks contain the greatest amount of calcium and magnesium, but as they are not so common in Scotland, much of the drinking water supply there is classified as soft. The Royal Lochnagar water source, with a pH value close to 9, also belongs to this soft water classification since it picks up relatively low levels of calcium and magnesium from the igneous and metamorphic rocks of the Cairngorms. However, if you travel North for about an hour by car along the windy lanes enjoying views of the scraggy mountains, you will reach the village of Portsoy on the coast, an area where the granite is augmented by more metamorphic rock. There at the Glenglassaugh Distillery, the renowned whisky maker Dr. Rachel Barrie will wax lyrical about the quality of the local water that they use for the production of their local single malt. *"The water we use at Glenglassaugh has the highest mineral content of that at any distillery in Scotland,"* she declares, going on to describe how because of this, the yeast produces more esters affecting the fermentation, adding pear-drop characteristics and leading to the sweetest new-make spirit she has ever tasted. *"You get tropical and candied fruits straight off the still."*[775]

Thus, for those professionally 'in the know', choosing the right water is fundamental, and dependent on the minerals present. Just as the Romans began taking the waters in spa towns 2,000 years ago, the right kind of water has been reputed to cure all sorts of ailments whether you are bathing in it or drinking it. And the quality and taste of the two whiskies in question is very different, mostly because of their selected natural water supply. Whereas safe tap water is still a dream in parts of Africa, many having to walk long distances to fill up containers and carry them home, most of us carry plastic bottles home from the supermarket in spite of the high purity of our tap water. Impurities in the water supply come of course in many forms, and news stories such as the excessive lead in the water supply provided for the citizens of Flint Michigan justifiably scare us. That was a terrible story and led to outbreaks of skin rashes, hair loss and worse. But considering the whole United States, it really was an exception. There can be so much goodness in our drinking water, but lead is definitely the wrong mineral to find there. What makes that case so sad, and what made it so dangerous for the citizens of Flint Michigan, is that a perfectly safe water source from Detroit was swapped out for drawing water from the polluted Flint river. It was a pure cost saving initiative.

The word whisky is apparently a corruption of the Scottish Gaelic word 'uisquebaugh', which translates as 'water of life', so where better to begin than by taking a look at the factors at play in your regular drinking water. After that, we will look at the influence of other minerals, many found in trace amounts in water, and what you can do to optimize your daily intake. These minerals perform many functions including activating the enzymes throughout your body and the essential minerals such as calcium, chloride, magnesium, phosphorus, potassium, sodium and sulfur can only be obtained from what we eat and drink. That's why they are called essential - we need them because we are unable to manufacture them in our body. You will discover how some of these are quite easy for you to obtain, while others are much harder. You can then decide whether your personal mineral intake is adequate for promoting good health or whether, like us, you choose to be particular with certain foods and add selected supplements where necessary.

Why Drink Water with Minerals?

With an aging infrastructure and more than 151,000 public water systems across the United States, the percentage of water systems in full compliance with health standards hovers between 90% and 93%. Researchers have estimated that there are as many as 32 million cases of waterborne disease occurring every year, and that is enough to cause concern[776,777].

It is a sign of our times that bottled water became the most widely sold beverage product in the U.S. in 2017, overtaking carbonated soft drinks[778]. Whereas whiskey manufacturers are looking for certain minerals but not necessarily calcium (which is the main reason for classifying water as hard or soft), commercial bottled water brands such as the popular San Pellegrino would be classed as both very hard and mineral rich, having a total mineral content of over one gram per litre[779]. For other brands it can be even higher, so when we review the importance of these minerals in our complete diet, it is usually worth considering your starting point. Do you know much about the content of your local water supply? If you have a hard water supply with lots of calcium and you enjoy eating pasta, then also consider the fact that your pasta more than doubles in weight as it absorbs that cooking water. If on the other hand, you have a water filter which removes the calcium, you have a quite different outcome when it comes to considering your daily intake and needs.

There are many benefits to drinking water with minerals compared to regular plain water:

- **Improved Digestion and Gut Health** – Stomach acid and digestion require salt and other minerals. Gastric juice is composed of hydrochloric acid, potassium and sodium chloride, which help to break down food and assimilate the nutrients. Other stomach cells produce bicarbonate that buffers against the acidity and regulates the pH.

- o Lack of stomach acid can promote digestive problems, indigestion, heartburn, small intestinal bacterial overgrowth and an increased risk of infections[780,781]. Low stomach acid may also reduce the absorption of other minerals. Acid-suppressing drugs decrease how much iron and zinc get absorbed[782]. Aging also lowers stomach acid production, which is why the elderly commonly have a zinc deficiency[783]. Drinking plain water without salt dilutes the stomach acid, making it less acidic. It shouldn't matter much in between meals, but if you drink plain water right before, during or after meals you will have less digestive power to break down your food, making it more likely you'll have bloating or other similar problems. At the same time, chloride-sulphate, calcium-sodium mineral water improves chronic gastritis with increased acid formation[784]. So, minerals regulate both low acidity as well as high acidity. Mineral water can improve dyspepsia, which is a condition of indigestion[785,786,787].

- o Constipation may also result from insufficient electrolytes. Electrolytes can improve bowel function in constipation[788]. Mineral water supplementation in patients with functional dyspepsia has been shown improve gastric emptying of solids[789]. **Magnesium- and sulphate-rich natural mineral water have been found to improve stool consistency and regularity compared to low-mineral natural water**[790,791,792]. Drinking 1 liter/day of sulfate-rich mineral water for 3 weeks increased the frequency of bowel movements in patients with functional constipation compared to regular tap water[793]. However, the difference became less significant after 6 weeks.

- Mineral water consumption and baths help to treat patients with irritable bowel syndrome and improve their psycho-emotional status[794]. **Thermal mineral spring bathing improves mood and mental state**[795]. Mineral waters also have positive effects on the psychological status in children[796].
- Dietary calcium may reduce the risk of colon cancer by accelerating cytotoxic surfactants like bile acids in the colonic lumen[797]. This prevents the formation and proliferation of harmful species and inflammation in the gut. Calcium-sulfate mineral water is equally as bioavailable as cow's milk for calcium and retains as much of it[798,799]. **Bicarbonate-calcium mineral water improves inflammation of the stomach lining**[800].

- **May Help Chronic Diseases** – A higher intake of calcium and magnesium, aligned with the RDA, may be protective against many chronic diseases, such as osteoporosis, hypertension, sudden cardiac death and cardiovascular disease[801].

  - **Drinking 1 L/day of mineral water reduces cardiometabolic risk factors, such as blood lipids, lipid oxidation, glucose, insulin and cholesterol**[802]. Sodium-bicarbonate mineral water with a meal reduces postprandial lipaemia compared to a low mineral water[803,804]. High bicarbonate mineral water lowers triglycerides and VLDL cholesterol compared to low mineral water[805]. **Bathing in mineral-rich mud has been shown to improve lipidemia and flow mediated dilation in peripheral arterial occlusive disease**[806].

  - A low salt intake induces insulin resistance, even in healthy subjects[807,808]. By only drinking plain water and not salting your food, you may be excreting more salt through the urine and becoming deficient. **Thermal sodium bicarbonate therapy at Vals-les-Bains has been shown to improve symptoms of diabetes**[809].

  - Although meta-analyses and observational studies suggest that magnesium supplements improve glycemic control, more evidence is needed to convincingly show that mineral water has a similar benefit[810]. Drinking sodium-rich bicarbonated mineral waters with a meal does lower postprandial insulin compared to low mineral water in postmenopausal women[811]. Sodium is required for insulin to do its job and thus more salt in the diet can improve insulin sensitivity. High amounts of sodium (4,600 mg per day), if given to individuals with a poor diet, however, may impair insulin sensitivity[812]. Thus, sodium must always be balanced with potassium, magnesium and other base-forming substances in the diet.

o Spa therapy can improve plasma levels of adiponectin and leptin, which are important hormones for appetite regulation, satiety, weight loss as well as cartilage metabolism[813].

- **Carbonated water can lower hunger [814], which is important for not overeating calories during the day**. The effects appear to be mediated by enhanced postprandial gastric and cardiac activity[815]. Mineral waters are a calorie-free source of essential minerals that can prevent certain nutrient deficiencies[816].

o Drinking 500 ml/day of bicarbonate-rich Água Vitalis® for 7 weeks caused blood pressure lowering effects[817]. Sodium bicarbonate water consumption appears to decrease blood pressure in normal as well as hypertensive men, whereas regular sodium chloride water does not[818,819]. Mineral water intake lowers blood pressure especially in subjects with low urinary magnesium and calcium levels[820]. Head-out immersion in natural mineral water also appears to have positive effects on hypertensive patients, as assessed by 12 randomized controlled trials, involving 1,122 participants[821].

125

o **Spa mineral water treatment has been shown to reduce markers of stress.** After 2 weeks of geothermic water therapy, symptoms of stress declined 60%, intensity of stress reduced 41% and control of stress improved 32%[822]. As a result, the health risks caused by stress decreased 26%, health resources increased by 11%, and the probability of general health risk dropped by 18%. Functional water infused with herbs and minerals can reduce heart rate and restore parasympathetic activity[823]. Sodium restriction with a low salt diet does not lower glucocorticoid activity or its induced acidity[824]. It has been found that anxiety- or fear-induced sweating can make you lose trace minerals similar to exercise, although the two types of sweat have a slightly different composition[825,826]. Thus, you need more minerals if you are constantly stressed. At the same time, the loss of minerals will cause additional stress and sympathetic nervous system activity.

o Among 192 patients with chronic venous insufficiency receiving spa mineral therapy, 66% saw improvements compared to the 28% in the control group[827]. **Highly mineralized baths with a salt concentration of 20 g/L have been shown to reduce peripheral vascular resistance and hypertension**[828].

o **Drinking Sulfurous mineral water protects against lipid and protein oxidation**[829]. Oxidation of these molecules increases the risk of cardiovascular disease, cancer and aging.

- **Improve Lung and Respiratory Conditions.** Aerosol therapy using "Dovolenskaya" mineral water, improves bronchial drainage and inflammation in patients with occupational broncho-pulmonary diseases [830]. Inhaling aerosolized sulphurous mineral water has been shown to improve inflammation in 65% of the studied subjects who suffer from chronic inflammation of the upper respiratory airway[831]. **A meta-analysis of 13 clinical studies utilizing thermal water** inhalations and irrigations concluded, "Thermal water applications with radon or sulphur can be recommended as additional nonpharmacological treatment in upper airway diseases."[832]

- o Sanatorium and spa treatment have been shown to improve cystic fibrosis of the lungs and pancreatic lesions in children[833].
- o Thermal water nasal spray improves chronic rhinosinusitis pathologies better than just saline water spray[834]. Nasal irritation with sulfurous, salty, bromic, iodic (SSBI) thermal water improves non-allergic chronic rhinosinusitis[835]. Sulphurous thermal water inhalations have been shown to be effective in the treatment of chronic rhinosinusitis[836]. Thermal water nasal aerosol has also been shown to help with seasonal allergic rhinitis[837].
- o It is important to note than any nasal inhalation or irrigation using mineral waters should only be performed after the water has been sterilized (boiled for 5 minutes) and then allowed to cool off.

- **Natural mineral water intake improves skin hydration and dryness[838].** Purified thermal water can reduce skin irritation and reduce transepidermal water loss[839]. Spraying thermal spring water to the face after dermatological surgery, laser therapy or chemical peelings reduces local inflammatory symptoms and adverse effects associated with the procedure[840].
  - o A 10-minute hot bath at 42°C has been shown to improve symptoms of atopic dermatitis in 76% of studied subjects[841]. Application of deep-sea mineral water inhibits the development of atopic dermatitis-like skin lesions in mice[842].
  - o Mineral water solutions enhance the benefits of phototherapy and light therapy[843]. Dead Sea products have been shown to decrease skin and mucosal toxicity in head and neck cancer patients who are receiving radiochemotherapy[844]. A systematic review has

127

concluded that Dead Sea treatments could be beneficial for rheumatoid arthritis and psoriasis[845].

- **Rheumatoid Arthritis and Osteoarthritis** – Minerals, especially magnesium and calcium, have a crucial role in bone health and density. Your bones are made of calcium and they need minerals to maintain their integrity. Skeletal bone acts as a sodium-rich reservoir that can be depleted during sodium deficiency, which has adverse negative side-effects on bone quality and fracture risk[846].
    - Spa therapy has been used to treat physical pains and diseases of physical degeneration for centuries. Long-term mud therapy also appears to be beneficial for bone mineral density[847].
    - Consuming high calcium mineral water lowers bone remodeling in post-menopausal women on a low calcium intake[848]. Drinking alkaline mineral water has also been shown to lower bone resorption even in those with a normal calcium intake[849]. In the same study, calcium-rich *acidic* water had no effect on bone resorption, suggesting that the benefits are due to the alkalinity of the water. Another study found that consuming mineral water with a modest amount of calcium (172 mg) inhibited bone resorption and parathyroid activity[850].
    - Drinking sodium-rich bicarbonated mineral water with a meal increases urinary sodium excretion without changing the excretion of potassium and bone minerals[851]. This was due to a decrease in aldosterone, the hormone that regulates sodium retention, after 120 minutes of consumption.
    - **Bathing in mineral-rich bath waters has been found to improve fibromyalgia[852].**
      The effects of balneotherapy (bathing in mineral waters) on fibromyalgia appear to last for up to 3 months, whereas **mud-bath treatments give longer lasting results[853].**

Mud bathing in patients with fibromyalgia also lowers triglycerides and C-reactive protein[854].

- Magnesium citrate appears to be effective on pain and clinical parameters in people with fibromyalgia[855]. Magnesium citrate is also more available and easily absorbable compared to magnesium oxide[856]. Magnesium-rich mineral water can be as easily absorbed as magnesium supplements, perhaps slightly better[857]. With age, magnesium absorption decreases, and magnesium mineral water might be able to compensate for that[858].

- **Drinking magnesium-rich mineral water alone ensures that about 50% of the magnesium gets absorbed**[859]. Consuming high doses of magnesium all at once is not optimal for absorption. It turns out that **you can get 40% better absorption and retention of magnesium from mineral water if consumed at a lower dose but higher frequency,** as noted when drinking 7 oz. of mineral water seven times per day versus 25 oz. twice per day[860].

o Spa therapy improves pain, functionality and quality of life in patients with shoulder pain[861]. Magnesium-Calcium-Sulfur spa therapy shows significant improvements of non-specific chronic lower back pain[862]. Bathing in calcium-magnesium, bicarbonate thermal mineral water improves clinical parameters and quality of life in patients with chronic low back pain[863]. Mineral water baths also improve clinical parameters of back pain more than tap water baths[864,865].

o **Taking a 30-min thermal water bath at 34°C (93.2°F) five times a week for 3 weeks improves osteoarthritis**[866]. The same Szigetvár spa waters in Hungary have been seen to help with range of motion in osteoarthritis[867]. Exercise combined with a sulfur bath therapy for 12 weeks has shown more sustained, significant benefits on joint function and decreased pain in hip osteoarthritis, compared to just exercise alone[868].

o Compared to a bath with regular tap water, taking a sulphurous water bath for 15 to 20-min sessions significantly improves hand osteoarthritis after 3 months[869]. Bathing in mineral waters combined with drinking mineral water improves pain and function of hand osteoarthritis significantly more so than either treatment alone [870]. However, there is not enough evidence to claim that bathing in mineral waters alone is better than other treatments[871]. **A meta-analysis of 122 studies on Hungarian thermal mineral waters concludes it is an effective therapy for lower back pain, as well as knee and hand osteoarthritis**[872].

o Treatment with mud and mud baths with Sillene mineral water remarkably improves clinical conditions of patients with knee arthritis[873]. Daily mud packs and mineral baths are superior to short-wave therapy in treating knee osteoarthritis although both show improvements[874]. Mud-therapy maintains benefits on hand osteoarthritis for up to 3 to 6 months[875] and also improves lumbar spine osteoarthritis[876].

o **Thermal balneotherapy may provide pain relief, improve joint function, and increase walking speed in patients with knee osteoarthritis**[877,878,879,880,881,882]. Sulfurous baths have more long-lasting effects than non-sulfurous baths although both are therapeutic[883]. The benefits on pain relief appear to be increasingly better with up to 15 spa sessions[884]. Spa therapy for just 2 weeks maintains the benefits on rheumatoid arthritis for up to 3 to 12 months[885,886,887]. Studies between 1980 and 2014 show balneotherapy significantly improves clinical parameters of rheumatoid arthritis[888,889].

o A review of 27 double-blind randomized clinical trials, involving 1,118 patients, found that mineral balneology (bathing in mineral waters) improves pain, functionality and rheumatological diseases compared to baseline and non-mineral similar treatments[890]. In rheumatoid arthritis, taking 12 thermal mineral spa baths at 36-37°C (96.8-98.6°C) for 20 min over the course of 2 weeks increased antioxidant levels like superoxide dismutase and decreased oxidative stress markers[891]. Bathing in thermal mineral waters may lower free radicals[892]. Bathing in sulfur-rich thermal water also increases the anti-inflammatory cytokine IL-10 and regulates antioxidant enzymes, which can help to lower inflammation[893].

- **Maintain Kidney Health** – The body's fluid balance and electrolyte status are governed by the kidneys. Electrolyte imbalances are commonly seen in kidney disease[894]. Dehydration can cause elevated levels of blood sodium, which is often seen in diseases associated with kidney problems like diabetes[895,896]. Edema, which is characteristic to nephrotic syndrome, can cause low sodium levels in the blood due to fluid retention[897].

  - Drinking magnesium-calcium carbonate mineral water can benefit those with kidney disease[898]. Consuming sulfate-bicarbonate, calcium-magnesium mineral water has also shown efficacy in patients with chronic pyelonephritis[899], which is renal disorders characterized by chronic inflammation. Drinking water rich in sodium-bicarbonate is also used to help with gastrointestinal issues, metabolism, kidneys and the urinary pathways[900].

  - **Drinking mineral water can help with kidney stones**[901]. Calcium can bind to oxalates[902], which are what the majority of kidney stones are made of. Indeed, about 80% of kidney stones are made of oxalates and 20% calcium phosphate[903]. Oxalate, or oxalic acid, is an organic acid found in certain plants, such as leafy green vegetables, spinach, some fruit, nuts and seeds[904].

Too many oxalates can prevent calcium from being absorbed into the body[905] and they may also lead to kidney stones and chronic systemic pain. Eating calcium-rich foods like cheese, dairy, fish, and broccoli can actually reduce the oxalate load in your body by providing calcium that can bind with oxalates in the gut [906]. **Drinking calcium and magnesium rich mineral water can reduce calcium oxalate stone formation**[907].

- **Cognition and Neurological Health** - Drinking rosemary-infused water can improve cognition and cerebrovascular health [908]. Mineral water consumption can increase the excretion of silicic acid and aluminum in Alzheimer's disease[909,910].

Mineral water consumption	Mineral water bathing
Helps constipation Improves hydration status Raises mineral levels Reduces postprandial lipids Lowers postprandial insulin Lowers triglycerides and VLDL Prevents insulin resistance Better glycemic control Appetite reduction Lowers blood pressure Lowers heart rate Improves vascular health Benefits kidney health Improves cognition Raises heavy metal excretion	Improved mood Promotes relaxation Improves skin hydration Reduces stress markers Reduces inflammation Reduces physical pains Improves fibromyalgia Improves osteoarthritis Improves rheumatoid arthritis

- **Exercise Performance** – Electrolytes, especially sodium and magnesium, are especially important for physical activities and muscle contraction. Sodium generates action potentials of nerves and muscle cells by entering the cell. Physical exertion and exercise burn through minerals and electrolytes, while increasing the demand for them. **In professional sports, vitamin and mineral supplementation can provide a competitive advantage[911]. Athletes should be well-hydrated with fluids and electrolytes before and after exercise for optimal results[912].**

   o Consuming only water or dilute solutions with little to no sodium during prolonged exercise, such as a marathon or a race, can lower plasma sodium levels and increase the risk of swelling in the brain. Especially during events that last hours or where intense sweating will occur, foods and fluids that contain sodium should be consumed[913]. **If you exercise 1 hour per day, you may need 68 mg/kg of body weight of sodium to maintain a positive calcium and magnesium balance[914]. In other words, a 70 kg adult may need 4,760 mg of sodium/day just to prevent calcium and magnesium loss from the body.**

   o **Mineral waters can help with post-exercise rehydration by replenishing the minerals lost through sweat versus low mineral waters[915].** Deep sea minerals can also improve hydration recovery after dehydrating exercise, which benefits muscle strength and recovery[916].

   o Not getting enough electrolytes and salt can cause negative health effects, especially when performing physical activity. It has been found that soldiers working in the heat who only consumed 2,300 mg of sodium a day had worse outcomes vs. those who consumed 5,880 mg of sodium/day. Indeed, heat exhaustion, hypotension, tachycardia, dehydration, vertigo, nausea and vomiting occurred in 25% of the men on the low-salt intake but only 2.5% in men on the moderate salt intake. **Sweat loss during sports can**

133

cause heat cramps and decreased performance, which can be prevented with appropriate salt and fluid intake[917]. Thus, obtaining enough salt keeps your body cooler during physical exertion, especially in the heat.

- o **High heat exposure caused by either exercise, sauna or exercising in a hot climate raises the demand for sodium and potassium[918].** Some have argued that moderate sodium restriction (1/2 tsp of salt/day) does not impair the ability to exercise in a hot environment (35°C/95°F) compared to consuming 1 and ½ tsp of salt/day[919]. However, this is because the study did not acutely load sodium and fluids prior to exercise, which is where the benefits are derived.

  Exercise-induced sweating has been shown to promote the excretion of trace minerals[920,921]. Additional sodium supplementation while exercising in 40°C does not result in potassium deficiency[922].

  - ▪ Exposure to different temperatures and seasons has been shown to influence the amount of minerals being excreted through sweat[923,924]. However, results may be contradicting, depending on whether sweat is collected with an arm-bag technique or with whole-body collection methods[925]. There are reports that show decreased concentrations of magnesium and copper in people's sweat during the summer versus the winter[926]. In contrast, sweat calcium, copper and zinc does not appear to differ between individuals living in the tropics compared to those living in cooler regions[927]. There is also a difference between how much individuals will excrete based on their level of heat adaptation[928,929,930]. **The amount of sodium or chloride lost through sweat can be** as low as **292 mg/L**[931,932,933,934] **or up to 8,650 mg/L**[935,936,937,938].

- ▪ After 10 days of exercising on a treadmill in 39.5°C, sweat calcium reduced by about 29%, copper 50%, and magnesium 43%[939]. Exercise-heat acclimatization has been shown to preserve some minerals lost through sweat. It takes about 5-10 days for the body to acclimatize to heat whereby the sweat glands achieve maximal capacity for sodium conservation[940]. Regardless of heat adaptation, there can still be a significant loss of whole-body sodium levels because sweating rate increases independent of the temperature[941].

- ▪ There have been reported losses of 54% of sweat zinc concentrations over the first hour of exercise in a hot climate[942]. The second hour of exercise produces up to 38% reduction in sweat zinc[943]. Heat acclimatization also promotes the conservation of calcium and zinc[944,945].

- o **Numerous studies show that slowly consuming a salt solution that contains ~ 2,300-2,900 mg of sodium in 20 to 26 oz. of water over the course of 60 minutes, starting 90-105 minutes prior to competition, dramatically increases how long an individual can exercise (21 minutes longer), reduces core body temperature (-0.75°F), lowers heart rate (9-10 beats/min) and boosts plasma volume (up to +8%)**[946,947,948]. Drinking 2,300 mg of sodium/liter of fluid, vs. 115 or 1,150 mg/L, reduces dehydration (0.75 L less fluid loss)[949]. Drinking salt solutions that contain 680 mg of sodium/liter reduces the decrease in plasma sodium levels and lowers the incidence of mild/severe hyponatremia[950].

- o Oral consumption of deep-sea minerals increases high-intensity intermittent running capacity in soccer players

135

in a double-blind, placebo-controlled crossover trial[951]. Sodium helps to buffer lactic acid that gets produced during exercise. **Sulfurous mineral water may protect against exercise-induced muscle damage and promote recovery**[952]. These benefits may have been due to the hydrogen sulfide contained in the water. Regardless, it is important to note that sulfate in mineral water needs to be balanced with bicarbonate, as sulfate is acidic and contributes to the dietary acid load.

o Potassium and magnesium have an important role in physical performance[953]. Magnesium deficiency is associated with limited strength and power and athletes might be in more need of magnesium[954].

The benefits of electrolyte and bicarbonate waters for performance

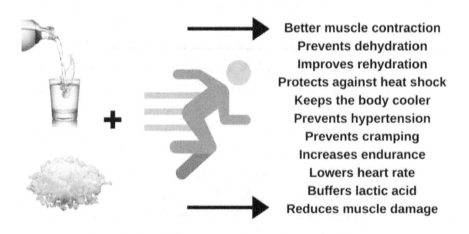

Better muscle contraction
Prevents dehydration
Improves rehydration
Protects against heat shock
Keeps the body cooler
Prevents hypertension
Prevents cramping
Increases endurance
Lowers heart rate
Buffers lactic acid
Reduces muscle damage

A blood sodium level of less than 135 mEq/L is considered low. It is called hyponatremia, which can be characterized by headaches, cramps, arrhythmia, and increased risk of seizures[955]. In certain cases, it is not a lack of sodium that is causing the problems but the excess water in relation to the amount of sodium, which dilutes the sodium concentration. That is why overhydration can easily cause hyponatremia[956], which has led to death and brain swelling[957,958]. There are more athletes being injured by hyponatremia than dehydration every year[959]. Overhydration is the primary cause of hyponatremia in athletes and an increase in sodium intake would help to mitigate these harms[960]. About 13% of Boston marathoners have been found to have hyponatremia and 0.6% of them had critical hyponatremia after finishing the race[961]. Generally, hyponatremia does not occur if you exercise less than hour, unless you're already dehydrated beforehand.

Here are the most common causes of low sodium levels

- Rapid loss of electrolytes from the body like during diarrhea, vomiting or excessive sweating
- Intestinal damage such as bariatric surgery, celiac's, IBS, Crohn's and ulcerative colitis
- Medications, particularly diuretics
- Prolonged exercise for several hours.
- Exercising in the heat or intense exercising causing significant sweating.
- Sauna sessions.
- Overhydration, i.e., drinking too much plain water without enough salt
- States of water retention such as congestive heart failure, cirrhosis and kidney failure
- Medications that cause water retention, such as selective serotonin reuptake inhibitors (SSRIs)
- Syndrome of inappropriate antidiuretic hormone production (SIADH). Anti-diuretic hormone is produced by the hypothalamus and it regulates water retention by the kidneys. When anti-diuretic hormone is produced in excess, it causes a drop in blood sodium levels.
- Hormonal imbalances affecting levels of aldosterone, thyroid hormones and cortisol

Treatment of hyponatremia depends on what is the cause of low sodium and how quickly it has developed[962]. Strategies can range from water restriction to replacement of sodium with salt tablets or with an IV infusion of saline solution.

Hypernatremia refers to a blood sodium level above 145 mEq/L. This most commonly happens because of water restriction that elevates the ratio of sodium to water. That is why hypernatremia is seen in diseases like diabetes and with excessive use of loop diuretics. Drinking water is the easiest and fastest way to lower hypernatremia, which is why it is often characterized by increased thirst.

Here are the most common causes of high sodium levels

- Lack of water intake
- Dehydration because of diarrhea or vomiting
- Diabetes
- Excess sodium consumption or supplementation

The body regulates and reduces the excretion of minerals out of urine when you are very deficient as a means of slowing down additional depletion. The absorption of minerals is also lowered when you reach excessive amounts of them in the body to prevent overload and toxicity. However, if you have a poor diet, metabolic syndrome, damaged kidneys or bad digestion, then your ability to absorb or reabsorb minerals is greatly diminished. There are additional things that can make you hold onto less minerals, like excess consumption of plain water without minerals or fasting (due to metabolic acidosis and mineral losses from bone). **Bicarbonate has been shown to reduce acute acidosis and improve exercise performance**[963].

Drink Mineral Spring Water: But Check the Label

There are hundreds, if not thousands of different water brands out in the market. One might think that water is water and there's no way to differentiate between them, but the truth is not all water is equal. Not only is there a drastic difference between plain water and mineral water in terms of the mineral content but also in the bicarbonate level and the way the waters are preserved and manufactured.

Among commercial bottled waters, there is a large variation of minerals – magnesium ranging from 0-126 mg/L, sodium 0-1,200 mg/L and calcium 0-546 mg/L. Generally, European bottled waters have a higher mineral content than North American ones. In North America, the average concentration of magnesium is 2.5 mg/L, sodium 5 mg/L and calcium 8 mg/L. In Europe, it is 23.5 mg/L for magnesium, 20 mg/L for sodium and 115 mg/L for calcium. There are some American brands like Adobe Springs and Mendocino that have magnesium levels comparable to European sparkling waters. According to the International Bottled Water Association, variation of minerals between individual bottles of the same brand are less than 5%.[964]

Mineral Content of Commercially Available North American Bottled Waters. Adapted from Garzon and Eisenberg (1998) 'Variation in the mineral content of commercially available bottled waters: implications for health and disease'. The American Journal of Medicine, 105(2), 125–130.

Brand	Magnesium (mg/L)	Sodium (mg/L)	Calcium (mg/L)
A Sante	1	160	4
Adobe Springs	96	5	3
Arrowhead	5	3	20
Black Mountain	1	8	25
Calistoga	2	164	8
Canadian Glacier	0	1	1
Canadian Spring	3	2	11
Carolina Mountain	0	5	6
Clairval	7	13	20

Crystal Geyser Alpine Spring	6	13	27
Crystal Geyser Sparkling Mineral	1	30	2
Deer Park	1	1	1
Great Bear	1	3	1
La Croix	22	4	37
Lithia Springs	7	680	120
Mendocino	120	260	240
Monclair	12	475	8
Mountain Valley Spring	7	1	160
Naya	20	6	38
Ozarka	1	5	18
Poland Spring	1	4	1
Pure Hawaiian	0	0	0
Sierra	0	0	0
Sparkletts	5	15	5
Talawanda Spring	0	3	0
Talking Rain	2	0	2
Vichy Springs	48	1,095	157
Zephyrhills	7	4	52

Mineral content is based on von Wiesenberger (1991) 'The Pocket Guide to Bottled Water', 1st edition, Chicago: Contemporary Press.[965]

Mineral Content of Commercially Available European Bottled Waters. Adapted from Garzon and Eisenberg (1998) 'Variation in the mineral content of commercially available bottled waters: implications for health and disease'. The American Journal of Medicine, 105(2), 125–130.

Brand	Magnesium (mg/L)	Sodium (mg/L)	Calcium (mg/L)
Apollinaris	126	572	95
Contrexéville	45	0	546
Evian	24	5	78
Ferrarelle	19	52	459
Gerolsteiner	112	134	368
Henniez	18	6	0
Levissima	1	2	17
Loka	4	139	4
Passuger	26	43	234
Pedras Saldadas	2	500	130
Perrier	5	15	143
Radenska	93	551	201
Ramlosa	0	0	0
San Pellegrino	57	47	204
Spa	1	3	4
Tipperary	23	25	37
Valser	55	10	436
Vichi Celestins	60	1,200	100
Vittel	38	4	181
Volvic	7	10	10

Mineral content is based on Green and Green (1994) 'The Good Water Guide' London, England: Rosendale Press. [966]

Most tap water has very little magnesium and trace amounts of calcium[967]. Unless you live in a region with plenty of magnesium in the water, you may be at risk of magnesium deficiency. Drinking even 1-2 liters of mineral water can provide 600-800 mg of calcium per day. Mineral waters high in sodium are considered harmful because of the perceived association between high salt intake and hypertension. However, low salt intake is actually associated with higher mortality from cardiovascular disease[968]. Additionally, the sodium in mineral waters is in most cases sodium bicarbonate, which has been shown to decrease blood pressure in hypertensive patients[969]. Regardless, it is much easier to obtain salt from other sources, such as food and seasoning, which is why magnesium would be the most valuable mineral in bottled water. Magnesium is also one of the biggest deficiencies people have, which is not the case with calcium.

Lithium is another important trace mineral that we obtain from certain natural mineral waters. Although high doses of lithium can be harmful and immunosuppressive, optimal amounts are linked to lower rates of mental disorders and increased longevity[970,971]. Doses of 0.3 mg/day of lithium have been shown to stabilize cognitive impairment in Alzheimer's disease[972]. Regions with less lithium in the tap water have higher rates of suicide and homicide. Most bottled waters have low amounts of lithium. Gerolsteiner is one that has 0.13 mg/L of lithium. Thus, getting about 0.2-0.3 mg of lithium a day from drinking water might have some therapeutic benefits.

San Pellegrino is a very popular water brand that's been around since the 12th century. Its mineral content and health effects were first investigated in 1748[973]. "San" means "Saint", which is named after the spring's said to be healing benefits. Coming from the foot of a dolomite mountain wall in the Italian Alps, San Pellegrino is carbonated and contains sulfate and bicarbonate. Sulfates are the 8th most common mineral in our bodies with benefits on the antioxidant system[974]. Getting the right amount of sulfate can help to support joints, the nervous system, the cardiovascular system and reduce inflammation[975]. Unfortunately, nowadays our food contains less sulfur and sulfates because of soil depletion[976]. However, sulfate is also acidic, and if you are looking to reduce metabolic acidosis or improve athletic performance, you need to be careful with overconsuming waters that are high in sulfate and low in bicarbonate.

Don't confuse sulfates with sulfites because the two are different. Sulfites are inorganic salts used for food preservation and in medications[977]. You can get sulfites mostly from processed foods, wine and processed meat. They can also inhibit the browning of fruit and vegetables[978]. Some people, especially asthmatics, are overly sensitive to sulfites, which cause gastrointestinal, cardiovascular, pulmonary and dermatological problems[979]. Nausea, abdominal cramps, diarrhea, and urticaria are commonly reported[980]. Although carcinogenic in laboratory animals, the FDA considers sulfites generally recognized as safe[981]. Most people don't experience any negative symptoms, but some can, particularly asthmatics.

Carbon dioxide (CO2) is an important molecule for tissue oxygenation, stress reduction and the metabolism. In the early 1900s, the Danish physician Christian Bohr discovered that carbon dioxide helps to separate oxygen from hemoglobin in the blood, thus allowing tissues, cells and organs to absorb oxygen better[982]. This phenomenon is called the Bohr Effect. Carbon dioxide in the blood will join with water to create carbonic acid. This lowers the blood pH and the nervous system responds by increasing your breathing rate, which is termed "respiratory compensation". During exhalation, CO2 gets exhaled and pH normalizes. Thus, CO2 is important for keeping your metabolic rate elevated and active. Hypothyroidism results in lower carbon dioxide production[983]. Lactic acidosis or metabolic acidosis is a medical condition caused by decreased tissue oxygenation (no Bohr Effect)[984]. It can cause inflammation, oxidative stress and growth of malignant cells, also known as The Warburg Effect[985].

Sparkling or carbonated water provides carbon dioxide (CO2), which can be an effective way to promote better oxygen levels throughout the body. However, in excess, it may also cause burping or bloating. If you do not stomach carbonation well, then stick to just plain mineral water but be aware that uncarbonated mineral waters tend to have slightly less minerals[986]. Naturally carbonated waters have more minerals because the carbonic acid allows the water to absorb the minerals from the rock better. Artificially flavored zero-calorie carbonated waters may have added sulfites, which you might have to be cautious of if sensitive.

When drinking bottled mineral water, it is better to have it in glass bottles to avoid the plastics and heavy metals in cans and plastic bottles. Most plastics leach hormone-mimicking agents called 'xenoestrogens' that mimic the hormone estrogen in the body[987]. Xenoestrogens can also disrupt natural hormone production, inhibiting testosterone[988,989]. Too much estrogen increases the risk of blood clots, heart attack, stroke, breast cancer, ovarian cancer and depression[990,991,992]. The observed decline in male testosterone levels might be explained by the increased use of plastics in our everyday life[993]. You can get exposed to xenoestrogens through water, food, soil and air[994]. Nearly 70% of 450 tested products release chemicals that act like estrogen. The most common xenoestrogens in plastics are bisphenol A (BPA), phthalates, parabens and dozens of others. We obviously can't avoid all plastics and xenoestrogens, but we should try to minimize it to the best of our ability by not drinking plastic bottled water on a daily basis. Instead, opt for glass bottles.

Here are the benefits of mineral waters:

- High bioavailability of minerals when consumed with food
- Lowers post-prandial lipids and insulin
- Fuels the body's physiological processes
- Helps to lower inflammation and stress
- Can relieve constipation, bloating, and digestion issues
- Improves insulin sensitivity and exercise performance
- Provides a zero-calorie source of essential trace minerals
- Covers the body's daily mineral demands for many elements
- Promotes skin hydration and health
- Decreases hunger levels
- Protects against lipid/protein oxidation

In essence, **our bodies are walking bags of salt water that contain various electrolytes and minerals.** Electrolytes are the ancient components of optimal cellular functioning used for centuries to improve health and treat certain conditions. The most frequent benefits of drinking mineral waters are better blood pressure and hydration. Spa therapy and thermal baths have more evidence for improving physical pains such as lower back pain, osteoarthritis and fibromyalgia. It requires almost no effort to implement mineral rich waters into your diet. Theoretically, you could get all the minerals you need from food, but as we've seen from research, adding mineral water and slowly consuming small amounts throughout the day provides a more bioavailable source of minerals. Thus, it is a prudent strategy for optimal results.

Chapter 6
Magnesium, Calcium and Phosphorus: Softening Up the Arteries and Hardening the Bones

The previous chapters have talked about the importance of magnesium quite extensively, especially in regard to its balance with calcium. This is because magnesium has a crucial role when it comes to overall bodily processes and cardiovascular disease (CVD) risk. It is also quite alarming to know how many people are deficient of this essential mineral. Not to mention the rates of soil depletion and its low presence in most commonly eaten foods.

Magnesium and calcium are particularly relevant to cardiovascular health, bone health and blood pressure. It is known that calcium build-up in the arteries contributes to atherosclerosis and heart disease risk[995]. Calcium supplementation has been associated with increased CVD mortality[996,997]. High calcium intake from supplements can offset the balance with magnesium[998,999]. Low magnesium is associated with an increased risk of cardiovascular disease, whereas high magnesium status is associated with a lower risk [1000, 1001, 1002, 1003, 1004, 1005]. Magnesium intake is also inversely associated with the risk of metabolic syndrome and diabetes [1006, 1007, 1008]. Magnesium also antagonizes the inflammation caused by increased intracellular calcium[1009, 1010], which is why it is often called 'nature's calcium blocker'[1011].

However, **increased *dietary* calcium intake has been found to be linked with a reduced incidence of atherosclerosis**[1012,1013,1014]. High intakes of calcium from food does not appear to increase vascular calcification either[1015]. Whole foods that contain calcium also bring some magnesium, which keeps the two in balance. Vitamin K1, and especially K2, also helps keeps calcium in check by directing calcium into the bones instead of the arteries[1016]. Thus, whether or not calcium becomes pathological or protective depends on the way it is used by the body and in what ratios you are getting it with other minerals, especially magnesium.

Adequate calcium intake is needed for maintaining bone mineral density and preventing osteoporosis. About 1.5 million hip fractures a year in the U.S. occur because of osteoporosis[1017]. Very little calcium from supplements will end up in the bones and high doses of calcium can lead to calcium overload in the blood and arterial calcifications[1018, 1019]. In older adults, osteoporosis co-exists with higher rates of arterial calcification[1020,1021]. Low bone mineral density is linked with vascular calcification[1022, 1023]. Hypercalcemia (high calcium in the blood) is associated with worse rheumatoid arthritis disease markers[1024]. However, vitamin K, magnesium and vitamin D are linked with better bone mineral density[1025, 1026, 1027]. Although calcium is particularly important for bone health, deficiencies in magnesium are likely more consequential for bone loss as we get older[1028].

This chapter will close the circle on magnesium and calcium by providing information about how you can get enough of them from dietary sources. We will also cover supplementation and how to fix your deficiencies.

Magnesium Deficiency and Calcium Overload

Magnesium is the 4th most common cation (positively charged ion) in the human body, the 2nd most common intracellular cation and the most common intracellular divalent cation[1029]. It is required for over 300 enzymes in the human body. The main functions of magnesium include regulation of sodium, calcium and potassium levels, ATP generation, modulation of inflammation, DNA/RNA protein synthesis and neurotransmitter production[1030,1031].

Extracellular magnesium contributes only ~1% of total body magnesium, which is concentrated primarily in the serum and red blood cells[1032]. The human body contains roughly 25 grams of magnesium with 50-60% of it being in bones and the remainder in soft tissue[1033,1034]. Out of that amount, 90% is bound and 10% is free[1035]. In the blood, 32% of magnesium is bound to albumin and 55% is free.

Here is how magnesium affects the pathogenesis of cardiovascular disease[1036]

- Magnesium activates ATP, which is essential for energy production and cell function. The sodium-potassium pump is magnesium-ATP-driven, and it affects blood pressure as well as sodium accumulation in the cell[1037]. ATP is required for heart muscle contraction and oxidative phosphorylation in heart mitochondria[1038].

- **Magnesium deficiency leads to intracellular sodium and calcium accumulation**, which promotes arterial vasospasms, blood vessel constriction and hypercoagulability[1039]. Increased intracellular calcium can lead to hypertension and vasospasms[1040]. Coronary vasospasms are thought to be one of the causes of sudden cardiac death[1041].

- Magnesium deficiency reduces membrane potential polarization through intracellular sodium accumulation, which can cause arrhythmias[1042].

- **Magnesium deficiency results in increased oxidative stress and low antioxidant defense**, which leaves the heart vulnerable to myocardial injury[1043,1044,1045,1046].

- Magnesium supports glutathione synthesis and glutathione deficiency promotes the accumulation of calcium[1047].

- Low magnesium status is associated with hypertension[1048,1049].

- Magnesium deficiency increases inflammatory cytokines and interleukins, which promotes metabolic syndrome, cardiovascular disease[1050] and endothelial dysfunction[1051].

- **Low magnesium promotes endothelial dysfunction, thrombosis and atherosclerosis**[1052].

- Magnesium lowers clotting factors and inhibits ADP-induced platelet aggregation[1053,1054].

- **Magnesium deficiency causes myocardial lesions through calcium overload** and catecholamine excess[1055,1056,1057].

- Magnesium depletion increases vasoconstriction and worsens cardiac contractility[1058].

- Vasoconstrictor hormones, such as angiotensin, serotonin and acetylcholine increase when extracellular magnesium is low[1059].

- **Low serum magnesium is associated with atrial fibrillation** in people without cardiovascular disease by modulating the inflow of calcium into the cell[1060]. Magnesium reduces the inhibition of plasmin, which is an enzyme that degrades fibrin clots[1061].

- **Magnesium deficiency results in an increase in triglycerides and blood lipids**[1062,1063]. Three months of magnesium therapy in patients with ischemic heart disease decreases apolipoprotein B concentrations by 15% and VLDL concentrations by 27%[1064].

- **Hypomagnesemia is the result and cause of insulin resistance**[1065,1066,1067]. Higher magnesium intake is associated with a reduced risk of diabetes[1068,].

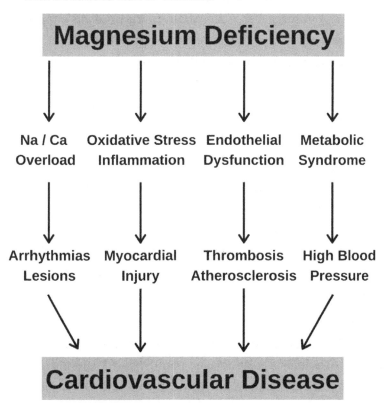

There is an inverse relationship between magnesium intake and arterial calcification [1069]. Deficient magnesium status promotes a pro-atherogenic phenotype in endothelial cells[1070]. In experimental studies, magnesium deficiency causes cardiac necrosis (death) and calcification[1071]. By calcifying the descending limb of the loop of Henle in the kidneys, magnesium deficiency can lead to dehydration and kidney disease[1072].

Hypomagnesemia impairs nitric oxide release from the coronary endothelium, whereas magnesium therapy improves endothelium-dependent vasodilation[1073]. **Magnesium supplementation in patients of coronary heart disease has been found to decrease platelet-dependent thrombosis, improve flow-mediated vasodilation and increase VO$_2$ max**[1074,1075,1076].

A meta-analysis among hypertensive and normotensive subjects discovered that 368 mg/d of magnesium for 3 months significantly reduced systolic blood pressure by 2.00 mmHg and diastolic blood pressure 1.78 mmHg [1077]. **Another meta-analysis among 1,173 people showed that magnesium supplementation decreased systolic blood pressure by 3–4 mmHg and diastolic blood pressure by 2–3 mmHg, with the effects being more significant when intakes exceeded 370 mg/d**[1078]. A meta-analysis of placebo-controlled studies on magnesium supplementation found a mean reduction of 18.7 mmHg and 10.9 mmHg in systolic and diastolic pressures, respectively, in hypertensive patients with a baseline systolic blood pressure > 155mmHg[1079]. The authors of the meta-analysis concluded, "the small effects reported in previous meta-analyses may reflect a blending of dissimilar studies, which acted to seriously underestimate the potential of magnesium in hypertension in some (but not all) subjects. Within studies, blending of non-, moderate and high-responder subjects in any one study might mask strong effects of magnesium treatment in some subjects."[1080]

Magnesium is also involved in bone formation by influencing the activity of osteoblasts, osteoclasts, parathyroid hormone and vitamin D[1081]. Higher magnesium intake is associated with better bone mineral density in both men and women[1082]. Women with osteoporosis have been found to have lower serum magnesium compared to those with osteopenia and healthy individuals[1083]. A short-term study on 20 postmenopausal women saw that 30 days of 290 mg/d of magnesium citrate suppressed bone turnover, indicating reduced bone loss[1084].

Magnesium has an important role in eggshell formation of domestic hens[1085]. Low magnesium intake leads to weaker eggshells and a high likelihood of them breaking. Before the extinction of dinosaurs, researchers noted a significant decrease in the magnesium content of fossil dinosaur eggshells, which might have played a part in their extinction [1086]. Ironically, magnesium deficiency may now be contributing to our early extinction on this planet, played out in shorter life spans and greater chronic disease.

Here are the magnesium-dependent enzymes, functions and consequences that may occur with a deficit:

Magnesium-Dependent Enzymes/Proteins	Function	Consequences of Deficit
ATP Synthase	Produce and activate ATP	Energy shortage, not enough energy to carry out vital bodily processes
Fatty Acid Oxidation	Burn triglycerides and lipids for fuel	Hyperlipidemia, hypercholesterolemia
Pyruvate Dehydrogenase	Convert pyruvate into acetyl-CoA and enable the burning of glucose for fuel	Hyperglycemia, insulin resistance
Glycolysis	Burn glucose for fuel	Hyperglycemia, glycation, insulin resistance

TCA Cycle	Direct acetyl-CoA into ATP production, NAD/NADH	Energy shortage, mitochondrial dysfunction
Insulin Production	Produce insulin to enable cells to pick up glucose from the blood	Insulin resistance, hyperglycemia
GLUT4 Translocation	Enable cells to pick up glucose without insulin	Hyperglycemia
Thyroid Hormones	Regulate metabolic rate and energy production	Hypothyroidism, chronic fatigue, brittle skin and hair, hypercholesterolemia
Glutathione Synthesis	Protect against oxidative stress	Increased oxidative stress and weaker immunity
Glutathione Peroxidase	Removes hydrogen peroxide	Increased oxidative stress and weaker immunity
Serotonin Production	Enable melatonin production, govern relaxation and docility	Chronic stress, anxiety and sleep problems
Melatonin Production	Promote sleep, relaxation and antioxidant repair	Oxidative stress, sleep problems, chronic stress
Dopamine Production	Regulate motivation, mood, attention and behavior	Depression, attention deficit disorders, procrastination

Steroid Hormone Production	Physical repair, protect against stress, regulate sex hormones	Frailty, aging and muscle loss, chronic stress
Testosterone Production	Affect bone density, muscle mass, fat burning, mood and stress	Increased risk of obesity, cardiovascular disease, frailty, and chronic stress
DNA Repair	Repair damaged DNA	Cell senescence, increased DNA mutations
T-cell Regulation	Balance anti-inflammatory and pro-inflammatory immune responses	Autoimmunity, inflammation, infection

Magnesium Food Sources

The recommended dietary amounts of magnesium have been set at 6 mg/kg/day[1087]. However, about 15-20% of the population is only consuming 4 mg/kg/day. **The RDA for magnesium in adults is approximately 350-420 mg per day, which around 50% of the population is not meeting**[1088]. Magnesium deficiency is widespread worldwide and should be considered a public health crisis[1089,1090]. Taiwanese men and women average 250 mg and 216 mg, respectively, which is only 68-70% of the RDA[1091]. In Germany, men get about 250 mg/d and women 200 mg/d of magnesium[1092]. A French study of 2,373 people found that 71.7% of men and 82.5% of women had an inadequate magnesium intake[1093]. **Magnesium deficiency has been found in 84% of postmenopausal women with osteoporosis**[1094].

Some studies indicate that 180-320 mg/d is enough to maintain a positive magnesium balance, but 107 mg/d is not enough[1095,1096,1097,1098]. A study on postmenopausal women showed they were able to maintain a positive magnesium balance by getting 399 mg of magnesium per day on a 2000 kcal diet whereas ~100mg of magnesium per 2000 kcal was inadequate[1099]. However, that would refer to an already homeostatic magnesium status, which most people are not at, as well as being without disease states that increase the demand for magnesium. People with marginal magnesium deficiencies are below the low end of the normal range, which predisposes them to many pathologies[1100]. In one study, they recorded the food intake of 34 men and women for 1 year and discovered their average magnesium intake was 323 mg/d and 234 mg/d, respectively, which is about 4 mg/kg/d[1101]. Despite that, they were still in negative magnesium balance (−32 and −25mg/day, respectively). Men with osteoporosis consuming 240 mg/d of magnesium were also in a negative magnesium balance [1102]. **Postmenopausal women on a low magnesium intake of 100 mg/d develop atrial fibrillation and elevated glucose levels**[1103]. Many studies find that at least 300 mg of magnesium needs to be supplemented in addition to the diet to increase serum magnesium levels[1104]. Thus, the RDA of 350-420 mg/d may not be adequate to reach that effect.

Optimal Intake of Magnesium (mg/d)

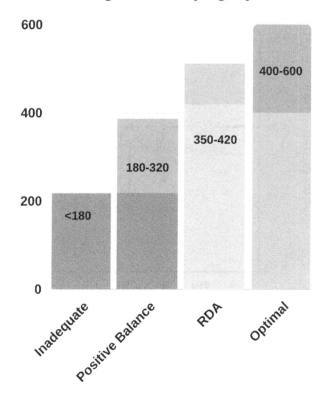

Adding an additional 100 mg of dietary magnesium a day has been associated with an 8% reduced risk of ischemic stroke among 241,378 subjects[1105]. A meta-analysis among 286,668 subjects and 10,912 cases of diabetes with a 6-17-year follow-up, saw that a 100 mg/d increase in magnesium intake lowered the risk of diabetes by 15%[1106]. The relative risk of type-2 diabetes is 23% lower in people with the highest magnesium consumption (360-770 mg/d) compared to the lowest (150-260 mg/d) [1107]. Foods high in magnesium are associated with cardioprotective properties[1108].

The Risk of Abdominal Aortic Calcification (AAC) and Coronary Artery Calcification (CAC) is lowest at 450 mg/d of magnesium intake

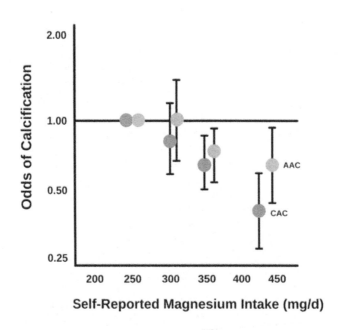

AAC = Abdominal Aortic Calcification; CAC = Coronary Artery Calcification

Adapted From: Hruby et al (2014) 'Magnesium Intake Is Inversely Associated with Coronary Artery Calcification: The Framingham Heart Study', JACC: Cardiovascular Imaging, Volume 7, Issue 1, January 2014, Pages 59-69.

The magnesium content of vegetables between 1940 and 1999 has decreased by 24%, in fruit by 17%, in meat by 15% and in cheese by 26%[1109]. In the UK, the decrease in magnesium concentrations in vegetables from 1930 to 1980 was approximately 35%[1110]. This is the result of soil erosion, pesticide use, inorganic fertilizers and chemicals. The reduction of magnesium from plants and soil is an increasingly bigger problem[1111]. Food processing such as the refinement of oils and grains removes minerals as well. In fact, it eliminates all magnesium. Even though safflower seeds contain 680 mg of magnesium per 1000 calories, safflower oil has zero magnesium[1112]. The same applies to sugar and refined grains or wheat, which reduces magnesium by 80-99%[1113].

Here are the foods highest in magnesium[1114]

Food	Mg of Magnesium per Serving	% of RDA
Pumpkin Seeds, 1 oz	156 mg	37%
Chia Seeds, 1 oz	111 mg	26%
Almonds, 1 oz	80 mg	19%
Spinach, ½ cup	78 mg	19%
Cashews, 1 oz	74 mg	18%
Lentils, 1 cup	71 mg	18%
Peanuts, ¼ cup	63 mg	15%
Soymilk, 1 cup	61 mg	15%
Black Beans, ½ cup	60 mg	14%
Edamame, ½ cup	50 mg	12%
Peanut Butter, 2 tbsp	49 mg	12%
Potato, 3.5 oz	43 mg	10%
Brown Rice, ½ cup	42 mg	10%
Yogurt, low fat, 8 oz	42 mg	10%
Fortified Cereal, 1 serving	42 mg	10%
Oatmeal, instant, 1 packet	36 mg	9%
Kidney Beans, canned, ½ cup	35 mg	8%
Banana, 1 medium	32 mg	8%
Mussels, 3 oz	31 mg	8%

157

Sardines, 3 oz	29 mg	7%
Salmon, 3 oz	26 mg	6%
Milk, 1 cup	24-27 mg	6%
Halibut, 3 oz	24 mg	6%
Liver, 3 oz	24 mg	6%
Raisins, ½ cup	23 mg	5%
Whole Wheat Bread, 1 slice	23 mg	5%
Avocado, ½ cup	22 mg	5%
Chicken Breast, 3 oz	22 mg	5%
Ground Beef, 90%, 3 oz	20 mg	5%
Broccoli, ½ cup	12 mg	3%
White Rice, ½ cup	10 mg	2%
Apple, 1 medium	9 mg	2%
Carrot, 1 medium	7 mg	2%
Egg, whole, 1 medium	5 mg	1%

About 20-40% of the dietary magnesium gets absorbed by the body[1115]. It is commonly thought that phytate-rich foods like beans, grains and legumes will lead to magnesium deficiency by binding to it and preventing its absorption. However, urinary magnesium excretion will reduce to compensate for a reduction in magnesium intake[1116]. Consuming 322 mg/d of magnesium on a high fiber diet has been noted to result in a negative magnesium balance, but that may be due to the inadequate magnesium intake itself[1117]. **A vitamin B6 deficiency will increase magnesium excretion and promote a negative magnesium balance[1118]. Combining vitamin B6 with magnesium increases its absorption rate and helps to drive magnesium into the cell[1119].** Increased protein and fructo-oligosaccharide consumption appear to improve magnesium absorption[1120].

Increased calcium and phosphorus intake can promote

magnesium deficiency and increase magnesium requirements [1121, 1122, 1123]. Calcitriol administration enhances the intestinal absorption of magnesium[1124,1125,1126,1127]. In physiological intracellular concentrations, magnesium competes with calcium for binding with calmodulin and other calcium-binding proteins, which is how magnesium downregulates nuclear factor kappa-beta activation and inflammation[1128,1129,1130].

Magnesium absorption can also be inhibited by antibiotics, such as ciprofloxacin, levofloxacin and demeclocycline, thus, antibiotics should be taken at least 2 hours before or 4-6 hours after magnesium supplementation [1131]. Magnesium decreases the absorption of bisphosphonates, such as alendronate, used to treat osteoporosis. Thus, magnesium supplements and bisphosphonates should be separated by at least 2 hours[1132].

Magnesium Excretion and Assessment

Magnesium excretion is mainly regulated by the kidneys, which excrete about 120 mg of magnesium every day through urine. Magnesium excretion increases during a surplus and falls down to ~12mg during deficits[1133]. When magnesium blood levels are low, magnesium will be pulled from muscles, organs and even bones [1134, 1135]. Renal magnesium wasting is diagnosed when magnesium excretion is higher than 24mg/day in the presence of hypomagnesemia (<0.7mmol/L) [1136]. It is caused by Bartter's syndrome, diabetes, hypercalcemia, diuretics, cisplatinum, aminoglycosides, pentamide, ciclosporin and calcitriol deficiency. Dietary aluminum can reduce magnesium retention in the body by 41%[1137].

Here are factors that contribute to magnesium deficiency and increase magnesium excretion[1138]:

- Kidney failure and kidney diseases[1139,1140,1141]
- Hemodialysis and peritoneal dialysis[1142,1143]
- Alcohol consumption[1144]
- Acetaminophen toxicity[1145]
- Antacids and diuretics[1146]
- Proton pump inhibitors[1147,1148]
- Aluminum exposure
- Metabolic syndrome[1149]
- Diabetes type 1 and 2[1150,1151]
- Calcium supplementation by competing with intestinal absorption[1152]
- Excessive vitamin D supplementation by increasing calcium absorption[1153]
- Physical exercise and exertion[1154]
- Increased sweating and sauna use
- High aldosterone[1155]
- Reduced stomach acid and low salt intake[1156]
- Malabsorption conditions[1157]
- Bariatric surgery, colon removal[1158]
- Aging[1159]
- Celiac disease[1160]
- Liver disease[1161]
- Cisplatin[1162,1163,1164,1165]
- Crohn's disease[1166]
- High sugar consumption[1167]
- High phosphorus intake
- Hyperinsulinemia[1168]
- Insulin resistance[1169]
- Emotional and psychological stress[1170]
- Enzymatic dysfunction by impairing magnesium distribution[1171]
- Estrogen therapy by shifting magnesium to soft and hard tissues, lowering serum magnesium[1172]

- Excessive or prolonged lactation[1173]
- Excessive menstruation
- Prolonged fasting[1174]
- Foscarnet, gentamicin and tobramycin[1175,1176,1177]
- Heart failure[1178]
- Diarrhea and laxatives
- Low selenium intake
- Vitamin B6 deficiency[1179]
- Metabolic acidosis[1180,1181]
- Pancreatitis (acute and chronic)[1182,1183,1184]

Normal serum magnesium is considered to be 0.7-1.0 mmol/L, but the optimal range has been proposed to be >0.80 mmol/L[1185]. Chronic subclinical magnesium deficiency usually sits at a serum magnesium level between 0.75 and 0.849 mmol/L[1186]. A serum magnesium below 0.82mmol/L (2.0mg/dL) with a 24-hour urinary magnesium excretion of 40–80mg/d suggests magnesium deficiency[1187]. If a person is experiencing symptoms of magnesium deficiency at a serum level below 0.9 mmol/L, then supplementation is recommended by the leading experts[1188]. Plasma magnesium <0.863mmol/L (despite 0.75mmol/L being considered normal) increases the risk of diabetes by 3.25-fold[1189]. **Among 14,323 Americans between the ages 45-64, the highest quartile of serum magnesium (at least 0.88 mmol/L) had a 38% reduced risk of sudden cardiac death compared to the lowest quartile (0.75 mmol/L or lower) over a 12-year follow-up**[1190]. The minimum suggested dose for fixing magnesium deficiency (defined as magnesium levels below 0.80 mmol/L) is 600 mg/d for one month, then continue with a dose that holds serum values no lower than 0.90 mmol/L[1191].

About 10-30% of a given population experiences subclinical magnesium deficiency based on serum magnesium levels below 0.80 mmol/L[1192]. One of the largest cross-sectional studies on 16,000 German subjects saw a 14.5% prevalence of hypomagnesaemia (magnesium levels below 0.80 mmol/L)[1193]. The 2006 National Health and Nutrition Survey found that 36.3% of Mexican females and 31% of males had low serum magnesium levels[1194]. Among apparently healthy university students in Brazil, 42% were discovered to have suboptimal magnesium status with an average magnesium intake of 215 mg/d[1195]. In patients with type 2 diabetes, 75% and 30.8% have magnesium depletion based on serum and intracellular magnesium status, respectively[1196].

A study on hospitalized patients found 42% of them had hypomagnesemia yet doctors request magnesium status in only 7% of these patients[1197]. Among intensive care unit (ICU) patients, 65% have been found to have hypomagnesaemia, which can contribute to the pathogenesis of hypocalcemia and cardiac arrhythmias [1198, 1199]. Another ICU study noted a hypomagnesemia rate of 52.5%[1200]. More than half of ICU patients are magnesium deficient[1201]. About 6.9-11% of hospitalized patients on routine exam without a recognized need have hypomagnesemia [1202]. Daily magnesium supplementation >1 gram/day is associated with lower mortality rates in critically ill patients in the intensive care unit[1203].

Magnesium deficiency can be present with normal serum magnesium levels[1204]. In one study, 20% of 381 elderly men and women were found to have low erythrocyte (red blood cell) potassium and magnesium levels[1205]. The current serum range of magnesium is inaccurate and serum magnesium levels at the lower normal end (0.75-0.85 mmol/L) likely suggests marginal magnesium deficiency. Muscle magnesium stores are a more accurate reflection of whole-body content of magnesium than the plasma, however muscle biopsy is an invasive procedure[1206]. **In hypertensive and heart disease patients, muscle magnesium and potassium levels are reduced in about 50% of patients**[1207].

Among hypertensive patients treated with hydrochlorothiazide or a non-diuretic drug for at least 6 months, 80% were found to have magnesium depletion based on the gold standard IV magnesium load test despite having normal serum magnesium levels[1208]. More troublingly, those treated with hydrochlorothiazide actually had high serum magnesium levels, showing that **you can still be magnesium**

depleted despite having high magnesium levels in the blood. Another study confirmed this whereby thiazide diuretics caused a magnesium deficiency undetectable by serum status[1209]. Thiazide diuretics deplete both magnesium and potassium [1210, 1211, 1212]. Potassium levels in muscle will not normalize until magnesium is restored even when serum potassium rises[1213,1214]. Diuretics may even contribute to ischemic heart disease through magnesium depletion[1215]. Potassium-sparing diuretics, however, such as amiloride and spironolactone, reduce magnesium excretion.

Here are the signs and symptoms of magnesium deficiency[1216]

- Hypokalemia and hypocalcemia[1217]
- Tremors and fascilations[1218]
- Arrhythmias[1219]
- Migraine headaches[1220].
   - Taking 300 mg of magnesium twice a day may prevent migraines[1221].
- Spontaneous spasms and muscle cramps[1222]
- Seizures[1223]
- Twitching of the facial muscles upon touch
- Aggression and irritability[1224]
- Confusion and disorientation
- Pain or hyperalgesia[1225]
- Photosensitivity[1226]
- Tinnitus (ringing in the ears)[1227]
- Hearing loss[1228]
- Vitamin D resistance
- Parathyroid resistance and impaired function[1229]
- Cataracts[1230]
- Coronary artery disease
- Cardiovascular disease
- Hypertension
- Mitral valve prolapse[1231]
- Weakened immune response[1232,1233]
- Depression[1234]

It is hard to diagnose magnesium deficiency because the symptoms are quite non-specific[1235]. **An elevated retention of an intravenous or oral magnesium load is likely the best way to test for magnesium deficiency**[1236]. It suggests that the body is trying to hold onto more magnesium because the tissues are depleted. However, the tests assume a normal kidney function for the IV test and normal gastrointestinal/kidney function for the oral test. If you do not have normal kidney function for the IV load or gastrointestinal/kidney function for the oral test, then the measurements can be inaccurate. Measuring hair, bone, lymphocyte, urinary or fecal magnesium excretion may be easier and cheaper, but they are less reliable methods [1237, 1238, 1239]. For the most reliable assessment, multiple methods need to be used[1240]. **The easiest way to identify magnesium deficiency is from a low-normal blood level (< 0.82 mmol/L), especially if the 24-hour urinary magnesium is low (< 80 mg/day).** This is not 100% accurate but it is highly suggestive of magnesium deficiency.

Thoren, using an intravenous magnesium loading test, suggested that when less than 70% of a 365-486mg of parenteral magnesium dose given to an adult over the course of an hour is excreted in the next 16 hours, it likely indicates magnesium deficiency[1241]. In other words, if you give ~400mg of IV magnesium over 1 hour and 70% or more of that dose (about 280mg or more) is not excreted in the urine over the following 16 hours, it implies magnesium deficiency even in the presence of normal magnesium levels. **Healthy magnesium-sufficient subjects have an IV magnesium load retention of just 2-8%** [1242, 1243]. Thus, even retaining around 10% or more of an IV magnesium load may indicate subclinical or marginal magnesium deficiency. The typical cut off is if someone retains 20% of an IV magnesium load, which suggests marginal magnesium deficiency and 50% for severe magnesium deficiency. On average elderly people retain around 28% of an IV magnesium load, suggesting that many older individuals have marginal magnesium deficiency[1244].

Intravenous magnesium retention in those with variant angina is 60% compared to 36% of controls despite both groups having a normal serum magnesium level of 2.1mg/dL. In patients with angina, magnesium deficiency can be improved with medications called calcium channel blockers[1245]. Gastrointestinal loss of magnesium may be found if there is increased conservation of magnesium by the kidneys[1246]. A urinary fractional magnesium excretion >2-4% suggests kidney magnesium wasting and kidney damage[1247, 1248]. When red blood cell magnesium levels are <1.65 mmol/L, this also may suggest magnesium deficiency[1249].

Measuring Magnesium Deficiency[1250]:

Test	Limitation
IV/oral magnesium load	High accuracy, Low availability
Mononuclear blood cell	High accuracy, Low availability
Tissue levels (intracellular)	High accuracy, invasive, research tool, low availability
Ionized serum magnesium	High accuracy, research tool, low availability
Serum	Low accuracy, but low-normal levels can suggest magnesium deficiency especially with low 24-hour urine magnesium levels.
Red Blood Cell	Low accuracy, Low availability

There are many different kinds of magnesium used in supplements with various effects. Here is an overview of them and for what condition they are best suited for[1251]:

- **Magnesium L-Threonate** is the best form of magnesium for increasing magnesium levels in the brain[1252]. It has been shown to improve cognition in those with cognitive impairment[1253], ADHD symptoms and IQ score in those with ADHD[1254] and memory in people with Alzheimer's disease[1255] and in mice with dementia[1256]. It has very good bioavailability and a low risk for diarrhea. Some people prefer taking magnesium L-threonate in the morning for focus and alertness, whereas others prefer to take it at night for relaxation and sleep. Different people experience different effects when taking magnesium L-threonate as the benefits will depend on a persons' baseline magnesium level in the brain.

- **Magnesium Glycinate** is one of the safest forms of magnesium with some of the least side-effects such as diarrhea[1257]. The added glycine, at least in children, may help with relaxation, pain and sleep by lowering body temperature[1258]. To be fair, the amount of glycine provided from magnesium glycinate supplements for adults is likely too low to have any real benefit. Doses of 125-300 mg of magnesium glycinate have been shown to rapidly resolve major depression in less than 7 days [1259]. Magnesium diglycinate seems to be a good alternative to magnesium oxide in patients with intestinal resection[1260].

- **Magnesium Malate** has been used for chronic fatigue syndrome and fibromyalgia[1261,1262]. Malic acid boosts ATP levels, which is a magnesium-dependent molecule [1263]. In animal studies, magnesium malate is highly bioavailable and stays elevated in the serum for hours[1264].

- **Magnesium Chloride** is the best magnesium for digestion issues because the extra chloride helps to produce stomach acid, which is why it is used to treat digestive disorders[1265]. Magnesium chloride has been shown to improve insulin sensitivity and metabolic control in type-2 diabetics[1266]. It has also been shown to improve symptoms of depression[1267]. Transdermal magnesium chloride may improve pain and quality of life in fibromyalgia[1268].

- **Magnesium Citrate** has fairly good bioavailability[1269]. It can withstand the acidic environment of the gut and can thus be absorbed over a longer period of time[1270]. Magnesium citrate has also been seen to improve arterial stiffness[1271]. Too much magnesium citrate can cause loose stool[1272].

- **Magnesium Taurate** is used for cardiovascular conditions as taurine helps the heart to work properly[1273]. Taurine can benefit congestive heart failure patients[1274]. Both magnesium and taurine have vascular-protective properties[1275].

- **Magnesium Sulfate** is mostly found in Epsom salt. It contains sulfur, which is a potent antioxidant needed for making glutathione. In pregnant women at imminent risk for delivery, magnesium sulfate supplementation has been shown to reduce the rate of cerebral palsy by 45%[1276].

- **Magnesium Arginate** helps with vasodilation and blood flow thanks to arginine.

- **Magnesium Lysine** contains the amino acid lysine, which has anti-viral effects. It can also support skin health.

- **Magnesium Ascorbate** contains vitamin C, which is why it can cause loose stool in large doses. It is a good bioavailable source of vitamin C and magnesium.

- **Magnesium Gluconate** is chelated with gluconic acid, which is the by-product of glucose fermentation. Together with potassium gluconate it has been shown to benefit myocardial function[1277].

- **Magnesium Orotate** is a magnesium salt of orotic acid. In patients with coronary heart disease, magnesium orotate improves heart function and exercise tolerance[1278]. It might be the best one for cardiovascular conditions[1279]. Even 25-50 mg/d of magnesium orotate has benefits in adolescents with syndromes of cardiac connective tissue dysplasia[1280]. Magnesium orotate has even been shown to improve survival in heart failure patients[1281].

- **Magnesium Oxide** has a fairly low bioavailability compared to other magnesium supplements. It is also one of the most commonly used forms of magnesium, but it can cause negative side-effects as it is not chelated and has poor water solubility [1282]. However, there is a case report of hypo-magnesaemia due to malabsorption wherein oral magnesium oxide supplementation elicited a response whereas magnesium glycerophosphate didn't[1283]. This may be because magnesium oxide is high in elemental magnesium compared to most magnesium supplements and if it does not cause diarrhea then it can provide a fairly large amount of magnesium.

When taking magnesium supplements, it is better to take smaller doses more frequently rather than large doses at once because of improved total absorption [1284]. In rats that are deficient in magnesium, magnesium supplements like magnesium chloride, aspartate, gluconate, citrate, and lactate have a similar bioavailability of 50-67% [1285]. However, the bioavailability will go down in states of magnesium sufficiency, where magnesium supplements are typically 40% bioavailable. Inorganic magnesium salts made in the U.S. may be equally bioavailable to organic magnesium salts [1286]. The best magnesium forms are L-threonate, sulfate, glycinate, citrate, malate and chloride. Magnesium oxide is the worst.

How to Restore Your Magnesium Levels: A 4 Step Plan

1.) Determine the factors that are causing you to become depleted in magnesium (see earlier in this chapter) and fix them.

2.) Eat a high magnesium diet.

3.) Determine if you are still magnesium deficient (low-end of normal serum magnesium levels plus low 24-hour urine magnesium level).

4.) Consider magnesium supplementation.

Hypermagnesemia or elevated magnesium levels is rare, but it can be the result of oversupplementation, kidney damage, inflammation or injury[1287,1288]. Animals challenged with an endotoxin see a significant increase in total and ionized magnesium[1289]. In healthy individuals with proper kidney function, too much magnesium does not pose a serious health risk because it will just get excreted in the urine[1290] or cause diarrhea[1291]. Large doses of magnesium-containing laxatives (over 5,000 mg of magnesium) are associated with magnesium toxicity as well as fatal hypermagnesemia[1292,1293,1294]. Hypermagnesemia is indicated by serum magnesium above 2.6 mg/dL, and severe hypermagnesemia (> 7 mg/dL) can be characterized by hypotension, nausea, vomiting, urine retention, muscle weakness, problems breathing and cardiac arrest.

Calcium Overload and Calcification

Calcium is the most abundant mineral in the human body. It is required for muscle contraction, vasodilation and bone health. However, only 1% of total body calcium is needed for carrying out these roles. The remaining 99% is stored in bones and teeth for structural support.[1295] The skeleton and bones are a readily available source of calcium to meet this baseline requirement[1296]. When calcium intake is low or malabsorbed, the body will pull stored calcium from bones to maintain normal functioning, which can eventually lead to osteoporosis and fractures. Low calcium levels in the body can cause muscle cramps, convulsions, abnormal heartbeat and eventually death[1297].

Calcium homeostasis is regulated by parathyroid hormone, calcitriol and calcitonin. When blood calcium levels drop, the parathyroid glands secrete parathyroid hormone (PTH), which stimulates the conversion of vitamin D in the kidneys into its active form calcitriol. This decreases urinary excretion of calcium but raises urinary excretion of phosphorus. Elevated PTH also promotes bone resorption or breakdown, which releases calcium and phosphorus into the serum from bones. Higher calcitriol concentrations increase intestinal absorption of calcium and phosphorus. As calcium levels normalize, PTH secretion stops and the thyroid gland secretes a peptide hormone

169

called calcitonin. Calcitonin inhibits PTH, reduces bone resorption as well as calcium absorption and promotes urinary calcium excretion.[1298]

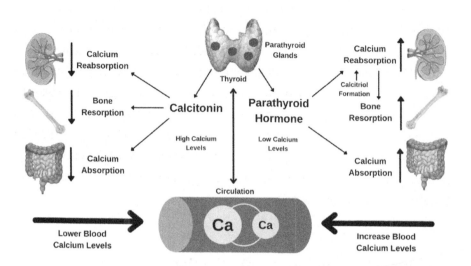

Adapted From: Linus Pauling Institute (2021) 'Calcium', Oregon State University, Accessed Online: https://lpi.oregonstate.edu/mic/minerals/calcium

Osteoporosis occurs when bone resorption is chronically higher than formation, which promotes the risk of fractures. Hip fractures are one of the most harmful consequences of osteoporosis with nearly 1/3rd of those who experience an osteoporotic hip fracture enter nursing homes and 1 in 4 dying within one year of the fracture[1299]. The risk of osteoporotic hip fracture is determined by one's peak bone mass and the rate of bone loss after that peak has been reached. Low calcium and low protein diets, age, female gender, estrogen deficiency, smoking, hyperthyroidism and high alcohol consumption increase the risk of developing osteoporosis[1300, 1301]. Postmenopausal women are at a higher risk of osteoporosis and fractures because of a drop in estrogen, which has a role in strengthening bones[1302]. Estrogen deficiency reduces the absorption of calcium,[1303] whereas estrogen therapy enhances calcium absorption[1304]. Low body mass index appears to be the strongest factors that promotes the development of osteoporosis-related sarcopenia[1305].

Lifelong physical activity, especially weight-bearing exercise, with adequate calcium and vitamin D slow the rate of bone loss later in life[1306]. Increased dietary calcium intake has been shown to increase bone mineral density with or without vitamin D[1307]. A meta-analysis of 20 randomized controlled trials has found that supplemental calcium reduced total fracture risk by 11%[1308]. Among 52,915 older people in the U.S., vitamin D (300-1,000 IU/day) and calcium (500-1,200 mg/day) supplementation for up to 7 years decreased the risk of a new fracture by 12% [1309]. The National Osteoporosis Foundation recommends a calcium intake of 1,000-1,200 mg/d and vitamin D 800-1,000 IU/d to middle-aged men and women[1310].

The FDA suggests that adequate calcium and vitamin D intake throughout life may reduce the risk of osteoporosis[1311]. However, the harms and benefits of supplementation need to be further assessed. **Excessive calcium intake (>1,500 mg/d) can decrease parathyroid hormone (PTH), which increases the risk of low bone turnover**[1312]. Too much calcium also reduces the bone growth stimulating effects of PTH[1313]. However, for the elderly or for someone with impaired calcium absorption, optimal calcium intake may be around 2,400 mg/d due to impaired absorption. Hyperparathyroidism is the most common cause of elevated calcium in the blood (hypercalcemia)[1314]. Patients with kidney disease on high calcium intakes experience low bone turnover and PTH suppression[1315]. Parathyroid hormone suppression caused by high calcium intake is also thought to reduce magnesium absorption[1316]. Sweden is the highest dairy and calcium consuming countries, but it also has the highest rate of hip fractures among developed nations[1317]. Meta-analysis find calcium supplementation does increase bone mineral density modestly but does not result in reduced incidence of fractures[1318,1319,1320]. Ultimately, the optimal level of calcium intake will also depend on the background intake of magnesium, vitamin D and vitamin K.

Extracellular calcium is constantly maintained at 1.25 mM by parathyroid hormone and 1,25-dihydroxyvitamin D (calcitriol) activity, except after supplementation over a 3-4-hour period[1321]. Intracellular calcium levels are maintained around 100 nM (nanomolar) and can rise up to 1 mcM (micromolar) upon activation, whereas extracellular calcium sits at 1.2 mM[1322]. When intracellular calcium reaches 1 mcM it is taken up by the mitochondria and through a uniporter it is released once levels drop below 1 mcM [1323]. Concentrations >1 mcM may inhibit mitochondrial respiration and trigger pro-cell death signals[1324]. The mitochondria can accumulate a lot of calcium, exceeding 1000 nmol/mg of mitochondrial protein[1325]. This ability is an intrinsic component of ATP production[1326]. Heart mitochondria have a sodium-calcium exchanger in addition to the calcium uniporter[1327,1328,1329]. Intracellular calcium is kept at a balance by the influx and efflux of calcium by voltage-operated channels or agonist binding (glutamate, ATP, acetylcholine) via receptor-operated channels. Calcium can also be released from internal stores such as the endoplasmic reticulum[1330].

Increased calcium intake decreases the gastrointestinal absorption of lead and can prevent it from being mobilized from bone during bone demineralization[1331]. Average dietary calcium intake of 900 mg/day and supplementation of 1,200 mg/d during pregnancy can reduce maternal lead concentrations by 8-14%[1332]. Similar results were found in the blood and breast milk[1333,1334]. In postmenopausal women, estrogen therapy and physical exercise is inversely associated with blood lead levels because they decrease bone demineralization and the release of lead from bone[1335]. Most calcium supplements contain some lead as they are typically sourced from oysters, shellfish, bone meal or dolomite[1336]. The FDA's provisional total tolerable intake (PTTI) level for lead is set at 7.5 mg/1,000 mg of elemental calcium[1337]. A review of 324 multivitamin/mineral supplements found lead exposure ranges from 1% to 4% of the PTTI[1338].

High calcium intake is also associated with a decreased risk of colon cancer[1339,1340,1341]. Calcium carbonate supplementation has also been shown to reduce the risk of adenoma in the colon, which is a precursor to cancer,[1342,1343] for even as long as 5 years after stopping the supplement[1344]. Two large prospective epidemiological trials found that consuming 700-800 mg of calcium per day lowered the risk of left-side colon cancer by 40-50% [1345], but these findings have seen conflicting results in other studies[1346,1347].

In 477,122 European subjects followed for an average of 11 years, dairy consumption was inversely associated with colorectal cancer risk [1348]. Among 36,282 postmenopausal women, daily supplementation with 1,000 mg of calcium and 400 IUs of vitamin D3 for 7 years has had no significant effect on colorectal cancer but it might help prevent colorectal adenomas (benign tumors)[1349,1350]. Dietary calcium intake of 1,000-1,250 mg/d in 41,403 women with a 16-year follow up is associated with a lower risk of developing colorectal adenomas by 76% compared to intakes equal to or below 500 mg/d[1351].

However, increased dairy and calcium intake (>1,500 mg/day) is weakly associated with an increased risk of prostate cancer[1352,1353,1354,1355,1356,1357]. Among 3,918 male health workers diagnosed with prostate cancer, the risk of prostate cancer death was higher in those who consumed whole milk > 4 servings/week compared to ≤ 3 servings/month[1358]. No increased risk was seen in the consumption of skim milk, low-fat or full-fat dairy products (excluding whole milk). **Non-dairy calcium does not appear to raise prostate cancer risk**[1359]. Dairy, in particular, promotes insulin-like growth factor (IGF-1), which regulates cell proliferation and growth[1360]. Circulating IGF-1 levels are positively correlated with cancer risk, especially prostate cancer[1361,1362,1363]. Prostate cancer risk has been observed to be the highest in people who consume the most dairy and animal protein[1364]. However, it has also been found that individuals with a higher dairy/calcium consumption are more likely to engage in healthy lifestyle practices like exercise or seeking of medical help, which might mitigate the association with increased prostate cancer risk[1365].

Higher calcium intakes are associated with lower bodyweight and less weight gain[1366,1367,1368]. Low calcium intake stimulates lipogenesis (growth of fat cells) and lipogenic gene expression[1369]. Higher calcium intake, however, promotes fat breakdown (lipolysis)[1370]. **A recent meta-analysis estimated that a high calcium intake (1,300 mg/d) increases fat oxidation by 11% compared to a low intake of 488 mg/d**[1371]. Dietary calcium may also bind to fat from food in the digestive tract and prevent its absorption[1372, 1373]. Vitamin D sufficiency could also help with lipolysis as vitamin D deficiency is associated with obesity[1374,1375]. According to a meta-analysis of 18 cross-sectional prospective studies, increasing calcium intake from 400 mg/d to 1,200 mg/d reduces BMI by 1.1 kg/m^2.[1376] Energy-restrictive diets of a 500-calorie deficit result in more weight loss when the calcium intake is higher (1,200 mg/d) compared to 800 mg/d on a standard diet[1377]. Dairy products appear to be more impactful for weight loss than calcium from other foods[1378,1379,1380]. Calcium supplementation (800-1,500 mg/d) has not been shown to have the same effects on fat loss[1381,1382]. Thus, it appears to be dairy foods that are associated with the greatest fat loss seen from increased calcium intake. Calcium may also regulate appetite and hunger levels, making the person eat fewer calories, and for that whole foods are superior to supplements[1383]. At the moment, more research is being done on the effects of calcium on fat metabolism[1384].

Higher calcium concentrations in the blood are associated with more cardiovascular events[1385,1386]. Several studies have indicated that calcium supplementation (>1,000 mg/day on top of diet) increases the risk of cardiovascular disease (CVD), myocardial infarction and coronary heart disease[1387,1388,1389,1390]. In a cohort of older Swedish women, calcium intake from diet and supplements of 1,400 mg/day and higher were associated with higher CVD death rates and ischemic heart disease compared to 600–1,000 mg/day[1391]. **Men taking 1,000 mg/d of supplemental calcium on top of their diet saw a 20% higher risk of CVD than those who didn't take it**[1392]. Finnish women aged 52-62 have a 14% higher risk of developing coronary artery disease compared to non-supplementers over the course of 6.75-years of follow-up[1393]. It is thought that calcium supplements override the homeostatic regulation of serum calcium, causing hypercalcemia[1394]. Hypercalcemia promotes blood coagulation, vascular calcification and arterial stiffness, which all elevate the risk of CVD[1395,1396]. CVD mortality is higher in those who obtain a total calcium intake (diet + supplements) of >1,500 mg/day[1397]. Based on a 2016 systematic review, the American Society for Preventive Cardiology and the National Osteoporosis Foundation have stated that calcium intake within the daily upper limit does not pose any harm[1398]. **The key take-away is that you should get your calcium from your**

diet, not from supplements, and most adults should aim for around 1,200 mg of calcium per day.

Phosphate has a role in the accumulation of calcium by activating the calcium uniporter and inhibiting calcium efflux[1399,1400,1401]. One of the contributing factors for arterial calcification is high serum phosphate, which has been shown to promote calcification in animal models and cell studies[1402,1403]. In humans, high serum phosphate is associated with increased cardiovascular disease events[1404]. For every 1 mg/dL increase above normal in phosphorus levels, the risk of coronary artery calcification has been seen to increase by 21%[1405]. A low calcium to phosphorus ratio in diet has adverse health effects, starting with arterial calcification and ending with bone loss[1406].

Excessive supplemental calcium can contribute to calcium overload, increasing urinary calcium excretion and possibly soft tissue calcification[1407]. It has been shown that about 9% of women taking calcium supplements had hypercalcemia and 31% had hypercalciuria[1408]. More than 50% of older men and 70% of older women in the U.S. are taking calcium supplements regularly to support their bone health[1409]. In total, 43% of U.S. adults are using calcium supplements[1410].

Excess calcium converts smooth muscle cells into bone-forming cells or osteoblasts that promote arterial calcification[1411]. High calcium intake also suppresses kidney synthesis of calcitriol, which raises cardiovascular risk[1412,1413].

Increased calcium intake has been inconsistently shown to lower blood pressure and the risk of hypertension[1414,1415,1416]. A meta-analysis of 23 large observational studies worldwide did find a reduction in systolic blood pressure of 0.34 mmHg and a 0.15 mmHg drop in diastolic blood pressure per 100 mg of calcium consumed per day[1417]. However, calcium supplementation has inconsistent results for reducing blood pressure and if it does the reductions tend to be small[1418,1419]. Calcium supplementation during pregnancy may reduce the risk of preeclampsia[1420], in which the pregnant woman develops hypertension and proteinuria after 20 weeks' gestation[1421]. Supplementing 1,000 mg/d of calcium may reduce the incidence of preeclampsia by 55%[1422].

However, it may only be effective in women with a low calcium intake (~314 mg/d) but not in those with more sufficient intakes (1,100 mg/d)[1423,1424]. There is an inverse relationship between calcium intake during pregnancy and the incidence of preeclampsia[1425].

Observational studies find that diets high in vegetables and minerals, including calcium, potassium and magnesium, tend to result in lower blood pressure[1426, 1427, 1428, 1429]. In the Dietary Approaches to Stop Hypertension (DASH) study, the low-fat dairy diet with added fruits and vegetables (1,200 mg/d of calcium) resulted in the biggest decrease in blood pressure (-11.4 mmHg and –5.5 mmHg systolic and diastolic blood pressure, respectively), compared to the control Standard American Diet and a fruit and vegetable only diet (800 mg/d of calcium, reducing systolic blood pressure by 7.2 mmHg and diastolic blood pressure by 2.8 mmHg)[1430]. **Thus, a daily intake of 1,000-1,200 mg of calcium might help to treat moderate hypertension**[1431].

Daily Calcium Intake

Low < 1,000 mg/d	Normal 1,000-1,200 mg/d	High > 1,500 mg/d
Osteoporosis Risk of Fractures Bone Loss Preeclampsia Hypertension Oxidative Stress CVD Risk Weight Gain	Weight Loss Bone Density Low Fracture Risk Low Osteoporosis Risk Low Colon Cancer Risk Reduced PMS Symptoms	Calcification Atherosclerosis Prostate Cancer Low Bone Turnover Osteoporosis Neuronal Death CVD Risk

Intracellular calcium homeostasis is regulated by the mitochondria's tightly regulated calcium transport system[1432]. The mitochondria also produce ATP, which generates reactive oxygen species as an inevitable by-product. In healthy subjects, this basal oxidative stress should be dealt with by the body's endogenous antioxidant systems. However, during pathophysiological states the balance is offset, causing calcium

176

dysregulation, oxidative stress and eventually cell death[1433,1434]. In vitro studies find that calcium in the brain inhibits mitochondrial respiration by inhibition of Complex I and thus reduces mitochondria-generated reactive oxygen species in a dose-dependent manner[1435,1436]. Calcium can also inhibit free radical production in the presence of ATP and magnesium[1437]. Calcium signaling also regulates autophagy, which is the recycling of cellular material that is beneficial in moderation but can also lead to cell death when in excess[1438].

Activation of the NMDA-selective glutamate receptors causes a massive influx of calcium into neurons, leading to their death[1439,1440,1441]. This is the result of excess mitochondrial superoxide production that damages organelles[1442,1443]. Beta-amyloid proteins involved in Alzheimer's disease cause sporadic intracellular calcium signaling and calcium influx that results in neuronal death[1444,1445].

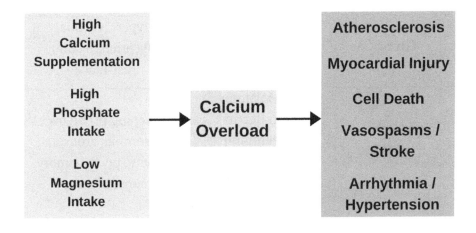

177

Here are the calcium-dependent enzymes, functions and consequences that may occur with a deficit

Calcium-Dependent Enzymes/Proteins	Function	Consequences of Deficit
ATP Synthase	Produce and activate ATP	Energy shortage, not enough energy to carry out vital bodily processes
Fatty Acid Oxidation	Burn triglycerides and lipids for fuel	Hyperlipidemia, hypercholesterolemia
Lipolysis	Breakdown of fat cells	Obesity, visceral adiposity
Glycolysis	Burn glucose for fuel	Hyperglycemia, glycation, insulin resistance
5-HTP	Melatonin production, serotonin production, relaxation, REM sleep	Sleeping problems, insomnia, arousal, anxiety, poor memory consolidation
Parathyroid Hormone (PTH)	Bone turnover, bone mineral density	Osteoporosis, increased bone loss, decreased bone density
Calcitriol	Active form of vitamin D, promote bone density, support immunity, govern hormone regulation	Osteoporosis, decreased bone density, increased risk of fractures, weaker immunity

	Regulate calcium balance, reduce calcium absorption	Calcium overload, calcification, atherosclerosis
Calcitonin		

Calcium Food Sources

The current RDA for calcium in women is 1,200 mg/d and for men 1,000 mg/d[1446,1447]. The tolerable upper limit is 3,000 mg/d for 9-18-year-olds, 2,500 mg/d for adults 19-50 years old and 2,000 mg/d for 51+ years of age[1448]. Healthy non-growing adults require 550-1,200 mg of calcium a day to maintain balance[1449]. For growing boys, the minimal intake to achieve maximal retention is 1,140 mg/d and 1,300 mg/d for growing girls[1450]. Intakes greater than 1,400 mg/d achieve a positive calcium balance in people with both normal renal function as well as in those with end-stage renal disease[1451,1452]. An intake of 2,000 mg/d has demonstrated a positive calcium balance of 450 mg/d in normal subjects and 750 mg/d in patients with mild chronic kidney disease (CKD)[1453]. Thus, calcium retention is higher in people with renal dysfunction and/or kidney disease. As a result, they may also need to aim for the lower end of the RDA and be more cautious with calcium supplementation to prevent soft tissue calcification [1454]. Among CKD patients, high calcium intake is associated with cardiovascular calcification[1455]. More than 29 million Americans have CKD[1456].

In the U.S., the average calcium intake for men is 871-1,266 mg/d and for women 748-968 mg/d [1457]. NHANES data from 2009-2012 indicated that 37.7% of non-supplemented adults and 19.6% of adults who supplement obtain inadequate calcium[1458]. Females, especially adolescent girls, are generally less likely to get adequate amounts of calcium from food[1459]. Dairy contributes to 75% of the calcium intake in the American diet. It is common for children to replace milk for sugary soft drinks during the most critical period of their peak bone mass development[1460]. Replacing milk with carbonated soft drinks high in phosphorus has been associated with a rise in bone mineral density loss and fracture risk[1461]. Soft drinks that contain phosphoric acid have been a major source of phosphorus over the past quarter century.

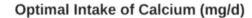

Optimal Intake of Calcium (mg/d)

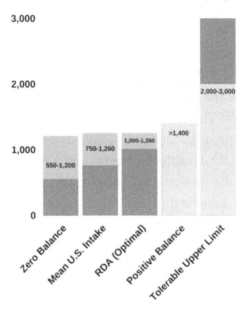

Calcium from food is not correlated with increased CVD risk, whereas supplemental calcium is[1462]. Among calcium supplement users, taking more than 1,400 mg/d of calcium total (from diet and supplements) is associated with higher all-cause mortality, including cardiovascular disease[1463]. Dietary calcium intake and the association with cardiovascular mortality follows a U-shaped pattern with intakes < 800 mg/d or > 1,200 mg/d sharply associated with an increased risk of cardiovascular mortality[1464]. Supplemental calcium >1,000 mg/d with or without vitamin D increases the risk of myocardial infarction slightly[1465]. The same applies to kidney stones – calcium from food decreases the risk while calcium supplementation increases it[1466]. It is thought that acute large boluses of calcium from supplements elevate serum calcium in a way that leads to transient vascular calcification[1467,1468]. There has not been an established link between moderate calcium intake and the coronary artery calcium (CAC) score[1469]. Thus, eating calcium-rich foods should not contribute to cardiovascular disease, unless magnesium deficiency occurs, or high-dose calcium supplements are taken.

The recommended ratio of calcium to magnesium is ~ 2:1 both for daily dietary intake and supplementation[1470]. In Western countries, the ratio of calcium to magnesium is much higher than it is in China (3 vs 1.7). A recent meta-analysis of prospective studies in Shanghai discovered that in people with a Ca/Mg ratio below 1.7, increased magnesium intake was associated with higher mortality, whereas in those with a ratio above 1.7, magnesium reduced mortality[1471]. Thus, high supplemental magnesium may not be advisable if calcium intake is low. Instead, it is better to aim for 500-600 mg/d of magnesium and 1,000-1,200 mg of calcium per day, which provides an optimal calcium to magnesium ratio of ~ 2:1. When calcium intake is 10 mg/kg/d, magnesium balance begins to decrease[1472]. So, when taking a calcium supplement, it would be optimal to have some magnesium in it as well. **Since the early 1900s, magnesium intake has reduced from 500 mg/d to about 250 mg/d, increasing the Ca/Mg ratio from 2/1 to 5/1**[1473]. There has been a sharp increase in type-2 diabetes in the U.S. between 1994-2001 when the Ca/Mg ratio from food sharply rose from < 3 to > 3[1474].

Optimal Calcium:Magnesium Ratio

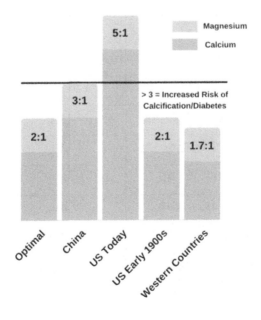

181

Here are the highest calcium food sources[1475]

Food	Mg of Calcium per Serving	% of RDA
Yogurt, low fat, 8 oz	415 mg	32%
Orange Juice, fortified, 1 cup	349 mg	27%
Mozzarella, 1.5 oz	333 mg	26%
Sardines, canned, with bones, 3 oz	325 mg	25%
Cheddar Cheese, 1.5 oz	307 mg	24%
Milk, nonfat, 1 cup	299 mg	23%
Soymilk, fortified, 1 cup	299 mg	23%
Milk, 2% fat, 1 cup	293 mg	23%
Whole Milk, 1 cup	276 mg	21%
Yogurt, low fat, 6 oz	258 mg	20%
Tofu, firm, ½ cup	253 mg	19%
Salmon, 3 oz	181 mg	14%
Cottage Cheese, 1% fat, 1 cup	138 mg	11%
Tofu, soft, ½ cup	138 mg	11%
Fortified Cereal, 1 serving	130 mg	10%
Sardines, without bones, 3 oz	110 mg	9%
Frozen Yogurt, ½ cup	103 mg	8%
Turnip Greens, ½ cup	99 mg	8%
Kale, cooked, 1 cup	94 mg	7%
Ice Cream, ½ cup	84 mg	6%
Chia Seeds, 1 tbsp	76 mg	6%

Bok Choi, 1 cup	74 mg	6%
White Bread, 1 slice	73 mg	6%
Corn Tortilla, 6" diameter	46 mg	4%
Flour Tortilla, 6" diameter	32 mg	2%
Sour Cream, reduced fat, 2 tbsp	31 mg	2%
Whole-Wheat Bread, 1 slice	30 mg	2%
Mussels, 3 oz	28 mg	2%
Egg, whole, 1 medium	25 mg	2%
Kale, raw, 1 cup	24 mg	2%
Broccoli, raw, ½ cup	21 mg	2%
Cream Cheese, 1 tbsp	14 mg	1%
Liver, 3 oz	5.6 mg	0.5%

The rate of gastrointestinal calcium absorption is about 10-30% for adults and as high as 60% for growing children[1476,1477,1478]. Antacids increase urinary calcium excretion and glucocorticoids promote calcium depletion[1479].

Urinary calcium excretion is limited to 4 mg/kg of bodyweight per day[1480]. For an average-weighing person that would equate to a limit of 280-350 mg per day. Because of that, the kidneys are not able to lower hypercalcemia during excess calcium intake. In the elderly and people with renal dysfunction, the arteries become a calcium sink because the kidneys are not able to excrete extra calcium. Hypercalcemia also increases the risk of developing kidney stones[1481].

Here are things that reduce calcium absorption and increase calcium demand

- **Certain plant foods**, even those rich in calcium like spinach and kale, inhibit calcium absorption due to their oxalic acid or oxalate content. Oxalates are found the most in spinach, rhubarb leaves, bok choy, sweet potato, cassava and beans. According to research, eating spinach and milk at the same time reduces the absorption of calcium from the milk[1482]. Citric acid or lemon juice helps to break down oxalate crystals.

- o **Supplemental calcium increases the risk of calcium oxalate kidney stones**[1483,1484]. Higher dietary calcium intake, however, does not appear to promote kidney stone formation and may even lower the risk[1485,1486,1487]. Adequate calcium intake reduces the absorption of dietary oxalate and reduces urinary oxalate by forming insoluble calcium oxalate salts[1488,1489]. Consuming large amounts of oxalate does not increase the risk of calcium oxalate stones when dietary calcium in the recommended amounts is present[1490].

- **Phytates** are weaker inhibitors of calcium absorption than oxalates. Wheat bran or dried beans can substantially reduce calcium absorption, whereas regular wheat does not appear to do so[1491]. To reduce the phytate and oxalate content of these foods, you can soak and sprout them beforehand. Yeast also contains a phytate-breaking enzyme called phytase that helps to break down phytate during fermentation.

- **High sodium and protein intake** can increase urinary calcium excretion but also calcium absorption[1492,1493,1494]. Sodium and calcium appear to compete in the kidneys for reabsorption. Every gram increment of sodium (2.5 g of sodium chloride) excretion by the kidneys has been found to draw 26.3 mg of calcium into the urine[1495]. However, higher sodium intakes are associated with fewer hip fractures[1496]. Thus, the increased absorption of calcium may offset any calcium loss out the urine. At the same time, high protein intake increases intestinal calcium absorption, nullifying the higher calcium excretion[1497]. No association has been found between higher protein intake and lower bone mineral density[1498]. In healthy subjects, high protein intake does not change calcium balance[1499]. Metabolic acidosis, which may result from excess animal protein or cereal consumption, also increases calcium excretion[1500]. Bicarbonate from fruits, vegetables or bicarbonate mineral water can help to offset that.

- **Lactose intolerance** increases the risk of calcium deficiency due to the avoidance of dairy[1501]. Some lactose intolerant people can tolerate small amounts of dairy, like an 8 oz glass of milk, without side-effects. Consuming dairy with other foods or spread throughout the day may improve tolerance[1502]. Low-lactose dairy products include aged cheeses, yogurt or lactose-free milk.

- **Vegan diets** may not provide adequate amounts of calcium due to the avoidance of dairy as well as the reduced bioavailability of calcium from the increased phytonutrient content of plants[1503,1504]. Bone fracture risk is higher in vegans compared to omnivores or vegetarians[1505]. Lacto-ovo-vegetarians (eggs and dairy) and non-vegetarians have similar calcium intakes[1506,1507]. So, having some dairy products in the diet appears to be enough to cover calcium needs.

- **Caffeine** from coffee, tea or soda can also raise urinary excretion while reducing the rate of absorption of calcium[1508]. However, one cup of coffee causes a loss of only 2-3 mg of calcium. Doses of 400 mg of caffeine do not change 24-hour urinary calcium excretion[1509,1510]. Moderate coffee consumption (1-2 cups a day) is not associated with poor outcomes on bone but when no milk or other calcium foods are consumed it is[1511]. Thus, habitual coffee consumption requires compensation in the form of increased calcium consumption from food. The increased urinary calcium excretion seen from the consumption of carbonated beverages is attributed to their caffeine content, not the carbonation or phosphorus[1512].

- **Alcohol** reduces calcium absorption directly and by inhibiting enzymes that convert vitamin D into its active form[1513]. However, moderate alcohol consumption (1-2 drinks or 30 grams per day) does not have a significant impact on bone health or vitamin D status[1514].

- **Menopause** promotes bone loss due to lower estrogen levels increasing bone resorption and reducing calcium absorption[1515,1516]. During the first year of menopause, bone mass may decrease 3-5% per year, but it drops down to 1% after the age of 65[1517]. Increasing calcium intake does not completely offset this loss[1518,1519]. To restore premenopausal bone remodeling, estrogen or hormone replacement therapy (HRT) may be needed[1520]. HRT is often prescribed to women at an increased risk of osteoporosis, but it must be balanced with a potential increased risk of cardiovascular events[1521].
  - Low calcium intake is associated with premenstrual syndrome (PMS) and supplemental calcium decreases the symptoms[1522]. Women in the highest quartile of dietary calcium (~1,283 mg/d) have a 30% reduced risk of developing PMS compared to those with the lowest intake (~529 mg/d)[1523]. Among 466 women with moderate-to-severe PMS symptoms, supplemental calcium of 1,200 mg/d for three menstrual cycles was associated with a 48% decrease in total symptoms compared to the 30% reduction of the placebo group[1524]. Similar results have been found with supplemental calcium of 400-500 mg/d and 1,000 mg/d[1525,1526,1527,1528].
- **Amenorrhea**, which is a condition wherein menstruation stops or fails to begin, causes a drop in circulating estrogen, which has a negative effect on calcium balance[1529]. Usually, it is associated with the "female athlete triad" – disordered eating or anorexia, amenorrhea and osteoporosis[1530,1531]. Menstrual irregularities and low bone mineral density are associated with the risk of future fractures[1532]. Calcium and vitamin D supplementation has been shown to reduce the incidence of stress fractures among female navy recruits[1533].

Calcium itself decreases the absorption of some drugs, such as bisphosphonates (used for osteoporosis), fluoroquinolones and tetracycline antibiotics, levothyroxine, phenytoin (an anticonvulsant), and tiludronate disodium (for Paget's disease)[1534,1535]. Consuming 600 mg of calcium with a meal cuts the absorption of zinc in half from that meal[1536]. Taking calcium supplements together with thiazide diuretics increases the risk of hypercalcemia because of increased calcium reabsorption by the kidneys. It can also promote abnormal heartbeat in people taking digoxin for heart failure[1537].

Calcium supplementation is not recommended for those who do not need it as dietary calcium comes in safer amounts and with other nutrients. However, it might be necessary for those who are having difficulties consuming calcium foods, like in those who are lactose intolerant or for postmenopausal women. To avoid calcium overload and increased urinary excretion, it is better to take no more than 500 mg per meal and not exceed 1,500 mg/d. Supplementing calcium (600-2,000 mg/d for 2-5 years) has been associated with gastrointestinal disturbance, constipation, cramping, bloating and diarrhea[1538]. The most cost-effective calcium supplement is calcium carbonate. Calcium citrate is best for those who have poor stomach acid or are on histamine-2 blockers or protein-pump inhibitors.[1539]

Phosphorus and Health

Phosphorus is another essential mineral component of bones and teeth as well as DNA and RNA[1540]. Calcium and phosphorus make up hydroxyapatite, which is the main structural component of bones, the collagen matrix and tooth enamel[1541]. In humans, phosphorus makes up ~1-1.4% of fat-free mass (approximately 700 grams). Out of this amount, 85% is located in bones and teeth as hydroxyapatite, 14% exists in soft tissue and 1% is present extracellularly.

Elemental phosphorus exists as red phosphorus and white phosphorus. White phosphorus begins to glow a bit when exposed to oxygen because of oxidation. Because of its luminescent properties, phosphorus gets its name from Greek mythology as "light-bearer" or Lucifer in Latin, which refers to the planet Venus. Phosphorus is never found as a free element on Earth, but it is found in the Earth's crust. In minerals, phosphorus is generally present as phosphate.

187

Inorganic phosphorus as phosphate (PO_4^{3-}) is required for all known life forms[1542]. Phosphorus is a part of cell membranes, ATP and phospholipids. Phosphorylation is the addition of a phosphoryl group to an organic molecule, which affects many proteins and sugars in the body. The phosphorylation of carbohydrates is involved with many steps in glycolysis[1543]. Glucose phosphorylation is needed for insulin-dependent mTOR activity in the heart, regulating cardiac growth[1544]. Thus, without phosphorus, or phosphorylation, glycogen resynthesis and glycolysis do not work as well. Phosphorylation also affects amino acids and proteins like histidine, lysine, arginine, aspartic acid and glutamic acid[1545,1546].

Phosphorus deficiency can cause anorexia, muscle wasting, rickets, hyperparathyroidism, kidney tubule defects, and diabetic ketoacidosis[1547]. Genetic phosphorus disorders include X-linked hypophosphatemic rickets, which promotes rickets, osteomalacia, pseudofractures, dental damage and enthesopathy (mineralization of ligaments and tendons)[1548]. Hypophosphatemic rickets may also be accompanied with hypercalciuria[1549]. In preterm infants, phosphorus and calcium deficiency are one of the main causes of osteopenia[1550]. Most of the fetal bone mineralization occurs during the third trimester of pregnancy, which is why preterm babies are born with low calcium and phosphorus in their bones[1551]. Fortified milk is commonly used to support the growth of these children[1552]. **Phosphorus deficiency occurs in 21.5% of chronic obstructive pulmonary disease patients, 30.4% chronic alcoholics, 33.9% of ICU patients, 75% of severe trauma or burn victims and up to 80% of people with sepsis**[1553].

Prolonged starvation or malnutrition can cause refeeding syndrome, which is characterized by hypophosphatemia but can also include abnormal balances in sodium and fluids, changes in metabolism, thiamine deficiency, hypokalaemia, and hypomagnesaemia[1554]. Out of 10,197 hospitalized patients, hypophosphatemia was found in 0.43% of people with malnutrition being one of the strongest risk factors[1555]. In early starvation, the body will shift from using carbs to using fat and protein for fuel, which can decrease metabolic rate by up to 20-25%[1556]. During refeeding, the increase in blood glucose increases insulin and decreases glucagon, which stimulates synthesis of glycogen, fat, and protein. This process requires phosphate, magnesium, and vitamin B1. Insulin stimulates the absorption of potassium, magnesium, and phosphate into the cells via the sodium-potassium ATPase pump, which also shuttles glucose into cells. This process decreases serum levels of these minerals because the body is already depleted of them. Refeeding syndrome can cause electrolyte deficiencies, fluid retention, cramps, heart palpitations, hypoventilation, respiratory failure, heart failure, impaired blood clotting, coma and even death[1557]. It is more likely to develop in patients who are underweight, anorexic, have a low-nutrient diet or with a history of drug/alcohol abuse[1558]. **Administration of phosphorus and thiamine can help to prevent refeeding syndrome.** However, electrolytes and sodium are also vital because an actual phosphorus deficiency is rare. For most people to become deficient in phosphorus, you would have to be ingesting close to zero phosphorus for a month or longer, which is why it most commonly occurs in third world malnutrition victims. Refeeding syndrome while fasting or calorie restriction occurs mostly because of dehydration, lack of potassium, sodium, and magnesium.

Normal serum phosphate in adults is 2.5-4.5 mg/dL or 0.81-1.45 mmol/L[1559]. Hypophosphatemia is defined when phosphate drops below the lower end of the normal range and hyperphosphatemia is when it is above the high end. However, serum or plasma phosphate does not necessarily reflect whole-body phosphorus content[1560].

High phosphate levels are linked to cardiovascular disease risk in people without a history of CVD[1561,1562]. Among 14,675 participants over a 20-year follow-up, every 1 mg/dL increase in serum phosphate has been associated with a 13% higher risk of atrial fibrillation[1563]. A meta-analysis involving 13,515 participants with a 6–29-year follow-up found a 36% higher CVD mortality in subjects at the highest phosphate levels (2.79–4.0 mg/dL) compared to those at 0.61–3.28 mg/dL[1564]. Every 1 mg/dL above 3.5 mg/dL increases the risk of death by 35% and CVD mortality by 45%[1565]. However, the literature doesn't show that restricting phosphorus intake prevents CVD[1566].

Optimal Serum Phosphate (mg/dL)

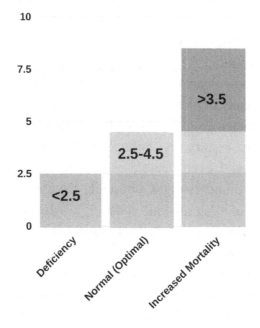

Here are the phosphorus-dependent enzymes, functions and consequences that may occur with a deficit

Phosphorus-Dependent Enzymes/Proteins	Function	Consequences of Deficit
ATP Synthase	Produce and activate ATP	Energy shortage, not enough energy to carry out vital bodily processes
Phosphorylation	Burn triglycerides and lipids for fuel	Hyperlipidemia, hypercholesterolemia
Glycolysis	Burn glucose for fuel	Hyperglycemia, glycation, insulin resistance

Glucokinase	Catalyze the phosphorylation of glucose	Risk of hyperglycemia and insulin resistance
Hexokinase	Catalyze the phosphorylation of glucose	Risk of hyperglycemia and insulin resistance
Glucose 6-Phosphate	Convert glucose into glycogen, glycogenolysis, glycolysis, gluconeogenesis	Risk of hyperglycemia and low glycogen storage
Fructose-6-Phosphate	Store glucose in the cells, glycolysis, gluconeogenesis	Risk of hyperglycemia and insulin resistance
Fructose-1-Phosphate	Store fructose in the cells, glycolysis, gluconeogenesis	Risk of hyperglycemia and insulin resistance
Parathyroid Hormone (PTH)	Bone turnover, bone mineral density	Osteoporosis, increased bone loss, decreased bone density
Calcitriol	Active form of vitamin D, promote bone density, support immunity, govern hormone regulation	Osteoporosis, decreased bone density, increased risk of fractures, weaker immunity
Calcitonin	Regulate calcium balance, reduce calcium absorption	Calcium overload, calcification, atherosclerosis

Phosphorus Food Sources

The RDA for phosphorus is 700 mg for adults, 1,250 mg for teens 9-18 years of age, 500 mg for 1-8-year-olds and < 275 mg for infants[1567,1568]. Tolerable upper intake levels (Uls) are set at 3,000-4,000 mg/d. Estimated Average Requirement (EARs) for basal requirements are deemed to be 580 mg/d for ages above 19[1569]. The RDA for phosphorus is being exceeded greatly and it may be even higher than currently estimated[1570,1571]. NHANES data from 2015-2016 shows that adults get on average 1,189 mg/d for women and 1,596 mg/d for men, while children and teens get 1,237 mg/d[1572]. In 2013-2014, NHANES showed the average phosphorus intake from both food and supplements was 1,744 mg/d for men and 1,301 mg/d for women. However, this may not be adequate as these surveys don't take into account the phosphate additives in many foods. **Prolonged phosphate intakes above 1,000 mg/d in adults are associated with adverse effects on the kidneys, bones and cardiovascular system**[1573,1574,1575]. Acute high doses of 6,600 mg of sodium phosphate twice a day can cause hyperphosphatemia, which can promote calcium overload and calcification of soft tissue[1576,1577].

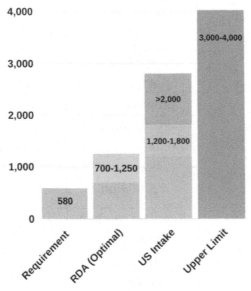

Optimal Intake of Phosphorus (mg/d)

192

High intake of phosphorus can contribute to calcium overload and magnesium deficiency.

Cell studies find excess phosphorus can cause vascular calcification and endothelial dysfunction[1578,1579,1580,1581,1582,1583]. A high intake of phosphorus (>1,400 mg/d) in relation to calcium keeps parathyroid hormone elevated constantly, which decreases bone mineral density[1584,1585,1586]. Over the long term, it can lead to an increased risk of skeletal fractures and cardiovascular disease mortality [1587]. However, if calcium intake is adequate, high intake of phosphorus doesn't seem to have a negative effect on bone mineral content[1588]. Excess phosphorus, however, may promote the formation of kidney stones and calcium oxalate[1589]. In animal models, high phosphorus intake can promote vascular and renal calcification, renal tubular injury and premature death[1590].

The recommended ratio of Ca/P is 1-2:1[1591]. That ratio in the U.S. between 1932-1939 was 1.2-1 and has risen to 1/4 in those who replaced soda with milk. Increased phosphoric acid consumption from soft drinks may have a negative effect on bone health[1592]. Diets with a low Ca/P ratio (≤0.5) have an increase in parathyroid hormone and urinary calcium excretion[1593,1594]. In Germany from 2006-2014, the average phosphorus consumption of 1,338 mg/d did not change but during that time calcium intake decreased from 1,150 to 895 mg/d (a ratio of < 1)[1595].

High dietary calcium and phosphate intake inhibit the absorption of magnesium[1596,1597]. People eating refined low magnesium diets also tend to get a lot of phosphorus from those same foods[1598]. **Since the early 1900s, the P/Mg ratio has increased from 1.2:1 to 7:1**[1599]. Dairy, especially cheese has a high phosphorus to magnesium ratio. For example, cheddar cheese has a P/Mg ratio of 18 and Ca/Mg ratio of 26[1600]. Pumpkin seeds, on the other hand, have a P/Mg ratio of 0.35 and a Ca/Mg ratio of 0.21[1601].

A diet providing 1,517 mg of calcium a day and 685 mg/d of phosphorus provides a fairly even phosphorus balance (+72 mg/d)[1602]. Supplementing that diet with glycerophosphate (1,549 mg of added total phosphorus/d) results in a positive phosphorus balance of +228 mg/d. Large loads of inorganic phosphorus (7-9 grams/d) cause a positive phosphorus balance of 2 grams/d[1603].

Optimal Phosphorus:Magnesium Ratio

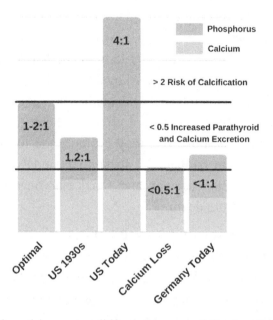

Phosphorus is found in many different types of foods, such as dairy, meats, fish, eggs, legumes, vegetables, grains and seeds[1604]. In the U.S., dairy contributes 20% of total phosphorus intake, bread products 10%, vegetables 5% and chicken 5%[1605]. The remaining 60% comes from a variety of foods, including eggs, meat, cereals, beef, beans and seafood. Infants fed cow-milk formulas have a 3x higher phosphorus intake and higher serum phosphate levels compared to those fed human milk[1606]. These levels seem to normalize after 6 weeks but less than 1 month old infants may be at a risk of hypocalcemia when fed exclusively high phosphorus formulas[1607,1608].

Phosphate additives like phosphoric acid, sodium phosphate and sodium polyphosphate are added to processed foods for preservation and they have been shown to reduce bone mineral density in humans[1609]. These additives can provide 300-1,000 mg to the total daily phosphorus intake with an average of 67 mg of phosphorus per serving[1610,1611,1612]. That is about 10-50% of the phosphorus intake in Western countries[1613,1614].

194

Here are the highest food sources of phosphorus[1615,1616]

Food	Mg of Phosphorus per Serving	% of RDA
Sardines, with bone, 3 oz	420 mg	34%
Liver, beef, 3 oz	392 mg	31%
Salmon, canned with bone, 3 oz	280 mg	24%
Yogurt, low fat, 6 oz	245 mg	20%
Mussels, 3 oz	242 mg	20%
Salmon, cooked, 3 oz	235 mg	19%
Milk, 2%, 1 cup	226 mg	18%
Ricotta, ½ cups	225 mg	18%
Beef, bottom round, 3 oz	217 mg	17%
Salmon, cold cut, 3 oz	214 mg	17%
American Cheese, 1 oz	211 mg	17%
Catfish, 3 oz	208 mg	16%
Tuna, fresh, cooked, 3 oz	208 mg	16%
Soybeans, ½ cups	206 mg	16%
Haddock, 3 oz	205 mg	16%
Scallops, 3 oz	201 mg	16%
Pork Loin, 3 oz	200 mg	16%
Veal, 3 oz	200 mg	16%
Cod, 3 oz	200 mg	16%
Mozzarella Cheese, 1.5 oz	197 mg	16%
Scallops, 3 oz	186 mg	15%
Turkey, white, 3 oz	184 mg	15%

Chicken Breast, 3 oz	182 mg	15%
Chicken, white, 3 oz	180 mg	15%
Greek Yogurt, ½ cups	178 mg	15%
Lentils, cooked, ½ cup	178 mg	14%
Northern Beans, ½ cups	178 mg	14%
Navy Beans, ½ cups	176 mg	14%
Crab, 3 oz	175 mg	14%
Duck, domestic, 3 oz	173 mg	14%
Beef Patty, 90%, 3 oz	172 mg	14%
Oysters, 3 oz	172 mg	14%
Swiss Cheese, 1 oz	172 mg	14%
Turkey, dark, 3 oz	171 mg	14%
Cottage Cheese, 2%, 1 oz	170 mg	14%
Black Eyed Beans, 1 cup	168 mg	13%
Ground Beef, 80%, 3 oz	165 mg	13%
Lamb Leg, 3 oz	162 mg	13%
Chicken, dark, 3 oz	157 mg	12%
Lobster, 3 oz	157 mg	12%
Cashews, 18 nuts	151 mg	12%
Cottage Cheese, 1%, 1 oz	151 mg	12%
Mozzarella, 1 oz	149 mg	12%
Roast Beef, 3 oz	145 mg	12%
Cheddar Cheese, 1 oz	145 mg	12%
Clams, 3 oz	144 mg	12%
Cashews, 1 oz	139 mg	11%
Tuna, in light water, 3 oz	139 mg	11%

Eggnog, ½ cups	139 mg	11%
Pistachios, 1 oz	137 mg	11%
Almonds, 24 nuts	134 mg	11%
Baked Beans, ½ cups	132 mg	11%
Chocolate, low fat, ½ cups	128 mg	11%
Skim Milk, ½ cups	124 mg	10%
Potatoes, baked, 1 medium	123 mg	10%
Black Beans, ½ cups	120 mg	9%
Shrimp, 3 oz	116 mg	9%
Milk, 1%, ½ cups	116 mg	9%
Kidney Beans, canned, ½ cup	115 mg	9%
Whole Milk, ½ cups	113 mg	9%
Pinto Beans, ½ cups	111 mg	9%
Blue Cheese, 1 oz	110 mg	9%
Buttermilk, ½ cups	109 mg	9%
Chickpeas, ½ cups	108 mg	8%
Brown Rice, cooked, ½ cup	102 mg	8%
Peanuts, 28 nuts	101 mg	8%
Lima Beans, ½ cups	100 mg	8%
Walnuts, 14 halves	98 mg	8%
Green Peas, boiled, ½ cup	94 mg	8%
Feta Cheese, 1 oz	94 mg	8%
Oatmeal, cooked, ½ cup	90 mg	7%
Egg, boiled, 1 large	86 mg	7%
Corn Tortilla, 1 medium	82 mg	7%

Parmesan Cheese, 2 tbsp	80 mg	7%
Pecans, 20 halves	79 mg	7%
Raisins, ½ cups	71 mg	7%
Ice Cream, vanilla, ½ cups	69 mg	6%
Whole Wheat Bread, 1 slice	60 mg	5%
Soy Milk, ½ cups	60 mg	5%
Sesame Seeds, 1 tbsp	57 mg	5%
Macadamia Nuts, 10-12 nuts	56 mg	5%
Whole Wheat Bread, 4" pita	50 mg	4%
Asparagus, boiled, ½ cup	49 mg	4%
Brazil Nuts, 1 nut	36 mg	3%
Dried Prunes, 5 prunes	33 mg	3%
Kiwifruit, 1 medium	30 mg	3%
Dried Figs, 2 figs	26 mg	2%
Banana, 1 medium	24 mg	2%
Mango, 1 medium	23 mg	2%
Tomatoes, chopped, ½ cup	22 mg	2%
Apple, 1 medium	20 mg	2%
Cauliflower, boiled, ½ cup	20 mg	2%
Carbonated Cola, 1 cup	18 mg	1%
Orange, 1 medium	18 mg	1%
Pear, 1 medium	18 mg	1%
Rice Milk, ½ cups	17 mg	1%
Clementine, 1 medium	16 mg	1%
Strawberries, ½ cups	16 mg	1%

Cream Cheese, 1 tbsp	15 mg	1%
Red Cherries, 10 cherries	13 mg	1%
Peach, 1 medium	12 mg	1%
Sour Cream, 1 tbsp	10 mg	1%
Apple, 1 medium	10 mg	1%
Raspberries, ½ cups	8 mg	0.5%
Apricot, 1 medium	7 mg	0.5%
Cranberries, ½ cups	7 mg	0.5%

Absorption of phosphorus from whole foods is anywhere from 40-70% with animal foods being more bioavailable than plants[1617]. The absorption rate of phosphate additives added to foods ais anywhere from 70-100%[1618,1619]. Unenriched meat and cottage cheese are better choices than hard cheeses or sausages that tend to have added phosphate additives[1620]. In seeds and grains, phosphorus is stored as phytic acid. Because humans lack the phytase enzyme, phytic acid is not absorbed and it actually inhibits the absorption of other nutrients. In rodents, calcium absorption is greater on a low-phytate diet and phytate availability is higher on the low calcium intake[1621]. Calcium from foods and supplements may bind to phosphorus and reduce its absorption. A high intake of calcium (2,500 mg/d) can bind 0.61–1.05 grams of phosphorus[1622]. Replacing high phosphorus foods like animal protein and phosphate additives with more calcium foods can reduce serum phosphate levels[1623].

Phosphorus homeostasis is regulated by the kidneys, bones and intestines. In kidney failure, the body cannot excrete phosphate efficiently and its levels rise[1624]. Phosphorus resorption by the kidneys also increases[1625]. Patients with moderate kidney dysfunction have higher serum phosphate levels (4.12 ml/dL) compared to those with normal kidney function (3.74 mg/dL)[1626]. Higher phosphorus retention promotes chronic kidney disease (CKD) and bone disorders[1627]. High as well as low bone turnover are common in CKD[1628].

CKD patients with high phosphate levels have a higher risk of death[1629,1630,1631]. A meta-analysis of 9 studies in 199,289 end-stage renal disease found that dialysis patients with the highest phosphate levels (>5.2–7.5 mg/dL) had a 39% greater risk of all-cause mortality during a 12-100-month follow-up compared to those with normal phosphate levels (3.0–5.5 mg/dL)[1632]. However, high phosphate does not seem to have the same mortality associations in mild CKD[1633]. Patients with mild CKD don't show higher rates of death despite high phosphate levels[1634]. This is likely because their CKD is not as severe. Patients with stage 3-5 CKD are recommended to limit their phosphorus intake[1635]. Reducing phosphorus containing foods, which are often high in protein, in CKD patients may not outweigh the benefit of controlling phosphorus levels and may lead to higher mortality because of protein restriction[1636]. Instead, getting higher calcium proteins foods like cottage cheese or whey protein might be a better approach.

Antacids can bind to phosphorus and over the long-term lead to hypophosphatemia[1637]. If the antacids contain calcium carbonate, they can also decrease the intestinal absorption of phosphorus[1638]. Laxatives that contain sodium phosphate can increase serum phosphate levels[1639]. When taken at high doses, laxatives that contain sodium phosphate may even lead to death, especially in those with kidney failure, heart disease or dehydration[1640].

Conclusion on Magnesium, Calcium and Phosphorus

Here is an overview of the mineral guidelines for this chapter:

- The optimal daily magnesium intake from food is around 400-600 mg/d. Pumpkin seeds, nuts, spinach, beans, seafood, fish and leafy greens are the most abundant sources of magnesium.

- Magnesium supplementation may be advisable, especially for people who suffer from kidney stones, diabetes, CVD or some other co-morbidity.

- Drinking mineral waters is the most bioavailable form of getting natural magnesium.

- The optimal daily intake of calcium is 1,000-1,200 mg/d from whole foods, preferably dairy and green vegetables.

- An optimal Ca/Mg ratio is ~ 2:1 and don't consume excessive amounts of phosphorus, especially phosphate additives.

- Taking calcium supplementation is not recommended unless you are eating a calcium deficient diet or are at a higher risk of osteoporosis. When taking calcium supplements, don't exceed 1,000 mg/d and 500 mg/d may be more optimal.

- The optimal phosphorus intake is ~ 700-1,250 mg/d. Don't exceed 1,400 mg/d chronically. You can find plenty of phosphorus from most foods, especially animal protein, which is why you more than likely do not and should not supplement with phosphorus.

- To maintain the optimal Ca/P ratio of 1-2:1, consume mineral waters high in calcium, green vegetables and/or some pastured milk or cheese. At the same time, make sure you are getting optimal intakes of magnesium. If you are consuming soda or processed foods with phosphate additives, replace them natural mineral waters.

In practice, you can find the optimal balance between these minerals by eating plenty of vegetables, some meat and dairy. Limit your consumption of soda and other phosphate additive-laden foods. Sardines and fish with the bones are an excellent source of all 3 of these nutrients.

Chapter 7
The History and Importance of Copper in the Diet

Our bodies are always generating and consuming energy, even during sleep. Without energy, life would not exist. As we found out in chapter two, minerals are essential for ATP production and activation, especially magnesium. One of the minerals known for its thermal and electrical conductivity is copper (Cu). It is one of the few metals found in nature in a directly usable metallic form.

Copper is a component of numerous enzymes in the body including cytochrome c oxidase in the electron transport chain. Copper helps with electron transport, energy production and oxygen transportation [1641]. It is also a very versatile catalyst for oxidation/reduction (redox) reactions [1642]. These roles of copper emerged in animals and plants after the appearance of oxygen in the Earth's atmosphere[1643]. As the Earth went from being anaerobic to aerobic due to the formation of oxygen from photosynthetic blue-green algae, the increase in atmospheric oxygen forced organisms to figure out a way to handle the highly reactive oxygen species such as hydroxyl radicals, peroxynitrite, superoxide anions and hydrogen peroxide. Thus, enzymes evolved like superoxide dismutase, which require copper, zinc and manganese in humans. In plants, copper is also needed for growth[1644].

As a trace mineral, copper is considered essential and needed for proper physical development. All organisms, including bacteria, have copper in their bodies[1645,1646,1647]. It represents the third most abundant trace mineral in humans[1648]. The human body contains roughly 1.4-2.1 mg of copper per kilogram of bodyweight[1649]. Thus, an average adult who weighs 70-90 kg has only about 1/8th to 1/10th of a single gram of copper. Although that may seem like a minuscule amount, it is still essential for carrying out many physiological processes. Low copper intake jeopardizes the immune response, which is not restored even after several weeks of high copper intake [1650]. A large part of the population is not meeting the RDA of 0.9 mg/day,[1651] not to mention the optimal intake for copper, which sits at around 2.6 mg/day[1652].

In this chapter, we will go through the history and origins of copper as a mineral and as a cofactor for numerous enzymatic reactions. There will be more information about the role of copper and how to ensure adequate intake of it.

The History and Ancient Utility of Copper

Copper was one of the first metals to be adopted by humans at around 8000 BC. It was also the first metal to be smelted and molded into shapes between 4000-5000 BC. At 3500 BC, copper was the first metal to be alloyed with another metal – tin – to create bronze. [1653] The name 'copper' originates from Roman times when it was mined primarily in Cyprus and called *aes Cyprium* (metal of Cyprus). Later it evolved into *cuprum* in Latin and *coper* in Old English[1654].

This reddish-brown metal is a common building material used to conduct heat and electricity. Because of that, copper vessels have been used for cooking food, which can be beneficial or harmful, depending on the dose[1655]. Excess copper can promote reactive oxygen species formation, [1656] whereas deficient copper promotes anemia [1657], neutropenia and ischemic heart disease[1658]. However, even 10 mg per day of copper has been found to be safe for most individuals. Copper excess is typically due to a loss in the control of copper utilization in the body and not due to an excessive intake. This is because copper is now a missing mineral in the diet. There are certain scenarios where some waters have high levels of copper, which may contribute to copper overload, but that does not appear to be an issue for most people anymore.

The medicinal uses of copper date back thousands of years to 2200-2600 BC Ancient Egypt[1659]. One of the ancient medical texts, The Smith Papyrus, notes that copper was used as a treatment for chest wound infections and to sterilize drinking water. Other records, such as Greek, Roman, Aztec, Hindu and Persian writings, and European medical literature, have revealed the many traditional healing properties and uses for copper, including antibacterial, anti-inflammatory, anti-arthritic, anti-cancer and anti-epileptic properties[1660]. Copper was even said to heal wounds and broken bones.

The Ebers Papyrus is the oldest book known to man (written circa 1550 BC). It documents medicinal practices that began hundreds of years before ancient Egypt. The Ebers Papyrus notes that copper compounds were used for treating headaches, epilepsy "trembling of limbs", burns, wounds, itching and boils[1661]. Various forms of copper, such as copper shavings, powders and copper salts and oxides were used for medicinal purposes. Green copper powders were combined with copper chips along with honey, cow-fat, and eye-salve (collyrium) to form a mesh to be applied over wounds to enhance healing. For the granulation of the eye, a remedy of collyrium, verdigris (the green pigment from metallic copper), onions, blue vitriol (copper sulfate) and powdered wood was mixed and applied to the eye. Indeed, copper was also used for treating bloodshot and bleary eyes, inflamed eyes, cataracts, and "fat in the eyes" (possibly indicating trachoma, i.e., a bacterial infection of the eye)[1662].

The ancient Egyptians were said to dip metallic copper into sea water and scrape off the green "rust", i.e., copper chloride, for use in the treatment of wounds[1663]. Malachite, also known as copper hydroxyl carbonate, is a bright green mineral composed of copper. This green copper ore was mined in the Sinai Peninsula, which links Africa with Asia, and in the eastern desert of Egypt. Along with chrysocolla, a greenish-blue mineral composed of copper silicate, **these copper metals were ground in a mortar and pestle to form "powders of green pigment", which were used for numerous medicinal purposes**.

The ancient Greek physician Pedanius Dioscorides, from the first century A.D., was said to have documented the oldest recorded method for preparing **verdigris, a green pigment, from metallic copper** by exposing the copper to rising vapors from concentrated vinegar forming the blue-green copper acetate[1664]. Powders from all three green powders, malachite, chrysocolla and copper acetate were demonstrated to have antibacterial properties by Majno, in 1975, when he saw that no bacteria grew in these powders with verdigris having the best antiseptic properties[1665]. Majno's experiment explains why **verdigris was the Ancient Greek antiseptic of choice**. In fact, the word verdigris means green-from-Greece[1666].

Copper was widely and easily accessible to the Ancient Greeks, as it was found in ample supply on the island of Cyprus. The Greek physician Hippocrates (460 to 380 B.C.) recommended copper for the treatment of leg ulcers in the Hippocratic Collection. Dolwett and Sorensen explained how this was used: "*After the wound had been cleaned, a dressing was applied to it consisting of verdigris, flower of copper (red copper oxide), lead oxide, roasted Egyptian alum, myrrh, frankincense, gall nuts, vine flowers, and lanolin, all dissolved in wine.*"[1667] The Greeks also sprinkled copper oxide and copper sulfate powders on wounds to prevent infection, and also applied a mixture of boiled honey and red copper oxide to wounds as a treatment[1668]. The antiseptic properties of copper are known to kill off bacteria and viruses like *E. coli*[1669], *Candida utilis*[1670], and poliovirus[1671], thus improving wound healing and reducing the risk of sepsis[1672].

By the time of the ancient Romans, copper was already well established as a medical treatment for numerous diseases. De Medicina, a series of books written by the ancient Roman physician Aulus Cornelius Celsus during the reign of Tiberius (14 to 37 AD), noted the many medicinal uses of copper and its derivatives[1673]. Powders of copper, along with pepper, myrrh, saffron and cooked antimony sulfide were pounded and combined, dried and then pounded again in raisin wine and then heated until dry. Honey and rose oil were also combined for similar treatments.

Galius Plinius Cecilius Secundus (23-79 A.D.), known as Pliny the Elder, a Roman scholar, noted in his Historia Naturalis: "*Copper ores and mines supply medicaments in a variety of ways...all kinds of ulcers are healed with the greatest rapidity.*"[1674] To remove intestinal worms, black copper oxide was given with honey. This mixture was also diluted and placed into nostrils as drops to clear the head and stop bleeding from the nostrils as well as hemorrhoid bleeds. This mixture was also given to purge the stomach, for eye pain, mouth ulcers, drawing out splinters of broken bones, arresting watery eyes, cleaning wounds and ulcers, decreasing swellings of the uvula, combined with linseed oil for relieving pain, and blown into ears via tubes to relieve ear issues. The astringent properties of copper were so strong, Pliny wrote: "*There has lately been discovered a plan of sprinkling in on the mouths of bears and lions in the Arena, and its astringent action is so powerful that they are unable to bite.*"[1675] Astringency indicates drying/shrinking/contracting effects on mucous membranes.

In a review paper covering these ancient writings, Sorenson and Dollwet concluded: "*Tracing the development of folk medicine and the many rediscoveries of the beneficial effects of copper compounds leads to the suggestion that serious consideration should be given to modern day medical uses of complexes of this essential metalloelement.*"[1676] "Metalloelement" referring to copper as a trace element and a metal.

The Aztecs also employed copper for medicinal uses. Explained in the Aztec manuscript Martinus de la Cruz, which was later translated into Latin, i.e., "*The Badianus Manuscript*", liquid from ground copper was to be held in the mouth within the teeth as a treatment for "*Faucium Calor*", i.e., heat of the throat[1677]. This suggests that copper was used to treat sore throats due to infections as the patient was also supposed to gargle the copper-containing liquid. In ancient India and Persia, copper was used to treat lung diseases [1678, 1679, 1680]. Paracelsus, a medieval Swiss-German physician prescribed copper to treat numerous conditions including parasites, especially nematodes. He was also the first recorded person to wear a copper bracelet and he did this to receive the goodwill of Mars, Saturn, Mercury, Venus, the Sun or the Moon, respectively[1681].

In the 1700s, Europeans noted that an ancient Chinese law existed for preventing the spread of bacterial infections. The law indicated that paper money was prohibited and instead **payments with copper coins were required**[1682]. Thus, the antiseptic properties of copper were well known even in ancient China. In the 1800s, Bergmann, who lived among a nomadic Mongolian tribe called the Kalmucken, reported that they treated and healed venereal ulcers with oral copper sulfate[1683]. And even during World War I, if the projectile from a copper-containing mantel was left in a wound longer, that wound would be better protected from infection.

The Modern Utilization of Copper

In 18th century France, copper was readily used for the treatment of nervous disorders. Hot baths lasting 8 to 12 hours long, that employed copper tubs, were noted to be particularly effective for those with "hardening of the nerves"[1684]. The surgeon to King Louis the XIV, Jacques Dalibour, used tinctures of copper, zinc and camphor to treat wounds, cuts and bruises. In France, this tincture was a first-line treatment for "impetigo" (a streptococcal skin infection) even until fairly recently.[1685] Thus, some of the most well-known uses of copper throughout the ancient and more modern world included treating bacterial and fungal infections and the promotion of wound healing.

The French physician Victor Burq was famous for employing metallotherapy (the external and internal applications of metals) to treat numerous conditions[1686]. Burq, using brass, which is a metal alloy made of copper and zinc, successfully treated those suffering from epileptic hysteria, anemia, neuralgia, hysteria, hypochondria and nervous paralysis of various sorts, such as hemiplegia, paraplegia, amaurosis, hysteria with amenorrhea, hysteria, beginning paralysis, complete hysteric paralysis with amenorrhea, neurosis of hysteric nature and hysterical shaking. Burq also orally administered copper oxide, one to three 2-gram tablets per day, to heal those with hysteric paralysis, anemia and persistent leucorrhea (yellowish/greenish vaginal discharge) along with the external application of two copper rings placed to each leg.[1687]

During the great European cholera epidemics, Burq noted the differences in morbidity and mortality among workers in the copper industry versus non-workers. There were no deaths due to cholera among the "*Bon Accord*" members (workers in the bronze industry) and only 16 deaths out of 30,000 copper workers of Paris during the epidemics of 1865 and 1866. In fact, several of the 16 deaths should not have been counted, as they were unemployed at the time. Thus, from the cholera epidemics in the mid-1800s in France, copper was documented to protect against cholera. Burq also noted that mortality was ten to forty-times higher in individuals working in non-copper manufacturing vocations[1688]. Apparently, copper played a role in improving the immunity of these workers. Later work by Kobert (1895)[1689], Schulz (1890)[1690] and von Linden (1935)[1691] confirmed Burq's observations regarding the benefits of copper in cholera.

In regions of India and Nepal, copper was used for treating a variety of disorders such as venereal diseases, fevers, diarrhea, skin diseases (such as ringworm, eczema and leprosy), colic, hemorrhoids, indigestion, spleen, liver and blood diseases and wound healing of ulcers and sores[1692,1693]. Copper was also noted to be a "destroyer of the whiteness of the skin" (vitiligo or perhaps due to anemia). The ancient Persians also used copper for treating boils, eye diseases and "yellow bile".[1694]

In Switzerland, a physician named Köchlin used copper to treat syphilis, rickets, tuberculosis, cholera, boils, skin eruptions, chorea, ulcers, epilepsy, hypochondria, hysteria, melancholy and other afflictions[1695]. Köchlin was said to be the first to publish an extensive review of metallocompounds in medicine noting that medieval physicians and the French physicians Gerbier and Gomet treated breast and uterine cancers with copper sulfate. Köchlin, reviewing Lieb's work, citing the healing of sexually transmitted disease-induced ulcers and that oral administration of copper dust from hammered copper metal, known as "*Hammerschlag*", promoted the healing of broken bones, muscle and bone wounds[1696]. Köchlin also noted that copper improved male fertility. In fact, there is even a link between copper deficiency and infertility in cows[1697].

Copper was first determined to be a constituent of blood in 1830. In 1848, the French chemist Auguste-Nicolas-Eugene Millon showed that copper was 'fixed' with iron in red blood cells, and based on these findings, was the first to suggest that chlorosis, or hypochromic anemia, was due to lack of copper[1698]. However, that same year (1848), Melsens of Belgium argued that Millon's conclusions about copper were wrong and that copper could not be found in any 21 tested samples of blood[1699]. Slightly over a decade later, in 1859, Béchamp, who reviewed the work of both Millon and Melsens, neither accepted nor refuted the idea that copper existed in blood[1700]. **Thus, it was not until the late 1800s that copper was even accepted to exist in human blood.** [1701]

Perhaps one of the first to note the low toxicity of copper was Rademacher. In the mid-1800s, he took 4 to 5 grains of copper oxide (~259-324 mg of copper oxide – a rather poorly absorbed form of copper) every morning for up to 8 months apparently without any harm[1702]. This amount would be around 100 times the average intake of copper nowadays, although we cannot extrapolate this poorly absorbable form of supplemental copper with dietary copper intake. Rademacher's confidence to dose himself with extremely large doses of copper came from his observations of copper hammerers of his time, who swallowed large amounts of copper and yet "were remarkably healthy."[1703] Rademacher treated his patients with muscular debility, delirium, weak memory, and acute fevers with dyspnea with black copper oxide and copper acetate. He claimed, "...*that copper not only could act as a curative drug but could render one's health more robust and increase both life span and virility.*"[1704] Rademacher also noted that copper cured neuralgias of the head, apoplexy, paralysis, angina (chest pain) and scarlatina (scarlet fever), pleurisy, dropsy, hematuria, acute and chronic rheumatism and asthma. Rademacher also used copper to kill and expel intestinal worms and utilized copper for treating numerous skin diseases such as eczema, itching, herpes and removal of warts. He even used a salve of copper carbonate to treat boils of the skin and noted that bones healed quicker when patients were given copper salts. It was not discovered until the late 1980s that copper is extremely important in the formation of bone[1705]. Indeed, lysyl oxidase, a copper-dependent enzyme is involved in the final step of collagen maturation into newly formed bone[1706].

Luton, a French physician practicing in the late 1800s, used copper acetate salve to treat ulcers, lupus-associated with tuberculosis and abscesses[1707,1708,1709]. He also prescribed 10 mg of copper acetate pills for numerous conditions and even rubbed copper acetate salve into the joins to treat arthritic conditions. It can be said that Luton was the first to use copper successfully in a clinical setting to treat lung tuberculosis as many of his patients were completely healed[1710]. The benefits of copper were later confirmed by Von Linden in 1920 in guinea pigs infected with tuberculosis [1711]. Sorgo-Alland (1913) [1712], Ritter (1937)[1713], Tüchler and Ranzenhofer (1940)[1714], and Goralewski (1940) [1715] performed clinical trials supporting coppers benefit in tuberculosis. **It is now established that copper is important for immune function.**[1716]

Dollwet and Sorenson concluded that ancient, medieval and nineteenth century physicians used copper for treating conditions such as "trembling limbs" and others, which have been more clearly defined as epileptic conditions by later physicians[1717]. Research nowadays reports that different copper chelates have anti-convulsant activity in animal models of epilepsy (Sorenson et al. 1979, 1980, 1983)[1718,1719,1720,1721].

Some of the earliest modern era studies were done by Strauss, who in 1912 Barmen, Germany treated facial epithelioma with a mix of copper chloride and lecithin[1722]. The effectiveness of his treatment was supported by before and after photographs of three women's faces. In 1913, Gelarie at the University of Liverpool, studied the effect of subcutaneous and intravenous copper salt and colloidal copper on Ehrlich carcinoma transplanted into mice[1723]. **The tumors began to soften and degenerate in response to copper therapy**. In 1918, Moullin reported a favorable effect of colloidal copper on women suffering from breast and liver cancer[1724]. In 1923, Sugiura and Benedict demonstrated the delaying of growth in Flexner-Jobling rat carcinoma with copper sulfate[1725]. In 1930, de Nabias told the French Cancer Association that **intramuscular injections of a copper preparation helped to expel tumor tissue**[1726]. He also noticed that during the repair, necrotic cells were replaced by healthy ones. In 1959, Voisin saw adequate results in mice with adenocarcinoma with intravenous injections of colloidal copper [1727]. The growth of adenocarcinoma was inhibited in all but two cases with daily injections.

Kobert, in 1895, published a review paper covering the benefits of copper compounds for treating acute and chronic diarrhea, dysentery, cholera, adenitis, eczema, impetigo, tuberculosis, lupus, syphilis, anemias, chorea (a neurological disorder hallmarked by jerky involuntary movements) and facial neuralgia [1728]. Heilmeyer and Stüwe, in 1938, were the first to suggest that **copper levels increase as a defense mechanism to combat diseases such as scarlet fever, diphtheria, tuberculosis, arthritis, malignant tumors, and lymphogranulomas** [1729]. Fenz, in 1941, noted that copper was effective for patients with polyarthritis, acute and chronic rheumatoid arthritis and ankylosing polyarthritis[1730]. Thus, these diseases may be caused or promoted by copper deficit.

After these early beneficial results, Forestier, a famous French rheumatologist, developed a copper compound known as Dicuprene, and published numerous papers spanning from 1944 to 1949 showing that when given as an intravenous or intramuscular injection copper compounds were effective for treating rheumatoid arthritis, chronic polyarticular synovitis, chronic polyarticular gout, ankylosing spondylitis and psoriasis arthropathica [1731, 1732, 1733, 1734]. Graber-Duvernay and Van Moorleghem, in 1950, obtained similar results using copper morrhuate in patients with chronic polyarthritis[1735].

In 1939, the German physician Werner Hangarter noted that Finnish copper miners were unaffected by arthritis while rheumatism was widespread across Finland at the time[1736]. Moreover, workers that were not in the copper industry had more rheumatic disease compared to those working in copper mines. Hangarter and Lübke would go on to show that copper chloride and sodium salicylate were effective for treating rheumatic fever, rheumatoid arthritis, neck and back problems and even sciatica[1737]. After Hangarter's retirement, the interest in copper as an antiarthritic, anti-inflammatory agent waned and stayed dormant. And **with the discovery of corticosteroids, which are now common day medications to treat inflammation, the interest in copper compounds for treating rheumatic and arthritic conditions died off.**[1738]

Copper Deficiency Anemia: The Copper/Iron Connection

Chlorosis (anemia thought to be caused by iron deficiency, causing a pale, faintly greenish complexion), also known as the 'green sickness', was first described by Hippocrates. Chlorosis was commonly diagnosed in European and American women in the mid-1500s up to the beginning of the 1900s. The absence of menstruation also gave it the name 'virgin's disease'.[1739] Iron deficiency anemia is one of the most widespread nutritional deficiencies today, affecting one quarter of the world's population [1740]. According to the World Health Organization, up to 47.4% of the world's 5- to 14- year-old children are anemic as well as 41.8% of pregnant women[1741]. Anemia is defined as a decrease in the oxygen carrying capacity of the blood[1742]. Anemia is suggested when levels are slightly below a normal hemoglobin level of around 13.8-17.2 g/dL in adult men and 12.1-15.1 g/dL in adult women[1743,1744].

Without enough iron you lack adequate amounts of red blood cells, which makes it harder to transport oxygen via hemoglobin. As a result, you can experience chronic fatigue, shortness of breath, weakness, pale skin, lightheadedness and other problems[1745,1746]. Both too much, as well as too little iron, can make people more susceptible to infections[1747]. Some amounts of iron are needed for fighting harmful bacteria, however, excess iron also promotes the growth of these pathogens[1748].

In 1580, iron was suggested as a treatment for chlorosis[1749], but later physicians noted only a 50% success rate with iron supplements[1750]. However, iron supplementation is not always necessary and sometimes can actually makes things worse. Individuals, especially children, who take supplements can overdose on iron[1751,1752]. In fact, you can get iron poisoning from doses as low as 10-20 mg/kg[1753]. **However, studies confirm that chlorosis can also be caused by a copper deficiency and administrating copper, instead of iron, could fix this condition of "iron-deficient anemia"**[1754]. A decrease in Cu,Zn-SOD has also been noted in those with "iron deficiency anemia"[1755].

In 1864, Pécholier and Saint-Pierre, who observed the robust health of young women working in copper factories, concluded that copper was helpful in preventing and overcoming chlorosis[1756]. The first direct experimental evidence for the theory was provided by the Italian physician Mendini, who in 1862 reported that supplementation of the diet with copper salts overcame chlorosis in young women[1757]. In 1877, Mendini's findings were confirmed by Levi and Barduzzi who used copper sulfate to treat several conditions, including chloroanemia[1758]. The subject's skin turned back to reddish and they regained normal menstruation, appetite and social behavior. Levi and Barduzzi hypothesized that **copper improves the ability of red blood cells to transport oxygen and nutrients, creating a 'hypernutritive state'.** Clinicians nowadays acknowledge that copper sulfate can increase the number of red blood cells. Copper can also protect against the oxidation of red blood cells, making them more resilient[1759].

In 1848, factory workers ingesting copper were described as having greenish hair and the walls on which they urinated also became green[1760]. These high-copper eating factory workers often lived to be octogenarians (living into their 80s). The green color of their hair and urine was caused by exposure to 'vert-de-gris' the green pigment produced from copper treated with vinegar, which was found to be safe in low amounts in rabbits and dogs but poisonous in very large amounts. In fact, women working in a vert-de-gris (copper) factory in Montpellier, France were said to exhibit a "healthy, fresh, corpulent appearance," whereas woman working at other factories in the area were noted to exhibit "lean, place faces."[1761]

Inhaling copper dust was noted to benefit anemia and chlorotic young women by Liégois (1891)[1762], Hare (1892)[1763] and Cervello and Barabini (1894)[1764]. Von Linden saw that soon after they began working in copper industries their anemic condition improved and their health was restored[1765]. Nowadays, it is well known that copper has an important role in liberating iron from liver stores, which is a process that precedes hemoglobin formation[1766]. Women working in copper factories were also reported to have regular menstruation and breast-fed their infants in the middle of the factory, even when their breasts where sometimes covered with copper salt[1767]. It was well known at the time that women suffering from chlorosis in the same city had their health restored in just a few months of working in a copper factory. There was no hesitation in advising chlorotic young ladies to start working as a vert-de-gris worker. Thus, **in the mid-1800s in France, it was common knowledge that chlorosis/anemia could be treated with exposure to copper.**

The essential role of copper in health was first discovered in 1928 when it was shown that rats fed a copper-deficient diet were unable to produce enough red blood cells[1768]. This was fixed by adding copper-containing foods back into their diet. The authors wrote: *"We think this is the first experiment in the literature giving to copper in association with iron the specific function of hemoglobin building in a mammal on an otherwise satisfactory diet."* [1769] Thus, **copper became the second discovered essential trace mineral for mammals after iron.**

Copper helps with iron uptake and a copper deficiency can cause symptoms of anemia [1770, 1771]. Edward Mills of Montreal treated hypochromic, microcytic 'idiopathic' anemia with copper and iron[1772]. Another 1928 study found that copper has an important role in the formation of hemoglobin and in the metabolism of animals with red blood[1773]. These two papers launched a spree of publications about copper and anemia with 29 articles being published by 1931 on the subject and more than 60 articles published in the following decade. Reviews released in the late 1920s until the 1940s confirmed the effectiveness of copper in several animals, such as chickens, pigs and dogs[1774,1775,1776]. **Although copper was not a major component of hemoglobin, it was considered a catalyst needed for hemoglobin synthesis**[1777]. Fixing a copper deficiency also improves erythropoietin unresponsiveness (erythropoietin is needed to make red blood cells) in anemic hemodialysis patients [1778]. In 1931, Cook and Spilles discovered that **copper stimulates the release of stored iron in tissues during the creation of red blood cells**[1779]. Thus, copper mobilizes iron, helping to shift iron storage into hemoglobin.

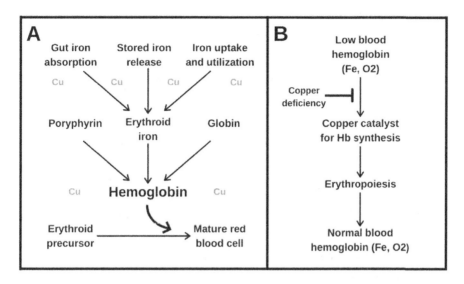

Erythropoietic pathways involving copper. (A) Iron-dependent and iron-independent pathways of hemoglobin formation and erythropoiesis. (B) Interdependence of iron and copper in erythropoiesis.

Adapted from: Fox (2003). '*The copper-iron chronicles: The story of an intimate relationship*'. Biometals, 16(1), 9–40. doi:10.1023/a:1020799512190

So how does copper play a role in iron deficiency anemia? Well, both iron and copper are absorbed in the upper small intestine and hepcidin controls the absorption of iron, by inhibiting iron export in the intestine. Hepcidin expression is decreased on a copper deficient diet, potentially leading to iron deficiency[1780,1781,1782]. In other words, **a low copper diet can lead to low iron absorption and iron deficiency anemia.** Giving more iron may help, however, the solution could also be giving more copper. In the case of "iron deficiency anemia" copper seems to be part of that solution. In fact, supplemental copper in copper-deficient rats increases iron absorption in the gut by about 25% [1783]. In anemic rats, copper doubles intestinal iron absorption[1784].

Hephaestin and its homologue ceruloplasmin, the latter being the major copper-carrying protein in blood, are required for efficient iron transformation into transferrin. Their synthesis and activity are positively correlated with copper levels in the cell. Thus, a copper deficiency can lead to a reduction in hepcidin, hephaestin and ceruloplasmin jeopardizing iron metabolism and restricting its movement out of the gut and liver to areas where it may be needed in the body.[1785] Additionally, copper is also needed for the synthesis of heme, which is a constituent of hemoglobin. Thus, in order to get iron where it needs to go in the body, it must be placed onto transferrin, which requires copper.

To sum it up, the absorption, export and transport of iron requires copper. All things regarding iron require adequate amounts of copper and **many issues that are thought to be caused by "iron deficiency" may actually be caused by copper deficiency.**

During the first half of the 20th century, it was claimed that copper was abundant in many foods and that copper was unlikely to help in anemia except in cases of severe copper deficiency. However, in 1931 it was discovered that using both copper and iron was superior in treating anemic infants than iron alone, especially in those with low hemoglobin[1786]. The same was reported by Milton Lewis in children with chronic nutritional anemia[1787]. In 1935, Elvehjem also showed that iron plus copper effectively raised hemoglobin in infants with severe nutritional anemia[1788], which was supported in 1938 by James Hutchinson's findings as well[1789]. It is suggested that patients with refractory anemia and leukopenia should have copper and ceruloplasmin levels measured as part of their diagnostic evaluation[1790].

In 1952, Wintrobe et al. showed that intravenous iron did not prevent anemia in copper-deficient pigs,[1791,1792] suggesting that certain cases of anemia may not be due to iron deficiency but to copper deficiency. They saw that intravenous **iron transport into hemoglobin was reduced by 75% in copper-deficient pigs**. Later it was found out that human ceruloplasmin increases the uptake of iron into red blood cells[1793]. Ceruloplasmin was discovered in 1948,[1794] and in 1960 it was found to be a ferroxidase enzyme, i.e., having the ability to convert $Fe2+$ (ferrous iron) to $Fe3+$ (ferric iron) through oxidation[1795]. One year later it was shown that this process was required for iron to bind to transferrin, which is the iron-binding protein that moves iron in the blood to different tissues[1796]. In 1966, Osaki and colleagues suggested to rename ceruloplasmin 'serum ferroxidase' because of its importance in iron metabolism[1797]. They showed how ceruloplasmin, which is the main copper-carrying protein in our blood, allowed iron to get into bone marrow by promoting iron transfer onto transferrin. Thus, numerous iron proteins need ceruloplasmin to work[1798,1799]. However, it wasn't even formally accepted until around 1984 that ceruloplasmin was an enzyme needed for iron to bind to transferrin[1800]. This is partly why so few doctors, or the lay public, knows about the benefits of copper in the body.

Only after Osaki's 1966 paper, was it confirmed that ceruloplasmin was important for moving iron from the gut to the blood and into bone marrow for the synthesis of hemoglobin and red blood cells. In other words, **for dietary iron to be used for synthesizing hemoglobin and red blood cells, it needs the copper carrying protein ceruloplasmin**. However, only around 10% of normal plasma ceruloplasmin levels are needed to enable a substantial iron flux, which might explain why most Wilson's disease patients have normal iron metabolism[1801]. Indeed, iron metabolism is not substantially affected until ceruloplasmin levels hit about 5% of normal levels[1802]. This was confirmed by Osaki and Johnson (1971) as well – ceruloplasmin works and promotes the release of iron from the liver at 10% of normal levels[1803]. Osaki and Johnson concluded in their 1971 paper: *"...ferroxidase (ceruloplasmin), due to its iron oxidase activity, generates a steep concentration gradient of Fe(II) between the iron storage cells and the capillary system, thus promoting efficient and maximum iron efflux."*[1804]

Ceruloplasmin and glycosylphosphatidylinositol (GPI)-ceruloplasmin are important in the release of iron from storage sites and from the central nervous system[1805]. Osaki and Johnson did an experiment on normal dogs' livers in 1969 and showed that the addition of ceruloplasmin increased the rate of iron release by up to 10-fold[1806]. **Thus, iron accumulation occurs in organs when ceruloplasmin is not functioning properly[1807].**

A copper deficiency can decrease iron levels and cause iron deficiency anemia in some tissues while resulting in iron overload in other tissues, such as the liver and intestine[1808]. **An absence or dysfunction of ceruloplasmin leads to the accumulation of iron in the brain, liver, intestine, pancreas and retina**[1809]. Tissue iron overload and very high serum ferritin levels have been seen in those with familial ceruloplasmin deficiency[1810]. Deficiencies in ceruloplasmin also cause iron to accumulate in the spleen, which leads to microcytic, hypochromic anemia, dementia, cerebellar ataxia and diabetes[1811,1812]. In 1999, Leah Harris and co-authors proved that ceruloplasmin is directly involved in stimulating iron release from tissue stores, by targeting ceruloplasmin via gene disruption[1813]. **Copper deficient diets lead to reduced ceruloplasmin activity and can cause iron overload in the liver**[1814]. Thus, iron release and storage are partially dependent on ceruloplasmin and copper status.

Patients with an acquired copper deficiency and lack of ceruloplasmin can get liver iron overload[1815], diabetes, neurological issues and retinal degeneration[1816]. **People with non-alcoholic fatty liver disease (NAFLD) have significantly lower copper levels in the liver**, which suggests that copper deficiency likely contributes to the iron accumulation in the liver of those with NAFLD[1817].

Iron overload is associated with many diseases like arthritis, cancer, tumor growth, diabetes, heart failure and liver damage[1818,1819]. Studies link excess heme iron with colon cancer[1820]. By reducing iron overload, copper may slow down the aging process[1821]. Furthermore, iron overload can induce copper deficiency[1822]. It's a vicious cycle.

The potential consequences of copper deficiency:

- **Iron deficiency anemia** - decreases absorption of iron by enterocytes, reduces iron release from storage sites, and reduces iron incorporation into transferrin reducing hemoglobin synthesis. Enterocytes are polarized epithelial cells lining the intestinal track that regulate the uptake of nutrients from the diet. Like all other cells, they have to balance copper metabolism to cover essential requirements without causing toxicity. Enterocytes actually need quite a lot of copper as a co-factor for hephaestin, which is essential for absorption of dietary iron[1823].

- **Iron overload -** in the liver (fatty liver disease), pancreas (diabetes), spleen (hypochromic anemia), brain (neurological disorders) and retina (retinopathy).

- **Lipofuscinogenesis** – lipofuscin is an age-related pigment that accumulates in the cells, promoting oxidative stress, cellular senescence and aging. Excess iron is one of the contributors for lipofuscin accumulation[1824].

Copper deficient diets can reduce cytochrome c oxidase activity and heme synthesis from iron and protoporphyrin[1825,1826]. This reduction in cytochrome c oxidase limits the reduction of $Fe3+$ iron to $Fe2+$ iron to form heme. Thus, **copper deficiency reduces iron utilization by the mitochondria**. Copper may also be involved in the cellular uptake of transferrin-bound iron, as copper deficient pigs have a red blood cell half-life of about half that of normal pigs (9 days vs 17 days)[1827]. Signs of iron deficiency, in copper-deficient rats, are not improved with iron supplementation[1828]. This further suggests that signs of iron deficiency in humans may actually be due to copper deficiency.

Sarata and Suzuki from the Tohuku Imperial University in Japan discovered that acute bleeding in rabbits causes a rapid rise in blood copper levels[1829]. They hypothesized that this increase in plasma copper is not only a by-product of the rapid plasma reformation, but it is an important factor in recovering from anemia as a stimulant for organs that produce blood cells. Similar findings were seen in dogs by

Sachs in 1938 who proposed that copper is brought into use from the body's reservoirs to stimulate blood cell formation[1830]. Elevated blood copper levels have also been found in iron-deficient children, which again suggests it's need by the body in anemias[1831,1832]. Those who are anemic, losing blood, or have a reduced ability to make red blood cells may need more dietary copper.

Why You Need Copper

Because of its role in energy production and tissue oxygenation, copper is vital for many other processes in the body. Here is an overview of the vital role of copper in many chronic diseases:

- **Cardiovascular Disease** – Copper deficiencies are seen animals and humans with a wide range of heart disease outcomes, such as aortic rupture, fissures, cardiac enlargement, abnormal lipid metabolism, and ischemic heart disease[1833]. It has been known for a few decades that disrupted copper metabolism plays a role in heart disease[1834]. Copper deficiency is one of the few nutrient shortages that elevates cholesterol, blood pressure, homocysteine, adversely affect the arteries, impairs glucose tolerance, and promotes thrombosis[1835]. People with hypertension tend to have lower copper than those with normal blood pressure[1836]. In men, copper deficiency can cause irregular heartbeat[1837].

  o Low copper and ceruloplasmin levels have been noted in a 13-year-old girl with coronary artery disease[1838]. According to a 1965 autopsy study, people who died from a heart attack, known as a myocardial infarction, had lower amounts of copper in their myocardium[1839]. Pigs fed a copper deficient diet have scarred blood vessels but exhibit atherosclerosis[1840]. The decrease of copper in the arteries appears to be linearly associated with an increase in atherosclerosis. **There are approximately 80 anatomical, chemical and physiological similarities between copper-deficient**

animals and humans and ischemic heart disease[1841,1842,1843].

o Atherosclerotic arteries have been shown to have lower copper and reduced cytochrome c oxidase activity than those without atherosclerosis [1844]. Cytochrome c oxidase is a copper-dependent enzyme. A shutdown of the copper-dependent cytochrome c oxidase is how cyanide leads to death, by inhibiting the production of ATP [1845]. Decreased cytochrome c oxidase in heart muscle has been noted after myocardial infarction[1846,1847]. There is an increase of copper levels in patients with myocardial infarction[1848,1849,1850,1851,1852], which may lead to copper depletion due an increase in copper need.

o A decline in the copper content of the aorta has been seen alongside increased atherosclerosis [1853]. Among Nigerians, in both older men and women, significant reductions of arterial copper are observed[1854]. Similar observations have been made in African Americans and Minnesota Caucasians, although their copper levels are higher[1855].

o Copper deficiency and low ceruloplasmin raises iron levels and can cause iron overload. High iron is a risk factor for heart disease and is associated with cardiovascular events[1856,1857]. **Elevated iron raises the demand for copper by inducing a mild copper deficiency**[1858]. Finland has abandoned the fortification of food with iron most likely because of the association of iron with heart disease.

o Copper is needed to strengthen collagen, and hence, **a lack of copper may reduce the health of the arteries and the heart**[1859]. Copper is needed as a cofactor for lysyl oxidase which cross-links collagen and elastin giving it tensile strength [1860]. High homocysteine increases homocysteine thiolactone, which inhibits lysyl oxidase [1861]. As a result, your arteries can get damaged and become more susceptible to atherosclerosis. **Aneurysms and blood vessels are more likely to rupture/tear with high blood pressure on a diet deficient in copper due to decreased collagen/elastin strength.** Low lysyl oxidase, a marker of reduced copper status, is associated with ischemic heart disease[1862]. Homocysteine alone is a risk factor for cardiovascular disease, stroke, and ischemic heart disease[1863,1864]. **Homocysteine can bind copper and induce copper deficiency**[1865,1866].

o Copper is important for neovascularization or angiogenesis (the process of growing new blood vessels). Thus, copper is also important in wound healing, whether that be ulcers, cuts, bruises or organ damage[1867]. The repair of collaterals, which are new blood vessels that supply the heart when larger arteries become blocked due to atherosclerosis, may not occur if the diet is low in copper. Copper ions also activate endothelial nitric oxide synthase (eNOS)[1868,1869], which explains its importance in vasodilation and better endothelial function.

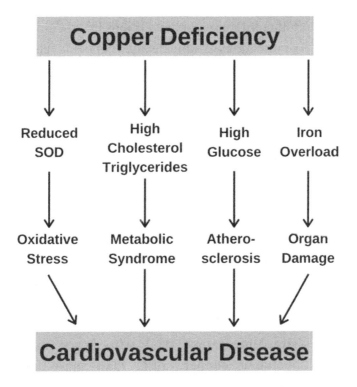

- **Inflammatory Conditions** – Many times elevated copper levels in the blood indicate inflammation[1870], which itself is a cardiovascular disease risk factor. That's why it is more accurate to look at enzyme activity or leukocyte copper levels than just blood copper levels.
  - Diabetics have a reduction in liver copper content[1871]. In fact, **diabetes itself can cause an imbalance of copper and a loss in copper utilization in the heart**[1872]. That can contribute to the pathogenesis of diabetic arteriopathy. Inflammation is also raised during hyperglycemia, hyperinsulinemia, glucose intolerance and diabetes [1873, 1874, 1875]. Patients with peripheral arterial disease show higher blood pressure, high triglycerides, lipids and elevated serum copper because inflammation raises copper[1876]. Thus, **diabetes can cause copper dysregulation and lead to cardiovascular disease development.**

- Other inflammatory conditions like rheumatoid arthritis or infections exhibit elevated copper levels[1877]. It is also known that **diets low in copper can cause osteoporosis**[1878,1879,1880]. **Copper deficiency reduces bone integrity,**[1881,1882] **leading to brittle bones and fractures**[1883] **by decreasing lysyl oxidase**[1884]. Low serum copper, iron and zinc are a risk factor for osteoporosis[1885]. Excessive intake of milk, high in calcium and low in copper, may exacerbate this problem instead of mitigating it[1886].

  - There is an epidemiologic association between osteoporosis, ischemic heart disease and a diet low in copper[1887,1888]. Osteoblast activity, osteoblasts are the cells that build our bone, is decreased in copper deficiency[1889] and human osteoporosis[1890,1891,1892]. **A supplementation trial with trace minerals that included copper, zinc, manganese and calcium improved bone density compared to either calcium only or trace minerals only**[1893]. Decreased copper has been found in people with bone spurs[1894], ischemic necrosis of the arteries[1895], fractures[1896] and decreased lumbar bone density[1897].

- **Oxidative Stress** – Copper inhibits oxidative stress and reactive oxygen species (ROS) via superoxide dismutase (SOD)[1898]. The superoxide anion causes lipid peroxidation in addition to other problems[1899], which can be neutralized primarily by copper-zinc superoxide dismutase (Cu,Zn SOD). Excessive oxidative stress is a key contributor to the pathogenesis of many diseases, primarily by raising inflammation[1900].

  - Endothelial dysfunction, which is when the lining of the arteries is damaged and there is decreased arterial relaxation, precedes cardiovascular disease and is caused by reduced nitric oxide availability[1901]. **A low copper intake can be a major contributor to reduced nitric oxide status.** This is because copper is a cofactor

224

for the function of superoxide dismutase, which inhibits the free radical superoxide anion, which sequesters nitric oxide to form the toxic peroxynitrite. Thus, **a copper deficiency can result in a "nitric oxide steal", transforming it into a damaging and inflammatory molecule.** Polyphenol-rich blackcurrant powder/juice may improve nitric-oxide mediated relaxation of coronary arteries via a copper- and iron-dependent antioxidant effect[1902].

o **Low dietary copper intake increases free radical production in healthy men, which may increase the risk of colon cancer**[1903]. Elevated reactive oxygen species cause death of endothelial cells, which also leads to cardiovascular disease. Reperfusion injury, which occurs after a blocked artery is re-opened, is also driven by ROS[1904]. Maintaining adequate copper intake helps to reduce the amount of ROS by regulating extracellular SOD[1905].

o **Copper seems to increase the activity of glutathione peroxidase, which is needed for handling hydrogen peroxide**[1906]. In fact, copper deficiency has been shown to decrease glutathione peroxidase[1907]. **Through an overall reduction in oxidative stress, ensuring adequate levels of copper can boost glutathione levels, which is the main antioxidant in the body that protects against oxidative stress.** Thus, copper acts as an antioxidant mineral[1908]. In fact, a lack of glutathione may reduce the ability of the body to store copper as a complex with metallothionein[1909]. Hence, a low copper status can increase oxidative stress, resulting in a reduction in glutathione, which leads to further loss of copper and dysfunctional copper utilization. In other words, a low intake of copper can lead to an increased loss of copper.

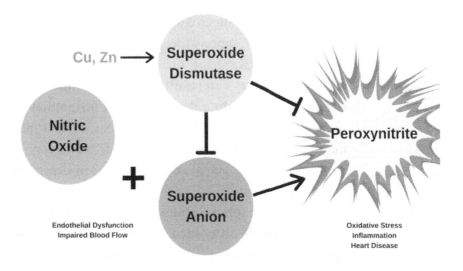

- **Mitochondrial Function** – Copper is a co-factor for respiratory complex IV in the mitochondria. A copper deficiency impairs immature red blood cell bioenergetics, which alters the metabolic pathways, turning off the mitochondria and switching over to more glycolysis (sugar burning) [1910]. As a result, there is a reduction in energy production and excessive lactate production from glycolysis. Lactic acidosis or the build-up of lactic acid is associated with several cancers and inflammatory diseases[1911]. During oxygen shortage, which can accompany copper deficiency anemia, lactic acid can begin to accumulate.
    - Copper also plays a role in burning fat[1912]. Now that a large proportion of the population is overweight, they may need more copper to help with fat loss. The estimated average requirement for copper is around 0.9 mg/day and around 31% of U.S. adults are not meeting the RDA for copper[1913, 1914]. Obese patients require more copper than the RDA (typically exceeding 1.23 mg/day) [1915]. Norepinephrine, the hormone that promotes fat burning and alertness, requires copper for its synthesis [1916]. The transcription factor in the hypothalamus called HIF-1 alpha, is also copper-dependent, and it has a role in preventing obesity[1917].

- **Metabolic Syndrome** – Copper deficiency has a detrimental role on your metabolic health and condition. Metabolic syndrome is a condition in which at least three or more of the five are present: high blood pressure, central obesity, high fasting triglycerides, high blood sugar and low serum HDL cholesterol[1918]. It is associated with cardiovascular disease and type 2 diabetes by causing inflammation [1919]. Metabolic syndrome doubles the risk of cardiovascular disease and increases all-cause mortality by 1.5-fold[1920].
  - In rats, **copper deficiency leads to impaired glucose tolerance** [1921], [1922], [1923]. Lower copper intake is associated with increased blood sugar levels in humans [1924] as well as rats [1925]. **Copper deficiency, induced by high fructose intakes, impairs insulin binding and reduces insulin sensitivity**[1926]. Diabetes can disrupt copper metabolism and copper deficiency can alter glucose metabolism[1927]. Accumulation of iron ions in the pancreas, due to copper deficiency and a lack of ferroxidase activity, is thought to cause diabetes[1928].
  - **Low copper intake also raises cholesterol and triglycerides**[1929,1930] and copper supplementation can lower their levels in the blood[1931,1932]. This association has been confirmed in multiple laboratories[1933]. In rats, there is an inverse relationship between serum copper and ceruloplasmin and levels of cholesterol and triglycerides [1934]. **Copper deficiency increases** the activity of hydroxymethylglutaryl-coenzyme A reductase (HMGA-CoA reductase), which is **the rate-controlling enzyme for cholesterol synthesis**, and hence increases cholesterol levels[1935]. In rats, a copper deficiency increases hepatic fatty acid biosynthesis two-fold[1936].
  - **Copper deficiency also impairs thyroid hormone production**[1937]. The thyroid is central to regulating metabolic rate and energy balance. There is a positive correlation between serum copper and thyroid

227

hormones in children with congenital hypothyroidism[1938]. The ratio of copper and selenium influences thyroid functioning in patients with hypothyroidism[1939]. In thyroid disease, the metabolism of zinc, copper, manganese and selenium is abnormal[1940]. In newborn rats, **copper deficiency reduces the active thyroid hormone T3 by 48% and T4 by 21%**[1941]. **Low copper status also reduces the conversion of T4 into T3**[1942]. Among the U.S. general population, a higher copper status is associated with elevated thyroid hormones[1943]. Serum copper is also regulated by thyroid hormones, which stimulates the synthesis and the export of ceruloplasmin[1944]. Less thyroid hormones (hypothyroidism) = decreased ceruloplasmin = copper deficit. Thus, thyroid hormones are important for copper absorption and improving copper status[1945]. In fact, thyroid hormones are known to be needed for kidney sodium reabsorption[1946]. Ironically, sodium is needed to bring iodine into the thyroid gland (as well as other tissues such as lactating breast, salivary glands, stomach and intestines) to make thyroid hormones[1947,1948]. Indeed, two sodium ions are needed to transport one iodide molecule into these tissues[1949]. Thus, thyroid hormone production and sodium status are interdependent on one another.

- **Kidney Health -** Ceruloplasmin protects the kidneys as it acts as an antioxidant. The development of kidney dysfunction may occur in part due to a lack of copper, with **kidney function improving upon copper supplementation**[1950]. One group of authors concluded, *"Copper deficiency can worsen nephrotic syndrome by decreasing the ceruloplasmin activity, which protects the glomeruli."*[1951] Additionally, **kidney damage can increase the loss of copper in the urine**. Patients with kidney damage tend to develop moderate copper deficiency[1952]. An easy indication of copper loss is spillage of albumin (protein) into the urine. This is because most copper in the blood is bound to the protein ceruloplasmin. **The urinary losses of copper can be 8-32 times higher than normal in those with kidney damage.**[1953,1954]

- **Reproductive Health** – Both copper transport as well as ceruloplasmin's ferroxidase activity are exhibited in the testicles, primarily helping in the processes of spermatogenesis[1955]. Thus, **copper is important for male reproductive systems.** Additionally, the copper-dependent cytochrome c oxidase has an integral role in energy metabolism in the testes, enabling the production of ATP needed for sperm motility[1956]. Essentially, if a man is deficient in copper, their sperm does not swim as well. On top of that, **a copper deficiency can also make the sperm more vulnerable to oxidative stress and DNA damage**[1957]. When couples are having difficulties getting pregnant, it might be due to inadequate copper status. Foods high in copper like liver, oysters and clams are also considered fertility-boosting foods.

- **Immune System** – Micronutrients, including copper and iron, are needed for modulating immune function and reducing the severity of infections[1958]. A copper deficiency has been shown to cause thymus (one of the main organs that produces immune cells) atrophy[1959], reducing the amount of circulating neutrophils and decreasing the ability of macrophages to kill pathogens. Repletion of copper appears to be able to reverse this[1960]. By causing iron deficiency, a copper deficiency can also reduce phagocytosis and lymphocyte proliferation. In fact, **infants with copper deficiency have been documented to have recovery in their immune health with copper supplementation**[1961]. Copper is also essential for the production of interleukin-2[1962], which is a cytokine that helps us fight infections.

Here are the enzymes and functions that are dependent on copper and the consequences of a copper deficit

Copper-Dependent Enzymes/Proteins	Function	Consequences of Deficit
Cytochrome c oxidase[1963]	Cellular respiration	Decreased energy production
Superoxide dismutase[1964]	Dismutation of superoxide anion radical	Increased oxidative stress
Catalase[1965]	Catalyze the conversion of hydrogen peroxide into water	Increased oxidative stress and lipid peroxidation in the heart
Glutathione	Scavenge free radicals	Increased oxidative stress
Glutathione peroxidase	Eliminates hydrogen peroxide	Increased oxidative stress
NADPH	Free radical protection and increase nitric oxide	Reduction in glutathione and increased oxidative stress
Tyrosinase[1966]	Converts tyrosine to dopamine	Depression
Dopamine-B-hydroxylase[1967]	Converts dopamine to norepinephrine	Depression, decreased "fight or flight response" potentially decreased ability to survive

		stressful events, obesity
Peptidylglycine alpha-amidating monooxygenase[1968,1969]	Neuropeptide synthesis and peptide hormone processing	Brain processing problems
Lysyl oxidase[1970,1971]	Conversion of procollagen to tropocollagen and of pro-elastin to elastin in the connective tissues	Decreased strength of blood vessels, cartilage, heart, bones, enamel, ligaments and damage to these tissues
Cartilage matrix glycoprotein[1972,1973,1974]	Formation of extracellular matrix and copper transport in cartilage cells	Decreased tendon strength, loss of cartilage tissue and osteoarthritis
Soluble pyridoxal-dependent monoamine oxidase[1975]	Oxidation of catecholamines to aldehydes	Reduced glucose uptake in fat cells[1976] and reduced leukocyte transmigration into endothelium decreasing pathogen killing
Ceramide galactosyl transferase[1977]	Myelinogenesis	Myelopathies and neurological disorders

Prostaglandin GG2 or GH2 reductase	Synthesis of prostaglandin F2-alpha	Inflammation, growth deficiency
Beta-oxidation	Governs fat burning	Metabolic syndrome, obesity & insulin resistance
Ceruloplasmin	Copper and iron transportation	Anemia, fatigue, iron overload
Hemoglobin	Tissue oxygenation and energy production	Anemia, fatigue, poor energy production
Hepcidin/Hephaestin	Intestinal iron absorption/oxidation of ferrous to ferric iron	Anemia

In humans, copper levels are high in the organs during childhood and start declining throughout later stages of life. During old age, hepatic and aortic copper decreases substantially, which is inversely associated with the concentration of calcium in the arteries.

The functions of copper are listed below

1.) Energy production (cytochrome c oxidase, composed of copper and iron)
2.) Detoxification of superoxide anions (superoxide dismutase converts superoxide to oxygen and hydrogen peroxide)
3.) Synthesis of collagen and elastin (copper makes up lysyl oxidase)
4.) Production of hemoglobin (ceruloplasmin catalyzes the oxidation of iron, which is necessary for iron to bind to its transport protein, transferrin)

5.) Melanin production (tyrosinase converts tyrosine to melanin and is a copper containing enzyme)[1978]

6.) Myelin production (the synthesis of phospholipids in myelin sheaths in peripheral nerves are dependent on copper)[1979]

7.) Fat burning and beta oxidation

8.) Inhibition of inflammation through antioxidants

9.) Synthesis of thyroid hormones (thyroxine)

In conclusion, copper has a central role in energy production and energetic processes. Copper deficiencies can cause many health problems, including anemia, chronic oxidative stress, cardiovascular disease and metabolic syndrome. Now that we've covered the extensive history and origins of copper in medical practice, we shall turn to covering how to obtain the right amounts of copper in balance with the other minerals for optimal health.

Chapter 8
Getting the Right Amount of Copper, Zinc and Iron

Iron deficiency is considered one of the most widespread nutrient deficiencies in the world, affecting nearly 1/4th of the population[1980,1981]. However, the problem might not be inadequate iron intake as we found out in the previous chapter. In fact, excess iron can have seriously negative health outcomes that increase the risk of cardiovascular disease and aging. Iron overload is more of an issue for men, whereas women tend to be iron deficient (at least up until menopause). There are also genetic conditions that can cause iron overload such as hemochromatosis.

In cases of anemia, low ferritin and malnutrition are often present, making it easy to assume that the issue is due to low iron. Fortunately, in the last decades, an increasing number of copper-responsive anemias have been documented[1982,1983,1984]. In fact, hypocupremia (low copper levels in the blood) has been associated with anemia since the 1940s[1985,1986,1987]. Patients with megaloblastic anemia and tropical sprue have also been reported to have hypocupremia[1988]. Copper-binding proteins regulate intestinal iron absorption with hephaestin and iron release from storage sites with the help of ceruloplasmin[1989,1990]. Copper deficiency impairs iron absorption, reduces heme synthesis and causes iron accumulation in the body[1991].

"Iron deficiency anemia" is not necessarily a disease of iron deficiency. In fact, it can be caused by copper deficiency. Unfortunately, most doctors and medical practitioners are not aware of this as they try to fix symptoms of anemia with supplemental iron. Making matters worse, high iron intakes can block copper absorption, increasing copper requirements and causing copper deficiency in the process[1992]. On the flip side, chelation or binding of iron, has been shown to reverse copper deficiency[1993].

The Western diet tends to be loaded with iron. There are many foods fortified with iron, such as milk, cereal and grains. In fact, dietary iron intake in the U.S. has never been higher. The average iron intake has gone from just 14 mg/day in the early 1930s to ~ 23 mg/day by the year 2000[1994]. There are many other factors that can cause an iron deficiency anemia, such as inflammation (as found in those with obesity or metabolic syndrome), bleeding, malnutrition, copper deficiency, infections, and lack of other nutrients but a lack of dietary iron tends to make all the headlines[1995]. On the flip side, insulin resistance can lead to liver iron overload[1996] and frequent blood donations can improve hyperinsulinemia.

Nutrition textbooks did not acknowledge copper deficiency in humans until around the 1960s[1997,1998]. The first mainstream report of copper deficiency in humans was reported in 1964 at the British-American Hospital in Lima, Peru[1999]. There, four infants who were fed exclusive milk diets (which completely lacked copper) had repeated bouts of diarrhea and/or vomiting. By 1969, data estimated that 8% of malnourished children were copper deficient upon hospital admission with another 63% becoming copper deficient in the hospital on a milk diet with nearly absent levels of ceruloplasmin in their blood[2000]. Nowadays, copper deficiency anemia is considered rare in children, but it is occasionally found in infants reared on a cow's milk only diet[2001]. Copper is in higher concentrations and is more bioavailable from breast milk vs. cow's milk[2002].

In this chapter, we are going to talk about getting the right amount of copper, zinc and iron. The reason being – they are all co-dependent of each other for anemia and cardiovascular disease risk management. All three of these minerals are essential, and an excess, as well as a deficiency, can be harmful to your health. That's why they need to be consumed in the appropriate dose and in balanced ratios.

The Copper-Iron-Deficiency Anemia Epidemic

What was your favorite childhood cereal? Fruit Loops? Frosted Flakes? Cocoa Pebbles? Cinnamon Toast Crunch? Or did you prefer regular granola? Whatever the answer might be, you definitely obtained a lot of iron from those grains. Food fortification or enrichment with vitamins and minerals has been practiced for decades with the goal of preventing large-scale nutrient deficiencies and associated diseases[2003]. The most commonly fortified foods are cereal, grain-based foods, milk, dairy products, infant formulas and some oils. The most common vitamins and minerals that are fortified into the food supply are vitamins A, B vitamins (especially folic acid), D and iron[2004]. Many breakfast cereals or muesli bars are loaded with 100% of the RDA for iron. Thus, it is almost impossible to become iron deficient unless you experience prolonged calorie restriction, bleeding or some other malnourishment.

Increasing iron intake does not seem to eliminate iron deficiency anemia. It might work in some people who are severely deficient in iron, such as during pregnancy or infections, but most of the population is already getting plenty of iron. Many iron toxicologists have expressed their concern about the excessive amount of iron in our food supply, recommending for us to reduce iron intake, except under specific circumstances that demand more iron[2005]. Unfortunately, these warnings are ignored by the grain lobbyists who push further increases in iron enrichment[2006]. See the problem? The idea that we need more iron comes from the food industry. It wasn't really about solving a medical problem or figuring out why it was happening. **In fact, the entire concept that iron deficiency anemia is solely due to a low intake of iron is one of the biggest medical myths ever!** And it has prevented the medical community from discovering the other important cause of "iron deficiency" anemia, that being copper deficiency. The reason why food manufacturers like to only focus on fortifying iron in food is because the government encourages manufacturers to only add enrichments for the deficiencies that are blatant and obvious. By completely ignoring copper, food manufacturers don't seem to really care about solving the global anemia problem, so long as they can say their food is a "good source of iron" in marketing materials.

It has been known since at least the 1930s that certain iron deficiency anemias can be cured by increasing copper intake[2007]. Additionally, we may be inadvertently diagnosing people with iron and/or zinc deficiency because those levels can drop with an increase in inflammation and overdiagnosing copper overload because copper levels increase with inflammation (see the problem here). Indeed, one group of authors wrote: *"Copper metabolism is altered in inflammation, infection, and cancer. In contrast to iron levels, which decline in serum during infection and inflammation, copper and ceruloplasmin levels rise."* [2008] This is why so many doctors fear "copper overload" and don't take copper deficiency seriously, i.e., because they rarely see low copper levels on a blood draw.

The Western diet is often low in copper, especially when compared to other fortified nutrients like iron. In the last century, there was a long period where an established RDA for copper did not exist but there had been RDAs for less studied micronutrients like magnesium, selenium and zinc. The 10th edition of the Recommended Dietary Allowances (RDA) in 1998 did not include copper, only an adequate daily intake was suggested [2009]. Nowadays, the daily dietary requirements for copper in adults ranges from 0.9-1.3 mg/day[2010]. In the United States, there are many who argue that the 0.9 mg RDA is too low for adequate copper status and optimal intakes have been suggested to sit around 2.6 mg/day[2011]. The estimated safe and adequate copper intake in 1989 was set at 1.5-3.0 mg/day[2012], which exceeded the previous required estimates of 1.2-2.0 mg/day. Why then is the current RDA set so low at just 0.9 mg at minimum? Even the World Health Organization recommends at least 1.3 mg a day. The reason is likely because if we kept the RDA at 1.2-3.0 mg/day, virtually no one in the United States would be meeting that requirement, and that would then require another mineral fortification. The required intake of any nutrient is defined as something that will maintain normal functioning and prevent failure [2013] but it should also include optimal health and longevity.

The Food and Nutrition Board suggests that the safe and adequate daily intake of copper is between 1.5-3.0 mg/day. Balance studies suggest that a daily intake of 0.8 mg leads to net copper loss whereas net gains are seen with 2.4 mg/day[2014]. Copper isotope studies reveal that a copper intake of only 0.8 mg is enough to maintain minimal body copper homeostasis[2015]. Thus, a minimal intake of copper just to remain in balance lies somewhere between 0.8-2.4 mg/day[2016]. A review of studies on copper deprivation in adult humans revealed that a copper intake of 1.0-1.25 mg/day is needed for copper maintenance for periods of up to 6 months[2017]. So why is the RDA for copper only 0.9 mg/day in the United States? Furthermore, even consuming 2.6 mg/day or greater of copper for up to 42 days is not sufficient to recover from copper deprivation[2018]. Recoveries of superoxide dismutase activity have been documented when either 3 mg/day or 4.3-6.4 mg/day of copper were consumed for 30 days or longer[2019,2020,2021]. That's quite a significant intake needed if you're already deficient in copper, i.e., you might need more than 2.6 mg/day for a long period of time just to recover from deficiency. Thus, **based on the scientific evidence, adults need at least 1.0-1.25 mg/day of copper and probably over 2.6 mg/day if you're already deficient.**

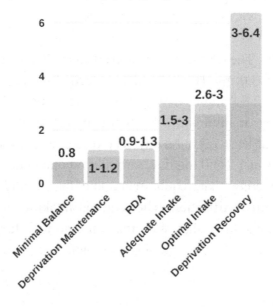

Optimal Intake of Copper (mg/d)

Nutrition surveys find that a significant proportion of the population get less copper than is recommended[2022]. Copper intake in the Western diet has been decreasing since the 1930s and some estimates suggest that half of the adult population obtains less than the RDA[2023]. In the U.S. and Canada, it may be less than $1/4^{th}$ of adults meeting the RDA. Not meeting the RDA for copper can be hazardous to health by increasing the risk of cardiovascular events and metabolic syndrome. It has also been shown to cause unexplained anemia in adults[2024]. **Men and women fed diets low in copper, around 1 mg/day, develop increases in blood pressure, cholesterol, glucose intolerance, and abnormal electrocardiograms**[2025]. This is an intake that many Americans don't even meet[2026].

Data from 10 dietary surveys shows that only 14% of typical diets in Belgium, Canada, the UK and the U.S. exceed 2 mg of copper a day[2027]. Only 3.2% of diets exceed 3 mg/day, 61% get less than 1.5 mg/day, and **$1/3^{rd}$ obtain less than 1 mg/day**[2028]. Surveyed hospital diets provide on average 0.76 mg of copper per day[2029], which means they do not even provide the RDA. The dietary intake of copper in Tehran is only 0.3 mg/day, three times less than the RDA[2030]. Preschool children in the Republic of Sprska (North-West Bosnia), get on average 0.19 mg of copper, 2.86 mg of iron, 1.71 mg of zinc, 0.21 mg of manganese, and 83.5 mg of calcium per meal[2031]. On a diet of 3 meals a day, that provides just 0.57 mg/day of copper. Diets low in copper, i.e., 0.64-1.02 mg/day, have been found to cause hypercholesterolemia[2032, 2033], abnormal electrocardiograms[2034], decreased glucose tolerance[2035] and elevations in blood pressure[2036].

Copper Intakes in Western Populations

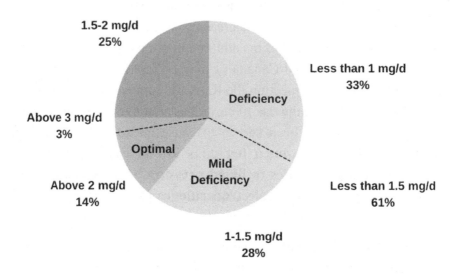

Adapted From: Klevay (1993) 'Copper in the western diet (Belgium, Canada, UK and USA)'. In Anke M, Meissner D, Mills CF (eds): "Proc. 8th Int. Symposium on Trace Elements in Man and Animals." Gersdorf, Germany: Verlag Media Tourishk, pp 207–210.

There is around 50-120 mg of copper in the human body[2037,2038]. Copper is mainly stored in the liver, but it is also found in the heart, brain, kidneys and muscle. About 1/3rd of total body copper is in the liver. However, copper is present in almost every tissue of the body. The daily copper turnover is estimated to be around 1 mg through fecal loss. Thus, total body copper stores can be depleted in a few months if daily intake is not near this level of intake. More importantly, this does not take into account copper losses in sweat, which can be quite significant.

Overweight people appear to require more copper than normal weight ones, generally needing more than 1.23 mg/day[2039]. In obese children, copper levels in the blood are lower, but slightly higher in the plasma, than in controls[2040]. They also have lower iron levels[2041], which may be due to inflammation caused by excess body fat. It is inflammation that raises copper and lowers iron in the blood. Obesogenic high-fat, high-carb diets in rats cause copper deficiency[2042].

More importantly, most human diets do not contain the 1.0-1.6 mg of copper that is lost from the body every day, which can eventually lead to copper deficiency. A healthy young adult will lose around 0.4-0.8 mg of copper per day through urine and stool plus around 0.33 mg of copper lost in sweat. Thus, healthy young adults need around 0.73 to 1.13 mg of copper just to remain in balance[2043]. This need would go up if exercising, living in hot climates, going into the sauna, etc. In fact, we can lose around 1.4-1.5 mg of copper per hour in sweat at $100°F$[2044]. Furthermore, certain medical conditions can also increase copper excretion. For example, patients with nephrotic syndrome have an 8-32-fold greater urinary loss of copper than normal patients[2045].

Fructose consumption also increases the need for copper and promotes copper deficiency, which increases oxidative stress, causes fatty liver and damages the intestine[2046,2047]. Added sugars, which contain fructose, have the same harmful effects[2048]. Compared to starch and sucrose, fructose depletes copper more significantly[2049]. In humans, copper status can suffer when the primary carbohydrate source in the diet is fructose[2050]. However, overconsumption of added sugars can still increase copper wasting by the kidneys. Patients with early diabetic neuropathy lose more ceruloplasmin in their urine[2051]. Damage to the glomerulus, which is a network of small blood vessels, located in the kidney, can also increase secretion of copper as seen in early IgA glomerulonephritis[2052]. Urinary ceruloplasmin could be a useful biomarker down the road to help diagnose kidney damage.

Things that are caused by copper deficiency and/or raise demand for or reduce copper levels:

- "Iron" deficiency anemia[2053]
- Sweating (exercise or sauna)
- Burn injuries[2054]
- Malabsorption diseases like celiac disease[2055], short bowel syndrome[2056] and IBS[2057]
- Pseudoscurvy[2058]
- Gastric bypass surgery[2059] and colon removal

- Nephrotic syndrome[2060], kidney damage and renal failure[2061]
- Neuropathy[2062], myelopathy[2063] and myelodysplastic syndrome[2064]
- Multiple sclerosis and hypomyelination[2065]
- Brain atrophy, damage or injury[2066]
- Muscle wasting or sarcopenia[2067]
- Cardiomyopathy[2068,2069]
- Progressive corneal thinning[2070]
- Liver damage, cirrhosis[2071] and fibrosis[2072]
- Non-alcoholic fatty liver disease and fatty liver[2073]
- Hemorrhages (subarachnoid hemorrhages, etc.)[2074]
- Aneurysms or blood vessel tears (aortic dissections, etc.)[2075]
- Pregnancy (for fetal neuropsychological and physical development)[2076,2077]
- High iron infant formulas
- Obesity and excess bodyweight
- High fructose consumption (e.g., added sugars)
- Processed food diet, iron fortified foods and refined grains
- Excess iron supplementation/consumption
- Excess zinc supplementation/consumption[2078,2079]
- Zinc denture adhesives[2080]
- Tooth wear[2081]
- Proton pump inhibitors, diuretics and antacids[2082]
- Hypothyroidism
- Osteopenia/osteoporosis and tendon injuries

Copper toxicity or overt deficiency is quite rare in humans. Documented copper toxicity has been observed after consuming copper through contaminated tap water [2083] and overusing copper supplements, causing liver cirrhosis[2084]. The upper safe threshold is deemed to be 10 mg/day for adults[2085]. Taking 10 mg/day of copper for 12 weeks has not been seen to cause liver damage[2086], but one case reports that a long-term intake of 60 mg/day resulted in acute liver failure[2087]. Intakes of 7-7.8 mg/day for 4-5 months in healthy male volunteers between the ages of 27-48 may cause some negative side effects, such as decreased antioxidant defense, suppressed immunity and increased excretion of copper[2088]. However, it seems that the body's own homeostatic regulation of copper absorption is being automatically regulated to minimize the amount of excess copper retention[2089]. In the same study of 7-7.8 mg/day for 4-5 months, apparent copper absorption was 29% on copper intakes of 1.6 mg/day and 16% at 7.8 mg/day. On 0.65 mg/day, true absorption was 40% and 29% at 2.2 mg/day. When copper intake was at 1.6 mg/day, copper retention was 0.06 mg/day but increased to 0.67 mg/day at intakes of 7.8 mg/day. So, as copper intake increases, its absorption levels slow down to prevent overload. High and low copper intakes exceed these regulatory mechanisms, causing either copper depletion or retention[2090]. A low copper consumption for 6 weeks does not appear to significantly change copper absorption compared to high copper consumption of 6 mg/day[2091]. In one study, supplementing copper at 6 mg/day for just 4 weeks did not have a significant effect on bone formation or bone absorption, although it's doubtful anything would in just a short period of time, however copper status in healthy young adult females was improved[2092].

Mammals and birds are 100-1000 times more resistant to copper than other species[2093]. They can accumulate copper in their liver under high exposure, but overt toxicity is rare. Thus, animal studies with extremely high copper intake will not necessarily translate over to humans. Multi-gastric mammals like sheep and cattle are known to experience copper toxicity but monogastric animals have a higher resistance[2094]. That might be because of the shorter transit time. Intoxication of copper by drinking water causes primarily gastrointestinal symptoms[2095].

Usually, copper deficiency occurs during malnutrition[2096], in patients receiving parental care with insufficient amounts of copper[2097], and when an individual ingests excess quantities of zinc on top of a low copper intake[2098,2099] (zinc is a copper absorption antagonist but zinc may not be an issue if the intake is 50 mg per day or less and copper intakes are at 1 mg or above). Copper deficiency has also been seen in infants fed only cow's milk[2100], lightweight preterm infants[2101] and the elderly[2102]. Pregnant and lactating women are also at risk of copper deficiency or people with malabsorption diseases[2103]. Bile eliminates most copper, whereas the kidneys typically only eliminate ionic or loosely bound copper.

Copper Deficiency Testing

The main symptoms of copper deficiency include anemia, secondary iron deficiency, neutropenia, and bone abnormalities. Additional signs include hypopigmentation, growth impairment, immune system suppression, abnormal electrocardiograms and dysregulated glucose and cholesterol metabolism[2104,2105]. Acute intake of copper between several milligrams to grams can cause headaches and gastrointestinal problems, such as vomiting or abdominal pain[2106]. Very large doses can lead to organ failure, shock, coma and death[2107].

Symptoms of copper deficiency include[2108]

- Anemia
- Defective keratinization of the oral cavity
- Neutropenia
- Hypopigmentation of hair and skin
- Abnormal bone formation/bone fragility
- Cartilage damage, joint pain and arthritis
- Reduced immunity
- Vascular/blood vessel issues
- Cardiac hypertrophy[2109]
- Heart murmurs and valvular regurgitation
- Fragile collagen/elastin (fragile organs/tissues) - tendon/tissue ruptures/tears
- Aneurysms of blood vessels (rupture of heart/blood vessels)
- Increased lipid accumulation in the heart
- Abnormal EKG - changes in ST segments, prolonged PR intervals and R wave duration and amplitude
- His Bundle electrical abnormalities

- Increased QT intervals, inversion of the T wave and increased QRS amplitudes and notching
- Decrease in ATP levels and energy
- Increased lactic acid[2110]
- Decreased ventricular contractility in the heart

How do you know if someone is copper deficient? A person with copper deficiency might have symptoms affecting several organ systems. Non-specific anemia may be one of the most obvious signs. It can appear either alone or with leukopenia and pancytopenia. Approximately 60-70% of symptomatic copper deficiency occurs with anemia and more than 50% are normocytic anemia[2111]. Excreting low amounts of copper can also indicate that copper intake is low.

Although serum copper levels can be measured directly, it is not a reliable marker because copper can be elevated with inflammation or infections[2112,2113,2114]. C-reactive protein has been associated with an elevation of copper[2115]. Usual plasma copper tests are insensitive and not entirely accurate[2116]. Low copper levels in the liver would likely be a better determinant but a more practical strategy would be to measure **leukocyte copper levels**, which **are more reflective of total body copper status and are depleted in those with significant atherosclerosis or coronary artery disease**[2117,2118]. Animals with fractures are three times more likely to have low levels of copper in their liver compared to the serum, with more than 50% of animals with fractures showing this copper deficiency pattern[2119,2120,2121]. Unfortunately, measuring copper levels in the liver requires a biopsy and hence it is not very practical.

Hair mineral analysis is a potential option to add to other measurements for an overall assessment of trace mineral status. In Chinese children, hair zinc, copper and iron are significantly lower during recurrent respiratory tract infections,[2122] which might be a contributing factor to the onset of the disease or the result of it[2123,2124,2125]. Scalp hair remains isolated from other metabolic activities and is a unique indicator of elements concentrated in an individual at a given time point[2126]. Hair analysis has been used for successful assessment of heavy metal toxicity.

Among Pakistani hypertensive patients, low levels of copper, iron, and zinc, measured with hair scalp hair, were similar to other controls with hypertension, but the levels of these minerals were high in the urine[2127]. Unlike urine or blood, the hair can give historical long-term data about trace elements and nutrients in the body [2128, 2129]. Measurements of heavy metals or minerals in the blood reflect only recent absorption and can vary daily. Thus, the hair can be a much more accurate evaluation of the actual element status than blood or urine[2130].

A high amount of copper (~95%) in the plasma is bound to ceruloplasmin, which can reflect total body copper status [2131]. Ceruloplasmin transports copper throughout the body and delivers it to deficient cells. Up to 60% of copper in red blood cells is contained in copper-zinc dependent superoxide dismutase and the other 40% is bound to proteins and amino acids. Thus, ceruloplasmin levels should be measured together with plasma copper. The validity of red blood cell copper concentration has not been established[2132]. However, in a population of 219 Brazilian babies aged 2-11-month-old, **5% of them were diagnosed with copper deficiency based on serum levels, however, 76% had copper deficiency when looking at their red blood cell copper levels**[2133]. Thus, red blood cell copper may also be a better indicator of copper status versus serum levels and may reveal an undiagnosed pandemic of copper deficiency. Further studies are still needed to validate red blood cell copper with total copper status.

Best to Worst Ways to Diagnose Copper Deficiency

1.) Liver copper levels

2.) Leukocyte copper levels

3.) Red blood cell copper levels

4.) Blood copper levels and ceruloplasmin

Copper and Iron in Food

The RDA for iron is 8 mg for adult men and 18 mg for adult women[2134]. During pregnancy, the RDA increases to 27 mg. Normal ranges for serum ferritin are 20-250 ng/ml for adult males and 10-120 ng/ml for women[2135]. A serum ferritin below 30 suggests iron deficiency[2136]. Numbers above the reference range may indicate oxidative stress or just iron overload. People, especially children, who take supplements may overdose on iron[2137,2138]. You can get iron poisoning from doses as low as 10-20 mg/kg[2139]. Hereditary hemachromatosis is a genetic disorder that makes you absorb too much iron from food. It's caused most often by a mutation in the gene called HFE[2140]. Patients who receive a lot of blood cell transfusions, like in myelodysplastic syndrome, thalassemia or sickle cell disease can develop iron overload. Drinking alcohol increases the absorption of iron. African iron overload is a condition that occurs in sub-Saharan populations who drink fermented beer with a high iron content[2141].

Foods highest in iron[2142]

Food	Mg of Iron per Serving	% of RDA
Breakfast Cereal (fortified with 100% of the iron RDA)	18 mg	100% for women, > 200% for men
Oysters, 3 oz	8 mg	44% for women, 100% for men
White Beans, canned, 1 cup	8 mg	44% for women, 100% for men
Dark Chocolate, 45-69%, 3 oz	7 mg	39% for women, 90% for men
Lentils, cooked, 1 cup	6 mg	34% for women, 80% for men
Spinach, cooked, 1 cup	6 mg	34% for women, 80% for men

Tofu, firm, 1 cup	6 mg	34% for women, 80% for men
Mussels, 3 oz	5.6 mg	30% for women 70% for men
Beef Liver, 3 oz	5 mg	28% for women, 65% for men
Kidney Beans, canned, 1 cup	4 mg	22% for women, 50% for men
Chickpeas, cooked, 1 cup	4 mg	22% for women, 50% for men
Sardines, canned, 3 oz	4 mg	22% for women, 50% for men
Beef, 3 oz	2 mg	11% for women, 25% for men
Potato, baked, medium size	2 mg	11% for women, 25% for men
Cashew Nuts, 1 oz (18 nuts)	2 mg	11% for women, 25% for men
Tomatoes, canned, ½ cup	2 mg	11% for women, 25% for men
Green Peas, cooked, 1 cup	2 mg	11% for women, 25% for men
White Rice, cooked, 1 cup	2 mg	11% for women, 25% for men
Sardines, 3 oz	1.4 mg	8% for women 18% for men
Chicken, with skin, 3 oz	1 mg	6% for women, 12% for men
Whole Wheat Bread, 1 slice	1 mg	6% for women, 12% for men

Whole Wheat Spaghetti, 1 cup	1 mg	6% for women, 12% for men
Tuna, canned, 3 oz	1 mg	6% for women, 12% for men
Turkey, roasted, 3 oz	1 mg	6% for women, 12% for men
Pistachio Nuts, 1 oz (49 nuts)	1 mg	6% for women, 12% for men
Broccoli, cooked, ½ cup	1 mg	6% for women, 12% for men
Egg, boiled, 1 large	1 mg	6% for women, 12% for men
Brown Rice, cooked, 1 cup	1 mg	6% for women, 12% for men

Our bodies have a hard time eliminating iron. Losses only occur, at least in a significant amount, during bleeding, blood donation, menstruation in women or through chelation. That is why females are more susceptible to anemia and iron deficiency, whereas men are more prone to iron overload. Common iron chelators include coffee, spirulina, chlorella, green tea, beans, whole grains and vegetables. That is why, although things like spinach and beans contain high amounts of iron, it is harder to reach iron overload eating them because a large proportion of the iron gets chelated and/or not absorbed. We now also cook with iron pots and pans instead of copper and this can increase our iron intake while raising the demand for copper. The situation is made worse by the fact that our overall diet is much higher in iron than it was in the past, especially due to foods fortified with iron and high intakes of muscle meat. Red meat is one of the most bioavailable sources of iron because it is in its heme form[2143]. Thus, it is easier to overload iron eating meat than veggies. Iron and zinc are copper antagonists. Foods are not fortified with copper, which contributes to this epidemic of copper deficiency. Unsaturated fats (omega-6 seed oils) are also lacking copper because transition metals are removed by chelation to increase shelf-life. At the same time, foods high in copper, such as liver, oysters, lobster and crab are eaten less frequently.

Here are the foods highest in copper[2144,2145,2146]

Food	Mg of Copper per Serving	% of RDA minimum (0.9 mg-s)
Beef Liver, 3 oz	12.4 mg	1378%
Mollusks, 3 oz	6.4 mg	600%
Oysters, 3 oz	4.8-6 mg	580%
Winged Beans, cooked, 1 cup	5.2 mg	530%
Lentils, cooked, 1 cup	2.5 mg	175%
Kidney Beans, 1 cup	2.0 mg	135%
Buckwheat, cooked, 1 cup	1.9 mg	130%
Seaweed, spirulina, 1 oz	1.7 mg	120%
Cocoa Powder, 1 oz	1.1 mg	110%
Pork, ham, 3 oz	0.8-1.1 mg	110%
Baking Chocolate, 1 oz	0.9 mg	104%
Beef Spleen, 3 oz	0.8 mg	90%
Spices, mace, 1 oz	0.7 mg	80%
Potatoes, cooked, medium	0.67 mg	75%
Thyme, 1 oz	0.67 mg	75%
Mushrooms, cooked, ½ cup	0.65 mg	72%
Cashew Nuts, 1 oz	0.62 mg	70%

Crab, cooked, 3 oz	0.62 mg	69%
Sunflower Seeds, ¼ cup	0.6 mg	68%
Black Pepper, 1 oz	0.59 mg	66%
Turkey, cooked, 3 oz	0.58 mg	65%
Dark Chocolate, 70-85%, 1 oz	0.5 mg	56%
Peanut Butter, 1 oz	0.5 mg	56%
Radishes, 1 oz	0.5 mg	56%
Game Meat, 3 oz	0.5 mg	56%
Pork Heart, 3 oz	0.5 mg	56%
Brazil Nuts, 1 oz	0.5 mg	56%
Tofu, firm, ½ cup	0.47 mg	53%
Beef Kidney, 3 oz	0.46 mg	50%
Beef Heart, 3 oz	0.45 mg	50%
Ham, 5% fat, 3 oz	0.45 mg	50%
Veal, cooked, 3 oz	0.45 mg	50%
Peanuts, oil-roasted, 1 oz (32 nuts)	0.4 mg	45%
Pecans, 1 oz (19 nuts)	0.3 mg	33%
Flaxseeds, 1 oz	0.3 mg	33%
Almonds, blanched, 1 oz	0.3 mg	33%
Chickpeas, ½ cup	0.29 mg	32%
Millet, cooked, 1 cup	0.28 mg	31%
Salmon, cooked, 3 oz	0.27 mg	30%
Whole Wheat Pasta, cooked, 1 cup	0.26 mg	29%

Turkey Breast, 3 oz	0.22 mg	28%
Chicken Breast, 3 oz	0.22 mg	28%
Beef Steak, 3 oz	0.1-2 mg	25%
Lamb, cooked, 3 oz	0.2 mg	24%
Pork, ribs, 3 oz	0.2 mg	24%
Avocado, ½ cup	0.2 mg	24%
Figs, dried, ½ cup	0.2 mg	24%
Spices, curry powder, 1 oz	0.2 mg	24%
Spinach, cooked, ½ cup	0.15 mg	17%
Asparagus, cooked, ½ cup	0.14 mg	17%
Sesame Seeds, ¼ cup	0.14 mg	16%
Turkey, cooked, 3 oz	0.13 mg	14%
Cream of Wheat, 1 cup	0.1 mg	12%
Gelatin, 1 oz	0.1 mg	12%
Egg, 1 medium	0.1 mg	12%
Fresh Garlic, 1 oz	0.1 mg	12%
Carrot, 1 oz	0.1 mg	12%
Mussels, 3 oz	0.1 mg	12%
Sardines, 3 oz	0.1 mg	12%
Tomatoes, raw, ½ cup	0.05 mg	6%
Greek Yogurt, 7 oz	0.042 mg	5%
Milk, no fat, 1 cup	0.027 mg	3%
Apples, raw, ½ cup	0.017 mg	2%

You can even get copper by breathing it in the air, but this would only supply at most around 0.02 mg/day, from areas with high atmospheric copper concentrations such as found in Boston, Massachusetts.

Vermont spring water appears to have the highest copper levels at 1.4 mg of copper per liter of water, whereas soft municipal tap water ranges from around 0.17-0.73 mg/liter. In other words, natural spring waters may be is 5 to 10-times higher in copper versus tap water.

Animal studies show that only eating muscle meat contributes to copper deficiency. High meat diets in mice cause hypercholesterolemia and weaker bones, which is thought to primarily be due to a copper deficiency[2147]. This is because muscle meat is extremely low in copper but high in zinc and iron. Heme iron, as found in meat, is particularly well absorbed compared to non-heme iron. The highly bioavailable iron in cooked meat may also reduce the absorption of copper[2148]. Excess cystine and cysteine consumption enhances copper deficiency in rats[2149]. Foods high in cystine/cysteine are animal proteins like poultry, beef, pork, eggs, fish, etc., and in smaller amounts in lentils and oatmeal[2150]. These foods are also highest in iron. Zinc absorption is also greater when eating animal protein compared to plant foods, which inhibits copper absorption[2151]. This might be why vegetarians or vegans may need more zinc than omnivores but less copper[2152].

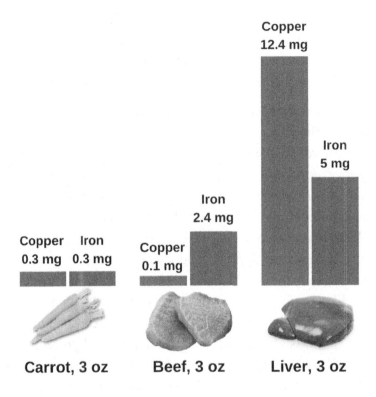

Carrot, 3 oz   Beef, 3 oz   Liver, 3 oz

Total copper absorption is higher with a lactoovovegetarian (dairy, eggs, and vegetarian) diet (0.48 mg/day) compared to a non-vegetarian diet (0.40 mg/day) because of its higher copper content[2153]. Moreover, the "antinutrients" in plants (phytic acid and phytates) can increase copper absorption by antagonizing zinc[2154]. In other words, increasing the intake of plants and reducing the intake of muscle meat can help to improve copper status; or simply eat other animal foods, such as liver and shellfish, which contain copper. Importantly, when you accumulate iron, your copper requirements increase. In other words, iron overload predisposes to copper deficiency. Thus, copper deficiency may be one of the most important and prevalence subclinical nutrient deficiencies affecting millions (if not billions) of people around the world. If we looked at red blood cell or leukocyte copper levels, it would be highly likely that most of the global population would be copper deficient.

It has been shown that the copper density of vegan meals is almost twice as much as that of an omnivorous diet (0.7 ± 0.29 *vs* 2.0 ± 0.34 mg/1000 kcal for the vegan and omnivorous diet respectively)[2155]. A higher copper intake may explain why some studies show that vegans live longer than those eating a Standard American Diet. Indeed, the daily copper intake is 27% higher in vegetarians compared to omnivorous adolescent females[2156]. These studies however are including people who do not frequently incorporate copper-rich organ meats like liver and rely mainly on high iron muscle meat, which is the issue. Despite the reduced bioavailability, the higher copper content of plant-based diets seems to at least provide an adequate amount of copper[2157]. Some fibers like locust bean, karaya gums, and carboxymethylcellulose have not been shown to have an effect on trace mineral bioavailability, including copper[2158]. Pinto beans have also been shown to be a great source of copper with good bioavailability [2159]. Foods rich in fructo-oligosaccharides like chicory root, blue agave, artichoke, asparagus, Yacon root, garlic, and green bananas, have also been shown to enhance the absorption of copper, zinc and selenium[2160]. Soybean protein, however, seems to reduce copper absorption[2161,2162]. A high fiber diet improves copper absorption because of fructo-oligosaccharides and inulin. The higher your intake of copper (up to around 7-8 mg/day) the more of it you retain (up to around 1 mg/day)[2163]. So, the more copper you eat, the more of it you will keep when consuming up to around 7-8 mg of copper a day. This suggests a large safety net when it comes to copper toxicity as the body controls copper homeostasis and it's hard to overdose on copper as it can be excreted in bile.

Zinc/Copper Ratio

In 1975, Leslie Klevay proposed the 'zinc-copper hypothesis' of coronary heart disease[2164]. He claimed that the imbalance of high zinc to copper in the diet leads to an absolute copper deficiency. Accordingly, too much zinc in relation to copper results in hypercholesterolemia and increased coronary heart disease mortality[2165]. Klevay concluded that the ratio of zinc to copper may be an important factor in the causation of coronary heart disease. However, a large cross-sectional study of 600 subjects found no significant association between the zinc/copper ratio and cholesterol or triglycerides[2166]. Zinc and copper levels have not been seen to be correlated with angiographically-defined coronary artery disease in Sudanese patients[2167]. However, that's because serum copper is not a good measure of copper status. When leukocyte copper levels are measured angiographically-defined coronary artery disease is highly correlated with low copper levels[2168,2169]. However, in a large Persian cohort, there was a weak association between lower serum copper and calculated 10-year coronary heart disease risk[2170]. And low zinc levels have been associated with cardiovascular disease risk factors like diabetes, hypertension and high triglycerides[2171,2172]. Serum copper, but not zinc, has been positively correlated with leptin (a satiety hormone)[2173], which may help to control some risk factors of cardiovascular disease like weight and metabolic syndrome.

Zinc is a copper antagonist, which is why ingesting large doses of zinc can lead to copper deficiency by inhibiting its absorption and increasing its secretion. A high concentration of zinc in the small intestine triggers the expression of metallothionines, which bind to copper[2174]. In fact, the popular use of zinc supplements may be a leading cause of subclinical copper deficiency, especially when used for prolonged periods of time[2175]. There are many documented cases of zinc-induced copper deficiency. In 70 anemic patients who were prescribed zinc, 62% of them received zinc doses large enough to cause a copper deficiency[2176]. The remaining 48% of patients showed low plasma zinc levels because of hypoalbuminemia or systemic inflammation. A woman with low white blood cells (neutropenia) and altered muscle movement (ataxia) experienced copper deficiency from taking 135 mg of zinc/day for seven years[2177]. After she stopped the zinc consumption, her copper and zinc normalized but her neurological status improved only partially. Total zinc intakes of 60 mg/day (50 mg from a zinc supplement plus 10 mg from diet) for 10 weeks has been shown to reduce copper status in females, assessed by decreased superoxide dismutase activity[2178]. Zinc supplementation has also been shown to cause adverse effects on lipid metabolism in humans with animal studies confirming this is due to the induction of a mild copper deficiency[2179]. Animal studies have also suggested that a moderate amount of zinc (when extrapolated to humans the dose of zinc equates to 22 mg/day for men and 16 mg/day for women) may induce mild copper deficiency[2180]. Of course, we are not animals, and zinc-induced copper deficiency will also depend on the background intake of copper. Indeed, supplemental zinc at 50 mg/day has been found to reduce indices of copper status (copper,zinc-SOD)[2181,2182]. However, human studies suggest that zinc intakes up to around 40-50 mg/day may not induce copper deficiency, at least in the short-term, as long as copper intakes are above 1 mg/day. However, these studies do not look at copper status using leukocyte or red blood cell copper levels and hence they should be interpreted with caution. **The golden rule when supplementing with zinc, is that at a minimum, for every 40 mg of zinc, 1 mg of copper should be employed.**

Based on these findings and other reports, the U.S.-Canadian upper limit for zinc for adults is set at 40 mg/day[2183]. The lowest median effective dose of supplementary zinc is deemed to be 24 mg/day[2184]. Currently, the US–Canadian RDA for zinc is 11 mg/day for adult men and 8 mg/day for adult women[2185]. Children 9-13 8 mg/d, children 1-8 years of age 3-5 mg/d, children <12 months 2-3 mg/d. Some suggest that 9 mg of zinc a day from supplements is safe for people weighting 60 kg[2186]. The more you weigh the higher your requirements tend to be. Although short-term use of high-dose zinc (80 mg/day for 4-5 days) is probably not going to cause copper deficiency[2187], overuse for weeks can cause copper deficiency, characterized by neurological complications [2188]. Hyperzincemia of unknown origin and gastrointestinal surgery have been shown to be associated with copper deficiency-induced myeloneuropathy[2189,2190].

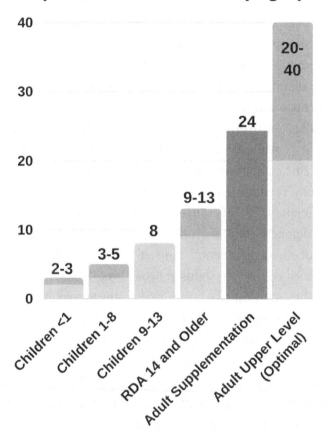

Optimal Intake of Zinc (mg/d)

Zinc denture adhesives and zinc-containing denture creams are another possible source of excess zinc that can lead to copper deficiency[2191,2192,2193]. The technology to stabilize denture adhesives with zinc salts was licensed in 1990[2194]. Many other manufacturers followed suit, but because of a large increase in the reported cases of hyperzincemia (high zinc levels in the blood) and hypocupremia (low copper levels in the blood), they stopped or modified the production of zinc adhesives since 2010. Despite that, zinc denture adhesives are still continued to be produced and marketed to common denture users. As of 2009, over 35 million Americans wear removable dentures. Thus, there needs to be more awareness and education about the situation by dentists, counselors and doctors.

Klevay noted that populations that have a higher rate of coronary heart disease eat higher amounts of fat and sugar and less vegetables, particularly fewer legumes, cereals and nuts. The phytic acid in these plant foods appears to limit the absorption of zinc but provides ample amounts of copper.[2195] This may explain why associational studies find that populations who consume more grains and vegetables, especially when compared to the Standard American Diet, have a lower risk of coronary heart disease[2196,2197,2198]. High copper and phytate intake may be a protective factor against the Standard American Diet high in zinc and iron (phytate can also bind free iron). Phytic acid decreases the ratio of zinc to copper that gets absorbed in the intestinal tract. This is not to say that you need to eat fiber or phytic acid, but it's important to balance the zinc/copper ratio, and that means sourcing more than just muscle meat and eggs.

The processing of wheat and grains increases the zinc to copper ratio. Klevay noted in 1975 that a Type A school lunch or a typical meal from McDonalds at the time had a zinc to copper ratio of 12/1 and 12-23/1, respectively[2199]. Out of 11 diets tabulated by Klevay, only two diets contained 2 mg of copper per day or more, but nine of the eleven diets contained at least 12 mg of zinc per day or more. In other words, diets consumed in the United States at the time lacked copper but were, in general, sufficient in zinc. It thus seems that the majority of fast-food or school lunch diets contain little copper, even for children. About 30% of Mexican children, 13% of adolescents and 17% of adults have low copper levels in their blood[2200]. Copper deficiency in Mexico has a high association with iron deficiency anemia[2201], which may also be driven by copper deficiency. Indeed, the Mexican food supply is high in copper-chelating foods that are high in iron and zinc[2202].

In lamb muscle meat, the nutrient composition per 3.5 oz is as follows: zinc (3.42 mg), iron (1.31 mg), copper (0.08 mg) with manganese being below the detection limit (0.025 mg). Based on that, lamb muscle tissue mineral ratios are as follows: Zn/Cu ~ 43 and Fe/Cu ratio ~ 16[2203]. Therefore, muscle meat is not a "well-balanced" food (at least when it comes Zn/Cu and Fe/Cu ratios) and hence its intake must be balanced by high-copper foods that have a low Zn/Cu and Fe/Cu ratio.

The approximate content of zinc, iron and copper in various types of meat (mg/3.5 oz.) are as follows:[2204,2205]

Type of Meat	Zinc	Iron	Copper	Zn/Cu Ratio	Fe/Cu Ratio
Beef	4.6 mg	1.8 mg	0.12 mg	38	15
Veal	4.2 mg	1.1 mg	0.08 mg	52.5	14
Lamb	3.42-4.5 mg	1.31-2.0 mg	0.08-0.12 mg	28.5-56	11-25
Mutton	3.9 mg	3.3 mg	0.22 mg	18	15

Organ meats like liver have a much more appropriate iron-zinc to copper ratio than muscle meat. Per ounce of beef liver, you get 4.1 mg of copper or 4.5 times the RDA for copper of 0.9 mg[2206]. Thus, just a little bit of liver goes a long way. However, this is also why it is not recommended to consume more than 1 oz. of beef liver per day as total intakes of copper at or over 10 mg for several months could cause unwanted side-effects. Although liver is high in cholesterol, it may be an antidote to the hypercholesterolemic effects of meat, which may actually be due to the low copper content of muscle meat[2207]. Liver, heart, kidney, suet, etc. have the fat-soluble vitamins like K2, A, D as well as CoQ10. Per calorie, liver is one of the most nutrient dense foods in the world. It is also relatively low in calories compared to muscle meat (~130-150 vs ~150-200 calories/3.5 oz). Eating a high nutrient diet with low calories has been shown to reduce hunger and help with weight loss[2208]. The standard Western diet is full of empty/harmful calories that do not have the essential nutrients our bodies need; thus, we are left hungry and unsatisfied. You can cover nearly all your needs for most vitamins and minerals by eating a single ounce of liver. Unfortunately, most people find organ meats disgusting but a simple way around this is to eat a blend of ground muscle meat with liver/heart (75% muscle meat/25% liver and heart). Organ meats and offal have been completely neglected in the modern industrialized diet landscape, whereas they are relatively common in France and other Mediterranean countries. Oysters are another example of this as they're high in copper, which seems more than sufficient to counteract the inhibitory effects of its high zinc content.

Part of the benefits of exercise may also be attributed to the fact that zinc needs dramatically increase when we exercise, as zinc is primarily found in muscle. Exercise stimulates the growth of muscle and bone, which are made-up of larger amounts of zinc compared to copper (zinc/copper ratios 56 and 120, respectively) and thus exercise tends to protect against a diet higher in zinc to copper (i.e., more zinc gets directed towards muscle and bone growth). This may be why weightlifters are somewhat protected from their high intake of meat, as the zinc is needed for muscle and bone growth. This also suggests that weightlifters need more zinc, in order to develop larger muscles and stronger bones[2209]. Thus, zinc requirements go up when building muscle, and this is likely why many weightlifters crave muscle meat (for the high zinc content).

Here are the foods highest in zinc[2210,2211,2212]

Food	Mg of Zinc per Serving	% of RDA minimum (11 mg)
Mollusks, 3 oz	154 mg	1029%
Oysters, 3 oz	74 mg	673%
Beef, chuck roast, 3 oz	7 mg	64%
Crab, cooked, 3 oz	6.5 mg	59%
Ground Beef, 80/20, 3 oz	5.4 mg	49%
Beef Patty, 3 oz	5.3 mg	48%
Wheat Germ, ¼ cup	4.8 mg	44%
Beef Liver, 3 oz	4.5 mg	41%
Buckwheat, cooked, 1 cup	4.1 mg	27%
Peanut Butter, 1 oz	4.0 mg	26%

Lamb, cooked, 3 oz	4.0 mg	26%
Beef Steak, 3 oz	4.0 mg	26%
Lobster, cooked, 3 oz	3.4 mg	31%
Pork Chop, cooked, 3 oz	2.9 mg	26%
Baked Beans, ½ cup	2.9 mg	26%
Breakfast Cereal, fortified with zinc, 1 serving	2.8 mg	25%
Lentils, cooked, 1 cup	2.5 mg	24%
Chicken, cooked, 3 oz	2.4 mg	22%
Mussels, 3 oz	2.3 mg	22%
Pumpkin Seeds, 1 oz	2.2-4.4 mg	20%
Cocoa Powder, 1 oz	1.9 mg	13%
Peanuts, oil-roasted, 1 oz (32 nuts)	1.9 mg	13%
Yogurt, low fat, 8 oz	1.7 mg	15%
Cashews, roasted, 1 oz	1.6 mg	15%
Chickpeas, cooked, ½ cup	1.3 mg	12%
Pecans, 1 oz (19 nuts)	1.3 mg	12%
Swiss Cheese, 1 oz	1.2 mg	11%
Flaxseeds, 1 oz	1.2 mg	11%
Sardines, 3 oz	1.2 mg	11%
Oatmeal, instant, 1 packet	1.1 mg	10%
Milk, low fat, 1 cup	1.0 mg	9%
Hemp Seeds, 1 tbsp	1.0 mg	9%
Baking Chocolate, 1 oz	1.0 mg	9%
Almonds, roasted, 1 oz	0.9 mg	8%

Brazil Nuts, 1 oz	0.9 mg	8%
Kidney Beans, cooked, ½ cup	0.9 mg	8%
Cheddar Cheese, 1 oz	0.9 mg	8%
Dark Chocolate, 70-85%, 1 oz	0.9 mg	8%
Mushrooms, cooked, ½ cup	0.7 mg	5%
Salmon, cooked, 3 oz	0.7 mg	5%
Seaweed, spirulina, 1 oz	0.6 mg	4%
Spices, mace, 1 oz	0.6 mg	4%
Egg, 1 medium	0.6 mg	4%
Green Peas, ½ cup	0.5 mg	4%
Flounder, cooked, 3 oz	0.3 mg	3%

The zinc to copper ratio of cow's milk is 38, whereas that of human milk is between 4 and 6, this might explain the health benefits of populations that breast feed for several years versus in the United States, where children are typically switched over to cow's milk at 9-12 months of age. A zinc/copper ratio of 38 leads to copper deficit in infants and is clearly not healthy for infants or adult humans. Additionally, a higher zinc to copper ratio (as found in cow's milk) positively correlates with mortality due to coronary heart disease in 47 cities in the United States[2213].

An optimal ratio of zinc/copper in adults should be based on optimal intakes of each. This depends on how well zinc is absorbed from the diet, i.e., more dietary fiber/phytate will necessitate more zinc, and what stage of adulthood you are in (elderly vs. middle age). **Thus, an optimal intake of zinc in an adult can range anywhere from 20-80 mg/day, depending on the person and the situation. The optimal intake of copper, however, seems to sit at around 3**

mg/day, providing an optimal Zn/Cu ratio of anywhere from 4-20:1. Hypercholesterolemia can be produced in rats with zinc to copper ratios of 14-20:1, however this depends on the background copper intake[2214]. Klevay (1975) noted from diets consumed in the United States, that the median zinc to copper ratio is 27:1, which is two-fold higher than the lowest ratio found to produce hypercholesterolemia in rats[2215]. Out of 71 analyzed foods, 31 of them had a zinc to copper ratio of 14 or above. In other words, 44% of the foods commonly consumed by Americans have a zinc to copper ratio could contribute to elevated cholesterol levels. Indeed, most animal foods consumed in the Western world (muscle meat, eggs, milk and cheese) have a high zinc to copper ratio. A zinc to copper ratio of 20:1 may seem high, but if the diet is providing 3 mg of copper, then this ratio could be optimal.

Here is the zinc to copper ratios for numerous foods (lowest to highest)[2216]

Food	Mg of Copper per Serving	Mg of Zinc per Serving	Zinc to Copper Ratio
Beef Liver, 3 oz	12.4 mg	4.5 mg	0.36
Seaweed, spirulina, 1 oz	1.7 mg	0.6 mg	0.36
Kidney Beans, 1 cup	2.0 mg	0.9 mg	0.45
Turkey, cooked, 3 oz	0.58 mg	0.4 mg	0.9
Spices, mace, 1 oz	0.7 mg	0.6 mg	0.9
Potatoes, cooked, medium	0.67 mg	0.6 mg	0.9
Mushrooms, cooked, ½ cup	0.65 mg	0.7 mg	1

Lentils, cooked, 1 cup	2.5 mg	2.5 mg	1
Baking Chocolate, 1 oz	0.9 mg	1.0 mg	1.1
Radishes, 1 oz	0.5 mg	0.6 mg	1.2
Spinach, cooked, ½ cup	0.15 mg	0.2 mg	1.3
Winged Beans, cooked, 1 cup	5.2 mg	8.2 mg	1.6
Cocoa Powder, 1 oz	1.1 mg	1.9 mg	1.7
Dark Chocolate, 70-85%, 1 oz	0.5 mg	0.9 mg	1.8
Brazil Nuts, 1 oz	0.5 mg	0.9 mg	1.8
Buckwheat, cooked, 1 cup	1.9 mg	4.1 mg	2.2
Asparagus, cooked, ½ cup	0.14 mg	0.35 mg	2.5
Pork, 3 oz	0.8-1.1 mg	2.9 mg	2.6
Cashew Nuts, 1 oz	0.62 mg	1.62 mg	2.6
Salmon, cooked, 3 oz	0.27 mg	0.7 mg	2.6
Almonds, blanched, 1 oz	0.3 mg	0.9 mg	3
Chickpeas, ½ cup	0.29 mg	1.2 mg	4
Flaxseeds, 1 oz	0.3 mg	1.2 mg	4
Pecans, 1 oz (19 nuts)	0.3 mg	1.3 mg	4.3
Avocado, ½ cup	0.2 mg	0.9 mg	4.5

Peanuts, oil-roasted, 1 oz (32 nuts)	0.4 mg	1.9 mg	4.75
Spices, curry powder, 1 oz	0.2 mg	1.1 mg	5.5
Egg, 1 medium	0.1 mg	0.6 mg	6
Peanut Butter, 1 oz	0.5 mg	4.0 mg	8
Crab, cooked, 3 oz	0.62 mg	6.5 mg	10.5
Chicken Breast, 3 oz	0.22 mg	2.4 mg	11
Oysters, 3 oz	4.8-6 mg	74 mg	15
Beef Steak, 3 oz	0.22 mg	4.0 mg	18
Lamb, cooked, 3 oz	0.2 mg	4.0 mg	20
Ground Beef, 80/20, 3 oz	0.25 mg	5.4 mg	21.6
Mollusks, 3 oz	6.4 mg	154 mg	24

The copper content of dark chocolate (70-90%) is significantly higher than that of milk chocolate. A 3 oz. bar of dark chocolate, for example, contains up to 0.75 mg of copper, which is over 100% of the RDA for children and nearly 80% of the RDA for teens and adults[2217]. This is because higher amounts of cacao provide more copper. Indeed, cocoa supplementation in infants with copper deficiency associated with tube feeding nutrition improves copper status[2218]. One study found that many people in the U.S. get more than 50% of their daily copper needs from chocolate foods[2219]. However, added sugars, especially fructose, increases copper demands. Thus, you should try and stick with high cacao dark chocolate (aim for 80% cacao) to reduce the amount of added sugars.

Foods with a high Zinc:Copper Ratio (these foods must be balanced with appropriate amounts of copper from other food sources):

- Oysters
- Muscle meat
- Breakfast cereal
- Cow's milk
- Prepackaged meat
- Mollusks/shellfish

Foods with a low Zinc:Copper Ratio (these will need to be paired with foods higher in zinc):

- Organ meats/liver
- Seaweed/spirulina
- Lentils/beans/chickpeas
- Dark chocolate/cacao
- Vegetables

Eating zinc-rich foods with a high zinc-copper ratio is not necessarily a bad thing. In fact, it can be great if you are deficient in zinc. It's a matter of context – how much, how often, the overall dietary intake and who is consuming it. The takeaway is that you shouldn't make these high zinc:copper ratio foods the only ones that you eat in your diet. Additionally, you should not overconsume high copper containing foods either, like eating 3 oz. of liver every day. As a rule of thumb, eat around 0.5 to 1 oz. of liver/day for copper and at least 12 oz. of red meat for zinc, iron, B12 and protein.

Copper and Molybdenum

Another copper inhibitor is molybdenum (Mo). It is a mineral found in foods like pork, lamb, beef, beans, eggs and cereal grains in small amounts. Molybdenum and copper have been found to have antagonistic roles with each other. Indeed, a Mo/Cu ratio of 2.5/1 in animals can lead to copper deficiency and altered immune responses during infection[2220]. Patients with type-2 diabetes have been shown to have higher serum and urine copper levels due to molybdenum removing it from tissues and eliminating it through urine[2221]. Those with severe nephropathy have a higher urine level of Cu/Mo. Thus, excess molybdenum, when combined with sulfur, may promote the excretion of copper through urine or bile via binding with protein-bound and free copper.

In animals, molybdenum overload has been shown to disrupt carbohydrate metabolism and increase oxidative stress by reducing copper-dependent enzymes like ceruloplasmin, superoxide dismutase, and myocardial cytochrome c oxidase[2222],[2223]. The glucose intolerance is a secondary symptom of copper deficiency. Since the mid-1980s, there was widespread "moose sickness" affecting the local moose population in south-western Sweden, characterized by symptoms of diabetes and muscle wasting[2224]. Studies found that the cause of this disease was molybdenum overload and secondary copper deficiency[2225]. The increased molybdenum consumption originated from an increased pH of the soil, which increased molybdenum content of vegetation, caused by liming and other practices. However, these effects may not be as pronounced in humans, as the formation of molybdenum-sulfur compounds that bind copper are believed to formed in the rumen.

Copper Absorption

Copper is absorbed in the gastrointestinal tract and is transported to the liver. However, there are many things that interfere with this process. Liver damage, cirrhosis or fibrosis increase the demand for copper and decrease its absorption[2226,2227]. Fibrate medications (such as bezafibrate, fenofibrate, gemfibrozil) may be able to restore low copper levels in NAFLD disease and increase concentrations of hepatic Cu-Zn SOD[2228]. Malabsorption diseases like celiac disease[2229], short bowel syndrome[2230] and IBS[2231] also reduce copper absorption. Copper deficiency has been seen in patients with celiac disease[2232] and it can cause anemia and thrombocytopenia[2233,2234]. Gastric bypass surgery or colon removal can cause copper deficiency. **Up to 70% of patients who have had gastric bypass surgery have low copper levels in their blood by three years** and almost 25% have low blood copper levels by 6 months[2235]. In the United States, around 113,000 bariatric surgeries are performed per year[2236].

The oral bioavailability of copper can range from 12-75%, depending on the amount of copper in the diet[2237]. The average bioavailability of most normal diets is between 30-40% on the typical Western diet[2238]. That number can be lower in the presence of excess zinc, molybdenum, iron or fructose/added sugars. **The refining of grains and cereals can reduce the copper content by up to 45%**[2239]. Indiscriminate use of multivitamins that often contain zinc and iron can be problematic for people low in copper. So, even if you are getting up to 10 mg/day of copper from food, it might be that you'll only end up absorbing $1/3^{rd}$ of it in the worst-case scenario and $2/3^{rds}$ at best.

Copper absorption occurs in the stomach and the small intestine, but the most efficient absorption takes place in the ileum and duodenum[2240,2241]. For optimal absorption, copper needs acid from the stomach to be liberated from food. During absorption, excess copper is transiently stored in the enterocytes by binding to metallothionine. Once inside the enterocyte, cuprous ions bind to different copper chaperones to be distributed to various organelles and cell compartments. Thus, damage to the microvilli of enterocytes, which contain micronutrient absorption transporters, will decrease copper absorption. It has been shown that the overconsumption of refined sugar and fructose damages the enterocytes[2242,2243], which will likely reduce copper absorption.

- Iron can compete with copper for absorption via the DMT1 (divalent metal transporter 1) transporter[2244,2245,2246]. Iron deprivation or iron deficiency due to chronic disease or malnutrition, can lead to copper overload, possibly due to absorption increases in ATP7A[2247], which brings copper into the portal circulation. Zinc also competes with copper absorption via DMT1[2248].

- Sodium may enhance copper absorption or retention and people on amiloride may need more copper as it appears to reduce copper and sodium absorption in the intestine[2249,2250]. Thus, low salt diets may reduce, whereas normal salt diets may improve copper absorption.

- In the presence of excess copper, CTR1 reduces copper absorption by enterocytes. However, when enterocytes are damaged because of intestinal tract injuries, copper deficiency may occur.

- Fructose increases the requirements for copper and exacerbates the effects of copper deficiency[2251,2252]. Thus, added sugars are a tax on copper status.

Approximately 0.5-2.5 mg of copper is excreted via feces every day. Biliary copper secretion cannot be reabsorbed, as it is prevented by the binding to bile salts and comes out in the feces. Thus, the body has the ability to get rid of copper excess through bile excretion, which is regulated by the liver (liver cells excrete excess copper into bile). Low blood copper levels, or low ferritin levels, leads to copper being released into the blood circulation. To prevent copper overload, surplus copper can be excreted through the natural shedding of the intestinal epithelial cells.

Copper absorption in the stomach is stimulated by an acidic pH and is inhibited by zinc and cadmium[2253,2254]. Stomach acid frees up copper bound to food and facilitates peptic digestion, which releases copper from natural organic complexes[2255]. That is why proton pump inhibitors or other acid suppressing over the counter therapies or medications can reduce copper absorption as it reduces the release of copper from natural organic complexes in food[2256]. Cadmium is a common toxic heavy metal that has accumulated in the environment due to pollution. Ironically, zinc helps to reduce the absorption of cadmium.

Vitamin C can enhance, or inhibit, copper absorption. If taken prior to (around 75 minutes before) or with copper, vitamin C reduces copper absorption by blocking the binding of copper to metallothionein. However, if vitamin C is taken after copper ingestion (75 minutes after) it increases ceruloplasmin and lysyl oxidase activity. Vitamin C also seems to help facilitate the transfer of copper ions into cells, reacting with the copper carrying protein ceruloplasmin, reducing cupric copper (CuII+) to cuprous copper (CuI+) making the bound copper atoms more freely available and facilitating their cross-membrane transport[2257]. Moreover, histidine, an amino acid, may aid the transport of copper from albumin into certain cells. Additionally, glutathione appears to help facilitate the transfer of copper to metallothionine and superoxide dismutase. Thus, cysteine and glycine, which help to increase glutathione levels, may also help with copper transport in the body. The below figure depicts the roles of vitamin C (ascorbate) and histidine in the transport of copper into cells and glutathione (and thus cysteine and glycine by default) in the transfer of copper to superoxide dismutase and metallothionein.

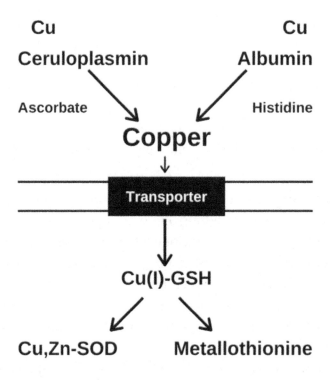

Klevay has previously suggested that large doses of ascorbic acid might increase the zinc-copper ratio and produce hypercholesterolemia. Hypercholesterolemia, caused by ascorbic acid overfeeding, has been documented in rats and is similar to the increase of cholesterol in patients with atherosclerosis caused by excessive ingestion of ascorbic acid[2258]. In guinea pigs, vitamin C doses of 25 mg per 100 grams of body weight per day, reduced liver copper levels 2-3-fold compared to those receiving 0.5 mg per 100 grams of body weight[2259]. Their iron and blood heme parameters also increased in proportion to the vitamin C intake. This is because ascorbic acid enhances iron absorption[2260]. Thus, in large doses, vitamin C may decrease copper status by increasing iron and zinc absorption. However, there may not be enough vitamin C in whole foods like fruit and vegetables to inhibit copper absorption or deplete it. Large doses of supplements, however, like 1-2 grams of vitamin C probably will but if you take vitamin C after copper intake there may not be any risk for copper depletion. That is why it is better to focus on getting vitamin C and potassium from whole foods and use supplemental doses only acutely during sickness or an infection. On the flip side, Vitamin C + E can also combat copper toxicity-induced lipid peroxidation and liver damage[2261]. They have also been shown to reduce the oxidation of HDL cholesterol caused by excess copper[2262].

Copper homeostasis is maintained in the liver[2263]. Importantly, the thyroid gland regulates more than 5% of all the genes expressed in the liver[2264,2265], including copper metabolism. Hypothyroid patients have significantly lower levels of zinc and copper, which are needed for normal thyroid functioning[2266]. Thyroid hormones stimulate the synthesis and export of ceruloplasmin from the liver into the serum[2267]. Thus, being hypothyroid may hinder copper homeostasis and utilization in the body.

The synthesis of ceruloplasmin by the liver appears to be very stable[2268]. Minor copper deficiency does not significantly alter serum copper levels[2269] nor does copper supplementation[2270]. Only certain genetic disorders, such as Wilson's disease (WD) or Menke's disease (MD) are known to disturb copper metabolism in a life-threatening way, by affecting the copper transporting proteins ATP7A and ATP7B[2271].

- Wilson's disease is characterized by autosomal recessive mutations in the gene encoding ATP7B, which affects 1 out of 30,000-100,000 people[2272]. WD patients suffer from excessive copper accumulation in the organs, mostly the liver and brain. This can be treated with copper-chelating agents like penicillamine, trientine and ammonium tetra-molybdate[2273,2274,2275]. Increased zinc intake or supp-lementation can also reduce the copper absorbed from diet[2276].

- Menke's disease is a condition of ATP7A mutations, which occurs in 1 out of 40,000-350,000 people[2277,2278]. Copper absorption is completely absent in Menkes disease, causing growth retardation, hypopigmentation, hypothermia and neurological problems[2279]. The bottleneck occurs in the intestines where copper absorption is blocked, which is why the only copper replacement strategy involves subcutaneous injection of copper-histidine[2280].

Copper chelating agents have been found to provide some benefit in certain medical conditions that are affected by copper overload. For example, penicillamine, trientine and tetrathiomolybdate can inhibit angiogenesis (the formation of new blood vessels) and decrease tumor progression and invasiveness [2281, 2282]. The expression of vascular endothelial growth factor (VEGF), which is an important angiogenic factor, has been found to be sensitive to copper[2283]. Forming new blood vessels is vital and necessary for physiological repair of the body, but in some cases, it can be hijacked by malignancies to direct themselves access to more blood flow and nutrients[2284]. You want blood flow in the healthy tissues, organs and muscles but not tumors. Copper chelators are currently being tested as potential anti-cancer agents in several clinical trials[2285,2286]. However, the risk to benefit ratio of them is not well understood yet. Trientine has also been recently used in type 2 diabetic humans to increase copper excretion[2287].

One of the biggest chelators of copper is glyphosate. Deficiencies in trace minerals like iron, molybdenum, copper and others is associated with celiac disease and it can also be attributed to glyphosate's ability to chelate these metals[2288]. Glyphosate is one of the most common pesticides in the U.S. used on almost all types of fruit and vegetables. Not only does it reduce the mineral content of the vegetation, but it also disrupts the microbiome potentially promoting malabsorption diseases[2289]. Glyphosate is a strong chelator thanks to its ability to form strong complexes with transition metals[2290,2291,2292]. Glyphosate has also been shown to decrease iron, magnesium, manganese and calcium levels in non-GMO soybeans[2293].

Estrogen and progesterone have been shown to increase serum copper and ceruloplasmin in rats and humans regardless of the dose, form or route, [2294] which may be due to increased copper need and mobilization. Thus, women who take oral hormonal contraceptives may actually need more copper despite having higher copper levels in their blood. Oral contraceptives also affect zinc status by either decreasing it or keeping it unchanged[2295].

In conclusion, most Americans are not getting optimal intakes of copper. It is not difficult to obtain the optimal amount of copper from diet, which we deem to be around 3 mg/day. If you are already deficient in copper, then intakes of above 2.6 mg/day are likely needed for several weeks if not months. Dietary copper intake should not exceed 10 mg/day. However, excess copper will typically be excreted or its absorption will be reduced. The highest copper-containing foods are beef liver, oysters, shellfish and beans. They also have a lower zinc-copper ratio (except oysters and mollusks), which improves copper absorption. Generally, it is recommended to eat liver at least once a week (3 oz. at a time), or if eaten several times per week, 0.5 to 1 oz. at a time. Eating plant fibers, phytate and phytonutrients can help to chelate iron and maintain a better copper status, but they can also reduce zinc absorption. Thus, it is important to balance plant foods with animal foods. To not impose additional demands for copper on the body, avoid added sugars and fructose-sweetened beverages.

Chapter 9
Zinc for the Immune and Endocrine System

The last chapter may have given you the idea that zinc is bad because it inhibits copper absorption. However, that is not the case, as zinc simply needs to be paired with appropriate amounts of copper. Zinc plays numerous roles in the body and most of us are not getting enough of it for optimal health and longevity.

Zinc is another essential mineral needed for many processes in the body, including postnatal development, protein synthesis, wound healing and immune system functioning[2296]. You also need zinc for a proper sense of taste and smell[2297].

Zinc acts as a catalyst for over 300 enzymatic reactions and over 1000 transcription factors [2298, 2299, 2300]. DNA/RNA transcription and replication factors are zinc-dependent, which will not work in the absence of zinc[2301,2302]. In rats, DNA synthesis is impaired by dietary zinc deficiency[2303]. Thus, zinc affects gene expression[2304]. Apoptosis, or programmed cell death, is regulated by zinc[2305,2306]. However, in some instances, zinc can protect against apoptosis during gamma irradiation, hyperthermia and cold shock[2307]. In other words, zinc can make our cells more resilient to certain stressors. This is a good thing if you are fighting off an infection or are dealing with a lot of oxidative stress.

Deficiencies in zinc cause growth retardation, hormonal imbalances, impotence, delayed wound healing, frailty, hair loss, diarrhea, skin lesions and increased susceptibility to infections[2308,2309,2310]. Zinc deficiency during pregnancy is associated with an increased risk of premature delivery and abortion[2311,2312]. Since the early 1960s, it has been noted that zinc deficiency can cause anemia, dwarfism, growth retardation and hypogonadism independent of iron deficiency[2313,2314]. Only 50 years later has it become apparent that zinc deficiency could be a factor driving many other problems[2315].

It is estimated that up to 25-40% of the world's population is zinc deficient, at least to some extent[2316]. Zinc deficiency is not widespread in Western countries, but it does affect a lot of people in the third world and most people in the Western world are not consuming *optimal* amounts of zinc. Stunted growth in childhood is typically caused by zinc deficiency, especially in low-income countries where the intake of animal foods tends to be lower[2317,2318].

In this chapter, we will cover the role of zinc in the body and what an optimal amount of zinc is per day. Zinc provides the delicate balance between other minerals like copper and iron.

Zinc and Health

Zinc (Zn) is the 24th most abundant element in the Earth's crust. Industrially, zinc is often used in electricity, batteries, organic chemistry and as anti-corrosive coating. Various zinc compounds can be found in deodorants, supplements, personal hygiene products and shampoos. It has a slightly bluish-silvery color and is quite brittle at room temperature.

The oldest ornaments of 80-90% zinc have been found to be 2500 years old[2319]. Use of zinc as a metal dates back to 10-14th century BC when zinc-copper alloy brass was employed in the Aegean region (Mesopotamia)[2320,2321]. Zinc, as a metal, was known to Ancient Greeks and Romans but its use was sparse[2322]. They used calamine brass (zinc silicate or carbonate, charcoal and copper) to make weapons, coins and food containers. An Ancient Roman ship that wrecked in 140 BC was found to contain zinc carbonates, hydrozincite and smithsonite pills, which were probably used for sore eyes[2323]. Zinc metal production became large scale in 12th century India[2324]. The zinc mines at Zawar, India have been estimated to produce 60,000 tons of zinc between the 12th-16th century[2325].

Paracelsus, the 16th century Swiss-German doctor, was the one to give zinc its name, calling it *zincum* or *zinken*[2326]. The word originates from the German word *zinke,* which means 'tooth-like or jagged' because metallic zinc crystals look like needles[2327]. Another description could be 'tin-like', as *zinn* in German means tin, which resembles zinc's color. Medieval alchemists would burn zinc metal and collect the zinc oxide. They called it *lana philosophica*, which is Latin for 'philosopher's wool' [2328]. The Ancient Roman physician Galen suggested treating ulcerating cancers with zinc oxide. Zinc oxide is also a typical ingredient in many natural sunscreens.

The essential role of zinc in growth development was first demonstrated by Raulin (1869), who showed that zinc is necessary for the growth of a type of fungus called *Aspergillus niger*[2329]. In 1934, Todd et al. discovered that zinc is needed for the growth and development of rats [2330]. One of the first human studies on the importance of zinc was published in 1957, where zinc was shown to be necessary for enzymatic functioning in the liver[2331]. Growth and mental retardation, hypogonadism and anemia from a zinc deficiency in Persian children was first described by Prasad and colleagues in 1961[2332].

Here are the main essential functions of zinc in health:

- **Zinc helps to catalyze the calcification of bone**[2333]. Zinc deficiency causes skeletal abnormalities by reducing parameters of calcium metabolism in the bone[2334]. Zinc is also needed for collagen synthesis and zinc deficiency can increase damage to the body's soft tissue[2335]. Supplementation with arginine, glutamine, vitamin C and zinc has been shown to increase collagen synthesis during the first 2 days after inguinal hernia repair[2336]. Zinc also helps those with bed sores[2337].

- **Zinc speeds up wound healing**[2338,2339]. Wounds do not heal as fast with zinc deficiency[2340,2341]. Oral zinc sulfate improves foot and leg ulcers[2342,2343,2344,2345]. Zinc deficiency exacerbates ulcers by increasing oxidative stress in the skin[2346]. Zinc sulfide nanoparticles improve skin regeneration[2347]. Healing of the aorta requires zinc[2348]. Think of zinc as a healing mineral. If you've ever watched X-men, then you would know that Wolverine has a unique ability to repair himself, and that he carries a unique metal inside of him called adamantium making him impervious to damage. **Zinc can be thought of as our adamantium and the source of our healing power.**

- **Zinc may help to protect against atherosclerosis.** The relationship between low zinc and atherosclerosis has been known since the 1990s[2349].
  - Zinc, especially when taken with appropriate amounts of copper, prevents the oxidation of LDL cholesterol, which is one of the main mechanisms for atherosclerosis [2350]. Excess iron promotes LDL oxidation, whereas zinc protects against this[2351]. Zinc supplementation at doses over 50 mg/day can reduce HDL cholesterol, however, if copper status is maintained, this will likely not occur [2352]. Atherosclerosis develops in parallel with the decrease of zinc absorption, greater prevalence of zinc deficiency and increased inflammation that happens during aging[2353].
  - The preventative effect of zinc on cardiomyopathy is mediated by metallothionine[2354], the main protein zinc is bound to. Metallothionine has an antioxidant effect, including in the heart[2355]. It controls the amount of zinc in tissues. Zinc deficiency causes a deficiency in metallothionine, which results in increased reactive oxygen species in the cell, enhanced oxidative stress, inhibition of cytochrome c oxidase activity, impaired mitochondrial function and eventually cellular death, especially in the liver, kidney and connective/collagenous tissues [2356]. Metallothionine expression protects against the toxicity of cancer treatment drugs like doxorubicin[2357]. In other words, if you are zinc deficient you will likely experience worse chemotherapy side effects. Zinc has also been shown to protect metallothionine-deficient mice from alcohol-induced myocardial fibrosis[2358]. Selenium promotes the release of zinc from metallothionine and their combination improves immunity in the elderly after influenza vaccination [2359]. Inflammation also makes metallothionine use zinc, which explains why zinc

levels are low in inflammatory conditions such as atherosclerosis[2360]. High homocysteine also impairs metallothionine and disrupts redox homeostasis[2361,2362].

- o Zinc supplementation may help heal unstable plaque by promoting calcification, which is less likely to rupture[2363,2364]. Statins work by reducing inflammation and promote the calcification of unstable plaques[2365]. Statin drugs, however, also reduce zinc levels by 8%[2366]. Thus, their benefits are limited and are they are not without side effects.

- o Elevated serum copper, with low zinc and magnesium, is associated with an increased risk of cardiovascular disease mortality[2367]. A low urinary zinc, which is indicative of zinc deficiency, is associated with atherosclerosis severity[2368]. In atherosclerosis, there is a significant decrease in plasma, aorta, liver, myocardium and pancreas zinc levels[2369]. Patients with myocardial infarctions have low plasma zinc levels, averaging just 67 mcg/dL, instead of the 75-125 mcg/dL that is considered normal[2370].

- **Zinc is important for brain development, learning and plasticity**[2371]. Zinc deficiencies are implicated in brain disorders[2372]. Zinc supplementation in malnourished schoolboys has been shown to increase cortical thickness significantly more than in those who have received all the essential amino acids, vitamins and minerals without zinc[2373].

  - o **Zinc is needed for synthesizing many neurotransmitters, such as serotonin and melatonin.** Taking zinc has been shown to improve sleep in humans[2374].

  - o Zinc homeostasis regulates the central nervous system[2375]. Dysregulated zinc homeostasis and excess synaptic zinc concentrations, typically induced by inflammation, can cause neurotoxicity and mitochondrial damage[2376]. Zinc also regulates the activity of the adrenal glands and cortisol levels[2377].

- **Zinc and other trace minerals like copper and selenium are needed for the production of thyroid hormones**. On the flip side, you need adequate amounts of thyroid hormones to absorb zinc, which is why **hypothyroidism can cause an acquired zinc deficiency. Hypothyroidism reduces zinc absorption in the intestine**[2378]. Zinc is required to activate the T3 receptor, hence zinc deficiency impairs T3 receptor action[2379]. Zinc deficiency is associated with hypothyroidism and severe alopecia, i.e., hair loss[2380]. Supplementing with zinc in those who are deficient improves thyroid function[2381,2382]. Thus, it's a vicious cycle of zinc deficiency impairing thyroid hormone function, which drives more zinc deficiency.

  o The overconsumption of sugar, especially in conjunction with copper deficiency, also drives zinc deficiency through the promotion of fatty liver disease. Indeed, since the liver produces the active thyroid hormone T3, and active thyroid hormones are required for the absorption of zinc, damage to the liver will reduce zinc status. Considering that millions of people have hypothyroidism, a zinc deficit may be more rampant than originally thought.

- **Zinc is important for glucose metabolism and insulin production**[2383,2384]. Zinc helps with the uptake of glucose into the cell and with insulin synthesis[2385,2386]. Zinc deficient rats and humans have impaired glucose tolerance[2387,2388,2389]. A 2012 systematic meta-analysis that included 22 studies concluded that zinc supplementation has a beneficial effect on glycemic control and lipids in patients with type-2 diabetes[2390]. In type-1 diabetes, a combination of zinc and vitamin A (10 mg zinc a day and 25,000 IU vitamin A every other day) can improve apolipoproteinB/A1 ratios (essentially LDL+VLDL/HDL ratios)[2391].

  o Zinc is required for pancreatic carboxypeptidase[2392], which may be needed for insulin maturation and secretion[2393]. Zinc deficient rats have lower insulin-like activity and glucose clearance[2394,2395]. Furthermore, zinc supplementation has been shown to improve insulin resistance and metabolic syndrome in obese children[2396].

o **Zinc deficiency may also lead to metabolic acidosis by reducing carbonic anhydrase activity.** Carbonic anhydrases are a family of enzymes that catalyze the conversion of carbon dioxide and water to bicarbonate and protons[2397]. Most carbonic anhydrases contain a zinc ion at their active site and are thus classified as metalloenzymes. **Without carbonic anhydrases, tissue oxygenation decreases, and lactic acidosis increases.** Zinc losses increase in urine and sweat during exercise[2398]. Additionally, zinc needs increase during exercise to help working muscle, as well as after exercise to repair and build muscle. Thus, **many athletes are at risk of zinc deficiency**, which can impair performance and decrease the lactate threshold (i.e., when lactate accumulates faster than it can be removed). In zinc-deficient rats, lactic acid buffering agents like lactic dehydrogenase (LDH), malic dehydrogenase (MDH), alcohol dehydrogenase (ADH) and NADH diaphorase are lower[2399].

Because zinc is a catalyst for hundreds of transcription factors, a deficiency in zinc can disrupt many metabolic pathways and protein folding[2400]. Thus, zinc deficiency has detrimental effects on many systems of the body, including immunity, physical development and cognition.

A zinc deficiency may lead to the following:

- A reduction in growth, development and maturation[2401,2402]
- Acne, dermatitis, psoriasis, eczema and dry skin[2403,2404,2405,2406]
- Loss of taste and smell[2407,2408]
- Reduced appetite[2409]
- Night blindness and vision impairment[2410]
- Frequent sickness and infections[2411]
- Frequent pneumonia and respiratory infections[2412]
- Frequent diarrhea and enteropathy[2413,2414]
- Loss of cognition and impaired learning[2415]
- Behavioral abnormalities, ADHD and depression[2416,2417,2418,2419]
- Schizophrenia and psychiatric disorders[2420]

Here are the zinc-dependent enzymes, functions and consequences that may occur with a deficit

Zinc-Dependent Enzymes/Proteins	Function	Consequences of Deficit
Metallothionine[2421]	Protection against oxidative stress	Increased oxidative stress and tissue damage
Zinc,Copper Superoxide Dismutase	Protect against oxidative stress	Increased oxidative stress and tissue damage
p53	DNA damage repair	DNA damage and DNA mutations
Poly (ADP-ribose) Polymerase	DNA damage repair	DNA damage and DNA mutations
Glutathione Synthesis	Protect against oxidative stress	Increased oxidative stress and weaker immunity

Glutathione Peroxidase	Removes hydrogen peroxide	Increased oxidative stress and weaker immunity
Nitric Oxide Synthase	Cardiovascular function, antiviral effects	Oxidative stress, atherosclerosis and hypertension
Thyroid Hormones[2422]	Regulate metabolic rate, body temperature and energy balance	Chronic fatigue, frailty, weight gain, metabolic syndrome and decreased immunity
Luteinizing Hormone[2423]	Precursor to testosterone	Hypogonadism and low sex hormones
Growth Hormone[2424]	Physical repair, fat burning	Frailty, aging and muscle loss
Insulin Secretion[2425]	Shuttle nutrients into the cells	Insulin resistance and metabolic syndrome
Serotonin	Promotes melatonin production and relaxation	Chronic stress, insomnia and altered mood
Melatonin	Promotes sleep onset and antioxidant activity	Sleeping problems, poor metabolic health, increased oxidative stress and neurodegeneration
Dopamine Transporter[2426]	Feeling of reward and motivation	Depression and apathy

Glycolysis	Oxidation of glucose and lactate	Lactic acidosis and glucose intolerance
Beta-Oxidation	Oxidation of lipids and triglycerides	Dyslipidemia and obesity
Autophagy[2427]	Removes cellular waste material and dysfunctional organelles	Mitochondrial dysfunction, excess inflammation and impaired immunity
Lysosomes[2428]	Engulf debris and mediates autophagy	Waste material accumulation
Carboxypeptidase[2429]	Digestive enzyme and digestion of protein	Digestion problems and nutrient deficiencies
Carbonic Anhydrase[2430]	Conversion of carbon dioxide and water to bicarbonate and protons	Anemia and reduced tissue oxygenation
Alkaline phosphatase[2431]	Helps to break down proteins	Liver dysfunction

Zinc and the Immune System

Zinc is an important nutrient for the immune system and zinc deficiency suppresses immunity[2432]. Even a modest zinc deficiency can impair the functions of macrophages, neutrophils, natural killer cells and the complement system, reducing their cytotoxicity[2433,2434,2435,2436]. Zinc is needed for the production of T cells[2437]. People with zinc deficiency show reduced natural killer cell cytotoxicity, which can be fixed with zinc supplementation[2438,2439]. In rats, zinc deficiency alters immunity, which persists in subsequent generations[2440,2441].

Zinc is an essential cofactor for thymulin, which is a thymic hormone[2442,2443]. Without zinc, thymulin can't bind to zinc and this impairs immunity[2444]. With the help of zinc, thymulin helps to differentiate immature T cells[2445], preserving the balance between killer T cells and helper T cells. Autoimmune diseases with a T cell imbalance, such as rheumatoid arthritis, are associated with a zinc deficiency[2446]. Thymulin also modulates the release of cytokines[2447]. Inflammatory responses are also exacerbated under zinc deficiency[2448]. Zinc deficiency decreases thymus hormones, [2449] whereas zinc supplementation can reverse these effects[2450].

Zinc is needed for the interaction between the natural killer cell inhibitory receptor p58 and major histocompatibility complex (MHC) class I molecules[2451]. A deficiency in zinc impairs natural killer cell activity, phagocytosis of macrophages, cytotoxicity of neutrophils and generation of the oxidative burst needed to kill pathogens[2452,2453]. Zinc ions have been shown to stimulate the production of lymphocytes [2454, 2455, 2456], which attack invading pathogens. The addition of zinc releases interleukin-1, interleukin-6, tumor necrosis factor-α and interferon gamma in human peripheral blood mononuclear cells, which help us fight infections[2457,2458,2459].

Low zinc status has been associated with an increased risk of pneumonia, respiratory tract infections, diarrhea and other infectious diseases[2460,2461,2462,2463]. Studies find that zinc supplementation (4-40 mg/day) shortens, and in many instances may prevent the course of infectious diarrhea among malnourished children in third world countries[2464,2465,2466]. Zinc administration helps patients with hepatitis C virus-induced chronic liver disease[2467]. It is also noted that zinc deficiency is related to different autoimmune diseases such as type-1 diabetes, rheumatoid arthritis, multiple sclerosis, systemic lupus, autoimmune hepatitis, celiac disease and Hashimoto's thyroiditis[2468]. **A significant number of COVID-19 patients are zinc deficient, which is associated with worse COVID-19 outcomes**[2469]. Zinc has been shown to inhibit the replication of viruses like SARS and arterivirus[2470].

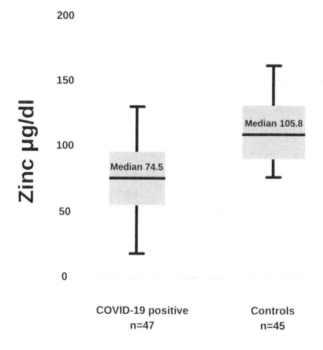

Adapted From: Jothimani et al (2020). 'COVID-19: Poor outcomes in patients with zinc deficiency'. International Journal of Infectious Diseases, 100, 343–349. doi:10.1016/j.ijid.2020.09.014

Zinc may reduce the severity and duration of common cold symptoms by inhibiting viral binding and replication[2471]. According to studies in children, regular use of zinc can prevent the flu[2472]. Taking 13.3 mg zinc acetate lozenges every 2-3 hours has been shown to significantly reduce the duration of cold symptoms compared to placebo[2473]. Zinc gluconate lozenges appear to reduce the duration of cold symptoms but not their severity[2474]. In asymptomatic patients, zinc gluconate nasal spray and zinc orotate lozenges (37 mg zinc every 2–3 hours) did not show a benefit after 7 days [2475]. Out of 14 randomized, placebo-controlled trials, 7 show that zinc has a beneficial effect on the common cold but 7 found no effect[2476]. Lozenges are beneficial only if taken within 24 hours of symptom onset, if the daily dose exceeds 75 mg and the optimal benefits occur when doses of 18 mg of ionic zinc are taken every 2-3 hours with at least four doses taken per day. The optimal dose in adults according to clinical studies is around 80-200 mg/day divided into multiple doses taken[2477]. In general, you should not exceed 200 mg of zinc per day, and doses above 40 mg per day should not be taken for any longer than one to two weeks unless copper is taken in conjunction with it. Avoid nasal sprays as they can cause a lingering loss of smell.

However, zinc may also help with bacterial infections. Zinc enables the calcium-binding protein calprotectin to inhibit the reproduction of bacteria through neutrophil degradation[2478,2479,2480].Prophylactic zinc intake before LPS treatment in a porcine sepsis model has been shown to reduce the inflammatory response[2481]. Thus, doses of zinc before an LPS infection may be protective[2482].

Extremely large doses of zinc (up to 400 mg/day) have been shown to impair immune function[2483,2484,2485]. In vitro, doses 7-8 times the physiological level inhibit T cell function and reduce interferon-alpha production[2486].

Zinc supplementation needs to be done in the right ratio with copper and other minerals. Typical ratios for the general population are 15-20 mg/1 mg zinc/copper or (30-40 mg/2 mg copper), in elderly populations usually 40 of zinc with 1 mg of copper is used once to twice daily. In the AREDs study, 40 mg/1mg of zinc/copper twice daily significantly lowered mortality by 27%, which was seemingly driven by a reduction from deaths from respiratory causes[2487].

Zinc Absorption and Bioavailability

The human body contains about 2-4 grams of zinc, out of which about 0.1% gets depleted every day[2488]. Only 1/1000 of the total zinc pool gets renewed on a daily basis. Zinc's biological half-life is 280 days[2489]. **Up to 57% of zinc in the body is located in muscle and 29% in bone[2490,2491]. There is no separate storage site for zinc in the body, which is why it needs to be obtained from dietary sources on a regular basis.**

The RDA for zinc is 11 mg/day for adult men and 8-9 mg/day for women[2492]. Severe zinc deficiency in the U.S. is currently not considered common, but many are likely subclinically zinc deficient[2493]. According to the U.S. Department of Agriculture, the average daily intake of zinc of men over 20 in 1994-1996 was 13.5 mg and 9.0 mg in women, respectively[2494]. During that same time period, subjects older than 60 obtained a mean 12.0 mg and 8.0 mg zinc a day, respectively[2495]. In people older than 60, 35-45% consume less than 6.8 mg/day of zinc for males and 9.4 mg/day for females[2496]. Most infants in the U.S. appear to consume the recommended amount of zinc per day (2-3 mg/day)[2497]. Zinc intakes seem to also be low in households that suffer from food scarcity[2498]. The elderly in those households get less than 50% of the RDA for zinc[2499].

Adults between the ages of 19-64 in the United Kingdom get on average 10.7 mg (men) and 7.9 mg (women) of zinc per day, which is less than the U.S. RDA[2500]. British children get a similar amount of zinc as adults[2501]. Diets providing only 2.6-3.6 mg/d of zinc for up to 6 months maintain plasma zinc concentrations within the normal range[2502]. However, that amount is considered inadequate for neurological function and can adversely affect cognition[2503]. The absolute minimum intake of zinc for compensating daily losses through urine and sweat has been suggested to be 2-3 mg/day[2504], which could easily be double that for athletes.

Optimal Intake of Zinc (mg/d)

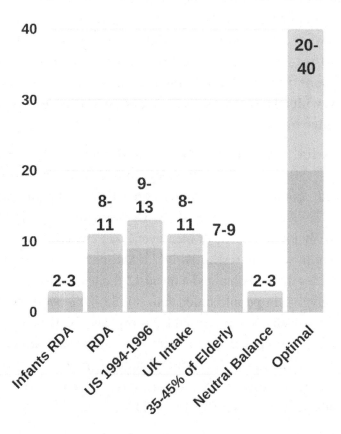

Cereals and pulses are the biggest sources of zinc for most people worldwide[2505]. In the U.S., 30% of zinc is obtained from cereal and pulses, 50% from meat and 20% from dairy[2506]. Red meat is one of the most commonly consumed high zinc foods. Mollusks and oysters are higher in zinc than muscle meat, but they are less frequently consumed. **Red meat avoidance is thought to contribute to iron and zinc deficiency, especially in young premenopausal women** [2507, 2508]. Vegetarian diets, as well as a preference of poultry, fish and dairy over red meat has been shown to increase the risk of zinc deficiency[2509]. The requirement of zinc for vegetarians is at least 50% higher than omnivores because zinc is not particularly bioavailable in plant-based foods[2510]. Thus, adult vegetarian males might need up to 16-20 mg/day and vegetarian females 12-14 mg/day of zinc.

The bioavailability of zinc from Western omnivorous diets has been deemed to be about 20-50%[2511,2512]. In young adults, consuming about 12 mg/day of zinc, this results in 6.6 mg absorbed[2513]. Children in certain U.S. middle- and upper-income families, have been seen to have impaired taste acuity, low hair concentrations of zinc and poor growth[2514]. This is due to "picky eating", but technically, it is due to not eating zinc-rich animal foods like red meat. When giving these children zinc at 2 mg/kg of body weight, their ability to taste, appetite and growth rate improves[2515,2516].

Phytate, phosphate and other phytonutrients are able to chelate zinc, including other minerals[2517]. Phytate is a mineral chelator that affects zinc bioavailability [2518]. In Korean adults, lower zinc bioavailability because of phytates is related to a higher risk of atherosclerosis[2519]. Foods high in phytates like grains bind to zinc, iron and calcium and reduce their absorption, which is why diets high in phytates can cause zinc and iron deficiency[2520,2521]. This is not to say that some unrefined grains cannot be incorporated into a well-balanced diet, but high phytate foods should not make up the majority of the diet. There has been a tendency to focus on iron deficiency but a lack of interest in zinc and copper deficiency, especially because iron levels are frequently low, whereas copper can even be high in serum despite significant deficiency. The demonization of all grains, especially in those who consume large amounts of muscle meat but not organ meats, may be a leading contributor of copper deficiency. On the flip side, a high intake of grains and low intake of animal protein can lead to dwarfism, as observed in Middle Eastern countries such as Turkey, Morocco, Tunisia, Iran and Egypt. The high phytate content of bread in some regions like Iran, where the diet is primarily made up of grains, contributes to zinc deficiency [2522,2523]. Unfortunately, it has been observed that the rising CO2 levels in the atmosphere can reduce the amount of zinc and iron in common crops, such as rice, wheat, peas and soybeans, with projections that a 10% drop in these minerals will occur by the end of the century[2524,2525]. This puts developing countries, which are particularly dependent of these crops, in greater danger of zinc/iron deficiencies.

Phosphates in clay bind to zinc, which is why geophagia (clay eating) is known to cause Iranian dwarfism[2526]. Zinc deficiency has been observed in regions like Egypt and Iran, who typically consume adequate amounts of zinc in their diet, but this is on top of excessive amounts of phytate and fiber[2527]. Thus, the bioavailability of iron, as well as zinc, is lower when eating plant-based diets compared to animal-based diets. Nevertheless, certain compounds in some plant foods, like polyphenols and folate, may help to reduce zinc loss. Indeed, supplementing 400 mcg of folic acid every other day for 4 weeks has been shown to reduce zinc excretion by 50%[2528]. However, polyphenols, such as resveratrol and quercetin, may enhance the uptake of zinc into certain cells via metallothionine[2529].

Another inhibitor of zinc absorption is calcium, which enhances phytate's ability to reduce zinc absorption[2530]. The ratios between phytate-zinc and phytate-zinc-calcium can predict the risk of zinc deficiency[2531]. Increasing dietary calcium increases the excretion of zinc in rats[2532]. In pigs, a high intake of dietary calcium has been shown to promote zinc deficiency[2533]. Pigs fed solely processed peanut meal protein develop zinc deficiency-associated dermatitis, which did not occur in animals who ate clover and alfalfa, or when given zinc supplements[2534]. A high intake of other minerals like copper, magnesium, calcium, iron and nickel also reduces the absorption of zinc[2535].

Ferrous iron (Fe^{2+}) supplements can reduce zinc absorption and lower plasma zinc levels[2536,2537,2538]. That is why experts recommend taking iron *supplements* away from food. However, when zinc and iron are consumed together in a meal, this effect does not seem to happen[2539]. It appears that ferric iron (Fe^{3+}) at a ratio of above 2:1 for iron/zinc reduces the plasma uptake of zinc, which is further reduced by ascorbic acid[2540]. In some studies, even a ratio of 1:1 decreases zinc absorption[2541]. No effect has been seen on zinc absorption with heme iron at a 3:1 iron/zinc ratio. Between 1970-1987, the fortification of food with zinc gluconate and zinc sulfate increased 3- and 27-fold, respectively[2542]. In contrast, addition of iron to food between that same time period increased 120-fold. That further creates a situation where we are getting too much iron that offsets the balance with other minerals, such as copper and zinc.

There are many medications that interact with zinc as well. Certain antibiotics can inhibit the absorption of zinc[2543,2544]. Taking these either 2 hours before, or 4-6 hours after zinc intake, can minimize this effect. Zinc reduces the absorption of penicillamine, which is used to treat rheumatoid arthritis [2545]. Diuretics like chlorthalidone and hydrochlorothiazide increase zinc excretion by as much as 60%[2546]. ACE inhibitors, like lisinopril and other blood pressure lowering medications in this class that end in "pril" deplete zinc [2547]. Omeprazole, a common antacid/heartburn medication, has been found to lower serum zinc levels.[2548] This is because proton pump inhibitors reduce zinc absorption from food due to a reduction in stomach acid.

How much zinc gets absorbed from the diet depends on age, intestinal health and the overall diet[2549]. Zinc deficiency primarily occurs due to reduced zinc absorption, increased zinc excretion or because of an increase in zinc demands[2550,2551]. Inflammation and certain disease states also promote zinc excretion[2552,2553]. Picolinate complexes are more easily absorbed by the body[2554]. Zinc picolinate has been seen to improve zinc status in children with a genetic mutation that prevents them from absorbing zinc from cow's milk[2555].

Factors that increase the demand for zinc:

- Intestinal malabsorption conditions and gut issues, like inflammatory bowel disease, Crohn's, sickle cell anemia, cystic fibrosis as well as diabetes, which can cause secondary zinc deficiency[2556,2557,2558,2559].
- Chronic diarrhea can lead to an excessive loss of zinc, whereas supplementation can help to offset these effects[2560,2561].
- Infections, like hookworm, can result in zinc deficiency, leading to physical and mental developmental problems in children[2562,2563]. Hookworms can also promote iron deficiency.
- Kidney diseases and liver diseases such as liver cirrhosis and non-alcoholic liver disease, alcoholism and chronic

inflammation can increase the urinary excretion of zinc[2564,2565,2566,2567]. Liver cirrhosis patients show abnormally high levels of zinc in the urine[2568].

- Mercury exposure and heavy metal toxicity can cause zinc deficiency[2569,2570]

- Zinc demand increases during pregnancy, nursing and growth periods[2571,2572,2573]. Pregnancy is hallmarked by an increased zinc retention and a lack of nutrition can lead to harm to the fetus that may have long lasting consequences.

- Bariatric surgery causes impaired zinc absorption and promotes zinc deficiency[2574]

- Obesity can increase zinc excretion due to kidney damage[2575,2576]. In obese subjects, plasma zinc concentrations are significantly lower[2577]. Low serum zinc levels in obese patients have been correlated with higher urinary zinc excretion[2578].

- Athletes also have a lower serum zinc level than non-athletes due to increased zinc demands and losses during exercise[2579].

Here is an overview of the things that either improve, inhibit or have no effect on zinc absorption:

Compound	Inhibits Zinc Absorption	Improves Zinc Absorption	No Significant Effect
Copper			X
Calcium	X		
Folic Acid		X	
Ferrous iron (Fe^{2+})	X		
Ferric iron (Fe^{3+})	X		
Heme Iron			X
Phytate	X		

Fiber/Phytonutrients	X		
Antibiotics	X		
Penicillamine	X		
Diuretics (increases zinc urinary losses)	X		
PPIs	X		
ACE Inhibitors	X		
Antacids	X		
Diarrhea	X		
Infections	X		
Inflammation	X		
Alcohol	X		
Intestinal Permeability	X		

A normal amount of zinc in sweat is around 0.15 mg/100 ml, which would equate to 1.5 mg/l lost in sweat per hour[2580]. In hot climates, you can lose up to 5 mg or more of zinc per day[2581]. If someone is already deficient in zinc, that loss may be half as much because zinc excretion decreases with lower zinc status. However, smaller sweat losses of zinc in someone who is zinc deficient can be more consequential due to the baseline zinc deficiency. Zinc is absorbed more efficiently in smaller amounts versus larger doses, and individuals with zinc deficiency tend to absorb it better than those with good status[2582]. This is because zinc homeostasis is tightly regulated with its absorption being adjusted based on influx and excretion[2583,2584].

Consuming up to 325-650 mg of zinc per day due to contamination issues causes zinc poisoning, nausea, abdominal cramping, vomiting and diarrhea[2585]. This high of a zinc overdose is quite rare from food and beverages. Ingesting 4 grams of zinc gluconate (570 mg elemental zinc) has been reported to cause severe nausea and vomiting[2586]. Taking zinc at 150-450 mg/day can lower copper status, alter iron metabolism, reduce immunity and decrease HDL cholesterol[2587]. Doses of zinc at 80 mg/day for up to 6 years is associated with an increased risk of hospitalization for genitourinary issues[2588]. Supplemental doses of 80-150 mg/day of zinc can be immunosuppressive if not taken with copper[2589,2590]. The lowest median effective dose of supplementary zinc is deemed to be 24 mg/day[2591]. Using zinc-containing nasal gels or sprays has been associated with a loss in the sense of smell[2592,2593], which is why the FDA has warned against the use of zinc-containing intranasal products[2594]. The U.S./Canadian upper safety limit for zinc for adults is set at 40 mg/day[2595]. This upper limit was set with a margin of error, as certain side effects began to occur at a total zinc intake of 60 mg/day in certain individuals (10 mg from diet and 50 mg from supplementation).

Zinc is not a mutagen nor a carcinogen[2596]. However, rat studies show that zinc deficiency can cause precancerous cell formation[2597]. However, men taking over 100 mg/day of zinc experience a 2.9-fold increase in the risk for metastatic prostate cancer, which is likely due to copper deficiency[2598]. In rats, zinc toxicity also reduces bone calcium and phosphorus levels, affecting bone mineralization[2599].

Best to worst ways to measure zinc status and zinc deficiency:

- **The best way to measure zinc deficiency is neutrophil zinc levels**[2600].

- **Zinc concentrations in leukocytes or lymphocytes can be much more reflective of zinc status** because they are associated with growth development and immunity[2601]. The ratio between CD4+ and CD8+ T cells has also been proposed as a test for zinc deficiency[2602].

- The levels of zinc in hair can reflect dietary intake of zinc, at least in animals[2603,2604,2605]. There is also a correlation between zinc concentrations in plasma and hair[2606]. The advantage of hair tests is that it can reflect intakes over several months, giving it a more accurate measurement of the body's zinc status. In Egyptian adolescents, zinc concentrations in hair of less than 70 ppm have been associated with symptomatic zinc deficiency[2607].

- Zinc-dependent enzyme activities such as superoxide dismutase, metallothionine and others in organs can be another way to measure zinc deficiency[2608]. In zinc-deficient animals, zinc-metalloenzymes and zinc itself are reduced[2609].

- Plasma and serum zinc levels are most commonly used to assess zinc deficiency, but they do not reflect cellular zinc status[2610]. Clinical symptoms of zinc deficiency can be seen even in the absence of low zinc indicators[2611]. What's more, plasma and serum zinc values fluctuate diurnally and drop after meals and exercise[2612,2613,2614].

The most accurate measurement of zinc deficiency is neutrophil zinc levels and possibly hair mineral analysis. Neutrophil zinc levels in healthy individuals tends to average around 108 ug of zinc/10^{10} cells, whereas those who are deficient in zinc average 82 ug of zinc/10^{10} cells[2615]. Normal zinc values range from 150-240 mcg/g of hair, whereas less than 70 mcg/g may indicate zinc deficiency. Zinc concentration in hair depends on the rate of hair growth and the delivery of zinc to the root, and hence, it is not 100% accurate.

Environmental contamination can also affect copper and zinc levels in hair[2616]. Thus, hair mineral analysis, in addition to neutrophil or perhaps lymphocyte or red blood cell zinc levels, and leukocyte copper levels, should be implemented for assessing suspected zinc and copper deficiency more accurately.

Getting the Right Amount of Zinc from Diet

Since zinc is a copper antagonist, too much dietary zinc can lead to copper deficiency[2617]. Accordingly, too much zinc in relation to copper is associated with hypercholesterolemia and increased coronary heart disease mortality[2618]. At the same time, excess iron supplementation inhibits zinc and copper absorption[2619,2620], which can weaken the immune system and cause copper-deficient anemia. Thus, it is necessary to balance these three minerals – iron, zinc and copper.

There is already an abundance of iron in our food supply, especially because of food fortification. The most commonly fortified foods like cereals, bread and dairy can also chelate zinc because of the phytates and calcium. Phytonutrients also chelate excess iron. Thus, it's not the particular food itself that is either good or bad but the relative amount in relation to your body's homeostatic requirements and how much of what you eat ends up getting absorbed.

Generally, most people should avoid iron supplements and focus on eating iron/zinc/copper rich foods. Here are some guidelines for meeting those guidelines:

- Consume copper-laden organ meats, such as liver, into your diet (0.5-1 oz. per day or 1-3 oz. two to three times per week). Oysters and mollusks are the highest sources of zinc and can be consumed perhaps 1-2 times per week. Other high copper foods include shellfish (lobster and crab), dark chocolate, certain seaweeds, nuts, lentils and beans.
- Daily zinc and iron requirements can be met with appropriate intakes of red meat based on your body's protein and iron/zinc requirements. The RDA for protein is 0.36 g/lb. of bodyweight or 0.8 g/kg, however, many experts consider this to be

inadequate[2621]. In fact, a higher protein intake has been found to be superior in terms of weight loss, satiety, body composition, wound healing and bone density[2622,2623,2624,2625,2626,2627,2628]. Thus, a more appropriate intake for most people is at least 0.6-0.7 g of protein/lb. of body weight or 1.2-1.4 g/kg. The optimal daily protein intake for muscle growth and hypertrophy appears to be 0.8-1.0 g/lb or 1.6-2.2 g/kg of body weight[2629].

- If you are eating a vegetarian diet, a diet high in phytates, and/or are using zinc inhibitors such as certain medications and antacids, then your zinc demand increases. Thus, you may need up to 50-100% more zinc every day.

Zinc supplementation is not needed when you are getting enough of it from diet. Zinc supplementation is mostly beneficial for fixing deficiencies quickly or trying to help with an acute infection. Chronic intakes of zinc over 80-100 mg/day can promote copper depletion, especially if dietary copper intake is not concomitantly increased. **The idea is to try and obtain anywhere from 20-80 mg of zinc, 8-18 mg of iron and 3 mg of copper each day.** This will of course depend on the person.

Chapter 10
Hypothyroidism and Hyperthyroidism:
The Sodium-Selenium-Iodine Connection

Your metabolism is always working, and the body is always producing energy. Metabolic rate and energy balance are regulated in large part by the thyroid gland, which is located at the base of your neck just below the Adam's apple. Thyroid cells absorb iodine from food and combine it with the amino acid tyrosine, which is used to create thyroid hormones such as thyroxine (T4) and triiodothyronine (T3). Most of the effects of thyroid hormones are performed by the active thyroid hormone T3[2630]. There are also T0, T1 and T2, which act as hormone precursors and byproducts. Thyroid hormones, primarily T3, are then released into the bloodstream to affect your body temperature, growth, daily caloric needs, heart rate and metabolic rate[2631]. The production of thyroid hormones requires certain minerals, in particular, iodine, selenium, sodium, zinc and magnesium. Only 20-50% of all iodine in the body is found in thyroid hormones or the thyroid gland, whereas the other 50-80% is concentrated in non-thyroid tissues.[2632,2633]

Thyroid dysfunction, or low thyroid function (hypothyroidism), can cause a wide variety of health problems. If your metabolic rate plummets because of inadequate thyroid hormone output or function, this can increase the risk of chronic diseases, such as insulin resistance, metabolic syndrome and cardiovascular disease[2634,2635]. These harms are not necessarily from overeating but from storing more calories as fat even when you are consuming the same amount of food. Having either excessive (hyperthyroidism) or deficient thyroid hormone function (hypothyroidism) can cause harm to your health. Thus, it is harder to stay at an optimal body composition and in good metabolic health if your thyroid, or your thyroid hormones, are not working properly. Symptoms of hypothyroidism include chronic fatigue, weight loss plateaus or weight gain, low testosterone and sex drive, cognitive dysfunction, intolerance to cold, joint pain, constipation, hair loss, brittle skin, water retention, depression and high cholesterol levels[2636,2637,2638,2639].

Virtually every cell in your body has a thyroid hormone receptor[2640,2641]. They are located in the nucleus of cells and on the cell wall. The thyroid hormones enter the cell with the help of a transporter. Since the 1960s, it was thought that the uptake of thyroid into cells depends on merely the concentration of free hormones (the "free hormone hypothesis")[2642,2643,2644], but this idea has been shown to be incorrect. It is now clear that thyroid activity in virtually all tissues and cells is rate-limited by the rate of thyroid hormone transportation into cells by transporters[2645,2646,2647,2648].

Cellular uptake of the thyroid hormones T4 and T3 is dependent on energy (ATP), magnesium and sodium[2649,2650,2651,2652,2653,2654]. One of the main thyroid hormone transporters is the sodium-iodide symporter (NIS)[2655]. The NIS transports two sodium cations (Na^+) and one iodide anion (I^-) into the thyroid gland. Albumin also appears to also have an essential role in thyroid hormone transportation[2656]. Indeed, ingested iodine gets put onto serum proteins, such as albumin, for its movement throughout the body.

In this chapter, we are going to look at optimizing thyroid function from a mineral perspective. This chapter will include information about the prevalence of thyroid diseases and the minerals needed for thyroid hormone transporters to work.

Iodine, Hypothyroidism and Goiter

Thyroid hormone levels are regulated by thyroid-stimulating hormone (TSH), also known as thyrotropin. TSH promotes the uptake of iodine by the thyroid and stimulates the synthesis and release of T4 and T3. Thyroid hormone production works in a negative feedback loop with TSH. In other words, when you have low thyroid hormones you will have an elevated TSH. This is why people with hypothyroidism have high TSH levels because their body is trying to make more thyroid hormones. In the presence of iodine, T4 gets synthesized and is transformed into T3 based on needs. The formation of thyroid hormones is initiated by thyroglobulin (Tg), which gets synthesized by TSH when thyroid hormones are low[2657]. If iodine is overconsumed, the activity of sodium-iodide symporter (NIS) decreases in order to slow down the synthesis of thyroid hormones[2658].

Iodine is an essential trace mineral needed for thyroid functioning, thyroid hormone synthesis, physical and mental development and metabolism[2659]. It can only be obtained from diet or supplements. Low iodine status is one of the biggest risk factors for hypothyroidism[2660]. Iodine is the heaviest, yet least abundant, element that occurs in several oxidation states, such as iodide (I^-) and iodate (IO^{-3})[2661]. The French chemist Bernard Courtois discovered iodine during the era of the Napoleonic wars in 1811[2662]. *'Iode'* comes from the Greek word ιοειδής, referring to the violet color of iodine vapor[2663]. In 1908, Antonio Grossrich came up with the idea for using iodine tinctures to rapidly sterilize human skin out in the field. Iodine has antimicrobial effects even in low concentrations, which is why it is commonly used in hospitals and for disinfecting medical wounds[2664]. Additionally, iodide combined to DHA and arachidonic acid in cell membranes protects them from oxidative damage[2665,2666]. Indeed, iodide acts as an electron donor in the presence of hydrogen peroxide and peroxidases. Thus, iodine/iodide is important for protecting against lipid peroxidation and oxidative stress. In fact, it is thought that the high levels of iodine in algae played an important antioxidant role when they first started to produce oxygen 3 billion years ago. Additionally, T4 and rT3 have been shown to be more potent at inhibiting lipid peroxidation compared to vitamin E, glutathione or vitamin C. Thus, iodide and thyroid hormones act as antioxidants.[2667]

Thyroid hormones like thyroxine (T4) and triiodothyronine (T3) need dietary iodine to carry out enzymatic reactions, regulate metabolic rate and body temperature. Iodine contributes to 65% of the molecular weight of T4 and 59% of T3. Only about 10-20% of T3 is secreted by the thyroid gland itself, whereas most of it is produced from T4[2668]. Up to 80% of T3 gets created outside of the thyroid gland through deiodination of T4 with the help of type I deiodinase in the liver and kidneys[2669,2670,2671]. Skeletal muscle can also initiate the conversion of T4 into T3[2672].

An iodine-replete adult contains about 25-50 mg of iodine out of which 20-50% is stored in the thyroid[2673]. The iodine gets transported into the thyroid as iodide by the sodium-iodide symporter (NIS). This NIS-mediated delivery of iodide into the follicular cells of the thyroid gland is the first step in the synthesis of thyroid hormones[2674]. That is why the concentration of iodine in the thyroid gland is 20-50 times greater than in the plasma[2675]. The remaining iodine that is left in the bloodstream will be excreted through urine.

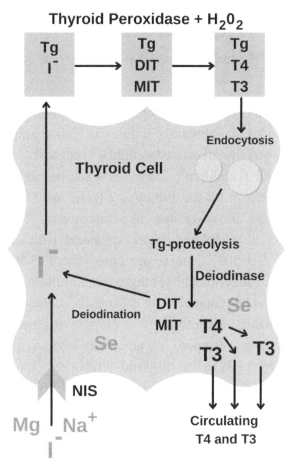

Adapted from: Zimmermann, M. B., Jooste, P. L., & Pandav, C. S. (2008). 'Iodine-deficiency disorders.' The Lancet, 372(9645), 1251–1262.

Figure description from the paper:

Iodide (I⁻) is transported into the thyrocyte by the sodium-iodide symporter (NIS) at the basal membrane and migrates to the apical membrane. I⁻ is oxidised by the enzymes thyroperoxidase (TPO) and hydrogen peroxidase (H_2O_2) and attached to tyrosyl residues in thyroglobulin (Tg) to produce the hormone precursors iodotyrosine (MIT) and di-iodotyrosine (DIT). Residues then couple to form thyroxine (T4) and triiodothyronine (T3) within the Tg molecule in the follicular lumen. Tg enters the cell by endocytosis and is digested. T4 and T3 are released into the circulation, and iodine on MIT and DIT is recycled within the thyrocyte.[2676]

The size of the thyroid gland is dependent on iodine intake, whereby an excessive or deficient intake of iodine can lead to goiter[2677]. Iodine-induced goiter was first described in the 19th century[2678] and it has also been documented in children[2679]. Excessive iodine intake is thought to contribute to goiter in Sudan, Ethiopia, Algeria and China.[2680,2681,2682] It can also lead to reversible hypothyroidism[2683]. Subclinical hypothyroidism is more predominant in areas with chronic excess iodine intake[2684]. A 2017 Chinese meta-analysis of 43 studies saw that the prevalence of subclinical hypothyroidism in those who consumed excess iodine was 8% compared to 3% and 2% of those with adequate or deficient intake, respectively[2685]. Hypothyroidism from excess iodine intake may happen because of thyroid autoimmunity, characterized by elevated antithyroid antibodies. Excess iodine is considered a risk factor for the development of thyroid autoimmune disease[2686,2687]. Autoimmune thyroiditis and hypothyroidism are more common the older you get with antibodies peaking at 45-55 years of age[2688,2689]. Urinary iodine levels > 300 µg/L are considered excessive in children and adults and levels > 500 µg/L are considered excessive in pregnant women.[2690]

The relationship between iodine intake and thyroid disorders is U-shaped[2691,2692]. Both too low, as well as excessive iodine intake, results in hypothyroidism, hyperthyroidism and potentially autoimmune thyroiditis[2693,2694]. Excess iodine can also cause hyperthyroidism, which happens after the iodine-deficient thyroid gland nodules escape the control of TSH and start overproducing thyroid hormones. Graves' disease is the most common form of hyperthyroidism [2695]. Other autoimmune thyroid disorders include Hashimoto's thyroiditis, post-partum thyroiditis and autoimmune arthritis [2696], [2697]. Hashimoto's thyroiditis is associated with a significantly higher risk of papillary thyroid carcinoma[2698]. Thyroiditis refers to inflammation of the thyroid gland. Inflammation also promotes hypothyroidism by blocking T4 conversion to T3[2699]. Low thyroid individuals have a higher risk of hip fractures and non-spine fractures[2700,2701].

Here are the iodine-dependent enzymes, functions and consequences that may occur with a deficit in iodine:

Iodine-Dependent Enzymes/Proteins	Function	Consequences of Deficit
Thyroid Hormones	Regulates metabolic rate, body temperature and energy balance	Chronic fatigue, frailty, weight gain, metabolic syndrome and decreased immunity
Thyroglobulin	Initiates thyroid hormone synthesis	Low thyroid function
Sodium-Iodine Symporter	Transports iodine into thyroid cells	Iodine deficiency and impaired thyroid function
Apoptosis[2702]	Programmed cell death and elimination of premalignancies	Accumulation of dysfunctional cells
Mucinase[2703]	Breaks down mucus and bacteria	Increased risk of infection

Brain Receptor Formation[2704]	Proper cognitive and mental development	Increased risk of cretinism and mental retardation

In Europe, the prevalence of undiagnosed thyroid dysfunction is 6.71% (4.94% hypothyroidism and 1.72% hyperthyroidism) [2705]. The prevalence of hyperthyroidism in the UK has been estimated at 2.7% in women and 0.23% in men [2706]. In the U.S., subclinical hyperthyroidism occurs in 1.3% of the population [2707]. In iodine-sufficient countries, hypothyroidism rates are rare at 1-2% [2708]. In Europe, it ranges from 0.2-5.3% and in the U.S. from 0.3-3.7% [2709,2710,2711]. Hypothyroidism is about 10 times more prevalent in women than in men because they have higher iodine requirements during lactation and pregnancy [2712].

Here are the risk factors for developing hypothyroidism or hyperthyroidism [2713]

- Pregnancy or lactation [2714]
- Iodine deficiency
- Iodine excess
- Rapid transition from iodine deficiency to sufficiency [2715]
- Autoimmune conditions [2716]
- Genetic risk factors [2717,2718]
- Smoking
- Selenium deficiency [2719]
- Drugs and pharmaceuticals
- Infections [2720]

There is also a link between excess iodine intake and thyroid cancer [2721]. However, these associations are not significant [2722]. A 2017 meta-analysis of 16 studies found a small correlation of an increased prevalence of papillary thyroid cancer from regions with high iodine intake based on urinary iodine level of $\geq$300 mcg/L [2723]. However, a

306

low intake of iodine can also increase the risk of hypothyroidism and thyroid cancer [2724]. Importantly, a meta-analysis discovered that consumption of iodine-rich seafood (>300 mcg/day of iodine) decreased the risk of thyroid cancer[2725]. Molecular iodine (I_2) at 3 mg/day has been proposed to be able to suppress benign and cancerous neoplasias due to its antioxidative effects[2726]. Radioactive iodine can increase the risk of thyroid cancer and its uptake is higher in iodine-deficient people[2727]. Thus, iodine-deficient people are at a higher risk of developing thyroid cancer. Potassium iodide is an FDA approved thyroid-blocking agent used to lower the risk of thyroid cancer[2728]. Iodine-131 is the primary component of nuclear reactors and fallouts [2729]. Ingesting large doses of non-radioactive iodine like potassium iodide at doses of 130 mg and 65 mg reduces the uptake of radioactive iodine by the thyroid[2730]. However, adults should not take potassium iodide unless they are expecting to get exposed to a large dose of radioactive iodine. The FDA recommends all children, young adults, newborns and pregnant women take potassium iodide when they have been contaminated or are expecting to get contaminated with radioactive iodide to protect their thyroid.[2731]

There's an interrelationship between thyroid dysfunction and hypogonadism or low testosterone in men[2732]. Free testosterone levels are reduced in subjects with hypothyroidism and thyroid hormone treatment normalizes that[2733]. Testosterone has protective effects on thyroid autoimmunity by reducing titres of thyroid peroxidase and thyroglobulin antibodies[2734]. There is an association between erectile dysfunction and hypothyroidism[2735]. Hypothyroidism increases the risk of gaining weight and developing obesity [2736,2737], which can promote metabolic syndrome and other chronic diseases.

Many people with low thyroid levels get an elevation in cholesterol as well as triglyceride levels[2738,2739]. The relationship between hypo-thyroidism and high cholesterol has been established since the 1930s[2740]. Hypothyroid patients have elevated lipoprotein(a) [Lp(a)], which is a risk factor for cardiovascular disease. Lp(a) attracts oxidized lipids and can cause inflammation[2741,2742]. Those with hypothyroidism also have higher phospholipase A2 (Lp-PLA2), which is a pro-inflammatory enzyme that moves with LDL particles[2743,2744]. C-reactive protein (CRP), one of the primary markers of inflammation has been found to be elevated in patients with subclinical hypothyroidism, which increases cardiovascular disease risk[2745].

The body needs thyroid hormones to use cholesterol and cholesterol is a precursor to testosterone and other steroid hormones like DHEA, pregnenalone and progesterone [2746]. Thyroid hormones influence cholesterol synthesis, catabolism, absorption and excretion by regulating cholesterol 7alpha-hydroxylase (CYP7A), the rate-limiting enzyme in the synthesis of bile acids [2747, 2748, 2749]. T3 stimulates lipoprotein lipase (LPL) to increase the breakdown of VLDL cholesterol[2750]. Furthermore, T3 increases the expression of LDL cholesterol receptors that enable LDL to enter cells to be used for its essential functions instead of staying in the bloodstream[2751,2752]. T3 can protect LDL from becoming oxidized by mopping up free radicals[2753]. In patients with hypothyroidism and hyperlipidemia, high cholesterol and blood lipids improve once thyroid function is restored[2754]. T4 therapy has been shown to reduce total cholesterol and LDL cholesterol[2755]. Those with higher TSH levels have a more drastic reduction in cholesterol. In people with subclinical hypothyroidism, T4 therapy drops total cholesterol by 8 mg/dL and LDL cholesterol by 10 mg/dL[2756]. However, if circulating free T4 is too high this can promote the oxidation of LDL[2757]. With optimal thyroid function, T4 will get converted into its active form T3, preventing any damaging effects on lipoprotein particles.

Studies also suggest that high TSH levels may directly raises cholesterol and triglyceride levels by decreasing hepatic lipase[2758]. Even TSH in the upper limits of normal (above 2.1 µU/ml) is associated with a less favorable cardiometabolic profile and a higher risk of developing cardiovascular diseases[2759]. Hyperthyroidism, or an over-active thyroid, has the opposite effect to hypothyroidism and is associated with low HDL and LDL levels[2760,2761,2762]. This is not ideal as very low cholesterol is associated with depression, memory loss and increased mortality[2763,2764,2765].

Subclinical hypothyroidism is associated with an increased risk of coronary heart disease events and mortality, especially in those

with a TSH level of 10 mIU/L or higher (normal range 0.5-5 mIU/L)[2766]. Thyroid hormones are important for the development of a healthy heart and abnormal thyroid hormone function can cause issues like cardiac hypertrophy and irregular heartbeat[2767]. Heart, endothelial and other cells have thyroid hormone receptors which regulate thyroid hormone function[2768]. Thyroid dysfunction can affect cardiac output, blood pressure, vascular resistance and heart rhythm[2769]. Iodine-deficient freshwater fish have a higher incidence of cancer and heart disease compared to marine animals[2770,2771]. Administration of iodide, the reduced form of iodine, has been shown to protect the heart tissue from myocardial ischemia reperfusion injury in mice[2772]. Smoking increases the risk of atherosclerosis, cardiovascular disease and autoimmune conditions like Graves' disease[2773]. Importantly, smokers appear to have lower levels of thyroid stimulating hormone activity than non-smokers[2774]. Smoking is also associated with an increased risk of thyroid disease[2775].

The RDA for iodine in schoolchildren is 120 mcg and 150 mcg for adults[2776]. During pregnancy, the RDA for iodine increases to 220-250 mcg[2777]. Despite the fact that the safe upper level of intake of iodine is 1,100 mcg/day[2778], intakes of ≥500 mcg/day of iodine for several weeks has been shown to cause an increase in TSH response to thyrotropin-releasing hormone (TRH), which is a hormone that stimulates the release of TSH from the pituitary gland[2779]. TSH tends to increase during hypothyroidism[2780]. Hypothyroid individuals may react worse to doses of iodine ≥750 mcg /day[2781]. In children, thyroid function tests have been seen to stay within the normal range even with intakes of iodine at 4,500 mcg/day for 2 weeks[2782]. The Joint Food and Agriculture Organization of the United Nations and WHO Expert Committee on Food Additives has suggested that the maximal upper limit of 1 mg/day of iodine from all sources would be safe for most people, except for those with iodine sensitivity or thyroid problems[2783]. However, Japanese people consume on average 25 times more than the safety upper limit of 1 mg/day and show no higher rates of autoimmune thyroiditis or hypothyroidism[2784].

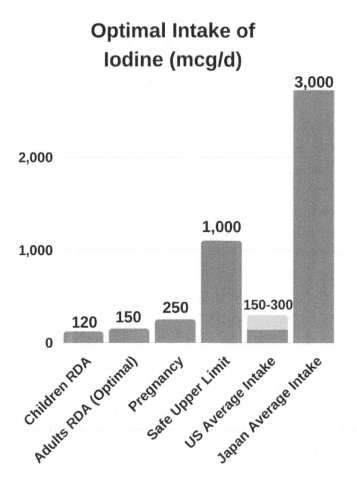

Optimal Intake of Iodine (mcg/d)

The World Health Organization estimates that 2 billion people worldwide have insufficient iodine intake [2785]. About 31.5% of schoolchildren worldwide are iodine deficient. In Europe, 44% of schoolchildren have insufficient iodine intake[2786,2787]. Tropical regions and many European countries have a fairly high prevalence of iodine deficiency[2788,2789]. Over the past 40 years, iodine deficiency has increased by four-fold in developed countries[2790]. In the 1970s, about 1 in 40 individuals in the U.S. had moderate to high iodine deficiency[2791]. By the 1990s, this number had risen to 1 in 9 people. Although urinary iodine levels have decreased by 50% since the early 1970s, most people in the United States are still considered iodine sufficient[2792]. The average daily iodine intake in the U.S. is 216 mcg/day, ranging from 141-296 mcg across all age groups, based on data from 2008-2012[2793]. Sub-Saharan African countries like Ethiopia, Sierra Leone and Angola suffer from iodine deficiency, whereas the Congo, Uganda and Kenya have iodine excess[2794,2795]. Nigeria was the first African country to successfully eliminate iodine deficiency[2796]. Attempts to implement iodine-salt programs in those countries have failed because of political instability and conflict[2797]. **Currently, there are 25 countries worldwide where iodine insufficiency is a public health concern**[2798].

Food and Other Sources of Iodine

Naturally, iodine is obtained from the diet, but this depends on the soil content. Importantly, many regions have low soil iodine content, especially those areas that are far inland from the coast[2799]. That is why iodine intake in the United States primarily comes from iodized salt, which is in the form of potassium iodide in North America but potassium iodate in other regions due to its better stability in hot/humid climates. Vaporized sea water coming as rainfall is not always able to enrich the soil with enough iodine. This is true even for some coastal areas like the Zanzibar Islands of Tanzania[2800]. Mountainous regions and river valleys have the most iodine-deficient soils in the world. Crops and animals grown on low iodine land and consuming low iodine foods become deficient in iodine, which leads to low iodine intakes and iodine deficiency in populations of that region.

Shrimp and especially seaweeds are rich in iodine. About 1-3% of seawater algae's dry weight is pure iodine[2801,2802]. If humans were to contain that large of a percentage of iodine, we would have up to 500 mg of iodine with us, contrasting to the 25-50 mg we currently have. Brown algae seaweed accumulate more than 30,000 times more iodine in seawater[2803,2804]. East-Asian countries like Japan and Korea include a lot of seaweeds into their diet[2805]. The average iodine intake in Japan is 1.2 mg/day from eating seaweeds like kelp, nori and kombu[2806]. Other studies support this high level of intake of iodine in Japan, which ranges between 1,000-3,000 mcg (1-3 mg)/day[2807]. However, the amount of iodine in commercially available seaweeds like kelp or nori

311

can range from 16-2,984 mcg per gram of food[2808]. Most foods eaten on traditional Western diets provide about 3–80 mcg of iodine per 3-5 oz serving[2809,2810]. The typical Swiss diet provides approximately 140 mcg/day of iodine, which is slightly below the RDA[2811]. In Lybia, the typical range of iodine intake is 100-180 mcg /day[2812]. According to the World Health Organization, based on estimates from 2002, the proportion of the population with insufficient iodine intake (measured as urinary iodine < 100 mcg/L) is as follows, Americas (9.8%), Western Pacific (24.0%), South-East Asia (39.8%), Africa (42.6%), Eastern Mediterranean (54.1%) and Europe (56.9%)[2813]. In other words, more than 1 out of 2 people in Europe is iodine insufficient, which is a major problem. This is driven by Europe's low intake of iodized salt and poor overall diet.

The Standard American Diet is typically low in iodine unless it includes things like pastured eggs, cranberries, milk, yogurt, shrimp, oysters, tuna/cod or seaweed[2814]. However, there has been reported cases of thyrotoxicosis due to accidental eating of thyroid tissue mixed with beef burgers[2815,2816,2817]. Acute thyrotoxicosis is usually treated with potassium iodide[2818]. Dairy and milk can also be a reliable source of iodine in many diets, including camel milk and goat milk[2819]. Vegan diets that lack seafood and dairy dramatically increase the risk of iodine deficiency unless seaweeds or two and a half medium sized potatoes are eaten on a daily basis.

Iodized bread and milk are the biggest sources of dietary iodine in the U.S. and Europe. The concentration of iodine in milk in industrialized countries ranges from 33-534 mcg/L, depending on the iodine intake of the dairy cows [2820 , 2821]. Iodine fortified foods and mineral supplements are often given to cattle to improve their iodine status[2822]. Iodophor disinfectants used for cleaning milk cans and cows' teats may also increase the iodine content of milk[2823]. Most commercial bread has extraordinarily little iodine, but it can be fortified with potassium iodate or calcium iodate [2824]. Pasta can contain iodine only when cooked in water with iodized salt or when made out of iodized dough. Most fruits and vegetables are a poor source of iodine.

Iodine is especially important during the first 1000 days of life, as infants in that timeframe are more vulnerable to hypothyroidism and developmental issues[2825,2826]. Thyroid hormones are needed for the brain's myelination and neuronal migration[2827]. An iodine deficiency during infancy can impair physical and neuromotor development[2828,2829]. It also increases the risk of stillbirths, abortions and developmental abnormalities[2830,2831]. Impaired thyroid function in iodine-deficient children is correlated with reduced insulin-like growth factor-1 (IGF-1) and IGF-binding protein-3 (IGFBP-3) and stunted growth[2832,2833]. Although severe iodine deficiency is rare in developed countries, even mild-to-modest deficiencies or insufficiencies could cause developmental complications to the child[2834,2835,2836].

A severe iodine deficiency in utero may lead to cretinism, which causes mental retardation, deaf-mutism (a person who is both deaf and unable to speak) and spasticity[2837]. Two meta-analysis have discovered that populations with chronic iodine deficiency have their intelligence quotient reduced by 12.5-13.5 points [2838, 2839]. In Baihuyaon, North-Eastern China, 72% of those born during severe iodine deficiency showed signs of neurological abnormalities, depressed intelligence and many had impaired neuromotor development[2840]. Similar findings have been observed in other areas of China and South America[2841]. However, it is difficult to differentiate the effects of in utero iodine deficiency and current iodine deficiency in later life. Iodine supplementation for 24 weeks in Albanian children has been shown to improve information processing, fine motor skills and visual problem solving[2842]. Iodine supplementation in iodine-deficient areas has had a positive effect on children's physical and mental development as well as reducing mortality[2843]. Thus, iodine intake is especially critical during the first developmental periods of life. Selenium deficiency is also thought to contribute to cretinism and lower intelligence as iodine and selenium work together in the formation of thyroid hormones[2844].

Most guidelines recommend an iodine intake of 220-290 mcg/day during pregnancy and lactation, respectively[2845,2846]. T4 production increases by 50% during pregnancy, which requires additional iodine intake[2847]. The American Thyroid Association recommends women planning pregnancy to add 150 mcg/day of iodine from potassium iodide[2848]. The American Academy of Pediatrics recommends the same dose of 150 mcg/day of iodine plus the use of iodized salt[2849]. According to the NHANES 2011–2014 data, 72.2% of pregnant woman took a dietary supplement, but only 17.8% of them took a product that contained iodine[2850]. However, iodine doses of ≥ 200 mcg/day can elevate TSH levels above 3 mU/mL in pregnant women as compared to those who took <100 mcg/day[2851]. Thus, high doses of supplemental iodine may lead to thyroid issues. It appears that getting more iodine naturally through diet, which also provides other nutrients like selenium, is safer compared to using bolus doses of iodine from supplements.

Women in regions with high dietary iodine intake have higher amounts of iodine in their breast milk[2852,2853]. In Korean preterm infants, subclinical hypothyroidism is associated with high iodine levels in breast milk[2854,2855]. Expression of the sodium-iodide symporter (NIS) in mammary glands regulates iodine absorption and contributes to the presence of iodine in breast milk. In the thyroid, NIS is regulated by thyroid stimulating hormone, whereas in breast tissue prolactin, oxytocin and β-estradiol regulate its expression. Some environmental chemicals like perchlorate, pertechnetate, nitrate and thiocyanate can compete with iodine absorption by hijacking the sodium-iodide cotransporter[2856,2857,2858,2859]. **Fluoride in drinking water may also inhibit the sodium-iodide symporter activity, causing iodine deficiency**[2860].

Infant formulas have to be fortified with iodine to mimic breast milk nutrition. The infant formulas in the U.S. are regulated to contain 5-76 mcg/100 kcal of iodine, whereas in the EU it is 15–29 mcg/100 kcal[2861]. If the mother is iodine deficient, their whole-body iodine stores will be more concentrated in their breast milk to safeguard infant dietary requirements[2862]. Prenatal supplements containing iodine are being recommended during pregnancy and lactation, but if the mother is already consuming too much iodine it may cause fetal complications[2863]. The iodine content of supplements is not labeled accurately across the board. Indeed, an Italian survey discovered that the labeled iodine content was inaccurate in over half of the tested supplements, ranging from 1.9-11 times higher than what was on the label[2864]. Out of 43 products, 17 didn't even have iodine labeled at all despite containing it. In 4 supplements, the maximal suggested daily dose exceeded the tolerable upper limit for iodine of 600 mcg (the upper limit adopted by the Scientific Committee for Food).

Here are the foods highest in iodine taken from the USDA, FDA and ODS-NIH Database for the Iodine Content of Common Foods Release 1.0 (2020)[2865,2866,2867]

Food	Mcg of Iodine per Serving	% of RDA (150 mcg)
Seaweed, Nori, 1 oz	664 mcg	440%
Haddock, fish, 3 oz	200 mcg	134%
Whole-Wheat Bread, iodate dough, 1 slice	198 mcg	132%
Lobster, 3.5 oz	185 mcg	123%
White Bread, iodate dough, 1 slice	185 mcg	123%
Cod, cooked, 3 oz	156 mcg	106%
Iodized Table Salt, 1/2 tsp	142-152 mcg	102%
Crab, cooked, 3 oz	32.5-150 mcg	100%
Iodized Sea Salt, 1/2 tsp	148 mcg	98%
Greek Yogurt, 1 cup	116 mcg	77%
Oysters, 3 oz	93 mcg	62%
Milk, nonfat, 1 cup	85 mcg	57%
Fish Sticks, cooked, 3 oz	58 mcg	39%
Mollusks, clam, 3 oz	50 mcg	31%
Pollock, fish, 3 oz	38 mcg	26%

Milk Chocolate, 3 oz	36 mcg	25%
Salmon, fish, 3 oz	30 mcg	21%
Egg, boiled, 1 large	26 mcg	17%
Protein Powder, 1 oz	25 mcg	16%
Chorizo, pork, 3 oz	22 mcg	12%
Pasta, enriched, boiled in water with iodized salt, 3 oz	22 mcg	12%
Bologna, beef/pork, 3 oz	20 mcg	10%
Beef Liver, 3 oz	14 mcg	9%
Cheddar Cheese, 1 oz	14 mcg	9%
Swordfish, 3 oz	12 mcg	8%
Tuna, 3 oz	7 mcg	5%
Beef Roast, 3 oz	3 mcg	2%
Chicken Breast, 3 oz	2 mcg	1%
Whole-Wheat Bread, without iodate dough, 1 slice	1 mcg	1%
White Bread, without iodate dough, 1 slice	1 mcg	1%
Brown Rice, cooked, 1 cup	1 mcg	1%
Sea Salt, non-iodized, ¼ tsp	<1 mcg	<1%
Broccoli, boiled, ½ cup	0 mcg	0%
Banana, 1 medium	0 mcg	0%
Lima Beans, boiled, ½ cup	0 mcg	0%

To get the right amount of iodine, you would want to consume a diet that provides anywhere from 150-300 mcg/day of iodine. That ensures there is circulating iodine in your system in adequate quantities to fuel thyroid hormones. The above foods also cover many other essential minerals that tend to be neglected like zinc and copper. For daily consumption, nutrient-dense foods like eggs, pork and dairy are great options. Fortified foods are great only if you do not have access to the above foods and should not be the staple of your diet.

Raw cruciferous vegetables contain goitrogenic compounds called glucosinolates that if overconsumed may inhibit iodine absorption and cause low thyroid function[2868]. Cruciferous vegetables include collard greens, broccoli, kale, cauliflower, cabbage and arugula. Soy, cassava, peanuts, corn, certain beans, millet, pine nuts and strawberries also contain goitrogens[2869]. Cooking lowers the amount of goitrogenic compounds, thus, if you consume these foods cooked, then its much less likely that there will be any issues[2870]. Indeed, in one study, the addition of 150 grams (5 oz.) of cooked Brussels sprouts daily for 4 weeks had no effect on thyroid function compared to controls[2871].

Most goitrogenic foods do not have a clinical effect in people who are getting adequate amounts of iodine from their food. It will have a bigger impact in those who are already iodine deficient or are consuming a diet low in iodine. If you have thyroid problems, then it's not a good idea to eat raw cruciferous vegetables. Nevertheless, the intake of cruciferous vegetables is associated with a reduced risk for cancer and cardiovascular disease[2872]. The breakdown products of glucosinolates activate anti-cancer pathways[2873,2874]. Thus, it is not necessarily recommended to stop eating cruciferous vegetables, as long as you are eating plenty of iodine-rich foods and cooking your vegetables properly.

Some amino acids can partially inhibit thyroid hormone transport by competing with the receptors[2875]. In rat small intestinal cells, tryptophan, phenylalanine and tyrosine inhibit T3 trans-portation[2876,2877]. Leucine has also been found to have inhibitory effects on T3 and T4 uptake by pituitary cells[2878]. Large doses of amino acids in isolation, like a tryptophan supplement or a branched chain/essential amino acid supplement, may have a competitive effect, but this may only be an issue for an hour after consumption. Whole food protein sources tend to be the most bioavailable sources of nutrients like iodine and selenium that are needed for good thyroid health.

Certain medications can inhibit thyroid hormone uptake into certain tissues by competing with them due to structural similarities[2879,2880]. These include certain antiarrhythmic drugs, calcium channel blockers (like nifedipine, verapamil and diltiazem), calmodulin antagonists and benzodiazepines[2881,2882,2883,2884]. Some anti-inflammatory drugs like diphenylhydantoin, meclofenamic acid, mefenamic acid, fenclofenac, flufenamic acid and diclofenac inhibit T3 uptake[2885]. Medications that have goitrogenic effects include antibiotics like ciprofloxacin and rifampin, steroids, statins and others[2886,2887,2888,2889,2890,2891]. However, diabetic drugs like metformin may reduce the goitrogenic effects of type-2 diabetes and obesity[2892,2893]. ACE inhibitors such as benazepril, lisinopril and fosinopril are blood pressure medications that can elevate potassium levels when taken together with potassium iodide. Taking potassium iodide with potassium-sparing diuretics can also cause hyperkalemia (high potassium). Certain food chemicals and flavor-enhancers like perchlorate block the thyroid's ability to absorb and utse dietary iodine[2894]. Perchlorate pervades food and water supplies throughout the U.S[2895].

Food deprivation and calorie restriction are known to reduce thyroid hormone output, thus lowering energy expenditure and mood[2896]. The hypothalamus-pituitary-thyroid (HPT) axis responds to environmental and nutritional challenges in a dynamic way by regulating thyroid hormones and metabolism to preserve energy during perceived starvation[2897]. Any form of chronic energetic stress and deprivation will reduce thyroid hormone output, increasing the risk of hypothyroidism. This is especially relevant for people who are trying to lose weight.

Chronic low calorie dieting can cause irreversible damage to the thyroid. A 2016 study on the Biggest Loser competitors discovered that 6 years after the show the participants had regained 70% of the

318

weight they initially lost and were burning 700 fewer calories per day compared to when they started the show[2898]. Despite gaining some lean muscle during the show, their metabolic rate didn't increase due to the severe calorie restriction they experienced, which mimicked starvation. This is the result of crash dieting and yo-yo dieting, which inevitably disrupts thyroid function. Studies have found that intermittent energy restriction vs. continuous energy restriction provides greater weight loss[2899]. At the end of the day you have to find out what gives you the best results but know that losing a lot of weight quickly could make it harder for you to keep the weight off.

Prolonged fasting for 72 hours has been shown to decrease serum T3 by 30% and thyroid-stimulating hormone by 70% in healthy men[2900]. Similar results have been noted with 4-day fasts[2901]. Men typically see greater changes than women. However, T3 and reverse T3 return to prefasting levels after refeeding and returning to eating a normal diet[2902]. Thus, alterations in thyroid hormones is an acute adaptive mechanism to food scarcity to preserve energy[2903]. Having a lower metabolic rate also protects against muscle loss during fasting[2904].

However, there's a difference between intermittent fasting and extended fasting. Shorter intermittent fasting isn't nearly as big of a stressor as extended fasting, and it also has less of an effect on thyroid functioning. Studies on Ramadan fasting have found that it doesn't significantly affect thyroid hormones and changes typically stay within normal ranges[2905,2906]. People with hypothyroidism don't typically need to change their thyroid medication dosage and can safely practice intermittent fasting. Serum T3 and T4 has dropped in some studies but the data is inconsistent[2907]. A decline in thyroid hormone levels with fasting is thought to be caused by alterations in protein binding because free thyroid indices stay the same[2908].

In rats, fasting reduces T3 uptake by the liver due to ATP depletion, which gets restored with refeeding[2909,2910]. However, similar reductions in ATP with a parallel T4 decrease has been seen in rats receiving IV fructose, which lowers cellular ATP stores[2911]. Fructose has been shown to reduce liver T4 uptake in humans and rats[2912]. This is thought to be caused by fructose raising lactic acid and uric acid levels, which consume ATP[2913,2914]. Physiological stress has also been noted to reduce T3 and T4[2915,2916]. Post-traumatic stress disorder is associated with higher rates of hypothyroidism[2917]. Thus, the synthesis and transport of thyroid hormones is energy-dependent and can be reduced with fasting, excessive fructose intake and magnesium deficiency.

It's also important to nourish and refeed properly after exercise or prolonged fasting. Calorie restriction in and of itself lowers thyroid functioning, especially if you combine it with fasting. A 1980 study saw that after a 10-day fast, eating 1500 calories for five days wasn't enough to restore depressed T3 levels in obese subjects[2918]. Therefore, it might be important to eat at least at maintenance for a little while after a fast to allow the thyroid to recover and transition out of metabolic slowdown.

Refeeding with a predominantly carbohydrate-rich diet has been shown to reverse changes in serum T3 and rT3 caused by fasting even when hypocaloric[2919]. Carbohydrates, and the glucose they are converted into, are the main fuel for the thyroid and brain, which can raise metabolic rate if insulin/leptin resistance is not induced[2920]. In fact, insulin is needed for converting T4 into T3 and raising metabolic rate. This can make exogenous carbohydrates important for certain people, especially those whose thyroid functioning does down on a low-carb diet. Acutely raising leptin by eating some whole food carbs and spiking insulin can improve insulin sensitivity and weight loss[2921]. Restoring normal leptin levels has been shown to normalize blood sugar and insulin resistance[2922]. Some ketogenic diets may reduce T3 and raise reverse T3[2923]. That is why chronic ketosis may not be optimal for thyroid function and insulin sensitivity because it can also induce mild short-term carbohydrate intolerance[2924]. Instead, cyclical keto can help to bypass this negative side-effect while still providing the other benefits of ketosis, such as an improved lipid profile and lower blood sugar[2925].

Here are 12 things that lower thyroid hormones or thyroid hormone uptake

- Low ATP/magnesium
- Low sodium
- Low iodine
- Chronic calorie restriction
- Prolonged starvation
- Extended fasting
- Severe illness[2926]
- Kidney damage[2927]
- Liver damage
- Chronic stress
- Excess fructose consumption
- Chronic sleep deprivation

Combating iodine deficiency worldwide is primarily done with universal salt iodization[2928]. Iodine deficiencies were endemic in the Great Lakes, Appalachians and Northwestern regions of the United States, a geographic area known as the "goiter belt", however, salt iodization has eliminated it almost entirely[2929]. The Morton company was the first one in the U.S. to add iodine to their salt in 1924[2930]. Before 1990, only a few countries like Canada, Switzerland, the U.S. and the Scandinavian countries were iodine sufficient, but this has been improved upon with the use of iodized salt[2931]. Iodized salt comes in the form of iodate/iodide, the former gets reduced to iodide and absorbed in the gut. The World Health Organization recommends salt iodization of ≥15 mg/kg and fortification of 20−40 mg/kg at a salt intake of about 10 g/day[2932]. In the U.S., iodized salt contains approximately 45 mcg of iodine per 1 gram of salt but most of the dietary salt in the U.S. diet comes from processed foods which is not made with iodized salt[2933]. Many salt manufacturers fail to add sufficient iodine to their salt. A reduction in salt intake may also have a negative effect on thyroid function by inhibiting iodine transport via the sodium-iodine symporter. Especially for people whose primary source of iodine is iodized salt, reducing salt intake would likely lead to negative consequences on thyroid function and metabolic health. Special salts, like sea salts, do not usually contain iodine, however, Himalayan and other pink rock salts typically do contain some naturally occurring iodine (note, these salts will state on their label that they are not a good source of *iodide* because they do not artificially add potassium iodide to their salt but that does not mean they do not contain *iodine*). However, salt fortification should be adapted to the local salt and iodine intake because it can create iodine excess[2934]. In tropical countries it is recommended to use potassium iodate instead of potassium iodide because it has a higher stability in the presence of heat and humidity[2935]. High humidity and porous packing can result in a 90% loss of iodine[2936]. Iodized salt loses about 14-64% of its iodine during cooking and boiling[2937].

Developing countries are said to lose $35.7 billion/year to iodine deficiency because of reduced cognition and higher rates of developmental problems. Salt iodization would cost only $0.5 billion/year, giving a cost to benefit ratio of 70 to 1[2938]. The cost of salt iodization for one child is $0.02-0.05 per year and the disability-adjusted life year gained is $34–36[2939]. **Salt iodization is the most cost-effective way to improve cognition in iodine-deficient populations**[2940].

Universal salt iodization has improved rates of goiter but excess iodine exposure from water or diet can promote hypothyroidism[2941]. In 1999, among 885 Slovenian adults, iodine-induced hypothyroidism had risen from 5% to 20% after 10 years of mandatory salt iodization from 10 to 25 mg/kg[2942]. Between that time period, hypothyroidism had also doubled in Slovenia[2943]. In rural Italy, thyroid antibody positivity rose 15 years after salt iodization[2944]. An increased incidence of thyroid autoimmunity has been noted after iodized salt was introduced in Poland, Sri-Lanka and Greece[2945,2946,2947]. However, other studies find a decrease in autoimmune thyroiditis when iodine status is within optimal levels[2948]. However, **abrupt intake of iodine after a period of deficiency, such as seen with salt iodization, can cause hyperthyroidism and raise thyroid antibodies, especially in young women**[2949,2950]. Thus, introducing too much iodine when you have been deficient beforehand might trigger autoimmunity against the thyroid[2951]. Thus, a more gradual re-introduction of iodine, and from more natural sources (salts or foods naturally containing iodine), may be optimal.

As of 2017, excess iodine intake has been reported in 11 countries, 114 countries report adequate intake, and 20 countries report an insufficient intake[2952]. Increased incidences of hyperthyroidism tend to occur after salt fortification with iodine[2953]. Iodine-induced hyperthyroidism has been seen to occur at daily doses of less than 300 mcg iodine a day[2954,2955]. However, this mainly occurs in those with long standing iodine deficiency or nodular goiter. In some U.S. brands, kelp and other seaweeds can often contain 3x the RDA for iodine per serving [2956]. Bread manufacturers put dough conditioner on the nutrition facts label but don't have to include iodine, which could mean you have no idea how iodized a particular dough product is[2957]. USDA data from 2019 shows that only 20% of labels for white bread, hamburger buns and hot dogs labels iodate[2958]. Thus, it is better to get iodine from whole foods because it comes in more appropriate amounts, along other important nutrients and is harder to overdose.

Drinking water contains on average 1-10 mcg/L of iodine[2959]. High levels of iodine in groundwater have been reported in Algeria, Argentina, China, Denmark, Djibouti, Somalia, Ethiopia and Kenya[2960,2961,2962,2963,2964,2965]. In some places like Somalia, drinking water is the only source of iodine[2966]. Long-term exposure to excess iodine from drinking water has been seen to cause hypothyroidism in children[2967]. Excess iodine from water is also thought to cause endemic goiter in some regions of China but not in others[2968,2969,2970]. Water purified with iodine has also been shown to cause thyroid dysfunction in a few cases of Nigerian workers and U.S. astronauts[2971,2972].

Iodine poisoning is quite rare and only happens when consuming exceptionally large doses in the 2-to-3-gram range for adults. Elemental iodine is harsh to the skin, causing skin damage and chemical burns[2973]. Importantly, excess iodine is more toxic in the presence of selenium deficiency[2974], which can lead to damage and oxidation of proteins. In fact, supplemental selenium alleviates the toxic effects of excess iodine, such as thyroid damage and thyroid hormone dysfunction[2975]. Acute symptoms of iodine poisoning include burning of the mouth, vomiting, diarrhea, coma and pain in the stomach and throat. Some people are also hypersensitive towards iodine-containing foods and products, which makes them experience rashes and allergies. However, there are no confirmed reports of actual iodine allergy[2976]. People with food allergies do not have an increased risk of contrast medium hypersensitivity against iodine[2977].

Assessing Iodine Status

Under normal circumstances, only 10% or less of circulating iodine gets taken up by the thyroid but during chronic deficiency it can be more than 80%[2978]. The half-life of plasma iodine is about 10 hours, but this is reduced in iodine deficiency. Over 90% of iodine is absorbed in the small intestine and 90% of it is excreted within the first 24-48 hours[2979]. The half-life of T4 is 5 days and for T3 it is roughly 1.5-3 days.

Urinary iodine concentration (UIC) is the most commonly used biomarker for measuring iodine status within a population [2980]. Intradiurnal rhythms will offset individual spot urine samples, which is why spot urinary iodine is not recommended for individual assessment[2981,2982]. These differences are thought to even out with large sample sizes. Estimating iodine intakes with 24-hour urine collections are more accurate but difficult to obtain. An average UIC between 100−199 mcg/L indicates adequate iodine status in adults and children but 200-299 is still safe. A 2009 New Zealand randomized, placebo-controlled study saw that giving an iodine supplement at 150 mcg/day for 28 weeks to iodine-deficient children with urinary iodine concentrations at 63 mcg/L raised median urinary iodine levels to 145 mcg/L[2983]. The threshold for iodine excess in adults and children is 300 mcg/L and 500 mcg/L for pregnant women.

Here are the urinary iodine concentration reference ranges for schoolchildren and pregnant women, based on the World Health Organization's guidelines[2984]

Median Urinary Iodine (mcg/L) for Schoolchildren	Iodine Intake	Iodine Status
<20	Insufficient	Severe iodine deficiency
20–49	Insufficient	Moderate iodine deficiency
50–99	Insufficient	Mild iodine deficiency
100–199	Adequate	Adequate iodine nutrition
200–299	Above requirements	Slight risk
>300	Excessive for preventing deficiency	Risk of hyperthyroidism, autoimmune thyroid disease, etc.
Median Urinary Iodine (mcg/L) for Pregnant Women	Iodine Intake	Iodine Status
<150	Insufficient	Mild iodine deficiency
150–249	Adequate	Adequate iodine nutrition
250–499	Above requirements	Slight risk

>500	Excessive	Risk of hyperthyroidism, autoimmune thyroid disease, etc.
Median Urinary Iodine (mcg/L) for Lactating Women	Iodine Intake	Iodine Status
<150	Insufficient	Mild iodine deficiency
≥150-250	Adequate	Adequate iodine nutrition
>500	Excessive	Risk of hyperthyroidism, autoimmune thyroid disease, etc.
Median Urinary Iodine (mcg/L) for Adults	Iodine Intake	Iodine Status
<100	Insufficient	Mild iodine deficiency
100–199	Adequate	Adequate iodine nutrition
200–299	Above requirements	Slight risk for hyperthyroidism
>300	Excessive for preventing deficiency	Risk of hyperthyroidism, autoimmune thyroid disease, etc.

Median urinary iodine in the U.S. is 145 mcg/L, which is still in the adequate zone, but this is half the median value seen in the 1970s which was 321 mcg/L [2985,2986]. Pregnant women in the U.S. are between 125-181 mcg/L, which is insufficient if below 150

326

mcg/L[2987,2988]. U.S. women of reproductive age are at 119 mcg/L, which is typically considered sufficient if not pregnant or lactating[2989]. In Australia, pregnant women taking iodine supplements are, on average, iodine insufficient, with levels at 138 mcg/L and 90 mcg/L when not taking supplements[2990]. Dairy consumption can play a role in iodine sufficiency. NHANES 2001-2006 data saw that pregnant women who did not consume dairy within the 24 hours of measurement had a mean urinary iodine concentration of only 100 mcg/L compared to 163 mcg/L of dairy consumers. **Women who restrict salt intake have lower urinary iodine than those who don't**[2991].

Thyroid-stimulating hormone (TSH) is often used to assess hypothyroidism, but it is not fully accurate due to individual differences and diurnal variations[2992]. Generally, TSH levels start to rise when iodine intake drops below 100 mcg/day. The normal range for TSH is between 0.45-4.5 mU/L and 95% of the disease-free population in the U.S. has their TSH at 0.45 and 4.12 mU/L[2993,2994]. T4 and T3 measure hormone levels but not necessarily thyroid hormone function (receptor activation and subsequent effects thereafter). TSH is not accurate for assessing iodine status in adults but it may be accurate for assessing iodine status in newborns because they have a higher rate of iodine turnover than adults[2995].

Here are the estimated ranges of TSH levels[2996]

Age Range	Low	Normal	High
0–4 days	<1 mU/L	1.6–24.3 mU/L	>30 mU/L
2–20 weeks	<0.5 mU/L	0.58–5.57 mU/L	>6.0 mU/L
20 weeks – 18 years	<0.5 mU/L	0.55–5.31 mU/L	>6.0 mU/L
18-30	<0.5 mU/L	0.5–4.1 mU/L	>4.1 mU/L
31–50 years	<0.5 mU/L	0.5–4.1 mU/L	>4.1 mU/L

51–70 years	<0.5 mU/L	0.5–4.5 mU/L	>4.5 mU/L
71–90 years	<0.4 mU/L	0.4–5.2 mU/L	>5.2 mU/L

The Sodium-Selenium-Iodine (SSI) Connection

Simply consuming nutrients does not guarantee that they are being delivered to or utilized by the right tissues. That is why simply consuming more iodine may not be the missing link for improving thyroid function. There are other nutrients, such as sodium and selenium, that help in the uptake of iodine and synthesis of thyroid hormones. The sodium-iodide cotransporter (NIS) being one of the main thyroid hormone cotransporters. As we discussed previously, two sodium ions are needed to bring one iodine into the thyroid gland and also into the breast tissue/breast milk. In addition, selenium is needed to activate the thyroid hormones.

Selenium is an essential mineral that protects against oxidative damage, promotes DNA synthesis and is needed for metabolism[2997]. Selenium is contained in over two dozen selenoproteins in the body, many of which have roles in cell redox homeostasis and antioxidant defense[2998]. Selenium has two forms: inorganic (selenate and selenite) and organic (selenomethionine and selenocysteine) both of which are good dietary sources of selenium[2999]. Selenoproteins are involved with thyroid hormone metabolism and antioxidant defense [3000], [3001]. Selenium is present in selenoproteins as selenocysteine, which is essential for enzymatic activities[3002]. In addition to iodine, the thyroid gland is also the highest concentrated source of selenium per gram of tissue in the body due to a high number of selenoproteins[3003].

The main selenoproteins, namely glutathione peroxidase, thioredoxin reductase and deiodinases are expressed in the thyroid gland in large quantities[3004]. Here is how they affect thyroid function:

- Glutathione peroxidases (GPx) are selenoenzymes that regulate thyroid hormone synthesis, contributing to the high content of selenium in the thyroid[3005,3006]. They also protect thyroid cells against hydrogen peroxide and other free radicals,

328

which would otherwise inhibit thyroid function [3007], [3008]. Selenium deficiency reduces glutathione peroxidase levels[3009]. A study noted that there was an association between higher TSH and decreased selenium/glutathione peroxidase activity[3010].

- Thioredoxin reductases (TrxR) are essential for antioxidant defense and regulation of certain transcription factors[3011]. So far, there have been three selenoenzymes in the thioredoxin reductase family identified – TrxR1, TrxR2 and TrxR3 [3012], [3013], [3014]. They help protect the thyroid against oxidative damage.

- Deiodinases (DIO) scavenge iodide from iodinated tyrosine inside the thyroid gland during thyroid hormone biosynthesis [3015], [3016] and are a family of thioredoxin proteins [3017]. The breakdown of thyroglobulin (Tg) during thyroid hormone biosynthesis produces 6-7 times more iodinated tyrosine than thyroid hormones; deiodinases are then available to salvage iodide from iodinated tyrosine[3018], [3019]. Without deiodinase, iodide and left-over iodinated tyrosine would be excreted through urine, reducing thyroid hormone biosynthesis[3020]. In fact, mutations in deiodinases causes iodine deficiency [3021] and selenium directly controls deiodinase activity[3022]. TSH stimulates the conversion of T4 into T3 via deiodinases[3023].

Thus, selenium is important for not only activating thyroid hormones but also recycling them. In other words, iodine does not work without selenium and sodium and a lack in any of these essential nutrients will worsen thyroid function.

The link between selenium deficiency and thyroid dysfunction was only recently appreciated beginning in the early 1990s[3024]. Giving 100 mcg/day of sodium selenite for three months to elderly subjects reduced T4, improving the T3/T4 ratio, improved selenium status and glutathione peroxidase levels[3025]. Similar results have been observed in patients receiving 10-40 mcg/day of selenium as L-selenomethionine for 5 months[3026]. It was estimated from this study that 90 mcg/day of selenium is required to maximize plasma glutathione peroxidase activity, well above the RDA of 55 mcg/day for most adults. Selenium administration with only one single Brazil nut per day ($\approx$ 5 grams, average 58.1 mcg Se/g) for 3 months has been shown to improve thyroid function and thyroid hormones in patients on hemodialysis, although T3 levels were not completely restored to normal[3027]. Sodium-selenium therapy improves thyroid status and the T3/T4 ratio in cystic fibrosis and congenital hypothyroidism[3028]. The more impactful effect seems to be that selenium supplementation improves thyroid parameters by increasing deiodinase activity[3029].

However, selenium supplementation without prior iodine replenishment may exacerbate hypothyroidism because there isn't enough glutathione peroxidase to clean up the hydrogen peroxide that gets created during iodine-deficient hypothyroidism[3030]. Those unleashed free radicals will then begin to damage thyroid cells and interfere with thyroid health. Thyroid function has not been shown to change in healthy subjects receiving additional supplemental selenium if they have no parameters of hypothyroidism[3031,3032,3033,3034]. This makes sense, i.e., you can't fix what isn't broken.

Selenium deficiency increases thyroid size and risk for goiter. Lower selenium levels are associated with increased thyroid volume and nodule formation [3035, 3036, 3037, 3038]. Thus, adequate selenium may protect against goiter as well as thyroid disease[3039]. The incidence of goiter in children is associated with the amount of selenium in the local soil – i.e., low selenium in soil → low selenium in food → selenium and iodine deficiency → hypothyroidism and goiter[3040]. Fixing iodine deficiency in children with goiter and selenium deficiency does not reduce the volume of goiter or improve thyroid function[3041].

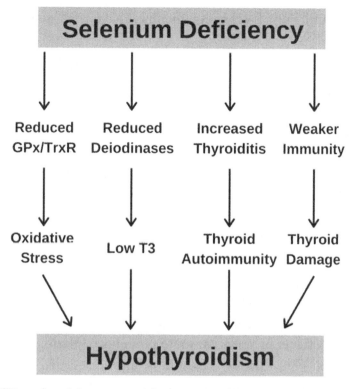

GPx, glutathione peroxidase, TrxR, thioredoxin reductase.

There is also some correlation between thyroid cancer and low selenium concentrations[3042]. Selenium appears to be decreased the most in subjects with Grave's disease and in thyroid cancer tissue[3043]. Selenium deficiency leads to the activation of oncogenes (cancer causing genes) due to an increased formation of reactive oxygen species[3044]. Thus, selenium might have a role in the prevention of cancer due to its antioxidant and immunomodulatory properties[3045]. Epidemiological studies and some meta-analyses find an inverse relationship between selenium levels and the risk of various cancers[3046, 3047]. A double-blind, randomized, controlled trial that included 1,312 U.S. adults with a history of non-melanoma skin cancer saw that consuming 200 mcg of selenium a day as high-selenium baker's yeast for 6 years was associated with a 49-65% reduced risk of prostate cancer, particularly in those with baseline selenium levels < 123.2 ng/mL or baseline PSA ≤ 4 ng/mL[3048]. Other similar trials, but this time utilizing L-selenomethionine, have not found similar benefits[3049,3050].

Chronic lymphocytic thyroiditis (CLT) can be improved with selenium at a dose of 200 mcg/day given for 3-12 months by decreasing anti-thyroperoxidase (TPO) antibodies[3051,3052,3053,3054,3055]. The suppression of antibodies appears to require doses above 100 mcg/day to maximize glutathione peroxidase[3056]. CLT is the most common autoimmune thyroid disease in which iodine status is adequate and where genetic factors of selenium deficiency are present[3057,3058]. Giving 200 mcg of selenium/day as selenomethionine might help to reduce postpartum thyroiditis by reducing thyroid antibodies[3059,3060]. Selenium given at 80 mcg/day for 12 months has also been observed to significantly lower anti-TPO antibodies in patients with Hashimoto's thyroiditis with normal T4 and TSH levels[3061]. Anti-TPO antibodies promote the production of inflammatory cytokines by thyroid lymphocytes, making the effects of selenium more pronounced during episodes of inflammation[3062]. Graves' disease is also correlated with lower selenium levels and selenium is necessary for protecting against the increased oxidative stress that occurs during this condition[3063,3064,3065]. Selenium supplementation has also been shown to improve the quality of life in patients with Graves' orbitopathy[3066]. Some studies find that these benefits on autoimmunity remain stable after discontinuation of the selenium supplementation whereas others do not. Regardless, maintaining an optimal selenium status with help support a strong immune system and thyroid function.

Selenium deficiency, in combination with an RNA viral infection called coxsackie virus, can lead to Keshan disease, which is a type of cardiomyopathy[3067]. Keshan disease originated from parts of China where people got on average 11 mcg/day of selenium. An intake of at least 20 mcg/day is needed to prevent Keshan disease. Observational studies have found an association between lower selenium in people with HIV and increased risk of cardiomyopathy and death[3068,3069]. Selenium deficient women also have a higher chance of transmitting the virus to their offspring[3070,3071]. Selenium supplementation can reduce hospitalization and HIV viral load[3072,3073].

Some meta-analyses have found an inverse association between serum selenium levels and risk of coronary heart disease[3074]. However, other studies have not seen this effect and in some cases higher selenium levels are associated with an increased risk of cardiovascular disease mortality [3075], [3076], [3077]. Selenium supplementation has not been found to have a significant effect on the primary prevention of cardiovascular disease[3078]. However, in elderly patients, the combination of selenium from yeast (200 mcg/day) and coenzymeQ10 (200 mg/day) significant reduced cardiovascular mortality[3079,3080]. Thus, selenium supplementation in those who have a baseline deficiency likely provides significant benefits, whereas consuming over 300 mcg/day of selenium may potentially lead to negative consequences.

- Generally, the majority of observational studies and meta-analyses see an inverse relationship between selenium/selenoprotein status and cardiovascular disease risk[3081,3082,3083,3084,3085]. The main mechanism appears to be due to selenoproteins' ability to inhibit oxidative stress, lower inflammation and protecting vascular cells against apoptosis or calcification[3086]. Selenoproteins regulate redox and calcium homeostasis [3087]. Selenoproteins increase resistance to oxidative stress, whereas selenium deficiency increases damage from oxidative stress[3088].

- Selenoproteins can prevent the oxidation of lipids, which reduces the potential for atherosclerosis[3089]. The oxidation of LDL is a bigger risk factor for atherosclerosis and heart disease than total or LDL cholesterol levels alone. Furthermore, lipoproteins become oxidized when oxidative stress exceeds the body's antioxidant capacity[3090]. Supplemental selenium at doses of 100-300 mcg/day has been shown to lower total cholesterol and raise HDL cholesterol, which may help clear the blood from potentially oxidizable lipids [3091]. In hypercholesterolemic rabbits, selenium with vitamin E inhibits atherosclerosis, independent of the effects on plasma cholesterol levels[3092]. Selenium deficiency in rats increases myocardial injury and lipid peroxidation after myocardial

333

ischemia/reperfusion (this is what occurs after surgeons re-open a clogged artery after a heart attack) [3093]. Adequate selenium intake also protects against post-myocardial ischemia/reperfusion arrhythmias in rats[3094].

- Glutathione peroxidase-3 (GPx3) deficiency, which is a selenium-dependent enzyme, promotes platelet thrombosis and vascular dysfunction[3095]. GPx3 can also inhibit the oxidation of LDL cholesterol by eliminating hydroperoxides, thus preventing vascular inflammation and atherogenesis[3096]. GPx4 has similar effects[3097]. Selenium levels are directly correlated with GPx activity[3098].

- Impairment of selenoproteins during selenium deficiency may be a contributing factor in congestive heart failure and cardiomyopathy[3099]. Low selenium status is associated with future cardiovascular death in patients with acute coronary syndrome (someone who has had a heart attack)[3100]. Selenium deficiency in heart failure patients is independently associated with impaired exercise tolerance and a 50% higher mortality rate[3101].

- Thioredoxins also regulate cardiac function and cardiovascular disease risk[3102]. They also affect cardiac remodeling[3103]. Trx-1 has been shown to reduce oxidative stress and cardiac hypertrophy in response to oxidative stress[3104].

Low-selenium regions in China, Tibet and Siberia have a higher prevalence of Kashin-Beck disease, which is a type of osteoarthritis[3105,3106]. In those areas, iodine deficiency is also a risk factor. Both selenium and iodine affect autoimmune and arthritic disorders by regulating thyroid function and the immune system.

Selenium deficiency is associated with cognitive decline and age-related brain dysfunction[3107,3108]. People with lower selenium status are more likely to experience cognitive decline and neurodegeneration because of increased oxidative stress[3109,3110]. Low selenium in the elderly also correlates with worse memory [3111]. In France, supplementation with antioxidants, including selenium, has been shown to improve episodic memory and semantic fluency in subjects aged 45-60[3112].

Selenium has detoxifying effects on several heavy metals, such as cadmium, mercury and lead [3113, 3114, 3115]. The mechanisms are mediated by glutathione peroxidases and other antioxidants that help to eliminate these toxic compounds. Mercury toxicity can inhibit selenoenzymes that are needed to combat oxidative stress[3116]. Thus, selenium might be a cornerstone mineral for preventing the damage that occurs from heavy metal toxicity. This is also one of the reasons why seafood that has higher levels of selenium poses a lower risk for mercury toxicity. Tuna actually contains selenoneine, which is a potent antioxidant[3117]. The ratio of selenium to mercury matters more as selenium counteracts the harms from mercury. The consumption of fish can contribute up to 16.7% of the dietary protein intake for humans worldwide[3118]. The addition of selenium fertilizers has been shown to reduce the accumulation of cadmium and lead into crops like lettuce. Fruit stays firm and ripe longer if sprayed with foliar selenium, possibly due to an increased protecting against oxidation. Selenium also protects plants against environmental stressors like UV-B radiation and extreme temperatures.[3119] However, in large amounts, selenium can act as an environmental pollutant, killing fish[3120]. In most cases, high selenium in the environment is the result of activities like coal burning and mining.

Here are the selenium-dependent enzymes, functions and consequences that may occur with a deficit

Selenium-Dependent Enzymes/Proteins	Function	Consequences of Deficit
Glutathione Peroxidase	Removes hydrogen peroxide	Increased oxidative stress and weaker immunity
Thioredoxin reductase	Antioxidant defense, peroxynitrite protection	Oxidative stress, atherosclerosis and lipid peroxidation
Deiodinases	Convert T4 into T3 and iodine transport in thyroid cells	Hypothyroidism
Thyroid Hormones[3121]	Regulate metabolic rate, body temperature and energy balance	Chronic fatigue, frailty, weight gain, metabolic syndrome and decreased immunity
Glutathione	Scavenge free radicals	Increased oxidative stress

Getting Enough Selenium from the Diet

Selenium was discovered in 1817 by Jöns Jacob Berzelius and Johan Gottlieb Gahn in Sweden[3122]. 'Selene' is derived from the Greek word 'σελήνη', referring to the moon-bright and grey color of melted selenium[3123]. In 1873, Willoughby Smith observed that the electrical resistance properties of selenium were dependent on ambient light[3124]. The amount of electrical current transmitted by selenium is in proportion to how much light is falling onto its surface. This is why it was used in electronics, light meters and other similar devices[3125].

How much selenium is in food depends on the amount of selenium in the soil. The soil consists of inorganic selenium that the plants obtain and convert into the organic form. Selenocysteine and selenite promote selenoprotein biosynthesis by getting reduced to hydrogen selenite, which is then converted to selenophosphate which supports selenoprotein biosynthesis[3126]. In animal and human tissues, selenium is in the form of selenomethionine and selenocysteine. Methionine is one of the most abundant amino acid in our bodies and in animal protein. Skeletal muscle accounts for about 28-46% of the body's total selenium pool[3127]. Ocean waters and rivers also contain quite a lot of selenium[3128], which is why meat, fish and seafood are generally much higher in selenium than plants.

The RDA for selenium is 15 mcg for infants, 20-40 mcg for children and 55 mcg for adults[3129]. During pregnancy and lactation, the RDA for selenium increases to 60-70 mcg/day, respectively. Selenium toxicity or selenosis generally occurs if you exceed 400 mcg/day (although the actual level that induces toxicity is likely at 800mcg/day or higher)[3130,3131]. This usually happens in regions with high amounts of selenium in the soil[3132,3133]. Acute selenium toxicity can trigger gastrointestinal and neurological problems[3134]. A 1992 study considered the maximum safe dietary selenium intake to be about 800 mcg/day (15 mcg/kg) but suggested the 400 mcg/day upper limit as a margin of safety[3135]. Large doses of selenium in individuals without selenium deficiency may promote hyperglycemia and insulin resistance[3136]. Symptoms of too much selenium consumption include a metallic taste in the mouth, garlic odor, hair and nail loss and brittleness[3137]. Diarrhea, nausea, fatigue and skin lesions are also common.

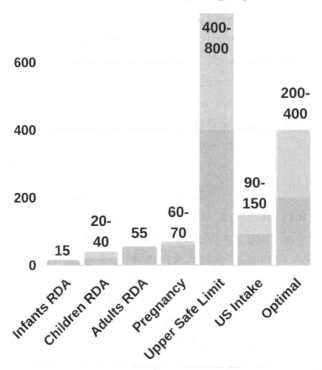

Optimal Intake of Selenium (mcg/d)

Most people in the U.S. get an adequate amount of selenium. The average daily intake of selenium for people over 2 years of age is 108.5 mcg from food and 120.8 mcg if supplements are considered[3138]. Adult men on average get 134 mcg of selenium per day from food and 151 mcg from food plus supplements. Adult women on average obtain 93 mcg of selenium/day from food and 108 mcg from food and supplements. Selenium intake varies between regions and depends on the selenium content of the soil. In the U.S., Mid-West and West residents have higher selenium concentrations than those in the South or North-East[3139]. Fortunately, this shortcoming can be easily overcome with food transportation or selenium supplementation. The low selenium content of New Zealand's diet was fixed by increasing the import of high-selenium wheat[3140]. Selenium levels are well known to be lower in smokers and the elderly[3141].

338

Here are the foods highest in selenium[3142]

Food	Mcg of Selenium per Serving	% of RDA
Brazil Nuts, 1 oz, 6-8 nuts	544 mcg	989%
Kidney, ruminant, 3 oz	125 mcg	200%
Tuna, cooked, 3 oz	92 mcg	167%
Mussels, 3 oz	76 mcg	140%
Crab Meat, 3 oz	75 mcg	140%
Halibut, cooked, 3 oz	47 mcg	85%
Sardines, canned, 3 oz	45 mcg	82%
Ham, 3 oz	42 mcg	76%
Shrimp, canned, 3 oz	40 mcg	73%
Macaroni, enriched, cooked, 1 cup	37 mcg	67%
Beef Steak, roasted, 3 oz	33 mcg	60%
Turkey, cooked, 3 oz	31 mcg	56%
Beef Liver, fried, 3 oz	28 mcg	51%
Chicken, roasted, 3 oz	22 mcg	40%
Cottage Cheese, 1%, 1 cup	20 mcg	36%
Brown Rice, cooked, 1 cup	19 mcg	35%
Ground Beef, 75-25, 3 oz	18 mcg	33%
Egg, hard boiled, 1 large	15 mcg	27%
Whole-Wheat Bread, 1 slice	13 mcg	24%
Beans, canned, 1 cup	13 mcg	24%
Oatmeal, cooked, 1 cup	13 mcg	24%

Milk, 1%, 1 cup	8 mcg	15%
Yogurt, low fat, 1 cup	8 mcg	15%
Lentils, boiled, 1 cup	6 mcg	11%
White Bread, 1 slice	6 mcg	11%
Spinach, cooked, ½ cup	5 mcg	9%
Spaghetti Sauce, 1 cup	4 mcg	7%
Cashew Nuts, roasted, 1 oz	3 mcg	5%
Corn Flakes, 1 cup	2 mcg	4%
Green Peas, boiled, ½ cup	1 mcg	2%
Bananas, ½ cup	1 mcg	2%
Potato, baked, 1 medium	1 mcg	2%

You can meet your daily selenium requirements by eating 2-3 Brazil nuts a day. However, there is great variability in the amount of selenium in foods, especially Brazil nuts, which obtain all their selenium from the soil. Assessment of UK foods has found that 3.5 ounces of Brazil nuts contains only 254 mcg of selenium, compared to much higher levels found in Brazil nuts from other areas [3143]. Nevertheless, Brazil nuts are by far the highest source of selenium and you should not eat more than 1 oz. per day. Since Brazil nuts are so high in selenium, they can cause selenium toxicity if consumed all the time or in excess. Other options for daily selenium consumption are consuming seafood 2-3 times per week since that will also provide iodine, omega-3s and protein.

The majority of selenium is absorbed in the small intestine (50-80%) and excreted by kidneys (60%). Thus, your selenium status is also determined by the state of your digestive and excretory organs.

Here are things that raise the requirement for selenium:

- Hemodialysis removes selenium from blood[3144]
- HIV patients have lower levels of selenium because of malabsorption[3145]
- Certain medications like cisplatin lower selenium in hair and serum[3146,3147]
- Malabsorption conditions like IBS, intestinal permeability, etc.
- Aging
- Heavy metal toxicity and pollution
- Living in a low selenium soil environment
- Hypothyroidism
- Chronic inflammatory conditions like diabetes and cardiovascular disease

Selenium supplements mostly come in the form of selenomethionine, selenium-enriched yeast, sodium selenite or sodium selenate. The human body can absorb up to 70-90% of selenomethionine but only 50% of selenium from selenite[3148]. Thus, selenomethionine is the best organic selenocompound for improving selenium status because it is incorporated into proteins in a non-specific way. However, selenomethionine needs to be reduced to hydrogen selenide (H_2Se) by selenocysteine beforehand, making it less efficient metabolically[3149]. Nevertheless, organic selenocompounds like selenomethionine cause less acute toxicity, which is why they are more preferred in short-term therapy. Inorganic selenocompounds have been proven to be most efficacious for optimizing selenoenzyme activity.[3150] Naturally, selenomethionine is mostly found in animal tissue and protein, which is why meat and fish tend to be far more bioavailable sources of selenium.

Selenium status is most commonly measured using plasma and serum selenium levels. Plasma or serum selenium levels at 8 mcg/dL or above are enough to meet the requirements for selenoprotein biosynthesis[3151]. The average serum selenium concentration in U.S. adults over 40 years old is 13.67 mcg/dL[3152]. Males tend to have higher selenium levels than females and whites more than African Americans[3153,3154]. Blood and urine selenium reflect only recently consumed selenium. Measuring glutathione peroxidase can be an indirect measurement of selenium status. Selenoprotein P may be one of the best markers for measuring total body selenium status[3155].

Other Minerals for Thyroid Health

The thyroid gland needs many minerals for the creation and distribution of thyroid hormones throughout the body. Deficiencies in iodine and selenium can cause hypothyroidism directly by inhibiting thyroid hormone biosynthesis as well as indirectly by leaving the thyroid more vulnerable to autoimmunity and oxidative stress. There are also other minerals relevant to thyroid function, which are summarized below.

- **Sodium** transports iodide into thyroid cells in order to make thyroid hormones via the sodium-iodide symporter.
- **Iodine** is essential for making thyroid hormones and governing physical and mental development. It is the main resource for optimal thyroid function, but it cannot work without the other minerals.
- **Selenium** helps to initiate thyroid hormone biosynthesis, activate thyroid hormones, catalyze the conversion of T4 into T3 and support the recycling of iodide to make more thyroid hormones. It also protects against thyroid damage by inhibiting oxidative stress and heavy metal contamination.
- **Zinc** also helps to activate thyroid hormones[3156]. Zinc deficiency impairs T3 production[3157]. Supplementing with zinc has been shown to improve the status of thyroid hormones and promote the conversion of T4 into T3[3158,3159]. Zinc deficiency enhances the expression of thyroxine-5'-monodeiodinase, which inactivates thyroid hormones[3160]. Hair loss is common in both zinc deficiency and hypothyroidism[3161]. However, excess zinc can also cause hyperthyroidism.

- **Iron** helps to convert inactive T4 into active T3[3162]. Iron deficiency also disrupts thyroid hormone synthesis by reducing heme-dependent thyroid peroxidase activity[3163]. There is an association between low thyroid and iron deficiency[3164]. Disruption in thermogenesis during iron deficiency could be caused by low thyroid function[3165]. However, iron overload can also impair thyroid function and promote thyroid autoimmune disease[3166,3167]. The importance for iron for thyroid health automatically means that copper is also important, as copper is needed to move iron around the body.
- **Magnesium** protects against oxidative stress and inflammation which damages the thyroid gland. Magnesium is also essential for making ATP that enables the sodium-iodide symporter to transport iodine into thyroid cells and kickstart thyroid hormone biosynthesis.
- **Insulin** is the hormone that is responsible for shuttling nutrients into cells. Thus, insulin resistance and chronically suppressed insulin, may lead to nutrient deficiencies and/or excessive loss of minerals through urine. With excessively low insulin levels you may excrete more of minerals out the urine, especially sodium. Carbohydrates and a healthy physiological insulin spike are important for maintaining normal thyroid function. As with everything, chronic excessive intakes of refined carbohydrates can cause many problems, but consuming normal amounts of healthy carbohydrate sources can provide unique health benefits.

In conclusion, minerals must be obtained from the diet in the right amounts on a regular basis. For more information about that, refer back to chapters 5 through 8. In general, this means eating mineral-dense superfoods like liver, oysters, spinach and seaweed at least 1-2 times per week and foods like pastured meat and eggs on a daily basis. Pay attention to the inhibitors and chelators like phytates and goitrogens but deliberate avoidance is not necessary, unless you already have existing clinical hypothyroidism.

Chapter 11
Potassium, Sodium and Hypertension

Elevated blood pressure or hypertension is the leading cause of cardiovascular disease, contributing to stroke, coronary heart disease, myocardial infarction (which is a heart attack), heart failure, atrial fibrillation and kidney disease[3168,3169]. Worldwide, hypertension is the primary cause of mortality and morbidity[3170]. About 1.13 billion people in the world have hypertension with 2/3rds of them living in low- and middle-income countries[3171]. NHANES data from 2005-2008 found that 33.5% of U.S. adults over the age of 20 have hypertension! That is essentially 1 in 3 adults living with elevated blood pressure. There are many more who have 'pre-hypertension' or who are at risk of developing hypertension down the line. If you live in America and reach the age of 70 or older, hypertension is found in 50% of people[3172]. African American adults have the highest rates of hypertension in the world at around 44%.[3173]

Most people are not aware that they have hypertension because they do not experience any visible symptoms, which is why it is called the "silent killer". However, if you do experience symptoms of elevated blood pressure, it can include headache, nosebleed, arrhythmia, heart pounding, blurry vision, buzzing in the ears, fatigue, nausea, chest pain, anxiety and tremors. Having your blood pressure monitored regularly is the only reliable method for assessing your condition.

Blood pressure is measured using two indicators. Systolic blood pressure represents the pressure in blood vessels while the heart contracts or beats. Diastolic blood pressure the pressure in the vessels during rests between heart beats. Hypertension is diagnosed if your systolic blood pressure is ≥ 140 mmHg (millimeters of mercury) and diastolic blood pressure is ≥ 90 mmHg on two different days.

There are many things that cause hypertension, such as obesity, aging, lack of exercise, excess alcohol consumption, smoking and electrolyte imbalances[3174,3175,3176,3177]. Insulin resistance and metabolic syndrome are also associated with hypertension[3178,3179] Consumption of more fruit and vegetables has been consistently shown to be associated with lower blood pressure[3180,3181,3182,3183]. Part of that is deemed to be because of a higher potassium content that regulates the body's fluid volume and leads to blood vessel dilation. Consuming excess sodium, typically on top of a low potassium intake, is associated with an increased risk of hypertension[3184,3185]. As many of you already know, salt is extremely important for health, but if it is not balanced with potassium, many people can see increases in blood pressure. In industrialized cultures, higher potassium intake is associated with lower blood pressure[3186,3187]. High potassium intake may protect against stroke mortality, hypertension, arterial endothelial injury, cardiac hypertrophy and kidney damage[3188,3189]. The American Heart Association suggests that increasing potassium intake may reduce hypertension by 17% and lengthen lifespan by 5.1 years in Americans[3190].

In this chapter, we will talk about the role of potassium in regulating blood pressure, insulin sensitivity and other risk factors for disease. Like with all the other minerals, potassium has to be consumed and looked upon in relation to other electrolytes, especially sodium. Sodium and potassium are intrinsically interdependent of each other and their balance has a major impact on your overall health.

Effects of Potassium on Health

Potassium is the most abundant intracellular cation (an ion with a positive charge) that helps to maintain intracellular fluid volume. The adult human body contains around 1,755 mg of potassium per kg of body weight[3191]. Out of that amount, only 2% is located in the extracellular fluid with most of it being found in skeletal muscle[3192,3193].

The concentration of potassium in the cell is 30 times higher than outside the cell. This difference creates a transmembrane electrochemical gradient that is regulated by the sodium-potassium ATPase pump (Na^+-K^+ ATPase)[3194,3195]. The gradient of potassium across cell membranes determines the cells' membrane potential. The resting membrane potential and the electro-chemical differences across cell membranes are critical for normal cellular function and biology[3196]. Transfer of potassium ions across nerve membranes is essential for nerve function and transmission.

Once activated, the sodium-potassium pump exchanges 2 extracellular potassium ions for 3 intracellular sodium ions. Other channels responsible for maintaining differences in cell membrane potential are the sodium-potassium chloride (Cl) symporter and sodium-calcium (Ca) exchanger. The ATPase is also stimulated by activation of β-adrenergic and insulin receptors, which are stimulated by epinephrine/norepinephrine and insulin, respectively. Consequently, simultaneous stimulation of both the β-adrenergic and insulin receptors increases the influx of potassium into the cell but causes sodium to leave the cell via the Na^+-K^+ ATPase. The thyroid hormones triiodothyronine (T3) and thyroxine (T4) increase Na-K-ATPase subunits by increasing gene expression (although the effect is the opposite in the thyroid gland, as thyroid hormones will have a negative feedback effect on the Na-K-ATPase). The Na-K-ATPase provides the sodium gradient to absorb iodide via the sodium-iodide symporter, thus reducing its activity will reduce iodine transport into the thyroid gland, thus reducing thyroid hormone synthesis[3197,3198,3199]. Insulin substrate receptor-1 (IRS1) and intracellular glucose transport proteins (GLUT4) facilitate the influx of glucose into the cell. Downstream signaling events to that, involving cyclic adenosine-monophosphate (cAMP), protein kinase A (Akt), and IRS1-phosphatidylinositide-3-kinase (PI3-K) regulated pathways also mediate the influx of glucose as well as potassium into the cell[3200]. The fastest potassium exchange occurs in the kidneys and the slowest in muscles and the brain[3201].

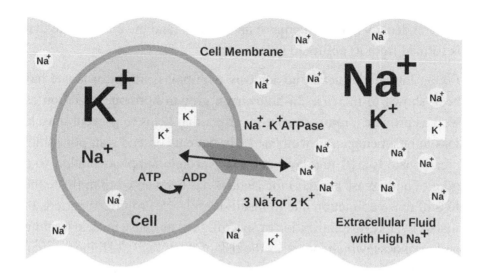

Metabolic acidosis, or a drop in *extracellular* pH, increases the loss of intracellular potassium into the extracellular space via transporters that regulate pH in skeletal muscle[3202]. Organic acidosis, caused by an accumulation of lactic acid or uric acid, lowers *intracellular* pH, which stimulates the movement of hydrogen out of the cell via the sodium-hydrogen transporter and bicarbonate into the cell via the sodium-bicarbonate transporter. As a result, intracellular sodium increases, which maintains Na+-K+ ATPase activity limiting the loss of potassium from the cell. Thus, organic acidosis, say from lactic acid build up from excessive exercise, causes a much smaller loss of intracellular potassium than does metabolic acidosis.

Metabolic acidosis promotes a net efflux of calcium from bone by increasing osteoclastic resorption and decreasing osteoblast formation[3203]. Neutralization of acidosis with potassium bicarbonate (KHCO3), but not sodium bicarbonate, improves calcium and phosphorus balance, reduce bone resorption, reduces calcium excretion through urine and reduce the age-related decrease in growth hormone secretion without salt restriction[3204,3205]. Potassium citrate has been shown to have beneficial calcium-retaining effects in bone[3206]. Increasing potassium consumption improves bone density in elderly women and may prevent osteoporosis[3207]. Greater potassium intake from fruits and vegetables is associated with higher bone mineral density thanks to potassium citrate's (and the bicarbonate that is formed from it) ability to balance acid[3208,3209].

Fixing low grade metabolic acidosis with potassium bicarbonate has been shown to increase 24-hour mean growth hormone secretion as well as provide a nitrogen sparing effect that helps to prevent muscle loss in postmenopausal women[3210]. In patients on bed rest, potassium bicarbonate (3,510 mg/day) and whey protein supplementation (0.6 g/kg of body mass per day) for 19 days has been noted to mitigate the loss of muscle function due to inactivity[3211,3212]. Prolonged periods of inactivity, like hospitalization or spaceflight, can cause muscle wasting and weakness, which increases the risk of fractures[3213]. Higher protein intake has been shown to mitigate muscle loss and catabolism[3214]. Taking whey protein alone, without balancing it with some form of base, might create a net acidic environment promoting bone demineralization. Thus, increased protein consumption, particularly from protein powders, would likely warrant increased intake of alkaline foods or beverages. To be clear, the body tries to maintain a normal pH in the blood, even with a surplus of acid. Thus, measuring blood pH levels is not the best way to determine acid-base balance. Typically, levels of bicarbonate in the blood will drop faster than blood pH and are a better marker of overall acid-base balance, as is urinary pH levels[3215]. You can have an acidic urine (indicating acid surplus) but a normal blood pH. Importantly, diet can affect whole body pH status (such as interstitial pH levels for example) even if the blood pH is normal, which supports some of the ideas promoted by the "alkaline theory".[3216] The particular notion that consuming a higher acid load will lead to calcium being pulled from bone is much more contentious, as in the face of normal kidney function, especially with adequate calcium intake, this is less likely to occur.[3217] However, this does not mean that there are no potential negative consequences from eating a highly acidic diet (i.e., connective tissue/cartilage damage, joint pain, insulin resistance, etc.). It will take a long time before the alkaline theory is proved/disproved in normal healthy individuals, but until then, there is enough data to at least consider balancing dietary acid load (e.g., dairy, especially cheese, grains, animal protein, protein supplements and salt) with some form of base (e.g., alkaline waters, bicarbonate, fruits and/or vegetables). The alkaline theory has already been tested in several studies of patients with kidney disease showing that consuming an alkaline diet (either via fruits/vegetables or sodium bicarbonate supplementation) over several months can improve metabolic acidosis and kidney function[3218,3219,3220]. In postmenopausal women, an alkaline treatment (potassium bicarbonate supplementation) improved calcium and phosphorus balance, reduced bone resorption and increased bone formation[3221] and reduces their urinary nitrogen (i.e., muscle) loss[3222]. These findings have been confirmed in middle-aged and elderly men, whereby alkaline therapy (potassium bicarbonate) has a muscle protein-sparing effect[3223,3224]. Additionally, a bone-sparing effect has been shown in older men and women[3225]. Thus, alkaline treatments may reduce muscle and bone breakdown in both older and middle-aged individuals. In healthy young people, studies may have to last years or even decades to potentially show any benefits, something that has yet to been done. Hence, the alkaline theory is still somewhat of a hypothesis, at least in young healthy people. However, clear benefits have been shown with alkaline treatments in older men and women and in patients with stage 2 or greater kidney disease.

The take-home message? Balance your animal food intake with some type of alkaline therapy (fruits/vegetables or alkaline waters/supplements).

Fruits and vegetables have a lot of potassium salts of organic anions and/or citric acid that can be metabolized into bicarbonate, providing that acid neutralizing effect[3226,3227,3228]. Animal proteins, when broken down, release their sulfur-containing amino acids that provide an acidic load (sulfuric acid), which cannot simply be breathed out of the body. Long-term high protein diet in rats without potassium citrate causes chronic low-grade metabolic acidosis and an increased loss of calcium and magnesium in the urine[3229]. The authors stated that an adequate intake of calcium protected their skeletons from long-term damage. Thus, eating a carnivore diet for example, may not cause any skeletal issues, especially if the calcium/magnesium intake is adequate and/or if alkaline waters are consumed. The alternative would be to couple animal foods and animal protein with an adequate amount of potassium from vegetables or citric acid from low-sugar fruits. This is also consistent with ancestral human diets that originated from equatorial Africa where there was an abundance of potassium/citric acid-rich foods[3230]. Added sugars and grains also contribute to the dietary acid load and are typically overconsumed in the Western world. The lack of potassium/bicarbonate-forming foods in the western diet exacerbates the metabolic acidosis caused by eating the processed, industrialized foods, promoting osteoporosis, inflammation and kidney stones [3231]. Chronic diet-induced metabolic acidosis is associated with hip fractures and accelerated bone loss in humans [3232, 3233]. Supplementation with alkaline-rich minerals like potassium, magnesium and calcium has been shown to raise blood and urinary pH, creating a more alkaline environment[3234]. A diet higher in fruits and vegetables can reduce kidney injury and improve metabolic acidosis[3235]. This seems to be particularly important for those with kidney issues.

Bicarbonate-forming and potassium-rich foods are thought to improve bone health, thanks to regulating the acid-base homeostasis as well as their antioxidant content. Fruits and vegetables are the only foods that contain both potassium and bicarbonate-forming substances, giving them a negative potential renal acid load (PRAL). Eating acidic foods isn't necessarily harmful as long as other variables like potassium/calcium/magnesium intake, bicarbonate-forming foods, metabolic and kidney health are taken into account.

Here is a chart of the potential renal acid load (PRAL) values of certain foods by Lanham-New (2008)[3236]

Food	Potential Renal Acid Load (PRAL)
Cheddar Cheese	26.4 mEq/100g
Egg Yolks	23.4 mEq/100g
Brown Rice	12.5 mEq/100g
Oat Flakes	10.7 mEq/100g
Liver Sausage	10.6 mEq/100g
Chicken Meat	8.7 mEq/100g
Cottage Cheese	8.7 mEq/100g
Pork Meat	7.9 mEq/100g
Beef Meat	7.8 mEq/100g
Spaghetti, White	6.5 mEq/100g
Cornflakes	6.0 mEq/100g
Bread, White	3.7 mEq/100g
Yogurt, Plain	1.5 mEq/100g
Milk, Whole	0.7 mEq/100g
Coca Cola	0.4 mEq/100g
Tea	-0.3 mEq/100g
Grape Juice	-1.0 mEq/100g
White Wine	-1.2 mEq/100g
Broccoli	-1.2 mEq/100g
Coffee	-1.4 mEq/100g
Apples	-2.2 mEq/100g
Red Wine	-2.4 mEq/100g

Lemon Juice	-2.5 mEq/100g
Potatoes	-4.0 mEq/100g
Carrots	-4.9 mEq/100g
Bananas	-5.5 mEq/100g
Spinach	-14 mEq/100g
Raisins	-21 mEq/100g

Potassium, Sodium and Blood Pressure

The blood pressure lowering effects of potassium were first described in 1928[3237]. In 1972, it was shown that increasing the potassium to sodium ratio of salt-sensitive hypertensive rats lowered their blood pressure[3238]. Recent studies have demonstrated how increasing potassium bicarbonate intake from 1,170 mg/day to 4,680 mg/day for 6 weeks can reduce rising blood pressure caused by excess sodium loading[3239].

Excess sodium intake has been traditionally associated with increased blood pressure, which is called the "salt-blood pressure hypothesis"[3240,3241,3242,3243,3244]. However, there hasn't been any definite proof that a reduction in blood pressure with a low salt diet reduces cardiovascular events or death and it can even be detrimental due to blood volume reduction and impaired kidney perfusion[3245,3246]. About 80% of people with normal blood pressure and 75% of people with prehypertension are not salt-sensitive. Even 55% of subjects with full-blown hypertension are essentially immune to the effects of salt on blood pressure[3247]. That's more than half of those with the highest blood pressure being unaffected by salt. Thus, the low salt guidelines are not really warranted for most people and may actually cause other problems, such as insulin resistance, hypothyroidism, increased heart rate, heart failure, kidney damage, high triglycerides and cholesterol[3248]. Low blood sodium and chloride have been independently known to increase the risk of death for a long time[3249].

352

Chronic salt restriction may cause "internal starvation", making the body raise insulin levels because insulin helps the kidneys retain sodium[3250]. That is why a high salt intake can be more dangerous if you are diabetic or have insulin resistance because your body is holding onto more sodium. On the flip side, healthy kidneys can handle excess sodium with ease. Salt sensitivity is primarily driven by insulin resistance and sympathetic overdrive[3251]. In fact, sugar is the real culprit when it comes to hypertension and metabolic syndrome, not salt. The body needs sodium for nerve function, muscle contraction and cell metabolism. You would be fine without ever eating another gram of sugar, but you wouldn't survive very long without salt.

Regular table salt (sodium chloride) can raise blood pressure significantly more than sodium bicarbonate or sodium acetate[3252]. Table salt is 100% sodium chloride, whereas many unrefined salts are anywhere from 92-97% sodium chloride, where the other 2-8% are composed of other minerals like calcium, magnesium and iodine. Sodium bicarbonate has actually been shown to lower blood pressure slightly in hypertensive individuals[3253]. In stroke-prone spontaneously hypertensive rats, potassium chloride administration significantly increases hypertension and plasma renin activity compared to those rats given potassium bicarbonate[3254]. Thus, the anion that comes along with sodium or potassium can determine the blood pressure response. The incidence of strokes and vascular lesions in the rats was also higher in the group receiving potassium chloride vs. potassium bicarbonate. Modern diets that are high in salt wouldn't be such a big issue if they also didn't lack bicarbonate and potassium. Thus, it isn't the dietary salt that's the problem, it is the lack of the other alkaline minerals (calcium, magnesium and potassium) and base-forming substances/bicarbonate. Fruit and vegetables contain potassium phosphate, sulfate, citrate, bicarbonate and others, but not chloride, which can be added to salt substitutes and supplements (think magnesium chloride)[3255]. Potassium bicarbonate has a natural sodium-excreting effect, reversing sodium chloride-induced increases in blood pressure[3256].

In men, a high potassium intake of about 4,300 mg/day has been found to lower the risk of stroke by 38% compared to those who consume

353

only 2,400 mg/day[3257]. Studies find that consuming less than 1,353 mg/day of potassium increases the risk of stroke by 28% and an intake between 3,500-4,700 mg/day is associated with a 24% reduced risk of stroke compared to an intake of less than 3,500 mg/day[3258]. Low potassium levels in the blood usually occurs alongside with low magnesium levels, both of which can promote cardiovascular complications[3259]. This is because low potassium levels can be caused by magnesium deficiency.

There are many ways potassium can help with hypertension and cardiovascular disease[3260,3261,3262]

- Inhibits free radical production in vascular endothelial cells and macrophages
- Inhibits proliferation of vascular smooth muscle cells
- Inhibits platelet aggregation and arterial thrombosis
- Reduces renal vascular resistance
- Reduces atherosclerotic lesion formation
- Lowers blood pressure and water retention
- Increases endothelial vasodilation
- Reduces inflammation, oxidative stress
- Improves insulin sensitivity
- Reduces catecholamine related vasoconstriction

Potassium also has a beneficial effect on blood sugar management and insulin resistance. These problems may become a bigger issue for hypertensive people who are prescribed potassium excreting thiazide diuretics. Thiazide diuretics are the preferred pharmacological treatment for hypertension but have a tendency to reduce glucose tolerance and increase the risk of type 2 diabetes[3263]. Thiazide diuretics lower serum potassium, which may actually be caused by an increased urinary loss of magnesium, and diuretic-induced hypokalemia has been shown to reduce glucose tolerance by reducing insulin secretion[3264]. Giving potassium supplements to patients receiving diuretics can improve the defective insulin response[3265]. Potassium-sparing diuretics, such as amiloride and spironolactone, however,

354

reduce potassium and magnesium excretion and in some instances can even cause hyperkalemia (too high potassium), particularly in those with kidney issues[3266].

Potassium depletion impairs insulin production and promotes carbohydrate intolerance in humans[3267,3268]. Insulin production by the pancreatic beta-cells results from potassium-induced cell depolarization[3269]. Potassium is an essential activator of pyruvate kinase, which is the enzyme involved with the last step of glycolysis, whereby energy is produced from glucose[3270]. One of the binding sites of pyruvate is dependent on potassium ions[3271]. High dietary potassium intake is also associated with a reduced risk of type 2 diabetes[3272,3273]. There is also an inverse relationship between serum potassium and fasting insulin levels[3274]. In young healthy men, insulin infusions increase the absorption of potassium into abdominal gastrointestinal organs and muscle, with a dose-dependent decrease in plasma potassium.[3275,3276]. This is the result of sodium-potassium ATPase activation and increased potassium influx into the cell. These associations are more pronounced in African Americans who tend to have lower potassium intakes[3277,3278]. In Koreans, a higher potassium intake is associated with a reduced risk of metabolic syndrome and diabetes[3279].

Here are the potassium-dependent enzymes, functions and consequences that may occur with deficient potassium[3280]

Potassium-Dependent Enzymes/Proteins	Function	Consequences of Deficit
Sodium-Potassium ATPase	Regulates transmembrane electrochemical gradient, nerve function and fluid volume	Sodium/calcium overload, hypertension, arterial calcification and nerve dysfunction
Pyruvate	The end-product of glycolysis and glucose metabolism	Hyperglycemia, diabetes and loss of ATP
Pyruvate Kinase[3281]	Glycolysis/glucose metabolism	Hyperglycemia, diabetes and loss of ATP
Pyruvate Dehydrogenase Kinase[3282]	Inactivate pyruvate dehydrogenase during glycolysis	Impaired energy production and loss of ATP
Ribokinase[3283]	Production of ATP and D-ribose, glucose metabolism	Impaired energy production and glucose intolerance
Branched-chain α-ketoacid dehydrogenase kinase[3284]	Catalyzation of the oxidative decarboxylation of branched, short-chain alpha-ketoacids	Iodine deficiency and impaired thyroid function
Fructose 1,6-bisphosphatase[3285]	Converts fructose-1,6-bisphosphate to fructose 6-	Inadequate glucose production and energy shortage in certain

	phosphate in gluconeogenesis	glucose-dependent orans
Diol Dehydratase[3286]	Catalyze the B12-dependent conversion of 1,2-diols to the corresponding aldehydes. Glycerol-lipid metabolism	Impaired alcohol and fatty acid metabolism
Heat Shock Cognate Protein (Hsc70)[3287,3288]	Regulate proper protein folding, autophagy, apoptosis and cell stability	Cell senescence, DNA damage, carcinogenesis and neurodegeneration
Pyridoxal Kinase[3289]	Vitamin B6 metabolism	Impaired serotonin, melatonin and dopamine production. Nerve dysfunction
Histone Deacetylase (HDAC) Inhibition[3290]	DNA binding and DNA expression	Accelerated aging, cardiac defects and neurodegeneration
IMP dehydrogenase or Inosine-5-monophosphate dehydrogenase (IMPDH)[3291]	Guanine de novo biosynthesis, DNA/RNA synthesis, and energy transfer	Impaired cellular function and weaker immunity
Serine Dehydratase (SDH)	Gluconeogenesis, pyruvate production	Hyperglycemia and impaired glucose tolerance

	and release of ammonia	
Tryptophanase[3292]	Tryptophan and nitrogen metabolism and neurotransmitter production	Ammonia build-up and low melatonin and serotonin
Tyrosine Phenol-Lyase[3293]	Tyrosine and nitrogen metabolism, protein synthesis, thyroid hormone production	Impaired neurotransmitter production, low thyroid

Because low potassium impairs calcium reabsorption by the kidneys, it can increase urinary calcium, which can cause kidney stones. Indeed, observational studies see an association between higher potassium intake and lower risk of kidney stones[3294,3295]. Potassium citrate may prevent kidney stones from forming and it also helps to break down kidney stones[3296,3297]. However, it is primarily citrate that seems to be responsible for this effect[3298]. Nevertheless, a low potassium intake is still a potential contributor to kidney stone formation. Consumption of fruit and/or vegetables or supplementation with sodium or potassium bicarbonate has been shown to reduce kidney injury in hypertensive kidney disease patients[3299,3300]. Thus, a higher sodium intake does not appear to be harmful to the kidneys as long as the diet is alkaline enough. This doesn't mean that you have to consume fruits and/or vegetables, as you can simply drink mineral waters that naturally contain bicarbonate.

You can ask your doctor to assess your kidney health and functioning using the below methods.

- **Blood Pressure** – hypertension damages small blood vessels in the kidneys. Most people are below 140/90. If you have kidney failure, most doctors will say that blood pressure should be lower than 130/80 but 120/80 is considered normal.

- **Protein in Urine** – traces of albumin protein in urine is an early sign of kidney disease. Optimally, you want to have less than 30 mg of albumin per gram of urinary creatinine.

- **Serum Creatinine** – poor kidney functioning leads to the accumulation of creatinine in the blood, typically a waste product. A normal serum creatinine is 0.7-1.3 mg/dL for men and 0.6-1.1 mg/dL for women. However, it can vary, depending on other variables, as having more muscle can increase serum creatinine.

- **Glomerular Filtration Rate (GFR)** – this is a calculation of kidney functioning based on creatinine levels, age, race, gender, etc. A score over 90 is good, 60-89 should be monitored, and less than 60 for three months indicates kidney damage.

- **Cystatin C** – is one of the best ways to estimate kidney function as muscle mass, exercise and creatinine levels will not affect the results, unlike GFR. A normal cystatin C is 0.6-1 mg/L.

To improve kidney health, you want to eat a healthy diet, maintain an active lifestyle, consume an adequate amount of salt, potassium and magnesium, consume bicarbonate or fruits/vegetables, stay hydrated and avoid refined carbs/sugars/omega-6 seed oils. You should also avoid smoking and excessive alcohol intake.

Getting Potassium from Food and Supplements

Potassium is found in both plants, as well as animal tissues, although fruits and vegetables tend to have more potassium than meat or fish. Up to 90% of the potassium consumed gets absorbed in the small intestine by passive diffusion[3301]. Malabsorption conditions, such as bariatric surgery, IBS and inflammatory bowel disease (ulcerative colitis and Crohn's) can reduce potassium absorption[3302].

There is large geographical variation when it comes to the foods that contribute to potassium intake. In Nordic countries, fruit and vegetables contribute 17.5% of overall potassium intake, whereas in Greece they provide 39%[3303]. Vegetables and potatoes typically provide about 24.5% of the total potassium intake in the UK[3304]. In the U.S., potatoes contribute up to 19-20% of the total daily potassium intake[3305,3306]. There is an inverse relationship between both raw, as well as cooked, vegetables and blood pressure, although the relationship is slightly greater with raw vegetables[3307]. Monocropping, and other non-regenerative farming methods, depletes the soil of potassium, reducing the potassium content of the food that is grown on it[3308].

The old RDA for potassium set by the Food and Nutrition Board of the Institute of Medicine is 4,700 mg/day[3309]. This number is based on meta-analyses investigating the effects of potassium supplementation on lowering blood pressure. However, the World Health Organization has their guidelines at 3,150 mg/day of potassium[3310]. In 2019, it was decided that there was insufficient data to set an RDA for potassium and thus an adequate intake for potassium was decided on 3,400 mg/day for men and 2,600 mg for women. However, as you know adequate intakes and RDAs are not optimal intakes. For primary prevention of hypertension, it has been recommended to get over 3,500 mg/day of potassium, which is above the adequate intake for men and women[3311]. How much potassium a person should consume per day depends on many factors, such as blood pressure, genetics and sodium intake. There is also a lot of variability in people's blood pressure responses to low and high sodium/potassium intake. In fact, many "salt sensitive" people simply need more potassium, magnesium or calcium instead of sodium restriction[3312]. It's very likely that the higher the magnesium intake, the less potassium is needed, as the former helps prevent potassium loss from the cell. On average, American adults only get around 200-250 mg of magnesium per day and less than 2,800 mg/day of potassium[3313], which is why potassium is considered a "nutrient of public health concern" in the U.S. Dietary Guidelines[3314]. It's possible that getting around 4,700 mg of potassium per day is optimal but that is probably only true for those consuming a standard American diet with a low background intake of magnesium. In those individuals, only 3% of adults in the U.S. reach that level of potassium intake[3315,3316]. In the U.S., potatoes and fruit are the primary sources of potassium[3317]. In Europe, Greece has the lowest potassium intake at 3,536 mg/day for men and 2,730 mg/day for women, which is above the adequate intake for potassium in the U.S. The highest average intake of potassium is in Spain, at 4,870 mg/day for men and 3,723 mg/day for women.[3318] In China, potassium intake is quite low, at 1,800 mg/day, which does not even meet the Chinese RDA of 2,000 mg/day[3319,3320]. Koreans get slightly more potassium at 2,900 mg/day, which primarily comes from rice, vegetables and fruit[3321].

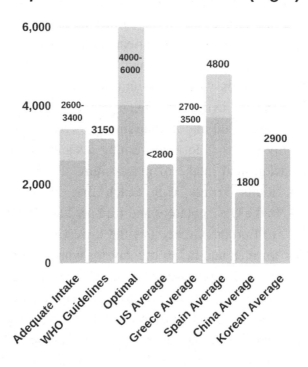

Optimal Intake of Potassium (mg/d)

Hunter-gatherer tribes that eat only whole foods have been estimated to consume anywhere from 5,850-11,310 mg/day of potassium[3322,3323]. Sodium intake was estimated at 1,131-2,500 mg/day but this did not take into account sodium consumed from blood, interstitial fluids, salt licks and salty/brackish water. Thus, the sodium intake is an underestimation. To be fair, the potassium to sodium ratio of our ancestors likely sits somewhere between 2-3:1. On the other hand, industrialized societies that consume a lot of processed foods get about 2,100-2,730 mg/day of potassium and about 3,400 mg/day of sodium or a K/Na ratio of 0.7:1 [3324,3325,3326]. If you eat a predominantly processed food diet composed of pre-packaged and/or canned foods, your sodium intake can be upwards of 10,000 mg. Thus, the ratio of potassium-to-sodium in the Western Diet is < 1, whereas it is typically thought to be > 2-3 but potentially as high as 10 among foragers[3327,3328]. In reality, if the ancestral diet was more meat heavy and the organs and blood were consumed, the true K/Na ratio sits closer to 1:1. Some papers by Eaton and Konner (1985) figure this ratio was as high as 16:1 based on low sodium intakes[3329]. However, as Dr. DiNicolantonio covers in his book *The Salt Fix*, estimates for ancestral sodium intake did not take into account the sodium content of aquatic vegetation/seafood, organs, blood, interstitial fluids, salt licks and salt/brackish water, which would have increased the estimated sodium intake that would have occurred during Paleolithic times. Indeed, blood contains 3,200 mg of sodium per liter and interstitial fluids can be even higher in salt. Our Paleolithic ancestors would have found areas that contained salt deposits. Just as animals seek out salt licks, humans would have consumed salt directly from these sources. Bottom line, we really have no idea how much salt our Paleolithic ancestors consumed because it is found in other sources besides land vegetation and muscle meat (which again were the only sources that were looked at by Eaton and Konner when estimating the "paleolithic" intake of sodium in 1985). The authors didn't take into account aquatic vegetation (such as seaweed), which can be 500-times higher in sodium than land vegetation, or aquatic animals (shellfish), both being a very rich source of salt. In fact, in their 25-year update these authors concluded:

> *Finally, it has become clear since our initial publications that marine, lacustrine, and riverine species were important sources of animal flesh during the evolution of modern Homo sapiens and may have played a role in the evolution of brain ontogeny. In any case, shellfish and other aquatic animal species must be considered part of the spectrum of ancestral nutrition adaptations. Thus, there have been changes in the way we estimate the likely diets of ancestral hunter-gatherer populations, admitting more variability. However, the best current estimates restrict most of that variability to a range from 35% to 65% animal flesh, including substantial marine animal resources for at least 0.2 million years. [3330]*

It's true that higher primates were predominantly plant-based with the addition of insects and some meat. Fossil evidence has discovered this pattern to have continued to be true with early hominids as well. However, meat consumption increased 2 million years ago during the development of Homo habilis and Homo erectus. The smaller size of the human gut compared to primates is mostly the result of cooking foods both plant and animal based, which decreased the demand for digestion[3331,3332]. Humans have gut features of both herbivores/frugivores as well as carnivores, which is why we are omnivores. This is probably why some people feel best on a plant-based diet, while others feel better on an animal-based diet.

The Dietary Approaches to Stop Hypertension (DASH) study concluded that a diet rich in fruit and vegetables has a much more beneficial effect on blood pressure than the Standard American Diet high in sugar, fat and added salt[3333]. They took 459 adults with systolic blood pressure at less than 160 mm Hg and diastolic blood pressures at 80-95 mm Hg who were assigned to a control diet low in fruits, vegetables and dairy for three weeks. After that, the subjects were randomly assigned to either the control diet, a diet high in fruits and vegetables or a combination diet high in fruits, vegetables and low-fat dairy. The subjects on the combination diet saw a 5.5 and 3.0 mmHg drop in systolic and diastolic blood pressure, respectively. Among 133 of the participants, the combination diet reduced systolic and diastolic blood pressure by 11.4 and 5.5 mmHg, respectively. The fruit and vegetables diet reduced systolic blood pressure by 2.8 mmHg and diastolic blood pressure by 1.1 mmHg. Thus, dietary patterns that include more fruit and vegetables and less processed foods can have a beneficial effect on blood pressure, but it is not the only diet that can do this. The largest benefits from any diet comes from the elimination of refined foods. That is why any diet that is composed of whole foods, including plant based or animal-based diets, are far better than your standard American diet.

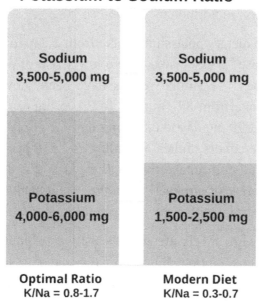

Optimal Dietary Potassium to Sodium Ratio

| Sodium 3,500-5,000 mg | Sodium 3,500-5,000 mg |

Optimal Ratio
K/Na = 0.8-1.7

Modern Diet
K/Na = 0.3-0.7

It is not necessary to add very large amounts of potassium on top of the diet to see a benefit on blood pressure. Increasing potassium by 700-1,200 mg/day can result in a 2-3 mmHg reduction in systolic blood pressure[3334]. Results from 33 randomized, controlled trials have shown that potassium supplementation, in patients with a high sodium intake, leads to a -2.53 to -6.36 mmHg drop in systolic blood pressure and a -0.74 to -4.16 mmHg drop in diastolic blood pressure[3335]. Compare that to the meager 0.8/0.2mmHg reduction in blood pressure with salt restriction in normotensive patients[3336]. A 2017 meta-analysis of 25 randomized controlled trials, including 1,163 subjects with hypertension, found that potassium chloride at doses 1,173-4,692 mg/day for 4-15 weeks reduced systolic blood pressure by 4.48 mmHg and diastolic blood pressure by 2.96 mmHg[3337]. In people with normal blood pressure, taking potassium chloride (2,346-2,541 mg/day for 4-24 weeks) reduced systolic blood pressure by about 6.8 mmHg and diastolic blood pressure by 4.6 mmHg[3338]. Potassium supplementation (1,560 mg for 16 weeks), but not magnesium or calcium (330 and 1,200 mg, respectively), causes a modest drop in blood pressure in normotensive people with a low potassium intake[3339]. However, there are reviews that find nonsignificant differences in potassium supplementation in normotensive subjects[3340].

Increasing the dietary potassium intake from 2,340 to 3,120 mg/day (a 400 mg increase) is associated with a lower risk of death from stroke in adult women[3341]. Similar results have been shown when raising potassium intake from 897 mg/day to 2,106 mg/day; 1,482 to 2,769 mg/day and 2,379 mg/day to 6,513 mg/day[3342,3343]. A meta-analysis of 15 prospective cohort studies, including 247,510 people, showed that increasing potassium intake by 1,640 mg/day was associated with a 21% reduced risk of stroke[3344]. Another meta-analysis found a 24% lower risk of stroke with higher potassium intake[3345].

Plasma potassium levels are more sensitive to potassium depletion than to overconsumption. Indeed, increasing potassium intake from 3,120 to 7,800 mg/day for 8 weeks only raised fasting potassium from 4.2 mmol/L to 4.4 mmol/L[3346]. Even a rapid dramatic increase of potassium intake from 0 to 11,700 mg/day only raised plasma potassium by 0.8 mmol/L over the 5-day period[3347]. Eating 15,000 mg/day of potassium for 20 days has shown to keep serum potassium levels still within the normal range[3348]. However, lowering potassium intake from just 3,744 to 624 mg/day for 10 days lowers plasma potassium from 4.2 to 3.4 mmol/L[3349]. Thus, it is more important to have a regularly adequate intake of potassium. Even fairly large daily doses of potassium do not seem to be an issue for those with normal kidney function. The ratio of dietary potassium to sodium also affects potassium concentrations. For example, reducing the dietary potassium to sodium ratio from 0.343 to 0.245 can decrease potassium levels from 4.26 to 3.85 mmol/L[3350].

Here is the potassium content of certain foods[3351,3352,3353,3354]

Food	Mg of Potassium per Serving	% of RDA
Carrot, dehydrated, 1 cup	1880 mg	47%
Apricots, dried, ½ cups	1,101 mg	23%
Potato, baked, 1 medium	1,000 mg	23%
Swiss Chard, 1 cup	961 mg	20%
Acorn Squash, 1 cup	896 mg	18%
Lentils, cooked, 1 cup	731 mg	16%
Prune Juice, 1 cup	707 mg	16%
Prunes, dried, ½ cup	699 mg	15%
Carrot Juice, 1 cup	689 mg	15%
Passion-Fruit Juice, 1 cup	687 mg	15%
Edamame, 1 cup	676 mg	14%
Tomato Paste, canned, ¼ cup	669 mg	14%
Pomegranate, 1 medium	666 mg	14%
Beet Greens, cooked, ½ cup	654 mg	14%
Squash, mashed, 1 cup	644 mg	14%
Raisins, ½ cups	618 mg	13%
Adzuki Beans, cooked, ½ cup	612 mg	13%
Kidney Beans, canned, 1 cup	607 mg	13%
Coconut Water, 1 cup	600 mg	13%

White Beans, canned, ½ cup	595 mg	13%
Butternut Squash, 1 cup	582 mg	13%
Parsnips, 1 cup	572 mg	13%
Tomato Puree, ½ cup	549 mg	12%
Sweet Potato, 1 medium	541 mg	12%
Spinach, 1 cup	540 mg	12%
Salmon, wild, 3 oz	534 mg	12%
Clams, canned, 3 oz	534 mg	12%
Pomegranate Juice, 1 cup	534 mg	12%
Tomato Juice, 1 cup	527 mg	12%
Beetroot, boiled, 1 cup	518 mg	11%
Baking Powder, 1 tsp	505 mg	11%
Orange Juice, 1 cup	496 mg	11%
Cream of Tartar, 1 tsp	495 mg	11%
Swiss Chard, cooked, ½ cups	481 mg	11%
Lima Beans, cooked, ½ cups	478 mg	11%
Mackerel, 3 oz	474 mg	11%
Artichoke, 1 medium	472 mg	11%
Vegetable Juice, 1 cup	468 mg	11%
Chili with Beans, ½ cups	460 mg	10%
Yams, cooked, ½ cups	456 mg	10%
Onions, dehydrated, 1 oz	454 mg	10%
Halibut, cooked, 3 oz	449 mg	9%

Soybeans, boiled, ½ cups	445 mg	9%
Snapper, cooked, 3 oz	444 mg	9%
Mushrooms, shiitake, 1 oz	430 mg	9%
Porn, loin, 3 oz	425 mg	9%
Banana, 1 medium	422 mg	9%
Cocoa Powder, 0.5 oz	405 mg	9%
Peaches, dried, ¼ cups	399 mg	9%
Rainbow Trout, 3 oz	383 mg	9%
Spirulina, dried, 1 oz	382 mg	9%
Milk, 1%, 1 cup	366 mg	8%
Avocado, ½ cups	364 mg	8%
Plantain Slices, ½ cups	358 mg	8%
Kidney Beans, cooked, ½ cups	357 mg	8%
Navy Beans, cooked, ½ cups	354 mg	8%
Green Peas, 1 cup	354 mg	8%
Brussels Sprouts, cooked, 1 cup	342 mg	8%
Sardines, 3 oz	340 mg	8%
Spinach, raw, 2 cups	334 mg	7%
Chicken Breast, grilled, 3 oz	332 mg	7%
Yogurt, non-fat, 6 oz	330 mg	7%
Salmon, farmed, 3 oz	326 mg	7%
Beef, sirloin, 3 oz	315 mg	7%
Seaweeds, 1 oz	325 mg	7%

Molasses, 1 tbsp	308 mg	7%
Cauliflower, 1 cup	303 mg	7%
Kale, raw, 1 cup	302 mg	7%
Carrots, 1 cup	300 mg	7%
Liver, 3 oz	300 mg	7%
Pistachio Nuts, 1 oz (49 kernels)	294 mg	6%
Tomato, raw, 1 medium	292 mg	6%
Beet Greens, 1 oz	290 mg	6%
Soymilk, 1 cup	287 mg	6%
Pumpkin Seeds, 1 oz	260 mg	6%
Greek Yogurt, nonfat, 6 oz	240 mg	5%
Sunflower Seeds, 1 oz	238 mg	5%
Broccoli, cooked, ½ cups	229 mg	5%
Mussels, 3 oz	227 mg	5%
Red Cabbage, 1 cup	216 mg	5%
Cantaloupe, ½ cups	214 mg	5%
Turkey Breast, roasted, 3 oz	212 mg	5%
Almonds, 1 oz	209 mg	4%
Asparagus, cooked, 3 oz	202 mg	4%
Apple, with skin, 1 medium	195 mg	4%
Cashew Nuts, 1 oz	187 mg	4%
Ham, pork, 1 slice	175 mg	4%
Watermelon, 1 cup	173 mg	4%
Bacon, pork, 1 oz	165 mg	4%

Brown Rice, 1 cup	154 mg	3%
Tuna, canned, 3 oz	153 mg	3%
Coconut Meat, 1 oz	152 mg	3%
Coffee, 1 cup	116 mg	2%
Pecans, 1 oz, 19 kernels	116 mg	2%
Macadamia Nuts, 1 oz, 12 kernels	103 mg	2%
Iceberg Lettuce, 1 cup	102 mg	2%
Dill Herb, 1 tbsp	99 mg	2%
Peanut Butter, 1 tbsp	90 mg	2%
Black Tea, 1 cup	88 mg	2%
Flaxseed, 1 tbsp	84 mg	2%
Bread, whole-wheat, 1 slice	81 mg	2%
Egg, 1 large	69 mg	1%
Brazil Nuts, 2 kernels	65 mg	1%
White Rice, cooked, 1 cup	54 mg	1%
Bread, white, 1 slice	81 mg	1%
Cheese, mozzarella, 1½ oz	36 mg	1%
Basil, 1 tsp	17 mg	0.5%
Parsley, 1 tbsp	15 mg	0.5%
Garlic, 1 clove	12 mg	0.5%
Ginger, 1 tsp	8 mg	0.5%
Oil (olive, corn, canola, soybean)	0 mg	0%

In the movie The Martian, Matt Damon plays a botanist named Mark Watney who gets stranded on Mars. The planet of red rocks and sand with nothing to eat. As they say: "*Necessity is the mother of innovation*" and like Mark said: "*Mars will come to fear my botany powers.*" He starts growing potatoes and successfully creates himself a sustainable source of food. In theory, you could survive eating just potatoes for an awfully long time. However, because of a lack in certain micronutrients, you'd eventually become deficient. Sorry Mark, dipping a potato in some crushed Vicodin won't work either. Potatoes are a fairly good source of potassium and they are quite ubiquitous in the Western diet food supply. Potatoes have even been shown to have beneficial effect on blood pressure, lipid profiles and glycemic control[3355]. This may have something to do with their high potassium content. Consider eating lightly cooked and cooled potatoes. Lightly cooking and cooling potatoes maintains the resistant starch, helping to reduce the spike in glucose and insulin that occurs after you eat it. Perhaps more importantly, eating a steak with your potato, will also reduce the glucose/insulin spike. Steak and potatoes are actually a great combination dish.

Potassium gluconate supplementation provides a similar bioavailability of potassium (~94% absorbed) as regular white potatoes[3356]. Several meta-analyses show that potassium supplementation can significantly lower blood pressure[3357,3358,3359,3360]. Giving potassium at 3,300 mg/day for 39 days can reduce systolic blood pressure by 5.9 mmHg and diastolic blood pressure by 3.4 mmHg[3361]. Meta-analyses suggest that the optimal supplemental dose for blood pressure reduction is between 1,900-3,700 mg/day of potassium, lowering systolic blood pressure by approximately 2-6 mmHg and diastolic blood pressure by 2-4 mmHg[3362,3363,3364]. Most potassium supplements are potassium chloride, citrate, phosphate, aspartate, bicarbonate and gluconate. The FDA has stated that some drugs that contain potassium chloride and provide 100 mg potassium are not safe because of their association with small-bowel lesions[3365]. Potassium salts that contain more than 100 mg of potassium per tablet are required to have a label that warns about the danger of small-bowel lesions[3366]. Enterically coated potassium chloride tablets are not as easily absorbed as liquid forms[3367].

Using salt substitutes has its risks and benefits. On one hand, salt substitutes that have more potassium and less sodium can be great for increasing dietary potassium intake without the need for supplementation[3368]. However, it can also cause hyperkalemia and do harm in patients with chronic renal failure whose kidneys are working at near maximum capacity to excrete potassium[3369]. This effect is exacerbated further by sodium restriction. For people without damaged kidneys, hyperkalemia from using salt substitutes is rare although the name 'substitute' may give off the wrong idea that salt is to be avoided completely and all you need is potassium. In reality, you need both sodium and potassium but in the right ratios. Most salt substitutes contain potassium chloride with the potassium content ranging from 440 mg to 2,800 mg per teaspoon[3370].

Potassium Absorption and Excretion

Approximately 90% of the consumed potassium is lost in the urine and 10% of it is excreted in the stool[3371]. A small amount of potassium is lost through sweat. With zero potassium intake, serum potassium can reach deficient levels of 3.0-3.5 mmol/L in about a week[3372]. Potassium excretion is regulated by the kidneys in response to dietary potassium intake. Unless you are potassium deficient, excretion of potassium increases rapidly after consuming potassium[3373]. After administration of large doses of potassium, only half of the dose appears in the urine 4-6 hours later[3374]. Potassium turnover in skeletal muscle is much slower (~70 h)[3375]. Excessive loss of potassium is rare and usually happens in diarrhea, severe burns, prolonged sweating from ultra-endurance sports or magnesium deficiency.

The kidneys regulate the excretion of potassium to maintain homeostasis based on increased or decreased intake[3376]. This is why people with healthy kidneys are able to consume a lot of potassium without toxicity. The glomerulus of the kidneys freely filters potassium and 70-80% of it is reabsorbed in the proximal tubule and loop of Henle. The two major factors that contribute to potassium loss are the renal handling of sodium and mineralocorticoid activity. Reabsorption of potassium in the proximal tubule is mostly passive and happens in proportion to the reabsorption of solute and water[3377]. In the Henle's loop of the kidney, a small amount of potassium is excreted in the descending limb, whereas reabsorption of potassium and sodium occurs in the thick ascending limb.

A lot of the potassium excretion/regulation happens in the late distal convoluted tubule (DCT) and the early connecting tubule of the kidney[3378]. Dietary potassium intake inhibits the sodium-chloride transporter in the distal convoluted tubule, reducing the absorption of salt by the kidneys. In other words, potassium consumption promotes salt excretion and helps people handle higher salt loads. Low potassium, however, causes salt retention and contributes to hypertension through activation of the sympathetic nervous system.

Aldosterone is a major mineralocorticoid that increases the excretion of potassium out in the urine by increasing sodium reabsorption in the lumen. It stimulates epithelial sodium channels and Na^+-K^+ ATPase activity. Primary aldosteronism is associated with an increased risk of cardiovascular disease [3379]. The diurnal rhythm of aldosterone expression can affect renal potassium excretion, which should be kept in mind when taking urine samples. Aldosterone tends to be highest in the morning between 6-9 AM together with cortisol and drops down in the afternoon [3380]. **Salt restriction increases aldosterone, which promotes sodium reabsorption and potassium/magnesium excretion,** creating the opposite desired effect[3381]. Normal or even excess sodium intake results in suppressed or delayed aldosterone activity[3382]. Thus, reducing sodium intake may not be the most effective long-term strategy for lowering blood pressure.

A normal serum potassium concentration is 3.6-5.0 mmol/L. Hypokalemia or low potassium levels occur below 3.6 mmol/L and hyperkalemia (elevated potassium) is above 5.0 mmol/L [3383]. Hypokalemia and hyperkalemia are rare in healthy people with normal kidney function, but it can occur due to diarrhea, kidney failure or vomiting. Hypokalemia affects up to 1/5th of hospitalized patients because of the use of diuretics and other pharmaceuticals[3384,3385]. Mild hypokalemia can cause constipation, muscle cramps, weakness and malaise. Moderate hypokalemia causes encephalopathy, glucose intolerance, paralysis, arrhythmias and dilute urine. Severe hypokalemia can be fatal due to the induction of arrythmias. Magnesium deficiency can promote hypokalemia by increasing excretion of potassium[3386]. Hypokalemia and magnesium deficiency are associated with each other. Thus, fixing potassium deficiency would also require improving magnesium deficiency. Hyperkalemia can result from the use of ACE inhibitors, such as benazepril, and ARBs, such as losartan because they reduce potassium excretion[3387,3388]. Potassium-sparing diuretics can also increase the risk of hyperkalemia. The side-effects of hyperkalemia include arrhythmias, palpitations, muscle pain and weakness[3389]. In severe cases hyperkalemia can cause cardiac arrest and death.

Here are the things that increase potassium demand or excretion

- Sodium overload
- Magnesium deficiency
- Metabolic acidosis
- Diabetes, insulin resistance
- A drop in extracellular pH levels
- A drop in extracellular bicarbonate
- Diarrhea, vomiting or extreme sweating
- Inflammatory bowel disease
- Diuretics or proton pump inhibitors (PPIs)
- Kidney damage or kidney injury

Here are the things that improve potassium status

- Sodium
- Magnesium
- Insulin
- Bicarbonate
- Citrate
- Potassium-sparing diuretics

Assessing potassium status is difficult because most of the body's potassium is located in the cell. Blood potassium levels do not correlate accurately with tissue potassium stores[3390]. Muscle biopsies can be used to look at tissue potassium status but measuring net potassium retention and excretion can also be an indicator.

Ways to Optimize Potassium Intake without Causing Hyperkalemia
Assess your blood pressure and kidney health
Include 4-5 cups of fruit and vegetables into your daily diet or consume land animal meat plus fish
Include more high-potassium foods (Fish, greens, potatoes, tomatoes and beans) in the diet if tolerated
Aim for a daily potassium intake of at least 4,000 mg and optimally 4,500 mg
Aim for a daily sodium intake of 3,500-4,000 mg
Increase sodium intake if you are sweating a lot and potassium intake if you have diarrhea or are suffering from some malabsorption diseases
Minimize packaged foods and processed foods
Salt to taste with natural salt sources like sea salt or rock salt
Be careful with using salt substitutes. Especially, if they're the only source of sodium in your diet.
Add potassium or sodium bicarbonate if you suffer from metabolic acidosis
Add potassium citrate if you suffer from kidney stones or kidney damage
Drinking alkaline mineral waters can help to keep you hydrated and reduce chronic latent metabolic acidosis
Before potassium supplementation, assess your potassium status

Check potassium levels 1 week after increasing potassium intake to see if there is a baseline risk for hyperkalemia.

Always work with your doctor before implementing any dietary change or adding a supplement.

In conclusion, potassium and sodium are important minerals for cardiovascular health and the prevention of hypertension and insulin resistance. Traditionally, all the blame has been put on sodium when really it is sugar that's the problem. Insulin resistance and diabetes can cause sodium retention and accumulation and raise blood pressure. At the same time, salt restriction comes with an array of negative side-effects that perpetuate insulin resistance and cardiac complications. Thus, it is more important to fix the underlying cause of hypertension, i.e., metabolic syndrome and obesity, which is due to an overconsumption of refined carbohydrates and sugars. Keeping potassium intake high by eating more muscle meat, fish, potatoes, fruit and green leafy vegetables alongside other mineral-dense foods is a great way to prevent glucose intolerance and ensure a healthy sodium to potassium ratio. Reaching an intake of potassium of 4,000-4,500 mg/day may seem like a daunting task but it is possible if you replace the processed foods with whole animal foods and fresh produce.

Chapter 12
Boron and Other Possibly Essential Trace Minerals

When people talk about minerals, the most common ones that get the spotlight are magnesium, potassium, sodium and calcium. Selenium, zinc and iodine also get their fair share of attention when it comes to specific conditions things like hypothyroidism or immunity. However, there are many other essential minerals that tend to fly under the radar, although they too have an important role. As a reminder, there are a total of 17 essential minerals our bodies need. In addition to that, there are 5 possibly essential trace minerals that have not been deemed to be absolutely mandatory. However, there is enough evidence to show that deficiencies in them can jeopardize health.

One of the lesser-known minerals is boron. Rest assured, there is nothing boring about boron because it has some unique benefits on the body that influence our overall health, such as improved vitamin D status, enhanced bone density and hormonal balance.

In humans, boron has not been established to be an essential nutrient. However, there are many new studies revealing the health benefits of nutritional boron[3391,3392]. **Boron intake is associated with a reduced risk of cancer, improved brain function, bone mineralization and reduced inflammation**[3393,3394,3395,3396,3397,3398]. It also seems to have anti-inflammatory, anti-osteoporotic, anti-coagulating, anti-neoplastic and hypolipemic (blood lipid lowering) effects[3399,3400,3401].

Boron is a trace element that is found in nature bound to oxygen and sodium[3402]. Boron is found in many foods, especially vegetation, as it is a structural component of plant cell walls, providing cell wall rigidity. In plants, boron also has important roles in nucleic acid, carbohydrate and protein metabolism[3403]. Awareness about the presence of boron in plants has been known since 1857[3404]. Boron is required for plant pollination, flowering, seed formation and growth[3405]. Deprivation of boron causes immediate death in the growing roots of *Arabidopsis thaliana* or thale cress[3406]. Boron deprivation in animals causes growth abnormalities and a higher prevalence of embryonic death[3407,3408,3409].

In this chapter, we will talk about the effects of boron on health and how to get enough of it from the diet. Additionally, we will give a brief overview of the other less commonly referred to trace minerals, such as lithium, vanadium, nickel and silicon. Because there is more evidence about the importance of getting enough boron than there is for lithium or nickel, we will be focusing predominantly on boron.

Boron's Effects on Health and Vitality

The first recorded use of boron as sodium tetraborate (or borax) dates back to the 8th century Arabian Peninsula where it was used to purify gold and silver[3410]. However, borax had been used in pottery as tincal glazes back in 300 AD China. Borax reacts with hydrochloric acid to form boric acid, whereas boron is the mineral found in the Earth's crust. Nowadays, the majority of boron is used in ceramics as boron carbide because of its increased hardness[3411]. Marco Polo brought boron glazes to Europe in the 13th century. In the 1600s, borax was used in metallurgy as a purifying agent. The first medicinal use of boric acid occurred in Italy in 1777 near the hot springs of Florence[3412]. In that region (Sasso, Italy), sassolite, or the mineral form of boric acid, was the main source of European borax during the 19th century[3413]. It wasn't until 1808 when boron was considered an element by Sir Humphry Davy who conducted an experiment in which he sent an electric current through a solution of borates[3414]. Nowadays, boron is used in different preservatives, fertilizers, antiseptics, fire retardants, cleaning agents as well as in industrial glass production, porcelain enamel, ceramic glazes and metal alloys[3415].

More than 90% of boron consumed is absorbed and distributed as boric acid with 98% getting excreted through urine within 120 hours[3416]. Nearly 96% of the boron in an organism is uncharged boric acid $[B(OH)_3]$ and a small amount of it is the borate anion $[B(OH)_4^-]$[3417,3418]. **Boric acid or borate forms ester complexes with many important sugars in energy production and stabilizes them, such as ribose,**

helping to produce energy and combat fatigue[3419,3420]. Because of that, boron can regulate ribose-containing enzymes and catalysts, such as S-adenosylmethionine (SAMe), diadenosine phosphate, NAD+, and the NAD+ metabolite cyclic ADP ribose (cADPR)[3421,3422]. These enzymes are involved with energy production, neurological function, cardiovascular health and bone formation. S-adenosylmethionine (SAMe) and diadenosine phosphates have a high affinity for boron[3423]. S-adenosylmethionine is one of the most common enzymatic substrates in the body, used primarily in methylation reactions[3424]. Boron also binds to oxidized NAD+ and cyclic ADP ribose, which can prevent the release of intracellular calcium[3425,3426].

Boron status is correlated with reduced prostate, cervical and lung cancer[3427,3428]. Among women with lung cancer, low boron intake (less than 0.78 mg/day) doubles the risk of lung cancer compared to those with an intake of more than 1.25 mg/day[3429]. Turkish men with a boron intake of 6 mg/day have significantly smaller prostate glands than men who consume 0.64–0.88 mg/day [3430]. Physiological concentrations of boric acid have been shown to inhibit prostate cancer cell growth in a dose-dependent manner through controlled apoptosis [3431], [3432]. Tumor suppressor p53 function requires the activation of activating transcription factor 4 (ATF4) and binding immunoglobulin protein (BiP) also known as glucose-regulated protein (GRP-78) or heat shock 70 kDa protein 5 (HSPA5), which get increased by physiological doses of boric acid[3433]. Boric acid inhibits cADPR, reducing endoplasmic reticulum Ca^{2+}. This reduction in endoplasmic reticulum Ca^{2+} activates ATF4 and nuclear factor erythroid 2 like 2 (Nrf2), which increases antioxidant response element genes[3434]. Thus, **supplemental doses of boron likely act as an Nrf2 booster, which activates our body's overall antioxidant defense enzymes.** This is why boron has been suggested to protect against oxidative stress and DNA damage. Boron compounds (such as boric acid and borax) can increase total glutathione levels, total antioxidant capacity and numerous antioxidant enzyme activities in red blood cells, such as superoxide dismutase, catalase, glutathione peroxidase, glutathione-S-transferase (GST) and glucose-6-phosphate dehydrogenase (G-6-PDH)[3435]. If you recall, superoxide dismutase prevents tissue damage from superoxide anions and catalase can prevent lipid and protein oxidation in red blood cell membranes against peroxide radicals. G-6-PDH provides the NADPH for increasing reduced glutathione, which prevents hemoglobin denaturation, preserves red blood cell membrane sulfhydryl group integrity and detoxifies oxidants in red blood cells. Thus, maintaining adequate boron intake may help to preserve the integrity of red blood cells and increase oxygenation throughout the body.

In postmenopausal women, boron intake at 3 mg/day versus 0.25 mg/day, increases red blood cell superoxide dismutase, serum enzymatic ceruloplasmin and serum copper levels (suggesting better antioxidant defenses and copper status), reduces urinary calcium and magnesium loss and increases 17 beta-estradiol and testosterone levels[3436]. The authors concluded, "...*boron is most likely an essential element in the human diet...Because of its apparent nutritional importance in calcium metabolism and utilization, humans should consume foods luxuriant in boron (fruits, vegetables, legumes and nuts)*."[3437] Unfortunately, many people do not tolerate these foods nowadays, so boron may need to be supplemented, especially considering that around 3 mg/day seems to be optimal. Another study confirmed these findings, showing that boron supplementation increases superoxide dismutase activity in red blood cells[3438]. Thus, boron seems to act as a master antioxidant by increasing glutathione levels and numerous antioxidant enzymes, likely through Nrf2 activation. In cell studies, boron compounds also protect against heavy metal-induced DNA damage[3439].

Boron might be useful for reducing symptoms of osteoarthritis by reducing inflammation[3440]. By binding to 6-phosphogluconate, boron inhibits the 6-phosphogluconate dehydrogenase enzyme and reduces the inflammatory response and reactive oxygen species[3441]. Boron also inhibits other inflammatory enzymes like lipoxygenase that triggers the inflammatory responses of prostaglandins, leukotrienes and thromboxanes[3442,3443]. Supplementing with calcium fructoborate at 112 mg/day reduces LDL, triglycerides, total cholesterol, interleukin-6, monocyte chemoattractant protein-1, c-reactive protein and the pro-inflammatory cytokine IL-1beta[3444]. Boron intake helps to regulate osteoblast and osteoclast proteins [3445]. Boron deprivation inhibits protein synthesis,[3446] which can result in delayed wound healing and soft tissue repair.

In regions with boron intake at less than 1.0 mg/day, the estimations of arthritis range from 20-70%, whereas in areas with 3-10 mg/day, the estimates for arthritis are 0-10%[3447]. It is thought that boron deficiency might also contribute to Kashin-Beck disease osteoarthritis in China[3448]. A small pilot study found that, 6 mg of boron for 8 weeks reduced symptoms of osteoarthritis in 50% of subjects compared to the 10% of placebo[3449]. A double-blind, placebo-controlled clinical trial saw that supplementing 6 mg of boron for 2 weeks reduced knee discomfort significantly in 60 adults over the age of 50[3450]. In animals, boron deficiency causes abnormal limb development and reduced bone strength[3451]. However, among Korean women, a boron intake of 0.9 mg/day does not appear to show any associations with bone mineral density[3452].

Boron also controls calcium and magnesium metabolism, which are vital for bone health [3453]. Boron supplementation reduces calcium excretion[3454]. In postmenopausal women, a low boron diet (0.25 mg boron/2,000 kcal) can raise urinary calcium and magnesium excretion [3455]. At the same time, a low boron diet promotes hyperabsorption of calcium for compensation [3456]. That can cause cardiovascular and bone health complications. Supplementing with 3 mg of boron a day for 10 months in sedentary female college students reduces serum phosphorus, increases serum magnesium and may slow the loss in bone mineral density (+0.012 g/cm^2 vs. -0.024 g/cm^2 in the boron and placebo groups, respectively)[3457]. A significant number of people do not consistently consume more than 1 mg of boron/day, suggesting that boron may be a nutrient of concern[3458].

Boron affects the function of many hormones, including vitamin D. Bone abnormalities, bone marrow sprout distortions and cartilage calcification are exacerbated by boron deficiency in vitamin D deficient chickens[3459,3460]. In rats, boron deficiency increases vitamin D deficiency-induced reduction in calcium and phosphorus absorption[3461]. Boron supplementation has been seen to increase the active vitamin D hormone (1,25-OH$_2$-vitamin D [calcitriol]) concentrations in rats[3462]. Boron also increases vitamin D3 levels in animals and vitamin-D deficient humans[3463,3464]. Supplementing 3 mg/day of boron after 63 days of boron deprivation (0.25 mg/day) raises 25-OH-vitamin D (calcidiol) levels in older men and women[3465]. Boron also increases the half-life of active vitamin D likely through inhibition of 24-hydroxylase, which is the primary enzyme that inactivates calcitriol[3466].

Boron affects sex hormones like estrogen and testosterone. By inhibiting sex hormone binding globulin (SHBG), boron prevents testosterone from being bound up, resulting in higher free testosterone. Instead of increasing estrogen directly, boron inhibits its breakdown and enhances estrogen receptor beta activity. Both estrogen and testosterone levels have been shown to double in women and men, respectively, after an increase in boron intake in individuals who were previously on a low boron diet[3467,3468]. In healthy men, supplementing with boron at 10 mg/d for only a week can raise free testosterone from 11.83 pg/mL to 15.18 pg/mL and decrease estrogen from 42.33 pg/mL to 25.81 pg/mL[3469] (although in some studies boron increases both testosterone and estradiol levels in men)[3470]. All inflammatory markers (high-sensitivity c-reactive protein, IL-6 and TNF-alpha) decreased. The increase in testosterone with boron supplementation may also be due to improved vitamin D status, which does have an effect on sex hormones[3471].

Boron deficiency might reduce mental alertness and impair executive brain function[3472]. In older men and women, boron supplementation after a period of deprivation improves cognitive processes, attention, psychomotor control and short-term memory[3473,3474]. Adding 3.25 mg/day of boron to one's diet improves memory and hand-coordination tasks compared to a boron intake of 0.25 mg/day[3475]. Boron deprivation in rats affects brain electrical activity, similar to malnutrition and heavy metal toxicity[3476]. Boron-deficient zebrafish develop photophobia (light sensitivity) caused by photoreceptor dystrophy[3477]. Thus, it's possible that people who suffer from light sensitivity may have boron deficiency (although magnesium deficiency has also been implicated in this phenomenon). There is also an association between macular degeneration and arthritis, conditions that can be driven by boron deficiency[3478].

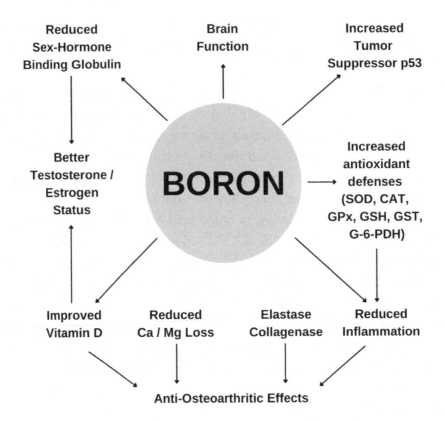

The health benefits of boron: Superoxide dismutase (SOD), catalase (CAT), glutathione peroxidase (GPx), glutathione-S-transferase (GST) and glucose-6-phosphate dehydrogenase (G-6-PDH)

Here are the boron-dependent enzymes, functions and consequences that may occur with deficient boron intake

Boron-Dependent Enzymes/Proteins	Function	Consequences of Deficit
Superoxide Dismutase	Removes superoxide anions	Increased tissue damage and oxidative stress
Catalase	Removes hydrogen peroxide	Increased tissue damage and oxidative stress
NAD+ (Nicotinamide Dinucleotide)	Energy production and governs most enzymatic reactions	Accelerated aging and onset of disease
D-Ribose	Component of ribonucleotides in RNA, energy production	Chronic fatigue and impaired gene expression
S-adenosyl-methionine (SAMe)	Methylation donor, wide enzymatic substrate	High homocysteine, inflammation and depression
Vitamin D	Hormone production, immune system function, bone density, physical growth	Increased risk of autoimmunity, weaker immune system, loss of bone density and mood disorders
Cyclic ADP Ribose (cADPR)	Calcium signaling, functions of ribose	Low blood calcium levels, intracellular calcium accumulation

6-Phosphogluconate	Regulates respiratory burst mechanisms and inflammation	Excess inflammation and reactive oxygen species
Collagenase	Degrades calcified collagen barriers	Bed sores, arthritis and tissue calcifications
Calcitonin	Reduces calcium levels and inhibits osteoclast activity	Excess calcification and reduced bone health
Estradiol	Female reproduction and fertility, neuroprotection	Infertility, neurodegeneration and impaired cognition
Gcn4	Transcription factor for gene expression and protein synthesis	Muscle mass and soft tissue deterioration
Delta-aminolevulinic acid dehydratase (ALA-D)[3479]	Heme synthesis, precursor to hemoproteins and cytochromes	Anemia, low heme and poor tissue oxygenation

Boron Food Sources

Boron does not have an established RDA or an adequate intake value, but the World Health Organization recommends an acceptable safe range of 1-13 mg of boron per day for adults[3480,3481]. A diet "high in boron" is considered to be 3.25 mg per 2,000 calories[3482]. The U.S. Institute of Medicine Food and Nutrition Board has set the upper tolerable limit for boron at 20 mg/day but no adequate intake[3483]. The WHO has increased their safe upper limit for boron to 0.4 mg/kg of body weight, which would be about 28 mg/day for a 70 kg person[3484]. The EU's upper limit, based on body weight, results in about 10 mg/day[3485]. According to data from the NHANES III (1988-1994) and the Continuing Survey of Food Intakes by Individuals (1994–1996), the median dietary boron intakes in American adults ranges from 0.87 to 1.35 mg/day[3486]. Reported intakes of boron ranges from 0.89-1.11 mg/d in the U.S., 1.75-2.12 mg/d in Mexico, 0.8-1.9 mg/d in the EU and 0.93 mg/d in Korea[3487,3488]. It seems an intake of 1-2 mg of boron a day is enough to prevent frank deficiencies, but an optimal intake is likely around 3 mg/day or more. That means that the average American adult may need to consume two to three-times more boron each day to reach optimal intake levels.

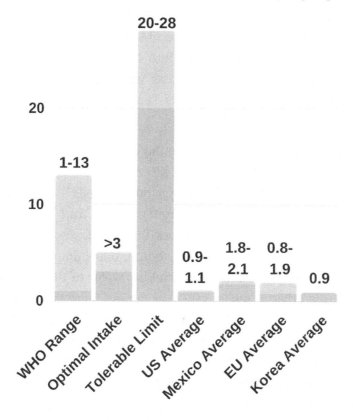

Boron is found the most in plant foods, such as legumes, vegetables, tubers and fruit. Alcoholic beverages like wine, beer and cider also have some boron. Personal-care products like toothpaste, lip balm, baby oil and deodorants also have trace amounts of boron[3489]. **Prunes are an excellent source of boron, providing 1.5 to 3.0 mg of boron per 3 oz serving**[3490]. A study found that eating 3 ounces of prunes a day for a year improved bone mineral density in postmenopausal women, but dried apples did not[3491]. Boron does not accumulate in fish or land animals, but it does in algae, seaweed and plants[3492]. Many people following an animal-based diet like to eat avocadoes to boost their boron intake (8 oz. provides ~ 2 mg of boron).

The amount of boron in plants depends on the soil boron content. Brazil, Japan and most of the U.S. have low boron in the soil because of high rainfall. California, Chile, Russia, China, Argentina, Turkey and Peru, however, have higher boron levels.[3493] Excessive levels of boron in the soil also reduce crop yields. One estimate suggested that up to 17% of the barley loss in Southern Australia was caused by boron toxicity[3494]. Borate deposits form into the ground when boric acid reacts with steam, which is why areas with hot springs and geysers tend to have more boron[3495] and why Turkey has the largest mineable borate reserves in the world[3496].

The main sources of dietary boron in the U.S. are coffee, milk, apples, beans and potatoes although they are relatively low in boron[3497]. Vegetarians have a marginally higher boron intake[3498]. For toddlers, the primary intake of boron comes from milk and fruit juices. In breast milk, boron concentrations are about 0.27 mg/L and 0.33 mg/L in cow's milk[3499]. Water also contains boron, depending on the region. The average boron amount in the drinking water of the U.S. is 0.031 mg/L[3500]. In northern France, water containing more than 0.3 mg/L of boron has been seen to significantly reduce mortality compared to less than 0.3 mg/L[3501]. That is why the World Health Organization raised its upper tolerable limit for boron in water from 0.3 mg/L to 0.5 mg/L[3502]. However, high boron in drinking water has not been shown to have adverse health effects[3503]. Living in an area with boron concentrations in drinking water of 2.05-29.00 mg/L has not caused negative health outcomes[3504].

Here are the top boron-containing foods[3505,3506,3507,3508]

Food	Mg of Boron per Serving	% of 3 mg/d
Prunes (dried plum), 1 cup	7.2 mg	240%
Red Kidney Beans, 1 cup	2.48 mg	83%
Avocado, 1 cup	2.06 mg	68%
Black Currants, 1 cup	1.74 mg	58%
Lentils, 1 cup	1.47 mg	49%
Prune Juice, 1 cup	1.43 mg	47%
Raisins, 1 oz	1.28-1.40 mg	42-46.6%
Chickpeas, 1 cup	1.05 mg	35%
Plum, 1 cup (3.5 plums)	1 mg	33%
Peaches, 1 medium	0.80 mg	26%
Almonds, 1 oz	0.80 mg	26%
Hazelnuts, 1 oz	0.79 mg	26%
Dates, 1 oz	0.26 mg	11.5%
Grape Juice, 1 cup	0.76 mg	25%
Celery, 1 cup	0.75 mg	25%
Apples, 1 medium	0.66 mg	22%

Apricots, 1 oz	0.59 mg	19%
Red Wine, 5 oz glass	0.54 mg	18%
Pears, 1 medium	0.50 mg	16%
Honey, 3 oz	0.50 mg	16%
Brazil Nuts, 1 oz	0.49 mg	16%
Peanuts, 1 oz	0.48 mg	16%
Broccoli, boiled, 1 cup	0.48 mg	16%
Walnuts, 1 oz	0.46 mg	15%
Apple Juice, 1 cup	0.45 mg	15%
Chili Con Carne with Beans, 1 cup	0.41 mg	13%
Grapes, ½ cup	0.37 mg	12%
Oranges, 1 medium	0.37 mg	12%
Lima Beans, cooked, ½ cup	0.35 mg	11%
Applesauce, ½ cup	0.34 mg	11%
Cashews, 1 oz	0.33 mg	11%
Orange Juice, 1 cup	0.18 mg	6%
Spinach, cooked, ½ cup	0.16 mg	5%
Banana, 1 medium	0.16 mg	5%

Spaghetti Sauce, ½ cup	0.16 mg	5%
Carrots, 1 medium	0.14 mg	4%
Peas, cooked, ½ cup	0.10 mg	3%
Egg, 1 medium	0.08 mg	3%
Coffee, 1 cup	0.07 mg	2%
Lettuce, 1 cup	0.06 mg	2%
Tomatoes, ½ cup	0.06 mg	2%
Tuna, canned, 3 oz	0.05 mg	2%
Milk, whole, 1 cup	0.04 mg	1%
Corn, cooked, ½ cup	0.04 mg	1%
White Rice, cooked, ½ cup	0.03 mg	1%
Chicken Breast, 3 oz	0.03 mg	1%
Tea, 1 cup	0.02 mg	0.6%
Lamb, 3 oz	0.02 mg	0.6%
White Bread, 1 slice	0.01 mg	0.3%

Boron does not easily accumulate in the body. Bone, nails and hair have higher levels of boron than fat tissue[3509]. Other tissues have a fairly even distribution of boron. Urine, blood and other bodily fluids primarily contain boric acid. The absorption of boron occurs in the intestine but not through the skin[3510]. Boron homeostasis is regulated primarily by the kidneys and urinary excretion similar to sodium[3511]. The excretion of boron happens mostly through urine, feces, bile or sweat[3512]. Up to 92-94% of boron gets excreted in the urine after 96 hours of consumption[3513]. If dietary intake of boron is high, excretion is also higher and vice versa[3514].

Environmental exposure of boron does not appear to have a significant effect on a person's boron status. A study on men working in a large boric acid borax factory saw no difference between boron levels in people working long hours versus less[3515]. Boron mine workers have a mean blood boron level of 224 ng/g and experience no symptoms of boron toxicity[3516]. Reports suggest that environmental boron exposure is not a threat to human health. However, accidental consumption of borax found in household chemicals and pesticides (at doses of 18 to 9,713 mg) causes nausea, gastrointestinal distress, vomiting, convulsions, diarrhea, rashes and vascular collapse[3517]. Oral doses of 88 grams of boric acid was not shown to be toxic[3518]. However, taking over 84 mg/kg of boron has caused gastrointestinal, cardiovascular and renal adverse effects, dermatitis and death[3519,3520,3521].

In the 1870s, it was discovered that sodium borate and boric acid can be used to preserve food[3522]. However, in 1904, it was reported by Wiley that boric acid in doses above 500 mg/day (77 mg/day of boron) for longer than a month caused disturbances in digestion and appetite[3523]. By the 1950s, boron was forbidden to be used as a food preservative. Excess borax is toxic to kidneys and other organs by causing DNA damage[3524,3525]. The reason why boron in physiological amounts is not toxic is because it is less directly absorbed compared to borax that can cause irritation on the skin and in the airways[3526]. However, the tolerance level for borax may be higher than expected. Intravenous borax at doses of 20 g (2.12 g of boron) has not been found to cause toxic side-effects in patients receiving brain tumor treatment[3527]. In excess amounts, boron can also contribute to the development of goiter by competing with iodine absorption[3528]. High concentrations of boron are used to eliminate bacterial and fungal infections by causing mitochondrial dysfunction[3529].

Supplemental boron usually comes in the form of sodium borate, sodium tetraborate, boron amino acid chelate, boron gluconate, boron glycinate, boron picolinate, boron ascorbate, boron aspartate, boron citrate and calcium fructoborate. Taking 10 mg of boron as sodium tetraborate for 7 days can reduce sex hormone binding globulin (SHBG), resulting in higher testosterone, lower high sensitivity CRP (hsCRP) and TNF-alpha 6 hours after supplementation[3530]. Boron supplementation does not seem to effect lean body mass or strength in young male bodybuilders already engaged in resistance training[3531]. Calcium fructoborate has been shown to reduce inflammation in osteoarthritis and cardiovascular disease[3532,3533]. Higher dose boron supplementation, compared to marginal amounts of boron, show improvements in bone density in animals[3534,3535,3536]. There is limited research about the bioavailability or efficacy of other forms of boron supplements.

High intakes of boric acid (over 3 grams) must be ingested to acutely increase the excretion of riboflavin (vitamin B2). Thus, there is likely nothing to worry about if consuming boron from whole foods or boron supplementation at typical intake levels[3537]. Boric acid can form complexes with thiamine (vitamin B1) and pyridoxine (vitamin B6), the consequences of which are still undetermined[3538]. When taking boron supplements, it might be worthwhile to consume away from foods that contain b-vitamins and/or consume more foods with B-vitamins like beef, fish, eggs, vegetables and beans. Boron has a high affinity for riboflavin and ingesting high doses of boron may lead to side effects due to riboflavin deficiency (dry skin, photosensitivity and inflammation of the mouth and tongue)[3539]. Thus, to be safe, it may be best to space boron supplementation away from your B-complex supplement or B-vitamin intake.

Other Possibly Essential Trace Minerals

Although boron is not considered an essential mineral, it is still particularly important and has numerous beneficial effects, especially in regard to bone density and hormonal balance. In addition to boron, there are other possibly essential trace minerals that have some benefits, such as lithium, vanadium, nickel and silicon. They may not be required to be consumed all the time, but they may be helpful for certain situations.

Here are the other possibly essential trace minerals our bodies need in small amounts:

- **Lithium** – Lithium is an element used in electronics, but it is also present in living organisms as well as plants[3540]. There is a lot of evidence to show that lithium benefits mental conditions like bipolar disorder, schizophrenia and depression[3541]. Lithium can also benefit cluster headaches[3542]. These benefits are partially due to increased serotonin transmission but also from enhanced folate and vitamin B12 transport[3543].

  o Areas with low lithium in drinking water have higher rates of crime, violence and suicides[3544]. Lithium deficiency can also promote aggression and rates of homicide[3545,3546]. Supplemental lithium for 4 weeks in former drug users increases positive mood scores, happiness and friendliness steadily over the course of the treatment compared to placebo[3547].

  o In animals, lithium deficiency causes low birth weight, depressed fertility and weaning weight[3548,3549,3550]. However, women who take lithium during pregnancy increase the risk of their infants developing Ebstein's cardiac anomaly[3551].

  o Lithium also has insulin mimetic properties, making it beneficial for blood sugar management[3552]. However, treating mental disorders with large doses of lithium can cause nephrogenic diabetes insipidus[3553]. Mild symptoms of lithium toxicity cause gastrointestinal problems, tremors and muscle weakness. Severe toxicity can result in coma, convulsions and death.[3554] This is why ingesting low doses of lithium contained naturally in mineral waters seems to be a better way to get lithium for the general population compared to large pharmaceutical doses.

  o Grains and vegetables are the predominant food sources of lithium, but fish, eggs and meat also contain it[3555]. The RDA for lithium is suggested to be 1 mg/day[3556].

The minimum adult requirement for lithium is estimated to be less than 100 mcg/day[3557]. The daily need for lithium can typically be covered with food and water intake but this usually falls short of an optimal intake. Supplementation with lithium should only be done with the provision of a medical professional.

- **Vanadium** is another trace metal with many biological functions[3558]. In animals, vanadium deficiency causes low thyroid, depressed fertility and lactation[3559].
  - Cell studies show that vanadium has insulin-mimetic properties and anti-diabetic effects in animals[3560,3561,3562]. Because of this potent insulin mimicry, excessive intakes of vanadium can cause hypertension and death[3563]. However, oral vanadyl sulfate at 100 mg/day for 3 weeks improves liver and peripheral insulin sensitivity in type 2 diabetic patients[3564]. Supplemental vanadyl sulfate (100 mg/d) or sodium metavanadate (125 mg/d) has not been shown to improve glycemic control in type 1 diabetics but their daily insulin requirements did decrease[3565,3566].
  - The threshold for vanadium toxicity in humans is around 10-20 mg/d or only 1/5th of the observed beneficial dosage for insulin reduction, causing mild gastrointestinal disturbance and green tongue[3567]. In mice, the lethal dose has been estimated to be 1000 mg/kg body weight[3568]. Vanadium deficiency is not considered common in humans and most diets provide 15-30 mcg/day[3569,3570]. Foods with vanadium include shellfish, mushrooms, herbs and some seeds[3571]. Fruit and vegetables contain little vanadium.
- **Nickel** is circumstantially essential for growth, reproduction and glucose regulation in animals[3572]. It also influences iron metabolism, increasing its concentrations in the liver[3573]. Vitamin B12 and folic acid are also connected to nickel status[3574,3575]. These vitamins are important for regulating

homocysteine and thus affecting cardiovascular disease risk[3576].

    o   Estimated daily requirements for nickel have been thought to be 25-35 mcg/d[3577]. Doses of 0.6 mg from water can cause skin irritation and rashes[3578]. Food sources of nickel include chocolate, nuts, beans, peas and grains[3579]. Most diets provide less than 150 mcg/d.

- **Silicon** is a mineral important for connective tissue, blood vessels and bones[3580]. Animals deprived of silicon show abnormal cartilage and collagen[3581]. Reports since the 1970s suggest deficient silicon intake contributes to hypertension, atherosclerosis, bone disorders, arthritis and Alzheimer's disease[3582]. Silicon might have antiatheroma activity, reducing the accumulation of plaque in the inner wall of arteries[3583].

    o   There is no RDA for silicon because of limited data. Athletes are recommended to get 30-35 mg/d and non-athletes 5-10 mg/d[3584]. Thus, the more physically active you are or the older you are, the more silicon you might need to compensate for the damage to the joints and tendons. On average, people get around 20-50 mg of silicon a day[3585]. Foods that contain silicon include vegetables, high bran grains, oats, fruit and beans[3586]. However, you may want to couple that with foods that contain collagen, such as animal meat tendons and ligaments. The vitamin C from plant foods will also help with collagen synthesis[3587].

- **Cobalt** is an essential mineral that we haven't touched upon much so far. It is a key component of cobalamin or vitamin B12, which is an essential vitamin[3588]. Vitamin B12 deficiency can cause hyperhomocysteinemia, which is associated with cardiovascular disease and Alzheimer's[3589,3590,3591]. Ruminants convert cobalt into vitamin B12 in their stomachs.

    o   Grazing animals in areas with low cobalt in the soil experience "bush sickness" and other wasting diseases[3592,3593]. Cobalamin neuropathy causes nervous system abnormalities[3594]. In experimental acrylamide neuropathy, ultra-high doses of vitamin B12 (500 mcg/kg of body weight, intraperitoneally) promotes nerve regeneration in rats[3595].

o Cobalt deficiency can lead to pernicious anemia, which is disease wherein not enough red blood cells are produced due to a vitamin B12 deficiency[3596]. It can be treated with oral B12 replacement at doses of 1,000 mcg/d or with injections[3597].

o There is no established RDA for cobalt, but adults are suggested to get 10-20 mcg/d. The upper limit is 250 mcg and therapeutic range 50-100 mcg/d.[3598] You can get cobalt from liver, buckwheat, cereal grains, meat, seafood and vegetables.

o The RDA for vitamin B12 is 2.4 mcg[3599]. You can get vitamin B12 only from animal foods. Clams and liver are the richest source of vitamin B12 with a dose of 70-84 mcg/3oz serving. Fish like salmon and trout provide 4.8-5.4 mcg/3oz. Nutritional yeast provides around 2.4 mcg of B12 per serving.

o The median lethal dose for soluble cobalt salts is estimated to be 150-500 mg/kg[3600]. Soluble cobalt salts are considered possibly carcinogenic to humans. Addition of cobalt compounds to stabilize beer foam in 1966 Canada caused a type of cardiomyopathy called *drinker's cardiomyopathy*[3601].

In addition to the ones already mentioned, there are many other trace minerals that play some biological role in the body (bad or good), such as bromine, germanium, rubidium, tin and others. Their requirements, however, are just so small that there is no need to specifically try to increase intake. The toxic heavy metals aluminum, cadmium, arsenic and lead should be avoided, as many of us are getting too much due to environmental contamination. In regard to cadmium toxicity, oysters and scallops are the most contaminated, thus, their intakes should be kept to a minimum[3602,3603,3604,3605,3606].

Chapter 13
Sulfur, Glutathione and Organosulfur Compounds: Fueling Up the Body's Antioxidant Defenses

Sulfur, after calcium and phosphorus, is the 3rd most abundant mineral in the human body[3607]. Elemental sulfur is non-toxic and soluble sulfate salts come packaged in things like Epsom salts, which are typically used in baths for helping with muscle recovery and muscle soreness. Burning sulfur (power plants) creates sulfur dioxide (SO_2), which can be harmful to the eyes and lungs in large concentrations. When SO_2 reacts with atmospheric water and oxygen, it produces sulfuric acid (H_2SO_4) and sulfurous acid (H_2SO_3), which make up acid rain. Sulfuric acid is also a powerful dehydrant that can be used to dehydrate sugar or organic tissue[3608]. Sulfuric acid can also be produced in the body by eating sulfur-rich amino acids found in animal protein.

Elemental sulfur has a bright yellow color and it is solid at room temperature. By mass, sulfur is the 5th most common element on Earth. Historically, it has also been called brimstone, which means "burning stone". It is used in making matches, pesticides, explosives and fireworks.

- Sulfur (S) is the chemical element with an atomic number of 16 and a neutral charge.
- Sulfate (SO_4^{2-}) and sulfite (SO_3^{2-}) are oxy-anions (an oxygen-containing negative ion) of sulfur with a negative charge[3609]. Sulfate is a salt found in some foods as well as cleaning products, but sulfite is used for food preservation and processing.
- Sulfur oxide is the smelly substance found in volcanoes and thermal springs, whereas organic sulfur is used by the body to carry out a wide range of processes, especially antioxidant defense.

Sulfur was used in Ancient Egypt, Greece, China and India for medicine, dermatology as well as gunpowder[3610,3611]. Historically, sulfur has been used to treat skin conditions, dandruff, improve wound healing and protect against acute radiation[3612,3613]. Today, organic sulfur has been seen to improve rosacea and psoriasis[3614]. Sulfur springs and water have been known to have therapeutic effects for centuries.[3615]. Studies show that spa therapy with sulfur water improves osteoarthritis and inhaling aerosolized sulfur-containing water improves respiratory conditions[3616,3617]. Sulfur-containing foods like broccoli may protect against inflammatory conditions like vascular complications from diabetes and heart disease[3618,3619].

In this chapter, we will talk about the many different forms of sulfur and how to obtain it from food. Sulfur can be found in various food sources and compounds. Many of these substances have a similar effect in promoting the body's detoxification systems, methylation and antioxidant defense through boosting glutathione.

Effects of Sulfur on the Body

Next to hydrogen, CO2 (carbon dioxide) and nitrogen, sulfur was probably one of the first nutrients organisms used as a building block of life and for energy production[3620]. These organisms can be divided into sulfur reducing or sulfur oxidizing[3621,3622]. Sulfur-reducing anaerobic bacteria are believed to trace back to 3.5 billion years ago, making them one of the oldest living microorganisms on Earth[3623]. They obtain energy through a process called sulfate respiration, during which the oxidation of organic compounds or molecular hydrogen gets coupled to the reduction of sulfate[3624].

Sulfur-oxidizing microorganisms oxidize hydrogen sulfide (H_2S) into elemental sulfur or sulfate to generate reducing power[3625]. Sulfur acts as a signaling nutrient for hydrogen sulfide[3626], which is a colorless gas that has many therapeutic effects when generated in the body[3627,3628,3629]. Many invertebrates need sulfur to grow and to avoid some of the potential harmful effects of hydrogen sulfide[3630,3631]. At low concentrations, hydrogen sulfide stimulates the electron transport chain increasing energy production[3632].

One of the most important roles of sulfur is serving as a precursor in glutathione synthesis and promoting detoxification[3633]. The sulfur amino acids (SAA) methionine and cysteine promote protein synthesis as well as glutathione synthesis [3634]. In plants, sulfur partitioning between glutathione and protein synthesis determines growth[3635]. Eating a sulfur-rich diet in humans increases glutathione levels and reduces oxidative stress[3636,3637,3638]. Glutathione regulates prostaglandin biosynthesis and thus has anti-inflammatory effects[3639]. It also has detoxifying properties that support liver health[3640]. Sulfur baths and sulfur mineral water consumption have been shown to increase antioxidant defense status, lower oxidative stress and improve lipids [3641, 3642]. **Most of the sulfur in our bodies is stored as glutathione in the liver and because inflammation depletes glutathione it will also deplete sulfur.** Reactive oxygen species oxidize sulfur-containing amino acid residues as well[3643]. Cysteine is the rate-limiting factor in glutathione synthesis and a cysteine deficiency will result in low glutathione levels. Thus, suboptimal cysteine levels can lead to low glutathione and increased oxidative stress. The increased oxidative stress seen in aging is even thought to be the result of cysteine deficiency[3644,3645]. Eating more sulfur in the diet can help spare the losses of glutathione.

Iron-sulfur (Fe-S) cluster proteins partake in many cellular processes that involve electron transfer, DNA synthesis and energy production[3646]. Defects in Fe-S cluster biogenesis cause numerous mitochondrial issues, anemia and problems with fatty acid and/or glucose metabolism[3647]. Mammalian target of rapamycin (mTOR), the body's master growth pathway responsible for growth, regulates iron metabolism through iron-sulfur cluster assembly [3648]. Prolonged elevation of iron-sulfur cluster assembly enzyme (ISCU) protein levels enhanced by mTOR can inhibit iron-responsive element and iron-regulatory protein binding activities that are involved in iron uptake. Thus, sulfur is important for keeping iron levels in check and preventing iron overload. Protein and amino acids that contain sulfur (which also tend to contain the most leucine) are the most mTOR-stimulating food sources that promote growth[3649,3650]. **Under low sulfur amino acid intake, protein synthesis is maintained at the**

expense of sulfate and glutathione synthesis[3651]. Low serum levels of cysteine and glutathione are associated with muscle wasting diseases[3652] and mitochondrial damage[3653].

Alzheimer's disease patients have low levels of sulfur and selenium[3654]. These reductions are implicated in the lower glutathione levels seen in these patients and the increased oxidative stress and neuroinflammation, which promote neurodegeneration[3655,3656]. **Sulfur is also a potent aluminum antagonist that can reduce aluminum accumulation.** Aluminum is a neurotoxin and considered a causative factor in Alzheimer's disease[3657]. High amounts of aluminum in the brain tissue are associated with familial Alzheimer's disease and other neurological disorders[3658].

Connective tissue, the skin, ligaments and tendons require sulfur for proper cross-linking and extracellular matrix proteins like glycosaminoglycans (chondroitin sulfate, dermatan sulfate, keratan sulfate and heparan sulfate). **Extracellular matrix proteins are highly sulfonated. They strengthen the bone structure and retain moisturization.** Sulfur is needed to make bile acid for fat digestion and is a constituent of bone, teeth and collagen. The hair and nails are made of a sulfur-rich protein called keratin.[3659] **Sulfur is also a component of insulin and hence is needed for blood glucose regulation.**

Vitamin D3 sulfate is a water-soluble form of vitamin D3, unlike un-sulfated vitamin D3, and as a result of that, it can travel the bloodstream more freely without needing to be carried in LDL lipoproteins[3660]. Vitamin D3 sulfate has less than 5% of the ability of vitamin D to mobilize calcium from bones and about 1% of the ability to stimulate calcium transport, raise serum phosphorus or cause bone calcification[3661,3662]. The form of vitamin D in human milk and raw cow's milk is vitamin D3 sulfate[3663] but pasteurization destroys it. The origins of vitamin D3 sulfate are not clear, but a sulphated precursor may be needed for its synthesis. Cholesterol sulfate is considered a potential precursor as it's widely distributed throughout the body[3664]. Instead of being just a metabolic end-product, cholesterol sulfate is found in all cell membranes and epidermal barriers, but mostly in skin tissue[3665,3666]. Sunlight hitting the skin also appears to be a source of vitamin D3 sulfate. Regardless, adequate sulfur status is required to make vitamin D3 sulfate.

Cholesterol sulfate helps to create a barrier against harmful bacteria and fungi in the skin as well as support platelet adhesion[3667]. It regulates the gene for a protein called profilaggrin, which is a precursor to filaggrin that protects the skin[3668,3669,3670]. By interacting with phospholipids, cholesterol sulfate can stabilize biological membranes[3671,3672]. Perhaps it is plausible that for optimal protection against the UV radiation from the sun you need adequate cholesterol sulfate and sulfur from diet. During sperm maturation, cholesterol sulfate stabilizes sperm cell membranes[3673]. In cultured skin fibroblasts, cholesterol sulfate inhibits sterol synthesis at the level of 3-hydroxy-3-methylglutaryl-CoA reductase, the rate-limiting step in cholesterol synthesis[3674]. This affects epidermal lipid metabolism. Atherosclerosis may develop because of a cholesterol sulfate deficiency[3675]. Cholesterol sulfate is also a substrate for the synthesis of sulfonated steroid hormones, such as pregnenolone sulfate and DHEA sulfate[3676,3677,3678].

Vitamin D induces sulfotransferase enzyme SULT2B1b activity, which governs cholesterol sulfurylation[3679]. **Sunlight exposure triggering eNOS sulfate production increasing sulfate availability for heparan sulfate proteoglycan (HSPG) synthesis, which buffers against glycation damage and coagulation**[3680]. Hyperinsulinemia reduces cholesterol sulfurylation into cholesterol sulfate by lowering calcitriol bioavailability, thus contributing to thrombosis seen in COVID-19[3681]. Platelets will respond to cholesterol sulfate but not other forms of cholesterol or steroid sulfates under the same conditions[3682]. Like vitamin D3 sulfate, cholesterol sulfate is also water-soluble and doesn't have to be packed in LDL particles to be delivered to tissues. **It has been shown that cholesterol sulfate inhibits enzymes involved in blood clotting, such as thrombin and plasmin, which may prevent coagulation in the arteries**[3683]. Additionally, sulfate promotes oxygen delivery to oxidative phosphorylation dependent cells. Thus, **a lack of sulfur in the diet**

may worsen COVID-19 outcomes by increasing protein glycation and coagulation and reducing tissue oxygenation.

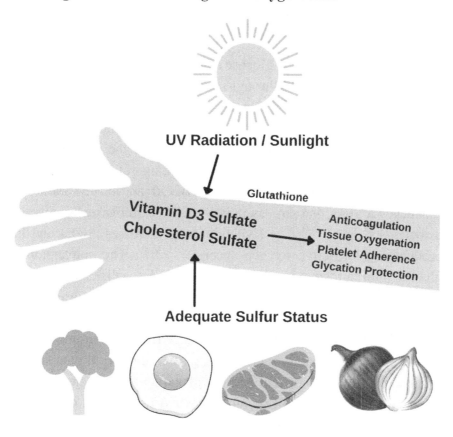

Sulfur is needed for transporting free fatty acids from chylomicrons/VLDL/LDL into the capillary endothelium. Lipoprotein lipase (LPL), which is an enzyme that governs the uptake of free fatty acids from lipoproteins into cells, works with heparan sulfate proteoglycans (HSPGs)[3684]. Abnormal or dysfunctional LPL expression is associated with various conditions like atherosclerosis, hypertriglyceridemia, obesity, diabetes, heart disease, stroke, Alzheimer's and chronic lymphocytic leukemia[3685,3686,3687]. **A low sulfur intake could lead to a decrease of free fatty acids into tissues that express LPL, such as the heart, skeletal muscle and brown adipose tissue, leading to an increase in free fatty acids in the blood**

and reduced supply to these tissues for energy[3688]. Those who are obese are known to have a reduction in free fatty acid uptake into brown adipose tissue resulting in lower heat production and reduced energy disposal[3689].

Sulfur is also involved with glucose metabolism via cholesterol sulfate. Glucose can enter the cells through specific cholesterol-rich sites in the cell wall called lipid rafts that also control GLUT-4's actions[3690]. GLUT4 is a receptor that sits on our cellular membranes to bring glucose into muscle cells. Cholesterol sulfate in the cell membrane reduces the risk of oxidation. Overconsuming refined glucose and fructose can promote the formation of advanced glycation end products (AGEs) that are associated with cardiovascular disease, diabetes and aging[3691,3692]. Hyperglycemia increases AGEs and the production of reactive oxygen species[3693,3694]. The conversion of glucose into fat storage also glycates the fat cells and damages them[3695]. As a result of that, cholesterol can't be transported to the membrane and it accumulates in the cell, leading to macrophage accumulation that contributes to atherosclerosis and thrombosis[3696]. Sulfur can be in oxidation states ranging from -2 to +6. If glucose gets reduced by sulfur +6, it will prevent glycating the muscle cells and protect against AGEs. **Sulfate ions attached to oxidized cholesterol have been shown to be protective against atherosclerosis**[3697]. Glutathione, the sulfur antioxidant, also eliminates AGEs and AGEs are more dangerous when glutathione levels are low[3698].

Here are the sulfur-dependent enzymes, functions and consequences that may occur with deficient sulfur intake

Sulfur-Dependent Enzymes/Proteins	Function	Consequences of Deficit
Glutathione	Protects against oxidative stress and inflammation	Increased oxidative stress and reduced immunity
Nrf2/ARE	Promotes glutathione synthesis and other antioxidants	Increased oxidative stress and reduced immunity
Heparan Sulfate Proteoglycans (HSPGs)	Anticoagulation and protection against glycation damage	Increased risk of thrombosis and atherosclerosis
Lipoprotein Lipase	Promotes the uptake of cholesterol and free fatty acids into tissues	Hyperlipidemia. atherosclerosis and decreased skeletal muscle/heart function
S-adenosyl-methionine (SAMe)	Methylation donor, wide enzymatic substrate	High homocysteine, inflammation and depression
Vitamin D3 Sulfate	Hormone production, immune system function, Anticoagulation	Increased risk of autoimmunity, weaker immune system, blood clots
Cholesterol Sulfate	Stabilizes cell membranes, protects the skin, promotes vitamin D3 sulfate	Increased risk of coagulation, thrombosis and platelet aggregation. Cell membranes

	synthesis, platelet adherence, anticoagulation	more vulnerable to oxidation.
Hydrogen Sulfide	Cell signaling, antioxidant defense, glutathione	Increased oxidative stress, cardiovascular complications, inflammation
Methylation	Moves methyl groups around, prevents high homocysteine	High homocysteine, neuronal complications and inflammation
Endothelial NO Synthase (eNOS)	Promotes nitric oxide and endothelial function	Atherosclerosis and hypertension
Trans-sulfuration Pathway	Mediates glutathione pathways and hydrogen sulfide production	Increased oxidative stress and reduced glutathione

Sulfur-Containing Compounds and Organosulfur Compounds

Sulfur exists in all cells and extracellular compartments as part of the amino acids cysteine and methionine. **Covalent bonds of sulfhydryl groups between molecules form disulfide bridges that are required for the structure of proteins that govern the function of enzymes, insulin and other proteins.** Sulfur is also a component of chondroitin in bones and cartilage, thiamine (vitamin B1), biotin (vitamin B7), pantothenic acid (vitamin B5) and S-adenosyl methionine (SAM-e), methionine, cysteine, homocysteine, cystathione (an intermediate in the formation of cysteine), coenzyme A, glutathione, chondroitin sulfate, glucosamine sulfate, fibrinogen, heparin, methallotheionein and inorganic sulfate.[3699,3700] In nature, sulfur is found in volcanic rocks and unrefined salt. Certain hard water sources like San Pellegrino (~500 mg/L) and Gerolsteiner (35 mg/L) also have some sulfur. With the exception of thiamine and biotin, all of these substances are synthesized utilizing methionine or cysteine. The vast majority of the sulfur demands of the body are met with methionine and cysteine consumption. **Glutathione, taurine, N-acetylcysteine, MSM (methylsulfonylmethane) and inorganic sulfate can spare the dietary need for methionine and cysteine**.

Here is an overview of the effects of sulfur-containing compounds[3701]:

- **Glucosamine Sulfate** - Glucosamine sulfate is an amino-monosaccharide (a combination of glutamine and glucose). It is required for cartilage glycosaminoglycan (GAG) synthesis[3702]. Glucosamine has many trials showing efficacy for osteoarthritis[3703]. It has been found that glucosamine supplementation was associated with a 39% reduction in overall mortality among 16,686 U.S. subjects[3704]. Among 466,039 participants without cardiovascular disease in the UK, habitual glucosamine use was linked to a lower risk of cardiovascular disease events[3705].

- **Chondroitin Sulfate** – Chondroitin sulfate is found in human cartilage, bone, skin, cornea and the arterial wall. It is believed to increase water retention and elasticity in cartilage. Sulfur in the diet provides sulfates for glycosaminoglycan synthesis and glutathione in cartilage[3706].

- **Glutathione** – Glutathione is the main antioxidant that regulates free radicals, immunity and redox homeostasis[3707]. **A low protein diet with inadequate sulfur amino acids can induce a glutathione deficiency. Cysteine and N-acetylcysteine are glutathione precursors**[3708].

- **Cysteine** – Oral cysteine supplementation increases glutathione levels[3709]. It can also chelate certain trace minerals and alleviate potential heavy metal toxicity.

- **N-acetylcysteine (NAC)** – Oral NAC increases intracellular cysteine and glutathione levels[3710]. Administration of the glutathione precursor N-acetylcysteine increases glutathione synthesis and improves hydrogen sulfide clearance[3711]. NAC can increase the release of histamine from mast cells and peripheral mononuclear blood cells and lower nitric oxide levels[3712,3713,3714,3715]. In certain susceptible individuals this may increase the contraction of the pulmonary vascular bed leading to what's commonly referred to as "wheezing in the lungs". Thus, NAC is not for everyone, and supplementation may need to be cycled on and off or necessitate the administration of nitric oxide boosters (beetroot powder, dietary nitrates, citrulline/arginine) and/or antihistamines.

- **Taurine** – Taurine regulates detoxification, bile acid conjugation, membrane stabilization and cellular calcium modulation[3716]. It is important for muscle contractions, energy production, hydrogen sulfide synthesis and more.

- **Alpha-Lipoic Acid (ALA)** – ALA regulates antioxidant activity and oxidative stress[3717]. It has also been shown to increase CoQ10 and glutathione levels[3718,3719]. ALA also activates Nrf2.

- **Dimethyl Sulfoxide (DMSO)** – DMSO can scavenge free radicals and pass-through membranes easily[3720,3721]. It can also protect against the breakdown of joint tissue in inflammatory arthritic conditions[3722].

- **Methyl-sulfonyl-methane (MSM)** – In humans, MSM is used to treat arthritic conditions, muscle pains, allergies and for immunomodulation, although its effectiveness is not considered clinically significant[3723,3724,3725,3726,3727]. MSM inhibits inflammation through suppressing NLRP3 inflammasome activation[3728]. It has been found to be safe and effective for hemorrhoids[3729]. In mice, MSM can be therapeutic against obesity-induced metabolic disorders, such as hyperglycemia, hyperinsulinemia and insulin resistance[3730].

- **S-adenosylmethionine (SAMe)** – SAMe is a metabolite of methionine and an important methyl donor that can lower homocysteine[3731]. The body can make all the SAMe it needs from methionine, but defective methylation or inadequate consumption of SAMe cofactors (methionine, choline, folate) would reduce SAMe production. SAMe also increases the production of hydrogen sulfide.

- **Methionine** – Methionine is one the main protein-creating amino acids needed for methylation and protein synthesis. As a methyl donor, it helps to prevent fatty liver[3732]. AIDS patients have low methionine, and it can be effective for treating Parkinson's disease and acute pancreatitis[3733,3734].

Here is an overview of the sulfur-containing compounds that have therapeutic indications (Adapted from Parcell 2002)

Sulfur Nutrient	Therapeutic Indications	Dosage
N-acetylcysteine	Acetaminophen toxicity and hepatoprotection[3735,3736]	250–1500 mg/day Oral or IV
	Chronic bronchitis[3737,3738]	200 mg two to three times a day or 400-600 mg/d
	HIV infection [3739,3740,3741,3742]	800-7,000 mg/day
Cysteine	Increase glutathione and chelates excess minerals[3743,3744]	Eat foods high in sulfur-containing amino acids, such as whey protein or eggs
Methionine	Precursor to SAMe, which supports methylation	Adequate daily intake 1,500-9,000 mg. Take together with B12, folate,

		glycine or trimethylglycine to avoid elevation of homocysteine.
	Acetaminophen poisoning[3745]	2.5 g orally every 4 hours up to a dose of 10 grams
	Parkinson's disease[3746]	Initially 1 g/d, then increase to 5 g/d. Decrease dose as improvements occur
	Ethanol detoxification[3747]	500 mg three times a day
	Fatty liver (helps to transmethylate choline, which prevents fatty liver)	500 mg three times a day
Taurine	Congestive heart failure[3748,3749]	1.5-4 g/day
	Diabetes[3750,3751]	1.5-4 g/day
	Prevention against macular degeneration and other age-related eye problems[3752,3753,3754]	1.5-4 g/day
	Inhibition of platelet aggregation[3755,3756]	1.5-4 g/day
	Hypercholesterolemia[3757,3758]	1.5-4 g/day
	Epilepsy[3759,3760]	200 mg/kg IV
	Alzheimer's disease[3761,3762]	1.5-4 g/day

	Cystic fibrosis[3763,3764,3765]	30 mg/kg/d for steatosis
Glutathione	Adjunct to cisplatin treatment for cancer[3766,3767,3768]	1.5g-2.5 g/m2 IV or 600 mg IM
	Optimal aging[3769]	600-1,200 mg/day of reduced glutathione orally
	Cardiovascular disease	600-1,200 mg/day of reduced glutathione orally
	Male infertility[3770]	600 mg/day IM
Alpha Lipoic Acid	Diabetic neuropathy [3771,3772,3773,3774]	600 mg three times daily
	Diabetes, inhibits glycosylation (in vitro)[3775]	Unknown but likely anywhere from 300-1,800 mg/day
	Daily use as an antioxidant	300-600 mg/day[3776]
MSM	Degenerative arthritis[3777,3778]	2,000-3,000 mg/day for at least six weeks
	Interstitial cystitis and other bladder disorders[3779]	30-50 cc instilled into the bladder
	Healing athletic injuries and muscle/joint pain[3780,3781,3782]	1,200-4,000 mg/day

	Depression[3783,3784,3785]	400-1,600 mg/day
S-adenosyl-methionine (SAMe)	Fibromyalgia[3786,3787]	800-1,200 mg/day
	Arthritis[3788,3789,3790]	400-1,200 mg/day
	Alcohol detoxification[3791]	400 mg/day
	Alcoholic cirrhosis[3792]	1,200 mg/day

Adapted from: Parcell S. (2002). 'Sulfur in human nutrition and applications in medicine.' Alternative Medicine Review: A Journal of Clinical Therapeutic, 7(1), 22–44.

Organosulfur compounds (OSCs) found in allium vegetables like garlic, shallots, onions and artichoke have therapeutic potential for cancer via anticarcinogenic and antigenotoxic properties[3793]. OSCs from allium vegetables contain various chemical structures, such as diallyl sulfide (DAS), diallyl disulfide (DADS), allylmethylsulfide (AMS), allicin, alliin, S-allylcysteine (SAC), S-allylmercaptocysteine (SAMC), dipropyl sulfide (DPS) and dipropyl disulfide (DPDS), that inhibit carcinogenesis. Alliums were recorded to be able to suppress tumor growth even by Ancient Egyptians, Indians and Hippocrates[3794]. Organic sulfur can even suppress cancerous cell growth[3795,3796,3797]. Sulfur-containing compounds and foods have been shown to be protective against radiation[3798].

Consumption of allium vegetables is associated with reduced cancer risk, especially stomach and colon cancer[3799,3800,3801,3802]. **Eating a half of an onion or more per day may lower the incidence of stomach cancer**[3803]. In Northeast China, consumption of fresh cabbage and onions is inversely associated with brain cancer risk[3804]. More than one serving of garlic per week is inversely associated with the risk of colon cancer in postmenopausal women[3805]. Onion and garlic also possess antidiabetic, antibiotic, cholesterol-lowering and fibrinolytic effects[3806]. **Garlic can lower mild hypertension and blood lipids, potentially reducing the risk of cardiovascular** disease[3807,3808,3809,3810]. **Allium-containing vegetables like garlic, shallots and onions can raise glutathione levels via their organosulfur compounds**[3811,3812,3813].

To activate the beneficial compounds of garlic, you have to first crush it and let it sit for a few minutes. Heat inactivates the enzyme alliinase (which catalyzes the synthesis of allicin), reducing the beneficial effects of garlic[3814]. An in vitro study found that heating or boiling inhibited the anti-platelet aggregation properties of crushed and uncrushed garlic, but the crushed garlic maintained more of its anti-aggregatory activity compared to uncrushed garlic[3815]. Microwaving uncrushed garlic for 60 seconds or for 45 minutes in a regular oven blocks the DNA damage protective effects against a carcinogen in rats[3816]. **Some of garlic's beneficial compounds can be retained if you crush it and leave it out in the open for 10 minutes before heating.**

Sulforaphane (SFN) is another sulfur-containing compound that has a long record of health benefits[3817]. Research has shown sulforaphane to be beneficial in managing Type-2 diabetes[3818], improving blood pressure[3819], Alzheimer's disease[3820], liver detoxification[3821], LDL cholesterol[3822], the immune system[3823], bacterial and fungal infections[3824], inflammation[3825], liver functioning[3826], brain derived neurtrophic factor (BDNF)[3827] and may reduce cancer risk[3828,3829,3830]. A lot of these effects are mediated by increased glutathione production as SFN promotes glutathione synthesis through the activation of the Nrf2/ARE antioxidant defense system[3831]. Sulforaphane is produced when we eat cruciferous vegetables like broccoli, cauliflower, cabbage and Brussels sprouts[3832]. **Eating cruciferous vegetables have been shown to raise glutathione S-transferase activity (a family of phase II detoxification enzymes), which binds glutathione to a wide variety of toxic compounds for their elimination**[3833,3834].

Sulforaphane primarily inhibits Histone Deacetylase (HDAC), which is a group of enzymes that interact with DNA. HDAC deacetylizes or unravels DNA proteins called histones that keep it compact.

Sulforaphane inhibits HDAC enzymes, which increases the activity of another pathway called Nrf2[3835]. This stimulates the production of important antioxidants like glutathione, thioredoxin, and NQO-1. The same HDAC inhibition leads to the activation of autophagy as well[3836]. Sulforaphane promotes energetic stress, autophagy, and cell death[3837]. It will kill both cancerous cells but may scavenge some weaker healthy cells in the process.

SFN causes mild oxidative stress, lipid peroxidation, and generates ROS[3838], which are considered to be a part of its chemo-protective properties by up-regulating glutathione and autophagy[3839]. Excessive sulforaphane can cause some genome instability and over-activation of white blood cells[3840]. In mice, sulforaphane increases the susceptibility to seizures and other symptoms of toxicity[3841]. However, that was done with a dose at 200 mg/kg, which is pretty hard to reach by eating just vegetables or broccoli. The optimal intake of sulforaphane is around 20-40 mg/day in humans.

When certain plants get damaged from either chewing or cutting, they produce myrosinase that transforms glucoraphanin into sulforaphane. After this process, SFN starts to degrade quite rapidly[3842]. Cooking at temperatures below 284°F (140°C) also produces sulforaphane[3843] but higher temperatuures starts to destroys it. Adding mustard seeds to cooked broccoli increases the bioavailability of sulforaphane[3844]. Sprouting cruciferous vegetables increases their glucoraphanin content by 10-100 times. Broccoli sprouts are the highest in glucoraphanin and sulforaphane[3845]. Raw cruciferous vegetables, if overconsumed, can inhibit iodine absorption because of the goitrogens. Uncooked Brussels sprout juice in rats causes DNA damage and apoptosis or programmed cell death[3846]. Thus, it is better to cook or steam your vegetables slightly to get the best benefits but not overcook them.

There is no RDA for sulfur specifically[3847]. Regardless, a significant amount of the population, especially the elderly, may not be getting enough sulfur[3848]. Sulfur-containing compounds like methionine and cysteine are mostly found in animal protein sources with some in legumes and cereal. Sulfur is the 6th most abundant micromineral in breast milk[3849]. A small amount of sulfur can be obtained from the organosulfur compounds found in foods like broccoli, garlic and onions. However, the actual content of sulfur in a food depends on the soil quality[3850]. Unfortunately, most U.S. soils are reported to be sulfur depleted, which promotes deficiencies in the population[3851]. The sulfur content of food will also reduce with storage and time. Grain-based diets will also result in sulfur deficiency because they are naturally low in sulfur, unless other sulfur-rich foods are eaten. You can recognize sulfur for its gassy smell that resembles rotten eggs, as eggs also contain this mineral.

Here are the highest sulfur-containing foods[3852]

Food	Mg of Sulphur per 100 Grams
Scallops, steamed	570 mg
Lobster, boiled	510 mg
Crab, boiled	470 mg
Peanuts, roasted	380 mg
Prawns, boiled	370 mg
Mussels, boiled	350 mg
Veal Cutlet, fried	330 mg
Veal Fillet, roast	330 mg
Milk, dried, skimmed	320 mg
Haddock, steamed	300 mg
Chicken, boiled	300 mg
Lamb Heart, roast	300 mg
Lamb Kidney, roast	290 mg
Haddock, fried	290 mg
Brazil Nuts	290 mg

Lamb Liver, fried	270 mg
Peanuts, raw in shells	260 mg
Sardines, canned	260 mg
Oysters, raw	250 mg
Cod, poached	250 mg
Chicken Liver, fried	250 mg
Parmesan Cheese	250 mg
Cod Roe, fried	240 mg
Milk, dried, whole	240 mg
Beef, corned, canned	240 mg
Peach, dried	240 mg
Cod, baked	230 mg
Stilton Cheese	230 mg
Cheddar Cheese	240 mg
Salmon, canned	220 mg
Beef, minced	220 mg
Beefburger	220 mg
Cod, steamed	210 mg
Lamb Tongue, stewed	190 mg
Salami, 3 slices	190 mg
Ham, canned	180 mg
Wholemeal, brown, 1 roll	170 mg
Apricots, dried	160 mg
Chicken Leg Quarter	160 mg
Pork, fried, grilled	160 mg
Wholemeal, white, 1 roll	150 mg

Almonds	150 mg
Beef Sausage, fried	140 mg
Tripe, stewed	140 mg
Chicken Wing Quarter	130 mg
Rabbit, stewed	130 mg
Liver Sausage	130 mg
Luncheon Meat, canned	120 mg
Meringue	110 mg
Pork Pie	100 mg
Walnuts	100 mg
Black Pepper	100 mg
Milk, skimmed	90 mg
Spinach Leaves	90 mg
Cabbage, raw	90 mg
Onions, fried	90 mg
Peach, stewed	90 mg
Bread, brown, 1 slice	90 mg
White Bread, 1 slice	80 mg
Wholemeal, 1 slice	80 mg
Figs, dried	80 mg
Chickpeas	80 mg
Milk, whole	80 mg
Coconut, desiccated	80 mg
Hazelnuts	80 mg
Brussels Sprouts	80 mg
Mushrooms, fried	70 mg

Bran, wheat	65 mg
Doughnut	60 mg
Mung Beans, cooked	60 mg
Roast Potatoes	60 mg
Dates, dried	50 mg
Onions, raw	50 mg
Spring Onions	50 mg
Kidney Beans, boiled	50 mg
Leeks, boiled	50 mg
Lentils, boiled	40 mg
Milk Pudding	40 mg
Sultanas	40 mg
Radishes	40 mg
Beans, baked in tomato sauce	40 mg
Peas, boiled	40 mg
Custard	40 mg
Barley, boiled	35 mg
Pasta, boiled	30 mg
Spaghetti, boiled	30 mg
Swede, boiled	30 mg
Mushrooms, raw	30 mg
White Rice	30 mg
Black Currants	30 mg
Cabbage, boiled	30 mg
Endive, raw	30 mg
Olives, in brine	30 mg

Potato, baked	30 mg
Mashed Potatoes	20 mg
Porridge, cooked	20 mg
Loganberries	20 mg
Sweet Potato, boiled	20 mg
Turnip, boiled	20 mg
Prunes	20 mg
Raisins	20 mg
Raspberries	20 mg
Asparagus, boiled	20 mg
Beetroot, boiled	20 mg
Celery, raw	20 mg
French Beans, boiled	10 mg
Banana	10 mg
Blackberries	10 mg
Strawberries	10 mg
Artichoke, boiled	10 mg
Apple, raw	5 mg

Whole foods appear to be a more bioavailable source of sulfur than supplements. A study found that sulfur-methyl-L-methionine (SMM) from kimchi was more bioavailable than SMM by itself and it led to better digestion[3853]. Fresh vegetables and plants also contain more organosulfur compounds than processed foods. **Taurine, which spares cysteine and hence the utilization of sulfur in the body for other functions, is found in animal foods but not in plants.**

Benefits of Hydrogen Sulfide (H_2S)

Inorganic sulfur compounds can also accept electrons to create hydrogen sulfide (H_2S). Hydrogen sulfide was long considered an environmental toxin produced by swamps or volcanos, but it has been observed to also have therapeutic benefits on the cardiovascular system and intestines [3854, 3855, 3856, 3857]. Overproduction of H_2S is implicated in cancer, whereas deficiency can cause vascular disease[3858]. Hydrogen sulfide is involved in multiple cell signaling processes, such as the regulation of reactive oxygen species, reactive nitrogen species, glutathione and nitric oxide[3859].

- **Hydrogen sulfide has cardioprotective effects that prevent atherosclerosis and hypertension**[3860,3861,3862,3863]. Hydrogen sulfide has vasorelaxant effects and acts as an endogenous potassium-ATP channel opener [3864, 3865]. H_2S stimulates endothelial cells to facilitate smooth muscle relaxation[3866]. Disrupted H_2S production has been suggested to promote endothelial dysfunction[3867].
  - **Hydrogen sulfide enhances the effects of nitric oxide by increasing endothelial NO synthase (eNOS)**[3868]. H_2S and nitric oxide are mutually dependent in regulating angiogenesis and endothelium-dependent vasorelaxation [3869, 3870]. Formation of NO and H_2S creates a novel compound called nitrosothiol that has vasodilating effects[3871,3872]. The cytoprotective effects of hydrogen sulfide are dependent of nitric oxide[3873]. Thus, **you need sufficient NO and the minerals required for its synthesis to gain the benefits of H_2S**. Next to carbon monoxide and nitric oxide, **hydrogen sulfide is thought to be the third biological gas**[3874,3875]. The benefits on vasoactivity of garlic are also mediated by H_2S, which is a food relatively high in sulfur[3876].
  - Hydrogen sulfide is an endogenous stimulator of angiogenesis or the growth of new blood vessels[3877,3878]. Patients with coronary artery occlusion or multivessel lesions have lower H_2S levels[3879]. In

mice and human umbilical vein endothelial cells, H_2S exerts antiatherogenic effects [3880]. It also protects against endoplasmic reticulum stress[3881]. **Some of the cardioprotection is also mediated through Nrf2 signaling**[3882]. Hydrogen sulfide alleviates myocardial ischemia-reperfusion injury by maintaining mitochondrial function[3883].

○ Hydrogen sulfide plays a role in kidney homeostasis and may provide kidney protection[3884,3885]. It affects glomerular filtration and sodium reabsorption[3886]. H_2S regulates blood pressure and vascular tone through activating the renin angiotensin aldosterone system (RAAS)[3887]. During renal hypoxia, H_2S can help to restore oxygen balance by increasing blood flow to the medulla [3888]. Tubulointerstitial hypoxia has been recognized as the final pathway from chronic kidney disease (CKD) to end-stage renal disease (ESRD)[3889]. Sodium hydrogen sulfide (NaHS) has been shown to attenuate fibrosis and inflammation in obstructive kidney disease at doses starting at 5.6 mcg/kg/d and optimally at 56 mcg/kg/d[3890,3891,3892].

- **H_2S may have neuroprotective effects by increasing glutathione and suppressing oxidative stress**[3893,3894]. There is a high level of hydrogen sulfide in the brain and it may act as an endogenous neurotransmitter[3895,3896]. H_2S might be able to scavenge peroxynitrite and prevent oxidative stress, especially in the brain where there is low extracellular glutathione[3897]. In mice and rats, H_2S is released from bound sulfur in neurons and astrocytes[3898]. Alzheimer's patients have lower hydrogen sulfide levels in the brain[3899].

- **Hydrogen sulfide is involved in cell-death and inflammatory signaling as an endogenous mediator**[3900,3901]. Elevation of H_2S accompanies inflammation, infection and septic shock[3902,3903,3904]. Inhibiting H_2S production contributes to the gastric injury caused by non-steroidal anti-inflammatory drugs (NSAIDS)[3905].

- Endogenous gases (CO, NO, H_2S) regulate mitochondrial biogenesis during inflammation and oxidative[3906]. Hydrosulfide anions HS^- (80% of H_2S dissociates to HS^- in the extracellular space but are essentially equal in the cell) are strong reducing agents of reactive oxygen species[3907]. In cardiomyocytes, **hydrogen sulfide activates Mn-SOD and Cu,Zn-SOD and decreases ROS during ischemia/reperfusion**[3908]. However, in the presence of oxygen (O_2), H_2S can generate free radicals.
- Nitric oxide and hydrogen sulfide protect gastrointestinal integrity and promote ulcer healing[3909]. However, H_2S produced by gut microbes is associated with ulcerative colitis, Crohn's disease and irritable bowel syndrome[3910]. Thus, having an overabundance of bacteria that produce H2S in the gut could be detrimental.

- **Hydrogen sulfide has a beneficial effect on longevity and lifespan.** Nematodes that live in an environment of 50 ppm H_2S exhibit higher thermotolerance and a 70% longer lifespan[3911]. They also have higher antioxidant and stress-response gene activity[3912]. In bacteria, endogenous hydrogen sulfide and nitric oxide protects against antibiotic-induced oxidative stress and death[3913]. In mice, H_2S exposure inhibits cytochrome c oxidase, lowers metabolic rate and body temperature, putting them in a suspended hibernation state[3914]. Calorie restriction is one of the few known ways of reliably extending lifespan in virtually all species[3915]. **Endogenous production of hydrogen sulfide appears to be essential for the benefits of restricting calories by mediating the enhanced stress resistance**[3916]. However, humans who are chronically exposed to exogenous sources of hydrogen sulfide from working in an industrial setting show signs of accelerated aging[3917].

Hydrogen sulfide gets synthesized by three enzymes: cystathionine γ-lyase (CSE), cystathionine β-synthetase (CBS) and 3-

mercaptopyruvate sulfurtransferase (3-MST)[3918,3919]. CSE and CBS go through the trans-sulfuration pathway during which a sulfur atom gets transferred from methionine to serine, forming a cysteine molecule[3920]. Thus, dietary amino acids like methionine and cysteine are the main substrates in the production of hydrogen sulfide. They are also needed for glutathione and taurine synthesis[3921,3922].

After consumption, methionine reacts with adenosine triphosphate (ATP) with the help of methionine adenosyltransferase to produce S-adenosylmethionine (AdoMet), a universal transmethylation methyl donor. The transfer of AdoMet creates S-adenosylhomocysteine (AdoHcy), which gets rapidly hydrolyzed into adenosine and homocysteine by AdoHcy hydrolase. Homocysteine can be either methylated into methionine or used to synthesize cysteine and hydrogen sulfide. About 50% of the methionine taken up by hepatocytes gets regenerated[3923]. The remaining 50% is metabolized by the trans-sulfuration pathway. In the first step of the trans-sulfuration pathway, homocysteine is condensed with serine to form cystathionine by cystathionine β-synthase (CBS). Then, cystathionine is cleaved into α-ketobutyrate, ammonia and cysteine by cystathionine γ-lyase (CSE). Cysteine cannot be converted back into methionine by mammals, making methionine an essential amino acid. However, cysteine can be created from methionine via the trans-sulfuration pathway.[3924,3925,3926]

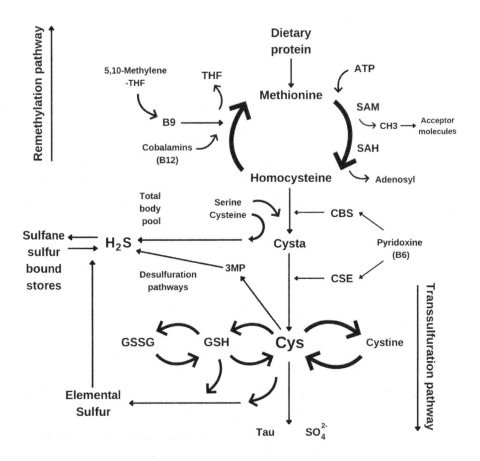

Abbrevations: THF – tetrahydrofolate; SAM - S-adenosyl methionine; SAH - S-adenosyl homocysteine; CH3 – methyl group; CBS - cystathionine β-synthase; Cysta – cystathionine; CSE - cystathionine γ-lyase; 3MP - 3-mercaptopyruvate; Cys – cysteine; GSH – glutathione; GSSG - glutathione disulfide; H_2S – hydrogen sulfide; Tau – taurine; SO_4^{2-} - sulfate oxyanions.

Adapted From: Ingenbleek, Y., & Kimura, H. (2013). Nutritional essentiality of sulfur in health and disease. Nutrition reviews, 71(7), 413–432.[3927]

The trans-sulfuration pathway is present in many tissues, such as the kidney, liver and pancreas[3928]. It does not appear to take place in the spleen, testes, heart and skeletal muscle[3929]. Inhibition of the trans-sulfuration pathway results in a 50% decrease in glutathione levels in cultured cells and tissues[3930,3931,3932,3933,3934]. Oxidative stress can activate the trans-sulfuration pathway and antioxidants downregulate it[3935,3936]. The synthesis of glutathione from cysteine depends on ATP and thus magnesium[3937].

Sulfates and Sulfites

Sulfites are food preservatives derived from sulfur added to packaged foods, hair colors, topical medications, eye drops, bleach and corticosteroids to prevent spoilage[3938,3939]. They can also develop naturally during fermentation, such as in sauerkraut, kimchi, beer or wine. Thus, alcohol can be a significant source of sulfites, which in excess can promote inflammation and gastrointestinal problems[3940]. About 1% of people, and 3-10% of asthmatics, are sulfite sensitive and they experience swelling, rashes, nausea and possibly seizures or anaphylactic shock when consuming large amounts of sulfites[3941,3942]. Some people are allergic to sulfur and sulfur-containing foods like garlic or eggs, causing them to experience swelling, rashes and low blood pressure[3943]. Consumption of high-sulfite wine has been linked to a higher occurrence of headaches among people with a history of wine-induced headaches[3944]. Roughly 10% of migraine patients report alcohol as a migraine trigger[3945].

Sulfate is a source of sulfur for amino acid synthesis. Sulfate-reducing bacteria in the gut can promote ulcerative colitis through hydrogen sulfide[3946]. Patients of ulcerative colitis have elevated levels of fecal sulfide and sulfate-reducing bacteria [3947],[3948]. Sodium sulfate supplementation has been shown to stimulate the growth of sulfate-reducing bacteria[3949]. Excess sulfide can overburden the detoxification systems, impairing butyrate oxidation and causing colonic epithelial inflammation.

Consumption of drinking water naturally high in sulfate (above 500 mg/L) is generally well tolerated, although large doses in certain susceptible individuals may cause diarrhea and gastrointestinal stress[3950]. Most public drinking water in the U.S. is below 250 mg/L and only 3% is greater than 250 mg/L[3951]. Most demineralized bottled water contains less than 250 mg/L of sulfate[3952,3953]. Ingesting 3.6 grams of sulfate from water with 1,200 mg/L of sulfate over the course of 3 days does not cause diarrhea in healthy adults[3954]. This was confirmed in a longer-term study showing that ingesting sulfate water at a concentration of 1,200 mg/L in healthy men does not induce diarrhea over the course of 6 days[3955]. Giving 18.1 grams of sodium sulfate in a single dose has been shown to cause severe diarrhea but not when given in four divided doses[3956].

Food sources of sulfate[3957]

Food	Mg of Sulfate per gram
Apples, dried	4.9 mg
Apricots, dried	3.0 mg
Potato, dried	2.0 mg
Brown Wheat Bread	1.5 mg
White Bread	1.3 mg
Raisins	1.3 mg
Soya Flour	1.2 mg
Dates, dried	1.1 mg
Currants	1.1 mg
Water Cress	1.1 mg
Prunes	1.0 mg
Sausage	1.0 mg

Sultanas	1.0 mg
Almonds	0.9 mg
Hazelnuts	0.9 mg
Broccoli	0.9 mg
Brussels Sprouts	0.9 mg
Mustard Cress	0.9 mg
Coconut, desiccated	0.9 mg
Rye Bread	0.8 mg
Crab, tinned	0.8 mg
Cabbage	0.8 mg
Jam	0.7 mg
Pectin	0.7 mg
Peanuts	0.7 mg
Sesame Seeds	0.7 mg
Swede	0.7 mg
Sauerkraut	0.7 mg
Shellfish	0.7 mg
Sunflower Seeds	0.6 mg
Muesli	0.6 mg
Turnip	0.6 mg

Avocado	0.5 mg
Okra	0.5 mg
Cauliflower	0.5 mg
Potato Chips	0.5 mg
Coconut Milk	0.5 mg
Parsley	0.4 mg
Snow Peas	0.4 mg
Figs, dried	0.4 mg
Red Wine	0.4 mg
Biscuits	0.35 mg
White Wine	0.3 mg
Corn Flakes	0.3 mg
Brazil Nuts	0.3 mg
Celery	0.3 mg
Potato	0.3 mg
Radish	0.3 mg
Cider	0.27 mg
Wheat Flour	0.26 mg
Beer	0.26 mg
Tomato Juice	0.25 mg

Corned Beef	0.24 mg
Chocolate	0.24 mg
Yoghurt	0.2 mg
Baker's Yeast	0.2 mg
Grapes, fresh	0.2 mg
Guava, fresh	0.2 mg
Kiwi Fruit, fresh	0.2 mg
Ice Cream	0.2 mg
Grape Juice	0.2 mg
Butter	0.14 mg
Cheese	0.13 mg
Egg	0.12 mg
Milk	0.1 mg
Coffee, Tea	0.1 mg
Coconut Flesh	0.1 mg
Bacon	0.1 mg
Sugar	0.1 mg
Cola	0.08 mg
Banana, fresh	0.07 mg
Apricot, fresh	0.06 mg

Apple, fresh	0.03 mg
Honey	0.02 mg

Gastrointestinal absorption of sulfate happens in the stomach, small intestine and colon[3958,3959,3960,3961]. The absorption process is sodium-dependent[3962, 3963]. Heat and cooking reduce the digestibility of cysteine because heating oxidizes cysteine into cystine, which is absorbed more poorly[3964]. More than 80% of oral sulfate taken as soluble sulfate salts like sodium sulfate or potassium sulfate gets absorbed[3965]. Insoluble sulfate salts like barium sulfate barley get absorbed[3966]. The sulfate that does not get absorbed in the upper gastrointestinal tract will be passed to the large intestine and colon where it is either excreted in the feces, reabsorbed or reduced to hydrogen sulfide[3967].

Getting Enough Sulfur-Containing Amino Acids from the Diet

While sulfur from soils and subsequently in food has seen a decline over the past few decades, sulfur-containing amino acids, especially methionine, are easily found in the Western food supply with the exception of vegan diets. The daily requirement for sulfur amino acids in humans is ~13–15 mg/kg, which for an average person weighing 80 kg would be 1,040-1,200 mg or 1-1.2 grams[3968,3969,3970]. However, some authorities believe this to be inadequate and recommend 25 mg/kg/d[3971,3972]. Getting about 3 grams of sulfur amino acids per day may be needed to avoid deficiency[3973]. These values may be 2-3 times higher after physical trauma, injury or healing[3974]. About 89% of sulfur amino acids are obtained as cystine, which is the oxidized disulfide of cysteine[3975]. Ingesting ample amounts of cysteine will also have a sparing effect on methionine[3976]. Safe minimum methionine requirements in the presence of excess dietary cysteine have been found to be 5.8-7.3 mg/kg/d compared to the 12.9-17.2 mg/kg/d in the absence of dietary cysteine (a 55-58% sparing effect)[3977].

Optimal Intake of
Sulfur-Containing Amino Acids

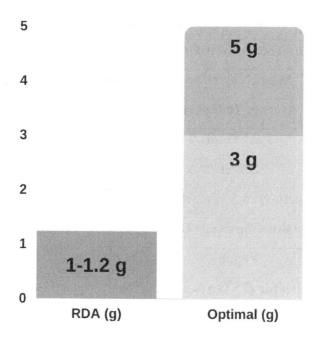

An analysis of long-term vegans in California revealed they get on average 64 grams of protein a day and 15 mg/kg/d of sulfur-containing amino acids[3978]. This meets the lower recommendations but may be inadequate for growing children, athletes or HIV patients. Not all plant foods are low in methionine. Corn, sunflower seeds, oats, chocolate, cashews, almonds and sesame seeds are relatively high in methionine although still lower than animal proteins[3979]. Oats and corn also have plenty of cysteine.

Here is an estimated intake of sulfur amino acids (SAA) on different diets[3980]

Group	SAA (g/d)
High Protein	6.8
High Protein, Low Calorie	5.0
Asian-American	4.8
Average Balanced	4.3
Fast Food	4.1
Dieter	3.5
Lacto-Ovo-Vegetarian	3.0
"Health-Conscious Diet"	2.6
Vegan	2.3
Elderly People (75 years and older)	1.8

Sulfur amino acids are not maintained in the body for the long-term. They either get excreted through urine, oxidized into sulfate or stored as glutathione. Sulfur is excreted primarily as sulfate with urinary sulfate reflecting the overall intake of sulfur from inorganic sources or amino acids[3981]. The 24-hour urinary excretion of urea, the final end-product of protein metabolism, reflects the 24-hour urinary excretion of sulfate because methionine and cysteine are the primary sources of body sulfate stores[3982,3983,3984]. Urinary sulfate excretion is inversely associated with all-cause mortality in the general population with higher excretion rates linked with mortality[3985]. In kidney transplant recipients, high urinary sulfate excretion also increases the risk of graft failure[3986], which is a life-threatening complication of hematopoietic stem cell transplantation (HSCT). Tylenol and laxatives increase the excretion of sulfur compounds and increase sulfur needs[3987,3988]. An excess of sulfur-containing amino acids promotes urinary calcium excretion, but this can be offset by increasing the alkalinity of the diet[3989].

Many drugs used in the treatment of joint diseases and pain like acetaminophen require a lot of sulfate for their excretion[3990]. Up to 35% of acetaminophen is excreted conjugated with sulfate and 3% is conjugated with cysteine[3991]. The rest is conjugated with glucuronic acid, which is a major component of glycosaminoglycans that is essential for the integrity of cartilage. Thus, acetaminophen depletes the body of sulfur. Added methionine or cysteine can overcome methionine deficiency induced by acetaminophen[3992]. Doses of acetaminophen at 3-4 g/d are commonly used in patients and this will tax their sulfur status.

The RDA for protein is 0.36 g/lb or 0.8 g/kg of bodyweight. That would be enough to cover your daily bare essentials for survival but a lot of experts also consider this to be inadequate[3993]. Average daily protein intake in Western countries falls somewhere between 12-17%, whereas in hunter-gatherer tribes it's somewhere around 19-35%, depending on the location[3994]. Eating around 20-25% of your calories in protein is considered safe and a good range to aim for[3995].

To maintain nitrogen balance and not lose muscle mass, the elderly need a minimum of protein intake of 0.8 g/kg of bodyweight a day but values of 1.0-1.25 g/kg have been suggested[3996,3997,3998]. Older people are recommended to get 15% of their daily calories as protein, which would equate to about 70-80 grams per day, providing about 3.5-4.0 grams of sulfur amino acids a day[3999]. Unfortunately, the majority of folks do not meet that requirement and are replacing protein foods with carbohydrates and fats[4000]. This can lead to age-related muscle loss or sarcopenia and metabolic syndrome as a result of that. Adequate protein intake prevents muscle loss or sarcopenia, frailty, and dependence on caretaking later in life[4001]. Maintaining adequate protein intake promotes bone health and reduces risk of hip fractures in old people[4002,4003]. A higher protein intake may be more important for the aging population amongst whom it's been found that the RDA for protein may be inadequate for maintaining skeletal muscle[4004].

Higher protein intake during a caloric deficit promotes weight loss, helps to maintain more muscle, and keeps the metabolic rate up[4005]. Compared with standard weight loss diets with normal protein and low-fat intake, high-protein diets have been found to be more effective[4006]. When people are allowed to eat as much as they want on a diet consisting of 30% protein, they end up consuming on average 441 fewer calories a day than when eating only 10% protein[4007]. Higher protein intake also promotes muscle growth and strength[4008]. Current research has seen that the maximum effects of protein on muscle growth appears to be around 0.8-1.0 grams of protein per pound of lean body mass, which would be roughly 1.0-1.2 grams per pound of total body weight[4009].

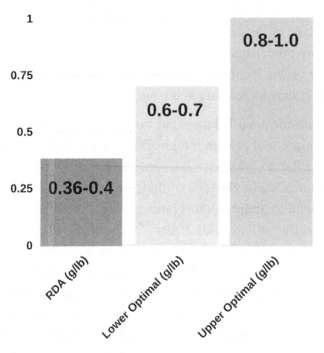

Glutathione status is compromised in various disease states and an increased supply of sulfur amino acids can reverse many of these changes[4010]. A restriction in dietary sulfur amino acids slows down the rate of glutathione synthesis and diminishes its turnover[4011].

Fruit and vegetables contribute up to 50% of dietary glutathione, whereas meat contributes 25% for an average diet[4012]. Direct food sources high in glutathione are freshly prepared meat, fruit and vegetables are moderate sources and dairy and cereal are low in glutathione[4013]. Freezing foods maintains relatively the same amount of glutathione as fresh food, but other preservation methods, such as fermentation or canning, lead to extensive losses. Whey protein is also a good source of cysteine and hence glutathione and has been shown to lower oxidative stress[4014,4015]. Milk thistle can raise glutathione levels and has antioxidant properties [4016, 4017, 4018]. Turmeric and curcumin can also promote glutathione synthesis and inhibit inflammation[4019].

Here is a table of the glutathione, methionine and cysteine content of common foods

Food	Glutathione mg/100g	Methionine mg/100g	Cysteine mg/100g
Apples	1.5	2	3
Pears	3.3	2	3
Bananas	3.3	11	17
Peaches	1.2	11	4
Cantaloupe	6.1	6	2
Watermelon	5.0	6	2
Strawberries	5.1	1	5
Oranges	4.8	20	10
Grapefruit	6.5	2	0
Green Beans	0.0	14	11
Green Peas	5.2	67	26
Pinto Beans	0.5	69	50

Corn	0.6	55	21
Winter Squash	11	14	10
Tomatoes	7.5	8	12
Broccoli	5.5	36	21
Cauliflower	4.0	26	22
Spinach	11.4	53	35
Carrots	5.9	7	8
Avocado	20.6	37	21
Asparagus	21.8	25	31
Potatoes	10.2	39	22
Sweet Potatoes	1.4	32	10
White Rice	0.8	56	49
Hamburger Beef	11.8	612	268
Steak Beef	12.3	639	279
Liver Beef	0.8	675	410
Pork Chop	18.9	666	350
Chicken Breast	6.5	716	348
Veal	26.3	639	279
Pollock	1.5	424	227
Tuna, canned	1.1	470	172
Shrimp, canned	1.0	650	259
Cod and Perch	5.7	715	259
Liverwurst	7.0	287	152
Boiled Ham	13.7	524	298
Chicken Soup	1.4	32	19

Tofu	0.0	153	165
White Bread	0.0	144	174
Whole Wheat Bread	0.0	130	178
Cornbread	0.0	152	117
Peanut Butter	1.1	302	315
Butter	0.0	21	8
Bran Flakes	0.5	177	229
Corn Cereal	0.4	173	190
Oatmeal	1.5	43	64
Sugar	0.0	0.0	0.0
Eggs	0.0	377	278
Bacon	2.2	72	312
Pork Sausage	2.4	478	196
Cottage Cheese	0.0	579	143
Flavored Yogurt	0.0	129	40
Whole Milk	0.0	82	30
Milk, 2%	0.0	84	31
Milk, 1%	0.0	83	30
Beer	1.1	1	3
Red Wine	0.7	0.0	0.0
White Wine	2.3	0.0	0.0
Coffee	0.0	0.0	0.0
Tea	0.0	0.0	0.0

Excess methionine intake may lead to harmful side-effects, such as brain lesions and retinal degeneration, especially if not balanced with glycine intake. High dietary methionine intake (5-6 g/d compared to the 1-1,2 g RDA) can also raise homocysteine levels, even on top of adequate B-vitamin intake [4020, 4021, 4022]. High homocysteine is an independent risk factor for cardiovascular disease[4023]. Mutations in the cystathionine β-synthase (CBS) are the most common causes of homocystinuria, which causes an accumulation of homocysteine[4024]. Thus, elevated homocysteine levels may reflect deficient H2S levels. Human deficiencies in CSE and CBS are associated with an increased risk of cardiovascular disease[4025,4026,4027,4028]. This too may reflect low H2S levels.

Methionine restriction (MR) is thought to increase lifespan and slow down aging[4029]. Additionally, it's possible that those effects can happen without caloric restriction, which so far is the only known way of lengthening life in many species. Restricting methionine in Baker's yeast extends their lifespan, which was accompanied by an increase in autophagy[4030]. However, when autophagy genes were deleted, the extension in lifespan was also prevented. It's thought that restricting just protein can give the same effect on life-extension than caloric restriction without needing to restrict calories. However, a large 2016 meta-analysis demonstrated that calorie restriction combined with protein restriction had an identical effect on life-extension as just calorie restriction without restricting protein[4031]. There are also many studies in which rodents who are under calorie restriction are fed a higher percentage of protein, including methionine, to keep it at the same level as those who eat without caloric restriction[4032,4033]. With protein being matched, the rodents under calorie restriction still gain the benefits of calorie restriction and do better than the ones eating with no restriction. Compared to caloric restriction, protein restriction does not contribute to the benefits of caloric restriction. The benefits of reduced protein intake are caused primarily by decreased caloric consumption. Restricting protein and methionine may actually cause other problems related to poor detoxification, methylation and glutathione synthesis. Improper methylation is linked with autoimmune conditions[4034].

Long-term methionine restrictive diets are impractical and not worth the costs of muscle loss and sarcopenia, which accelerates aging[4035]. Loss of methionine promotes the greying of hair[4036]. Methionine and cysteine are also important for alleviating oxidative stress[4037]. In rats, sulfur amino acid sufficiency ensures glutathione synthesis and glutathione-dependent enzyme activity during inflammation [4038]. Furthermore, **glycine supplementation has been found to have the same effects on life-extension as methionine restriction**[4039]. Glycine is found in organ meats, ligaments, drumsticks, skin and collagen supplements. Bone broth or chicken soup (especially ones that contain collagenous meats), rich in glycine, glucosamine and sulfur, has been found to lower inflammation, infections and reduce joint pain[4040,4041].

You can get sulfur from both animal and plant foods, but animal protein is by far the more predominant source. Methionine and cysteine are the most widespread sulfur amino acids that support glutathione and protein synthesis. A low intake of them can promote muscle wasting and inflammation.

- The minimal optimal intake of sulfur amino acids per day is roughly 3.0 grams, but this demand increases up to 5.0 grams during disease states and/or injury. Generally, you can obtain that amount from eating 0.6-1.0 grams of protein per pound of body weight every day. To prevent the negative side-effects of excess methionine, ensure an adequate intake of B vitamins and glycine (3-5 grams per meal) or get your protein from glycine-rich organ meats/tendons/ligaments.

- Organosulfur compounds in allium vegetables like garlic and onions are also beneficial for the body's antioxidant systems. They may have protective effects on cardiovascular disease and cancer. Eating only a half of an onion per day and a single serving of garlic per week may be enough to provide the benefits.

- Sulforaphane-containing vegetables like broccoli and cabbage give an additional boost in glutathione and anti-cancer defenses. To activate the beneficial compounds, you have to cut and slightly cook the vegetables at temperatures below 284°F (140°C). Eating cruciferous raw will begin to inhibit iodine absorption and promote hypothyroidism. How many vegetables you need to eat is hard to know but the general recommendation of 3-5 cups of vegetables a day should be more than enough. You also have to pay attention to how you individually react because sulforaphane may cause digestive problems for some people.

In conclusion, sulfur is a central mineral for the body's detoxification and antioxidant defense systems. It is needed for preventing oxidative stress-related conditions like atherosclerosis, cardiovascular disease, neurodegeneration, arthritis and aging in general.

Chapter 14
Chromium and Blood Sugar Management

One of the oldest diseases ever described is diabetes – an Egyptian manuscript from 1500 BC referred to it as "too frequent emptying of the urine". [4042] Diabetes was given its name by the Greek Apollonius Memphites in 230 BC[4043]. The technical term nowadays is diabetes mellitus, which is derived from the Greek word 'diabetes' meaning siphon or 'to pass through' and the Latin word 'mellitus' meaning honeyed or sweet[4044]. The term mellitus is due to the fact that the urine of diabetics contains excess sugar and tastes sweet. Around 400-500 AD, the Indian physicians Sushruta and Charaka discovered that there were two different types of diabetes. They called the disease *honey urine* because it would attract ants. [4045] One of the symptoms of diabetes is increased urination with a sweet odor. In Ancient Rome, diabetes was reported to be quite rare as the Roman physician Galen encountered only two such cases during his entire career[4046]. Galen called diabetes "diarrhea of the urine" ("diarrhea urinosa") as he contributed it to the weakening of the kidneys[4047]. The Swiss doctor Paracelsus confused the white residue in the urine of diabetics as excess salt instead of sugar[4048]. However, in 1776, the British physiologist Matthew Dobson demonstrated that the sweetness of the urine and serum of patients with diabetes was from excess sugar[4049].

More than 392 million people worldwide have diabetes[4050,4051]. More than half of U.S. adults have diabetes or pre-diabetes[4052]. Type-1 diabetes is an autoimmune disorder with a genetic basis wherein the pancreas produces almost no insulin[4053,4054]. Without treatment, blood sugar can stay continuously elevated in Type 1 diabetics. Type 2 diabetes is where the body becomes resistant to the effects of insulin. In other words, the body can make insulin, but it doesn't respond to it as well. It is estimated that 3.4 million people globally died in 2004 due to consequences from a high fasting blood sugar[4055]. More than 80% of diabetes-related deaths occur in low- to middle-income countries[4056]. The World Health Organization predicts diabetes will be the 7th leading cause of death by the year 2030[4057].

Diabetes increases the risk of cardiovascular disease and stroke by up to 1.8 to 6-fold[4058,4059,4060]. Nearly 50% of diabetics die due to cardiovascular disease[4061]. Diabetes is also the leading cause of kidney disease and kidney failure[4062]. The overall risk of death in diabetics is twice that compared to those without diabetes[4063]. Diabetic retinopathy can cause blindness and impaired vision, whereas diabetic neuropathy in the limbs can lead to a lack of feeling in the extremities resulting in untreated wounds, which can lead to amputation[4064,4065]. Furthermore, diabetes is associated with impaired cognition and neurodegenerative diseases like Alzheimer's disease[4066].

One of the most predominant chronic diseases is Type 2 diabetes or adult-onset diabetes. It is characterized by insulin resistance, high blood sugar and high insulin levels[4067]. Type 2 diabetes is caused by poor lifestyle habits, i.e., eating refined carbohydrates, sugars, seed oils, processed foods, lack of exercise and overeating. Rates of Type 2 diabetes have risen in parallel with obesity as the two are interrelated[4068]. Type 2 diabetes contributes to 90% of the diabetes cases in adults worldwide[4069]. Conversely, Type 1 diabetes makes up only 5-10% of all diabetic cases[4070]. Up to 87% of the elderly have impaired glucose tolerance[4071], which can be fixed with dietary changes. However, impaired glucose tolerance has already started to occur at higher rates in younger people[4072].

The first sign of Type 2 diabetes is hyperinsulinemia. However, this can only be picked up by measuring insulin levels after an oral glucose tolerance test,[4073,4074] which most doctors do not order. Thus, by the time someone is diagnosed with having impaired glucose tolerance and/or impaired fasting glucose, they have already lost ~ 50% of their beta-cells that are needed to produce insulin[4075]. Both Type 1 and Type 2 diabetes are diagnosed as a fasting blood glucose ≥ 7.0 mmol/l (126 mg/dl) or when plasma glucose after a glucose challenge is ≥ 11.1 mmol/l (200 mg/dl) two hours later[4076,4077]. Glycated hemoglobin (HbA1c) of ≥ 48 mmol/mol (6.5%) is another diagnosis method[4078]. Symptoms of diabetes include dry mouth, increased thirst, fatigue, hair loss, blurred vision, peripheral neuropathy and frequent urination.

	Fasting Glucose		2-Hour Glucose		HbA1C	
Unit	mmol/L	mg/dL	mmol/L	mg/dL	mmol/mol	%
Normal	<5.6	<100	<7.8	<140	<42	<5.7
Impaired Glucose Tolerance	5.6–7.0	100–125	≥7.8	>140	42–46	5.7-6.4
Diabetes Mellitus	≥7.0	≥126	≥11.1	≥200	≥48	≥6.5

Strategies that are employed to improve glucose tolerance include regular exercise, avoidance of refined carbohydrates/sugars/seed oils/smoking and eating lower glycemic foods[4079,4080,4081]. Both resistance training and aerobic exercise improve metabolic syndrome and diabetes[4082]. The benefits of exercise occur even when the person's weight does not initially drop[4083]. High levels of physical activity can reduce the risk of diabetes by up to 28%[4084]. In 1930, it was also proposed that prolonged periods of fasting can help lower blood sugar in diabetics[4085]. Consumption of low-glycemic fruit (berries) and vegetables and limiting sugar-sweetened beverages is associated with a reduced risk of diabetes[4086,4087]. This risk reduction does not apply to 100% fruit juice[4088]. Dietary fiber can help lower the blood sugar response after meals and is associated with a lower risk of diabetes, however, this must be carefully balanced with how much sugar is being provided[4089]. If blood sugar does not drop with diet and exercise, most doctors will prescribe the blood sugar lowering medication metformin[4090]. Insulin injections are typically a last resort treatment[4091]. However, lifestyle changes are more effective in the long-term than pharmaceuticals because the drugs stop working after their cessation and do not fix the underlying issue[4092].

Besides diet and exercise, certain minerals and nutrients are important for managing blood sugar and insulin levels. Most of them have at least some role in either facilitating an insulin response or helping to lower blood sugar after eating. For example, magnesium is required for insulin action and people with type-2 diabetes have low magnesium [4093] . Magnesium deficiency has been implicated in pancreatic beta-cell function, reduced DNA repair capacity, insulin resistance, cardiovascular disease, type-2 diabetes, osteoporosis, hyperglycemia and hyperinsulinemia[4094,4095]. Copper, zinc, potassium and sodium are also needed for proper glucose metabolism.

There is one specific mineral called chromium that is known for its effects on blood sugar and insulin. There is good evidence to indicate that chromium supplementation could benefit those with diabetes and impaired insulin sensitivity[4096,4097]. In this chapter, we will look at the effects of chromium on blood sugar parameters and how to get enough of it from diet.

Here are the main causes of Type 2 diabetes and/or impaired glucose intolerance:

- Overconsumption of added sugars and sugar-sweetened beverages[4098,4099,4100,4101]
- Overconsumption of omega-6 seed oils[4102,4103]
- Overconsumption of hydrogenated fats[4104]
- Overconsumption of refined carbohydrates[4105]
- Physical inactivity[4106]
- Obesity and excess body fat[4107]
- Visceral fat accumulation[4108]
- Low magnesium[4109,4110,4111,4112,4113,4114]
- Low chromium[4115,4116]
- Smoking and tobacco[4117]
- Persistent organic pollutants and plastics[4118]
- Lack of sleep and sleep deprivation[4119]
- Testosterone deficiency[4120,4121]
- Low vitamin D levels[4122]

Chromium Benefits

In 1959, a novel protein was discovered in Brewer's yeast that was termed 'glucose tolerance factor' (GTF)[4123]. The substance was later identified to be trivalent chromium bound to a complex in Brewer's yeast that also contains glycine, glutamic acid, cysteine and nicotinic acid.[4124]. Chromium 3+, or trivalent chromium, was found to be the main active component of the 'glucose tolerance factor' in rats that alleviated their glucose intolerance caused by high sucrose consumption[4125]. In diabetic patients, chromium-enriched yeast can decrease fasting blood glucose and insulin[4126,4127,4128]. Chromium is required for the binding of insulin to the cell surface so it can exert its effects[4129]. However, chromium appears to require the synergy with nicotinic acid to work in lowering blood sugar through the glucose tolerance factor[4130]. GTF enhances the activity of insulin. Chromium-deficient rats have diabetic-like glucose levels and stunted growth[4131, 4132]. Chronic maternal chromium restriction in rats promotes visceral adiposity and hyperlipidemia[4133]. Rats fed a chromium-rich diet have higher levels of glutathione peroxidase and Cu,Zn superoxide dismutase[4134].

GLUCOSE TOLERANCE FACTOR (GTF)

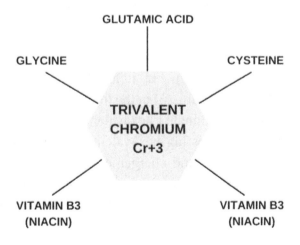

Adapted From: NutriPlex Formulas 'Glucose Tolerance Factor, Chromium, Diabetes & Balancing Blood Sugar', Accessed Online Jan 18th, 2021: http://nutriplexformulas.com/

One review paper by Balk et al (2007) summarized why brewer's yeast may be one of the best supplemental sources of chromium:

> *Among participants with type 2 diabetes, the effects of brewer's yeast, chromium chloride, and chromium picolinate on fasting glucose were each significantly different from each other (P < 0.02), such that* ***studies of brewer's yeast had the greatest net effect*** *(−1.1 mmol/l), followed by chromium picolinate (−0.8 mmol/l) and chromium chloride (−0.3 mmol/l). Similarly, among studies of participants with normal glucose tolerance,* ***brewer's yeast was significantly more likely to reduce fasting glucose than chromium chloride*** *(−0.2 vs. +0.1 mmol/l, P = 0.01)* ***and to raise HDL cholesterol than chromium picolinate*** *(+0.21 vs. −0.02, P = 0.002).* [4135]

Around the 1970s, chromium deficiency was noted to impair glucose tolerance, elevate triglycerides, prevent the use of glucose as energy and cause neuropathy in patients with normal insulin levels on long-term total parental nutrition[4136,4137]. Intravenous nutrition without chromium can cause chromium deficiency and glucose regulation problems[4138]. Administrating 150-250 mcg of chromium to patients on total parental nutrition alleviates glucose intolerance, neuropathy and hyperglycemia[4139,4140]. This is why high dose chromium is routinely given to patients on total parental nutrition[4141].

Chromium found in foods and supplements is a trace element trivalent (Cr^{3+} or trivalent chromium), but it also exists in the form of a hexavalent (Cr^{6+} or chromium +6) in the toxic by-products of steel and metal manufacturing.[4142] Inhaled hexavalent chromium is mutagenic and carcinogenic[4143]. Ingesting hexavalent chromium has also been linked to stomach tumors and allergenic contact dermatitis[4144]. The movie Erin Brockovich is based on the contamination of a water supply with hexavalent chromium in the Southern Californian town of Hinkley.

Chromium is the main component of stainless steel because of its anti-corrosive qualities. The name is derived from the Greek word *chrōma*, meaning color. Because of that, chromium is used in dyes, paints and leather products. People working in such factories often have allergies to chromate solutions because of chronic exposure[4145]. Trivalent chromium is generally non-toxic and is considered to have numerous health benefits[4146].

Chromium has been deemed an essential nutrient in the U.S., India and several other countries based on its ability to affect insulin, lipid and carbohydrate metabolism[4147]. However, the European Food Safety Authority claimed in 2014 there was not enough evidence to consider chromium essential[4148].

The most recent adequate intake (AI) for chromium in the U.S. has been set at 25-35 mcg/d for adults[4149]. In 1969, it was estimated that humans only need 1 mcg/d of chromium, but the absorption of chromium chloride is only 1-3%[4150] and dietary chromium absorption is only 0.4-2.5%[4151]. To reach the 1 mcg/d recommendation you would have to ingest about 33-100 mcg/d. In 1980, the Estimated Safe and Adequate Daily Dietary Intake (ESADDI) for chromium was set at 50-200 mcg/d for adults[4152]. According to the World Health Organization, an approximate chromium intake of 33 mcg/d is likely to meet normal requirements[4153]. In Australia and New Zealand, the AI for chromium is 35 mcg/d for men, 25 mcg/d for women, 30 mcg/d for pregnant women and 45 mcg/d for lactating women. India's recommended daily intake of chromium for adults is 33 mcg/d. Despite considering chromium an essential nutrient, Japan promotes a daily AI of just 10 mcg[4154]. In the U.S., the daily value for chromium on food labels has been set at 35 mcg by the FDA[4155].

Optimal Intake of Chromium (mcg/d)

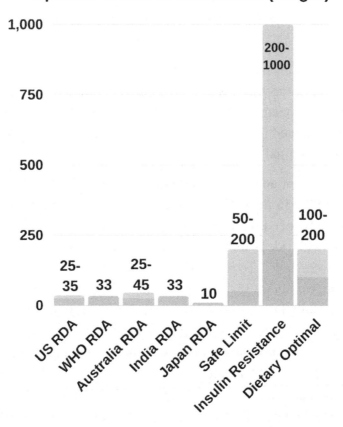

The FDA suggests that chromium picolinate may reduce the risk of insulin resistance and Type 2 diabetes, but these claims are not definitive[4156]. They also reject claims that chromium could treat cardiovascular disease, retinopathy or kidney disease caused by high blood sugar[4157]. Based on the same uncertainty, the American Diabetes Association does not recommend chromium supplementation either[4158,4159]. In 2010, the European Food Safety Authority (EFSA) approved claims that chromium helps to maintain normal blood sugar levels but rejected claims for helping to lose weight or combat fatigue[4160].

Based on a recent 2021 study, chromium picolinate supplementation of 400 mcg a day for 3 months improved glycemic control, reduced triglycerides, HOMA-IR, inflammation and insulin levels [4161].

Supplementing 600 mcg of chromium picolinate a day for 4 months has shown a beneficial effect on the glycemic control of Type 2 diabetics without affecting the lipid profile [4162]. Some scientists speculate that taking 600 mcg chromium picolinate for 5 years could lead to tissue accumulation and chromosomal damage[4163]. In Jordanian and Nigerian malnourished infants, chromium has been found to improve glucose removal rates after 18 hours of administration[4164]. Similar results have been observed in protein and calorie-deprived infants[4165,4166]. Taking a chromium supplement at around 600 mcg two to three times per week may help to ensure optimal chromium status in the body.

Most multivitamin supplements contain 25-120 mcg of chromium, but chromium-specific products can have anywhere from 200-500 mcg up to 1,000 mcg. About 31% of U.S. adults take a multivitamin or mineral supplement that contains chromium[4167]. Chromium in supplements is used in the form of chromium chloride, chromium citrate, chromium (III) picolinate, chromium (III) polynicotinate and others.

Chromium supplementation does not appear to improve insulin sensitivity in healthy non-obese people,[4168,4169,4170] which makes sense, i.e., you can't fix what isn't broken. In rat studies, a low chromium diet may not alter glucose or insulin tolerance, but the insulin response is lower after a glucose challenge with higher chromium in the diet[4171]. Taking 1,000 mcg of chromium compared to 100 mcg a day has been found to significantly lower fasting glucose (128 mg/dl vs 159 mg/dl) in type-2 diabetics[4172]. Their response to a glucose challenge and HbA1c was also lower. Thus, even if you consider chromium to not be absolutely essential, chromium can still provide a beneficial effect on metabolic health. Many researchers believe that an abnormally high fasting blood glucose without any apparent reason should be deemed chromium deficiency until proven otherwise.

The exact mechanisms by which chromium improves blood sugar management is complex. The current understanding is that chromium binds to an oligopeptide to form chromodulin that activates the insulin receptor to mediate the actions of insulin[4173]. Chromodulin stimulates insulin-dependent tyrosine kinase activity that activates the insulin receptor[4174]. Thus, chromodulin functions as an amplifier of insulin signaling. Another oligopeptide called low-molecular-weight chromium-binding substance (LMWCr) carries chromium around the body as a second messenger for insulin signaling[4175,4176]. In vitro, cobalt and chromium ions have been shown to increase glycolytic flux[4177]. A reduction in glycolytic flux may lead to glucose intolerance, metabolic inflexibility, lactic acid accumulation and lack of energy. **Chromium deficiency will thus reduce the insulin response and promote insulin resistance[4178].**

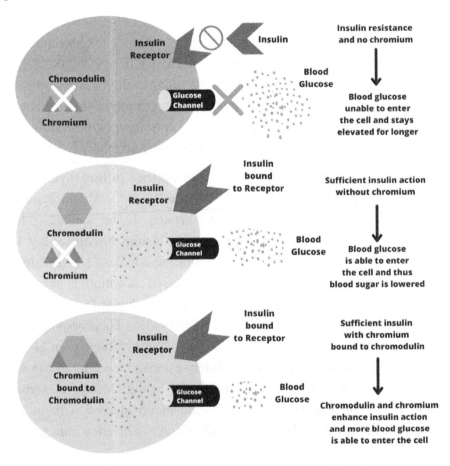

Adapted From: Phung et al (2010) 'Improved Glucose Control Associated with i.v. Chromium Administration in Two Patients Receiving Enteral Nutrition', Am J Health Syst Pharm. 2010;67(7):535-541[4179].

Because of its effects on insulin and glucose metabolism, chromium is thought to help with polycystic ovary syndrome (PCOS), which is characterized by insulin resistance and dyslipidemia [4180,4181,4182]. Chromium supplementation of 200-1,000 mcg/d for 8-24 weeks has not been found to have a significant effect on fasting glucose, but it did lower fasting insulin and bodyweight [4183]. Among diabetic PCOS patients, chromium supplementation improved HOMA-IR scores (a marker of insulin resistance) [4184]. However, due to mixed results, more studies are needed. Out of 84 Canadian postmenopausal women, 60% get less than the adequate intake of chromium a day [4185].

Thanks to improving insulin sensitivity, chromium may help with body composition and weight loss [4186,4187,4188], but evidence is conflicting [4189]. A 2019 meta-analysis showed that chromium doses of 200-1,000 mcg/d for 9-24 weeks in 1,316 obese participants produced a weight loss of 0.75 kg compared to placebo [4190]. Most dietary supplements do not produce a weight loss effect of greater than 2 kg, especially in the long-term [4191] and typically only work when combined with a calorie restricted diet. Chromium intake can reduce appetite and food intake [4192]. Reduced hunger and less energy consumption are probably the most important variables for sustainable weight loss.

By increasing insulin sensitivity, chromium supplementation has also been promoted as a way to increase muscle mass and athletic performance [4193]. With higher insulin action, nutrients would be stored and utilized faster, which is why bodybuilders use injectable insulin. The potential benefits of chromium on muscle anabolism are thought to be marginal, however, many athletes are thought to be deficient in this nutrient [4194]. A double-blind study on 10 male college students saw that 200 mcg of chromium picolinate a day resulted in a 3.4 kg fat loss and a 2.6 kg lean body weight gain after 24 days of weight training, whereas the placebo group only lost 1 kg of fat and gained only 1.8 kg of lean body weight [4195]. The authors speculated this was due to chromium's ability to potentiate the uptake of amino acids and nutrients into the muscles. A randomized, double-blind, placebo-controlled study in 154 patients showed that 72 days of supplementing with 200 or 400 mcg of chromium/day improves body composition vs. placebo [4196]. Other studies have not shown a benefit of chromium on body composition, which might be due to subjects that were not depleted in chromium[4197,4198]. According to the International Olympic Committee, there is no need for high-level athletes to supplement chromium because they are thought to consume enough dietary chromium[4199]. However, consuming "enough" chromium to live, is not the same thing as consuming an optimal intake. For example, most people can live on just 180 mg/day of magnesium, but optimal intakes are more than twice this amount[4200].

Indeed, because you lose more chromium during exercise through urine and sweat, it might be a needed nutrient, especially for athletes who aren't getting enough from diet. Right after a 6-mile run, serum chromium levels have been seen to increase by 30% and stay elevated for 2 hours[4201]. This is thought to be due to chromium mobilization from storage sites during exercise. As a result, urinary chromium concentrations increase by almost 5-fold compared to pre-run levels with an approximate 2-fold greater 24-hour chromium excretion through urine[4202]. Since the kidneys reabsorb less than 5% of chromium in the blood, once chromium gets released from tissues almost all of it is lost in the urine. An elevated blood chromium after exercise may occur to facilitate the entry of glucose into muscle for glycogen replenishment.

An 8-week study showed that urinary chromium excretion increased steadily over the course of a workout program up to 20% above baseline[4203]. Untrained people who engage in periodic strenuous exercise or who follow calorie-restricted diets would likely not be able to offset the losses of chromium from exercise[4204,4205]. In other words, the more you exercise the more chromium depleted you may become. Currently, it is not known whether or not the body can adapt to an increased loss of chromium from exercise, but it is likely that the body will slowly become depleted if someone is consuming a marginal amount of chromium and does not replace what is lost. The average urinary chromium level is 0.2-0.4 mcg/day but exercise doubles this[4206]. Since an average person only absorbs 0.4-2.5% of dietary chromium, you would have to consume an extra 8-100 mcg of chromium in the diet to replace the 0.2-0.4 mcg lost from exercise. The body does try to compensate for these losses by reducing urinary chromium losses on non-exercise days. However, exercise also increases chromium loss through sweat. One study indicated that simply being at 100°F for 8 hours causes 60 mcg of chromium lost through sweat[4207]. If we assume an equal loss of chromium in sweat per hour, and that a similar loss of chromium occurs with intense exercise as being maintained at 100°F, then **one hour of intense exercise may induce a loss of 7.5 mcg of chromium in sweat, which could necessitate anywhere from 600-750 mcg of dietary chromium to replace that loss.** A second study showed that **wrestlers lose ~100 mcg of chromium per hour of exercise through sweat**[4208] (using a typical sweat loss of 1 liter per hour). However, this study used the arm bag method versus whole body washdown to collect mineral losses which overestimates the mineral losses in sweat. Since, to our knowledge, there are only 2 studies on chromium losses in sweat, we can't definitively say how much chromium gets lost per hour of exercise in sweat. However, the estimate that 7.5 mcg of chromium gets lost in sweat after 1 hour of exercise is more reasonable versus 100 mcg. Thus, **athletes who train at an intense level and sweat for around 60 minutes per training session, should consider supplementing with an extra 600 mcg of chromium picolinate (which has a 1.2% bioavailability, providing 7.2 mcg of chromium) or another chromium supplement with a similar bioavailability (such as Brewer's yeast chromium) on exercise days**[4209]. Wrestlers who use body sweat bags to lose water weight may be causing a significant loss of minerals through sweat, especially chromium, which could necessitate much more than 600 mcg of chromium to replace losses. Going into a sauna for 30 minutes may also necessitate around 300 mcg of chromium to replace losses through sweat.

Minerals lost in sweat after 1 hour of exercise*

Mineral	Amount lost
Salt	½ teaspoon of salt (1,150 sodium and 1,725 mg chloride)
Potassium	140 mg
Calcium	40 mg
Magnesium	8-10 mg
Iron	0.16-0.63 mg
Copper	0.4 mg (up to 1.5 mg at temperatures of 100°F)
Zinc	0.4 mg
Iodine	52 mcg**
Selenium	40 mcg
Chromium	7.5 mcg **(this would necessitate ~600-750 mcg of chromium from diet or supplementation due to a bioavailability of only ~1%)**

*(These are estimates and will change depending on many factors)
**(At 89.6-98.6°F)

Diets high in simple sugars increase urinary chromium excretion by 300%[4210]. Athletes tend to consume more simple sugars to fuel their workouts and for post-exercise glycogen replacement. This would lead to further chromium losses out the urine and increase the risk of chromium deficiency. On the flip side, athletes also tend to eat more food. Thus, if an athlete is eating an overall healthy diet, they will be getting more chromium, which will help to replace losses from eating simple sugars and exercise. As a precautionary note, caffeine or coffee may increase urinary chromium losses. Thus, **it may not be a bad idea for those consuming caffeine/coffee to get extra chromium in their diet.**

Evidence of chromium benefiting lipids and cholesterol have also been reported with significant reductions in serum triglycerides and total cholesterol[4211]. Chromium picolinate at 200 mcg/d for 42 days can lower blood lipids[4212]. However, there are mixed results in this area as well[4213]. Overall, meta-analyses in those with PCOS and diabetes have not shown that chromium significantly lowers cholesterol levels[4214,4215]. Some studies however do show that chromium raises the "good" cholesterol called HDL cholesterol and reduces triglycerides[4216,4217]. Both of those markers (HDL and triglycerides) are a fairly good marker of insulin sensitivity. Supplementation of 200 mcg of chromium for 12 weeks can raise HDL cholesterol from 35 to 39 mg/dl in insulin resistant subjects[4218]. Both chromium deficiency and elevated blood lipids are often seen in candidates for bariatric surgery[4219].

A prospective study involving 3,648 subjects found an inverse association between the occurrence of metabolic syndrome and toenail chromium concentrations[4220]. Low toenail chromium concentration has also been associated with an increased risk of a heart attack[4221]. In Korean males, insulin resistance is associated with lower chromium hair concentrations and higher Ca/Mg ratio[4222]. Type 1 and Type 2 diabetes are correlated with blood chromium deficiency[4223].

Here are the chromium-dependent enzymes, functions and consequences that may occur with deficient chromium intake

Chromium-Dependent Enzymes/Proteins	Function	Consequences of Deficit
Glucose Tolerance Factor (GTF)	Enhances insulin activity	High blood sugar, reduced muscle gains
Chromodulin	Activates the insulin receptor	High blood sugar, insulin resistance & reduced muscle gains
Tyrosine Kinase	Activates the insulin receptor	High blood sugar, insulin resistance & reduced muscle gains
Low-Molecular-Weight Chromium-Binding Substance (LMWCr)	Carry chromium around the blood, mediate insulin signaling	Elevated blood sugar, insulin resistance and reduced muscle gains
Glycolytic Flux	Conversion of glucose into pyruvate and ATP	Glucose intolerance, metabolic in-flexibility, lactic acid accumulation & lack of energy
Superoxide Dismutase	Removes superoxide anions	Increased tissue damage & oxidative stress
Glutathione Peroxidase	Removes hydrogen peroxide	Increased oxidative stress and weaker immunity
DNAzymes[4224]	RNA cleavage, catalyst of enzymes	Inadequate enzymatic reactions

Chromium Foods

Most foods contain on average 1-13 mcg of chromium per serving[4225]. Chromium is found in many foods, starting with meat and ending with vegetables. Many medicinal plants like sand immortelle, foxglove, Alexandrian laurel, Greek valerian, marsh cudweed, adenostilis and lobelia have high amounts of chromium [4226]. However, not all chromium in foods has glucose tolerance factor (GTF) and thus total chromium content may not be a valid indicator of the insulin sensitizing benefits of a given food. Foods with the highest amount of chromium as GTF are brewer's yeast, black pepper, liver, cheese, bread and beef, whereas the lowest ones are skim milk, chicken breast, flour and haddock[4227]. Supplementation with 9 grams of Brewer's yeast per day for 8 weeks can improve impaired glucose tolerance, reduce serum cholesterol and lower the insulin response to a glucose load in humans[4228]. Polyphenolic herbs and spices like cinnamon have also been shown to improve insulin sensitivity together with chromium[4229].

The richest sources of chromium are mussels and oysters, probably because of environmental contact. Fresh water fish living in areas of stainless-steel manufacturing, chrome plating or rubber processing have nearly 5 times more chromium than normal[4230]. They also get more of the toxic hexavalent chromium, which causes mutagenic gene damage. Out of 35 cities in the U.S., 25 have more hexavalent chromium than expected in their drinking water[4231]. In Africa, areas with more naturally occurring trivalent chromium in drinking water appear to have a lower rate of diabetes and vascular occlusive disease[4232].

Many staple foods in Western diets like wheat, potatoes and milk are quite low in chromium[4233]. How much chromium is in plants depends on the soil's mineral content. Agricultural practices and food processing can also affect the amount of chromium in a given food. The chromium content of oatmeal can vary 50-fold because of product differences.[4234] **Refining grains and wheat reduces the amount of chromium by up to 8-fold**[4235]. Peeling apples and eating them without the skin reduces their chromium content by 70% (from 1.4 mcg to 0.4 mcg per apple).

Human milk also contains small amounts chromium, which ranges from 0.25-60 mcg/L, depending on the nutrient and lactation status of the mother[4236,4237]. Infants of less than 6 months of age need less than 0.5 mcg/d of chromium[4238]. Finnish infants who are exclusively breast-fed and get 0.27 mcg/d of chromium do not show any abnormalities[4239]. Exposure to excess environmental chromium during pregnancy increases the risk of delivering low birth weight babies[4240]. Chromium levels in the body are higher at birth than later in life[4241], which might explain why infants need much less chromium.

Food tracking studies in the U.S., Finland, England and Canada find that women and men get on average 25 mcg and 33 mcg of chromium per day, respectively, which is a borderline adequate intake[4242]. In Mexico, the average daily intake of chromium is around 30 mcg, coming from primarily tortillas, cheese, pasta, milk and meat[4243]. Turkey, Denmark and Switzerland get around 50 mcg/d of chromium[4244,4245]. In France, the average intake of chromium is around 40 mcg/d, which is lower than their national RDA of 60 mcg/d[4246]. In Spain, the average intake is 58 mcg of chromium per day from cereal, vegetables/tubers, dairy and seafood[4247]. Chromium intake appears to be higher in developing countries like Sudan than in developed countries like Sweden (105 mcg/d vs 22 mcg/d)[4248,4249].

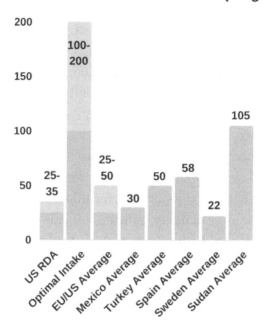

Chromium Intake in Countries (mcg/d)

NHANES does not have data about chromium intake, which makes assessing its status more complicated among Americans. However, based on food tracking studies people in the United States are barley meeting the adequate intake. People in the U.S. see a significant drop in their tissue levels of chromium the older they get, which is not observed in subjects in Near and Far East and Europe[4250]. That is probably due to poor dietary habits, which is why older people may also need a higher chromium intake. **Supplementing 150 mcg of chromium per day for 4 months restores glucose tolerance in 50% of elderly subjects**[4251]. However, it is not age per se that contributes to chromium deficiency, as older people eating nutritious diets do not show low chromium levels. Thus, the true cause of chromium deficiency is likely driven by diet, not by age.

Consuming less than 50 mcg of chromium a day does not mean you will become deficient, but it does increase your risk of deficiency. In one study, 22 elderly men and women had an average chromium intake of 24.5 mcg/d, out of the 22 subjects, 3 showed a negative chromium balance and 16 were in equilibrium (just maintaining balance, meaning the amount lost in the urine and feces equaled the amount absorbed)[4252]. However, this study did not look at chromium losses in sweat. Thus, this study suggests that 19 out of the 22 subjects were likely in negative chromium balance (losing more chromium than was being absorbed). Importantly, balance studies cannot determine if someone is deficient in a mineral (especially if sweat losses aren't taken into account) because they typically only look at urinary and fecal losses after a particular dietary intake. Additionally, in deficiency the body tends to shut down urinary/fecal losses and increase mineral absorption. Thus, it may appear that someone is in positive mineral balance (less urinary/fecal losses than what is being absorbed) but this may actually indicate mineral deficiency. This is why you typically need to give an oral or IV loading dose of a mineral to see how much gets excreted out in the urine (at least for minerals that are regulated by the kidney) to determine deficiency. This is because if the body does not excrete much of a high loading dose of a mineral, this suggests a deficiency, as the body is trying to hold onto the mineral. People who already have impaired glucose tolerance see a further decrease in their glucose control when going on a low chromium intake of less than 20 mcg/d for 4 weeks[4253]. Therefore, a daily intake of chromium less than 20 mcg is likely suboptimal, especially in those with impaired glucose tolerance.

Here are the foods with the most chromium[4254,4255,4256,4257]

Food	Mcg of Chromium per Serving	% of AI
Mussels, 3 oz	120 mcg	390%
Oysters, 3 oz	52 mcg	120%
Lobster, 3 oz	29 mcg	71%
Shrimp, 3 oz	24 mcg	67%
Broccoli, 1 cup	22 mcg	65%
Barley, ½ cup	12 mcg	36%
Turkey Ham, 3 oz	10.4 mcg	30%
Oats, ½ cup	10 mcg	30%
Grape Juice, 1 cup	7.5 mcg	21%
Waffles, 1 (75 g)	6.7 mcg	18%
Ham, 3 oz	3.6 mcg	10%
Muffin, whole wheat	3.6 mcg	10%
Chocolate Chip Cookies (4)	3.4 mcg	9%
Brewer's Yeast, 1 tbsp	3.3 mcg	9%
Potatoes, 1 cup	3.0 mcg	9%
Orange Juice, 1 cup	2.2 mcg	6%

Beef, 3 oz	2.0 mcg	6%
Lettuce, 5 oz	1.8 mcg	5%
Turkey Breast, 3 oz	1.7 mcg	5%
Barbeque Sauce, 1 tbsp	1.7 mcg	5%
Tomato Juice, 1 cup	1.5 mcg	4%
Apple, unpeeled, 1 medium	1.4 mcg	4%
White Rice, 1 cup	1.2 mcg	3%
Green Beans, ½ cup	1.1 mcg	3%
Banana, 1 medium	1.0 mcg	3%
Brazil Nuts, 1 nut	1.0 mcg	3%
Red Wine, 1 glass	1.0 mcg	3%
Whole Wheat Bread, 1 slice	1.0 mcg	3%
Ketchup, 1 tbsp	1.0 mcg	3%
Oatmeal Raisin Cookies (4)	0.94 mcg	3%
Tomato, 1 medium	0.9 mcg	3%
American Cheese, 1½ oz	0.8 mcg	2%
Peanut Butter, 1 tbsp	0.6 mcg	2%
Brown Rice, 1 cup	0.6 mcg	2%

Haddock, 3 oz	0.6 mcg	2%
Beer, 1 glass	0.6 mcg	2%
Chicken Breast, 3 oz	0.5 mcg	1%
Apples, peeled, 1 medium	0.4 mcg	1%
Peas, ½ cup	0.4 mcg	1%
Orange, 1 medium	0.4 mcg	1%
Vinegar, 1 tbsp	0.38 mcg	1%
Spaghetti, 1 cup	0.3 mcg	1%
Carrots, 1 medium	0.3 mcg	1%
Egg, 1 medium	0.2 mcg	1%
Lima Beans, cooked, ½ cup	0.35 mcg	11%
Applesauce, ½ cup	0.34 mcg	11%
Cashews, 1 oz	0.33 mcg	11%
Egg, 1 medium	0.2 mcg	7%
Orange Juice, 1 cup	0.18 mcg	6%
Spinach, cooked, ½ cup	0.16 mcg	5%
Banana, 1 medium	0.16 mcg	5%
Spaghetti Sauce, ½ cup	0.16 mcg	5%

Carrots, 1 medium	0.14 mcg	4%
Peas, cooked, ½ cup	0.10 mcg	3%
Coffee, 1 cup	0.07 mcg	2%
Lettuce, 1 cup	0.06 mcg	2%
Tomatoes, ½ cup	0.06 mcg	2%
Tuna, canned, 3 oz	0.05 mcg	2%
Milk, whole, 1 cup	0.04 mcg	1%
Corn, cooked, ½ cup	0.04 mcg	1%
White Rice, cooked, ½ cup	0.03 mcg	1%
Chicken Breast, 3 oz	0.03 mcg	1%
Tea, 1 cup	0.02 mcg	0.6%
Lamb, 3 oz	0.02 mcg	0.6%
Whole Milk, 1 cup	0.12 mcg	
White Bread, 1 slice	0.01 mcg	0.3%

Chromium can also be obtained from the use of stainless-steel cookware during cooking[4258]. Cooking acidic foods like tomato sauce for several hours promotes the leaching of nickel and chromium from the cookware into the food[4259]. Preparing fresh meat in a food processor equipped with stainless-steel blades nearly doubles its chromium content and it does so 10-fold for liver after 3 minutes of blending[4260]. Canned and processed foods may be higher in chromium than fresh foodstuff because of this reason[4261]. The exception is refined white sugar that is incredibly low in chromium, whereas brown sugar and molasses are high in chromium[4262]. Consuming refined sugar as it comes in candies, pastries or other processed foods will thus contribute to excretion of chromium, especially if it is not being replaced. The average person in the U.S. consumes up to 50 kg of sugar a year[4263].

Here is the chromium content of different sugars (mcg/g)[4264]:

Sugar	Chromium (mcg/g)
Corn Syrup	3.42
Maple Syrup	3.07
Raw Sugar (Philippines)	1.59
Raw Sugar (Columbian)	1.58
Brown Sugar	1.19
Black-Strap Molasses	0.43
Honey (Refined)	0.41
Molasses (Refinery)	0.35
Grape Juice	0.34
Orange Juice	0.25
Refined Granulated Sugar	Not detectable to 0.09

The rate of dietary chromium absorption is quite low at 0.4-2.5%. That number is similar to chromium supplements. Increased chromium intake or supplementation will decrease chromium absorption. A study found that going from 10 mcg/d to 40 mcg/d or 240 mcg/d decreased dietary chromium absorption from 2% to 0.5%[4265]. There is no established threshold of low chromium intake at which chromium supplementation could induce significant changes. The majority of chromium is excreted through urine, making urinary chromium levels a potentially valid indicator of chromium intake. After a glucose challenge, plasma chromium levels rise higher and this is dependent of chromium intake from diet [4266]. Increased insulin resistance is associated with higher urinary chromium excretion[4267].

Vitamin C (ascorbic acid) and prostaglandin inhibitors, such as aspirin, increase chromium absorption, whereas antacids and oxalates decrease it[4268,4269]. Taking 100 mg of vitamin C together with 1,000 mcg of chromium raises plasma chromium levels more than taking 1,000 mcg of chromium alone[4270]. High sugar and fructose intake increases chromium excretion[4271]. Simple sugars excrete more chromium than complex carbohydrates[4272]. Thus, hyperglycemia and insulin resistance will also promote chromium elevation in blood and its excretion. Diabetics show a 3-fold increase in urinary chromium excretion[4273]. Physical exercise, sweating and injury will also promote chromium losses[4274]. Infections such as viruses promote the excretion of chromium[4275].

Trivalent chromium competes with iron for absorption[4276]. It can then either prevent iron (Fe^{3+}) accumulation or promote iron deficiency, depending on the person's iron intake[4277]. Transferrin is responsible for maintaining Cr^{3+} levels in the blood and shuttling it into tissues in an insulin-responsive manner[4278]. Thus, a copper deficiency could affect chromium binding to transferrin and cause a decrease in chromium delivery to insulin sensitive tissues. It would be interesting to know if chromium also inhibits the absorption of other +3 metals like aluminum. Aluminum toxicity and accumulation has been seen in Alzheimer's, epilepsy, autism, kidney disease and chronic fatigue[4279,4280,4281,4282].

Taking chromium together with insulin can trigger hypoglycemia because of the increased insulin sensitivity[4283]. The same applies to metformin or other blood sugar lowering medication. One study found that chromium picolinate reduces the absorption of levothyroxine, which is a drug used to treat hypothyroidism [4284]. Thus, it is recommended to not take levothyroxine of other thyroid medications with food or together with a chromium supplement. Instead, it would be best to take levothyroxine before eating and chromium at least 2 hours after levothyroxine. Chromium supplementation has been shown to reverse corticosteroid-induced diabetes[4285,4286].

Chromium toxicity from dietary or supplements is rare. There are a few cases wherein oral chromium picolinate can cause dermatitis[4287]. In rats, it could also cause anemia, weight loss, thrombocytopenia, liver dysfunction, renal failure, rhabdomyolysis, and hypoglycemia, but these effects have not been seen in humans[4288].

Normal serum chromium levels range from 0.05-0.5 mcg/mL (50-500 ng/mL) or ≤1.4 mcg/L (≤1.4 ng/mL)[4289,4290]. The majority of specimens submitted for analysis to the Mayo Clinic contain 0.3 ng/mL to 0.9 ng/mL of chromium[4291]. Proposed acceptable upper limits for blood chromium have been said to be 2.56 mcg/L[4292]. Hexavalent chromium enters red blood cells, but trivalent doesn't. Thus, having an elevated red blood cell chromium level may suggest hexavalent chromium overload[4293]. Prosthetic joints can increase serum chromium levels because of the metal leaching[4294]. To avoid external contamination, metal-free serum collection procedures must be followed, and centrifuged serum must be aliquoted into a metal-free vial.

In conclusion, chromium is considered an essential nutrient, especially because of its effects on insulin, glucose and lipid metabolism. However, healthy individuals do not need to deliberately be eating a high chromium diet to prevent metabolic syndrome as there are other more important variables, such as overall energy intake and body composition. Chromium has a more beneficial effect in people who have diabetes, insulin resistance or prediabetes. For them, chromium picolinate supplementation of 200-1,000 mcg/d may improve glycemic control and fasting insulin levels. An adequate consumption of 25-35 mcg/d from whole foods would probably be enough to prevent prediabetes in already healthy subjects but optimally most people would benefit from 33-100 mcg/d. To obtain that amount, you can get the most chromium from animal foods, especially mussels, oysters and lobster, but nutritional yeast and potatoes also have quite a lot. The demand for chromium increases with diabetic comorbidities, exercise and sweating.

Chapter 15
Manganese and Molybdenum: Hidden Players of the Body's Antioxidant Defense

The most commonly known minerals for detoxification and antioxidant defense are magnesium, selenium, zinc and sulfur. However, there are some minerals that fly under the radar and do not receive much attention. These minerals are manganese and molybdenum. In fact, manganese has its own superoxide dismutase – manganese superoxide dismutase (MnSOD) – which functions to protect our mitochondria and endothelium from oxidative stress. If our mitochondria and endothelium are not protected against oxidative stress this can lead to their damage and dysfunction and a whole host of diseases.

It is worthwhile to remember that many of the chronic diseases that plague society are caused by excess inflammation and oxidative stress. That oxidative stress needs to be bolstered against and dealt with on a regular basis because living itself causes oxidative stress. Molybdenum is also an interesting mineral that plays a part in a lot of enzymatic reactions in the body, involving detoxification of sulfites, purines and alcohol. So, if you do have a few drinks every once in a while, you want to make sure you are getting enough molybdenum.

Although molybdenum deficiencies are much rarer than the other minerals mentioned beforehand, there is still an optimal amount that needs to be consumed. Additionally, the data suggests that many of us are not getting optimal intakes of manganese, which we will cover in this chapter.

Manganese, MnSOD and the Body's Antioxidant Defense

Manganese (Mn) is an essential mineral involved in the function of many enzymes, the immune system, blood clotting, bone formation and metabolism[4295]. In nature, it is found in combination with iron. Deficiencies in manganese impair growth, lead to skeletal defects, reduce fertility and alter glucose tolerance [4296, 4297]. Manganese metalloenzymes include arginase, glutamine synthetase, phosphoenolpyruvate decarboxylase and MnSOD, all of which have an important role in antioxidant defense and metabolic reactions. Manganese superoxide dismutase deficiency triggers mitochondrial uncoupling and the Warburg effect[4298], which may promote cancer and metastasis.

The historical origins of manganese trace back to Ancient Greece where it was called *magnes*. Spartans used manganese to strengthen their steel[4299]. Magnetite or lodestone was considered the male *magnes* that could attract iron, hence the term magnet. The female *magnes* was used to decolorize glass, which was later named *magnesia* or manganese dioxide. Manganese dioxide was called *manganesum* by 16th century glassmakers. Egyptian and Roman glassmakers also used manganese compounds to add or remove color from glass[4300]. The metal isolated from *magnesia* became known as *manganese*, which comes from the German word *mangan*. Manganese pigments were used in the 24-30,000-year-old cave paintings in Gargas, France[4301]. The 18th century Swedish chemist Carl Wilhelm Scheele used manganese dioxide to create chloride by reacting hydrochloric acid, or a mixture of dilute sulfuric acid and sodium chloride with manganese dioxide[4302]. Nowadays, manganese is used to make stainless steel and aluminum alloys[4303].

Manganese deficiency reduces bone mineral density, whereas supplementation improves bone health[4304]. Women with osteoporosis have been observed to have lower serum manganese levels than those without osteoporosis[4305]. In postmenopausal women, higher serum manganese levels have been correlated with better bone mineral density and reduced fracture rates[4306,4307]. However, other studies have not found such associations[4308,4309]. These discrepancies may have to do with the study population or the fact that measuring mineral levels in blood does not necessarily reflect total body mineral status. However, manganese deficiency in rats does cause skeletal deformities and reduced bone formation[4310,4311]. Thus, based on studies that induce deficiency or that supplement with manganese, it is clear that it does have a role in bone health.

One of primary functions of manganese is that it makes up Mn superoxide dismutase (MnSOD), which scavenges free radicals and reactive oxygen species (ROS) in the mitochondria, endothelium and even in atherosclerotic plaque [4312]. MnSOD protects the mitochondria against ROS and free radicals that contribute to metabolic syndrome[4313]. Manganese intake is inversely associated with metabolic syndrome, abdominal obesity and high triglycerides in Chinese men, but positively correlated with low HDL cholesterol in both men and women[4314]. In Korean women with metabolic syndrome, the dietary intake of manganese is significantly lower than in healthy controls[4315]. Among Chinese adults, a higher daily manganese intake is associated with a lower number of metabolic syndrome components. [4316] However, blood and urine concentrations of manganese are not necessarily associated with metabolic syndrome[4317].

The initiation of atherosclerotic lesions (plaque in the arteries) results from excess ROS production [4318]. Atherosclerosis is a disease of chronic inflammation that damages the blood vessel wall[4319] and oxidizes LDL cholesterol[4320]. Superoxide dismutase protects against the oxidation of lipids [4321]. Manganese protects against heart mitochondria lipid peroxidation in rats through MnSOD[4322]. MnSOD can reduce oxLDL-induced cell death of macrophages[4323], inhibit LDL oxidation and protect against endothelial dysfunction[4324]. There is an association between decreased MnSOD and atherogenesis [4325]. Manganese compounds given in animals can reduce vascular inflammation[4326]. Interestingly, higher blood manganese levels have been found in people with atherosclerosis[4327]. This may suggest greater manganese recruitment in blood to inhibit the higher inflammation and to help heal the damaged endothelium.

ROS production also impairs the antioxidant capacity of the adipose tissue, whereas SOD has a beneficial effect on obesity-related conditions [4328,4329]. Mice fed an obesogenic diet show decreased MnSOD status[4330]. MnSOD mimetics may help to prevent and treat non-alcoholic fatty liver disease in humans[4331,4332]. In Polish men aged 50-75, there was a positive correlation between manganese intake and BMI, waist-to-hip ratio, abdominal circumference and HOMA-IR (a marker of insulin resistance) but not metabolic syndrome[4333]. Higher manganese intake (> 5.12 mg/d) has been associated with a reduced risk of abdominal obesity in Chinese men [4334]. However, U.S. NHANES data 2011–2014 found the highest blood Mn concentrations to be associated with obesity in children[4335].

Insulin resistance can be thought of as a cellular antioxidant defense mechanism against oxidative stress in the absence of other antioxidant defense systems, such as manganese superoxide dismutase or glutathione[4336]. In other words, a lack of manganese may be a direct cause of insulin resistance. Indeed, insulin resistance appears to be a compensatory response to inadequate antioxidant defenses in the face of excess oxidative stress. In mice, MnSOD protects against diabetic complications, such as cardiomyopathy, retinopathy and neuropathy[4337,4338,4339,4340]. In animals, manganese treatment improves glucose tolerance and insulin secretion[4341,4342,4343]. In rats, dietary and acute manganese exposure reduces plasma insulin and hyperglycemia, causing reactionary hypoglycemia[4344,4345]. What's more, a manganese deficiency significantly decreases tissue selenium levels in pigs[4346], which might mean that manganese is also important for maintaining adequate glutathione status through maintenance of selenium status.

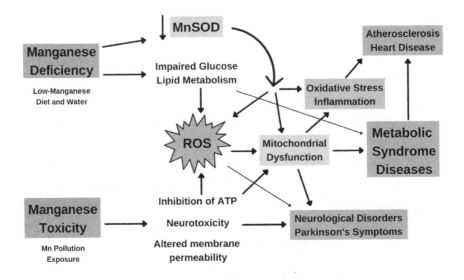

Adapted From: Li, Longman; Yang, Xiaobo (2018). 'The Essential Element Manganese, Oxidative Stress, and Metabolic Diseases: Links and Interactions'. Oxidative Medicine and Cellular Longevity, 2018(), 1–11.

Epidemiological studies find a U-shaped correlation between blood manganese levels and type-2 diabetes[4347,4348]. Among 122 Chinese adults with newly diagnosed diabetes and 429 adults without diabetes, subjects in the highest tertile of serum manganese (> 2.42 mcg/L) were 7.88 times more likely to have diabetes compared to those in the lowest tertile (< 1.67 mcg/L)[4349]. A higher manganese level in the blood, likely suggests increased inflammation, something that is also seen with copper blood levels.

Manganese is required for creating oxaloacetate from pyruvate via pyruvate carboxylase[4350]. In mammals, oxaloacetate is needed for gluconeogenesis, the urea cycle, neurotransmitter synthesis, lipogenesis and insulin secretion[4351]. Gluconeogenesis is the process of creating new glucose from non-carbohydrate substrates and is required for maintaining stable blood sugar levels throughout the day or when fasting[4352]. It's possible that people who do not tolerate low-carb diets have poor gluconeogenesis, which may be driven by a poor manganese status. Oxaloacetate also synthesizes aspartate, which then gets converted into other amino acids, asparagine, methionine, lysine and threonine. During gluconeogenesis, pyruvate is converted first into oxaloacetate by pyruvate carboxylase, which is then simultaneously decarboxylated and phosphorylated into phosphoenolpyruvate (PEP)[4353]. This is the rate-limiting step in gluconeogenesis. Pyruvate carboxylase is expressed the most in gluconeogenic tissues, such as the liver, kidneys, pancreatic islets and lactating mammary glands. There is a moderate amount of activity in the brain, heart and adrenal glands[4354].

Arginase is another manganese-containing enzyme and the final enzyme in the urea cycle, during which the body gets rid of ammonia. Arginase converts L-arginine into L-ornithine and urea[4355]. Manganese ions are required for stabilizing water and hydrolyzing L-arginine into L-ornithine and urea[4356]. Arginase is also involved with nitric oxide synthase. Disorders in arginase metabolism are implicated with neurological impairment, dementia and hyperammonemia[4357]. Excess ammonia is not acutely harmful to humans as it will either be converted into amino acids or excreted through urine[4358]. However, high ammonia is associated with upper gastrointestinal bleeding in cirrhosis and kidney damage[4359,4360]. Urea cycle disorders cause delirium, lethargy and even strokes in adults[4361].

Manganese is a co-factor for glutamine synthetase (GS), which is an enzyme that forms glutamine from ammonia and glutamate[4362,4363]. Glutamine is used by activated immune cells[4364]. It supports lymphocyte proliferation and helps to produce cytokines by lymphocytes and macrophages[4365]. Additionally, glutamine may help people with food hypersensitivities by reducing inflammation on the gut surface[4366]. It can thus protect against and repair leaky gut, hence improving immunity[4367]. Getting enough glutamine from the diet or by using a supplement may help to protect intestinal epithelial cell tight junctions, which prevents intestinal permeability[4368]. Glutamine synthetase is most predominantly found in the brain, astrocytes, kidneys and liver[4369]. In the brain, glutamine synthetase regulates ammonia detoxification and glutamate the excitatory neuro-transmitter[4370]. Manganese gets in the brain with the help of the iron-carrying protein transferrin, but manganese doesn't seem to compete with iron absorption[4371].

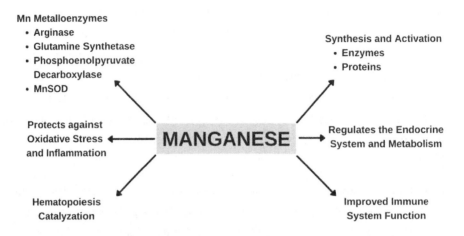

Mn Metalloenzymes
- Arginase
- Glutamine Synthetase
- Phosphoenolpyruvate Decarboxylase
- MnSOD

Synthesis and Activation
- Enzymes
- Proteins

Protects against Oxidative Stress and Inflammation

MANGANESE

Regulates the Endocrine System and Metabolism

Hematopoiesis Catalyzation

Improved Immune System Function

Adapted From: Li, Longman; Yang, Xiaobo (2018). 'The Essential Element Manganese, Oxidative Stress, and Metabolic Diseases: Links and Interactions'. Oxidative Medicine and Cellular Longevity, 2018(), 1–11.

Acute manganese toxicity causes manganism, characterized by neurological symptoms, mood swings, compulsive behavior and decreased response speed[4372]. Manganese overexposure can also impair cardiovascular function and heartbeat[4373]. Chronic exposure leads to a more permanent dysfunction that resembles Parkinson's disease[4374]. Unlike Parkinson's, manganism does not appear to cause a loss of sense of smell and patients do not respond to L-DOPA treatment[4375]. The neurotoxic effects appear to be caused by disturbed iron and aluminum metabolism and iron overload that causes oxidative stress[4376,4377,4378,4379,4380]. Oxidative stress is one of the main factors of manganese-induced neurotoxicity[4381]. It is important to note that a lack copper in the body leads to iron overload[4382], which can lead to manganese overload in tissues[4383]. Thus, a lack of one mineral, such as copper, can lead to the harmful accumulation and dysregulation of other minerals in the body.

Manganese accumulation in the mitochondria can also cause mitochondrial dysfunction by inhibiting complex I and II[4384,4385,4386]. The highest accumulation rate is observed in the mitochondria of astrocytes and neurons compared to other organelles after chronic manganese exposure[4387]. Excessive manganese gets excreted out of the mitochondrial lumen through sodium-independent mechanisms, but it gets imported mainly by the calcium uniporter[4388,4389,4390]. Manganese inhibits calcium efflux, which increases the probability of mitochondrial permeability transition associated with brain injury and stroke[4391]. This goes to show that a dysregulation in manganese metabolism, which can be caused by many factors, can lead to manganese accumulation and damage to tissues.

Manganese poisoning can occur due to drinking contaminated water or when exposed to the fuel additive methylcyclopentadienyl manganese tricarbonyl (MMT) and the pesticide manganese ethylene-bis-dithiocarbamate (Maneb)[4392,4393,4394,4395]. Permanganate (Mn^{7+}) is much more toxic than Mn^{2+} with potassium permanganate having a lethal dose of 10 grams[4396,4397]. Mining and processing manganese causes air and water pollution, which threatens the health of workers and local residence, especially in South Africa, China and Australia where most of the world's manganese is mined from. Factory workers exposed to manganese dust have been found to have significantly fewer children[4398]. Inhaling airborne manganese is the most common exposure route for occupational workers, such as miners, smelters and welders[4399,4400,4401]. The U.S. Occupational Safety and Health Administration (OSHA) has set the permissible limit for manganese exposure in the workplace as 5 mg/m3 over an 8-hour workday[4402]. Doses of 500 mg/m^3 are immediately hazardous to health and life[4403]. Tobacco smoke also has some manganese and other metals but at concentrations not dangerous to human health[4404,4405], aside from the long-term consequences on cancer and atherosclerosis risk.

The brain is the most vulnerable organ to manganese toxicity, exemplified by the neurological complications seen in manganese poisoning. The olfactory tract is the most direct pathway for manganese to get into the brain[4406]. By using two zinc transporters ZIP8 and ZIP14, it can bypass the blood-brain barrier[4407]. Infants have an immature blood-brain barrier, making them more vulnerable to manganese toxicity[4408]. MRI studies show that manganese accumulates predominantly in the globus pallidus located in the basal ganglia[4409]. Dopamine oxidation by manganese causes oxidative stress[4410]. Chronic manganese exposure has been seen to reduce choline levels in the hypothalamus and thalamus[4411].

Here are the manganese-dependent enzymes, functions and consequences that may occur with deficient manganese intake

Boron-Dependent Enzymes/Proteins	Function	Consequences of Deficit
Superoxide Dismutase	Removes superoxide anions	Increased tissue and mitochondrial damage and oxidative stress
Arginase	Participates in the urea cycle to remove harmful ammonia	Ammonia accumulation, kidney damage
Pyruvate Carboxylase	Converts glucose into oxaloacetate, gluconeogenesis, lipogenesis, neurotransmitter biosynthesis, insulin secretion	Impaired insulin production, low-carb intolerance, ammonia accumulation
Glutamine Synthetase	Glutamine formation, nitrogen metabolism, ammonia detoxification	Weaker immunity, intestinal permeability, ammonia accumulation, neurotoxicity
Divalent Metal Transporter 1 (DMT1)	Transports ferrous iron, regulates iron homeostasis, absorption and transportation of manganese,	Poor iron homeostasis, manganese deficiency

	binds to divalent metals	
Transferrin Receptor (TfR)	Imports iron into the cell, manganese influx and efflux	Poor iron homeostasis, manganese overload or deficiency

Manganese Food Sources

There is no established RDA for manganese. The estimated safe and adequate daily intake for manganese has been set at 2-5 mg/d[4412]. Adequate intakes for adult males are 2.3 mg/d and 1.8 mg/d for females. Men on experimentally manganese-deficient diets (< 0.74 mg/d) have been shown to develop erythematous rashes[4413]. Women consuming < 1 mg of manganese per day experience altered mood and increased pain during their premenstrual phase of the estrous cycle[4414]. During pregnancy or lactation, the demand for manganese increases to 2.0-2.6 mg/d. Children that are 1-3 years old should get 1.2 mg/d, 4-8 years old 1.5 mg/d and boys 9-13 years old should get 1.9 mg/d and girls 1.6 mg/d. Newborns that are 6 months old or younger should get 0.003 mg/d and 7–12-month-olds should obtain 0.6 mg/d[4415]. The tolerable upper intake levels for manganese have been set at 9-11 mg for adults and 2-9 mg for children 12 months of age or older.[4416]

Optimal Intake of Manganese (mg/d)

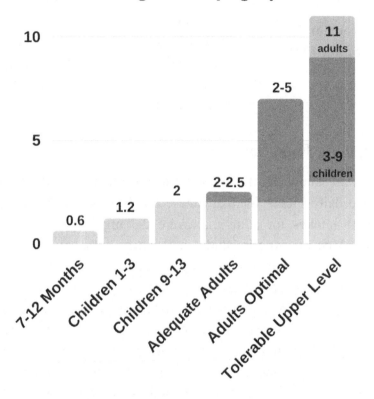

The average intake of manganese on Western diets is 0.7-10.9 mg/d[4417,4418]. In the U.S., data from 1982-1989 indicates an average manganese intake of 1.1 mg/d in infants, 1.48 mg/d in 2-year-old children, 1.78-2.76 mg/d in teenagers, 2.14-2.23 in adult females and 2.64-2.81 mg/d in adult males[4419]. A 2018 Italian study in adults showed an average intake of 2.34 mg/d in Northern Italy[4420].

Manganese is found in many foods, including grains, clams, oysters, legumes, vegetables, tea and spices. One of the most commonly consumed sources of dietary manganese are rice, nuts and tea[4421]. Dietary and non-experimental manganese deficiency is quite rare, and toxicity occurs mostly due to environmental exposure. Some supplements are also fortified with manganese, ranging from 5 to 20 mg[4422].

The amount of manganese in human breast milk ranges from 3-10 mcg/L. Cow's milk-based infant formulas contain 30-100 mcg/L[4423]. Soy-based formulas have the highest concentration of manganese (200-300 mcg/L), which might lead to manganese accumulation. The absorption of manganese from human milk is the highest (8.2%) compared to soy formulas (0.7%) and cow's milk formula (3.1%)[4424]. Intravenous absorption of manganese, however, is close to 100%, which can cause manganese toxicity. Infants have a much higher absorption and retention of manganese than adults, making them more susceptible to manganism[4425,4426]. They also have a higher total amount of manganese in the body than older children and adults[4427]. The amount of manganese in the hair of newborn babies increases from 0.19 mcg/g at birth to 0.965 mcg/g at 6 weeks of age and 0.685 mcg/g at 4 months when they're fed infant formulas. Normal children at age 8 have a hair manganese concentration of 0.268 mcg/g and those with learning disability (hyperactive) have 0.434 mcg/g.[4428] In rat pups, a high intake of dietary manganese is neurotoxic and results in developmental deficits[4429]. Both high and low manganese intake during pregnancy impairs birth weight and infant health[4430,4431,4432,4433]. In 1985, the recommended manganese intake for exclusively parenterally fed preterm infants was set at 2-10 mcg/kg/d[4434], but this was revised down to 1 mcg/kg/d in 2003[4435,4436].

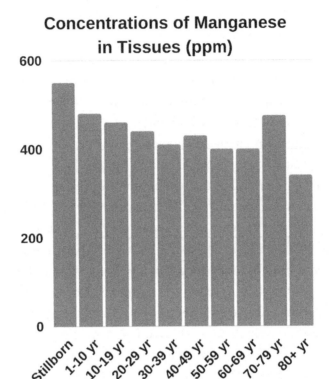

Concentrations of Manganese in Tissues (ppm)

Adapted From: Schroeder, H. A., Balassa, J. J., & Tipton, I. H. (1966). Essential trace metals in man: Manganese. Journal of Chronic Diseases, 19(5), 545–571.

Drinking water also contains some manganese. For an average 70 kg-weighing adult, the lowest amount of manganese in drinking water with adverse effects is 4.2 mg/d[4437]. The World Health Organization recommends manganese concentrations in drinking water to be < 400 mcg/L[4438] whereas in the U.S. the benchmark is 300 mcg/L[4439]. In Bangladesh, the amount of manganese in drinking water ranges from 1 mcg/L to 2 mg/L[4440], with the higher concentrations having been noted to alter classroom behavior in school-aged children[4441]. Higher exposure to manganese through drinking water has also been associated with intellectual impairment in Canadian (Quebec) school-aged children[4442]. People who drink water with manganese as high as 28 mg/L have developed manganese toxicity[4443].

480

Here are the main food sources of manganese[4444,4445]

Food	Mg of Manganese per Serving	% of RDA
Mussels, blue, cooked, 3 oz	5.8 mg	252%
Hazelnuts, dry roasted, 1 oz	1.6 mg	70%
Pecans, dry roasted, 1 oz	1.1 mg	48%
Brown Rice, cooked, ½ cup	1.1 mg	48%
Oysters, cooked, 3 oz	1.0 mg	43%
Clams, cooked, 3 oz	0.9 mg	39%
Chickpeas, cooked, ½ cups	0.9 mg	39%
Spinach, boiled, ½ cups	0.8 mg	35%
Pineapple, raw, ½ cups	0.8 mg	35%
Soybeans, boiled, ½ cups	0.7 mg	30%
Whole Wheat Bread, 1 slice	0.7 mg	30%
Oatmeal, cooked, ½ cups	0.7 mg	30%
Peanuts, oil-roasted, 1 oz	0.5 mg	22%
Black Tea, 1 cup	0.5 mg	22%
Lentils, cooked, ½ cups	0.5 mg	22%
Potato, baked, 1 medium	0.3 mg	13%
White Rice, cooked, ½ cups	0.3 mg	13%
Kidney Beans, canned, ½ cups	0.3 mg	13%
Acorn Squash, cooked, ½ cups	0.3 mg	13%

Blueberries, raw, ½ cups	0.3 mg	13%
Sesame Seeds, dried, 1 tbsp	0.2 mg	9%
Kale, raw, 1 cup	0.2 mg	9%
Black Pepper, ½ tsp	0.2 mg	9%
Asparagus, boiled, ½ cups	0.1 mg	4%
Apple, raw with skin, 1 medium	0.1 mg	4%
Romaine Lettuce, 1 cup	0.1 mg	4%
Coffee, 1 cup	0.1 mg	4%
Liver, 1 oz	0.1 mg	4%
Sardines, 3 oz	0.1 mg	4%
Shrimp, cooked, 3 oz	0.0 mg	0%
Tuna, canned, 3 oz	0.0 mg	0%
Chicken Breast, 3 oz	0.0 mg	0%
Ground Beef, cooked, 3 oz	0.0 mg	0%
Whole Egg, 1 large	0.0 mg	0%
Milk, 1%, 1 cup	0.0 mg	0%
Yogurt, low-fat, 1 cup	0.0 mg	0%

Manganese absorption and influx is mostly mediated by the divalent metal transporter 1 (DMT1) and transferrin receptor (TfR) on the cell surface that also transport other divalent cations, such as iron and calcium[4446,4447]. Iron deficiency can increase the risk of manganese poisoning because manganese absorption will increase under low iron states[4448]. In iron-deficient rats and pigs, manganese levels in the brain are upregulated[4449,4450]. About 75% of the manganese in human milk is bound to lactoferrin[4451]. Excess ferric lactoferrin could inhibit the absorption of this manganese complex[4452]. The addition of calcium to human milk significantly decreases manganese absorption, while addition of phytates, phosphate and ascorbic acid to infant formulas, as well as iron and magnesium to wheat bread has no significant effect[4453]. High manganese intake leads to adaptive changes that include reduced gastrointestinal absorption of manganese, enhanced liver metabolism and increased manganese excretion[4454,4455].

In adults, 3-5% of manganese is absorbed through the gastrointestinal (GI) tract with women absorbing slightly more than men, possibly due to poorer iron status[4456,4457]. After GI absorption, manganese enters the bloodstream and is distributed throughout different tissues. Intravenous administration of manganese bypasses GI regulation and results in 100% of absorption. Aging decreases manganese absorption and retention[4458,4459]. Thus, we need more manganese as we get older.

The primary manganese excretion pathway is biliary secretion. More than 95% of manganese is excreted through bile so the threshold for dietary manganese toxicity is quite high[4460,4461]. However, in rats, mice and kittens, there is almost no biliary excretion of manganese during the neonatal period, making them again more susceptible to manganism[4462]. Some manganese can also be lost through urine, milk and sweat[4463,4464]. Tracing radiomanganese (^{54}Mn) whole-body elimination shows it is a biphasic dose-dependent process with an elimination rate of 70% and a half-life of 39 days[4465,4466]. During low manganese intake, the half-life increases up to 90 days[4467]. Consumed manganese has an average retention of 10 days[4468].

The liver regulates whole-body manganese levels through endogenous gut losses by expressing various manganese transporters on cell membranes, including DMT1, transferrin, TfR, ZIP14 and citrate transporters[4469,4470,4471,4472,4473]. Hepatic dysfunction, liver damage and cholestasis are risk factors for accumulating manganese in the brain[4474,4475,4476,4477]. **Liver damage impairs manganese excretion, causing high levels of manganese in the blood**[4478]. Patients with portosystemic shunts (also known as liver shunts) and biliary atresia (narrowed or blocked bile ducts) exhibit hypermanganesemia, even without increasing dietary manganese intake[4479,4480,4481]. Autopsies of chronic hepatic encephalopathy patients reveal they have elevated manganese levels in the basal ganglia[4482]. Children with cholestasis on total parental nutrition show movement disorders and high manganese levels in the blood[4483]. Cessation of parental manganese supplements rapidly decreases plasma manganese levels and improves liver function[4484].

Normal blood manganese levels are 4-15 mcg/L[4485], but this is highly variable and dependent of manganese intake[4486]. Some healthy adults have an average plasma concentration of 1.28 mcg/L [4487]. Females tend to have ~30% higher levels than men because of higher iron retention[4488]. **Lymphocyte manganese is thought to be better than whole blood manganese for measuring manganese deficiency.** Based on one animal study, a group of authors concluded: "*These results suggest that, for assessment of manganese nutritional status, measurement of manganese in lymphocytes is better than that in whole blood*"[4489].

Most of blood manganese gets distributed in soft tissue (~60%), with the remainder being in the liver (30%), kidney (5%), pancreas (5%), colon (1%), bone (0.5.%), urinary system (0.2.%), brain (0.1.%) and erythrocytes (0.0.2%)[4490]. Divalent Mn^{2+} is the predominant form of blood manganese and it is complexed with different molecules, such as albumin (84% of total Mn^{2+}), hexahydrated ion (6%), bicarbonate (6%), citrate (2%), and transferrin (Tf) (1%), whereas almost all trivalent Mn^{3+} is bound to transferrin[4491,4492,4493]. Mn^{3+} is more reactive and gets reduced to Mn^{2+} and Mn^{2+} can be oxidized to Mn^{3+} by ceruloplasmin the active form of copper[4494]. Mn^{3+}, typically coming in the form of manganese(III) fluoride, manganese(III) oxide and manganese(III) acetate, is more effective at inhibiting the mitochondrial complex I [4495]. The reduction of Mn^{3+} to $Mn2^{+}$ is mediated by ferrireductase, which helps to avoid oxidative stress[4496,4497].

Normal tissue manganese concentrations in mammals are around 0.3-2.9 mcg of Mn/g of wet tissue weight[4498,4499]. Whole-body manganese can be an indicator of blood manganese[4500]. **Tissues with a high energy demand like the brain and liver as well as high pigment**

regions such as the retina and skin have the highest concentrations of manganese. Approximately 40% of total body manganese is stored in the bones (1 mg/kg)[4501,4502]. It has been found that the hand bone manganese levels of welders exposed to high manganese environments are significantly higher compared to non-occupationally exposed individuals[4503]. In rats, it takes 6 weeks of manganese exposure to raise and stabilize bone manganese 2-3-fold higher than initially[4504]. The half-life of manganese in the femur, tibia and humerus in rats is 77, 263 and 429 days, respectively. In humans, that would be the equivalent of a few years.

Low hair manganese levels could indicate a manganese deficiency. Infants with congenital malformations and their mothers have low hair manganese levels compared to full-term and preterm infant-mother controls[4505]. Thus, the manganese status of the mother controls that of the fetus and prenatal manganese analysis might be a tool for assessing the risk of intrauterine malformations.

Molybdenum for Fixing Nitrogen and Detoxifying Toxins

In nature, molybdenum (Mo) does not appear as a free metal but is found in various oxidation states in minerals. Do not confuse molybdenum for lead. There are no significant elemental similarities between molybdenum and lead, except for how they look, which is why molybdenum ores were confused with lead ores, giving it such a name[4506]. In Ancient Greek, *molybdos*, means lead, which gives the basis to *molybdaenum* in Neo-Latin. Molybdenite, which is the primary ore from which molybdenum is now extracted from, was often confused with and used as graphite to blacken surfaces[4507]. The 18th century Swedish chemist Carl Wilhelm Scheele was the first to differentiate molybdenum from other metals in 1778[4508]. Another Swedish chemist Peter Jacob Hjelm isolated molybdenum in 1781 using carbon and linseed oil[4509]. Because of its high smelting point, molybdenum is used in steel alloys and in high-pressure applications. Before World War I, molybdenum was not commonly used but its industrial demand rose because of its function in armor plating for tanks, replacing manganese steel plating that was much heavier and less maneuverable[4510].

Molybdenum cofactors (Moco) are complexed to a pterin, forming molybdopterin, which is a cofactor for many important enzymes in the body including sulfite oxidase, xanthine oxidase, dimethyl sulfoxide (DMSO) reductase, aldehyde oxidase, carbon monoxide dehydrogenase (CODH), nitrate reductase and mitochondrial amidoxime reducing component (mARC)[4511]. They metabolize sulfur-containing amino acids and heterocyclic compounds, including purines and pyrimidines. Xanthine oxidase, aldehyde oxidase, and mARC also help to metabolize drugs, alcohol and toxins[4512,4513,4514,4515]. The only molybdenum enzyme that does not contain molybdopterin is nitrogenases that fix nitrogen (protein) in all life forms[4516]. The cofactor for nitrogenase is called FeMoco (iron-molybdenum cofactor) that converts atmospheric nitrogen into ammonia[4517].

Genetic mutations of a molybdenum cofactor deficiency cause an absence of molybdopterin, which leads to the accumulation of sulfite and neurological damage due to lack of sulfite oxidase[4518]. Some people with blatant molybdenum deficiency may also have troubles dealing with sulfites in food because of a poorly functioning sulfite oxidase[4519]. Molybdenum cofactor deficiency is not the same as molybdenum deficiency with just over 100 reported cases as of 2010[4520]. In most cases, it leads to death within days or months of birth[4521]. However, there are cases where intravenous purified cyclic pyranopterin monophosphate (cPMP) at doses of 80 to 160 microg of cPMP/kg of body weight for 1-2 weeks has been used to normalize all urinary markers of sulfite oxidase and xanthine oxidase deficiency for longer than 2 years [4522,4523]. Cyclic pyranopterin monophosphate (cPMP) is a precursor to molybdenum cofactor derived from *E. coli*. There is one 1981 case report of nutritional molybdenum deficiency due to receiving total parental nutrition without added molybdenum, causing tachycardia, tachypnea, headache, night blindness and coma that were resolved with molybdenum administration[4524].

Molybdenum cofactors cannot be obtained as a nutrient from dietary sources and need to be synthesized by the body (*de novo* biosynthesis)[4525]. One of the enzymes that catalyzes this process is radical SAM[4526,4527] (an enzyme that uses iron-sulfur clusters to cleave S-adenosyl-L-methionine (SAM) to generate a radical[4528,4529]. The other option for molybdopterin, besides molybdenum-sulfur pairing, is to complex with tungsten(wolfram)-using enzymes, which requires selenium for its action[4530]. Thus, it appears that the minerals that help with the production of molybdenum cofactors are iron, sulfur and selenium.

Here are the molybdenum-dependent enzymes, functions and consequences that may occur with deficient molybdenum intake[4531,4532]

Molybdenum-Dependent Enzymes/Proteins	Function	Consequences of Deficit
Molybdopterin	Molybdenum cofactor used in molybdenum- and tungsten-containing enzymes	Sulfite accumulation and toxin buildup
Sulfite Oxidase	Oxidize sulfite and sulfate via cytochrome C, transfer electrons to the electron transport chain and allow the generation of ATP[4533]	Sulfite and sulfate accumulation, poor energy production
Xanthine Oxidase	Break down xanthine and purines into uric acid, generate	Insufficient ROS signaling, in excess promotes gout

	reactive oxygen species and superoxide	
Dimethyl Sulfoxide (DMSO) Reductase	Catalyze the reduction of dimethyl sulfoxide (DMSO) to dimethyl sulfide (DMS)	Excess sulfoxide accumulation
Aldehyde Oxidase	Oxidize aldehydes into carboxylic acid, eliminate alcohol toxicity	Alcohol toxicity, liver damage
Carbon Monoxide Dehydrogenase (CODH)	Partake in the carbon cycle as a source of energy and fixate CO_2	Poor energy metabolism and growth
Nicotinate Dehydrogenase	Partake in nicotinate and nicotinamide (NAM) metabolism. NAM and nicotinate are forms of vitamin B3, like niacin and NAD+	Poor energy production, lack of enzymatic reactions
Nitrate Reductase	Reduce nitrate to nitrite, which is critical for producing protein in plants	Poor nutritional quality and low protein crops
Nitrogenase	Fixate nitrogen, facilitate growth, biosynthesis of	Poor growth, physical deterioration

	nucleotides and amino acids	
Mitochondrial Amidoxime Reducing Component (mARC)	Reduce amidoximes to amidines, help with cholesterol metabolism	Poor lipid profile, liver damage

Molybdenum Food Sources

The RDA for molybdenum is 45 mcg/d for adults 19 years of age and older and 43 mcg/d for teenagers 14-18 years of age[4534]. During pregnancy and lactation, it is recommended to get 50 mcg/d of molybdenum and for children 9-13 years old 34 mcg/d. Infants from birth to 6 months of age should get 2 mcg/day and from 6 to 12 months of age 3 mcg/d. Children aged 1-3 years of age should get 17 mcg/day and children 4-8 years of age should get 22 mcg/day. The tolerable upper intake level (UL) for adults 19 years of age and older is 2,000 mcg/d. The UL for children 1-3 years old is 300 mcg/d, 4-8 years old is 600 mcg/d, 9-13 years old is 1,100 mcg/d and 14-18 years old is 1,700 mcg/d.[4535] Consuming a reasonably high molybdenum diet does not pose a threat to health because it gets rapidly excreted through urine[4536]. The minimum requirement for molybdenum for adults is deemed to be 22-25 mcg/d and estimated average requirement is 34 mcg/d[4537,4538].

Excess molybdenum intake has been reported to cause copper deficiency in ruminants by forming a thiomolybdate complex with copper[4539]. Doses of 25 mg/kg/d in rabbits can reduce hemoglobin concentrations and hematocrit [4540,4541,4542,4543], possibly due to interfering with copper metabolism. This interaction is not considered to be significant enough for humans. Furthermore, one of the highest sources of copper (liver and beans) are also naturally high in molybdenum. There is one report of increased urinary copper excretion with a molybdenum intake of 500-1,500 mcg from sorghum [4544].

However, these findings were not confirmed in a controlled study with equal levels of dietary molybdenum intake[4545].

Low soil concentrations of molybdenum, ranging from Iran to Northern China cause a dietary molybdenum deficiency, which is associated with an increased rate of esophageal cancer[4546,4547,4548]. There is no evidence that excess molybdenum causes cancer in humans or animals[4549].

Exposure to prolonged high intakes of molybdenum can raise uric acid levels because xanthine oxidase breaks down purines into uric acid[4550]. Armenians from two towns consuming 10-15 mg/d of molybdenum and 5-10 mg/d of copper from food have been observed to experience increased uric acid in plasma and urine, correlating with serum molybdenum concentrations[4551]. In those two towns, where the soil contained 77 mg/kg of molybdenum, 18 and 31% of people, respectively, showed symptoms of gout with elevated uric acid and xanthine oxidase activity. In a control area where molybdenum intake was 1-2 mg/d and copper intake was 10-15 mg/d, no increased uric acid or incidence of gout-like disorders was observed[4552]. Other studies find no change in uric acid excretion or copper metabolism with intakes of 1.5 mg/d[4553]. Thus, it might be that molybdenum toxicity depends on copper status and a high molybdenum intake would require an adequate copper intake as well.

Mining and metal workers chronically exposed to 60 to 600 mg Mo/m^3 report an increased incidence of weakness, fatigue, headaches, anorexia and muscle pain [4554]. Exposure to molybdenum in molybdenum-copper plants can raise serum bilirubin and decrease blood albumin/globulin ratios, which is interpreted to indicate liver dysfunction [4555]. The U.S. Occupational Safety and Health Administration (OSHA) set an 8-hour total weight average permissible exposure limit of molybdenum at 15 mg/m^3. [4556]

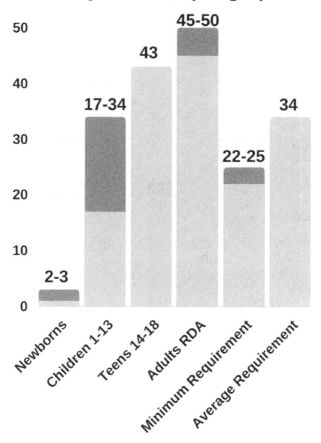

Optimal Intake of Molybdenum (mcg/d)

Foods high in molybdenum include legumes, beans, whole grains, nuts and liver[4557]. They are also the top sources of molybdenum in the U.S. diet. For teenagers and children, the top sources are milk and cheese.[4558] Molybdenum deficiency is quite rare because it can be found in a lot of different foods[4559]. Thus, most Americans are thought to consume enough molybdenum, which is probably why National surveys no longer collect data about molybdenum intake. The FDA's 1984 Total Diet Study estimated an average molybdenum intake of 109 mcg/d in men and 76 mcg/d in women[4560]. Another 1980 study reported an average intake of 180 mcg/d, which was lower than the 300-400 mcg/d seen in previous studies[4561]. NHANES 1988–1994 showed that the average molybdenum intake from supplements was 23-24 mcg/d[4562].

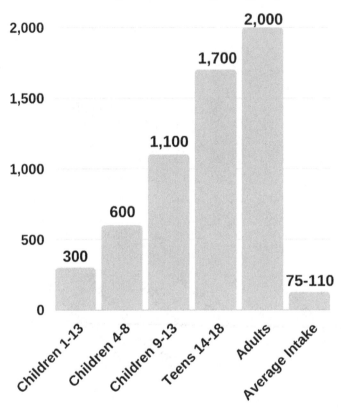

Tolerable Upper Level Intake of Molybdenum (mcg/d)

Infants get their molybdenum from breast milk. There are no reported cases of full-term infants exclusively fed human milk with any signs of molybdenum deficiency. The concentrations of molybdenum in the milk of mothers of premature infants ranges from 2.1-23 mcg/L, with an average level of 5 mcg/L[4563]. Infants and newborns absorb close to 100% of the molybdenum from breast milk or baby formula[4564,4565]. Daily average consumption of 0.5-0.8 liters of milk should cover the 2-3 mcg/d molybdenum requirement and prevent excessive intake[4566]. After birth, molybdenum in breast milk rapidly decreases from 15 mcg/L on day 1, to 4.8 mcg/L at 7-10 days postpartum, and 2.6 mcg/L by 1 month[4567]. At 42-60 days postpartum, human milk contains around 1.42 mcg/L of molybdenum and 1.78 mcg/L at day 97-293[4568]. Cow's milk contains more molybdenum than human milk.

Drinking water is generally a low source of molybdenum. In 100 of the largest cities in the U.S., the consumption of molybdenum from drinking water is estimated to be about 3 mcg/d based on an intake of 2 liters of water per day[4569]. The U.S. Environmental Protection Agency stated in their 2017 report that 0.8% of drinking water samples contained molybdenum levels above 40 mcg/L[4570]. In rabbits, 5 mg/kg/d of molybdenum from water causes histological changes in the liver and kidneys but not at lower doses[4571].

Here are the highest sources of molybdenum[4572]

Food	Mcg of Molybdenum per Serving	% of RDA
Black-Eyed Peas, boiled, ½ cup	288 mcg	640%
Beef Liver, fried, 3 oz	104 mcg	231%
Lima Beans, boiled, ½ cup	104 mcg	231%
Yogurt, low-fat, 1 cup	26 mcg	58%
Milk, 2%, 1 cup	22 mcg	49%
Potato, baked with skin, 1 medium	16 mcg	36%
Cheerios Cereal, ½ cup	15 mcg	33%
Shredded Wheat Cereal, ½ cup	15 mcg	33%
Banana, 1 medium	15 mcg	33%
White Rice, cooked, ½ cup	13 mcg	29%

Whole Wheat Bread, 1 slice	12 mcg	27%
Peanuts, dry roasted, 1 oz	11 mcg	24%
Chicken, roasted, 1 oz	9 mcg	20%
Egg, soft-boiled, large	9 mcg	20%
Spinach, boiled, ½ cup	8 mcg	18%
Ground Beef, fried, 3 oz	8 mcg	18%
Pecans, dry roasted, 1 oz	8 mcg	18%
Sweet Corn, cooked, ½ cup	6 mcg	13%
Cheddar Cheese, 1 oz	6 mcg	13%
Tuna, canned, 3 oz	5 mcg	11%
Potato, boiled without skin, ½ cup	4 mcg	9%
Orange, 1 medium	4 mcg	9%
Green Beans, boiled, ½ cup	3 mcg	7%
Carrots, raw, ½ cup	2 mcg	4%
Asparagus, boiled, ½ cup	2 mcg	4%

Molybdenum is absorbed at a rate of 40-100% from dietary sources in adults[4573,4574,4575,4576]. Soy contains relatively high amounts of molybdenum but is a less bioavailable source (56.7% absorption rate), whereas foods like kale are as bioavailable as other foods (86.1%)[4577]. Dietary tungsten reduces the amount of molybdenum in tissues and sodium tungsten is a competitive inhibitor of molybdenum [4578]. You can get exposed to tungsten in cities by breathing in industry-polluted air and drinking water, but most vegetables contain extraordinarily little of it (17 mcg/kg)[4579].

The human body contains roughly 0.07 mg of molybdenum per kilogram of bodyweight[4580]. Molybdenum is stored in the liver, kidneys, adrenal glands and bones in the form of molybdopterin[4581]. It is also found in tooth enamel, helping to prevent tooth decay[4582]. The ability to synthesize molybdopterin, which is an iron-sulfur and selenium-dependent process, seems to be necessary for retaining molybdenum in tissues[4583].

Molybdenum status is not usually clinically assessed because it is not thought to be a common deficiency. It is also difficult to measure because of big fluctuations based on dietary intake. A small 30 subject study saw that serum molybdenum levels in healthy adults ranges from 0.28-1.17 ng/mL[4584]. Plasma molybdenum peaks an hour after a meal and returns to baseline afterwards[4585,4586]. Infused molybdenum tracers disappear rapidly from the blood with only 2.5-5% remaining after an hour[4587].

The kidneys are the main organs regulating molybdenum levels in the body and promote its excretion through urine. Urinary excretion of molybdenum directly reflects dietary molybdenum intake. During low molybdenum intake, about 60% of consumed molybdenum gets excreted through urine and 90% is excreted when molybdenum intake is high[4588,4589]. The average U.S. urinary molybdenum concentration is 69 mcg/L[4590]. In molybdenum cofactor deficiency and in that single case of molybdenum deficiency, urinary sulfate and serum uric acid were low, but urinary xanthine, hypoxanthine and plasma methionine increased[4591]. However, these indicators have not been associated with molybdenum intake in normal healthy people.

Getting Enough Manganese and Molybdenum

As you can see, manganese and molybdenum are quite fascinating minerals with some important roles in the body. It is likely that you do not have frank deficiency in them, but you would still want to avoid chronic deficiencies and many people are ingesting suboptimal intakes, especially with manganese. Here is a brief overview of the daily requirements:

- **The optimal intake of manganese is 2-5 mg/d with a tolerable upper limit of 11 mg/d for adults.** Average Western diets may not provide an optimal intake of manganese but eating mussels and oysters once a week can help you reach those levels. Other manganese-rich foods include beans, vegetables, unrefined whole grains, nuts and spices.
- The tolerable upper limit of manganese for children is 3-9 mg/d, which they are not likely to hit eating an average diet, unless they eat a lot of mussels daily. Children 7-12 months old should consume around 0.6 mg/d, which can be obtained from breast milk. Be cautious with manganese-fortified baby formulas.
- The RDA for molybdenum in adults 19 years of age and older is 45-50 mcg/d with a tolerable upper limit of 2,000 mcg/d. Infants should get 2-3 mcg/d, which can be easily obtained from 0.5-0.8 liters of breast milk.
- The highest sources of molybdenum are beans, legumes and liver. Getting enough copper from these foods also prevents copper deficiency that may happen due to excess molybdenum intake. Other minerals needed for molybdenum to work are iron, sulfur and selenium.
- Molybdenum and manganese toxicity and frank deficiency are rare with the former usually occuring because of industrial exposure. Excess manganese and molybdenum are rapidly excreted from the body.

In conclusion, manganese and molybdenum are hidden players in the body's antioxidant defense system that provide protection against free radicals, oxidative stress and inflammation. It is hard to become deficient in them, but many people are not getting optimal intakes, especially for manganese.

Chapter 16
Eating for the Minerals and Preventing Deficiencies

Throughout human history, food scarcity has been quite common and frequent. Although the preconceived idea of the chronically starving hunter-gatherer is false and misleading, it is true that foragers are forced to skip a meal more often than people in industrialized societies. Despite having access to food 24/7, the average person still suffers from many health problems and nutrient deficiencies. This is because the food that we eat is less nutritious compared to just 50 years ago. Additionally, the chronic diseases that many of us suffer from reduces the absorption of nutrients into the body and into our cells. Many of the vitamins and minerals that we are deficient in can be obtained by eating large amounts of calories but that will come with the additional consequences of weight gain and insulin resistance. So, it is the quality of what you eat and the micronutrients you get from it that matter more than just the overall caloric content. If you want to appropriately absorb the nutrients from your diet, then you must fix any intestinal permeability or damage, and if you want to get nutrients into the cell then you must improve insulin resistance.

The Mineral Fix has revealed the intrinsic function of all the essential and possibly essential minerals in the human body. By now you should have realized how vital these elements are for creating optimal health. Having optimal health does not mean that you are meeting the bare minimal requirements or adequate intake. Instead, it is about getting the amount of minerals that leads to optimal bodily functions, depending on your physical state and lifestyle. Some people need more minerals due to certain medical conditions or just by virtue of being larger. As you have already learned, a lot of people in developed countries are deficient in at least one of these minerals. What's more, just a blanket approach of taking supplements may not work because of poor bioavailability or limited absorption. Thus, a more precise dietary strategy is needed to cover all your bases.

This chapter will bring together all the information about getting the right amount of minerals from our food and how to improve their status in the body. It serves both as an overview as well as a collection of guidelines. We will also talk about supplementation.

Optimal Daily Intake of Minerals

As you recall from chapter one, there are a total of 17 essential minerals with an additional 5 that could be considered essential. They include 7 essential macrominerals and 10 essential trace minerals. Essential minerals cannot be produced by the body and thus have to be obtained from the diet on a regular basis. Chronic deficiencies in essential minerals leads to physiological defects and/or disease.

To give you an example of the importance of non-essential nutrients let's take a look at the long-chain omega-3 fatty acids known as eicosapentaenoic acid (EPA) and docosahexaenoic acid (DHA). Both EPA and DHA can be created by the body by converting the essential omega-3 fatty acid alpha-linoleic acid (ALA) into EPA and DHA. So technically, EPA and DHA are not essential nutrients. However, the conversion of ALA to EPA and DHA in the body is low and taking preformed EPA and DHA has numerous health benefits[4592]. Hence, despite the fact that EPA and DHA are not considered 'essential', a lack of these nutrients in the diet can lead to poor health, especially during pregnancy, malnourishment, childhood growth and during some diseases[4593]. And this is likely to be the case for numerous 'non-essential' minerals. In fact, the situation is likely grimmer as there isn't a mechanism in the body to produce non-essential minerals. Thus, **both essential and non-essential minerals must be obtained through diet on a regular basis to maintain optimal nutrient status and health.**

Here is a list of the minerals and what primary function they have

7 Macrominerals		
Mineral	**Health Function**	**Risk of Deficiency/ Excess**
Calcium	Improves bone mineral density Promotes fat breakdown	**Deficiency**: osteoporosis, weight gain **Excess**: calcification, atherosclerosis
Chloride	Creates stomach acid Fights infections Maintains electrolyte balance	**Deficiency**: lack of nutrient absorption, illness **Excess**: hypertension, vascular damage and metabolic acidosis
Magnesium	Improves bone mineral density Regulates blood pressure Maintains insulin sensitivity	**Deficiency**: atherosclerosis, hypertension, insulin resistance, osteoporosis **Excess**: diarrhea
Phosphorus	Improves bone mineral density Gycolysis gluconeogenesis	**Deficiency**: osteoporosis, anorexia, rickets **Excess**: atherosclerosis, cardiovascular disease

Potassium	Regulates blood pressure Maintains insulin sensitivity Reduces atherosclerotic lesions	**Deficiency**: hypertension, atherosclerosis, insulin resistance **Excess**: Impaired kidney function, electrolyte imbalance, arrhythmia
Sodium	Regulates blood pressure Electrolyte balance Transports iodine into the thyroid Transports nutrients into the cell	**Deficiency**: hypotension, insulin resistance, cramping, hypothyroidism **Excess**: hypertension
Sulfur	Promotes antioxidant systems, Cholesterol and vitamin D sulfate Manages inflammation Detoxification, Methylation	**Deficiency**: low glutathione, low protein synthesis, weaker immunity, hypercholesterolemia, atherosclerosis, vascular damage **Excess**: gut disturbance, rashes, inflammation, high methionine levels

10 Trace Minerals		
Mineral	**Health Function**	**Risk of Deficiency/Excess**
Chromium	Enhances insulin action Improves glycemic control Supports lipid metabolism Lowers blood sugar Supports antioxidant defense	**Deficiency:** insulin resistance, hyperglycemia, hyperlipidemia, hyperinsulinemia, diabetes **Excess:** hypoglycemia, low birth weight in infants, anemia, iron deficiency
Cobalt	Vitamin B12 function Nerve function and regeneration Myelination and cognition	**Deficiency:** neuropathy, anemia, muscle wasting, cognitive impairment **Excess:** cardiomyopathy, lethal toxicity
Copper	Regulates iron status Improves lipid profile Maintains glycemic control Supports antioxidant defense Helps with energy production Collagen and soft tissue synthesis Thyroid function Immune system function Reproductive system Kidney health	**Deficiency:** anemia, cardiovascular disease, atherosclerosis, vascular damage, hyperglycemia, hypothyroidism, iron overload, collagen damage **Excess:** Angiogenesis/survival of malignant cells and tumors, inflammation

Fluoride	Prevents tooth decay Dental mineralization Fights infections	**Deficiency:** tooth decay, bacterial infections, bone demineralization, weight gain, impaired growth **Excess:** cognitive impairment, nausea, abdominal pain, gastrointestinal distress, dental fluorosis
Iodine	Maintains thyroid function Produces thyroid hormones Supports metabolic health Mental development Immune system function Protects against lipid peroxidation	**Deficiency:** hypothyroidism, hypogonadism, low energy, frailty, osteoporosis, goiter, hypercholesterolemia, obesity **Excess:** autoimmunity, thyroiditis, muscle wasting
Iron	Tissue oxygenation Regulates oxidative stress Nitrogen fixation Electron transfer	**Deficiency:** anemia, fatigue, low energy, infection risk, physical deterioration **Excess:** Atherosclerosis, inflammation, infection risk, organ damage, oxidative stress

Manganese	Antioxidant defense MnSOD activity Immune system function Glycolysis, gluconeogenesis Nitrogen metabolism Removes excess ammonia Bone mineral density	**Deficiency:** atherosclerosis, endothelial dysfunction, insulin resistance, diabetes, kidney damage, cirrhosis **Excess:** neurological complications, mitochondrial dysfunction, metabolic syndrome, atherosclerosis
Molybdenum	Nitrogen fixation Removes excess sulfites Metabolizes toxins and alcohol Metabolizes purines and sulfur	**Deficiency:** neurological damage, poor physical development, toxin accumulation **Excess:** reduces copper absorption, increases urea levels, promotes gout, liver dysfunction,
Selenium	Supports thyroid function Produces thyroid hormones Immune system function Protects against oxidative stress Prevents lipid peroxidation Detoxifies heavy metals	**Deficiency:** hypothyroidism, weaker immune system, atherosclerosis, oncogenesis, low glutathione, hyperlipidemia **Excess:** hyperglycemia, insulin resistance, nausea

| Zinc | Immune system function
Antioxidant defense
Calcification of bone
Wound healing
Produces thyroid hormones
Insulin production
Glucose metabolism
Brain development
and plasticity
Sex hormone production
Melatonin/serotonin
production
Glutathione synthesis
DNA damage repair | **Deficiency:**
hypothyroidism,
hypogonadism,
hyperglycemia,
atherosclerosis,
osteoporosis, mental
impairment,
weak immunity

Excess: decreased HDL
cholesterol, reduced
immunity, altered iron
metabolism, nausea,
diarrhea, cramping |

5 Possibly Essential Trace Minerals		
Mineral	**Health Function**	**Risk of Deficiency/Excess**
Boron	Brain function Tumor suppression Antioxidant defense Improves vitamin D status Better testosterone/estrogen status Elastase/collagenase activity Anti-osteoarthritic effects	**Deficiency:** vitamin D deficiency, osteoarthritis, hypogonadism, inflammation, impaired brain function **Excess:** gastrointestinal distress, kidney damage, goiter, reduced iodine absorption

Lithium	Neurotransmitter balance Brain function Mimics the effects of insulin Improves glucose metabolism	**Deficiency:** depression, increased suicide rate, mental impairment, aggression **Excess:** inhibits iodine absorption, gastrointestinal stress, nausea, convulsions, coma, death
Nickel	Regulates glucose metabolism Regulates homocysteine metabolism Supports reproduction and growth	**Deficiency:** hyperglycemia, hyperhomocysteinemia, impaired growth, infertility **Excess:** rashes and skin irritation
Silicon	Support connective tissue, blood vessels and arteries Reduces plaque formation Protects against atherosclerosis	**Deficiency:** atherosclerosis, osteoarthritis, plaque formation, hypertension **Excess:** calcification, impaired tissue mobility
Vanadium	Mimics the effects of insulin Improves glucose metabolism Supports metabolic health	**Deficiency:** hypothyroidism, depressed fertility and growth, hyperglycemia, insulin resistance **Excess:** hypertension, gastrointestinal stress, death

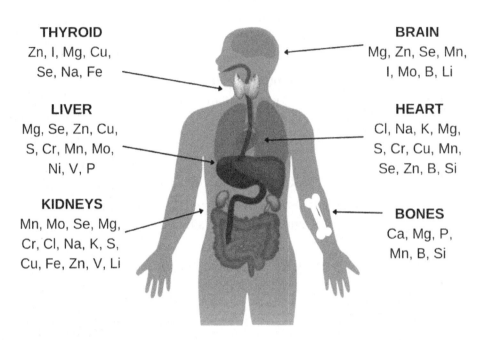

THYROID
Zn, I, Mg, Cu,
Se, Na, Fe

BRAIN
Mg, Zn, Se, Mn,
I, Mo, B, Li

LIVER
Mg, Se, Zn, Cu,
S, Cr, Mn, Mo,
Ni, V, P

HEART
Cl, Na, K, Mg,
S, Cr, Cu, Mn,
Se, Zn, B, Si

KIDNEYS
Mn, Mo, Se, Mg,
Cr, Cl, Na, K, S,
Cu, Fe, Zn, V, Li

BONES
Ca, Mg, P,
Mn, B, Si

Zn=Zinc, I=Iodine, Mg=Magnesium, Ca=Calcium, Cu=Copper, Se=Selenium, Na=Sodium, Fe=Iron, S=Sulfur, Cr=Chromium, Mn=Manganese, Mo=Molybdenum, Ni=Nickel, V=Vanadium, P=Phosphorus, Cl=Chloride, K=Potassium, Li=Lithium, B=Boron, Si=Silicon.

THE MINERAL FIX PYRAMID

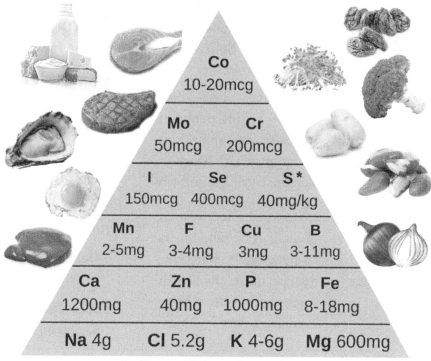

| Co 10-20mcg |
Mo 50mcg	Cr 200mcg
I 150mcg	Se 400mcg	S* 40mg/kg
Mn 2-5mg	F 3-4mg	Cu 3mg	B 3-11mg
Ca 1200mg	Zn 40mg	P 1000mg	Fe 8-18mg
Na 4g	Cl 5.2g	K 4-6g	Mg 600mg

*sulfur-containing amino acids

Na=Sodium, Cl=Chloride, K=Potassium, Mg=Magnesium, Ca=Calcium, Zn=Zinc, P=Phosphorus, Fe=Iron, Mn=Manganese, F=Fluoride, Cu=Copper, B=Boron, I=Iodine, Se=Selenium, S=Sulfur, Cr=Chromium, Mo=Molybdenum, Co=Cobalt.

Here is an overview of these same minerals, their recommended dietary sources and recommended daily intakes for adults

7 Macrominerals		
Mineral	**Recommended Dietary Sources**	**Optimal/Deficiency/ Excess Intake**
Calcium	Milk, cottage cheese, curd, cheese, yogurt, pumpkin seeds, nuts, spinach, sardines with bones, salmon, cartilage, soft ribs	**Optimal**: 1,000-1,200 mg/d **Deficiency**: < 550 mg/d **Excess Intake:** >1,500-2,000 mg/d
Chloride	Sea salt, rock salt, mineral waters, celery, tomatoes, lettuce, meat, olives, fish, seaweeds, kelp, whole grains, beans, legumes	**Optimal**: 5,200 mg/d **Deficiency**: < 1,000 mg/d **Excess Intake:** >7,500 mg/d
Magnesium	Pumpkin seeds, nuts, legumes, beans, lentils, spinach, chia seeds, salmon, halibut, avocado, dark chocolate, coffee	**Optimal**: 400-600 mg/d **Deficiency**: < 180 mg/d **Excess Intake:** >1,000 mg/d (however some people may benefit from high amounts, i.e., 1,800 mg/day for high blood pressure for example)
Phosphorus	Sardines with bones, salmon with bones, liver, yogurt, fish, meat, cheese, seafood, beans	**Optimal**: 750-1,250 mg/d **Deficiency**: < 580 mg/d

		Excess Intake: >2,000 mg/d
Potassium	Potatoes, carrots, apricots, swiss chard, bok choy, broccoli, cauliflower, collard greens, squash, beans, legumes, strawberries, cherries, blueberries, oranges, apples, seafood, fish	**Optimal**: 4,000-6,000 mg/d **Deficiency**: < 2,400 mg/d **Excess Intake:** >15,000 mg/d
Sodium	Sea salt, rock salt, mineral waters, celery, tomatoes, lettuce, meat, olives, fish, seaweeds, kelp, whole grains, beans, legumes	**Optimal**: 3,500 mg/d **Deficiency**: < 1,000 mg/d **Excess Intake:** >5-6,000 mg/d (intake will depend on needs and losses, some people will need more than 5,000 mg/d)
Sulfur	Seafood, fish, eggs, meat, cruciferous vegetables, garlic, shallots, leaks, onions, organ meats	**Sulfur-containing amino acids** **RDA**: 13-15 mg/kg body weight **Optimal:** 3-4X higher than the RDA. Taking 1 gram of MSM 3X/d for extra sulfur has shown numerous benefits on joint health and allergies

10 Trace Minerals		
Mineral	**Recommended Dietary Sources**	**RDA/Deficiency/ Excess Intake**
Chromium	Mussels, clams, oysters, brewer's yeast, broccoli, meat, fish, shrimp, oats, barley, maple syrup, apples with the skin	**RDA**: 33-50 mcg/d **Optimal:** 200-1,000 mcg/d **Deficiency**: < 24 mcg/d **Excess Intake:** >1,000 mcg/d
Cobalt	Liver, seafood, clams, oysters, buckwheat, meat, beef, vegetables	**Optimal**: 10-20 mcg/d **Deficiency**: < 2.4 mcg/d **Excess Intake:** > 1 g/d
Copper	Liver, kidneys, mollusks, oysters, beans, lentils, seaweeds, buckwheat, dark chocolate, cocoa powder, potatoes	**Optimal**: 2.6-3.0 mg/d **Deficiency**: < 0.8 mg/d **Excess Intake:** >10 mg/d
Fluoride	Toothpaste, fluorinated drinking water, bottled water, tea, coffee, shrimp, seafood	**Optimal**: 3-4 mg/d **Deficiency**: < 2 mg/d **Excess Intake:** >5 mg/d
Iodine	Seaweeds, kelp, nori, spirulina, salmon, fish, oysters, clams, whole milk, cheese, yogurt, iodized salt, fortified bread, eggs	**Optimal**: 150-200 mcg/d **Deficiency**: <100 mcg/d **Excess Intake:** >300-1,000 mcg/d

Iron	Red meat, beef, pork, oysters, clams, dark chocolate, beans, lentils, beetroot, spinach	**Optimal**: 8-18 mg/d **Deficiency**: < 8 mg/d **Excess Intake:** >45 mg/d
Manganese	Mussels, oysters, hazelnuts, pecans, rice, beans, legumes, chickpeas, clams, spinach, pineapple	**Optimal**: 2-5 mg/d **Deficiency**: < 2 mg/d **Excess Intake:** >11 mg/d
Molybdenum	Beans, liver, peas, legumes, yogurt, chickpeas, eggs, potatoes	**Optimal**: 45-50 mcg/d **Deficiency**: < 22 mcg/d **Excess Intake:** >2,000 mcg/d
Selenium	Brazil nuts, kidney, clams, oysters, sardines, shrimp, salmon, beef, eggs, liver, beans	**Optimal**: 300-400 mcg/d **Deficiency**: < 50 mcg/d **Excess Intake:** >800 mg/d
Zinc	Oysters, mollusks, clams, eggs, meat, beef, lamb, mutton, pork, wheat germ, buckwheat	**Optimal**: 20-80 mg/d **Deficiency**: < 8 mg/d **Excess Intake:** >80 mg/d (technically safe upper limit is set at 40 mg based on 60 mg/day causing some side effects but this also included supplemental zinc)

5 Possibly Essential Trace Minerals		
Mineral	**Recommended Dietary Sources**	**RDA/Deficiency/ Excess Intake**
Boron	Legumes, beans, lentils, vegetables, dried prunes, raisins, avocado, black currants, plums, almonds	**Optimal**: 3-11 mg/d **Deficiency**: < 1 mg/d **Excess Intake:** >28 mg/d
Lithium	Mineral water, grains, vegetables, mustard, kelp, pistachios, dairy, fish and meat	**Optimal**: 1 mg/d **Deficiency**: < 100 mcg/d **Excess Intake:** >2 mg/d
Nickel	Black tea, nuts and seeds, cacao, chocolate, meat, fish and grains	**Optimal**: 25-150 mcg/d **Deficiency**: < 25 mcg/d **Excess Intake:** 500mcg/d or higher
Silicon	Whole grains, fruits, vegetables	**Optimal**: 5-35 mg/d **Deficiency**: <5 mg/d **Excess Intake:** >35 mg/d
Vanadium	Mushrooms, shellfish, black pepper, beer, wine, grains and certain unrefined salts	**Optimal**: 10-15 mcg/d **Deficiency**: <10 mcg/d **Excess Intake:** >10-20 mg/d

Guidelines for Eating Superfoods

Not all foods are created equal in terms of their nutrient values, especially their mineral content. Some of them, like beef liver and pastured eggs, contain virtually all the nutrients your body needs while others, like prunes are an excellent source of primarily one thing – boron. Then there are a bunch of foods that are moderately good for getting a wide range of minerals, such as beans or potatoes. Regardless, there are specific "superfoods" that you may want to keep in your diet on a regular basis to cover your bases for some of the more common deficiencies. However, you shouldn't be eating things like liver, cruciferous vegetables, dairy or legumes in excess either because they can cause imbalances with other minerals or reduce their absorption.

Here is a list of the more frequently referred to superfoods that you should know in what amounts and how often to eat:

- **Liver** – Arguably the most nutrient-dense food on the planet is liver, whether from beef, lamb, pork, chicken or game. It is an excellent source of the commonly deficient minerals, especially copper, iron, chromium, molybdenum, selenium and zinc. However, because liver is so packed with vitamins and minerals, eating it in excess will lead to increased urinary excretion and overload of certain nutrients.
  - o You can either eat 0.5-1 oz. per day or 1-3 oz. two to three times per week. Theoretically, more frequent smaller intakes throughout the week are more beneficial and will result in greater absorption compared to large boluses in a single sitting.
  - o There is the concern that the liver of conventionally raised animals is full of toxins and chemicals. Liver can store dioxins and kidneys tend to store cadmium. However, if you source quality organs from reputable companies consuming organs in the above amounts should not pose any problems. In fact, the fat tissue can have more toxins because the adipose tissue is the primary storage site for calories as well as toxins. So, eating liver, even from conventionally raised animals,

should have less toxins, unlike the fatty marbled meat. Kidneys do taste funny and weird because of their filtration role. You can soak both the liver and kidneys in water or milk to draw out their gnarly taste. Buying ground blends of meat that contain muscle meat, liver, heart and kidney will help mask the taste. You can cook the ground meats on the stove top and add taco spices to further mask the taste.

- **Heart** – Although not as nutrient-dense as liver, heart is still packed with a lot vitamins and minerals, in comparison to regular muscle meat. The most noticeable nutrient in heart is CoQ10, which is a coenzyme involved with many mitochondrial processes as well as participates in the electron transport chain and ATP generation[4594]. It also has antioxidant properties and is has been used in cardiovascular diseases including those with heart failure[4595,4596]. Heart also contains high amounts of protein and amino acids, zinc, selenium and elastin. However, it is slightly higher in iron than regular red meat. Consuming about 0.5-1 oz. of heart daily or 2-3 oz. of heart two to three times per week would suffice.

- **Oysters/Clams/Mollusks** – Just a single 3 oz. serving of oysters or mollusks can cover your entire weekly zinc demand (75-150 mg vs the 8-11 mg RDA). However, it is likely your body doesn't absorb all of it in a single sitting and responds by increasing urinary excretion. Regardless, eating oysters/clams/mollusks every day is probably not a good idea as it could lead to zinc overload, which reduces copper absorption. Thus, eating seafood like oysters once a week is sufficient enough to help boost your zinc RDA.
    - o Remember, it is beneficial to include 1 mg of copper for every 20-40 mg of zinc. So, if you do eat large amounts of zinc in a given meal, have more copper-rich foods, like liver.

- **Red Meat/Beef/Pork/Chicken/Game** – Meat is also an excellent source of many minerals, especially zinc, iron and sulfur. It is the best way to get all the sulfur amino acids, like methionine and cysteine, but because of that same reason can lead to a high methionine to glycine ratio.

- o Too much zinc and iron can inhibit copper absorption, elevating cholesterol levels and causing symptoms of anemia. That is why a diet high in muscle meat should be balanced with liver or other sources of copper such as Ezekiel bread.

- o Eating excessive amounts of processed meat has been linked with an increased risk of colon cancer but the evidence isn't definitive and does not apply to pastured meat [4597]. Cooking meat and protein at high temperatures does create carcinogenic compounds like heterocyclic amines and polycyclic aromatic hydrocarbons[4598]. Consuming cooked meat with certain spices, coffee and other plant compounds seems to offset these harms. In fact, drinking coffee is associated with a lower risk of numerous cancers including liver cancer[4599].

- o The tendons, ligaments and cartilage from ribs, drumsticks and wings is also a better way to get some glycine, which would balance the methionine, while still getting a high amount of sulfur amino acids. Eating pastured meat every day is actually important for optimal health, however you want to make sure that overall dietary acid load is balanced. This means that the diet should include some berries, dates, dark greens and/or bicarbonate-containing mineral waters.

- **Beans/Legumes/Lentils** – Beans, legumes and lentils are one of the top nutrient-dense foods in developing countries that don't have as much access to meat. They are the highest sources of plant-based protein, making them essential for any vegetarian/vegan diet.

  - o Beans and lentils are also relatively high in copper, boron, molybdenum, magnesium and potassium. However, because of their phytate content, they will also chelate things like zinc, iron and calcium. That can either be a good or bad thing, depending on the person's nutrient status. Excess iron, zinc and calcium can all be harmful to your health by causing calcification, oxidative stress and by inhibiting copper absorption. In that case, the phytates in beans and legumes will improve your health. On the other hand, if you are deficient in zinc (hypothyroid, hypogonadism) or deficient in calcium (osteoporosis), the antinutrients are exacerbating the deficiency of these minerals. Regardless, if you tolerate them, adding some beans and legumes to your iron/zinc-rich meals is an excellent way to prevent their excess intake.

- o You will likely realize whether or not you are eating too many beans and legumes by paying attention to your digestion and gastrointestinal condition. Cooking, soaking and sprouting beans/legumes/lentils greatly reduces their antinutrient content.

- **Broccoli/Cauliflower/Cabbage** – Cruciferous vegetables are great for increasing glutathione through sulforaphane and Nrf2. They are also good for getting more potassium, boron, chromium, calcium and magnesium. Compared to beans, broccoli and cauliflower do not contain phytates or phytonutrients that chelate iron or zinc. However, their goitrogenic content does reduce iodine absorption if high amounts are consumed raw, which may cause goiter and hypothyroidism. To prevent that, you should not eat a high amount of these vegetables raw or in smoothies. Instead, cooking, heating, frying and steaming them reduces their goitrogenic properties without losing a lot of micronutrients.

- **Kale/Spinach/Collard Greens** – All kinds of greens like kale and spinach can have some health properties, especially in terms of their magnesium, potassium and calcium content. However, they can also harm the thyroid when eaten raw. That is why you should cook them beforehand. They are also high in oxalates that can promote kidney stones and gastrointestinal distress in those who are susceptible, however, their high calcium content tends to make them fairly low in bioavailable oxalates. Citric acid (lemon juice) and increased calcium intake helps to break down oxalates. So, if you are making a salad, adding some lemon juice, vinegar and eating it with some dairy can prevent potential negative effects.

- **Eggs** – Similar to liver, eggs contain nearly all the vitamins and minerals your body needs. Eggs have all the amino acids both essential and non-essential. Because of that, eating 2-4 pastured eggs a day is an easy way to meet your daily sulfur requirements, while simultaneously hitting a lot of the other minerals, such as iodine, magnesium, molybdenum, selenium, zinc and phosphorus. You should avoid eating conventional eggs as they will have less omega-3s and other health promoting nutrients. To avoid a high methionine/glycine ratio, either stick to eating around 4 eggs a day or ensure you are consuming additional sources of glycine such as hydrolyzed collagen peptides.
  - The egg itself doesn't contain calcium but the eggshells do. Eating eggshells isn't necessary, but they can be a more natural and moderate-dose calcium supplement for those at a higher risk of osteoporosis or when overall calcium intake is low. You can wash the eggshells carefully, dry them and then grind them up into a powder and take around 1 tsp/d. However, it may be easier to consume calcium from natural mineral waters, which will also have a better bioavailability versus eggshells.

- **Dairy/Cheese/Milk** – One of the most bioavailable and common sources of calcium is dairy. Milk is probably more bioavailable than cheese and curds because it's a liquid and, similar to mineral waters, minerals get absorbed better when consumed in a liquid form. It is hard to get excess calcium (>1,500 mg/d) by eating dietary calcium, unless you are following the Swiss Alps' goat herder meal plan. Regardless, you may want to add a little bit of dairy/calcium to your larger meals because it also reduces the total absorption of fat, helping

517

with body composition. Consuming more calcium from sardines (with the bones) or a glass of pastured milk with salads will also protect against oxalates. On a daily basis, you can meet your calcium requirements by drinking either 1 glass of milk per meal or having 3 oz of fish with the bones next to 1.5-3 oz of cheese. Many people do not tolerate dairy, thus dairy consumption should be individualized.

- **Fish/Salmon/Sardines** – Everyone has heard that fatty fish is good for your health because of the omega-3 fatty acids. It is true that omega-3s are greatly beneficial for reducing inflammation and improving lipid profile. Fish itself is also a great source of other minerals, such as magnesium, iodine, selenium, zinc, manganese and potassium. You can also get calcium from the bones of small fish, like sardines or sprats.

    o Wild fish are more exposed to heavy metals and environmental pollution than farmed fish. However, they also have a higher selenium content that detoxifies some of these toxins. So, unless you are eating high-mercury fish like tuna or swordfish every day, you don't have a lot to worry about in terms of heavy metal toxicity. The increased iodine content in open water fish also protects against lipid peroxidation, which can occur during cooking and damage the healthy fats.

    o Overheating farmed fish turns the omega-3s inflammatory and more harmful than good because it has fewer protective minerals and antioxidants. Getting enough copper will also provide enough protection through superoxide dismutase. Both caffeine and coffee melanoidins inhibit lipid peroxidation and reduce the absorption of secondary lipoxidation products[4600,4601].

    o Fish consumption has been linked with reduced risk of cardiovascular disease and better metabolic health for a long time[4602]. People who eat fish once or twice a week have 50% fewer strokes, 50% lower cardiovascular (CVD) risk and a 34% lower CVD mortality risk compared to those eating no fish[4603,4604]. Wild salmon is an excellent source of omega-3s and the antioxidant astaxanthin.

- **Coffee/Tea** – The most consumed beverages in the world after water are coffee and tea. They have a long history of culinary and recreational use. However, research also finds these drinks have some health benefits. There's evidence that habitual tea drinking has positive effects on brain efficiency and slows down neurodegeneration.[4605] The polyphenols in coffee have also shown to reduce the risk of diabetes[4606], Alzheimer's[4607], dementia[4608], and even liver cancer[4609].

  - There is not a high amount of minerals in teas but there can be a fair amount of manganese in tea and some potassium and chromium in coffee. However, coffee, and teas, are potent chelators of other minerals, such as calcium, iron and zinc. Thus, their intake must be individualized.

  - Chelation of iron and zinc can be a good thing, depending on the context. For example, chelating iron can protect against the oxidation of fats when we eat cooked meat. If you are eating a low calcium diet, you may want to consume some calcium, like cheese or milk, with coffee to prevent calcium deficiency or better yet natural mineral waters that contain calcium.

  - Contrary to popular belief, coffee does not make you lose magnesium directly, unless you overdose and induce diarrhea or overactivate the sympathetic nervous system, both of which can promote magnesium excretion[4610].

  - The biggest minerals that get excreted due to coffee and caffeine are sodium and chloride. So, drinking mineral waters or consuming a bit more salt while drinking coffee can help prevent sodium and chloride deficiency.

  - On a daily basis, 1-2 cups of coffee or tea a day is a good moderate dose. It should prevent the caffeine dependency and anxiety a lot of people are suffering form. The upper limit should be 3 cups a day. Any more than that may start to interfere with sleep quality. If you feel like you need caffeine to wake up and start the day, you should look into improving the quality of your sleep. Learning to function on less caffeine, such as ½ cup of coffee twice daily, is a great option for preventing the caffeine blues and other side effects.

- **Chocolate/Cacao** – One of the best-known superfoods of South America is cacao found in chocolate. It is true that chocolate actually has a significant amount of some minerals, such as magnesium, copper, iron and chromium.
  - o Chocolate and cacao do contain some oxalates, but they do not contain phytates that chelate minerals. However, most conventional chocolates are high in sugars and fats that actually promote the excretion of minerals, especially magnesium. If you become insulin resistant or obese because of overindulging on chocolate and candy, then you will also increase the overall demand for these minerals. Thus, you should stick to dark chocolate (≥70%) and/or raw cacao powders. Eating 1 oz. of 80% cacao dark chocolate can be a great savory treat for dessert.

- **Fruit/Berries/Juices** – Fruits and berries are naturally high in potassium, which is hard to come by in other foods. You can also get citrate, which helps to buffer against the dietary acid load from meat and eggs. However, added fructose as a sweetener tends to promote the excretion of minerals. Added fructose can also induce insulin resistance, which places an additional demand for certain minerals, such as magnesium and chromium.
  - o Fructose-sweetened beverages are linked with insulin resistance[4611]. Drinking juices from natural fruit is also not the best idea because you are getting a very large dose of fructose in one sitting, which overburdens the liver. Thus, it is best to stick to whole food sources of

fructose from lower sugar fruit and berries, such as strawberries, blueberries and raspberries.

o Vitamin C enhances the absorption of iron and chromium from the diet.

- **Shilajit (mumie, moomiyo or mummiyo)** also called mineral pitch is a black-colored substance, consisting of paleohumus and vegetation fossils, that's high in fulvic acid and has been used in Ayurvedic medicine for thousands of years[4612]. It is collected from steep rock faces at altitudes 1000-5000 meters. Shilajit is not an actual food per se but instead an herb that can be taken as a supplement. Typical doses range from 200-2,000 mg/d. We haven't covered shilajit in the book so far, but it is worthwhile to mention it here.

  o Research has shown that shilajit improves mitochondrial respiration and oxidative phosphorylation, which promotes ATP production[4613]. Animal and human studies show it enhances spermatogenesis, testosterone levels and physical performance[4614,4615]. It also has a beneficial effect on lipid profile, cholesterol levels, cognition and antioxidant status[4616,4617,4618].

  o Shilajit has anti-inflammatory and antiulcerogenic properties[4619]. In obese patients, shilajit improves the function and regeneration of skeletal muscle[4620].

  o Shilajit has been shown to have anti-addictive effects with fewer side-effects than alpha2-adrenergic or opioid agonists[4621]. By interacting with GABA levels in the brain, shilajit can also reduce the sensation of pain[4622,4623]. In mice, ashwagandha and shilajit prevents ethanol withdrawal and alcohol addiction[4624].

  o Shilajit powder contains some iron, calcium, magnesium, selenium, zinc and other minerals. The predominant fulvic acid makes the minerals more bioavailable. Humic acids in shilajit also acts as a heavy metal chelator[4625].

More is not always better, especially when it comes to some of the superfoods like liver or oysters. Fortunately, the vast majority of people are not eating these foods because of preconceived notions and cultural norms. However, these foods are the most sought after and most valued foods among hunter-gatherer tribes. It is a shame to let them go to waste and miss out on all the vitamins and minerals that our bodies need. Instead of taking supplements for things we could get naturally, we ought to widen the nutrient-density of our diet. There are also spices and other preparation methods that can make even liver taste great. For example, if you can't tolerate organ meats by themselves, you can grind or mince them together with ground beef and make patties or pate.

Generally, cooking and overheating destroys some nutrients, which for goitrogens, lectins or phytates may actually be a good thing. Lightly cooking broccoli and cabbage triples their sulforaphane content vs. fully cooked[4626]. Steaming cruciferous vegetables leads to the highest nutrient content versus other cooking methods[4627]. Other foods like meat can become more hazardous from high heat cooking through the formation of carcinogens and oxidized lipids/cholesterol. For that, vinegars, plant polyphenols and spices and chelators like phytate can help offset any harms. Fortunately, marinating meat before cooking reduces the formation of these carcinogens by up to 90%[4628]. Regardless, animal foods are more adversely affected by cooking than plant foods. Vegetables and legumes actually need to be cooked to a reasonable degree to make them safer to eat, while the fats and protein in meat or fish can become oxidized. As a rule of thumb, cook your animal foods on light to moderate or sear them shortly and boil/roast the plants for longer. The other alternative to make meat healthier is to cut off the char.

Lightly cooking and cooling starch like potatoes and rice also increases their resistant starch content. There are many studies showing that resistant starch can improve insulin sensitivity, lower blood sugar, reduces appetite and help with digestion[4629]. Resistant starch also stimulates the bacteria in your gut to produce short-chain fatty acids (SCFAs) like acetic acid, propionic acid, and butyric acid[4630]. The SCFAs can feed the cells that line the colon and help with nutrient absorption[4631]. Some studies show that 15-30 grams of resistant starch/day for 4 weeks can improve insulin sensitivity by 33-50%[4632,4633]. An average American consumes about 3-8 grams of resistant starch a day from cereals and bread, which are not the best sources[4634]. One medium cooked and cooled potato contains about 3 grams of resistant starch while 100 grams of cooked and cooled rice has 5 grams. To keep the resistant starch intact, you can reheat the food at low temperatures under less than 130 degrees[4635]. You don't have to eat them cold but too high heat will convert it into regular starch.

Fresh foods tend to have more nutrients as storage can reduce nutrient content. Freezing, however, can help reduce the loss of the nutrients if the food is frozen right after harvest. Unfortunately, frozen veggies deactivate myrosinase, which is an enzyme that creates sulforaphane. Regardless, you would still get plenty of potassium, vitamin C and sulfur from vegetables. Organic foods also have more bioavailable nutrients, as pesticides and glyphosate can bind to minerals reducing their presence in the food and their bioavailability once consumed.

The US Department of Agriculture's Pesticide Data Program publishes an annual report on the most pesticide-rich foods. They divide it into **The Dirty Dozen and The Clean 15**. Here's a list for the year 2018:

- **The Dirty Dozen (Buy Organic and avoid conventional)** – strawberries, spinach, nectarines, apples, grapes, peaches, cherries, pears, tomatoes, celery, potatoes, sweet bell peppers.

- **The Clean 15 (Safer to buy but still aim for organic)** – avocados, sweet corn, pineapples, cabbages, onions, sweet peas, papayas, asparagus, mangoes, eggplants, honeydews, kiwis, cantaloupes, cauliflower and broccoli.

Making healthy food cheaper and more accessible to the entire population should be one of the primary concerns of the healthcare systems. As Hippocrates said: *"Let food be thy medicine and medicine be thy food."* Cheap processed foods are devoid of essential nutrients, but they have a lot of harmful calories that if overconsumed can cause metabolic syndrome and diabetes. Overconsuming processed foods leads to a vicious cycle of disease that keeps people dependent on medications and their quality of life low. It is sad that lower income households in food deserts are forced to buy the cheapest food they can get just to make ends meet while seeing their health deteriorate. Of course, everything cannot be blamed on the inaccessibility or cost of healthy food as some personal responsibility is also required. However, the majority of the public lacks the knowledge about nutrition and even still, most tend to opt in for the immediate gratification versus a healthy food option.

Fixing Mineral Deficiencies

You are not what you eat – you are what you end up absorbing – because not everything that you put into your mouth gets assimilated and metabolized. That is why there are a lot of people who may develop some nutrient deficiencies not because of their poor diet but because of other factors that inhibit the absorption of their food. The poor health condition of Western countries cannot be solely caused by inadequate nutrition. Instead, it is the environment and lifestyle that leads to additional losses of these minerals that are not recovered from dietary intake.

Based on the National Health and Nutrition Examination Survey (NHANES) 2007-2010 (2009-2014 for potassium) and the United States Department of Agriculture 2009 data, **1 out of every 3 people in the United States has at least 10 minerals that they are deficient in.** Those 10 minerals are potassium, manganese, magnesium, calcium, zinc, iron, copper, selenium, chromium, molybdenum and boron.

Thus, **about a third of the U.S. population is likely to be deficient in the below 10 minerals** (estimated % not hitting RDA/AI or estimated % deficient)[4636,4637,4638]:

1. Boron (> 75%)
2. Manganese (~ 75%)
3. Magnesium (52.2-68%)
4. Chromium (56%)
5. Calcium (44.1-73%)

524

6. Zinc (42-47%)
7. Iron (25-34%)
8. Copper (25-31%)
9. Selenium (15-40%)
10. Molybdenum (15%)

Here is how to prevent your body from becoming deficient of essential minerals by protecting against their excretion or improving their absorption:

- **Limit Added Sugar and Refined Food Intake** – Hyperglycemia and high sugar consumption places an additional burden on the liver and kidneys, which also makes the body increase excretion of certain minerals, namely magnesium, chromium and copper.
  - Added sugars drive coronary heart disease by inducing insulin resistance and hyperinsulinemia [4639]. Sugar, especially fructose, is worse than starch or other whole foods carbohydrate sources[4640]. The overconsumption of fructose-sweetened beverages is linked with insulin resistance[4641].
  - Animal and human studies have shown that replacing starch and glucose with sucrose or fructose, despite isocaloric eating, raises fasting insulin[4642,4643], reduces insulin sensitivity[4644,4645] and increases fasting blood sugar[4646]. Compared to a diet containing less than 10% of calories from added sugars, a diet that consists of 25% calories or more from added sugars triples the risk of cardiovascular disease mortality[4647].
  - Overconsuming added sugars can promote to copper deficiency, which contributes to fatty liver and insulin resistance [4648]. Most refined foods are also virtually non-existent of vitamins and minerals because the processing methods removes them. The more refined foods and sugar you consume the more minerals you need, especially magnesium, chromium and copper.

- **Fix Insulin Resistance and Improve Glycemic Control –** During insulin resistance, the body either is not producing enough insulin (like in type-1 diabetes), keeping the blood sugar elevated for longer, or the cells are not responsive to the actions of insulin and don't allow the entry of nutrients into the cell[4649]. In either case, hyperglycemia ensues that makes you burn through minerals while increasing their excretion.
  - Abdominal visceral fat is strongly correlated with insulin resistance and type 2 diabetes [4650]. Thus, reducing the intake of added fructose, especially when combined with fat bombs such as heavy cream and butter, which can lead to visceral fat accumulation, is advised. Reducing the intake of calories shouldn't happen at the expense of decreased nutrient intake, which means you have to focus more on eating nutrient dense foods as mentioned earlier.
  - Physical activity is one of the biggest predictors of overall insulin sensitivity and glucose tolerance[4651]. Resistance training and having more muscle mass are the best things for improving glucose tolerance[4652]. Skeletal muscle acts like a sponge for glucose and the more muscle you have the higher your carbohydrate tolerance is.
  - A lack of sleep impairs glucose tolerance, raises blood sugar and cortisol and promotes insulin resistance. Even one single night of bad sleep has been shown to induce the biomarkers of a pre-diabetic in the short term[4653].
  - Trans fats and vegetable oils like margarine, corn, soybean, safflower, cottonseed and canola oil promote oxidative stress, inflammation and insulin resistance[4654]. People who consume high amounts of omega-6 seed oils have a worse lipid profile and markers of insulin resistance [4655], [4656], [4657].Chronic inflammation also promotes insulin resistance[4658].

- Minerals that support glycemic control and insulin production are chromium, magnesium, potassium, sodium, copper and zinc. Insulin mimetics are lithium, nickel and vanadium although their supplementation requires consultation with your medical professional.

- **Improve Gut Health and Fix Malabsorption Conditions** – Your gut is where most of the absorption of minerals from food occurs. Having a healthy gut is vital for assimilating and retaining nutrients. Many malabsorption conditions, such as intestinal permeability (leaky gut), IBS, Crohn's and ulcerative colitis can reduce the absorption of certain minerals. If you have any gut condition, you will need to hit at least the RDA for magnesium, potassium, zinc, copper and selenium. If you already show signs of deficiencies in these minerals, you may need to increase your intake further in the short term.
  - Chloride is used by our body to make hydrochloric acid, helping to form stomach acid for killing pathogens and absorbing nutrients. Acid-suppressing drugs decrease how much stomach acid gets produced and, as a result, fewer minerals are absorbed[4659]. Thus, a low salt intake can reduce stomach acid production and inhibit the absorption of nutrients from food because of inadequate digestion.
  - Drinking mineral waters improves mineral absorption by 40-50% compared to food.
  - Zinc supplementation improves intestinal barrier function and may even help to resolve intestinal permeability in patients with Crohn's disease [4660]. Sufficient amino acid intake from protein is also required for repairing the gut lining. Certain allergenic foods like gluten or eggs may damage the intestinal lining and lead to intestinal permeability.

- **Improve Liver and Kidney Health** – Most of the metabolic processes are regulated by the liver and kidneys. They also determine the homeostatic balance and excretion of all minerals. Poor kidney function tends to promote the urinary loss of magnesium, chromium, manganese, zinc, copper and many others.

- o Excess iron damages the liver through oxidative stress and promotes fatty liver (visceral fat)[4661]. Production of ROS during iron metabolism causes lipid peroxidation [4662]. Too much ferritin also supports lipofuscin formation, which is an age-related pigment that slows down cellular processes and promotes fatty liver[4663]. Replacing some of your muscle meat with organ meats or beans/legumes will help to lower iron overload and prevent liver damage.

- o Studies find that coffee can reduce risk of liver cirhhosis by 25-70%[4664]. It can also reduce risk of non-alcoholic fatty liver disease (NAFLD) by 30-60%[4665]. NAFLD results primarily from metabolic syndrome. Losing some weight and improving insulin resistance can help improve NAFLD.

- o Liver detoxification pathways require zinc, selenium, magnesium and molybdenum [4666]. Sulfur- and glutathione-rich foods like cruciferous vegetables, garlic, onions, eggs, and leeks support phase 2 detoxification.

- o The kidneys affect electrolyte balance the most. Kidney damage increases the demand for potassium, copper, zinc and chromium. Excess ammonia, resulting from deficient manganese and potassium, can overburden the kidneys. Proper hydration and drinking adequate amounts of water are also important for filtrating out waste products that would otherwise accumulate in the body.

- **Avoid Heavy Metal Exposure** – Environmental pollutants, especially heavy metals, also increase the excretion of some minerals and compete with their absorption. What's more, mineral deficiencies like iron deficiency can increase the absorption of heavy metals, such as cadmium, lead and aluminum[4667].

528

- Zinc deficiency has been shown to promote the accumulation of cadmium in the liver whereas iron and copper deficiency raise cadmium intake by the kidneys[4668]. Cadmium is a toxic metal with a half-life of 10-30 years that antagonizes zinc[4669]. Animal studies show that cadmium promotes the urinary excretion of copper, zinc and iron[4670,4671]. Supplementation with copper and zinc has helped to prevent against the adverse effects of cadmium[4672].
- Sauna therapy also helps to eliminate heavy metals like arsenic, cadmium, lead and mercury[4673] as well as persistent organic pollutants (POPs)[4674]. Sauna use in combination with niacin and exercise can result in a 25-30% decrease in POP levels in fat tissue and blood by heat-induced sweating[4675]. Sweating alone has actually been used to improve uremia, or the accumulation of toxins in the blood of patients with kidney disease[4676].
- You can't avoid all heavy metal exposure in an industrialized world. However, you can support your body with additional detoxification methods, such as exercise and sauna. Getting enough selenium, zinc and copper are also important for the body's antioxidant defense systems.

- **Avoid Drugs/Medications That Promote Mineral Loss** – Pharmaceuticals tend to reduce the absorption of minerals and promote their excretion. Antacids and diuretics affect magnesium and potassium the most. When taking a prescription drug for a certain medical condition that cannot be avoided, look up to see what nutrients they may deplete and make sure you obtain enough of them in the diet or through supplementation.

- **Eat Mineral-Dense Foods Regularly** – You should be eating things like liver, oysters and/or clams on a fairly regular basis, at least once a week. This way your requirement for supplements will greatly reduce as you'll be getting the nutrients from your food. It is not necessary to be eating "superfoods" daily with every meal. However, you could also "microdose" (1 oz/d) foods like liver to spread your intake across the entire week. Large acute doses of minerals tend to make the body increase urinary excretion or reduce their absorption. It is also harder to catch up on deficiencies compared to having a consistent intake of minerals from foods.

- **Add Some Mineral Waters to Your Diet** – One of the best ways to get more magnesium and calcium into your diet is to drink mineral waters. Mineral waters have a better bioavailability while providing other health benefits. Because they lack calories, mineral water is one of the healthiest ways to simultaneously improve your mineral status and metabolic health. Consuming about 1/3-2/3^{rds} of your daily water intake as mineral water would contribute greatly to your daily mineral requirements.

  Supplement Your Deficiencies – Taking supplements is a quick way to overcome severe nutrient deficiencies that are causing health problems. However, they may also have negative side-effects. For example, taking an iron or zinc supplement will impair copper absorption. Likewise, a chromium supplement for someone who is already metabolically healthy may be just a waste of money. Thus, you should supplement only those minerals you are deficient or suboptimal in. First, test your mineral status and then consult with a medical professional about the appropriate course of action in terms of supplementation. Minor deficiencies can easily be fixed by improving diet or metabolic health.

There is something that does make you excrete minerals and make you more prone to deficiencies regardless of your health status. That is sweating and exercise. People who exercise or sweat a lot due to either being physically more active, sunbathing, or taking saunas frequently are more prone to electrolyte imbalances. When you sweat you lose water, sodium, chloride, copper, chromium, selenium and iodine. Because sweating is an essential way for humans to regulate their body temperature, we can't avoid it and thus may be prone to becoming deficient or at least suboptimal in different minerals.

It's estimated that sweat contains on average 920-1,380 mg of sodium per liter[4677]. However, that would depend on your own electrolyte status and how hydrated you are[4678]. The RDA for sodium is 2300 mg, which is 6 grams or 1 teaspoon of salt. **Vigorous exercise in hot weather for a prolonged period of time such as an endurance race or marathon may make you lose up to 4-10 liters and 3500-7000 mg of sodium through sweat[4679].**

It is ironic to think about how many people are trying to exercise harder to lose weight and get fit. Indeed, physical activity, both resistance training and cardio, are very beneficial for long-term health and body composition. However, few tend to think about the role of minerals lost in sweat. If you are going for a long run, you do burn calories and fat, but you also lose sodium and other minerals through sweat. To keep the weight off, maintain insulin sensitivity and ensure optimal nutrient intakes. If you're vigorously exercising or sweating without replacing minerals you may find yourself in a vicious cycle of nutrient deficiencies, mild insulin resistance, increased stress and enhanced cravings for salty/sugary junk foods.

Fluid and electrolyte balance post-exercise can be restored when significant amounts of salt are ingested after exercise. There are very few commercially available products capable of achieving this[4680]. Compared to oral rehydration fluids known to be effective in cholera, coconut water was found to have adequate potassium and glucose content, however, was relatively deficient in sodium, chloride and bicarbonate. The addition of salt to the coconut water is suggested to compensate for the sodium and chloride deficiency. In areas of the world where coconuts are plentiful, the advantages of sterility, availability and acceptability make coconut water theoretically feasible for the oral rehydration of patients with severe gastroenteritis when conventional fluids are unavailable. [4681]

Concluding Remarks

We have now reached the end of this book. Our goal for writing The Mineral Fix was to provide you with the most comprehensive and up to date collection of information about the function and importance of minerals in human health. We also wanted to provide practical real-life recommendations that you can implement, starting today. Even minor changes to your diet or supplementation can result in drastic improvements in your vitality and longevity.

How many people have ever thought that maybe their sleeping problems or cardiovascular issues are due to a deficiency in either magnesium or selenium? Whose physician has considered improving copper status to fix symptoms of anemia, instead of giving additional iron tablets as a supplement? Although the importance of iodine in thyroid function is well known, when did someone mention that you need sodium to get iodine into the thyroid in the first place? All these examples show that there is a general lacking in understanding of the importance of minerals in the body's physiological processes among the general public as well as medical professionals. What's more, the vast majority of people have at least one nutrient deficiency that may cause chronic health problems down the line. Even worse, the general decline in the nutrient content of our food supply should be an increasingly bigger concern for our entire society. Hopefully, this book helps to fix this issue and brings more light to this situation.

To finish off on a brighter note, you now have the toolkit for improving the quality of your diet and nutrient status. The devil is in the details, but you do not need to fall into the weeds, trying to micromanage everything. At the end of the day, our bodies are constantly changing and our requirement for certain minerals differs on a daily basis. What we can do is eat a whole food-based diet on a regular basis, fix our mineral-depletions and implement more superfoods like liver and other organs into our weekly menu.

We wish you a successful journey in figuring out what nutrients you need more of and how to obtain the right amount of them from diet. Because, after all, it is a constant process of exploration and implementation.

References

[1] Gernand, A. D., Schulze, K. J., Stewart, C. P., West, K. P., & Christian, P. (2016). Micronutrient deficiencies in pregnancy worldwide: health effects and prevention. Nature Reviews Endocrinology, 12(5), 274–289. doi:10.1038/nrendo.2016.37

[2] Tucker K. L. (2016). Nutrient intake, nutritional status, and cognitive function with aging. Annals of the New York Academy of Sciences, 1367(1), 38–49. https://doi.org/10.1111/nyas.13062

[3] Fisher, Z., Hernandez Prada, J. A., Tu, C., Duda, D., Yoshioka, C., An, H., Govindasamy, L., Silverman, D. N., & McKenna, R. (2005). Structural and kinetic characterization of active-site histidine as a proton shuttle in catalysis by human carbonic anhydrase II. Biochemistry, 44(4), 1097–1105. https://doi.org/10.1021/bi0480279

[4] J X Chipponi, J C Bleier, M T Santi, D Rudman; Deficiencies of essential and conditionally essential nutrients, The American Journal of Clinical Nutrition, Volume 35, Issue 5, 1 May 1982, Pages 1112–1116.

[5] Underwood EJ. (1971) 'Introduction'. In: Underwood EJ, ed. 'Trace Elements in Human and Animal Nutrition 3rd ed'. Academic Press, New York, NY, pp. 1-13.

[6] Nielsen, F. H. (2000). Possibly Essential Trace Elements. Clinical Nutrition of the Essential Trace Elements and Minerals, 11–36. doi:10.1007/978-1-59259-040-7_2

[7] Mertz W. (1981). The essential trace elements. Science (New York, N.Y.), 213(4514), 1332–1338. https://doi.org/10.1126/science.7022654

[8] Mertz W. (1970). Some aspects of nutritional trace element research. Federation proceedings, 29(4), 1482–1488.

[9] DiNicolantonio, J. J., Mangan, D., & O'Keefe, J. H. (2018). Copper deficiency may be a leading cause of ischaemic heart disease. Open Heart, 5(2), e000784. doi:10.1136/openhrt-2018-000784

[10] Ordman, A. R. (2010). Vitamin C twice a day enhances health. Health, 02(08), 819–823. doi:10.4236/health.2010.28123

[11] DiNicolantonio, J. J., O'Keefe, J. H., & Wilson, W. (2018). Subclinical magnesium deficiency: a principal driver of cardiovascular disease and a public health crisis. Open Heart, 5(1), e000668. doi:10.1136/openhrt-2017-000668

[12] Campbell, J. D. (2001). Lifestyle, minerals and health. Medical Hypotheses, 57(5), 521–531. doi:10.1054/mehy.2001.1351

[13] MedlinePlus (2020) 'Boron', Herbs and Supplements, Accessed Online Nov 6 2020: https://medlineplus.gov/druginfo/natural/894.html

[14] Campbell, J. D. (2001). Lifestyle, minerals and health. Medical Hypotheses, 57(5), 521–531. doi:10.1054/mehy.2001.1351

[15] Wallace, T. C., McBurney, M., & Fulgoni, V. L., 3rd (2014). Multivitamin/mineral supplement contribution to micronutrient intakes in the United States, 2007-2010. Journal of the American College of Nutrition, 33(2), 94–102. https://doi.org/10.1080/07315724.2013.846806

[16] Berardi (2020) 'How to fix a broken diet: 3 ways to get your eating on track.', Precision Nutrition, Accessed Online Nov 11 2020: https://www.precisionnutrition.com/fix-a-broken-diet

[17] National Academies of Sciences, Engineering, and Medicine; Health and Medicine Division; Food and Nutrition Board; Committee to Review the Dietary Reference Intakes for Sodium and Potassium; Oria M, Harrison M, Stallings VA, editors. Dietary Reference Intakes for Sodium and Potassium. Washington (DC): National Academies Press (US); 2019 Mar 5. Potassium: Dietary Reference Intakes for Adequacy. Available from: https://www.ncbi.nlm.nih.gov/books/NBK545428/

[18] Campbell, J. D. (2001). Lifestyle, minerals and health. Medical Hypotheses, 57(5), 521–531. doi:10.1054/mehy.2001.1351

[19] DiNicolantonio, J. J., & Berger, A. (2016). Added sugars drive nutrient and energy deficit in obesity: a new paradigm. Open Heart, 3(2), e000469. doi:10.1136/openhrt-2016-000469

[20] Sakamaki, Y., Goto, K., Watanabe, Y., Takata, T., Yamazaki, H., Imai, N., Ito, Y., & Narita, I. (2014). Nephrotic syndrome and end-stage kidney disease accompanied by bicytopenia due to copper deficiency. Internal medicine (Tokyo, Japan), 53(18), 2101–2106. https://doi.org/10.2169/internalmedicine.53.2338

[21] DiNicolantonio, J. J., Bhutani, J., & O'Keefe, J. H. (2016). Added sugars drive chronic kidney disease and its consequences: A comprehensive review. Journal of Insulin Resistance, 1(1). doi:10.4102/jir.v1i1.3

[22] DiNicolantonio, J. J., O'Keefe, J. H., & Wilson, W. (2018). Subclinical magnesium deficiency: a principal driver of cardiovascular disease and a public health crisis. Open Heart, 5(1), e000668. doi:10.1136/openhrt-2017-000668

[23] Thomas, D. (2007). The Mineral Depletion of Foods Available to US as A Nation (1940–2002) – A Review of the 6th Edition of McCance and Widdowson. Nutrition and Health, 19(1-2), 21–55. doi:10.1177/026010600701900205

24 Thomas D. (2007). The mineral depletion of foods available to us as a nation (1940-2002)--a review of the 6th Edition of McCance and Widdowson. Nutrition and health, 19(1-2), 21–55. https://doi.org/10.1177/026010600701900205

25 Mayer, A. (1997), "Historical changes in the mineral content of fruits and vegetables", British Food Journal, Vol. 99 No. 6, pp. 207-211. https://doi.org/10.1108/00070709710181540

26 Davis, D.R. (2011). Impact of Breeding and Yield on Fruit, Vegetable, and Grain Nutrient Content. In Breeding for Fruit Quality (eds M.A. Jenks and P.J. Bebeli). doi:10.1002/9780470959350.ch6

27 Moore, J. X., Chaudhary, N., & Akinyemiju, T. (2017). Metabolic Syndrome Prevalence by Race/Ethnicity and Sex in the United States, National Health and Nutrition Examination Survey, 1988–2012. Preventing Chronic Disease, 14. doi:10.5888/pcd14.160287

28 CDC (2020) 'Adult Obesity Facts', Overweight & Obesity, Accessed Online: https://www.cdc.gov/obesity/data/adult.html

29 WHO Obesity and Overweight [Online]. World Health Organization (2019). Available online at: https://www.who.int/news-room/fact-sheets/detail/obesity-and-overweight (accessed September 18, 2020).

30 Mayer, A. (1997), "Historical changes in the mineral content of fruits and vegetables", British Food Journal, Vol. 99 No. 6, pp. 207-211. https://doi.org/10.1108/00070709710181540

31 Davis, D.R. (2011). Impact of Breeding and Yield on Fruit, Vegetable, and Grain Nutrient Content. In Breeding for Fruit Quality (eds M.A. Jenks and P.J. Bebeli). doi:10.1002/9780470959350.ch6

[32] Guo, W., Nazim, H., Liang, Z., & Yang, D. (2016). Magnesium deficiency in plants: An urgent problem. The Crop Journal, 4(2), 83–91. doi:10.1016/j.cj.2015.11.003

[33] Guo, W., Nazim, H., Liang, Z., & Yang, D. (2016). Magnesium deficiency in plants: An urgent problem. The Crop Journal, 4(2), 83–91. doi:10.1016/j.cj.2015.11.003

34 Garvin, D.F., Welch, R.M. and Finley, J.W. (2006), Historical shifts in the seed mineral micronutrient concentration of US hard red winter wheat germplasm. J. Sci. Food Agric., 86: 2213-2220. doi:10.1002/jsfa.2601

35 Farnham, M.W., Keinath, A.P. and Grusak, M.A. (2011), Mineral Concentration of Broccoli Florets in Relation to Year of Cultivar Release. Crop Science, 51: 2721-2727. doi:10.2135/cropsci2010.09.0556

[36] Cakmak, I., Yazici, A., Tutus, Y., & Ozturk, L. (2009). Glyphosate reduced seed and leaf concentrations of calcium, manganese, magnesium, and iron in non-glyphosate resistant soybean. European Journal of Agronomy, 31(3), 114–119. doi:10.1016/j.eja.2009.07.001

[37] Goyer, R. A. (1997). TOXIC AND ESSENTIAL METAL INTERACTIONS. Annual Review of Nutrition, 17(1), 37–50. doi:10.1146/annurev.nutr.17.1.37

[38] Ralston, N. V. C., Blackwell, J. L., & Raymond, L. J. (2007). Importance of Molar Ratios in Selenium-Dependent Protection Against Methylmercury Toxicity. Biological Trace Element Research, 119(3), 255–268. doi:10.1007/s12011-007-8005-7

[39] Campbell, J. D. (2001). Lifestyle, minerals and health. Medical Hypotheses, 57(5), 521–531. doi:10.1054/mehy.2001.1351

[40] Freedman, A. M., Mak, I. T., Stafford, R. E., Dickens, B. F., Cassidy, M. M., Muesing, R. A., & Weglicki, W. B. (1992). Erythrocytes from magnesium-deficient hamsters display an enhanced susceptibility to oxidative stress. American Journal of Physiology-Cell Physiology, 262(6), C1371–C1375. doi:10.1152/ajpcell.1992.262.6.c1371

[41] Mills, B. J., Lindeman, R. D., & Lang, C. A. (1986). Magnesium Deficiency Inhibits Biosynthesis of Blood Glutathione and Tumor Growth in the Rat. Experimental Biology and Medicine, 181(3), 326–332. doi:10.3181/00379727-181-42260

[42] DiNicolantonio, J. J., O'Keefe, J. H., & Wilson, W. (2018). Subclinical magnesium deficiency: a principal driver of cardiovascular disease and a public health crisis. Open Heart, 5(1), e000668. doi:10.1136/openhrt-2017-000668

[43] DiNicolantonio, J. J., O'Keefe, J. H., & Wilson, W. (2018). Subclinical magnesium deficiency: a principal driver of cardiovascular disease and a public health crisis. Open Heart, 5(1), e000668. doi:10.1136/openhrt-2017-000668

[44] Pace, N. R. (2001). The universal nature of biochemistry. Proceedings of the National Academy of Sciences, 98(3), 805–808. doi:10.1073/pnas.98.3.805

[45] Wesselink, E., Koekkoek, W. A. C., Grefte, S., Witkamp, R. F., & van Zanten, A. R. H. (2019). Feeding mitochondria: Potential role of nutritional components to improve critical illness convalescence. Clinical Nutrition, 38(3), 982–995. doi:10.1016/j.clnu.2018.08.032

[46] Stern, M. (2017). Evidence that a mitochondrial death spiral underlies antagonistic pleiotropy. Aging Cell, 16(3), 435–443. doi:10.1111/acel.12579

[47] Ames, B. N., Atamna, H., & Killilea, D. W. (2005). Mineral and vitamin deficiencies can accelerate the mitochondrial decay of aging. Molecular Aspects of Medicine, 26(4-5), 363–378. doi:10.1016/j.mam.2005.07.007

[48] Bratic, I., & Trifunovic, A. (2010). Mitochondrial energy metabolism and ageing. Biochimica et Biophysica Acta (BBA) - Bioenergetics, 1797(6-7), 961–967. doi:10.1016/j.bbabio.2010.01.004

[49] Jiroutková, K., Krajčová, A., Ziak, J., Fric, M., Waldauf, P., Džupa, V., … Duška, F. (2015). Mitochondrial function in skeletal muscle of patients with protracted critical illness and ICU-acquired weakness. Critical Care, 19(1). doi:10.1186/s13054-015-1160-x

[50] Batt, J., Mathur, S., & Katzberg, H. D. (2017). Mechanism of ICU-acquired weakness: muscle contractility in critical illness. Intensive Care Medicine, 43(4), 584–586. doi:10.1007/s00134-017-4730-3

[51] Brealey, D., Brand, M., Hargreaves, I., Heales, S., Land, J., Smolenski, R., … Singer, M. (2002). Association between mitochondrial dysfunction and severity and outcome of septic shock. The Lancet, 360(9328), 219–223. doi:10.1016/s0140-6736(02)09459-x

[52] Weber-Carstens, S., Schneider, J., Wollersheim, T., Assmann, A., Bierbrauer, J., Marg, A., … Spuler, S. (2013). Critical Illness Myopathy and GLUT4. American Journal of Respiratory and Critical Care Medicine, 187(4), 387–396. doi:10.1164/rccm.201209-1649oc

[53] Wolf, F. (2003). Cell physiology of magnesium. Molecular Aspects of Medicine, 24(1-3), 11–26. doi:10.1016/s0098-2997(02)00088-2

[54] Ha, B. G., Park, J.-E., Cho, H.-J., & Shon, Y. H. (2015). Stimulatory Effects of Balanced Deep Sea Water on Mitochondrial Biogenesis and Function. PLOS ONE, 10(6), e0129972. doi:10.1371/journal.pone.0129972

[55] Takaya, J., Higashino, H., & Kobayashi, Y. (2004). Intracellular magnesium and insulin resistance. Magnesium research, 17(2), 126–136.

[56] Carré, J. E., Orban, J.-C., Re, L., Felsmann, K., Iffert, W., Bauer, M., … Singer, M. (2010). Survival in Critical Illness Is Associated with Early Activation of Mitochondrial Biogenesis. American Journal of Respiratory and Critical Care Medicine, 182(6), 745–751. doi:10.1164/rccm.201003-0326oc

[57] Killilea, D. W., & Ames, B. N. (2008). Magnesium deficiency accelerates cellular senescence in cultured human fibroblasts. Proceedings of the National Academy of Sciences, 105(15), 5768–5773. doi:10.1073/pnas.0712401105

[58] Ha, B. G., Moon, D.-S., Kim, H. J., & Shon, Y. H. (2016). Magnesium and calcium-enriched deep-sea water promotes mitochondrial biogenesis by AMPK-activated signals pathway in 3T3-L1 preadipocytes. Biomedicine & Pharmacotherapy, 83, 477–484. doi:10.1016/j.biopha.2016.07.009

[59] Waldenström, J. G. (2009). Biochemistry. By Lubert Stryer. Acta Medica Scandinavica, 198(1-6), 436–436. doi:10.1111/j.0954-6820.1975.tb19571.x

[60] Zorova, L. D., Popkov, V. A., Plotnikov, E. Y., Silachev, D. N., Pevzner, I. B., Jankauskas, S. S., … Zorov, D. B. (2018). Mitochondrial membrane potential. Analytical Biochemistry, 552, 50–59. doi:10.1016/j.ab.2017.07.009

[61] Cantó, C., Menzies, K. J., & Auwerx, J. (2015). NAD+ Metabolism and the Control of Energy Homeostasis: A Balancing Act between Mitochondria and the Nucleus. Cell Metabolism, 22(1), 31–53. doi:10.1016/j.cmet.2015.05.023

[62] Garrett and Grisham (2010) 'Biochemistry', Brooks/Cole, 2010, pp 598-611

[63] Garrett R, Grisham CM (2016). biochemistry. Boston: Cengage. p. 687. ISBN 978-1-305-57720-6.

[64] Jonckheere, A. I., Smeitink, J. A. M., & Rodenburg, R. J. T. (2011). Mitochondrial ATP synthase: architecture, function and pathology. Journal of Inherited Metabolic Disease, 35(2), 211–225. doi:10.1007/s10545-011-9382-9

[65] Okuno, D., Iino, R., & Noji, H. (2011). Rotation and structure of FoF1-ATP synthase. Journal of Biochemistry, 149(6), 655–664. doi:10.1093/jb/mvr049

[66] Brookes, P. S., Yoon, Y., Robotham, J. L., Anders, M. W., & Sheu, S.-S. (2004). Calcium, ATP, and ROS: a mitochondrial love-hate triangle. American Journal of Physiology-Cell Physiology, 287(4), C817–C833. doi:10.1152/ajpcell.00139.2004

[67] Wesselink, E., Koekkoek, W. A. C., Grefte, S., Witkamp, R. F., & van Zanten, A. R. H. (2019). Feeding mitochondria: Potential role of nutritional components to improve critical illness convalescence. Clinical Nutrition, 38(3), 982–995. doi:10.1016/j.clnu.2018.08.032

[68] Huskisson, E., Maggini, S., & Ruf, M. (2007). The Role of Vitamins and Minerals in Energy Metabolism and Well-Being. Journal of International Medical Research, 35(3), 277–289. doi:10.1177/147323000703500301

[69] Lukaski, H. C. (2000). Magnesium, zinc, and chromium nutriture and physical activity. The American Journal of Clinical Nutrition, 72(2), 585S–593S. doi:10.1093/ajcn/72.2.585s

[70] Krishna, B. H. R., & Sreenivasaya, M. (1928). The determination of pyruvic acid. Biochemical Journal, 22(5), 1169–1177. doi:10.1042/bj0221169

[71] Sokolove, P. M. (1994). Interactions of Adriamycin aglycones with mitochondria may mediate Adriamycin cardiotoxicity. International Journal of Biochemistry, 26(12), 1341–1350. doi:10.1016/0020-711x(94)90176-7

[72] Whitacre, M. E., & Combs, G. F. (1983). Selenium and Mitochondrial Integrity in the Pancreas of the Chick. The Journal of Nutrition, 113(10), 1972–1983. doi:10.1093/jn/113.10.1972

[73] Laughlin, M. R., & Thompson, D. (1996). The Regulatory Role for Magnesium in Glycolytic Flux of the Human Erythrocyte. Journal of Biological Chemistry, 271(46), 28977–28983. doi:10.1074/jbc.271.46.28977

[74] Römer-Lüthi, C. (2006). Mineralstoffe und Spurenelemente im Kohlenhydratstoffwechsel. Ihre potenzielle Bedeutung für die Prävention und Therapie von Krankheiten. Schweizerische Zeitschrift Für Ganzheitsmedizin / Swiss Journal of Integrative Medicine, 18(4), 207–212. doi:10.1159/000282053

[75] Otto and Ontko (1978) 'Activation of Mitochondrial Fatty Acid Oxidation by Calcium', The JOUSNAL or BIOLOGICAL CHEMISTRY, Vol. 253, No. 3, Issue of February 10, pp. 189-799. Accessed Online Nov 14 2020: https://www.jbc.org/content/253/3/789.full.pdf

[76] Ha, B. G., Park, J.-E., Cho, H.-J., & Shon, Y. H. (2015). Stimulatory Effects of Balanced Deep Sea Water on Mitochondrial Biogenesis and Function. PLOS ONE, 10(6), e0129972. doi:10.1371/journal.pone.0129972

[77] Let's Talk Academy (2018) 'https://www.letstalkacademy.com/publication/read/electron-transport-chain-the-components-of-the-electron-transport-chain-copper-proteins', https://www.letstalkacademy.com/publication/read/electron-transport-chain-the-components-of-the-electron-transport-chain-copper-proteins, Accessed Online Nov 14 2020: https://www.letstalkacademy.com/publication/read/electron-transport-chain-the-components-of-the-electron-transport-chain-copper-proteins

[78] Touyz, R., M. (2004). Magnesium in clinical medicine. Frontiers in Bioscience, 9(1-3), 1278. doi:10.2741/1316

[79] Lin et al (1993) 'The subunit location of magnesium in cytochrome c oxidase', J. Biol. Chem., 268: 22210-22214.

[80] Wolf, F. (2003). Cell physiology of magnesium. Molecular Aspects of Medicine, 24(1-3), 11–26. doi:10.1016/s0098-2997(02)00088-2

[81] Toto, K. H., & Yucha, C. B. (1994). Magnesium: homeostasis, imbalances, and therapeutic uses. Critical care nursing clinics of North America, 6(4), 767–783.

[82] Aithal, H. N., & Toback, F. G. (1978). Defective mitochondrial energy production during potassium depletion nephropathy. Laboratory investigation; a journal of technical methods and pathology, 39(3), 186–192.

[83] Cox, I. M., Campbell, M. J., & Dowson, D. (1991). Red blood cell magnesium and chronic fatigue syndrome. The Lancet, 337(8744), 757–760. doi:10.1016/0140-6736(91)91371-z

[84] Laurberg, P., Knudsen, N., Andersen, S., Carlé, A., Pedersen, I. B., & Karmisholt, J. (2012). Thyroid Function and Obesity. European Thyroid Journal, 1(3), 159–167. doi:10.1159/000342994

[85] Samuels, M. H. (2014). Psychiatric and cognitive manifestations of hypothyroidism. Current Opinion in Endocrinology & Diabetes and Obesity, 21(5), 377–383. doi:10.1097/med.0000000000000089

[86] Bennett, W. E., & Heuckeroth, R. O. (2012). Hypothyroidism Is a Rare Cause of Isolated Constipation. Journal of Pediatric Gastroenterology and Nutrition, 54(2), 285–287. doi:10.1097/mpg.0b013e318239714f

[87] Joffe, R.T., Pearce, E.N., Hennessey, J.V., Ryan, J.J. and Stern, R.A. (2013), Subclinical hypothyroidism, mood, and cognition in older adults: a review. Int J Geriatr Psychiatry, 28: 111-118. doi:10.1002/gps.3796

[88] Afhami, S., Haghpanah, V., Heshmat, R. et al. Assessment of the Factors Involving in the Development of Hypothyroidism in HIV-infected Patients: A Case-Control Study. Infection 35, 334–338 (2007). https://doi.org/10.1007/s15010-007-6163-3

[89] Jara, E. L., Muñoz-Durango, N., Llanos, C., Fardella, C., González, P. A., Bueno, S. M., … Riedel, C. A. (2017). Modulating the function of the immune system by thyroid hormones and thyrotropin. Immunology Letters, 184, 76–83. doi:10.1016/j.imlet.2017.02.010

[90] Karkhaneh, M., Qorbani, M., Ataie-Jafari, A., Mohajeri-Tehrani, M. R., Asayesh, H., & Hosseini, S. (2019). Association of thyroid hormones with resting energy expenditure and complement C3 in normal weight high body fat women. Thyroid Research, 12(1). doi:10.1186/s13044-019-0070-4

[91] Aihara, K., Nishi, Y., Hatano, S., Kihara, M., Yoshimitsu, K., Takeichi, N., … Usui, T. (1984). Zinc, copper, manganese, and selenium metabolism in thyroid disease. The American Journal of Clinical Nutrition, 40(1), 26–35. doi:10.1093/ajcn/40.1.26

[92] Wu, Q., Rayman, M. P., Lv, H., Schomburg, L., Cui, B., Gao, C., … Shi, B. (2015). Low Population Selenium Status Is Associated With Increased Prevalence of Thyroid Disease. The Journal of Clinical Endocrinology & Metabolism, 100(11), 4037–4047. doi:10.1210/jc.2015-2222

[93] Soldin, O. P., & Aschner, M. (2007). Effects of manganese on thyroid hormone homeostasis: potential links. Neurotoxicology, 28(5), 951–956. https://doi.org/10.1016/j.neuro.2007.05.003

[94] Khatiwada, S., Gelal, B., Baral, N., & Lamsal, M. (2016). Association between iron status and thyroid function in Nepalese children. Thyroid Research, 9(1). doi:10.1186/s13044-016-0031-0

[95] Moncayo, R., & Moncayo, H. (2015). The WOMED model of benign thyroid disease: Acquired magnesium deficiency due to physical and psychological stressors relates to dysfunction of oxidative phosphorylation. BBA Clinical, 3, 44–64. doi:10.1016/j.bbacli.2014.11.002

[96] Maxwell, C., & Volpe, S. L. (2007). Effect of Zinc Supplementation on Thyroid Hormone Function. Annals of Nutrition and Metabolism, 51(2), 188–194. doi:10.1159/000103324

[97] Huskisson, E., Maggini, S., & Ruf, M. (2007). The Role of Vitamins and Minerals in Energy Metabolism and Well-Being. Journal of International Medical Research, 35(3), 277–289. doi:10.1177/147323000703500301

[98] Lewis (2020) 'Overview of Electrolytes', MSD Manual Consumer Version, Accessed Online Feb 18 2021: https://www.msdmanuals.com/home/hormonal-and-metabolic-disorders/electrolyte-balance/overview-of-electrolytes

[99] Lee J. W. (2010). Fluid and electrolyte disturbances in critically ill patients. Electrolyte & blood pressure : E & BP, 8(2), 72–81. https://doi.org/10.5049/EBP.2010.8.2.72

[100] Weglicki, W., Quamme, G., Tucker, K., Haigney, M., & Resnick, L. (2005). Potassium, magnesium, and electrolyte imbalance and complications in disease management. Clinical and experimental hypertension (New York, N.Y. : 1993), 27(1), 95–112. https://doi.org/10.1081/ceh-200044275

[101] Tello, L., & Perez-Freytes, R. (2017). Fluid and Electrolyte Therapy During Vomiting and Diarrhea. The Veterinary clinics of North America. Small animal practice, 47(2), 505–519. https://doi.org/10.1016/j.cvsm.2016.09.013

[102] Dhondup, T., & Qian, Q. (2017). Electrolyte and Acid-Base Disorders in Chronic Kidney Disease and End-Stage Kidney Failure. Blood Purification, 43(1-3), 179–188. doi:10.1159/000452725

[103] Winston A. P. (2012). The clinical biochemistry of anorexia nervosa. Annals of clinical biochemistry, 49(Pt 2), 132–143. https://doi.org/10.1258/acb.2011.011185

[104] Hauhouot-Attoungbre, M. L., Mlan, W. C., Edjeme, N. A., Ahibo, H., Vilasco, B., & Monnet, D. (2005). Intérêt du ionogramme chez le brûlé thermique grave [Disturbances of electrolytes in severe thermal burns]. Annales de biologie clinique, 63(4), 417–421.

[105] Olivero J. J., Sr (2016). Cardiac Consequences Of Electrolyte Imbalance. Methodist DeBakey cardiovascular journal, 12(2), 125–126. https://doi.org/10.14797/mdcj-12-2-125

[106] Bara, M., Guiet-Bara, A., & Durlach, J. (1993). Regulation of sodium and potassium pathways by magnesium in cell membranes. Magnesium research, 6(2), 167–177.

[107] NISHIMUTA, M., KODAMA, N., YOSHITAKE, Y., SHIMADA, M., & SERIZAWA, N. (2018). Dietary Salt (Sodium Chloride) Requirement and Adverse Effects of Salt Restriction in Humans. Journal of Nutritional Science and Vitaminology, 64(2), 83–89. doi:10.3177/jnsv.64.83

[108] NISHIMUTA, M., KODAMA, N., MORIKUNI, E., YOSHIOKA, Y. H., MATSUZAKI, N., TAKEYAMA, H., … KITAJIMA, H. (2005). Positive Correlation between Dietary Intake of Sodium and Balances of Calcium and Magnesium in Young Japanese Adults-Low Sodium Intake Is a Risk Factor for Loss of Calcium and Magnesium-. Journal of Nutritional Science and Vitaminology, 51(4), 265–270. doi:10.3177/jnsv.51.265

[109] KODAMA, N., NISHIMUTA, M., & SUZUKI, K. (2003). Negative Balance of Calcium and Magnesium under Relatively Low Sodium Intake in Humans. Journal of Nutritional Science and Vitaminology, 49(3), 201–209. doi:10.3177/jnsv.49.201

[110] DiNicolantonio, J. J., O'Keefe, J. H., & Wilson, W. (2018). Subclinical magnesium deficiency: a principal driver of cardiovascular disease and a public health crisis. Open Heart, 5(1), e000668. doi:10.1136/openhrt-2017-000668

[111] Ahmad, A., & Bloom, S. (1989). Sodium pump and calcium channel modulation of Mg-deficiency cardiomyopathy. The American journal of cardiovascular pathology, 2(4), 277–283.

[112] Dyckner, T., & Wester, P. O. (1979). Ventricular extrasystoles and intracellular electrolytes before and after potassium and magnesium infusions in patients on diuretic treatment. American Heart Journal, 97(1), 12–18. doi:10.1016/0002-8703(79)90108-x

[113] Dyckner, T., & Wester, P. O. (2009). Relation between Potassium, Magnesium and Cardiac Arrhythmias. Acta Medica Scandinavica, 209(S647), 163–169. doi:10.1111/j.0954-6820.1981.tb02652.x

[114] Boyd, J. C., Bruns, D. E., DiMarco, J. P., Sugg, N. K., & Wills, M. R. (1984). Relationship of potassium and magnesium concentrations in serum to cardiac arrhythmias. Clinical Chemistry, 30(5), 754–757. doi:10.1093/clinchem/30.5.754

[115] Shafique, S., Sellen, D. W., Lou, W., Jalal, C. S., Jolly, S. P., & Zlotkin, S. H. (2016). Mineral- and vitamin-enhanced micronutrient powder reduces stunting in full-term low-birth-weight infants receiving nutrition, health, and hygiene education: a 2×2 factorial, cluster-randomized trial in Bangladesh. The American journal of clinical nutrition, 103(5), 1357–1369. https://doi.org/10.3945/ajcn.115.117770

[116] Oxenkrug G. F. (2010). Tryptophan kynurenine metabolism as a common mediator of genetic and environmental impacts in major depressive disorder: the serotonin hypothesis revisited 40 years later. The Israel journal of psychiatry and related sciences, 47(1), 56–63.

537

[117] Sikander, A., Rana, S. V., & Prasad, K. K. (2009). Role of serotonin in gastrointestinal motility and irritable bowel syndrome. Clinica Chimica Acta, 403(1-2), 47–55. doi:10.1016/j.cca.2009.01.028

[118] Maes, M. (1995). Evidence for an immune response in major depression: A review and hypothesis. Progress in Neuro-Psychopharmacology and Biological Psychiatry, 19(1), 11–38. doi:10.1016/0278-5846(94)00101-m

[119] Majewski, M., Kozlowska, A., Thoene, M., Lepiarczyk, E., & Grzegorzewski, W. J. (2016). Overview of the role of vitamins and minerals on the kynurenine pathway in health and disease. Journal of physiology and pharmacology : an official journal of the Polish Physiological Society, 67(1), 3–19.

[120] Duff, J. (2014). Nutrition for ADHD and Autism. Clinical Neurotherapy, 357–381. doi:10.1016/b978-0-12-396988-0.00014-3

[121] Tan, D., Manchester, L. C., Reiter, R. J., Qi, W., Zhang, M., Weintraub, S. T., ... Mayo, J. C. (1999). Identification of highly elevated levels of melatonin in bone marrow: its origin and significance. Biochimica et Biophysica Acta (BBA) - General Subjects, 1472(1-2), 206–214. doi:10.1016/s0304-4165(99)00125-7

[122] Manchester, L. C., Coto-Montes, A., Boga, J. A., Andersen, L. P. H., Zhou, Z., Galano, A., ... Reiter, R. J. (2015). Melatonin: an ancient molecule that makes oxygen metabolically tolerable. Journal of Pineal Research, 59(4), 403–419. doi:10.1111/jpi.12267

[123] Acuña-Castroviejo, D., Escames, G., Venegas, C., Díaz-Casado, M. E., Lima-Cabello, E., López, L. C., ... Reiter, R. J. (2014). Extrapineal melatonin: sources, regulation, and potential functions. Cellular and Molecular Life Sciences, 71(16), 2997–3025. doi:10.1007/s00018-014-1579-2

[124] Favero, G., Franceschetti, L., Bonomini, F., Rodella, L. F., & Rezzani, R. (2017). Melatonin as an Anti-Inflammatory Agent Modulating Inflammasome Activation. International journal of endocrinology, 2017, 1835195. https://doi.org/10.1155/2017/1835195

[125] Reiter, R. J., Rosales-Corral, S., Tan, D. X., Jou, M. J., Galano, A., & Xu, B. (2017). Melatonin as a mitochondria-targeted antioxidant: one of evolution's best ideas. Cellular and Molecular Life Sciences, 74(21), 3863–3881. doi:10.1007/s00018-017-2609-7

[126] Mooney, S., Leuendorf, J.-E., Hendrickson, C., & Hellmann, H. (2009). Vitamin B6: A Long Known Compound of Surprising Complexity. Molecules, 14(1), 329–351. doi:10.3390/molecules14010329

[127] Billyard et al (2006) 'Dietary magnesium deficiency decreases plasma melatonin in rats', Magnesium research: official organ of the International Society for the Development of Research on Magnesium 19(3):157-61

[128] Abbasi, B., Kimiagar, M., Sadeghniiat, K., Shirazi, M. M., Hedayati, M., & Rashidkhani, B. (2012). The effect of magnesium supplementation on primary insomnia in elderly: A double-blind placebo-controlled clinical trial. Journal of research in medical sciences : the official journal of Isfahan University of Medical Sciences, 17(12), 1161–1169.

[129] Rondanelli, M., Opizzi, A., Monteferrario, F., Antoniello, N., Manni, R., & Klersy, C. (2011). The Effect of Melatonin, Magnesium, and Zinc on Primary Insomnia in Long-Term Care Facility Residents in Italy: A Double-Blind, Placebo-Controlled Clinical Trial. Journal of the American Geriatrics Society, 59(1), 82–90. doi:10.1111/j.1532-5415.2010.03232.x

[130] Medical News Today 'Insomnia: Studies Suggest Calcium And Magnesium Effective', Accessed Online Nov 15 2020: https://www.medicalnewstoday.com/releases/163169#1

[131] Grandner et al (2014) 'Sleep Symptoms Associated with Intake of Specific Dietary Nutrients', J Sleep Res. Author manuscript; available in PMC 2015 Feb 1.

[132] Drennan et al (1991) 'Potassium affects actigraph-identified sleep', Sleep. 1991 Aug;14(4):357-60.

[133] Markham, G. D., & Pajares, M. A. (2008). Structure-function relationships in methionine adenosyltransferases. Cellular and Molecular Life Sciences, 66(4), 636–648. doi:10.1007/s00018-008-8516-1

[134] Hamon et al (1978) 'Activation of Tryptophan Hydroxylase by Adenosine Triphosphate, Magnesium, and Calcium', Molecular Pharmacology January 1978, 14 (1) 99-110.

[135] Wasserbauer (2017) 'Does Dietary Melatonin Play a Role in Bone Mineralization?', Theses - ALL. 120.

[136] Billyard et al (2006) 'Dietary magnesium deficiency decreases plasma melatonin in rats.', Magnesium Research, 01 Sep 2006, 19(3):157-161.

[137] Rondanelli, M., Opizzi, A., Monteferrario, F., Antoniello, N., Manni, R., & Klersy, C. (2011). The Effect of Melatonin, Magnesium, and Zinc on Primary Insomnia in Long-Term Care Facility Residents in Italy: A Double-Blind, Placebo-Controlled Clinical Trial. Journal of the American Geriatrics Society, 59(1), 82–90. doi:10.1111/j.1532-5415.2010.03232.x

[138] Peuhkuri, K., Sihvola, N., & Korpela, R. (2012). Dietary factors and fluctuating levels of melatonin. Food & Nutrition Research, 56(1), 17252. doi:10.3402/fnr.v56i0.17252

[139] Sugden, D. (1989). Melatonin biosynthesis in the mammalian pineal gland. Experientia, 45(10), 922–932. doi:10.1007/bf01953049

[140] Schultz W. (2015). Neuronal Reward and Decision Signals: From Theories to Data. Physiological reviews, 95(3), 853–951. https://doi.org/10.1152/physrev.00023.2014

[141] Dobryakova, E., Genova, H. M., DeLuca, J., & Wylie, G. R. (2015). The Dopamine Imbalance Hypothesis of Fatigue in Multiple Sclerosis and Other Neurological Disorders. Frontiers in Neurology, 6. doi:10.3389/fneur.2015.00052

[142] Wang, Y., Chan, G. L., Holden, J. E., Dobko, T., Mak, E., Schulzer, M., Huser, J. M., Snow, B. J., Ruth, T. J., Calne, D. B., & Stoessl, A. J. (1998). Age-dependent decline of dopamine D1 receptors in human brain: a PET study. Synapse (New York, N.Y.), 30(1), 56–61. https://doi.org/10.1002/(SICI)1098-2396(199809)30:1<56::AID-SYN7>3.0.CO;2-J

[143] Moraga-Amaro, R., Gonzalez, H., Pacheco, R., & Stehberg, J. (2014). Dopamine receptor D3 deficiency results in chronic depression and anxiety. Behavioural Brain Research, 274, 186–193. doi:10.1016/j.bbr.2014.07.055

[144] Di Chiara G. (1997). Alcohol and dopamine. Alcohol health and research world, 21(2), 108–114.

[145] Volkow, N. D., Fowler, J. S., Wang, G.-J., Swanson, J. M., & Telang, F. (2007). Dopamine in Drug Abuse and Addiction. Archives of Neurology, 64(11), 1575. doi:10.1001/archneur.64.11.1575

[146] Frantom, P. A., Seravalli, J., Ragsdale, S. W., & Fitzpatrick, P. F. (2006). Reduction and oxidation of the active site iron in tyrosine hydroxylase: kinetics and specificity. Biochemistry, 45(7), 2372–2379. https://doi.org/10.1021/bi052283j

[147] Kim, J., & Wessling-Resnick, M. (2014). Iron and mechanisms of emotional behavior. The Journal of Nutritional Biochemistry, 25(11), 1101–1107. doi:10.1016/j.jnutbio.2014.07.003

[148] Cardoso, C. C., Lobato, K. R., Binfaré, R. W., Ferreira, P. K., Rosa, A. O., Santos, A. R. S., & Rodrigues, A. L. S. (2009). Evidence for the involvement of the monoaminergic system in the antidepressant-like effect of magnesium. Progress in Neuro-Psychopharmacology and Biological Psychiatry, 33(2), 235–242. doi:10.1016/j.pnpbp.2008.11.007

[149] Musayev, F. N., di Salvo, M. L., Ko, T. P., Gandhi, A. K., Goswami, A., Schirch, V., & Safo, M. K. (2007). Crystal Structure of human pyridoxal kinase: structural basis of M(+) and M(2+) activation. Protein science : a publication of the Protein Society, 16(10), 2184–2194. https://doi.org/10.1110/ps.073022107

[150] Markham, G. D., & Pajares, M. A. (2008). Structure-function relationships in methionine adenosyltransferases. Cellular and Molecular Life Sciences, 66(4), 636–648. doi:10.1007/s00018-008-8516-1

[151] Wasserbauer (2017) 'Does Dietary Melatonin Play a Role in Bone Mineralization?', Theses - ALL. 120.

[152] Billyard et al (2006) 'Dietary magnesium deficiency decreases plasma melatonin in rats.', Magnesium Research, 01 Sep 2006, 19(3):157-161.

[153] Rondanelli, M., Opizzi, A., Monteferrario, F., Antoniello, N., Manni, R., & Klersy, C. (2011). The Effect of Melatonin, Magnesium, and Zinc on Primary Insomnia in Long-Term Care Facility Residents in Italy: A Double-Blind, Placebo-Controlled Clinical Trial. Journal of the American Geriatrics Society, 59(1), 82–90. doi:10.1111/j.1532-5415.2010.03232.x

[154] Peuhkuri, K., Sihvola, N., & Korpela, R. (2012). Dietary factors and fluctuating levels of melatonin. Food & Nutrition Research, 56(1), 17252. doi:10.3402/fnr.v56i0.17252

[155] Sugden, D. (1989). Melatonin biosynthesis in the mammalian pineal gland. Experientia, 45(10), 922–932. doi:10.1007/bf01953049

[156] Tarleton, E. K., & Littenberg, B. (2015). Magnesium intake and depression in adults. Journal of the American Board of Family Medicine : JABFM, 28(2), 249–256. https://doi.org/10.3122/jabfm.2015.02.140176

[157] Li, B., Lv, J., Wang, W., & Zhang, D. (2016). Dietary magnesium and calcium intake and risk of depression in the general population: A meta-analysis. Australian & New Zealand Journal of Psychiatry, 51(3), 219–229. doi:10.1177/0004867416676895

[158] Barragán-Rodríguez, L., Rodríguez-Morán, M., & Guerrero-Romero, F. (2008). Efficacy and safety of oral magnesium supplementation in the treatment of depression in the elderly with type 2 diabetes: a randomized, equivalent trial. Magnesium research, 21(4), 218–223.

[159] Boyle, N.B.; Lawton, C.; Dye, L. The Effects of Magnesium Supplementation on Subjective Anxiety and Stress—A Systematic Review. Nutrients 2017, 9, 429.

[160] Sartori, S. B., Whittle, N., Hetzenauer, A., & Singewald, N. (2012). Magnesium deficiency induces anxiety and HPA axis dysregulation: Modulation by therapeutic drug treatment. Neuropharmacology, 62(1), 304–312. doi:10.1016/j.neuropharm.2011.07.027

[161] Heiden, A., Frey, R., Presslich, O., Blasbichler, T., Smetana, R., & Kasper, S. (1999). Treatment of severe mania with intravenous magnesium sulphate as a supplementary therapy. Psychiatry Research, 89(3), 239–246. doi:10.1016/s0165-1781(99)00107-9

[162] Chouinard, G., Beauclair, L., Geiser, R., & Etienne, P. (1990). A pilot study of magnesium aspartate hydrochloride (Magnesiocard®) as a mood stabilizer for rapid cycling bipolar affective disorder patients. Progress in Neuro-Psychopharmacology and Biological Psychiatry, 14(2), 171–180. doi:10.1016/0278-5846(90)90099-3

[163] Mauskop, A., & Altura, B. M. (1998). Role of magnesium in the pathogenesis and treatment of migraines. Clinical neuroscience (New York, N.Y.), 5(1), 24–27.

[164] Peikert, A., Wilimzig, C., & Köhne-Volland, R. (1996). Prophylaxis of Migraine with Oral Magnesium: Results From A Prospective, Multi-Center, Placebo-Controlled and Double-Blind Randomized Study. Cephalalgia, 16(4), 257–263. doi:10.1046/j.1468-2982.1996.1604257.x

[165] Piñero, D. J., & Connor, J. R. (2000). Iron in the Brain: An Important Contributor in Normal and Diseased States. The Neuroscientist, 6(6), 435–453. doi:10.1177/107385840000600607

[166] Atamna, H. (2004). Heme, iron, and the mitochondrial decay of ageing. Ageing Research Reviews, 3(3), 303–318. doi:10.1016/j.arr.2004.02.002

[167] Hurtado, E. K., Claussen, A. H., & Scott, K. G. (1999). Early childhood anemia and mild or moderate mental retardation. The American Journal of Clinical Nutrition, 69(1), 115–119. doi:10.1093/ajcn/69.1.115

[168] Beard, J. L., & Connor, J. R. (2003). IRONSTATUS ANDNEURALFUNCTIONING. Annual Review of Nutrition, 23(1), 41–58. doi:10.1146/annurev.nutr.23.020102.075739

[169] Damulina, A., Pirpamer, L., Soellradl, M., Sackl, M., Tinauer, C., Hofer, E., … Langkammer, C. (2020). Cross-sectional and Longitudinal Assessment of Brain Iron Level in Alzheimer Disease Using 3-T MRI. Radiology, 296(3), 619–626. doi:10.1148/radiol.2020192541

[170] Pfeiffer, C. C., & Braverman, E. R. (1982). Zinc, the brain and behavior. Biological psychiatry, 17(4), 513–532.

[171] Duke University Medical Center. (2011, September 21). Zinc regulates communication between brain cells. ScienceDaily. Retrieved November 15, 2020 from www.sciencedaily.com/releases/2011/09/110921132334.htm

[172] Marcellini, F., Giuli, C., Papa, R., Gagliardi, C., Dedoussis, G., Herbein, G., … Mocchegiani, E. (2006). Zinc status, psychological and nutritional assessment in old people recruited in five European countries: Zincage study. Biogerontology, 7(5-6), 339–345. doi:10.1007/s10522-006-9048-4

[173] Markiewicz-Żukowska, R., Gutowska, A., & Borawska, M. H. (2015). Serum Zinc Concentrations Correlate with Mental and Physical Status of Nursing Home Residents. PLOS ONE, 10(1), e0117257. doi:10.1371/journal.pone.0117257

[174] Bilici, M., Yıldırım, F., Kandil, S., Bekaroğlu, M., Yıldırmış, S., Değer, O., … Aksu, H. (2004). Double-blind, placebo-controlled study of zinc sulfate in the treatment of attention deficit hyperactivity disorder. Progress in Neuro-Psychopharmacology and Biological Psychiatry, 28(1), 181–190. doi:10.1016/j.pnpbp.2003.09.034

[175] Sensi, S. L., Paoletti, P., Koh, J.-Y., Aizenman, E., Bush, A. I., & Hershfinkel, M. (2011). The Neurophysiology and Pathology of Brain Zinc. Journal of Neuroscience, 31(45), 16076–16085. doi:10.1523/jneurosci.3454-11.2011

[176] DiNicolantonio, J. J., Liu, J., & O'Keefe, J. H. (2018). Magnesium for the prevention and treatment of cardiovascular disease. Open Heart, 5(2), e000775. doi:10.1136/openhrt-2018-000775

[177] Purvis, J. R., & Movahed, A. (1992). Magnesium disorders and cardiovascular diseases. Clinical Cardiology, 15(8), 556–568. doi:10.1002/clc.4960150804

[178] Fischer, P. W. F., & Giroux, A. (1987). Effects of Dietary Magnesium on Sodium-Potassium Pump Action in the Heart of Rats. The Journal of Nutrition, 117(12), 2091–2095. doi:10.1093/jn/117.12.2091

[179] Madden, J. A., Willems, W. J., Smith, G. A., & Mueller, R. A. (1984). Sodium kinetics and membrane potential in aorta of magnesium-deficient rats. Magnesium, 3(2), 73–80.

[180] Houston, M. (2011). The Role of Magnesium in Hypertension and Cardiovascular Disease. The Journal of Clinical Hypertension, 13(11), 843–847. doi:10.1111/j.1751-7176.2011.00538.x

[181] Hruby, A., O'Donnell, C. J., Jacques, P. F., Meigs, J. B., Hoffmann, U., & McKeown, N. M. (2014). Magnesium Intake Is Inversely Associated With Coronary Artery Calcification. JACC: Cardiovascular Imaging, 7(1), 59–69. doi:10.1016/j.jcmg.2013.10.006

[182] Stühlinger, H. G., Kiss, K., & Smetana, R. (2000). Der Stellenwert von Magnesium bei Herzrhythmusstörungen [Significance of magnesium in cardiac arrhythmias]. Wiener medizinische Wochenschrift (1946), 150(15-16), 330–334.

[183] Yang, Q. (2011). Sodium and Potassium Intake and Mortality Among US Adults. Archives of Internal Medicine, 171(13), 1183. doi:10.1001/archinternmed.2011.257

[184] Krishna G. G. (1990). Effect of potassium intake on blood pressure. Journal of the American Society of Nephrology : JASN, 1(1), 43–52.

[185] D'Elia, L., Barba, G., Cappuccio, F. P., & Strazzullo, P. (2011). Potassium Intake, Stroke, and Cardiovascular Disease. Journal of the American College of Cardiology, 57(10), 1210–1219. doi:10.1016/j.jacc.2010.09.070

[186] Khan, E., Spiers, C., & Khan, M. (2013). The heart and potassium: A banana republic. Acute Cardiac Care, 15(1), 17–24. doi:10.3109/17482941.2012.741250

[187] Piazza (2017) 'How too little potassium may contribute to cardiovascular disease', NIH National Institute of Health, NIH Research Matters, Accessed Online Nov 15 2020: https://www.nih.gov/news-events/nih-research-matters/how-too-little-potassium-may-contribute-cardiovascular-disease

[188] Stone, M. S., Martyn, L., & Weaver, C. M. (2016). Potassium Intake, Bioavailability, Hypertension, and Glucose Control. Nutrients, 8(7), 444. https://doi.org/10.3390/nu8070444

[189] Iimura, O., Kijima, T., Kikuchi, K., Miyama, A., Ando, T., Nakao, T., & Takigami, Y. (1981). Studies on the Hypotensive Effect of High Potassium Intake in Patients with Essential Hypertension. Clinical Science, 61(s7), 77s–80s. doi:10.1042/cs061077s

[190] Technical University of Munich (TUM). (2017, April 18). Zinc supply affects cardiac health: Study shows link between zinc levels and cardiac health. ScienceDaily. Retrieved November 15, 2020 from www.sciencedaily.com/releases/2017/04/170418094238.htm

[191] Giacconi, R., Cai, L., Costarelli, L., Cardelli, M., Malavolta, M., Piacenza, F., & Provinciali, M. (2017). Implications of impaired zinc homeostasis in diabetic cardiomyopathy and nephropathy. BioFactors, 43(6), 770–784. doi:10.1002/biof.1386

[192] Li, B., Tan, Y., Sun, W., Fu, Y., Miao, L., & Cai, L. (2012). The role of zinc in the prevention of diabetic cardiomyopathy and nephropathy. Toxicology Mechanisms and Methods, 23(1), 27–33. doi:10.3109/15376516.2012.735277

[193] Yu, X., Huang, L., Zhao, J., Wang, Z., Yao, W., Wu, X., … Bian, B. (2018). The Relationship between Serum Zinc Level and Heart Failure: A Meta-Analysis. BioMed Research International, 2018, 1–9. doi:10.1155/2018/2739014

[194] Koşar, F., Sahin, I., Taşkapan, C., Küçükbay, Z., Güllü, H., Taşkapan, H., & Cehreli, S. (2006). Trace element status (Se, Zn, Cu) in heart failure. Anadolu kardiyoloji dergisi : AKD = the Anatolian journal of cardiology, 6(3), 216–220.

[195] Nazem, M. R., Asadi, M., Jabbari, N., & Allameh, A. (2019). Effects of zinc supplementation on superoxide dismutase activity and gene expression, and metabolic parameters in overweight type 2 diabetes patients: A randomized, double-blind, controlled trial. Clinical biochemistry, 69, 15–20. https://doi.org/10.1016/j.clinbiochem.2019.05.008

[196] Dhalla, N. S., Temsah, R. M., & Netticadan, T. (2000). Role of oxidative stress in cardiovascular diseases. Journal of hypertension, 18(6), 655–673. https://doi.org/10.1097/00004872-200018060-00002

[197] California Institute of Technology. (2015, April 9). Microbes help produce serotonin in gut. ScienceDaily. Retrieved November 16, 2020 from www.sciencedaily.com/releases/2015/04/150409143045.htm

[198] Pachikian, B. D., Neyrinck, A. M., Deldicque, L., De Backer, F. C., Catry, E., Dewulf, E. M., … Delzenne, N. M. (2010). Changes in Intestinal Bifidobacteria Levels Are Associated with the Inflammatory Response in Magnesium-Deficient Mice. The Journal of Nutrition, 140(3), 509–514. doi:10.3945/jn.109.117374

[199] Liu, Y., Han, R., Wang, J., Yang, P., Wang, F., & Yang, B. (2020). Magnesium Sensing Regulates Intestinal Colonization of Enterohemorrhagic Escherichia coli O157:H7. mBio, 11(6). doi:10.1128/mbio.02470-20

[200] Winther et al (2015) 'Dietary magnesium deficiency alters gut microbiota and leads to depressive-like behaviour', Acta Neuropsychiatrica 18(03):1-9, DOI: 10.1017/neu.2015.7

[201] Pal et al (2019) 'Enterochromaffin cells as the source of melatonin: key findings and functional relevance in mammals', Melatonin Research. 2, 4 (Dec. 2019), 61-82. DOI:https://doi.org/https://doi.org/10.32794/mr11250041.

[202] Lovenberg, W., Jequier, E., & Sjoerdsma, A. (1967). Tryptophan Hydroxylation: Measurement in Pineal Gland, Brainstem, and Carcinoid Tumor. Science, 155(3759), 217–219. doi:10.1126/science.155.3759.217

[203] Balemans, M. G., Bary, F. A., Legerstee, W. C., & van Benthem, J. (1978). Estimation of the methylating capacity in the pineal gland of the rat with special reference to the methylation of N-acetylserotonin and 5-hydroxytryptophol separately. Experientia, 34(11), 1434–1435. https://doi.org/10.1007/BF01932333

[204] Voisin, P., Namboodiri, M. A., & Klein, D. C. (1984). Arylamine N-acetyltransferase and arylalkylamine N-acetyltransferase in the mammalian pineal gland. The Journal of biological chemistry, 259(17), 10913–10918.

[205] Axelrod, J., & Weissbach, H. (1960). Enzymatic O-Methylation of N-Acetylserotonin to Melatonin. Science, 131(3409), 1312–1312. doi:10.1126/science.131.3409.1312

[206] Morton, D. J., & James, M. F. M. (1985). Effect of Magnesium Ions on Rat Pineal N-Acetyltransferase (EC 2. 3 1.5) Activity. Journal of Pineal Research, 2(4), 387–391. doi:10.1111/j.1600-079x.1985.tb00718.x

[207] Morton D. J. (1989). Possible mechanisms of inhibition and activation of rat N-acetyltransferase (EC 2.3.1.5.) by cations. Journal of neural transmission, 75(1), 51–64. https://doi.org/10.1007/BF01250643

[208] Turgut, M., Yenisey, Ç., Akyüz, O., Özsunar, Y., Erkus, M., & Biçakçi, T. (2006). Correlation of Serum Trace Elements and Melatonin Levels to Radiological, Biochemical, and Histological Assessment of Degeneration in Patients with Intervertebral Disc Herniation. Biological Trace Element Research, 109(2), 123–134. doi:10.1385/bter:109:2:123

[209] Zaouali-Ajina, M., Gharib, A., Durand, G., Gazzah, N., Claustrat, B., Gharib, C., & Sarda, N. (1999). Dietary Docosahexaenoic Acid-Enriched Phospholipids Normalize Urinary Melatonin Excretion in Adult

(n-3) Polyunsaturated Fatty Acid-Deficient Rats. The Journal of Nutrition, 129(11), 2074–2080. doi:10.1093/jn/129.11.2074

[210] Lavialle, M., Champeil-Potokar, G., Alessandri, J. M., Balasse, L., Guesnet, P., Papillon, C., Pévet, P., Vancassel, S., Vivien-Roels, B., & Denis, I. (2008). An (n-3) polyunsaturated fatty acid-deficient diet disturbs daily locomotor activity, melatonin rhythm, and striatal dopamine in Syrian hamsters. The Journal of nutrition, 138(9), 1719–1724. https://doi.org/10.1093/jn/138.9.1719

[211] ROSS, J. R. (2001). A case of hypomagnesaemia due to malabsorption, unresponsive to oral administration of magnesium glycerophosphate, but responsive to oral magnesium oxide supplementation. Gut, 48(6), 857–858. doi:10.1136/gut.48.6.857

[212] Fine, B. P., Barth, A., Sheffet, A., & Lavenhar, M. A. (1976). Influence of magnesium on the intestinal absorption of lead. Environmental Research, 12(2), 224–227. doi:10.1016/0013-9351(76)90029-3

[213] Sturniolo, G. C., Di Leo, V., Ferronato, A., D'Odorico, A., & D'Incà, R. (2001). Zinc Supplementation Tightens "Leaky Gut" in Crohn's Disease. Inflammatory Bowel Diseases, 7(2), 94–98. doi:10.1097/00054725-200105000-00003

[214] Bothe, G., Coh, A., & Auinger, A. (2015). Efficacy and safety of a natural mineral water rich in magnesium and sulphate for bowel function: a double-blind, randomized, placebo-controlled study. European Journal of Nutrition, 56(2), 491–499. doi:10.1007/s00394-015-1094-8

[215] Morishita, D., Tomita, T., Mori, S., Kimura, T., Oshima, T., Fukui, H., & Miwa, H. (2020). Senna Versus Magnesium Oxide for the Treatment of Chronic Constipation. American Journal of Gastroenterology, Publish Ahead of Print. doi:10.14309/ajg.0000000000000942

[216] Turecky, L., Kupcova, V., Szantova, M., Uhlikova, E., Viktorinova, A., & Czirfusz, A. (2006). Serum magnesium levels in patients with alcoholic and non-alcoholic fatty liver. Bratislavske lekarske listy, 107(3), 58–61.

[217] Wu, L., Zhu, X., Fan, L., Kabagambe, E. K., Song, Y., Tao, M., Zhong, X., Hou, L., Shrubsole, M. J., Liu, J., & Dai, Q. (2017). Magnesium intake and mortality due to liver diseases: Results from the Third National Health and Nutrition Examination Survey Cohort. Scientific reports, 7(1), 17913. https://doi.org/10.1038/s41598-017-18076-5

[218] Dongiovanni, P., Fracanzani, A. L., Fargion, S., & Valenti, L. (2011). Iron in fatty liver and in the metabolic syndrome: a promising therapeutic target. Journal of hepatology, 55(4), 920–932. https://doi.org/10.1016/j.jhep.2011.05.008

[219] Grant, D. M. (1991). Detoxification pathways in the liver. Journal of Inherited Metabolic Disease, 14(4), 421–430. doi:10.1007/bf01797915

[220] HOFMANN, A. (1963). THE FUNCTION OF BILE SALTS IN FAT ABSORPTION. THE SOLVENT PROPERTIES OF DILUTE MICELLAR SOLUTIONS OF CONJUGATED BILE SALTS. Biochemical Journal, 89(1), 57–68. doi:10.1042/bj0890057

[221] Đanić, M., Stanimirov, B., Pavlović, N., Goločorbin-Kon, S., Al-Salami, H., Stankov, K., & Mikov, M. (2018). Pharmacological Applications of Bile Acids and Their Derivatives in the Treatment of Metabolic Syndrome. Frontiers in pharmacology, 9, 1382. https://doi.org/10.3389/fphar.2018.01382

[222] Eshraghi, T., Eidi, A., Mortazavi, P., Asghari, A., & Tavangar, S. M. (2015). Magnesium protects against bile duct ligation-induced liver injury in male Wistar rats. Magnesium Research, 28(1), 32–45. doi:10.1684/mrh.2015.0380

[223] Aydin, B., Önol, M., Hondur, A., Kaya, M., Özdemir, H., Cengel, A., & Hasanreisoglu, B. (2010). The Effect of Oral Magnesium Therapy on Visual Field and Ocular Blood Flow in Normotensive Glaucoma. European Journal of Ophthalmology, 20(1), 131–135. doi:10.1177/112067211002000118

[224] Ekici, F., Korkmaz, Ş., Karaca, E. E., Sül, S., Tufan, H. A., Aydın, B., & Dileköz, E. (2014). The Role of Magnesium in the Pathogenesis and Treatment of Glaucoma. International Scholarly Research Notices, 2014, 1–7. doi:10.1155/2014/745439

[225] Marcocci, C., Kahaly, G. J., Krassas, G. E., Bartalena, L., Prummel, M., Stahl, M., … Wiersinga, W. (2011). Selenium and the Course of Mild Graves' Orbitopathy. New England Journal of Medicine, 364(20), 1920–1931. doi:10.1056/nejmoa1012985

[226] Khong, J. J., Goldstein, R. F., Sanders, K. M., Schneider, H., Pope, J., Burdon, K. P., … Ebeling, P. R. (2014). Serum selenium status in Graves' disease with and without orbitopathy: a case-control study. Clinical Endocrinology, 80(6), 905–910. doi:10.1111/cen.12392

[227] Age-Related Eye Disease Study Research Group (2001). A randomized, placebo-controlled, clinical trial of high-dose supplementation with vitamins C and E, beta carotene, and zinc for age-related macular degeneration and vision loss: AREDS report no. 8. Archives of ophthalmology (Chicago, Ill. : 1960), 119(10), 1417–1436. https://doi.org/10.1001/archopht.119.10.1417

[228] George Mason University. (2007, August 28). Zinc Linked To Macular Degeneration, Study Suggests. ScienceDaily. Retrieved November 14, 2020 from www.sciencedaily.com/releases/2007/08/070827143203.htm

[229] Harris, E. D., Rayton, J. K., Balthrop, J. E., DiSilvestro, R. A., & Garcia-de-Quevedo, M. (1980). Copper and the synthesis of elastin and collagen. Ciba Foundation symposium, 79, 163–182. https://doi.org/10.1002/9780470720622.ch9

[230] DiSilvestro, R. A., Selsby, J., & Siefker, K. (2010). A pilot study of copper supplementation effects on plasma F2alpha isoprostanes and urinary collagen crosslinks in young adult women. Journal of trace elements in medicine and biology : organ of the Society for Minerals and Trace Elements (GMS), 24(3), 165–168. https://doi.org/10.1016/j.jtemb.2010.02.003

[231] Tengrup, I., Ahonen, J., & Zederfeldt, B. (1981). Influence of zinc on synthesis and the accumulation of collagen in early granulation tissue. Surgery, gynecology & obstetrics, 152(3), 323–326.

[232] Seo, H. J., Cho, Y. E., Kim, T., Shin, H. I., & Kwun, I. S. (2010). Zinc may increase bone formation through stimulating cell proliferation, alkaline phosphatase activity and collagen synthesis in osteoblastic MC3T3-E1 cells. Nutrition research and practice, 4(5), 356–361. https://doi.org/10.4162/nrp.2010.4.5.356

[233] Bonneaud et al. 'Assessing the cost of mounting an immune response'. Am Nat. 2003;161(3):367-379. doi:10.1086/346134

[234] Ray, S. D., Farris, F. F., & Hartmann, A. C. (2014). Hormesis. Encyclopedia of Toxicology, 944–948. doi:10.1016/b978-0-12-386454-3.00398-5

[235] Schneiderman, N., Ironson, G., & Siegel, S. D. (2005). Stress and health: psychological, behavioral, and biological determinants. Annual review of clinical psychology, 1, 607–628. https://doi.org/10.1146/annurev.clinpsy.1.102803.144141

[236] Stojanovich and Marisavljevich (2008). 'Stress as a trigger of autoimmune disease', Autoimmunity Reviews, 7(3), 209–213. doi:10.1016/j.autrev.2007.11.007

[237] Hayes, D. P. (2006). Nutritional hormesis. European Journal of Clinical Nutrition, 61(2), 147–159. doi:10.1038/sj.ejcn.1602507

[238] Dmitrašinović et al (2016). ACTH, Cortisol and IL-6 Levels in Athletes Following Magnesium Supplementation. Journal of Medical Biochemistry, 35(4), 375–384. doi:10.1515/jomb-2016-0021

[239] Boyle, N. B., Lawton, C., & Dye, L. (2017). The Effects of Magnesium Supplementation on Subjective Anxiety and Stress-A Systematic Review. Nutrients, 9(5), 429. https://doi.org/10.3390/nu9050429

[240] Meltem et al (2009) 'A hypokalemic muscular weakness after licorice ingestion: a case report', Cases J. 2009 Sep 17;2:8053. doi: 10.1186/1757-1626-0002-0000008053.

[241] Olivero, J. J. (2016). Cardiac Consequences Of Electrolyte Imbalance. Methodist DeBakey Cardiovascular Journal, 12(2), 125–126. doi:10.14797/mdcj-12-2-125

[242] Stone, M., Martyn, L., & Weaver, C. (2016). Potassium Intake, Bioavailability, Hypertension, and Glucose Control. Nutrients, 8(7), 444. doi:10.3390/nu8070444

[243] Feldman, R. (1999). Moderate dietary salt restriction increases vascular and systemic insulin resistance. American Journal of Hypertension, 12(6), 643–647. doi:10.1016/s0895-7061(99)00016-3

[244] Jürgens, G., & Graudal, N. A. (2003). Effects of low sodium diet versus high sodium diet on blood pressure, renin, aldosterone, catecholamines, cholesterols, and triglyceride. The Cochrane database of systematic reviews, (1), CD004022. https://doi.org/10.1002/14651858.CD004022

[245] Weinberger, M. H. (1996). Salt Sensitivity of Blood Pressure in Humans. Hypertension, 27(3), 481–490. doi:10.1161/01.hyp.27.3.481

[246] Adler, A. J., Taylor, F., Martin, N., Gottlieb, S., Taylor, R. S., & Ebrahim, S. (2014). Reduced dietary salt for the prevention of cardiovascular disease. Cochrane Database of Systematic Reviews. doi:10.1002/14651858.cd009217.pub3

[247] Alderman, M. H., Cohen, H., & Madhavan, S. (1998). Dietary sodium intake and mortality: the National Health and Nutrition Examination Survey (NHANES I). The Lancet, 351(9105), 781–785. doi:10.1016/s0140-6736(97)09092-2

[248] Cohen, H. W., Hailpern, S. M., Fang, J., & Alderman, M. H. (2006). Sodium Intake and Mortality in the NHANES II Follow-up Study. The American Journal of Medicine, 119(3), 275.e7–275.e14. doi:10.1016/j.amjmed.2005.10.042

[249] Thomas, M. C., Moran, J., Forsblom, C., Harjutsalo, V., Thorn, L., … Ahola, A. (2011). The Association Between Dietary Sodium Intake, ESRD, and All-Cause Mortality in Patients With Type 1 Diabetes. Diabetes Care, 34(4), 861–866. doi:10.2337/dc10-1722

[250] Stolarz-Skrzypek, K. (2011). Fatal and Nonfatal Outcomes, Incidence of Hypertension, and Blood Pressure Changes in Relation to Urinary Sodium Excretion. JAMA, 305(17), 1777. doi:10.1001/jama.2011.574

[251] O'Donnell, M. J., Yusuf, S., Mente, A., Gao, P., Mann, J. F., Teo, K., … Schmieder, R. E. (2011). Urinary Sodium and Potassium Excretion and Risk of Cardiovascular Events. JAMA, 306(20). doi:10.1001/jama.2011.1729

[252] Mottillo, S., Filion, K. B., Genest, J., Joseph, L., Pilote, L., Poirier, P., … Eisenberg, M. J. (2010). The Metabolic Syndrome and Cardiovascular Risk. Journal of the American College of Cardiology, 56(14), 1113–1132. doi:10.1016/j.jacc.2010.05.034

[253] Hunnicutt et al (2014) 'Dietary Iron Intake and Body Iron Stores Are Associated with Risk of Coronary Heart Disease in a Meta-Analysis of Prospective Cohort Studies, The Journal of Nutrition, Volume 144, Issue 3, March 2014, Pages 359–366, https://doi.org/10.3945/jn.113.185124

543

[254] Berg, J. (1990). Zinc fingers and other metal-binding domains. *Receptor* 29: 31.

[255] Barnett, J. & Hamer, D. & Meydani, S. (2010). Low zinc status: a new risk factor for pneumonia in the elderly? *Nutrition Reviews* 68 (1): 30–37.

[256] Frye C. A. (2009). Steroids, reproductive endocrine function, and affect. A review. Minerva ginecologica, 61(6), 541–562.

[257] Bose, H. S., Marshall, B., Debnath, D. K., Perry, E. W., & Whittal, R. M. (2020). Electron Transport Chain Complex II Regulates Steroid Metabolism. iScience, 23(7), 101295. doi:10.1016/j.isci.2020.101295

[258] Chung, B. C., Matteson, K. J., Voutilainen, R., Mohandas, T. K., & Miller, W. L. (1986). Human cholesterol side-chain cleavage enzyme, P450scc: cDNA cloning, assignment of the gene to chromosome 15, and expression in the placenta. Proceedings of the National Academy of Sciences, 83(23), 8962–8966. doi:10.1073/pnas.83.23.8962

[259] Duarte, A., Poderoso, C., Cooke, M., Soria, G., Cornejo Maciel, F., Gottifredi, V., & Podestá, E. J. (2012). Mitochondrial Fusion Is Essential for Steroid Biosynthesis. PLoS ONE, 7(9), e45829. doi:10.1371/journal.pone.0045829

[260] GARREN, L. D., GILL, G. N., MASUI, H., & WALTON, G. M. (1971). On the Mechanism of Action of ACTH. Proceedings of the 1970 Laurentian Hormone Conference, 433–478. doi:10.1016/b978-0-12-571127-2.50035-3

[261] Crivello, J. F., & Jefcoate, C. R. (1980). Intracellular movement of cholesterol in rat adrenal cells. Kinetics and effects of inhibitors. The Journal of biological chemistry, 255(17), 8144–8151.

[262] Privalle, C. T., Crivello, J. F., & Jefcoate, C. R. (1983). Regulation of intramitochondrial cholesterol transfer to side-chain cleavage cytochrome P-450 in rat adrenal gland. Proceedings of the National Academy of Sciences of the United States of America, 80(3), 702–706. https://doi.org/10.1073/pnas.80.3.702

[263] Prasad, A. S., Mantzoros, C. S., Beck, F. W. J., Hess, J. W., & Brewer, G. J. (1996). Zinc status and serum testosterone levels of healthy adults. Nutrition, 12(5), 344–348. doi:10.1016/s0899-9007(96)80058-x

[264] Cinar, V., Polat, Y., Baltaci, A. K., & Mogulkoc, R. (2010). Effects of Magnesium Supplementation on Testosterone Levels of Athletes and Sedentary Subjects at Rest and after Exhaustion. Biological Trace Element Research, 140(1), 18–23. doi:10.1007/s12011-010-8676-3

[265] Sheu, J.-R., Hsiao, G., Shen, M.-Y., Fong, T.-H., Chen, Y.-W., Lin, C.-H., & Chou, D.-S. (2002). Mechanisms involved in the antiplatelet activity of magnesium in human platelets. British Journal of Haematology, 119(4), 1033–1041. doi:10.1046/j.1365-2141.2002.03967.x

[266] Duarte, A., Castillo, A. F., Castilla, R., Maloberti, P., Paz, C., Podestá, E. J., & Cornejo Maciel, F. (2007). An arachidonic acid generation/export system involved in the regulation of cholesterol transport in mitochondria of steroidogenic cells. FEBS Letters, 581(21), 4023–4028. doi:10.1016/j.febslet.2007.07.040

[267] Katona, P. & Katona-Apte, J. (2008). The Interaction between Nutrition and Infection. *Clinical Infectious Diseases* 46 (10): 1582–1588.

[268] Tinggi, U. (2008). Selenium: its role as antioxidant in human health. *Environmental Health and Preventive Medicine* 13 (2): 102–108.

[269] Tam, M., Gómez, S., González-Gross, M., & Marcos, A. (2003). Possible roles of magnesium on the immune system. European Journal of Clinical Nutrition, 57(10), 1193–1197. doi:10.1038/sj.ejcn.1601689

[270] Weglicki, W. B., Phillips, T. M., Freedman, A. M., Cassidy, M. M., & Dickens, B. F. (1992). Magnesium-deficiency elevates circulating levels of inflammatory cytokines and endothelin. Molecular and Cellular Biochemistry, 110(2), 169–173. doi:10.1007/bf02454195

[271] Malpuech-Brugère C, Kuryszko J, Nowacki W, et al. Early morphological and immunological alterations in the spleen during magnesium deficiency in the rat. Magnesium Research. 1998 Sep;11(3):161-169.

[272] Li, F.-Y., Chaigne-Delalande, B., Su, H., Uzel, G., Matthews, H., & Lenardo, M. J. (2014). XMEN disease: a new primary immunodeficiency affecting Mg2+ regulation of immunity against Epstein-Barr virus. Blood, 123(14), 2148–2152. doi:10.1182/blood-2013-11-538686

[273] Prasad, A. S. (2008). Zinc in Human Health: Effect of Zinc on Immune Cells. Molecular Medicine, 14(5-6), 353–357. doi:10.2119/2008-00033.prasad

[274] Allan, G. & Arroll, B. (2014). Prevention and treatment of the common cold: making sense of the evidence. *CMAJ* 186 (3): 190–199.

[275] Hemilä, H. & Chalker, E. (2017). Zinc for preventing and treating the common cold. *Cochrane Database of Systematic* Reviews 2017 (9): CD012808.

[276] Köhler, Kerstin; Ferreira, Pedro; Pfander, Boris; Boos, Dominik (2016). *The Initiation of DNA Replication in Eukaryotes*. Springer, Cham. pp. 443–460.

[277] Bernstein H, Payne CM, Bernstein C, Garewal H, Dvorak K (2008). Cancer and aging as consequences of un-repaired DNA damage. In: New Research on DNA Damages (Editors: Honoka Kimura and Aoi Suzuki) Nova Science Publishers, Inc., New York, Chapter 1, pp. 1–47.

[278] Hoeijmakers JH (2009). "DNA damage, aging, and cancer". *New England Journal of Medicine*. **361** (15): 1475–1485.

[279] Bernstein, H; Payne, CM; Bernstein, C; Garewal, H; Dvorak, K (2008). "Cancer and aging as consequences of un-repaired DNA damage.". In Kimura, Honoka; Suzuki, Aoi (eds.). *New Research on DNA Damage*. Nova Science Publishers. pp. 1–47.

[280] Holmes, G. E., Bernstein, C., & Bernstein, H. (1992). Oxidative and other DNA damages as the basis of aging: a review. Mutation Research/DNAging, 275(3-6), 305–315. doi:10.1016/0921-8734(92)90034-m

[281] Narayanan, L., Fritzell, J. A., Baker, S. M., Liskay, R. M., & Glazer, P. M. (1997). Elevated levels of mutation in multiple tissues of mice deficient in the DNA mismatch repair gene Pms2. Proceedings of the National Academy of Sciences, 94(7), 3122–3127. doi:10.1073/pnas.94.7.3122

[282] Lahtz, C., & Pfeifer, G. P. (2011). Epigenetic changes of DNA repair genes in cancer. Journal of molecular cell biology, 3(1), 51–58. https://doi.org/10.1093/jmcb/mjq053

[283] Shah, N. C., Shah, G. J., Li, Z., Jiang, X. C., Altura, B. T., & Altura, B. M. (2014). Short-term magnesium deficiency downregulates telomerase, upregulates neutral sphingomyelinase and induces oxidative DNA damage in cardiovascular tissues: relevance to atherogenesis, cardiovascular diseases and aging. International journal of clinical and experimental medicine, 7(3), 497–514.

[284] Wolf, F. (2003). Chemistry and biochemistry of magnesium. Molecular Aspects of Medicine, 24(1-3), 3–9. doi:10.1016/s0098-2997(02)00087-0

[285] Wolf, F. (2003). Cell physiology of magnesium. Molecular Aspects of Medicine, 24(1-3), 11–26. doi:10.1016/s0098-2997(02)00088-2

[286] Bienkowski (2015) 'Heavy Metal May Age Cells Prematurely', Scientific American, Environmental Health News, January 6, 2015, Accessed Online: https://www.scientificamerican.com/article/heavy-metal-may-age-cells-prematurely/

[287] Song, Y., Leonard, S. W., Traber, M. G., & Ho, E. (2009). Zinc Deficiency Affects DNA Damage, Oxidative Stress, Antioxidant Defenses, and DNA Repair in Rats. The Journal of Nutrition, 139(9), 1626–1631. doi:10.3945/jn.109.106369

[288] Sharif, R., Thomas, P., Zalewski, P. and Fenech, M. (2015), Zinc supplementation influences genomic stability biomarkers, antioxidant activity, and zinc transporter genes in an elderly Australian population with low zinc status. Mol. Nutr. Food Res., 59: 1200-1212. doi:10.1002/mnfr.201400784

[289] Oteiza, P. (2000). Zinc deficiency induces oxidative stress and AP-1 activation in 3T3 cells. Free Radical Biology and Medicine, 28(7), 1091–1099. doi:10.1016/s0891-5849(00)00200-8

[290] Gomes, L., Menck, C., & Leandro, G. (2017). Autophagy Roles in the Modulation of DNA Repair Pathways. International Journal of Molecular Sciences, 18(11), 2351. doi:10.3390/ijms18112351

[291] Yang et al (2010) 'Defective Hepatic Autophagy in Obesity Promotes ER Stress and Causes Insulin Resistance', Cell Metab. 2010 Jun 9; 11(6): 467–478.

[292] Nakai, A., Yamaguchi, O., Takeda, T., Higuchi, Y., Hikoso, S., Taniike, M., ... Otsu, K. (2007). The role of autophagy in cardiomyocytes in the basal state and in response to hemodynamic stress. Nature Medicine, 13(5), 619–624. doi:10.1038/nm1574

[293] Hua, Y., Zhang, Y., Ceylan-Isik, A. F., Wold, L. E., Nunn, J. M., & Ren, J. (2011). Chronic Akt activation accentuates aging-induced cardiac hypertrophy and myocardial contractile dysfunction: role of autophagy. Basic research in cardiology, 106(6), 1173–1191. https://doi.org/10.1007/s00395-011-0222-8

[294] Liao et al (2012) 'Macrophage Autophagy Plays a Protective Role in Advanced Atherosclerosis', Cell Metabolism, Volume 15, Issue 4, 4 April 2012, Pages 545-553.

[295] Shi et al (2012) 'Activation of autophagy by inflammatory signals limits IL-1β production by targeting ubiquitinated inflammasomes for destruction', Nat Immunol. 2012 Jan 29;13(3):255-63.

[296] Henderson and Stevens (2012) 'The Role of Autophagy in Crohn's Disease', Cells. 2012 Sep; 1(3): 492–519.

[297] Deretic and Levine (2009) 'Autophagy, immunity, and microbial adaptations', Cell Host Microbe. 2009 Jun 18;5(6):527-49.

[298] Bossy et al (2008) 'Clearing the Brain's Cobwebs: The Role of Autophagy in Neuroprotection', Curr Neuropharmacol. 2008 Jun; 6(2): 97–101.

[299] Chu, Hiutung; Khosravi, Arya; Kusumawardhani, Indah P et al. (2016) Gene-microbiota interactions contribute to the pathogenesis of inflammatory bowel disease. Science 352:1116-20

[300] Khambu et al (2018) 'Autophagy in non-alcoholic fatty liver disease and alcoholic liver disease', Liver Research, Volume 2, Issue 3, September 2018, Pages 112-119.

[301] Liuzzi, J. P., & Yoo, C. (2013). Role of zinc in the regulation of autophagy during ethanol exposure in human hepatoma cells. Biological trace element research, 156(1-3), 350–356. https://doi.org/10.1007/s12011-013-9816-3

[302] Hwang, J. J., Kim, H. N., Kim, J., Cho, D. H., Kim, M. J., Kim, Y. S., Kim, Y., Park, S. J., & Koh, J. Y. (2010). Zinc(II) ion mediates tamoxifen-induced autophagy and cell death in MCF-7 breast cancer cell line. Biometals : an international journal on the role of metal ions in biology, biochemistry, and medicine, 23(6), 997–1013. https://doi.org/10.1007/s10534-010-9346-9

[303] Kawamata, T., Horie, T., Matsunami, M., Sasaki, M., & Ohsumi, Y. (2017). Zinc starvation induces autophagy in yeast. The Journal of biological chemistry, 292(20), 8520–8530. https://doi.org/10.1074/jbc.M116.762948

[304] Bootman et al (2018) 'The regulation of autophagy by calcium signals: Do we have a consensus?', Cell Calcium, Volume 70, March 2018, Pages 32-46.

[305] Sun et al (2017) 'Dietary potassium regulates vascular calcification and arterial stiffness', JCI Insight. 2017;2(19):e94920. https://doi.org/10.1172/jci.insight.94920.

[306] Yue, J., Jin, S., Gu, S., Sun, R., & Liang, Q. (2019). High concentration magnesium inhibits extracellular matrix calcification and protects articular cartilage via Erk/autophagy pathway. Journal of cellular physiology, 234(12), 23190–23201. https://doi.org/10.1002/jcp.28885

[307] Minich (2018) 'Vitamin-Mineral Interactions', Metagenics, Inc. Accessed Online Nov 15 2020: https://blog.metagenics.com/wp-content/uploads/2020/04/MET2557_Vitamin-Mineral_Interactions_Chart.pdf

[308] Ames (2012) 'The "triage theory": micronutrient deficiencies cause insidious damage that accelerates age-associated chronic disease', Accessed Online Nov 6 2020: http://www.bruceames.org/Triage.pdf

[309] Ames, B. N., McCann, J. C., Stampfer, M. J., & Willett, W. C. (2007). Evidence-based decision making on micronutrients and chronic disease: long-term randomized controlled trials are not enough. The American journal of clinical nutrition, 86(2), 522–524. https://doi.org/10.1093/ajcn/86.2.522

[310] Kirkwood T. B. (2008). Understanding ageing from an evolutionary perspective. Journal of internal medicine, 263(2), 117–127. https://doi.org/10.1111/j.1365-2796.2007.01901.x

[311] Shiraki, M., Tsugawa, N., & Okano, T. (2015). Recent advances in vitamin K-dependent Gla-containing proteins and vitamin K nutrition. Osteoporosis and Sarcopenia, 1(1), 22–38. doi:10.1016/j.afos.2015.07.009

[312] Heuvel, E. G. H. M. van den, van Schoor, N. M., Lips, P., Magdeleyns, E. J. P., Deeg, D. J. H., Vermeer, C., & Heijer, M. den. (2014). Circulating uncarboxylated matrix Gla protein, a marker of vitamin K status, as a risk factor of cardiovascular disease. Maturitas, 77(2), 137–141. doi:10.1016/j.maturitas.2013.10.008

[313] DiNicolantonio et al (2017) 'Subclinical magnesium deficiency: a principal driver of cardiovascular disease and a public health crisis', Open Heart 2018;5:e000668. doi:10.1136/openhrt-2017-000668

[314] O'Connell, B. S. (2001). Select Vitamins and Minerals in the Management of Diabetes. Diabetes Spectrum, 14(3), 133–148. doi:10.2337/diaspect.14.3.133

[315] Harman, D. (1956) 'Aging: A Theory Based on Free Radical and Radiation Chemistry', Journal of Gerontology, Vol 11(3), p 298-300.

[316] Harman, D. (1956) 'Aging: A Theory Based on Free Radical and Radiation Chemistry', Journal of Gerontology, Vol 11(3), p 298-300.

[317] Harman, D. (1972) 'The biologic clock: the mitochondria?', Journal of the American Geriatrics Society, April 20(4), p 145-147.

[318] Schriner, SE. et al (2005) 'Extension of murine life span by overexpression of catalase targeted to mitochondria', Science, Vol 308(5730), p 1909-1911.

[319] Miguel, J. et al (1980) 'Mitochondrial role in cell aging', Experimental Gerontology, Vol 15(6), p 575-591.

[320] Wei, YH. et al (2001) 'Mitochondrial theory of aging matures--roles of mtDNA mutation and oxidative stress in human aging', Zhonghua Yi Xue Za Zhi (Taipei), Vol 64(5), p 259-270.

[321] Giustarini, D., Dalle-Donne, I., Tsikas, D., & Rossi, R. (2009). Oxidative stress and human diseases: Origin, link, measurement, mechanisms, and biomarkers. Critical Reviews in Clinical Laboratory Sciences, 46(5-6), 241–281. doi:10.3109/10408360903142326

[322] D. Trachootham, W. Lu, M. A. Ogasawara, N. R.-D. Valle, and P. Huang, "Redox regulation of cell survival," *Antioxidants & Redox Signaling*, vol. 10, no. 8, pp. 1343–1374, 2008.

[323] Rahman K. (2007). Studies on free radicals, antioxidants, and co-factors. Clinical interventions in aging, 2(2), 219–236.

[324] Lobo, V., Patil, A., Phatak, A., & Chandra, N. (2010). Free radicals, antioxidants and functional foods: Impact on human health. Pharmacognosy Reviews, 4(8), 118. doi:10.4103/0973-7847.70902

[325] Ighodaro, O. M., & Akinloye, O. A. (2018). First line defence antioxidants-superoxide dismutase (SOD), catalase (CAT) and glutathione peroxidase (GPX): Their fundamental role in the entire antioxidant defence grid. Alexandria Journal of Medicine, 54(4), 287–293. doi:10.1016/j.ajme.2017.09.001

[326] Niki E. (1993) Antioxidant Defenses In Eukariotic Cells: An Overview. In: Poli G., Albano E., Dianzani M.U. (eds) Free Radicals: from Basic Science to Medicine. Molecular and Cell Biology Updates. Birkhäuser Basel. https://doi.org/10.1007/978-3-0348-9116-5_31

[327] Köhler, Kerstin; Ferreira, Pedro; Pfander, Boris; Boos, Dominik (2016). *The Initiation of DNA Replication in Eukaryotes*. Springer, Cham. pp. 443–460.

546

[328] Bernstein H, Payne CM, Bernstein C, Garewal H, Dvorak K (2008). Cancer and aging as consequences of un-repaired DNA damage. In: New Research on DNA Damages (Editors: Honoka Kimura and Aoi Suzuki) Nova Science Publishers, Inc., New York, Chapter 1, pp. 1–47.

[329] Hoeijmakers JH (2009). "DNA damage, aging, and cancer". *New England Journal of Medicine.* **361** (15): 1475–1485.

[330] Giglia-Mari, G., Zotter, A., & Vermeulen, W. (2011). DNA damage response. Cold Spring Harbor perspectives in biology, 3(1), a000745. https://doi.org/10.1101/cshperspect.a000745

[331] Zhang, L., & Yu, J. (2013). Role of apoptosis in colon cancer biology, therapy, and prevention. Current colorectal cancer reports, 9(4), 10.1007/s11888-013-0188-z. https://doi.org/10.1007/s11888-013-0188-z

[332] Ng, Y., Barhoumi, R., Tjalkens, R. B., Fan, Y.-Y., Kolar, S., Wang, N., … Chapkin, R. S. (2005). The role of docosahexaenoic acid in mediating mitochondrial membrane lipid oxidation and apoptosis in colonocytes. Carcinogenesis, 26(11), 1914–1921. doi:10.1093/carcin/bgi163

[333] Watkins and German (1998) 'Docosahexaenoic acid accumulates in cardiolipin and enhances HT-29 cell oxidant production', Journal of Lipid Research 39(8):1583-8.

[334] Lee, M., & Bae, M. A. (2007). Docosahexaenoic acid induces apoptosis in CYP2E1-containing HepG2 cells by activating the c-Jun N-terminal protein kinase related mitochondrial damage. The Journal of nutritional biochemistry, 18(5), 348–354. https://doi.org/10.1016/j.jnutbio.2006.06.003

[335] Giros, A., Grzybowski, M., Sohn, V. R., Pons, E., Fernandez-Morales, J., Xicola, R. M., Sethi, P., Grzybowski, J., Goel, A., Boland, C. R., Gassull, M. A., & Llor, X. (2009). Regulation of colorectal cancer cell apoptosis by the n-3 polyunsaturated fatty acids Docosahexaenoic and Eicosapentaenoic. Cancer prevention research (Philadelphia, Pa.), 2(8), 732–742. https://doi.org/10.1158/1940-6207.CAPR-08-0197

[336] Ding et al (2008) 'Association of Autophagy Defect with a Malignant Phenotype and Poor Prognosis of Hepatocellular Carcinoma', Cancer Research, Volume 68, Issue 22, DOI: 10.1158/0008-5472.CAN-08-1573

[337] Galati, S., Boni, C., Gerra, M. C., Lazzaretti, M., & Buschini, A. (2019). Autophagy: A Player in response to Oxidative Stress and DNA Damage. Oxidative Medicine and Cellular Longevity, 2019, 1–12. doi:10.1155/2019/5692958

[338] Gillespie, D. A., & Ryan, K. M. (2015). Autophagy is critically required for DNA repair by homologous recombination. Molecular & Cellular Oncology, 3(1), e1030538. doi:10.1080/23723556.2015.1030538

[339] Browner, W. S., Kahn, A. J., Ziv, E., Reiner, A. P., Oshima, J., Cawthon, R. M., … Cummings, S. R. (2004). The genetics of human longevity. The American Journal of Medicine, 117(11), 851–860. doi:10.1016/j.amjmed.2004.06.033

[340] Vazquez, B. N., Thackray, J. K., & Serrano, L. (2017). Sirtuins and DNA damage repair: SIRT7 comes to play. Nucleus (Austin, Tex.), 8(2), 107–115. https://doi.org/10.1080/19491034.2016.1264552

[341] Zhou et al (2014) 'CLOCK/BMAL1 regulates circadian change of mouse hepatic insulin sensitivity via SIRT1.', Hepatology 59(6), DOI: 10.1002/hep.26992

[342] Ramis et al (2015) 'Caloric restriction, resveratrol and melatonin: Role of SIRT1 and implications for aging and related-diseases', Mechanisms of Ageing and Development, Volumes 146–148, March 2015, Pages 28-41.

[343] Favero et al (2020) 'Sirtuin1 Role in the Melatonin Protective Effects Against Obesity-Related Heart Injury', Front. Physiol., 11 March 2020 | https://doi.org/10.3389/fphys.2020.00103

[344] Jung-Hynes, B., Reiter, R. J., & Ahmad, N. (2010). Sirtuins, melatonin and circadian rhythms: building a bridge between aging and cancer. Journal of pineal research, 48(1), 9–19. https://doi.org/10.1111/j.1600-079X.2009.00729.x

[345] Liu et al (2019) 'Melatonin ameliorates cerebral ischemia/reperfusion injury through SIRT3 activation', Life Sciences, Volume 239, 15 December 2019, 117036.

[346] Lourenço dos Santos, S., Petropoulos, I., & Friguet, B. (2018). The Oxidized Protein Repair Enzymes Methionine Sulfoxide Reductases and Their Roles in Protecting against Oxidative Stress, in Ageing and in Regulating Protein Function. Antioxidants, 7(12), 191. doi:10.3390/antiox7120191

347 Zheng, W., & Lee, S. A. (2009). Well-done meat intake, heterocyclic amine exposure, and cancer risk. Nutrition and cancer, 61(4), 437–446. https://doi.org/10.1080/01635580802710741

[348] Adhikari, S., Toretsky, J. A., Yuan, L., & Roy, R. (2006). Magnesium, Essential for Base Excision Repair Enzymes, Inhibits Substrate Binding ofN-Methylpurine-DNA Glycosylase. Journal of Biological Chemistry, 281(40), 29525–29532. doi:10.1074/jbc.m602673200

[349] Izumi, T., Wiederhold, L. R., Roy, G., Roy, R., Jaiswal, A., Bhakat, K. K., Mitra, S., & Hazra, T. K. (2003). Mammalian DNA base excision repair proteins: their interactions and role in repair of oxidative DNA damage. Toxicology, 193(1-2), 43–65. https://doi.org/10.1016/s0300-483x(03)00289-0

[350] Song, Y., Leonard, S. W., Traber, M. G., & Ho, E. (2009). Zinc deficiency affects DNA damage, oxidative stress, antioxidant defenses, and DNA repair in rats. The Journal of nutrition, 139(9), 1626–1631. https://doi.org/10.3945/jn.109.106369.

[351] Ames and Ho (2002) 'Low intracellular zinc induces oxidative DNA damage, disrupts p53, NFκB, and AP1 DNA binding, and affects DNA repair in a rat glioma cell line', PNAS December 24, 2002 99 (26) 16770-16775; https://doi.org/10.1073/pnas.222679399

[352] Song, Y., Chung, C. S., Bruno, R. S., Traber, M. G., Brown, K. H., King, J. C., & Ho, E. (2009). Dietary zinc restriction and repletion affects DNA integrity in healthy men. The American journal of clinical nutrition, 90(2), 321–328. https://doi.org/10.3945/ajcn.2008.27300

[353] Walsh, C. T., Sandstead, H. H., Prasad, A. S., Newberne, P. M., & Fraker, P. J. (1994). Zinc: health effects and research priorities for the 1990s. Environmental health perspectives, 102 Suppl 2(Suppl 2), 5–46. https://doi.org/10.1289/ehp.941025

[354] Ikejima M, Noguchi S, Yamashita R, et al. The zinc fingers of human poly(ADP-ribose) polymerase are differentially required for the recognition of DNA breaks and nicks and the consequent enzyme activation. Other structures recognize intact DNA. The Journal of Biological Chemistry. 1990 Dec;265(35):21907-21913.

[355] Zhang C. (2014). Essential functions of iron-requiring proteins in DNA replication, repair and cell cycle control. Protein & cell, 5(10), 750–760. https://doi.org/10.1007/s13238-014-0083-7

[356] Lukianova and David (2005) 'A role for iron-sulfur clusters in DNA repair.' Current Opinion in Chemical Biology, Volume 9, Issue 2, April 2005, Pages 145-151.

[357] Beckman, J. S., & Koppenol, W. H. (1996). Nitric oxide, superoxide, and peroxynitrite: the good, the bad, and ugly. American Journal of Physiology-Cell Physiology, 271(5), C1424–C1437. doi:10.1152/ajpcell.1996.271.5.c1424

[358] Pacher, P., Beckman, J. S., & Liaudet, L. (2007). Nitric Oxide and Peroxynitrite in Health and Disease. Physiological Reviews, 87(1), 315–424. doi:10.1152/physrev.00029.2006

[359] Thomson, L. (2015). 3-Nitrotyrosine Modified Proteins in Atherosclerosis. Disease Markers, 2015, 1–8. doi:10.1155/2015/708282

[360] Van der Loo et al (2000). Enhanced Peroxynitrite Formation Is Associated with Vascular Aging. The Journal of Experimental Medicine, 192(12), 1731–1744. doi:10.1084/jem.192.12.1731

[361] Pall (2016) 'Electromagnetic Fields Act Similarly in Plants as in Animals: Probable Activation of Calcium Channels via Their Voltage Sensor', Current Chemical Biology, Volume 10 , Issue 1 , 2016, DOI : 10.2174/2212796810666160419160433

[362] Yingxin et al (2012) 'Roles of oxidative stress in synchrotron radiation X-ray-induced testicular damage of rodents', Int J Physiol Pathophysiol Pharmacol. 2012; 4(2): 108–114.

[363] Fessel, J. P., & Oldham, W. M. (2018). Pyridine Dinucleotides from Molecules to Man. Antioxidants & Redox Signaling, 28(3), 180–212. doi:10.1089/ars.2017.7120

[364] Lassègue, B., & Griendling, K. K. (2010). NADPH Oxidases: Functions and Pathologies in the Vasculature. Arteriosclerosis, Thrombosis, and Vascular Biology, 30(4), 653–661. doi:10.1161/atvbaha.108.181610

[365] Block, M. L. (2008). NADPH oxidase as a therapeutic target in Alzheimer's disease. BMC Neuroscience, 9(S2). doi:10.1186/1471-2202-9-s2-s8

[366] Inoguchi, T., Li, P., Umeda, F., Yu, H. Y., Kakimoto, M., Imamura, M., … Nawata, H. (2000). High glucose level and free fatty acid stimulate reactive oxygen species production through protein kinase C-dependent activation of NAD(P)H oxidase in cultured vascular cells. Diabetes, 49(11), 1939–1945. doi:10.2337/diabetes.49.11.1939

[367] Jaspers, I., Zhang, W., Brighton, L. E., Carson, J. L., Styblo, M., & Beck, M. A. (2007). Selenium deficiency alters epithelial cell morphology and responses to influenza. Free Radical Biology and Medicine, 42(12), 1826–1837. doi:10.1016/j.freeradbiomed.2007.03.017

[368] Pannala, V. R., & Dash, R. K. (2015). Mechanistic characterization of the thioredoxin system in the removal of hydrogen peroxide. Free radical biology & medicine, 78, 42–55. https://doi.org/10.1016/j.freeradbiomed.2014.10.508

[369] Heo, S.; Kim, S.; Kang, D. The Role of Hydrogen Peroxide and Peroxiredoxins throughout the Cell Cycle. Antioxidants 2020, 9, 280.

[370] Trujillo, M., Ferrer-Sueta, G., & Radi, R. (2008). Peroxynitrite Detoxification and Its Biologic Implications. Antioxidants & Redox Signaling, 10(9), 1607–1620. doi:10.1089/ars.2008.2060

[371] Radi R. (2013). Peroxynitrite, a stealthy biological oxidant. The Journal of biological chemistry, 288(37), 26464–26472. https://doi.org/10.1074/jbc.R113.472936

[372] Riddell, D. R., & Owen, J. S. (1997). Nitric Oxide and Platelet Aggregation. Vitamins & Hormones, 25–48. doi:10.1016/s0083-6729(08)60639-1

[373] Hobbs, D. A., George, T. W., & Lovegrove, J. A. (2013). The effects of dietary nitrate on blood pressure and endothelial function: a review of human intervention studies. Nutrition Research Reviews, 26(2), 210–222. doi:10.1017/s0954422413000188

[374] Park, J. W., Piknova, B., Nghiem, K., Lozier, J. N., & Schechter, A. N. (2014). Inhibitory effect of nitrite on coagulation processes demonstrated by thrombelastography. Nitric oxide : biology and chemistry, 40, 45–51. https://doi.org/10.1016/j.niox.2014.05.006

548

[375] Matsushita, K., Morrell, C. N., Cambien, B., Yang, S.-X., Yamakuchi, M., Bao, C., … Lowenstein, C. J. (2003). Nitric Oxide Regulates Exocytosis by S-Nitrosylation of N-ethylmaleimide-Sensitive Factor. Cell, 115(2), 139–150. doi:10.1016/s0092-8674(03)00803-1

[376] O'Donnell, V. B., & Freeman, B. A. (2001). Interactions Between Nitric Oxide and Lipid Oxidation Pathways. Circulation Research, 88(1), 12–21. doi:10.1161/01.res.88.1.12

[377] McIntyre, M., & Dominiczak, A. F. (1997). Nitric oxide and cardiovascular disease. Postgraduate Medical Journal, 73(864), 630–634. doi:10.1136/pgmj.73.864.630

[378] Houston, M., & Hays, L. (2014). Acute Effects of an Oral Nitric Oxide Supplement on Blood Pressure, Endothelial Function, and Vascular Compliance in Hypertensive Patients. The Journal of Clinical Hypertension, n/a–n/a. doi:10.1111/jch.12352

[379] Zhang, S., Yang, T., Xu, X., Wang, M., Zhong, L., Yang, Y., … Wang, C. (2015). Oxidative stress and nitric oxide signaling related biomarkers in patients with pulmonary hypertension: a case control study. BMC Pulmonary Medicine, 15(1). doi:10.1186/s12890-015-0045-8

[380] Davies, K. P. (2015). Development and therapeutic applications of nitric oxide releasing materials to treat erectile dysfunction. Future Science OA, 1(1). doi:10.4155/fso.15.53

[381] Bivalacqua, T., Champion, H., Mehta, Y., Abdel-Mageed, A., Sikka, S., Ignarro, L., … Hellstrom, W. (2000). Adenoviral gene transfer of endothelial nitric oxide synthase (eNOS) to the penis improves age-related erectile dysfunction in the rat. International Journal of Impotence Research, 12(S3), S8–S17. doi:10.1038/sj.ijir.3900556

[382] Mayo Clinic Stafff (2019) 'High blood pressure and sex: Overcome the challenges', Mayo Clinic, Accessed Online Nov 11 2020: https://www.mayoclinic.org/diseases-conditions/high-blood-pressure/in-depth/high-blood-pressure-and-sex/art-20044209

[383] Musicki, B., Liu, T., Lagoda, G. A., Bivalacqua, T. J., Strong, T. D., & Burnett, A. L. (2009). Endothelial Nitric Oxide Synthase Regulation in Female Genital Tract Structures. The Journal of Sexual Medicine, 6, 247–253. doi:10.1111/j.1743-6109.2008.01122.x

[384] Reiss, C. & Komatsu, T. (1998). Does nitric oxide play a critical role in viral infections? *Journal of Virology* 72 (6): 4547-4551.

[385] Åkerström, S. et al. (2005). Nitric oxide inhibits the replication cycle of severe acute respiratory syndrome coronavirus. *Journal of Virology* 79 (3): 1966-1969.

[386] Åkerström, S., Gunalan, V., Keng, C. T., Tan, Y.-J., & Mirazimi, A. (2009). Dual effect of nitric oxide on SARS-CoV replication: Viral RNA production and palmitoylation of the S protein are affected. Virology, 395(1), 1–9. doi:10.1016/j.virol.2009.09.007

[387] Chen, L., Liu, P., Gao, H., Sun, B., Chao, D., Wang, F., … Wang, C. G. (2004). Inhalation of Nitric Oxide in the Treatment of Severe Acute Respiratory Syndrome: A Rescue Trial in Beijing. Clinical Infectious Diseases, 39(10), 1531–1535. doi:10.1086/425357

[388] Wu, G., & Morris, S. M., Jr (1998). Arginine metabolism: nitric oxide and beyond. The Biochemical journal, 336 (Pt 1)(Pt 1), 1–17. https://doi.org/10.1042/bj3360001

[389] Epstein, F. H., Moncada, S., & Higgs, A. (1993). The L-Arginine-Nitric Oxide Pathway. New England Journal of Medicine, 329(27), 2002–2012. doi:10.1056/nejm199312303292706

[390] Agarwal, U., Didelija, I. C., Yuan, Y., Wang, X., & Marini, J. C. (2017). Supplemental Citrulline Is More Efficient Than Arginine in Increasing Systemic Arginine Availability in Mice. The Journal of nutrition, 147(4), 596–602. https://doi.org/10.3945/jn.116.240382

[391] Knowles, R. G., & Moncada, S. (1994). Nitric oxide synthases in mammals. The Biochemical journal, 298 (Pt 2)(Pt 2), 249–258. https://doi.org/10.1042/bj2980249

[392] Spaans et al (2015). NADPH-generating systems in bacteria and archaea. Frontiers in microbiology, 6, 742. https://doi.org/10.3389/fmicb.2015.00742

[393] Spaans SK, Weusthuis RA, van der Oost J, Kengen SW (2015). "NADPH-generating systems in bacteria and archaea". *Frontiers in Microbiology.* 6: 742.

[394] Rush et al (1985). Organic hydroperoxide-induced lipid peroxidation and cell death in isolated hepatocytes. Toxicology and applied pharmacology, 78(3), 473–483. https://doi.org/10.1016/0041-008x(85)90255-8

[395] Luiking, Y. C., Engelen, M. P., & Deutz, N. E. (2010). Regulation of nitric oxide production in health and disease. Current Opinion in Clinical Nutrition and Metabolic Care, 13(1), 97–104. doi:10.1097/mco.0b013e328332f99d

[396] Wu, G., & Meininger, C. J. (2002). REGULATION OFNITRICOXIDESYNTHESIS BYDIETARYFACTORS. Annual Review of Nutrition, 22(1), 61–86. doi:10.1146/annurev.nutr.22.110901.145329

[397] Ochiai, M., Hayashi, T., Morita, M., Ina, K., Maeda, M., Watanabe, F., & Morishita, K. (2012). Short-term effects of l-citrulline supplementation on arterial stiffness in middle-aged men. International Journal of Cardiology, 155(2), 257–261. doi:10.1016/j.ijcard.2010.10.004

[398] Cormio, L., De Siati, M., Lorusso, F., Selvaggio, O., Mirabella, L., Sanguedolce, F., & Carrieri, G. (2011). Oral L-citrulline supplementation improves erection hardness in men with mild erectile dysfunction. Urology, 77(1), 119–122. https://doi.org/10.1016/j.urology.2010.08.028

[399] Gonzales, J. U., Raymond, A., Ashley, J., & Kim, Y. (2017). Does l-citrulline supplementation improve exercise blood flow in older adults?. Experimental physiology, 102(12), 1661–1671. https://doi.org/10.1113/EP086587

[400] Bailey et al (2010) 'Acute l-arginine supplementation reduces the O2 cost of moderate-intensity exercise and enhances high-intensity exercise tolerance', Journal of Applied Physiology, Volume 109 Issue 5, Pages 1394-1403.

[401] Orozco-Gutiérrez, J. J., Castillo-Martínez, L., Orea-Tejeda, A., Vázquez-Díaz, O., Valdespino-Trejo, A., Narváez-David, R., Keirns-Davis, C., Carrasco-Ortiz, O., Navarro-Navarro, A., & Sánchez-Santillán, R. (2010). Effect of L-arginine or L-citrulline oral supplementation on blood pressure and right ventricular function in heart failure patients with preserved ejection fraction. Cardiology journal, 17(6), 612–618.

[402] McKinley-Barnard, S., Andre, T., Morita, M., & Willoughby, D. S. (2015). Combined L-citrulline and glutathione supplementation increases the concentration of markers indicative of nitric oxide synthesis. Journal of the International Society of Sports Nutrition, 12, 27. https://doi.org/10.1186/s12970-015-0086-7

[403] Ghigo, D., Geromin, D., Franchino, C., Todde, R., Priotto, C., Costamagna, C., Arese, M., Garbarino, G., Pescarmona, G. P., & Bosia, A. (1996). Correlation between nitric oxide synthase activity and reduced glutathione level in human and murine endothelial cells. Amino acids, 10(3), 277–281. https://doi.org/10.1007/BF00807330

[404] Andrew, P. (1999). Enzymatic function of nitric oxide synthases. Cardiovascular Research, 43(3), 521–531. doi:10.1016/s0008-6363(99)00115-7

[405] Chen, G., Dunbar, R. L., Gao, W., & Ebner, T. J. (2001). Role of Calcium, Glutamate Neurotransmission, and Nitric Oxide in Spreading Acidification and Depression in the Cerebellar Cortex. The Journal of Neuroscience, 21(24), 9877–9887. doi:10.1523/jneurosci.21-24-09877.2001

[406] Okuda, Y., Kawashima, K., Sawada, T., Tsurumaru, K., Asano, M., Suzuki, S., ... Yamashita, K. (1997). Eicosapentaenoic Acid Enhances Nitric Oxide Production by Cultured Human Endothelial Cells. Biochemical and Biophysical Research Communications, 232(2), 487–491. doi:10.1006/bbrc.1997.6328

[407] Swartz-Basile, D. A., Goldblatt, M. I., Blaser, C., Decker, P. A., Ahrendt, S. A., Sarna, S. K., & Pitt, H. A. (2000). Iron Deficiency Diminishes Gallbladder Neuronal Nitric Oxide Synthase. Journal of Surgical Research, 90(1), 26–31. doi:10.1006/jsre.2000.5827

[408] Goldblatt, M. (2001). Iron deficiency suppresses ileal nitric oxide synthase activity,. Journal of Gastrointestinal Surgery, 5(4), 393–400. doi:10.1016/s1091-255x(01)80068-8

[409] ALDERTON, W. K., COOPER, C. E., & KNOWLES, R. G. (2001). Nitric oxide synthases: structure, function and inhibition. Biochemical Journal, 357(3), 593. doi:10.1042/0264-6021:3570593

[410] Persechini, A., McMillan, K., & Masters, B. S. S. (1995). Inhibition of Nitric Oxide Synthase Activity by Zn2+ Ion. Biochemistry, 34(46), 15091–15095. doi:10.1021/bi00046a015

[411] Spranger, M., Schwab, S., Desiderato, S., Bonmann, E., Krieger, D., & Fandrey, J. (1998). Manganese Augments Nitric Oxide Synthesis in Murine Astrocytes: A New Pathogenetic Mechanism in Manganism? Experimental Neurology, 149(1), 277–283. doi:10.1006/exnr.1997.6666

[412] Reddy GR, Chetty CS, Sajwan K, Desaiah D. (2001). 'Lead and manganese alters the activity and expression of nitric oxide synthase in rat brain'. FASEB J. 15:A222

[413] Kim, D.-H., Meza, C. A., Clarke, H., Kim, J.-S., & Hickner, R. C. (2020). Vitamin D and Endothelial Function. Nutrients, 12(2), 575. doi:10.3390/nu12020575

[414] Dawes M, Ritter JM. (2000). 'Mg2+-induced vasodilation in human vasculature is inhibited by NG-monomethyl-L-arginine but not by indomethacin'. J. Vasc. Res. 37:276–81

[415] Pearson, P. J., Evora, P. R. B., Seccombe, J. F., & Schaff, H. V. (1998). Hypomagnesemia Inhibits Nitric Oxide Release From Coronary Endothelium: Protective Role of Magnesium Infusion After Cardiac Operations11This article has been selected for the open discussion forum on the STS Web site: http://www.sts.org/annals. The Annals of Thoracic Surgery, 65(4), 967–972. doi:10.1016/s0003-4975(98)00020-4

[416] Wu, G., Haynes, T. E., Li, H., Yan, W., & Meininger, C. J. (2001). Glutamine metabolism to glucosamine is necessary for glutamine inhibition of endothelial nitric oxide synthesis. The Biochemical journal, 353(Pt 2), 245–252. https://doi.org/10.1042/0264-6021:3530245

[417] Williams, S. B., Goldfine, A. B., Timimi, F. K., Ting, H. H., Roddy, M. A., Simonson, D. C., & Creager, M. A. (1998). Acute hyperglycemia attenuates endothelium-dependent vasodilation in humans in vivo. Circulation, 97(17), 1695–1701. https://doi.org/10.1161/01.cir.97.17.1695

[418] Grundy, S. M., Benjamin, I. J., Burke, G. L., Chait, A., Eckel, R. H., Howard, B. V., ... Sowers, J. R. (1999). Diabetes and Cardiovascular Disease. Circulation, 100(10), 1134–1146. doi:10.1161/01.cir.100.10.1134

[419] Weksler-Zangen, S., Jörns, A., Tarsi-Chen, L., Vernea, F., Aharon-Hananel, G., Saada, A., ... Raz, I. (2013). Dietary copper supplementation restores β-cell function of Cohen diabetic rats: a link between

550

mitochondrial function and glucose-stimulated insulin secretion. American Journal of Physiology-Endocrinology and Metabolism, 304(10), E1023–E1034. doi:10.1152/ajpendo.00036.2013

[420] A scientific review: the role of chromium in insulin resistance. (2004). The Diabetes educator, Suppl, 2–14.

[421] Prabodh, S., Prakash, D. S. R. S., Sudhakar, G., Chowdary, N. V. S., Desai, V., & Shekhar, R. (2010). Status of Copper and Magnesium Levels in Diabetic Nephropathy Cases: a Case-Control Study from South India. Biological Trace Element Research, 142(1), 29–35. doi:10.1007/s12011-010-8750-x

[422] Takagawa, Y., Berger, M. E., Hori, M. T., Tuck, M. L., & Golub, M. S. (2001). Long-term fructose feeding impairs vascular relaxation in rat mesenteric arteries. American Journal of Hypertension, 14(8), 811–817. doi:10.1016/s0895-7061(01)01298-5

[423] DiNicolantonio, J. J., O'Keefe, J. H., & Wilson, W. (2018). Subclinical magnesium deficiency: a principal driver of cardiovascular disease and a public health crisis. Open Heart, 5(1), e000668. doi:10.1136/openhrt-2017-000668

[424] DiNicolantonio, J. J., Mangan, D., & O'Keefe, J. H. (2018). The fructose–copper connection: Added sugars induce fatty liver and insulin resistance via copper deficiency. Journal of Insulin Resistance, 3(1). doi:10.4102/jir.v3i1.43

[425] Pompella et al (2003). The changing faces of glutathione, a cellular protagonist. Biochemical Pharmacology, 66(8), 1499–1503. doi:10.1016/s0006-2952(03)00504-5

[426] McKinley-Barnard, S., Andre, T., Morita, M., & Willoughby, D. S. (2015). Combined L-citrulline and glutathione supplementation increases the concentration of markers indicative of nitric oxide synthesis. Journal of the International Society of Sports Nutrition, 12, 27. https://doi.org/10.1186/s12970-015-0086-7

[427] Barbagallo et al (1999) 'Effects of Glutathione on Red Blood Cell Intracellular Magnesium', Hypertension. 1999;34:76–82, https://doi.org/10.1161/01.HYP.34.1.76.

[428] Bede, O., Nagy, D., Surányi, A. et al. Effects of magnesium supplementation on the glutathione redox system in atopic asthmatic children. Inflamm. res. 57, 279–286 (2008). https://doi.org/10.1007/s00011-007-7077-3

[429] Tinggi, U. (2008). Selenium: its role as antioxidant in human health. *Environmental Health and Preventive Medicine* 13 (2): 102–108.

[430] Roy, M., Kiremidjian-Schumacher, L., Wishe, H. I., Cohen, M. W., & Stotzky, G. (1994). Supplementation with selenium and human immune cell functions. Biological Trace Element Research, 41(1-2), 103–114. doi:10.1007/bf02917221

[431] Kiremidjian-Schumacher, L., Roy, M., Wishe, H. I., Cohen, M. W., & Stotzky, G. (1994). Supplementation with selenium and human immune cell functions. Biological Trace Element Research, 41(1-2), 115–127. doi:10.1007/bf02917222

[432] Hawkes, W. C., Kelley, D. S., & Taylor, P. C. (2001). The Effects of Dietary Selenium on the Immune System in Healthy Men. Biological Trace Element Research, 81(3), 189–213. doi:10.1385/bter:81:3:189

[433] Nelson, H. K., Shi, Q., Van Dael, P., Schiffrin, E. J., Blum, S., Barclay, D., Levander, O. A., & Beck, M. A. (2001). Host nutritional selenium status as a driving force for influenza virus mutations. FASEB journal : official publication of the Federation of American Societies for Experimental Biology, 15(10), 1727–1738.

[434] Yu, L., Sun, L., Nan, Y., & Zhu, L.-Y. (2010). Protection from H1N1 Influenza Virus Infections in Mice by Supplementation with Selenium: A Comparison with Selenium-Deficient Mice. Biological Trace Element Research, 141(1-3), 254–261. doi:10.1007/s12011-010-8726-x

[435] Zhang, J., Taylor, E. W., Bennett, K., Saad, R., & Rayman, M. P. (2020). Association between regional selenium status and reported outcome of COVID-19 cases in China. The American Journal of Clinical Nutrition, 111(6), 1297–1299. doi:10.1093/ajcn/nqaa095

[436] Vašák, M. (2005). Advances in metallothionein structure and functions. Journal of Trace Elements in Medicine and Biology, 19(1), 13–17. doi:10.1016/j.jtemb.2005.03.003

[437] Coyle, P., Philcox, J. C., Carey, L. C., & Rofe, A. M. (2002). Metallothionein: the multipurpose protein. Cellular and Molecular Life Sciences (CMLS), 59(4), 627–647. doi:10.1007/s00018-002-8454-2

[438] Klaassen, C. D., Liu, J., & Diwan, B. A. (2009). Metallothionein protection of cadmium toxicity. Toxicology and Applied Pharmacology, 238(3), 215–220. doi:10.1016/j.taap.2009.03.026

[439] Templeton, D. M., & George Cherian, M. (1991). [3] Toxicological significance of metallothionein. Methods in Enzymology, 11–24. doi:10.1016/0076-6879(91)05079-b

[440] Karin, M., Cathala, G., & Nguyen-Huu, M. C. (1983). Expression and regulation of a human metallothionein gene carried on an autonomously replicating shuttle vector. Proceedings of the National Academy of Sciences of the United States of America, 80(13), 4040–4044. https://doi.org/10.1073/pnas.80.13.4040

[441] Kägi J. H. (1991). Overview of metallothionein. Methods in enzymology, 205, 613–626. https://doi.org/10.1016/0076-6879(91)05145-l

[442] Shaw, C. F., 3rd, Savas, M. M., & Petering, D. H. (1991). Ligand substitution and sulfhydryl reactivity of metallothionein. Methods in enzymology, 205, 401–414. https://doi.org/10.1016/0076-6879(91)05122-c

[443] Malaiyandi, L. M., Dineley, K. E., & Reynolds, I. J. (2004). Divergent consequences arise from metallothionein overexpression in astrocytes: zinc buffering and oxidant-induced zinc release. Glia, 45(4), 346–353. https://doi.org/10.1002/glia.10332

[444] Kröncke, K. D., Fehsel, K., Schmidt, T., Zenke, F. T., Dasting, I., Wesener, J. R., Bettermann, H., Breunig, K. D., & Kolb-Bachofen, V. (1994). Nitric oxide destroys zinc-sulfur clusters inducing zinc release from metallothionein and inhibition of the zinc finger-type yeast transcription activator LAC9. Biochemical and biophysical research communications, 200(2), 1105–1110. https://doi.org/10.1006/bbrc.1994.1564

[445] Andrews G. K. (2000). Regulation of metallothionein gene expression by oxidative stress and metal ions. Biochemical pharmacology, 59(1), 95–104. https://doi.org/10.1016/s0006-2952(99)00301-9

[446] Ruttkay-Nedecky, B., Nejdl, L., Gumulec, J., Zitka, O., Masarik, M., Eckschlager, T., Stiborova, M., Adam, V., & Kizek, R. (2013). The role of metallothionein in oxidative stress. International journal of molecular sciences, 14(3), 6044–6066. https://doi.org/10.3390/ijms14036044

[447] Kojima-Yuasa, A., Umeda, K., Ohkita, T., Opare Kennedy, D., Nishiguchi, S., & Matsui-Yuasa, I. (2005). Role of reactive oxygen species in zinc deficiency-induced hepatic stellate cell activation. Free radical biology & medicine, 39(5), 631–640. https://doi.org/10.1016/j.freeradbiomed.2005.04.015

[448] Cortese, M. M., Suschek, C. V., Wetzel, W., Kröncke, K. D., & Kolb-Bachofen, V. (2008). Zinc protects endothelial cells from hydrogen peroxide via Nrf2-dependent stimulation of glutathione biosynthesis. Free radical biology & medicine, 44(12), 2002–2012. https://doi.org/10.1016/j.freeradbiomed.2008.02.013

[449] Hayes, J. D., Dinkova-Kostova, A. T., & Tew, K. D. (2020). Oxidative Stress in Cancer. Cancer Cell, 38(2), 167–197. doi:10.1016/j.ccell.2020.06.001

[450] Ohl, K., Tenbrock, K., & Kipp, M. (2016). Oxidative stress in multiple sclerosis: Central and peripheral mode of action. Experimental Neurology, 277, 58–67. doi:10.1016/j.expneurol.2015.11.010

[451] Kattoor, A. J., Pothineni, N. V. K., Palagiri, D., & Mehta, J. L. (2017). Oxidative Stress in Atherosclerosis. Current Atherosclerosis Reports, 19(11). doi:10.1007/s11883-017-0678-6

[452] Zhao, Y., & Zhao, B. (2013). Oxidative Stress and the Pathogenesis of Alzheimer's Disease. Oxidative Medicine and Cellular Longevity, 2013, 1–10. doi:10.1155/2013/316523

[453] Martin, S. J. (2011). Mitochondrial Fusion: Bax to the Fussure. Developmental Cell, 20(2), 142–143. doi:10.1016/j.devcel.2011.01.016

[454] Nakada, K., Inoue, K., & Hayashi, J.-I. (2001). Interaction Theory of Mammalian Mitochondria. Biochemical and Biophysical Research Communications, 288(4), 743–746. doi:10.1006/bbrc.2001.5838

[455] Yu, T., Robotham, J. L., & Yoon, Y. (2006). Increased production of reactive oxygen species in hyperglycemic conditions requires dynamic change of mitochondrial morphology. Proceedings of the National Academy of Sciences, 103(8), 2653–2658. doi:10.1073/pnas.0511154103

[456] Makino, A., Scott, B. T., & Dillmann, W. H. (2010). Mitochondrial fragmentation and superoxide anion production in coronary endothelial cells from a mouse model of type 1 diabetes. Diabetologia, 53(8), 1783–1794. https://doi.org/10.1007/s00125-010-1770-4

[457] Willerson, J. T. (2004). Inflammation as a Cardiovascular Risk Factor. Circulation, 109(21_suppl_1), II-2–II-10. doi:10.1161/01.cir.0000129535.04194.38

458 Colotta, F., Allavena, P., Sica, A., Garlanda, C., & Mantovani, A. (2009). Cancer-related inflammation, the seventh hallmark of cancer: links to genetic instability. Carcinogenesis, 30(7), 1073–1081. doi:10.1093/carcin/bgp127

459 Grivennikov, S. I., Greten, F. R., & Karin, M. (2010). Immunity, Inflammation, and Cancer. Cell, 140(6), 883–899. doi:10.1016/j.cell.2010.01.025

[460] Pase, M. P., Himali, J. J., Beiser, A. S., DeCarli, C., McGrath, E. R., Satizabal, C. L., … Bis, J. C. (2019). Association of CD14 with incident dementia and markers of brain aging and injury. Neurology, 94(3), e254–e266. doi:10.1212/wnl.0000000000008682

461 Barbé-Tuana, F., Funchal, G., Schmitz, C.R.R. et al. The interplay between immunosenescence and age-related diseases. Semin Immunopathol (2020). https://doi.org/10.1007/s00281-020-00806-z

[462] Gross, O., Thomas, C. J., Guarda, G., & Tschopp, J. (2011). The inflammasome: an integrated view. Immunological Reviews, 243(1), 136–151. doi:10.1111/j.1600-065x.2011.01046.x

[463] García-Hernández, A. L., Muñoz-Saavedra, Á. E., González-Alva, P., Moreno-Fierros, L., Llamosas-Hernández, F. E., Cifuentes-Mendiola, S. E., & Rubio-Infante, N. (2018). Upregulation of proteins of the NLRP3 inflammasome in patients with periodontitis and uncontrolled type 2 diabetes. Oral Diseases. doi:10.1111/odi.13003

[464] Pirzada, R. H., Javaid, N., & Choi, S. (2020). The Roles of the NLRP3 Inflammasome in Neurodegenerative and Metabolic Diseases and in Relevant Advanced Therapeutic Interventions. Genes, 11(2), 131. doi:10.3390/genes11020131

552

[465] Freeman, L. C., & Ting, J. P.-Y. (2015). The pathogenic role of the inflammasome in neurodegenerative diseases. Journal of Neurochemistry, 136, 29–38. doi:10.1111/jnc.13217

[466] Spel, L., & Martinon, F. (2020). Inflammasomes contributing to inflammation in arthritis. Immunological reviews, 294(1), 48–62. https://doi.org/10.1111/imr.12839

[467] Carlström, M., Ekman, A.-K., Petersson, S., Söderkvist, P., & Enerbäck, C. (2012). Genetic support for the role of the NLRP3 inflammasome in psoriasis susceptibility. Experimental Dermatology, 21(12), 932–937. doi:10.1111/exd.12049

[468] Li, R., Wang, J., Li, R., Zhu, F., Xu, W., Zha, G., He, G., Cao, H., Wang, Y., & Yang, J. (2018). ATP/P2X7-NLRP3 axis of dendritic cells participates in the regulation of airway inflammation and hyper-responsiveness in asthma by mediating HMGB1 expression and secretion. Experimental cell research, 366(1), 1–15. https://doi.org/10.1016/j.yexcr.2018.03.002

[469] Kim, S. R., Kim, D. I., Kim, S. H., Lee, H., Lee, K. S., Cho, S. H., & Lee, Y. C. (2014). NLRP3 inflammasome activation by mitochondrial ROS in bronchial epithelial cells is required for allergic inflammation. Cell Death & Disease, 5(10), e1498–e1498. doi:10.1038/cddis.2014.460

[470] Contassot, E., & French, L. E. (2014). New Insights into Acne Pathogenesis: Propionibacterium Acnes Activates the Inflammasome. Journal of Investigative Dermatology, 134(2), 310–313. doi:10.1038/jid.2013.505

[471] Pope, R. M., & Tschopp, J. (2007). The role of interleukin-1 and the inflammasome in gout: Implications for therapy. Arthritis & Rheumatism, 56(10), 3183–3188. doi:10.1002/art.22938

[472] Rodrigues et al (2020). Inflammasome activation in COVID-19 patients. doi:10.1101/2020.08.05.20168872

[473] Shah, A. (2020). Novel Coronavirus-Induced NLRP3 Inflammasome Activation: A Potential Drug Target in the Treatment of COVID-19. Frontiers in Immunology, 11. doi:10.3389/fimmu.2020.01021

[474] Yu, Z.-W., Zhang, J., Li, X., Wang, Y., Fu, Y.-H., & Gao, X.-Y. (2020). A new research hot spot: The role of NLRP3 inflammasome activation, a key step in pyroptosis, in diabetes and diabetic complications. Life Sciences, 240, 117138. doi:10.1016/j.lfs.2019.117138

[475] Liang, X., Zhang, D., Liu, W., Yan, Y., Zhou, F., Wu, W., & Yan, Z. (2017). Reactive oxygen species trigger NF-κB-mediated NLRP3 inflammasome activation induced by zinc oxide nanoparticles in A549 cells. Toxicology and Industrial Health, 33(10), 737–745. doi:10.1177/0748233717712409

[476] He, M., Chiang, H.-H., Luo, H., Zheng, Z., Qiao, Q., Wang, L., … Chen, D. (2020). An Acetylation Switch of the NLRP3 Inflammasome Regulates Aging-Associated Chronic Inflammation and Insulin Resistance. Cell Metabolism, 31(3), 580–591.e5. doi:10.1016/j.cmet.2020.01.009

[477] Pétrilli, V., Papin, S., Dostert, C., Mayor, A., Martinon, F., & Tschopp, J. (2007). Activation of the NALP3 inflammasome is triggered by low intracellular potassium concentration. Cell Death & Differentiation, 14(9), 1583–1589. doi:10.1038/sj.cdd.4402195

[478] He, Y., Zeng, M. Y., Yang, D., Motro, B., & Núñez, G. (2016). NEK7 is an essential mediator of NLRP3 activation downstream of potassium efflux. Nature, 530(7590), 354–357. https://doi.org/10.1038/nature16959

[479] Huang, C.-L., & Kuo, E. (2007). Mechanism of Hypokalemia in Magnesium Deficiency. Journal of the American Society of Nephrology, 18(10), 2649–2652. doi:10.1681/asn.2007070792

[480] Nishimuta, M., Kodama, N., Yoshitake, Y., Shimada, M., & Serizawa, N. (2018). Dietary Salt (Sodium Chloride) Requirement and Adverse Effects of Salt Restriction in Humans. Journal of nutritional science and vitaminology, 64(2), 83–89. https://doi.org/10.3177/jnsv.64.83

[481] Nishimuta, M., Kodama, N., Morikuni, E., Yoshioka, Y. H., Matsuzaki, N., Takeyama, H., Yamada, H., & Kitajima, H. (2005). Positive correlation between dietary intake of sodium and balances of calcium and magnesium in young Japanese adults--low sodium intake is a risk factor for loss of calcium and magnesium--. Journal of nutritional science and vitaminology, 51(4), 265–270. https://doi.org/10.3177/jnsv.51.265

[482] Kodama, N., Nishimuta, M., & Suzuki, K. (2003). Negative balance of calcium and magnesium under relatively low sodium intake in humans. Journal of nutritional science and vitaminology, 49(3), 201–209. https://doi.org/10.3177/jnsv.49.201

[483] Mariathasan, S., Weiss, D. S., Newton, K., McBride, J., O'Rourke, K., Roose-Girma, M., … Dixit, V. M. (2006). Cryopyrin activates the inflammasome in response to toxins and ATP. Nature, 440(7081), 228–232. doi:10.1038/nature04515

[484] Katsnelson, M. A., Rucker, L. G., Russo, H. M., & Dubyak, G. R. (2015). K+ efflux agonists induce NLRP3 inflammasome activation independently of Ca2+ signaling. Journal of immunology (Baltimore, Md. : 1950), 194(8), 3937–3952. https://doi.org/10.4049/jimmunol.1402658

[485] Karmakar, M., Katsnelson, M. A., Dubyak, G. R., & Pearlman, E. (2016). Neutrophil P2X7 receptors mediate NLRP3 inflammasome-dependent IL-1β secretion in response to ATP. Nature communications, 7, 10555. https://doi.org/10.1038/ncomms10555

[486] Hewinson, J., Moore, S. F., Glover, C., Watts, A. G., & MacKenzie, A. B. (2008). A key role for redox signaling in rapid P2X7 receptor-induced IL-1 beta processing in human monocytes. Journal of

553

immunology (Baltimore, Md. : 1950), 180(12), 8410–8420. https://doi.org/10.4049/jimmunol.180.12.8410

[487] Feng, L., Chen, Y., Ding, R., Fu, Z., Yang, S., Deng, X., & Zeng, J. (2015). P2X7R blockade prevents NLRP3 inflammasome activation and brain injury in a rat model of intracerebral hemorrhage: involvement of peroxynitrite. Journal of Neuroinflammation, 12(1). doi:10.1186/s12974-015-0409-2

[488] Munoz, F. M., Patel, P. A., Gao, X., Mei, Y., Xia, J., Gilels, S., & Hu, H. (2020). Reactive oxygen species play a role in P2X7 receptor-mediated IL-6 production in spinal astrocytes. Purinergic signalling, 16(1), 97–107. https://doi.org/10.1007/s11302-020-09691-5

[489] Uwitonze, A. M., & Razzaque, M. S. (2018). Role of Magnesium in Vitamin D Activation and Function. The Journal of the American Osteopathic Association, 118(3), 181. doi:10.7556/jaoa.2018.037

[490] Ma, D., Zhang, R., Wen, Y., Yin, W., Bai, D., Zheng, G., ... Wen, J. (2017). 1, 25(OH) 2 D 3 -induced interaction of vitamin D receptor with p50 subunit of NF-κB suppresses the interaction between KLF5 and p50, contributing to inhibition of LPS-induced macrophage proliferation. Biochemical and Biophysical Research Communications, 482(2), 366–374. doi:10.1016/j.bbrc.2016.11.069

[491] Zhou, R., Tardivel, A., Thorens, B., Choi, I., & Tschopp, J. (2009). Thioredoxin-interacting protein links oxidative stress to inflammasome activation. Nature Immunology, 11(2), 136–140. doi:10.1038/ni.1831

[492] Patwari, P., Higgins, L. J., Chutkow, W. A., Yoshioka, J., & Lee, R. T. (2006). The Interaction of Thioredoxin with Txnip. Journal of Biological Chemistry, 281(31), 21884–21891. doi:10.1074/jbc.m600427200

[493] Hwang, J., Suh, H. W., Jeon, Y. H., Hwang, E., Nguyen, L. T., Yeom, J., Lee, S. G., Lee, C., Kim, K. J., Kang, B. S., Jeong, J. O., Oh, T. K., Choi, I., Lee, J. O., & Kim, M. H. (2014). The structural basis for the negative regulation of thioredoxin by thioredoxin-interacting protein. Nature communications, 5, 2958. https://doi.org/10.1038/ncomms3958

[494] Mustacich, D., & Powis, G. (2000). Thioredoxin reductase. The Biochemical journal, 346 Pt 1(Pt 1), 1–8.

[495] Allan, C. B., Lacourciere, G. M., & Stadtman, T. C. (1999). Responsiveness of selenoproteins to dietary selenium. Annual review of nutrition, 19, 1–16. https://doi.org/10.1146/annurev.nutr.19.1.1

[496] Ma, J., Zhu, S., Guo, Y., Hao, M., Chen, Y., Wang, Y., Yang, M., Chen, J., & Guo, M. (2019). Selenium Attenuates Staphylococcus aureus Mastitis in Mice by Inhibiting the Activation of the NALP3 Inflammasome and NF-κB/MAPK Pathway. Biological trace element research, 191(1), 159–166. https://doi.org/10.1007/s12011-018-1591-8

[497] Moghaddam, A., Heller, R. A., Sun, Q., Seelig, J., Cherkezov, A., Seibert, L., ... Schomburg, L. (2020). Selenium Deficiency Is Associated with Mortality Risk from COVID-19. Nutrients, 12(7), 2098. doi:10.3390/nu12072098

[498] Heller, R. A., Sun, Q., Hackler, J., Seelig, J., Seibert, L., Cherkezov, A., Minich, W. B., Seemann, P., Diegmann, J., Pilz, M., Bachmann, M., Ranjbar, A., Moghaddam, A., & Schomburg, L. (2020). Prediction of survival odds in COVID-19 by zinc, age and selenoprotein P as composite biomarker. Redox biology, 38, 101764. Advance online publication. https://doi.org/10.1016/j.redox.2020.101764

[499] Zhang, J., Taylor, E. W., Bennett, K., Saad, R., & Rayman, M. P. (2020). Association between regional selenium status and reported outcome of COVID-19 cases in China. The American journal of clinical nutrition, 111(6), 1297–1299. https://doi.org/10.1093/ajcn/nqaa095

[500] Campbell J. D. (2001). Lifestyle, minerals and health. Medical hypotheses, 57(5), 521–531. https://doi.org/10.1054/mehy.2001.1351

[501] Wallace, T. C., McBurney, M., & Fulgoni, V. L. (2014). Multivitamin/Mineral Supplement Contribution to Micronutrient Intakes in the United States, 2007–2010. Journal of the American College of Nutrition, 33(2), 94–102. doi:10.1080/07315724.2013.846806

[502] Jothimani, D., Kailasam, E., Danielraj, S., Nallathambi, B., Ramachandran, H., Sekar, P., ... Rela, M. (2020). COVID-19: Poor outcomes in patients with zinc deficiency. International Journal of Infectious Diseases, 100, 343–349. doi:10.1016/j.ijid.2020.09.014

[503] Campbell, J. D. (2001). Lifestyle, minerals and health. Medical Hypotheses, 57(5), 521–531. doi:10.1054/mehy.2001.1351

[504] Wallace, T. C., McBurney, M., & Fulgoni, V. L. (2014). Multivitamin/Mineral Supplement Contribution to Micronutrient Intakes in the United States, 2007–2010. Journal of the American College of Nutrition, 33(2), 94–102. doi:10.1080/07315724.2013.846806

505 Moi, P., Chan, K., Asunis, I., Cao, A., & Kan, Y. W. (1994). Isolation of NF-E2-related factor 2 (Nrf2), a NF-E2-like basic leucine zipper transcriptional activator that binds to the tandem NF-E2/AP1 repeat of the beta-globin locus control region. Proceedings of the National Academy of Sciences of the United States of America, 91(21), 9926–9930. https://doi.org/10.1073/pnas.91.21.9926

506 Pall, M. L., & Levine, S. (2015). Nrf2, a master regulator of detoxification and also antioxidant, anti-inflammatory and other cytoprotective mechanisms, is raised by health promoting factors. Sheng li xue bao : [Acta physiologica Sinica], 67(1), 1–18.

554

507 Xu, X., Zhang, L., Ye, X., Hao, Q., Zhang, T., Cui, G., & Yu, M. (2017). Nrf2/ARE pathway inhibits ROS-induced NLRP3 inflammasome activation in BV2 cells after cerebral ischemia reperfusion. Inflammation Research, 67(1), 57–65. doi:10.1007/s00011-017-1095-6

508 Han, D., Chen, W., Gu, X., Shan, R., Zou, J., Liu, G., … Han, B. (2017). Cytoprotective effect of chlorogenic acid against hydrogen peroxide-induced oxidative stress in MC3T3-E1 cells through PI3K/Akt-mediated Nrf2/HO-1 signaling pathway. Oncotarget, 8(9), 14680–14692. doi:10.18632/oncotarget.14747

509 Chaiprasongsuk, A., Onkoksoong, T., Pluemsamran, T., Limsaengurai, S., & Panich, U. (2016). Photoprotection by dietary phenolics against melanogenesis induced by UVA through Nrf2-dependent antioxidant responses. Redox Biology, 8, 79–90. doi:10.1016/j.redox.2015.12.006

510 Son, T. G., Camandola, S., & Mattson, M. P. (2008). Hormetic Dietary Phytochemicals. NeuroMolecular Medicine, 10(4), 236–246. doi:10.1007/s12017-008-8037-y

511 Huang, T.-C., Chung, Y.-L., Wu, M.-L., & Chuang, S.-M. (2011). Cinnamaldehyde Enhances Nrf2 Nuclear Translocation to Upregulate Phase II Detoxifying Enzyme Expression in HepG2 Cells. Journal of Agricultural and Food Chemistry, 59(9), 5164–5171. doi:10.1021/jf200579h

512 Kim, K. M., Lee, J. Y., Im, A.-R., & Chae, S. (2018). Phycocyanin Protects Against UVB-induced Apoptosis Through the PKC α/βII-Nrf-2/HO-1 Dependent Pathway in Human Primary Skin Cells. Molecules, 23(2), 478. doi:10.3390/molecules23020478

513 Patil, J., Matte, A., Nissbrandt, H., Mallard, C., & Sandberg, M. (2016). Sustained Effects of Neonatal Systemic Lipopolysaccharide on IL-1β and Nrf2 in Adult Rat Substantia Nigra Are Partly Normalized by a Spirulina-Enriched Diet. Neuroimmunomodulation, 23(4), 250–259. doi:10.1159/000452714

514 Gao, Y., Liu, C., Wan, G., Wang, X., Cheng, X., & Ou, Y. (2016). Phycocyanin prevents methylglyoxal-induced mitochondrial-dependent apoptosis in INS-1 cells by Nrf2. Food & Function, 7(2), 1129–1137. doi:10.1039/c5fo01548k

515 McCarty, M. F., Barroso-Aranda, J., & Contreras, F. (2010). Practical strategies for targeting NF-kappaB and NADPH oxidase may improve survival during lethal influenza epidemics. Medical Hypotheses, 74(1), 18–20. doi:10.1016/j.mehy.2009.04.052

516 Farruggia, C., Kim, M.-B., Bae, M., Lee, Y., Pham, T. X., Yang, Y., … Lee, J.-Y. (2018). Astaxanthin exerts anti-inflammatory and antioxidant effects in macrophages in NRF2-dependent and independent manners. The Journal of Nutritional Biochemistry, 62, 202–209. doi:10.1016/j.jnutbio.2018.09.005

517 Lee, H.-H., Park, S.-A., Almazari, I., Kim, E.-H., Na, H.-K., & Surh, Y.-J. (2010). Piceatannol induces heme oxygenase-1 expression in human mammary epithelial cells through activation of ARE-driven Nrf2 signaling. Archives of Biochemistry and Biophysics, 501(1), 142–150. doi:10.1016/j.abb.2010.06.011

518 Matzinger, M., Fischhuber, K., & Heiss, E. H. (2018). Activation of Nrf2 signaling by natural products-can it alleviate diabetes? Biotechnology Advances, 36(6), 1738–1767. doi:10.1016/j.biotechadv.2017.12.015

[519] McCarty, M. F., & Assanga, S. B. I. (2018). Ferulic acid may target MyD88-mediated pro-inflammatory signaling – Implications for the health protection afforded by whole grains, anthocyanins, and coffee. Medical Hypotheses, 118, 114–120. doi:10.1016/j.mehy.2018.06.032

[520] Liu, Y.-M., Shen, J.-D., Xu, L.-P., Li, H.-B., Li, Y.-C., & Yi, L.-T. (2017). Ferulic acid inhibits neuro-inflammation in mice exposed to chronic unpredictable mild stress. International Immunopharmacology, 45, 128–134. doi:10.1016/j.intimp.2017.02.007

[521] He, G. Y., Xie, M., Gao, Y., & Huang, J. G. (2015). Sichuan da xue xue bao. Yi xue ban = Journal of Sichuan University. Medical science edition, 46(3), 367–371.

[522] Bumrungpert, A., Lilitchan, S., Tuntipopipat, S., Tirawanchai, N., & Komindr, S. (2018). Ferulic Acid Supplementation Improves Lipid Profiles, Oxidative Stress, and Inflammatory Status in Hyperlipidemic Subjects: A Randomized, Double-Blind, Placebo-Controlled Clinical Trial. Nutrients, 10(6), 713. doi:10.3390/nu10060713

[523] Ren, Z., Zhang, R., Li, Y., Li, Y., Yang, Z., & Yang, H. (2017). Ferulic acid exerts neuroprotective effects against cerebral ischemia/reperfusion-induced injury via antioxidant and anti-apoptotic mechanisms in vitro and in vivo. International Journal of Molecular Medicine, 40(5), 1444–1456. doi:10.3892/ijmm.2017.3127

[524] Tan, Z.-X., Chen, Y.-H., Xu, S., Qin, H.-Y., Wang, H., Zhang, C., … Zhao, H. (2016). Calcitriol inhibits tumor necrosis factor alpha and macrophage inflammatory protein-2 during lipopolysaccharide-induced acute lung injury in mice. Steroids, 112, 81–87. doi:10.1016/j.steroids.2016.05.005

[525] Nonn, L., Peng, L., Feldman, D., & Peehl, D. M. (2006). Inhibition of p38 by vitamin D reduces interleukin-6 production in normal prostate cells via mitogen-activated protein kinase phosphatase 5: implications for prostate cancer prevention by vitamin D. Cancer research, 66(8), 4516–4524. https://doi.org/10.1158/0008-5472.CAN-05-3796

526 Beutler, B., & Cerami, A. (1988). Tumor Necrosis, Cachexia, Shock, and Inflammation: A Common Mediator. Annual Review of Biochemistry, 57(1), 505–518. doi:10.1146/annurev.bi.57.070188.002445

555

527 Rietschel, E. T., Kirikae, T., Schade, F. U., Mamat, U., Schmidt, G., Loppnow, H., … Brade, H. (1994). Bacterial endotoxin: molecular relationships of structure to activity and function. The FASEB Journal, 8(2), 217–225. doi:10.1096/fasebj.8.2.8119492

[528] Zhang, Y., Leung, D. Y. M., Richers, B. N., Liu, Y., Remigio, L. K., Riches, D. W., & Goleva, E. (2012). Vitamin D Inhibits Monocyte/Macrophage Proinflammatory Cytokine Production by Targeting MAPK Phosphatase-1. The Journal of Immunology, 188(5), 2127–2135. doi:10.4049/jimmunol.1102412

[529] Brown, D. I., & Griendling, K. K. (2009). Nox proteins in signal transduction. Free radical biology & medicine, 47(9), 1239–1253. https://doi.org/10.1016/j.freeradbiomed.2009.07.023

[530] Meijles, D. N., & Pagano, P. J. (2016). Nox and Inflammation in the Vascular Adventitia. Hypertension, 67(1), 14–19. doi:10.1161/hypertensionaha.115.03622

[531] Ogawa et al (October 2008). "The association of elevated reactive oxygen species levels from neutrophils with low-grade inflammation in the elderly". *Immunity & Ageing.* 5: 13.

[532] Zhang, M., & Ying, W. (2019). NAD+ Deficiency Is a Common Central Pathological Factor of a Number of Diseases and Aging: Mechanisms and Therapeutic Implications. Antioxidants & redox signaling, 30(6), 890–905. https://doi.org/10.1089/ars.2017.7445

[533] KAWAI, S., & MURATA, K. (2008). Structure and Function of NAD Kinase and NADP Phosphatase: Key Enzymes That Regulate the Intracellular Balance of NAD(H) and NADP(H). Bioscience, Biotechnology, and Biochemistry, 72(4), 919–930. doi:10.1271/bbb.70738

534 Bogan, K. L., & Brenner, C. (2008). Nicotinic acid, nicotinamide, and nicotinamide riboside: a molecular evaluation of NAD+ precursor vitamins in human nutrition. Annual review of nutrition, 28, 115–130. https://doi.org/10.1146/annurev.nutr.28.061807.155443

[535] Easlon (2018) 'Fermentation and Regeneration of NAD+', UC Davis Biological Sciences (BIS 2A), Introduction to Biology: Essentials of Life on Earth, Winter 2018, Accessed Online: https://bio.libretexts.org/Courses/University_of_California_Davis/BIS_2A%3A_Introductory_Biology_ (Easlon)/Readings/09.3%3A_Fermentation_and_Regeneration_of_NAD

536 Yang et al (2007) 'Nutrient-Sensitive Mitochondrial NAD+ Levels Dictate Cell Survival', Cell, Volume 130, Issue 6, 21 September 2007, Pages 1095-1107.

537 Hayashida, S., Arimoto, A., Kuramoto, Y. et al. Fasting promotes the expression of SIRT1, an NAD+-dependent protein deacetylase, via activation of PPARα in mice. Mol Cell Biochem 339, 285–292 (2010). https://doi.org/10.1007/s11010-010-0391-z

538 Chen, D., Bruno, J., Easlon, E., Lin, S. J., Cheng, H. L., Alt, F. W., & Guarente, L. (2008). Tissue-specific regulation of SIRT1 by calorie restriction. Genes & development, 22(13), 1753–1757. https://doi.org/10.1101/gad.1650608

[539] Brandauer, J., Vienberg, S. G., Andersen, M. A., Ringholm, S., Risis, S., Larsen, P. S., … Treebak, J. T. (2013). AMP-activated protein kinase regulates nicotinamide phosphoribosyl transferase expression in skeletal muscle. The Journal of Physiology, 591(20), 5207–5220. doi:10.1113/jphysiol.2013.259515

540 Cantó, C., Jiang, L. Q., Deshmukh, A. S., Mataki, C., Coste, A., Lagouge, M., Zierath, J. R., & Auwerx, J. (2010). Interdependence of AMPK and SIRT1 for metabolic adaptation to fasting and exercise in skeletal muscle. Cell metabolism, 11(3), 213–219. https://doi.org/10.1016/j.cmet.2010.02.006

541 Costford, S. R., Bajpeyi, S., Pasarica, M., Albarado, D. C., Thomas, S. C., Xie, H., Church, T. S., Jubrias, S. A., Conley, K. E., & Smith, S. R. (2010). Skeletal muscle NAMPT is induced by exercise in humans. American journal of physiology. Endocrinology and metabolism, 298(1), E117–E126. https://doi.org/10.1152/ajpendo.00318.2009

542 Raynes, Rachel Rene, "SIRT1 Regulation of the Heat Shock Response in an HSF1-Dependent Manner and the Impact of Caloric Restriction" (2013). Graduate Theses and Dissertations.

543 Maalouf et al (2007) 'Ketones inhibit mitochondrial production of reactive oxygen species production following glutamate excitotoxicity by increasing NADH oxidation', Neuroscience, Volume 145, Issue 1, 2 March 2007, Pages 256-264.

[544] Kanikarla-Marie, P., & Jain, S. K. (2015). Hyperketonemia (acetoacetate) upregulates NADPH oxidase 4 and elevates oxidative stress, ICAM-1, and monocyte adhesivity in endothelial cells. Cellular physiology and biochemistry : international journal of experimental cellular physiology, biochemistry, and pharmacology, 35(1), 364–373. https://doi.org/10.1159/000369702

[545] Newton, C. A., & Raskin, P. (2004). Diabetic ketoacidosis in type 1 and type 2 diabetes mellitus: clinical and biochemical differences. Archives of internal medicine, 164(17), 1925–1931. https://doi.org/10.1001/archinte.164.17.1925

[546] Fulco, M., Cen, Y., Zhao, P., Hoffman, E. P., McBurney, M. W., Sauve, A. A., & Sartorelli, V. (2008). Glucose Restriction Inhibits Skeletal Myoblast Differentiation by Activating SIRT1 through AMPK-Mediated Regulation of Nampt. Developmental Cell, 14(5), 661–673. doi:10.1016/j.devcel.2008.02.004

547 Schultz and Sinclair (2016) 'Why NAD+ Declines during Aging: It's Destroyed', Cell Metab. 2016 Jun 14; 23(6): 965–966.

[548] Wu, G., Haynes, T. E., Li, H., Yan, W., & Meininger, C. J. (2001). Glutamine metabolism to glucosamine is necessary for glutamine inhibition of endothelial nitric oxide synthesis. The Biochemical journal, 353(Pt 2), 245–252. https://doi.org/10.1042/0264-6021:3530245

[549] McCarty, M. F., Iloki-Assanga, S., Lujan, L. M. L., & DiNicolantonio, J. J. (2019). Activated glycine receptors may decrease endosomal NADPH oxidase activity by opposing ClC-3-mediated efflux of chloride from endosomes. Medical Hypotheses, 123, 125–129. doi:10.1016/j.mehy.2019.01.012

[550] Pizzorno J. (2014). Glutathione!. Integrative medicine (Encinitas, Calif.), 13(1), 8–12.

[551] McCarty et al (2019) 'Activated Glycine Receptors May Decrease Endosomal NADPH Oxidase Activity by Opposing ClC-3-Mediated Efflux of Chloride from Endosomes', Medical Hypotheses 123, DOI: 10.1016/j.mehy.2019.01.012

[552] Smith, M. E., & Morton, D. G. (2010). LIVER AND BILIARY SYSTEM. The Digestive System, 85–105. doi:10.1016/b978-0-7020-3367-4.00006-2

[553] Lanone, S., Bloc, S., Foresti, R., Almolki, A., Taillé, C., Callebert, J., … Boczkowski, J. (2005). Bilirubin decreases NOS2 expression via inhibition of NAD(P)H oxidase: implications for protection against endotoxic shock in rats. The FASEB Journal, 19(13), 1890–1892. doi:10.1096/fj.04-2368fje

[554] Jiang, F., Roberts, S. J., Datla, S. raju, & Dusting, G. J. (2006). NO Modulates NADPH Oxidase Function Via Heme Oxygenase-1 in Human Endothelial Cells. Hypertension, 48(5), 950–957. doi:10.1161/01.hyp.0000242336.58387.1f

[555] Fujii, M., Inoguchi, T., Sasaki, S., Maeda, Y., Zheng, J., Kobayashi, K., & Takayanagi, R. (2010). Bilirubin and biliverdin protect rodents against diabetic nephropathy by downregulating NAD(P)H oxidase. Kidney International, 78(9), 905–919. doi:10.1038/ki.2010.265

[556] McCarty, M. F. (2007). Clinical Potential of Spirulina as a Source of Phycocyanobilin. Journal of Medicinal Food, 10(4), 566–570. doi:10.1089/jmf.2007.621

[557] Terry MJ, Maines MD, Lagarias JC. Inactivation of phytochromeand phycobiliprotein-chromophore precursors by rat liver biliverdin reductase. J Biol Chem 1993;268:26099–106.

[558] Zheng, J., Inoguchi, T., Sasaki, S., Maeda, Y., McCarty, M. F., Fujii, M., … Takayanagi, R. (2013). Phycocyanin and phycocyanobilin fromSpirulina platensisprotect against diabetic nephropathy by inhibiting oxidative stress. American Journal of Physiology-Regulatory, Integrative and Comparative Physiology, 304(2), R110–R120. doi:10.1152/ajpregu.00648.2011

[559] Romay, C. h., González, R., Ledón, N., Remirez, D., & Rimbau, V. (2003). C-phycocyanin: a biliprotein with antioxidant, anti-inflammatory and neuroprotective effects. Current protein & peptide science, 4(3), 207–216. https://doi.org/10.2174/1389203033487216

[560] Liu, Q., Huang, Y., Zhang, R., Cai, T., & Cai, Y. (2016). Medical Application ofSpirulina platensisDerived C-Phycocyanin. Evidence-Based Complementary and Alternative Medicine, 2016, 1–14. doi:10.1155/2016/7803846

[561] Furukawa, S., Fujita, T., Shimabukuro, M., Iwaki, M., Yamada, Y., Nakajima, Y., Nakayama, O., Makishima, M., Matsuda, M., & Shimomura, I. (2004). Increased oxidative stress in obesity and its impact on metabolic syndrome. The Journal of clinical investigation, 114(12), 1752–1761. https://doi.org/10.1172/JCI21625

[562] Talior, I., Tennenbaum, T., Kuroki, T., & Eldar-Finkelman, H. (2005). PKC-delta-dependent activation of oxidative stress in adipocytes of obese and insulin-resistant mice: role for NADPH oxidase. American journal of physiology. Endocrinology and metabolism, 288(2), E405–E411. https://doi.org/10.1152/ajpendo.00378.2004

[563] Han, C. Y., Umemoto, T., Omer, M., Den Hartigh, L. J., Chiba, T., LeBoeuf, R., Buller, C. L., Sweet, I. R., Pennathur, S., Abel, E. D., & Chait, A. (2012). NADPH oxidase-derived reactive oxygen species increases expression of monocyte chemotactic factor genes in cultured adipocytes. The Journal of biological chemistry, 287(13), 10379–10393. https://doi.org/10.1074/jbc.M111.304998

[564] Prokudina et al (2017) 'The Role of Reactive Oxygen Species in the Pathogenesis of Adipocyte Dysfunction in Metabolic Syndrome. Prospects of Pharmacological Correction', Annals of the Russian academy of medical sciences, 2017;72:11–16.

[565] DiNicolantonio, J. J., McCarty, M. F., & O'Keefe, J. H. (2018). Antioxidant bilirubin works in multiple ways to reduce risk for obesity and its health complications. Open Heart, 5(2), e000914. doi:10.1136/openhrt-2018-000914

[566] Nano et al (2016) 'Association of circulating total bilirubin with the metabolic syndrome and type 2 diabetes: A systematic review and meta-analysis of observational evidence', Diabetes Metab 2016;42:389–97.

[567] Lee, M. J., Jung, C. H., Kang, Y. M., Hwang, J. Y., Jang, J. E., Leem, J., Park, J. Y., Kim, H. K., & Lee, W. J. (2014). Serum bilirubin as a predictor of incident metabolic syndrome: a 4-year retrospective longitudinal study of 6205 initially healthy Korean men. Diabetes & metabolism, 40(4), 305–309. https://doi.org/10.1016/j.diabet.2014.04.006

[568] Huang et al (2015) 'Serum Bilirubin Levels Predict Future Development of Metabolic Syndrome in Healthy Middle-aged Nonsmoking Men', The American Journal of Medicine, Volume 128, Issue 10, October 2015, Pages 1138.e35-1138.e41.

569 Bergman, R. N., Kim, S. P., Catalano, K. J., Hsu, I. R., Chiu, J. D., Kabir, M. , Hucking, K. and Ader, M. (2006), Why Visceral Fat is Bad: Mechanisms of the Metabolic Syndrome. Obesity, 14: 16S-19S.

557

570 Balkau et al (2008). Physical activity and insulin sensitivity: the RISC study. Diabetes, 57(10), 2613–2618. https://doi.org/10.2337/db07-1605

[571] Fan, J., Ye, J., Kamphorst, J. J., Shlomi, T., Thompson, C. B., & Rabinowitz, J. D. (2014). Quantitative flux analysis reveals folate-dependent NADPH production. Nature, 510(7504), 298–302. doi:10.1038/nature13236

[572] Centers for Disease Control and Prevention. Underlying Cause of Death, 1999–2018. CDC WONDER Online Database. Atlanta, GA: Centers for Disease Control and Prevention; 2018. Accessed Nov 10, 2020.

[573] Virani et al (2020) 'Heart Disease and Stroke Statistics—2020 Update: A Report From the American Heart Association, Circulation. 2020;141(9):e139–e596. https://doi.org/10.1161/CIR.0000000000000757

[574] Benjamin et al (2019) 'Heart Disease and Stroke Statistics—2019 Update: A Report From the American Heart Association', Circulation. 2019;139(10):e56–528. https://doi.org/10.1161/CIR.0000000000000659

[575] Fryar et al (2012) 'Prevalence of Uncontrolled Risk Factors for Cardiovascular Disease: United States, 1999–2010', NCHS data brief, no. 103. Hyattsville, MD: National Center for Health Statistics; 2012. Accessed Online Nov 10 2020: https://www.cdc.gov/nchs/data/databriefs/db103.pdf

[576] Grundy, S. M., Hansen, B., Smith, S. C., Cleeman, J. I., & Kahn, R. A. (2004). Clinical Management of Metabolic Syndrome. Arteriosclerosis, Thrombosis, and Vascular Biology, 24(2). doi:10.1161/01.atv.0000112379.88385.67

[577] Mottillo, S., Filion, K. B., Genest, J., Joseph, L., Pilote, L., Poirier, P., … Eisenberg, M. J. (2010). The Metabolic Syndrome and Cardiovascular Risk. Journal of the American College of Cardiology, 56(14), 1113–1132. doi:10.1016/j.jacc.2010.05.034

[578] SCHROEDER H. A. (1960). Relation between mortality from cardiovascular disease and treated water supplies: variations in states and 163 largest municipalities of the United States. Journal of the American Medical Association, 172, 1902–1908. https://doi.org/10.1001/jama.1960.03020170028007

[579] Schroeder, H. A. (1960). Relations between hardness of water and death rates from certain chronic and degenerative diseases in the United States. Journal of Chronic Diseases, 12(6), 586–591. doi:10.1016/0021-9681(60)90002-3

[580] Kobayashi (1957) 'On geographical relations between the chemical nature of river water and death rate from apoplexy. Ber Ohara Inst. 1957;11:12–21.

[581] MORRIS, J. (1961). HARDNESS OF LOCAL WATER-SUPPLIES AND MORTALITY FROM CARDIOVASCULAR DISEASE in the County Boroughs of England and Wales. The Lancet, 277(7182), 860–862. doi:10.1016/s0140-6736(61)90180-5

[582] Masironi, R., & Shaper, A. G. (1981). Epidemiological studies of health effects of water from different sources. Annual review of nutrition, 1, 375–400. https://doi.org/10.1146/annurev.nu.01.070181.002111

[583] Crawford, M. D., Gardner, M. J., & Morris, J. N. (1968). Mortality and hardness of local water-supplies. Lancet (London, England), 1(7547), 827–831. https://doi.org/10.1016/s0140-6736(68)90297-3

[584] Masironi, R., & Shaper, A. G. (1981). Epidemiological studies of health effects of water from different sources. Annual review of nutrition, 1, 375–400. https://doi.org/10.1146/annurev.nu.01.070181.002111

[585] Masironi, R., & Shaper, A. G. (1981). Epidemiological studies of health effects of water from different sources. Annual review of nutrition, 1, 375–400. https://doi.org/10.1146/annurev.nu.01.070181.002111

[586] Rubenowitz, E., Axelsson, G., & Rylander, R. (1996). Magnesium in drinking water and death from acute myocardial infarction. American journal of epidemiology, 143(5), 456–462. https://doi.org/10.1093/oxfordjournals.aje.a008765

[587] Rubenowitz, E., Axelsson, G., & Rylander, R. (1999). Magnesium and calcium in drinking water and death from acute myocardial infarction in women. Epidemiology (Cambridge, Mass.), 10(1), 31–36.

[588] Rubenowitz, E., Molin, I., Axelsson, G., & Rylander, R. (2000). Magnesium in Drinking Water in Relation to Morbidity and Mortality from Acute Myocardial Infarction. Epidemiology, 11(4), 416–421. doi:10.1097/00001648-200007000-00009

[589] Greathouse, D. G., & Osborne, R. H. (1980). Preliminary report on nationwide study of drinking water and cardiovascular diseases. Journal of environmental pathology and toxicology, 4(2-3), 65–76.

[590] Masironi, R., & Shaper, A. G. (1981). Epidemiological studies of health effects of water from different sources. Annual review of nutrition, 1, 375–400. https://doi.org/10.1146/annurev.nu.01.070181.002111

[591] Masironi, R., & Shaper, A. G. (1981). Epidemiological studies of health effects of water from different sources. Annual review of nutrition, 1, 375–400. https://doi.org/10.1146/annurev.nu.01.070181.002111

[592] Masironi, R., & Shaper, A. G. (1981). Epidemiological studies of health effects of water from different sources. Annual review of nutrition, 1, 375–400. https://doi.org/10.1146/annurev.nu.01.070181.002111

[593] DiNicolantonio, J. J., O'Keefe, J. H., & Wilson, W. (2018). Subclinical magnesium deficiency: a principal driver of cardiovascular disease and a public health crisis. Open Heart, 5(1), e000668. doi:10.1136/openhrt-2017-000668

[594] World Health Organization. Calcium and Magnesium in Drinking Water: Public health significance. Geneva: World Health Organization Press; 2009.

[595] Rosanoff A. (2005). [Magnesium and hypertension], Clinical calcium, 15(2), 255–260.

[596] Hénaut, L., & Massy, Z. A. (2018). Magnesium as a Calcification Inhibitor. Advances in Chronic Kidney Disease, 25(3), 281–290. doi:10.1053/j.ackd.2017.12.001

[597] Rodríguez-Ortiz, M. E., Gómez-Delgado, F., Arenas de Larriva, A. P., Canalejo, A., Gómez-Luna, P., Herencia, C., ... Almadén, Y. (2019). Serum Magnesium is associated with Carotid Atherosclerosis in patients with high cardiovascular risk (CORDIOPREV Study). Scientific Reports, 9(1). doi:10.1038/s41598-019-44322-z

[598] Sakaguchi, Y., Hamano, T., & Isaka, Y. (2018). Magnesium and Progression of Chronic Kidney Disease: Benefits Beyond Cardiovascular Protection? Advances in Chronic Kidney Disease, 25(3), 274–280. doi:10.1053/j.ackd.2017.11.001

[599] Stühlinger, H. G., Kiss, K., & Smetana, R. (2000). Der Stellenwert von Magnesium bei Herzrhythmusstörungen [Significance of magnesium in cardiac arrhythmias]. Wiener medizinische Wochenschrift (1946), 150(15-16), 330–334.

[600] An, G., Du, Z., Meng, X., Guo, T., Shang, R., Li, J., ... Zhang, C. (2014). Association between Low Serum Magnesium Level and Major Adverse Cardiac Events in Patients Treated with Drug-Eluting Stents for Acute Myocardial Infarction. PLoS ONE, 9(6), e98971. doi:10.1371/journal.pone.0098971

[601] Masironi, R., & Shaper, A. G. (1981). Epidemiological studies of health effects of water from different sources. Annual review of nutrition, 1, 375–400. https://doi.org/10.1146/annurev.nu.01.070181.002111

[602] Masironi, R., & Shaper, A. G. (1981). Epidemiological studies of health effects of water from different sources. Annual review of nutrition, 1, 375–400. https://doi.org/10.1146/annurev.nu.01.070181.002111

[603] Insights & Solutions, Inc. (2004) 'Survey of Water Softener Penetration Into the Residential Market in The Phoenix Metropolitan Area', Prepared for U.S. DEPARTMENT OF THE INTERIOR BUREAU OF RECLAMATION LOWER COLORADO REGION PHOENIX AREA OFFICE', Accessed Online: https://www.usbr.gov/lc/phoenix/programs/cass/pdf/Phase2/3BSalinityControlWWTPAppendixB.pdf

[604] Masironi, R., & Shaper, A. G. (1981). Epidemiological studies of health effects of water from different sources. Annual review of nutrition, 1, 375–400. https://doi.org/10.1146/annurev.nu.01.070181.002111

[605] Rosengren, A., Smyth, A., Rangarajan, S., Ramasundarahettige, C., Bangdiwala, S. I., AlHabib, K. F., ... Yusuf, S. (2019). Socioeconomic status and risk of cardiovascular disease in 20 low-income, middle-income, and high-income countries: the Prospective Urban Rural Epidemiologic (PURE) study. The Lancet Global Health, 7(6), e748–e760. doi:10.1016/s2214-109x(19)30045-2

[606] Havranek, E. P., Mujahid, M. S., Barr, D. A., Blair, I. V., Cohen, M. S., Cruz-Flores, S., ... Yancy, C. W. (2015). Social Determinants of Risk and Outcomes for Cardiovascular Disease. Circulation, 132(9), 873–898. doi:10.1161/cir.0000000000000228

[607] Veronesi, G., Tunstall-Pedoe, H., Ferrario, M. M., Kee, F., Kuulasmaa, K., ... Chambless, L. E. (2016). Combined effect of educational status and cardiovascular risk factors on the incidence of coronary heart disease and stroke in European cohorts: Implications for prevention. European Journal of Preventive Cardiology, 24(4), 437–445. doi:10.1177/2047487316679521

[608] Stringhini, S., Carmeli, C., Jokela, M., Avendaño, M., Muennig, P., Guida, F., Ricceri, F., d'Errico, A., Barros, H., Bochud, M., Chadeau-Hyam, M., Clavel-Chapelon, F., Costa, G., Delpierre, C., Fraga, S., Goldberg, M., Giles, G. G., Krogh, V., Kelly-Irving, M., Layte, R., ... LIFEPATH consortium (2017). Socioeconomic status and the 25 × 25 risk factors as determinants of premature mortality: a multicohort study and meta-analysis of 1·7 million men and women. Lancet (London, England), 389(10075), 1229–1237. https://doi.org/10.1016/S0140-6736(16)32380-7

[609] Petrovic, D., Haba-Rubio, J., de Mestral Vargas, C., Kelly-Irving, M., Vineis, P., ... Kivimäki, M. (2019). The contribution of sleep to social inequalities in cardiovascular disorders: a multi-cohort study. Cardiovascular Research, 116(8), 1514–1524. doi:10.1093/cvr/cvz267

[610] Koottatep, S., Karnchanawong, S., Karntawanichkul, S., & Shevasant, S. (1988). SOCIO-ECONOMIC STATUS AND WATER RESOURCES QUALITY. Water Pollution Control in Asia, 7–12. doi:10.1016/b978-0-08-036884-9.50008-9

[611] Root, E. D., Rodd, J., Yunus, M., & Emch, M. (2013). The Role of Socioeconomic Status in Longitudinal Trends of Cholera in Matlab, Bangladesh, 1993–2007. PLoS Neglected Tropical Diseases, 7(1), e1997. doi:10.1371/journal.pntd.0001997

[612] MORRIS, J. (1961). HARDNESS OF LOCAL WATER-SUPPLIES AND MORTALITY FROM CARDIOVASCULAR DISEASE in the County Boroughs of England and Wales. The Lancet, 277(7182), 860–862. doi:10.1016/s0140-6736(61)90180-5

[613] Seelig M, Rosanoff A. The Magnesium Factor. New York: Avery; 2003.

[614] Dean C. The Magnesium Miracle. New York: Ballantine Books; 2007.

[615] Masironi, R., & Shaper, A. G. (1981). Epidemiological studies of health effects of water from different sources. Annual review of nutrition, 1, 375–400. https://doi.org/10.1146/annurev.nu.01.070181.002111

[616] Masironi, R., & Shaper, A. G. (1981). Epidemiological studies of health effects of water from different sources. Annual review of nutrition, 1, 375–400. https://doi.org/10.1146/annurev.nu.01.070181.002111

[617] Xiao, Q., Murphy, R. A., Houston, D. K., Harris, T. B., Chow, W.-H., & Park, Y. (2013). Dietary and Supplemental Calcium Intake and Cardiovascular Disease Mortality. JAMA Internal Medicine, 173(8), 639. doi:10.1001/jamainternmed.2013.3283

[618] Bolland, M. J., Avenell, A., Baron, J. A., Grey, A., MacLennan, G. S., Gamble, G. D., & Reid, I. R. (2010). Effect of calcium supplements on risk of myocardial infarction and cardiovascular events: meta-analysis. BMJ, 341(jul29 1), c3691–c3691. doi:10.1136/bmj.c3691

[619] Dickinson, H. O., Nicolson, D., Cook, J. V., Campbell, F., Beyer, F. R., Ford, G. A., & Mason, J. (2006). Calcium supplementation for the management of primary hypertension in adults. Cochrane Database of Systematic Reviews. doi:10.1002/14651858.cd004639.pub2

[620] Cormick, G., Ciapponi, A., Cafferata, M. L., & Belizán, J. M. (2015). Calcium supplementation for prevention of primary hypertension. Cochrane Database of Systematic Reviews. doi:10.1002/14651858.cd010037.pub2

[621] Webb, R. C. (2003). SMOOTH MUSCLE CONTRACTION AND RELAXATION. Advances in Physiology Education, 27(4), 201–206. doi:10.1152/advan.00025.2003

[622] Paziana, K., & Pazianas, M. (2015). Calcium supplements controversy in osteoporosis: a physiological mechanism supporting cardiovascular adverse effects. Endocrine, 48(3), 776–778. doi:10.1007/s12020-015-0550-9

[623] Hauschka P. V. (1986). Osteocalcin: the vitamin K-dependent Ca2+-binding protein of bone matrix. Haemostasis, 16(3-4), 258–272. https://doi.org/10.1159/000215298

[624] Shea, M. K., & Holden, R. M. (2012). Vitamin K Status and Vascular Calcification: Evidence from Observational and Clinical Studies. Advances in Nutrition, 3(2), 158–165. doi:10.3945/an.111.001644

[625] Pérez-Barrios, C., Hernández-Álvarez, E., Blanco–Navarro, I., Pérez-Sacristán, B., & Granado-Lorencio, F. (2016). Prevalence of hypercalcemia related to hypervitaminosis D in clinical practice. Clinical Nutrition, 35(6), 1354–1358. doi:10.1016/j.clnu.2016.02.017

[626] Shea, M. K., & Holden, R. M. (2012). Vitamin K Status and Vascular Calcification: Evidence from Observational and Clinical Studies. Advances in Nutrition, 3(2), 158–165. doi:10.3945/an.111.001644

[627] Shea et al (2009). Vitamin K supplementation and progression of coronary artery calcium in older men and women. The American Journal of Clinical Nutrition, 89(6), 1799–1807. doi:10.3945/ajcn.2008.27338

[628] Forrest, K. Y. Z., & Stuhldreher, W. L. (2011). Prevalence and correlates of vitamin D deficiency in US adults. Nutrition Research, 31(1), 48–54. doi:10.1016/j.nutres.2010.12.001

[629] Uwitonze, A. M., & Razzaque, M. S. (2018). Role of Magnesium in Vitamin D Activation and Function. The Journal of the American Osteopathic Association, 118(3), 181. doi:10.7556/jaoa.2018.037

[630] RUDE, R. K., ADAMS, J. S., RYZEN, E., ENDRES, D. B., NIIMI, H., HORST, R. L., … SINGER, F. R. (1985). Low Serum Concentrations of 1,25-Dihydroxyvitamin D in Human Magnesium Deficiency. The Journal of Clinical Endocrinology & Metabolism, 61(5), 933–940. doi:10.1210/jcem-61-5-933

[631] Reddy, V., & Sivakumar, B. (1974). MAGNESIUM-DEPENDENT VITAMIN-D-RESISTANT RICKETS. The Lancet, 303(7864), 963–965. doi:10.1016/s0140-6736(74)91265-3

[632] Dai, Q., Zhu, X., Manson, J. E., Song, Y., Li, X., Franke, A. A., … Shrubsole, M. J. (2018). Magnesium status and supplementation influence vitamin D status and metabolism: results from a randomized trial. The American Journal of Clinical Nutrition, 108(6), 1249–1258. doi:10.1093/ajcn/nqy274

[633] Van Ballegooijen, A. J., Pilz, S., Tomaschitz, A., Grübler, M. R., & Verheyen, N. (2017). The Synergistic Interplay between Vitamins D and K for Bone and Cardiovascular Health: A Narrative Review. International Journal of Endocrinology, 2017, 1–12. doi:10.1155/2017/7454376

[634] Xiao, Q., Murphy, R. A., Houston, D. K., Harris, T. B., Chow, W. H., & Park, Y. (2013). Dietary and supplemental calcium intake and cardiovascular disease mortality: the National Institutes of Health-AARP diet and health study. JAMA internal medicine, 173(8), 639–646. https://doi.org/10.1001/jamainternmed.2013.3283

[635] Yang, B., Campbell, P. T., Gapstur, S. M., Jacobs, E. J., Bostick, R. M., Fedirko, V., … McCullough, M. L. (2016). Calcium intake and mortality from all causes, cancer, and cardiovascular disease: the Cancer Prevention Study II Nutrition Cohort. The American Journal of Clinical Nutrition, 103(3), 886–894. doi:10.3945/ajcn.115.117994

[636] Preidt (2016) 'Calcium Supplements May Not Be Heart Healthy', WebMD, Osteoporosis, News, Accessed Online Nov 2nd 2020: https://www.webmd.com/osteoporosis/news/20161011/calcium-supplements-may-not-be-heart-healthy#1

[637] Masironi, R., & Shaper, A. G. (1981). Epidemiological studies of health effects of water from different sources. Annual review of nutrition, 1, 375–400. https://doi.org/10.1146/annurev.nu.01.070181.002111

[638] WebMD 'Confused About Calcium Supplements?', Osteoporosis, References, Accessed Online Nov 2nd 2020: https://www.webmd.com/osteoporosis/calcium-supplements-tips#1

[639] Johnson, C. J., Peterson, D. R., & Smith, E. K. (1979). Myocardial tissue concentrations of magnesium and potassium in men dying suddenly from ischemic heart disease. The American Journal of Clinical Nutrition, 32(5), 967–970. doi:10.1093/ajcn/32.5.967

[640] Eisenberg, M. J. (1992). Magnesium deficiency and sudden death. American Heart Journal, 124(2), 544–549. doi:10.1016/0002-8703(92)90633-7

[641] Peacock, J. M., Ohira, T., Post, W., Sotoodehnia, N., Rosamond, W., & Folsom, A. R. (2010). Serum magnesium and risk of sudden cardiac death in the Atherosclerosis Risk in Communities (ARIC) Study. American heart journal, 160(3), 464–470. https://doi.org/10.1016/j.ahj.2010.06.012

[642] Yang, C.-Y. (1998). Calcium and Magnesium in Drinking Water and Risk of Death From Cerebrovascular Disease. Stroke, 29(2), 411–414. doi:10.1161/01.str.29.2.411

[643] DiNicolantonio, J. J., O'Keefe, J. H., & Wilson, W. (2018). Subclinical magnesium deficiency: a principal driver of cardiovascular disease and a public health crisis. Open Heart, 5(1), e000668. doi:10.1136/openhrt-2017-000668

[644] Masironi, R., & Shaper, A. G. (1981). Epidemiological studies of health effects of water from different sources. Annual review of nutrition, 1, 375–400. https://doi.org/10.1146/annurev.nu.01.070181.002111

[645] Masironi, R., & Shaper, A. G. (1981). Epidemiological studies of health effects of water from different sources. Annual review of nutrition, 1, 375–400. https://doi.org/10.1146/annurev.nu.01.070181.002111

[646] Schechter et al (2000) 'Low intracellular magnesium levels promote platelet-dependent thrombosis in patients with coronary artery disease', American Heart Journal, Volume 140, Issue 2, August 2000, Pages 212-218.

[647] Liao, F., Folsom, A. R., & Brancati, F. L. (1998). Is low magnesium concentration a risk factor for coronary heart disease? The Atherosclerosis Risk in Communities (ARIC) Study. American heart journal, 136(3), 480–490. https://doi.org/10.1016/s0002-8703(98)70224-8

648 Gromova, O. A., Torshin, I. Y., Kobalava, Z. D., Sorokina, M. A., … Villevalde, S. V. (2018). Deficit of Magnesium and States of Hypercoagulation: Intellectual Analysis of Data Obtained From a Sample of Patients Aged 18–50 years From Medical and Preventive Facilities in Russia. Kardiologiia, 17(4), 22–35. doi:10.18087/cardio.2018.4.10106

649 Çiçek, G., Açikgoz, S. K., Yayla, Ç., Kundi, H., & İleri, M. (2016). Magnesium as a predictor of acute stent thrombosis in patients with ST-segment elevation myocardial infarction who underwent primary angioplasty. Coronary Artery Disease, 27(1), 47–51. doi:10.1097/mca.0000000000000318

650 Shen, M. Y., Sheu, J. R., Hsiao, G., Lee, Y. M., & en, M. H. (2003). Antithrombotic Effects of Magnesium Sulfate in In Vivo Experiments. International Journal of Hematology, 77(4), 414–419. doi:10.1007/bf02982655

651 Rosique-Esteban, N., Guasch-Ferré, M., Hernández-Alonso, P., & Salas-Salvadó, J. (2018). Dietary Magnesium and Cardiovascular Disease: A Review with Emphasis in Epidemiological Studies. Nutrients, 10(2), 168. doi:10.3390/nu10020168

652 De Baaij, J. H. F., Hoenderop, J. G. J., & Bindels, R. J. M. (2015). Magnesium in Man: Implications for Health and Disease. Physiological Reviews, 95(1), 1–46. doi:10.1152/physrev.00012.2014

[653] Adeva-Andany, M. M., Martínez-Rodríguez, J., González-Lucán, M., Fernández-Fernández, C., & Castro-Quintela, E. (2019). Insulin resistance is a cardiovascular risk factor in humans. Diabetes & metabolic syndrome, 13(2), 1449–1455. https://doi.org/10.1016/j.dsx.2019.02.023

[654] DiNicolantonio, J. J., O'Keefe, J. H., & Wilson, W. (2018). Subclinical magnesium deficiency: a principal driver of cardiovascular disease and a public health crisis. Open Heart, 5(1), e000668. doi:10.1136/openhrt-2017-000668

[655] Neri, L. C., & Johansen, H. L. (1978). WATER HARDNESS AND CARDIOVASCULAR MORTALITY. Annals of the New York Academy of Sciences, 304(1 Mild Hyperten), 203–219. doi:10.1111/j.1749-6632.1978.tb25595.x

[656] Marier, J. R., Neri, L. C., Anderson, T. W. 1978. Water hardness, human health, and the importance of magnesium. Rep. ISSN 0316-0114 NRCC No. 17581 NatL Res. Counc. Canada, Ottawa, 119 pp.

[657] Galland L. (1991). Magnesium, stress and neuropsychiatric disorders. Magnesium and trace elements, 10(2-4), 287–301.

[658] Zoetman, B. C. J., Brinkmann, F. J. J. (1976) in Commission of the European Communities. 1976. Hardness of drinking water and public health. Report of a Symposium, Luxembourg 1975, pp. 173-202, Amavis, R., Hunter, W. J., Smeets, J.

[659] Masironi, R., & Shaper, A. G. (1981). Epidemiological studies of health effects of water from different sources. Annual review of nutrition, 1, 375–400. https://doi.org/10.1146/annurev.nu.01.070181.002111

[660] Guerrero-Romero, F., & Rodríguez-Morán, M. (2005). Complementary therapies for diabetes: the case for chromium, magnesium, and antioxidants. Archives of medical research, 36(3), 250–257. https://doi.org/10.1016/j.arcmed.2005.01.004

[661] A scientific review: the role of chromium in insulin resistance. (2004). The Diabetes educator, Suppl, 2–14.

[662] San Mauro-Martin, I., Ruiz-León, A. M., Camina-Martín, M. A., Garicano-Vilar, E., Collado-Yurrita, L., Mateo-Silleras, B. d., & Redondo Del Río, M. (2016). Nutricion hospitalaria, 33(1), 27. https://doi.org/10.20960/nh.v33i1.27

[663] Costello, R. B., Dwyer, J. T., & Bailey, R. L. (2016). Chromium supplements for glycemic control in type 2 diabetes: limited evidence of effectiveness. Nutrition reviews, 74(7), 455–468. https://doi.org/10.1093/nutrit/nuw011

[664] Coulston (2001) 'CHAPTER 29 - Nutritional Management for Type 2 Diabetes', Nutrition in the Prevention and Treatment of Disease, Pages 441-452.

[665] Centers for Disease Control and Prevention (2017) 'New CDC report: More than 100 million Americans have diabetes or prediabetes', CDC Newsroom Releases, Accessed Online Nov 2nd 2020: https://www.cdc.gov/media/releases/2017/p0718-diabetes-report.html

[666] Masironi, R., & Shaper, A. G. (1981). Epidemiological studies of health effects of water from different sources. Annual review of nutrition, 1, 375–400. https://doi.org/10.1146/annurev.nu.01.070181.002111

[667] Masironi, R., & Shaper, A. G. (1981). Epidemiological studies of health effects of water from different sources. Annual review of nutrition, 1, 375–400. https://doi.org/10.1146/annurev.nu.01.070181.002111

[668] Abraham, A. S., Sonnenblick, M., & Eini, M. (1982). The effect of chromium on cholesterol-induced atherosclerosis in rabbits. Atherosclerosis, 41(2-3), 371–379. doi:10.1016/0021-9150(82)90201-5

[669] Moradi et al (2021) 'A pilot study of the effects of chromium picolinate supplementation on serum fetuin-A, metabolic and inflammatory factors in patients with nonalcoholic fatty liver disease: A double-blind, placebo-controlled trial', Journal of Trace Elements in Medicine and Biology, Volume 63, January 2021, 126659.

[670] Masironi, R., & Shaper, A. G. (1981). Epidemiological studies of health effects of water from different sources. Annual review of nutrition, 1, 375–400. https://doi.org/10.1146/annurev.nu.01.070181.002111

[671] Liaugaudaite et al (2017) 'Lithium levels in the public drinking water supply and risk of suicide: A pilot study', Journal of Trace Elements in Medicine and Biology, Volume 43, September 2017, Pages 197-201.

[672] Zarse, K., Terao, T., Tian, J. et al. Low-dose lithium uptake promotes longevity in humans and metazoans. Eur J Nutr 50, 387–389 (2011). https://doi.org/10.1007/s00394-011-0171-x

[673] Masironi, R., & Shaper, A. G. (1981). Epidemiological studies of health effects of water from different sources. Annual review of nutrition, 1, 375–400. https://doi.org/10.1146/annurev.nu.01.070181.002111

[674] Dean (2017) 'Lithium in Our Tap Water Could Protect People From Dementia, New Study Suggests', Science Alert, Health, Accessed Online Nov 2nd 2020: https://www.sciencealert.com/lithium-in-our-tap-water-could-actually-protect-people-from-dementia-says-new-study

[675] Liaugaudaite, V., Mickuviene, N., Raskauskiene, N., Naginiene, R., & Sher, L. (2017). Lithium levels in the public drinking water supply and risk of suicide: A pilot study. Journal of Trace Elements in Medicine and Biology, 43, 197–201. doi:10.1016/j.jtemb.2017.03.009

[676] Cipriani et al (2005) 'Lithium in the Prevention of Suicidal Behavior and All-Cause Mortality in Patients With Mood Disorders: A Systematic Review of Randomized Trials', Am. J. Psychiatry, 162 (10) (2005), pp. 1805-1819

[677] Falhammar, H., Skov, J., Calissendorff, J., Lindh, J. D., & Mannheimer, B. (2020). Reduced risk for hospitalization due to hyponatraemia in lithium treated patients: A Swedish population-based case–control study. Journal of Psychopharmacology. https://doi.org/10.1177/0269881120937597

[678] McKnight, RF, Adida, M, Budge, K, et al. (2012) Lithium toxicity profile: A systematic review and meta-analysis. Lancet 379: 721–728.

[679] Tilkian, A. G., Schroeder, J. S., Kao, J. J., & Hultgren, H. N. (1976). The cardiovascular effects of lithium in man. A review of the literature. The American journal of medicine, 61(5), 665–670. https://doi.org/10.1016/0002-9343(76)90145-5

[680] Patorno, E., Huybrechts, K. F., Bateman, B. T., Cohen, J. M., Desai, R. J., Mogun, H., … Hernandez-Diaz, S. (2017). Lithium Use in Pregnancy and the Risk of Cardiac Malformations. New England Journal of Medicine, 376(23), 2245–2254. doi:10.1056/nejmoa1612222

[681] Ahad and Ganie (2010) 'Iodine, Iodine metabolism and Iodine deficiency disorders revisited.', Indian Journal of Endocrinology and Metabolism, 01 Jan 2010, 14(1):13-17.

682 Wang et al (2012). Thyroid-Stimulating Hormone Levels within the Reference Range Are Associated with Serum Lipid Profiles Independent of Thyroid Hormones. The Journal of Clinical Endocrinology & Metabolism, 97(8), 2724–2731. doi:10.1210/jc.2012-1133

[683] Moon (2013) 'Hypothyroidism and Metabolic Syndrome', Journal of Korean Thyroid Association 6(2):101.

[684] Wikipedia 'Iodised salt', Accessed Online Nov 2nd 2020: https://en.wikipedia.org/wiki/Iodised_salt

[685] Masironi, R., & Shaper, A. G. (1981). Epidemiological studies of health effects of water from different sources. Annual review of nutrition, 1, 375–400. https://doi.org/10.1146/annurev.nu.01.070181.002111

[686] Brazier (2018) 'Why do we have fluoride in our water?', Medical News Today, Accessed Online Nov 2nd 2020: https://www.medicalnewstoday.com/articles/154164

[687] Kim, J. K., Baker, L. A., Davarian, S., & Crimmins, E. (2013). Oral health problems and mortality. Journal of dental sciences, 8(2), 10.1016/j.jds.2012.12.011. https://doi.org/10.1016/j.jds.2012.12.011

[688] Moyer, V. A., & US Preventive Services Task Force (2014). Prevention of dental caries in children from birth through age 5 years: US Preventive Services Task Force recommendation statement. Pediatrics, 133(6), 1102–1111. https://doi.org/10.1542/peds.2014-0483

[689] National institute of Dental and Craniofacial Research (2020) 'Fluoride & Dental Health', Health Info, Accessed Online Feb 16 2021: https://www.nidcr.nih.gov/health-info/fluoride/

[690] IOM (Institute of Medicine). 2011. Advancing Oral Health in America. Washington, DC: The National Academies Press.

[691] Touger-Decker R, Radler DR, Depaola DP. Nutrition and dental medicine. In: Ross AC, Caballero B, Cousins RJ, Tucker KL, Ziegler TR, eds. Modern Nutrition in Health and Disease. 11th ed. Baltimore, MD: Lippincott Williams & Wilkins; 2014:1016-40.

[692] Rango, T., Vengosh, A., Jeuland, M., Whitford, G. M., & Tekle-Haimanot, R. (2017). Biomarkers of chronic fluoride exposure in groundwater in a highly exposed population. The Science of the total environment, 596-597, 1–11. https://doi.org/10.1016/j.scitotenv.2017.04.021

[693] Iheozor-Ejiofor, Z., Worthington, H. V., Walsh, T., O'Malley, L., Clarkson, J. E., Macey, R., Alam, R., Tugwell, P., Welch, V., & Glenny, A. M. (2015). Water fluoridation for the prevention of dental caries. The Cochrane database of systematic reviews, 2015(6), CD010856. https://doi.org/10.1002/14651858.CD010856.pub2

[694] Slade, G. D., Grider, W. B., Maas, W. R., & Sanders, A. E. (2018). Water Fluoridation and Dental Caries in U.S. Children and Adolescents. Journal of dental research, 97(10), 1122–1128. https://doi.org/10.1177/0022034518774331

[695] Slade, G. D., Sanders, A. E., Do, L., Roberts-Thomson, K., & Spencer, A. J. (2013). Effects of fluoridated drinking water on dental caries in Australian adults. Journal of dental research, 92(4), 376–382. https://doi.org/10.1177/0022034513481190

[696] Mahoney, G., Slade, G. D., Kitchener, S., & Barnett, A. (2008). Lifetime fluoridation exposure and dental caries experience in a military population. Community dentistry and oral epidemiology, 36(6), 485–492. https://doi.org/10.1111/j.1600-0528.2008.00431.x

[697] Peckham, S., & Awofeso, N. (2014). Water fluoridation: a critical review of the physiological effects of ingested fluoride as a public health intervention. TheScientificWorldJournal, 2014, 293019. https://doi.org/10.1155/2014/293019

[698] CDC (2020) 'Fluoridation Growth', Water Fluoridation Data & Statistics, Community Water Fluoridation, Accessed Online Nov 2nd 2020: https://www.cdc.gov/fluoridation/statistics/FSGrowth.htm

[699] Institute of Medicine, Food and Nutrition Board. Dietary Reference Intakes for Calcium, Phosphorus, Magnesium, Vitamin D, and Fluoride. Washington, DC: National Academies Press; 1997.

[700] U.S. Department of Health, Education, and Welfare. Public Health Service drinking water standards, revised 1962. Washington, DC: PHS Publication No. 956; 1962.

[701] U.S. Environmental Protection Agency.(2010) 'Fluoride: Exposure and Relative Source Contribution Analysis', Health and Ecological Criteria Division Office of Water, Accessed Online Feb 16 2021: https://www.epa.gov/sites/production/files/2019-03/documents/fluoride-exposure-relative-report.pdf

[702] Cressey, P., Gaw, S., & Love, J. (2010). Estimated dietary fluoride intake for New Zealanders. Journal of public health dentistry, 70(4), 327–336. https://doi.org/10.1111/j.1752-7325.2010.00192.x

[703] Tan, I., Lomasney, L., Stacy, G. S., Lazarus, M., & Mar, W. A. (2019). Spectrum of Voriconazole-Induced Periostitis With Review of the Differential Diagnosis. AJR. American journal of roentgenology, 212(1), 157–165. https://doi.org/10.2214/AJR.18.19991

[704] Barajas, M. R., McCullough, K. B., Merten, J. A., Dierkhising, R. A., Bartoo, G. T., Hashmi, S. K., Hogan, W. J., Litzow, M. R., Patnaik, M. M., Wilson, J. W., Wolf, R. C., & Wermers, R. A. (2016). Correlation of Pain and Fluoride Concentration in Allogeneic Hematopoietic Stem Cell Transplant Recipients on Voriconazole. Biology of blood and marrow transplantation : journal of the American Society for Blood and Marrow Transplantation, 22(3), 579–583. https://doi.org/10.1016/j.bbmt.2015.10.021

[705] Whitford G. M. (2011). Acute toxicity of ingested fluoride. Monographs in oral science, 22, 66–80. https://doi.org/10.1159/000325146

[706] Gutteridge, D. H., Stewart, G. O., Prince, R. L., Price, R. I., Retallack, R. W., Dhaliwal, S. S., Stuckey, B. G., Drury, P., Jones, C. E., Faulkner, D. L., Kent, G. N., Bhagat, C. I., Nicholson, G. C., & Jamrozik, K. (2002). A randomized trial of sodium fluoride (60 mg) +/- estrogen in postmenopausal osteoporotic vertebral fractures: increased vertebral fractures and peripheral bone loss with sodium fluoride; concurrent estrogen prevents peripheral loss, but not vertebral fractures. Osteoporosis international : a journal established as result of cooperation between the European Foundation for Osteoporosis and the National Osteoporosis Foundation of the USA, 13(2), 158–170. https://doi.org/10.1007/s001980200008

[707] Bhagavatula, P., Curtis, A., Broffitt, B., Weber-Gasparoni, K., Warren, J., & Levy, S. M. (2018). The relationships between fluoride intake levels and fluorosis of late-erupting permanent teeth. Journal of public health dentistry, 78(2), 165–174. https://doi.org/10.1111/jphd.12260

[708] Beltrán-Aguilar, E. D., Barker, L., & Dye, B. A. (2010). Prevalence and severity of dental fluorosis in the United States, 1999-2004. NCHS data brief, (53), 1–8.

[709] Wiener, R. C., Shen, C., Findley, P., Tan, X., & Sambamoorthi, U. (2018). Dental Fluorosis over Time: A comparison of National Health and Nutrition Examination Survey data from 2001-2002 and 2011-2012. Journal of dental hygiene : JDH, 92(1), 23–29.

[710] Waugh D. (2020). Association Between Maternal Fluoride Exposure and Child IQ. JAMA pediatrics, 174(2), 211–212. https://doi.org/10.1001/jamapediatrics.2019.5233

[711] Valdez Jiménez, L., López Guzmán, O. D., Cervantes Flores, M., Costilla-Salazar, R., Calderón Hernández, J., Alcaraz Contreras, Y., & Rocha-Amador, D. O. (2017). In utero exposure to fluoride and

563

cognitive development delay in infants. Neurotoxicology, 59, 65–70. https://doi.org/10.1016/j.neuro.2016.12.011

[712] Grandjean P. (2019). Developmental fluoride neurotoxicity: an updated review. Environmental health : a global access science source, 18(1), 110. https://doi.org/10.1186/s12940-019-0551-x

[713] Green, R., Lanphear, B., Hornung, R., Flora, D., Martinez-Mier, E. A., Neufeld, R., Ayotte, P., Muckle, G., & Till, C. (2019). Association Between Maternal Fluoride Exposure During Pregnancy and IQ Scores in Offspring in Canada. JAMA pediatrics, 173(10), 940–948. Advance online publication. https://doi.org/10.1001/jamapediatrics.2019.1729

[714] Duan, Q., Jiao, J., Chen, X., & Wang, X. (2018). Association between water fluoride and the level of children's intelligence: a dose–response meta-analysis. Public Health, 154, 87–97. doi:10.1016/j.puhe.2017.08.013

[715] Christakis, D. A. (2019). Decision to Publish Study on Maternal Fluoride Exposure During Pregnancy. JAMA Pediatrics, 173(10), 948. doi:10.1001/jamapediatrics.2019.3120

[716] National Research Council. 2006. Fluoride in Drinking Water: A Scientific Review of EPA's Standards. Washington, DC: The National Academies Press. https://doi.org/10.17226/11571.

[717] NIH (2020) 'Fluoride: Fact Sheet for Health Professionals', Accessed Online Feb 16 2021: https://ods.od.nih.gov/factsheets/Fluoride-HealthProfessional/

[718] Tubert-Jeannin, S., Auclair, C., Amsallem, E., Tramini, P., Gerbaud, L., Ruffieux, C., Schulte, A. G., Koch, M. J., Rège-Walther, M., & Ismail, A. (2011). Fluoride supplements (tablets, drops, lozenges or chewing gums) for preventing dental caries in children. The Cochrane database of systematic reviews, 2011(12), CD007592. https://doi.org/10.1002/14651858.CD007592.pub2

[719] Chou, R., Cantor, A., Zakher, B., Mitchell, J. P., & Pappas, M. (2013). Preventing dental caries in children <5 years: systematic review updating USPSTF recommendation. Pediatrics, 132(2), 332–350. https://doi.org/10.1542/peds.2013-1469

[720] APEC Water 'Silica in Drinking Water', Accessed Online Nov 2nd 2020: https://www.freedrinkingwater.com/water-education2/711-silica-water.htm

[721] Exley (2017) 'Why everyone should drink silicon-rich mineral water', Hippocratic Post, Accessed Online Nov 2nd 2020: https://www.hippocraticpost.com/nursing/why-everyone-should-drink-silicon-rich-mineral-water/

[722] Masironi, R., & Shaper, A. G. (1981). Epidemiological studies of health effects of water from different sources. Annual review of nutrition, 1, 375–400. https://doi.org/10.1146/annurev.nu.01.070181.002111

[723] Idrees, N., Tabassum, B., Abd_Allah, E. F., Hashem, A., Sarah, R., & Hashim, M. (2018). Groundwater contamination with cadmium concentrations in some West U.P. Regions, India. Saudi Journal of Biological Sciences, 25(7), 1365–1368. doi:10.1016/j.sjbs.2018.07.005

[724] Masironi, R., & Shaper, A. G. (1981). Epidemiological studies of health effects of water from different sources. Annual review of nutrition, 1, 375–400. https://doi.org/10.1146/annurev.nu.01.070181.002111

[725] Masironi, R., & Shaper, A. G. (1981). Epidemiological studies of health effects of water from different sources. Annual review of nutrition, 1, 375–400. https://doi.org/10.1146/annurev.nu.01.070181.002111

[726] Masironi, R., & Shaper, A. G. (1981). Epidemiological studies of health effects of water from different sources. Annual review of nutrition, 1, 375–400. https://doi.org/10.1146/annurev.nu.01.070181.002111

[727] Masironi, R., & Shaper, A. G. (1981). Epidemiological studies of health effects of water from different sources. Annual review of nutrition, 1, 375–400. https://doi.org/10.1146/annurev.nu.01.070181.002111

[728] NEAL, J. B., & NEAL, M. (1962). Effect of hard water and MgSO4 on rabbit atherosclerosis. Archives of pathology, 73, 400–403.

[729] Masironi, R., & Shaper, A. G. (1981). Epidemiological studies of health effects of water from different sources. Annual review of nutrition, 1, 375–400. https://doi.org/10.1146/annurev.nu.01.070181.002111

[730] Masironi, R., & Shaper, A. G. (1981). Epidemiological studies of health effects of water from different sources. Annual review of nutrition, 1, 375–400. https://doi.org/10.1146/annurev.nu.01.070181.002111

[731] Masironi, R., & Shaper, A. G. (1981). Epidemiological studies of health effects of water from different sources. Annual review of nutrition, 1, 375–400. https://doi.org/10.1146/annurev.nu.01.070181.002111

[732] Florida Energy, Water, and Air 'How Hard is the Water in Tampa, FL?', Accessed Online Nov 2 2020: https://www.myfewa.com/hard-water-tampa.html

[733] University of Bach (2014) 'The science behind the perfect coffee', Phys Org, Accessed Online Nov 2 2020: https://phys.org/news/2014-06-science-coffee.html

[734] Izaki (2014) '2014 World Barista Championship', Maruyamacoffee Co., Ltd., Japan, Accessed Online Nov 2 2020: https://www.worldbaristachampionship.org/wp-content/uploads/2015/02/2014-WBC-RANKINGS.pdf?x58757

[735] Chipperfield, B., & Chipperfield, J. R. (1977). Magnesium and the heart. American Heart Journal, 93(6), 679–682. doi:10.1016/s0002-8703(77)80061-6

[736] Héroux, O., Peter, D., & Tanner, A. (1975). Effect of a Chronic Suboptimal Intake of Magnesium on Magnesium and Calcium Content of Bone and on Bone Strength of the Rat. Canadian Journal of Physiology and Pharmacology, 53(2), 304–310. doi:10.1139/y75-043

[737] Heroux, O., Peter, D., & Heggtveit, A. (1977). Long-term effect of suboptimal dietary magnesium on magnesium and calcium contents of organs, on cold tolerance and on lifespan, and its pathological consequences in rats. The Journal of nutrition, 107(9), 1640–1652. https://doi.org/10.1093/jn/107.9.1640

[738] Kubena, K. S., & Durlach, J. (1990). Historical review of the effects of marginal intake of magnesium in chronic experimental magnesium deficiency. Magnesium research, 3(3), 219–226.

[739] Lehr, D., Chau, R., & Irene, S. (1975). Possible role of magnesium loss in the pathogenesis of myocardial fiber necrosis. Recent advances in studies on cardiac structure and metabolism, 6, 95–109.

[740] Masironi, R., & Shaper, A. G. (1981). Epidemiological studies of health effects of water from different sources. Annual review of nutrition, 1, 375–400. https://doi.org/10.1146/annurev.nu.01.070181.002111

[741] Anderson, T. W., Hewitt, D., Neri, L. C., Schreiber, G., & Talbot, F. (1973). Letter: Water hardness and magnesium in heart muscle. Lancet (London, England), 2(7842), 1390–1391. https://doi.org/10.1016/s0140-6736(73)93360-6

[742] Schwalfenberg, G. K., & Genuis, S. J. (2017). The Importance of Magnesium in Clinical Healthcare. Scientifica, 2017, 1–14. doi:10.1155/2017/4179326

[743] Greathouse, D. G., & Osborne, R. H. (1980). Preliminary report on nationwide study of drinking water and cardiovascular diseases. Journal of environmental pathology and toxicology, 4(2-3), 65–76.

[744] Hodge, A. (1981). Vitruvius, Lead Pipes and Lead Poisoning. American Journal of Archaeology, 85(4), 486 491. doi:10.2307/504874

[745] Delile, H., Blichert-Toft, J., Goiran, J. P., Keay, S., & Albarède, F. (2014). Lead in ancient Rome's city waters. Proceedings of the National Academy of Sciences of the United States of America, 111(18), 6594–6599. https://doi.org/10.1073/pnas.1400097111

[746] Nriagu J. O. (1983). Saturnine gout among Roman aristocrats. Did lead poisoning contribute to the fall of the Empire?. The New England journal of medicine, 308(11), 660–663. https://doi.org/10.1056/NEJM198303173081123

[747] GILFILLAN S. C. (1965). LEAD POISONING AND THE FALL OF ROME. Journal of occupational medicine. : official publication of the Industrial Medical Association, 7, 53–60.

[748] Lewis, J. (1985). "Lead Poisoning: A Historical Perspective". EPA Journal. 11 (4): 15–18. Accessed Online Dec 11 2020: https://archive.epa.gov/epa/aboutepa/lead-poisoning-historical-perspective.html

[749] Jackson, R. (1990). Waters and spas in the classical world. Medical History, 34(S10), 1–13. doi:10.1017/s0025727300070952

[750] Croutier AL. Taking the waters: spirit, art, sensuality. New York: Abbeville Publishing Group, 1992.

[751] Looman J, Pillen H. The development of the bathing culture [in Dutch]. Integraal1989;4:7–24..

[752] Schadewalt H. The history of Roman bathing culture [in Dutch]. Integraal1989;4:25–35..

[753] Routh, H. B., Bhowmik, K. R., Parish, L. C., & Witkowski, J. A. (1996). Balneology, mineral water, and spas in historical perspective. Clinics in dermatology, 14(6), 551–554. https://doi.org/10.1016/s0738-081x(96)00083-1

[754] Palmer, R. (1990). "In this our lightye and learned tyme": Italian baths in the era of the Renaissance. Medical History, 34(S10), 14-22. doi:10.1017/S0025727300070964

[755] Brockliss, L. W. B. (1990). The development of the spa in seventeenth-century France. Medical History, 34(S10), 23–47. doi:10.1017/s0025727300070976

[756] Bouchard (2009) 'Epsom Spa', Epsom and Ewell History Explorer, Accessed Online: https://eehe.org.uk/?p=31208

[757] Bouchard (2009) 'Epsom Spa', Epsom and Ewell History Explorer, Accessed Online: https://eehe.org.uk/?p=31208

[758] Epsom Salt Council 'What is Epsom salt?', Accessed Online: https://www.epsomsaltcouncil.org/about/

[759] Sukenik, S., Neumann, L., Buskila, D., Kleiner-Baumgarten, A., Zimlichman, S., & Horowitz, J. (1990). Dead Sea bath salts for the treatment of rheumatoid arthritis. Clinical and experimental rheumatology, 8(4), 353–357.

[760] Elkayam, O., Wigler, I., Tishler, M., Rosenblum, I., Caspi, D., Segal, R., Fishel, B., & Yaron, M. (1991). Effect of spa therapy in Tiberias on patients with rheumatoid arthritis and osteoarthritis. The Journal of rheumatology, 18(12), 1799–1803.

[761] Sukenik, S., Buskila, D., Neumann, L., Kleiner-Baumgarten, A., Zimlichman, S., & Horowitz, J. (1990). Sulphur bath and mud pack treatment for rheumatoid arthritis at the Dead Sea area. Annals of the Rheumatic Diseases, 49(2), 99–102. doi:10.1136/ard.49.2.99

[762] van Tubergen, A., Landewé, R., van der Heijde, D., Hidding, A., Wolter, N., Asscher, M., Falkenbach, A., Genth, E., Thè, H. G., & van der Linden, S. (2001). Combined spa-exercise therapy is effective in patients with ankylosing spondylitis: a randomized controlled trial. Arthritis and rheumatism, 45(5), 430–438. https://doi.org/10.1002/1529-0131(200110)45:5<430::aid-art362>3.0.co;2-f

[763] Gröber, U., Werner, T., Vormann, J., & Kisters, K. (2017). Myth or Reality—Transdermal Magnesium? Nutrients, 9(8), 813. doi:10.3390/nu9080813

[764] Borzelleca (2000) 'Paracelsus: Herald of Modern Toxicology', Toxicological Sciences, Volume 53, Issue 1, January 2000, Pages 2–4, https://doi.org/10.1093/toxsci/53.1.2

[765] Habashi (2015) 'Discovering the 8th Metal: A History of Zinc', International Zinc Association (IZA), www.zincworld.org, Accessed Online Nov 10 2020: https://web.archive.org/web/20150606210821/http://www.zinc.org/general/ZP-Discovering_the_8th_Metal1.pdf

[766] Pagel (1986) 'Paracelsus: An Introduction to Philosophical Medicine in the Era of the Renaissance', Journal of the History of Biology 19 (1):162-166.

[767] Paracelsus, De 9 Bächer De Natura rerum; Sudhoff, Paracelsus Werke, I/11:319.

[768] Hamlin, C. (2009). Paracelsus: Medicine, Magic and Mission at the End of Time. JAMA, 301(12), 1288. doi:10.1001/jama.2009.395

[769] Heywood, A. (1990). A trial of the Bath Waters: the treatment of lead poisoning. Medical History, 34(S10), 82–101. doi:10.1017/s0025727300071015

[770] O'Hare, J. P., Heywood, A., Summerhayes, C., Lunn, G., Evans, J. M., Walters, G., … Dieppe, P. A. (1985). Observations on the effect of immersion in Bath spa water. BMJ, 291(6511), 1747–1751. doi:10.1136/bmj.291.6511.1747

[771] Wikipedia (2020) 'Spa, Belgium', Accessed Online November 2nd 2020: https://en.wikipedia.org/wiki/Spa,_Belgium

[772] Thermes de Spa 'THE DIFFERENT KINDS OF WATER', Accessed Online: https://www.thermesdespa.com/all-about-spa-water/

[773] Rosanoff, A. (2013). The high heart health value of drinking-water magnesium. Medical Hypotheses, 81(6), 1063–1065. doi:10.1016/j.mehy.2013.10.003

[774] O'Hare, J. P., Heywood, A., Summerhayes, C., Lunn, G., Evans, J. M., Walters, G., … Dieppe, P. A. (1985). Observations on the effect of immersion in Bath spa water. BMJ, 291(6511), 1747–1751. doi:10.1136/bmj.291.6511.1747

[775] Glenkeir Whiskies Ltd (2018) 'Rachel Barrie & The Three Distilleries', The Whiskey Shop, Accessed Online Dec 17 2020: https://www.whiskyshop.com/blog/rachel-barrie

[776] Rose (2019) 'The US drinking water supply is mostly safe, but that's not good enough', The Conversation, Accessed Online Dec 11 2020: https://theconversation.com/the-us-drinking-water-supply-is-mostly-safe-but-thats-not-good-enough-115028

[777] CDC (2016) 'Magnitude & Burden of Waterborne Disease in the U.S.', Publications, Data, & Statistics, Accessed Online Dec 11 2020: https://www.cdc.gov/healthywater/burden/index.html

[778] Arthur (2018) "Bottled water is America's favorite drink!' Bottled water takes top spot in US', Beverage Daily, Accesse Online Dec 11 2020: https://www.beveragedaily.com/Article/2018/06/01/Bottled-water-takes-top-spot-in-US-in-2017

[779] Mineral Calculator, San Pellegrino, Compare Waters, Accessed Online Dec 11 2020: https://www.mineral-calculator.com/compare-waters/2203/

[780] Britton, E., & McLaughlin, J. (2013). Ageing and the gut. Proceedings of the Nutrition Society, 72(1), 173-177. doi:10.1017/S0029665112002807

[781] Iwai, W., Abe, Y., Iijima, K. et al. Gastric hypochlorhydria is associated with an exacerbation of dyspeptic symptoms in female patients. J Gastroenterol 48, 214–221 (2013). https://doi.org/10.1007/s00535-012-0634-8

[782] G C Sturniolo, M C Montino, L Rossetto, A Martin, R D'Inca, A D'Odorico & R Naccarato (1991) Inhibition of gastric acid secretion reduces zinc absorption in man., Journal of the American College of Nutrition, 10:4, 372-375, DOI: 10.1080/07315724.1991.10718165

[783] Miyata S. (2007). Nihon Ronen Igakkai zasshi. Japanese journal of geriatrics, 44(6), 677–689.

[784] Ishchenko, N. V., Nikitin, A. V., Verikovskiĭ, V. A., & Mordasova, V. I. (2007). Voprosy kurortologii, fizioterapii, i lechebnoi fizicheskoi kultury, (6), 29–30.

[785] BERTONI, M., OLIVERI, F., MANGHETTI, M., BOCCOLINI, E., BELLOMINI, M. G., BLANDIZZI, C., … DEL TACCA, M. (2002). EFFECTS OF A BICARBONATE-ALKALINE MINERAL WATER ON GASTRIC FUNCTIONS AND FUNCTIONAL DYSPEPSIA: A PRECLINICAL AND CLINICAL STUDY. Pharmacological Research, 46(6), 525–531. doi:10.1016/s1043661802002323

[786] Bortolotti, M., Turba, E., Mari, C., Lopilato, C., Porrazzo, G., Scalabrino, A., & Miglioli, M. (1999). Modificazioni indotte da un'acqua minerale sulla motilità gastrointestinale di pazienti con dispepsia cronica idiopatica [Changes caused by mineral water on gastrointestinal motility in patients with chronic idiopathic dyspepsia]. Minerva medica, 90(5-6), 187–194.

[787] Bortolotti, M., Turba, E., Mari, C., Lopilato, S., Scalabrino, A., & Miglioli, M. (1999). Effect of a mineral water on gastric emptying of patients with idiopathic dyspepsia. International journal of clinical pharmacology research, 19(2), 53–56.

[788] Nakajima, A., Shinbo, K., Oota, A., & Kinoshita, Y. (2019). Polyethylene glycol 3350 plus electrolytes for chronic constipation: a 2-week, randomized, double-blind, placebo-controlled study with a 52-week open-label extension. Journal of gastroenterology, 54(9), 792–803. https://doi.org/10.1007/s00535-019-01581-x

[789] Anti, M., Lippi, M. E., Santarelli, L., Gabrielli, M., Gasbarrini, A., & Gasbarrini, G. (2004). Effects of mineral-water supplementation on gastric emptying of solids in patients with functional dyspepsia assessed with the 13C-octanoic-acid breath test. Hepato-gastroenterology, 51(60), 1856–1859.

[790] Dupont, C., Constant, F., Imbert, A., Hébert, G., Zourabichvili, O., & Kapel, N. (2019). Time to treatment response of a magnesium- and sulphate-rich natural mineral water in functional constipation. Nutrition (Burbank, Los Angeles County, Calif.), 65, 167–172. https://doi.org/10.1016/j.nut.2019.02.018

[791] Dupont, C., Campagne, A., & Constant, F. (2014). Efficacy and safety of a magnesium sulfate-rich natural mineral water for patients with functional constipation. Clinical gastroenterology and hepatology : the official clinical practice journal of the American Gastroenterological Association, 12(8), 1280–1287. https://doi.org/10.1016/j.cgh.2013.12.005

[792] Bothe, G., Coh, A., & Auinger, A. (2015). Efficacy and safety of a natural mineral water rich in magnesium and sulphate for bowel function: a double-blind, randomized, placebo-controlled study. European Journal of Nutrition, 56(2), 491–499. doi:10.1007/s00394-015-1094-8

[793] Naumann, J., Sadaghiani, C., Alt, F., & Huber, R. (2016). Effects of Sulfate-Rich Mineral Water on Functional Constipation: A Double-Blind, Randomized, Placebo-Controlled Study. Forschende Komplementarmedizin (2006), 23(6), 356–363. https://doi.org/10.1159/000449436

[794] Kaĭsinova, A. S., Osipov, I., Litvinova, M. A., & Prosol'chenko, A. V. (2011). Voprosy kurortologii, fizioterapii, i lechebnoi fizicheskoi kultury, (2), 34–36.

[795] Baroni, S., Marazziti, D., Consoli, G., Picchetti, M., Catena-Dell'Osso, M., & Galassi, A. (2012). Modulation of the platelet serotonin transporter by thermal balneotherapy: a study in healthy subjects. European review for medical and pharmacological sciences, 16(5), 589–593.

[796] Polushina, N. D., Babina, L. M., & Shvedunova, L. N. (1994). Vliianie pit'evykh mineral'nykh vod na gormonal'nyĭ i psikhologicheskiĭ statusy (éksperimental'no-klinicheskoe issledovanie) [The effect of potable mineral waters on the hormonal and psychological status (experimental and clinical research)]. Voprosy kurortologii, fizioterapii, i lechebnoi fizicheskoi kultury, (2), 4–6.

[797] Govers, M. J., Termont, D. S., Lapré, J. A., Kleibeuker, J. H., Vonk, R. J., & Van der Meer, R. (1996). Calcium in milk products precipitates intestinal fatty acids and secondary bile acids and thus inhibits colonic cytotoxicity in humans. Cancer research, 56(14), 3270–3275.

[798] Couzy, F., Kastenmayer, P., Vigo, M., Clough, J., Munoz-Box, R., & Barclay, D. V. (1995). Calcium bioavailability from a calcium- and sulfate-rich mineral water, compared with milk, in young adult women. The American Journal of Clinical Nutrition, 62(6), 1239–1244. doi:10.1093/ajcn/62.6.1239

[799] Heaney, R. P., & Dowell, M. S. (1994). Absorbability of the calcium in a high-calcium mineral water. Osteoporosis International, 4(6), 323–324. doi:10.1007/bf01622191

[800] Grassi, M., Fraioli, A., Messina, B., Di Giulio, E., & Fragassi, G. (1988). Valutazione endoscopica e clinica dell'azione terapeutica di un'acqua bicarbonato-calcica in gastroduodenitici [Endoscopic and clinical evaluation of the therapeutic action of a bicarbonate-calcium mineral water in patients with gastroduodenitis]. La Clinica terapeutica, 126(2), 123–130.

[801] Caudarella and Vescini (2001) 'The role of some ion-containing mineral waters in the pathogenesis of common chronic diseases', Rivista Italiana di Biologia e Medicina 21(3):76-91

[802] Toxqui, L., & Vaquero, M. (2016). An Intervention with Mineral Water Decreases Cardiometabolic Risk Biomarkers. A Crossover, Randomised, Controlled Trial with Two Mineral Waters in Moderately Hypercholesterolaemic Adults. Nutrients, 8(7), 400. doi:10.3390/nu8070400

[803] Schoppen, S., Pérez-Granados, A. M., Carbajal, Á., Sarriá, B., Sánchez-Muniz, F. J., Gómez-Gerique, J. A., & Vaquero, M. P. (2005). Sodium bicarbonated mineral water decreases postprandial lipaemia in postmenopausal women compared to a low mineral water. British Journal of Nutrition, 94(4), 582–587. doi:10.1079/bjn20051515

[804] Toxqui, L., Pérez-Granados, A. M., Blanco-Rojo, R., & Vaquero, M. P. (2012). A sodium-bicarbonated mineral water reduces gallbladder emptying and postprandial lipaemia: a randomised four-way crossover study. European journal of nutrition, 51(5), 607–614. https://doi.org/10.1007/s00394-011-0244-x

[805] Zair, Y., Kasbi-Chadli, F., Housez, B., Pichelin, M., Cazaubiel, M., Raoux, F., & Ouguerram, K. (2013). Effect of a high bicarbonate mineral water on fasting and postprandial lipemia in moderately hypercholesterolemic subjects: a pilot study. Lipids in health and disease, 12, 105. https://doi.org/10.1186/1476-511X-12-105

[806] Quarto, G., Amato, B., Serra, R., Benassai, G., Monti, M. G., Salzano, A., D'Assante, R., & Furino, E. (2017). The effects of Crenotherapy and exercise in peripheral arterial occlusive disease. A comparison with simple exercise training. Annali italiani di chirurgia, 88, 469–477.

[807] Garg et al (2011) 'Low-salt diet increases insulin resistance in healthy subjects', Metabolism, Volume 60, Issue 7, July 2011, Pages 965-968.

[808] Garg, R., Sun, B., & Williams, J. (2014). Effect of low salt diet on insulin resistance in salt-sensitive versus salt-resistant hypertension. Hypertension (Dallas, Tex. : 1979), 64(6), 1384–1387. https://doi.org/10.1161/HYPERTENSIONAHA.114.03880

[809] Alland, A., & Vague, P. (1974). Vers une meilleure connaissance du mécanisme d'action de la cure thermale bicarbonatée sodique de Vals-les-Bains dans le diabète [Towards a better knowledge of the

action mechanism of thermal sodium bicarbonate therapy at Vals-les-Bains in diabetes]. Semaine des hopitaux. Therapeutique, 50(4), 291–295.

[810] Naumann, J., Biehler, D., Lüty, T., & Sadaghiani, C. (2017). Prevention and Therapy of Type 2 Diabetes-What Is the Potential of Daily Water Intake and Its Mineral Nutrients?. Nutrients, 9(8), 914. https://doi.org/10.3390/nu9080914

[811] Schoppen, S., Sánchez-Muniz, F. J., Pérez-Granados, M., Gómez-Gerique, J. A., Sarriá, B., Navas-Carretero, S., & Pilar Vaquero, M. (2007). Does bicarbonated mineral water rich in sodium change insulin sensitivity of postmenopausal women?. Nutricion hospitalaria, 22(5), 538–544.

[812] Donovan, D. S., Solomon, C. G., Seely, E. W., Williams, G. H., & Simonson, D. C. (1993). Effect of sodium intake on insulin sensitivity. American Journal of Physiology-Endocrinology and Metabolism, 264(5), E730–E734. doi:10.1152/ajpendo.1993.264.5.e730

[813] Fioravanti, A., Cantarini, L., Bacarelli, M. R., de Lalla, A., Ceccatelli, L., & Blardi, P. (2011). Effects of spa therapy on serum leptin and adiponectin levels in patients with knee osteoarthritis. Rheumatology international, 31(7), 879–882. https://doi.org/10.1007/s00296-010-1401-x

[814] SUZUKI, M., MURA, E., TANIGUCHI, A., MORITANI, T., & NAGAI, N. (2017). Oral Carbonation Attenuates Feeling of Hunger and Gastric Myoelectrical Activity in Young Women. Journal of Nutritional Science and Vitaminology, 63(3), 186–192. doi:10.3177/jnsv.63.186

[815] WAKISAKA, S., NAGAI, H., MURA, E., MATSUMOTO, T., MORITANI, T., & NAGAI, N. (2012). The Effects of Carbonated Water upon Gastric and Cardiac Activities and Fullness in Healthy Young Women. Journal of Nutritional Science and Vitaminology, 58(5), 333–338. doi:10.3177/jnsv.58.333

[816] Greupner, T., Schneider, I., & Hahn, A. (2017). Calcium Bioavailability from Mineral Waters with Different Mineralization in Comparison to Milk and a Supplement. Journal of the American College of Nutrition, 36(5), 386–390. doi:10.1080/07315724.2017.1299651

[817] Santos, A., Martins, M. J., Guimarães, J. T., Severo, M., & Azevedo, I. (2010). Sodium-rich carbonated natural mineral water ingestion and blood pressure. Revista portuguesa de cardiologia : orgao oficial da Sociedade Portuguesa de Cardiologia = Portuguese journal of cardiology : an official journal of the Portuguese Society of Cardiology, 29(2), 159–172.

[818] Luft, F. C., Zemel, M. B., Sowers, J. A., Fineberg, N. S., & Weinberger, M. H. (1990). Sodium bicarbonate and sodium chloride: effects on blood pressure and electrolyte homeostasis in normal and hypertensive man. Journal of hypertension, 8(7), 663–670. https://doi.org/10.1097/00004872-199007000-00010

[819] Toxqui, L., & Vaquero, M. P. (2016). Aldosterone changes after consumption of a sodium-bicarbonated mineral water in humans. A four-way randomized controlled trial. Journal of physiology and biochemistry, 72(4), 635–641. https://doi.org/10.1007/s13105-016-0502-8

[820] Rylander, R., & Arnaud, M. J. (2004). Mineral water intake reduces blood pressure among subjects with low urinary magnesium and calcium levels. BMC Public Health, 4(1). doi:10.1186/1471-2458-4-56

[821] Yuan, D., Yu, Z. X., Wang, W., & Chen, Y. (2019). Head-out immersion in natural thermal mineral water for the management of hypertension: a review of randomized controlled trials. International journal of biometeorology, 63(12), 1707–1718. https://doi.org/10.1007/s00484-019-01780-4

[822] Rapolienė, L., Razbadauskas, A., & Jurgelėnas, A. (2015). The Reduction of Distress Using Therapeutic Geothermal Water Procedures in a Randomized Controlled Clinical Trial. Advances in Preventive Medicine, 2015, 1–10. doi:10.1155/2015/749417

[823] Johansson B. (2009). Effects of functional water on heart rate, heart rate variability, and salivary immunoglobulin a in healthy humans: a pilot study. Journal of alternative and complementary medicine (New York, N.Y.), 15(8), 871–877. https://doi.org/10.1089/acm.2008.0336

[824] Buehlmeier, J., Remer, T., Frings-Meuthen, P., Maser-Gluth, C., & Heer, M. (2016). Glucocorticoid activity and metabolism with NaCl-induced low-grade metabolic acidosis and oral alkalization: results of two randomized controlled trials. Endocrine, 52(1), 139–147. https://doi.org/10.1007/s12020-015-0730-7

[825] Montagna and Parakkal (1974) 'The eccrine-sweat glands. The Structure and Function of the Skin. New York, Academic Press, pp. 366-411.

[826] Montagna and Parakkal (1974) 'The apocrine-s weat glands'. The Structure and Function of the Skin. New York, Academic Press, pp. 332-365.

[827] Forestier, R. J., Briancon, G., Francon, A., Erol, F. B., & Mollard, J. M. (2014). Balneohydrotherapy in the treatment of chronic venous insufficiency. Vasa, 43(5), 365–371. doi:10.1024/0301-1526/a000374

[828] L'vova, N. V., Tupitsyna, I., Badalov, N. G., Krasnikov, V. E., & Lebedeva, O. D. (2013). Voprosy kurortologii, fizioterapii, i lechebnoi fizicheskoi kultury, (6), 14–17.

[829] Benedetti, S., Benvenuti, F., Nappi, G., Fortunati, N. A., Marino, L., Aureli, T., … Canestrari, F. (2007). Antioxidative effects of sulfurous mineral water: protection against lipid and protein oxidation. European Journal of Clinical Nutrition, 63(1), 106–112. doi:10.1038/sj.ejcn.1602892

[830] Poteriaeva, E. L., Ivashchenko, I. E., Logvinenko, I. I., Nesina, I. A., Erzin, D. A., & Perminova, I. I. (2007). Meditsina truda i promyshlennaia ekologiia, (4), 18–22.

[831] Cristalli, G., Abramo, A., & Pollastrini, L. (1996). Trattamento delle flogosi croniche delle vie aeree superiori con crenoterapia inalatoria solfureo-solfato-bicarbonato-carbonica-alcalinoterrosa: studio della

citologia nasale [Treatment of chronic inflammation of the upper respiratory airways by inhalation thermal therapy with sulfur-sulfate-bicarbonate- carbonate-alkaline earth mineral water: a study of nasal cytology]. Acta otorhinolaryngologica Italica : organo ufficiale della Societa italiana di otorinolaringologia e chirurgia cervico-facciale, 16(6 Suppl 55), 91–94.

[832] Keller, S., König, V., & Mösges, R. (2014). Thermal Water Applications in the Treatment of Upper Respiratory Tract Diseases: A Systematic Review and Meta-Analysis. Journal of Allergy, 2014, 1–17. doi:10.1155/2014/943824

[833] Mesropian, S. K., Kaïsinova, A. S., Stanilevich, T. B., & Ter-Akopov, N. G. (2010). Voprosy kurortologii, fizioterapii, i lechebnoi fizicheskoi kultury, (1), 18–20.

[834] Passali, D., Lauriello, M., Passali, G. C., Passali, F. M., Cassano, M., Cassano, P., & Bellussi, L. (2008). Studio clinico per la valutazione dell'effi cacia terapeutica dello spray nasale con acqua termale salsobromoiodica isotonica delle Terme di Salsomaggiore nel trattamento delle patologie rinosinusali [Clinical evaluation of the efficacy of Salsomaggiore (Italy) thermal water in the treatment of rhinosinusal pathologies]. La Clinica terapeutica, 159(3), 181–188.

[835] Ottaviano, G., Marioni, G., Staffieri, C., Giacomelli, L., Marchese-Ragona, R., Bertolin, A., & Staffieri, A. (2011). Effects of sulfurous, salty, bromic, iodic thermal water nasal irrigations in nonallergic chronic rhinosinusitis: a prospective, randomized, double-blind, clinical, and cytological study. American Journal of Otolaryngology, 32(3), 235–239. doi:10.1016/j.amjoto.2010.02.004

[836] Salami, A. (2010). Sulphurous thermal water inhalations in the treatment of chronic rhinosinusitis. Rhinology Journal, 48(1). doi:10.4193/rhin09.065

[837] Del Giudice, M. M., Decimo, F., Maiello, N., Leonardi, S., Parisi, G., Golluccio, M., … Ciprandi, G. (2011). Effectiveness of Ischia Thermal Water Nasal Aerosol in Children with Seasonal Allergic Rhinitis: A Randomized and Controlled Study. International Journal of Immunopathology and Pharmacology, 24(4), 1103–1109. doi:10.1177/039463201102400431

[838] Mac-Mary, S., Creidi, P., Marsaut, D., Courderot-Masuyer, C., Cochet, V., Gharbi, T., … Humbert, P. (2006). Assessment of effects of an additional dietary natural mineral water uptake on skin hydration in healthy subjects by dynamic barrier function measurements and clinic scoring. Skin Research and Technology, 12(3), 199–205. doi:10.1111/j.0909-752x.2006.00160.x

[839] Ferreira, M. O., Costa, P. C., & Bahia, M. F. (2010). Effect of São Pedro do Sul thermal water on skin irritation. International journal of cosmetic science, 32(3), 205–210. https://doi.org/10.1111/j.1468-2494.2010.00527.x

[840] Barolet, D., Lussier, I., Mery, S., & Merial-Kieny, C. (2009). Beneficial effects of spraying low mineral content thermal spring water after fractional photothermolysis in patients with dermal melasma. Journal of cosmetic dermatology, 8(2), 114–118. https://doi.org/10.1111/j.1473-2165.2009.00432.x

[841] Kubota, K., Machida, I., Tamura, K., Take, H., Kurabayashi, H., Akiba, T., & Tamura, J. (1997). Treatment of refractory cases of atopic dermatitis with acidic hot-spring bathing. Acta dermato-venereologica, 77(6), 452–454. https://doi.org/10.2340/0001555577452454

[842] Bak, J.-P., Kim, Y.-M., Son, J., Kim, C.-J., & Kim, E.-H. (2012). Application of concentrated deep sea water inhibits the development of atopic dermatitis-like skin lesions in NC/Nga mice. BMC Complementary and Alternative Medicine, 12(1). doi:10.1186/1472-6882-12-108

[843] Boer, J. (1996). The influence of mineral water solutions in phototherapy. Clinics in Dermatology, 14(6), 665–673. doi:10.1016/s0738-081x(96)00102-2

[844] Matceyevsky, D., Hahoshen, N. Y., Vexler, A., Noam, A., Khafif, A., & Ben-Yosef, R. (2007). Assessing the effectiveness of Dead Sea products as prophylactic agents for acute radiochemotherapy-induced skin and mucosal toxicity in patients with head and neck cancers: a phase 2 study. The Israel Medical Association journal : IMAJ, 9(6), 439–442.

[845] Katz, U., Shoenfeld, Y., Zakin, V., Sherer, Y., & Sukenik, S. (2012). Scientific Evidence of the Therapeutic Effects of Dead Sea Treatments: A Systematic Review. Seminars in Arthritis and Rheumatism, 42(2), 186–200. doi:10.1016/j.semarthrit.2012.02.006

[846] Hannon, M. J., & Verbalis, J. G. (2014). Sodium homeostasis and bone. Current Opinion in Nephrology and Hypertension, 23(4), 370–376. doi:10.1097/01.mnh.0000447022.51722.f4

[847] Loi, A., Lisci, S., Denotti, A., & Cauli, A. (2013). Bone mineral density in women on long-term mud-bath therapy in a Salus per Aquam (SPA) environment. Reumatismo, 65(3). doi:10.4081/reumatismo.2013.121

[848] Meunier, P. J., Jenvrin, C., Munoz, F., de la Gueronnière, V., Garnero, P., & Menz, M. (2005). Consumption of a high calcium mineral water lowers biochemical indices of bone remodeling in postmenopausal women with low calcium intake. Osteoporosis International, 16(10), 1203–1209. doi:10.1007/s00198-004-1828-6

[849] Wynn, E., Krieg, M. A., Aeschlimann, J. M., & Burckhardt, P. (2009). Alkaline mineral water lowers bone resorption even in calcium sufficiency: alkaline mineral water and bone metabolism. Bone, 44(1), 120–124. https://doi.org/10.1016/j.bone.2008.09.007

[850] Guillemant, J., Le, H.-T., Accarie, C., du Montcel, S. T., Delabroise, A.-M., Arnaud, M. J., & Guillemant, S. (2000). Mineral water as a source of dietary calcium: acute effects on parathyroid function

and bone resorption in young men. The American Journal of Clinical Nutrition, 71(4), 999–1002. doi:10.1093/ajcn/71.4.999

[851] Schoppen, S., Pérez-Granados, A. M., Carbajal, A., Sarriá, B., Navas-Carretero, S., & Pilar Vaquero, M. (2008). Sodium-bicarbonated mineral water decreases aldosterone levels without affecting urinary excretion of bone minerals. International journal of food sciences and nutrition, 59(4), 347–355. https://doi.org/10.1080/09637480701560308

[852] Pérez-Fernández, M. R., Calvo-Ayuso, N., Martínez-Reglero, C., Salgado-Barreira, Á., & Muiño López-Álvarez, J. L. (2019). Efficacy of baths with mineral-medicinal water in patients with fibromyalgia: a randomized clinical trial. International journal of biometeorology, 63(9), 1161–1170. https://doi.org/10.1007/s00484-019-01729-7

[853] Bazzichi, L., Da Valle, Y., Rossi, A., Giacomelli, C., Sernissi, F., Giannaccini, G., Betti, L., Ciregia, F., Giusti, L., Scarpellini, P., Dell'Osso, L., Marazziti, D., Bombardieri, S., & Lucacchini, A. (2013). A multidisciplinary approach to study the effects of balneotherapy and mud-bath therapy treatments on fibromyalgia. Clinical and experimental rheumatology, 31(6 Suppl 79), S111–S120.

[854] Maeda, T., Kudo, Y., Horiuchi, T., & Makino, N. (2017). Clinical and anti-aging effect of mud-bathing therapy for patients with fibromyalgia. Molecular and Cellular Biochemistry, 444(1-2), 87–92. doi:10.1007/s11010-017-3233-4

[855] Bagis, S., Karabiber, M., As, I., Tamer, L., Erdogan, C., & Atalay, A. (2013). Is magnesium citrate treatment effective on pain, clinical parameters and functional status in patients with fibromyalgia?. Rheumatology international, 33(1), 167–172. https://doi.org/10.1007/s00296-011-2334-8

[856] Lindberg, J. S., Zobitz, M. M., Poindexter, J. R., & Pak, C. Y. (1990). Magnesium bioavailability from magnesium citrate and magnesium oxide. Journal of the American College of Nutrition, 9(1), 48–55. https://doi.org/10.1080/07315724.1990.10720349

[857] Karagülle, O., Kleczka, T., Vidal, C., Candir, F., Gundermann, G., Külpmann, W. R., ... Gutenbrunner, C. (2006). Magnesium Absorption from Mineral Waters of Different Magnesium Content in Healthy Subjects. Complementary Medicine Research, 13(1), 9–14. doi:10.1159/000090016

[858] Verhas, M., de La Guéronnière, V., Grognet, J.-M., Paternot, J., Hermanne, A., Van den Winkel, P., ... Rayssiguier, Y. (2002). Magnesium bioavailability from mineral water. A study in adult men. European Journal of Clinical Nutrition, 56(5), 442–447. doi:10.1038/sj.ejcn.1601333

[859] Sabatier, M., Arnaud, M. J., Kastenmayer, P., Rytz, A., & Barclay, D. V. (2002). Meal effect on magnesium bioavailability from mineral water in healthy women. The American journal of clinical nutrition, 75(1), 65–71. https://doi.org/10.1093/ajcn/75.1.65

[860] Sabatier, M., Grandvuillemin, A., Kastenmayer, P., Aeschliman, J.-M., Bouisset, F., Arnaud, M. J., ... Berthelot, A. (2011). Influence of the consumption pattern of magnesium from magnesium-rich mineral water on magnesium bioavailability. British Journal of Nutrition, 106(3), 331–334. doi:10.1017/s0007114511001139

[861] Chary-Valckenaere, I., Loeuille, D., Jay, N., Kohler, F., Tamisier, J. N., Roques, C. F., Boulange, M., & Gay, G. (2018). Spa therapy together with supervised self-mobilisation improves pain, function and quality of life in patients with chronic shoulder pain: a single-blind randomised controlled trial. International journal of biometeorology, 62(6), 1003–1014. https://doi.org/10.1007/s00484-018-1502-x

[862] Huber, D., Grafetstätter, C., Proßegger, J., Pichler, C., Wöll, E., Fischer, M., Dürl, M., Geiersperger, K., Höcketstaller, M., Frischhut, S., Ritter, M., & Hartl, A. (2019). Green exercise and mg-ca-SO4 thermal balneotherapy for the treatment of non-specific chronic low back pain: a randomized controlled clinical trial. BMC musculoskeletal disorders, 20(1), 221. https://doi.org/10.1186/s12891-019-2582-4

[863] Gáti, T., Tefner, I. K., Kovács, L., Hodosi, K., & Bender, T. (2018). The effects of the calcium-magnesium-bicarbonate content in thermal mineral water on chronic low back pain: a randomized, controlled follow-up study. International journal of biometeorology, 62(5), 897–905. https://doi.org/10.1007/s00484-017-1491-1

[864] Tefner, I. K., Németh, A., Lászlófi, A., Kis, T., Gyetvai, G., & Bender, T. (2012). The effect of spa therapy in chronic low back pain: a randomized controlled, single-blind, follow-up study. Rheumatology international, 32(10), 3163–3169. https://doi.org/10.1007/s00296-011-2145-y

[865] Kulisch, , Bender, T., Németh, A., & Szekeres, L. (2009). Effect of thermal water and adjunctive electrotherapy on chronic low back pain: A double-blind, randomized, follow-up study. Journal of Rehabilitation Medicine, 41(1), 73–79. doi:10.2340/16501977-0291

[866] Hanzel, A., Berényi, K., Horváth, K., Szendi, K., Németh, B., & Varga, C. (2019). Evidence for the therapeutic effect of the organic content in Szigetvár thermal water on osteoarthritis: a double-blind, randomized, controlled clinical trial. International journal of biometeorology, 63(4), 449–458. https://doi.org/10.1007/s00484-019-01676-3

[867] Hanzel, A., Horvát, K., Molics, B., Berényi, K., Németh, B., Szendi, K., & Varga, C. (2018). Clinical improvement of patients with osteoarthritis using thermal mineral water at Szigetvár Spa-results of a randomised double-blind controlled study. International journal of biometeorology, 62(2), 253–259. https://doi.org/10.1007/s00484-017-1446-6

[868] Kovács, C., Bozsik, Á., Pecze, M., Borbély, I., Fogarasi, A., Kovács, L., Tefner, I. K., & Bender, T. (2016). Effects of sulfur bath on hip osteoarthritis: a randomized, controlled, single-blind, follow-up trial: a pilot study. International journal of biometeorology, 60(11), 1675–1680. https://doi.org/10.1007/s00484-016-1158-3

[869] Kovács, C., Pecze, M., Tihanyi, Á., Kovács, L., Balogh, S., & Bender, T. (2012). The effect of sulphurous water in patients with osteoarthritis of hand. Double-blind, randomized, controlled follow-up study. Clinical Rheumatology, 31(10), 1437–1442. doi:10.1007/s10067-012-2026-0

[870] Horváth, K., Kulisch, Á., Németh, A., & Bender, T. (2011). Evaluation of the effect of balneotherapy in patients with osteoarthritis of the hands: a randomized controlled single-blind follow-up study. Clinical Rehabilitation, 26(5), 431–441. doi:10.1177/0269215511425961

[871] Verhagen, A. P., Bierma-Zeinstra, S. M., Boers, M., Cardoso, J. R., Lambeck, J., De Bie, R., & De Vet, H. C. (2015). Balneotherapy (or spa therapy) for rheumatoid arthritis. An abridged version of Cochrane Systematic Review. European journal of physical and rehabilitation medicine, 51(6), 833–847.

[872] Bender, T., Bálint, G., Prohászka, Z., Géher, P., & Tefner, I. K. (2013). Evidence-based hydro- and balneotherapy in Hungary—a systematic review and meta-analysis. International Journal of Biometeorology, 58(3), 311–323. doi:10.1007/s00484-013-0667-6

[873] Fraioli, A., Serio, A., Mennuni, G., Ceccarelli, F., Petraccia, L., Fontana, M., ... Valesini, G. (2010). A study on the efficacy of treatment with mud packs and baths with Sillene mineral water (Chianciano Spa Italy) in patients suffering from knee osteoarthritis. Rheumatology International, 31(10), 1333–1340. doi:10.1007/s00296-010-1475-5

[874] Cantarini, L., Leo, G., Giannitti, C., Cevenini, G., Barberini, P., & Fioravanti, A. (2007). Therapeutic effect of spa therapy and short wave therapy in knee osteoarthritis: a randomized, single blind, controlled trial. Rheumatology international, 27(6), 523–529. https://doi.org/10.1007/s00296-006-0266-5

[875] Fioravanti, A., Tenti, S., Giannitti, C., Fortunati, N. A., & Galeazzi, M. (2013). Short- and long-term effects of mud-bath treatment on hand osteoarthritis: a randomized clinical trial. International Journal of Biometeorology, 58(1), 79–86. doi:10.1007/s00484-012-0627-6

[876] Mennuni, G., Di Franco, M., Petraccia, L., Bietta, P., Lucchetta, M. C., Malkowski, M. L., Zingarini, A., Fontana, M., Nocchi, S., Scarno, A., Tanzi, G., Valesini, G., & Fraioli, A. (2009). La terapia termale nell'osteoartrosi: esperienza di Cervia [Spa therapy in osteoarthritis: experience in Cervia]. La Clinica terapeutica, 160(2), 115–119.

[877] Masiero, S., Vittadini, F., Ferroni, C., Bosco, A., Serra, R., Frigo, A. C., & Frizziero, A. (2018). The role of thermal balneotherapy in the treatment of obese patient with knee osteoarthritis. International journal of biometeorology, 62(2), 243–252. https://doi.org/10.1007/s00484-017-1445-7

[878] Kulisch, Á., Benkö, Á., Bergmann, A., Gyarmati, N., Horváth, H., Kránicz, Á., Mándó, Z. S., Matán, Á., Németh, A., Szakál, E., Szántó, D., Szekeres, L., & Bender, T. (2014). Evaluation of the effect of Lake Hévíz thermal mineral water in patients with osteoarthritis of the knee: a randomized, controlled, single-blind, follow-up study. European journal of physical and rehabilitation medicine, 50(4), 373–381.

[879] Fioravanti, A., Giannitti, C., Bellisai, B., Iacoponi, F., & Galeazzi, M. (2011). Efficacy of balneotherapy on pain, function and quality of life in patients with osteoarthritis of the knee. International Journal of Biometeorology, 56(4), 583–590. doi:10.1007/s00484-011-0447-0

[880] Bálint, G. P., Buchanan, W. W., Ádám, A., Ratkó, I., Poór, L., Bálint, P. V., ... Bender, T. (2006). The effect of the thermal mineral water of Nagybaracska on patients with knee joint osteoarthritis—a double blind study. Clinical Rheumatology, 26(6), 890–894. doi:10.1007/s10067-006-0420-1

[881] Harzy, T., Ghani, N., Akasbi, N., Bono, W., & Nejjari, C. (2009). Short- and long-term therapeutic effects of thermal mineral waters in knee osteoarthritis: a systematic review of randomized controlled trials. Clinical Rheumatology, 28(5), 501–507. doi:10.1007/s10067-009-1114-2

[882] Wigler, I., Elkayam, O., Paran, D., & Yaron, M. (1995). Spa therapy for gonarthrosis: a prospective study. Rheumatology international, 15(2), 65–68. https://doi.org/10.1007/BF00262710

[883] Branco, M., Rêgo, N. N., Silva, P. H., Archanjo, I. E., Ribeiro, M. C., & Trevisani, V. F. (2016). Bath thermal waters in the treatment of knee osteoarthritis: a randomized controlled clinical trial. European journal of physical and rehabilitation medicine, 52(4), 422–430.

[884] Özkuk, K., & Uysal, B. (2019). Is the Duration of Spa Cure Treatment Important in Knee Osteoarthritis? A Randomized Controlled Study. Ist die Dauer der Spa-Therapie bei Kniegelenksarthrose von Bedeutung? Eine randomisierte kontrollierte Studie. Complementary medicine research, 26(4), 258–264. https://doi.org/10.1159/000498890

[885] Karagülle, M., Kardeş, S., & Karagülle, M. Z. (2018). Long-term efficacy of spa therapy in patients with rheumatoid arthritis. Rheumatology international, 38(3), 353–362. https://doi.org/10.1007/s00296-017-3926-8

[886] Fioravanti, A., Iacoponi, F., Bellisai, B., Cantarini, L., & Galeazzi, M. (2010). Short- and Long-Term Effects of Spa Therapy in Knee Osteoarthritis. American Journal of Physical Medicine & Rehabilitation, 89(2), 125–132. doi:10.1097/phm.0b013e3181c1eb81

571

[887] Gaál, J., Varga, J., Szekanecz, Z., Kurkó, J., Ficzere, A., Bodolay, E., & Bender, T. (2008). Balneotherapy in elderly patients: effect on pain from degenerative knee and spine conditions and on quality of life. The Israel Medical Association journal : IMAJ, 10(5), 365–369.

[888] Santos, I., Cantista, P., & Vasconcelos, C. (2015). Balneotherapy in rheumatoid arthritis—a systematic review. International Journal of Biometeorology, 60(8), 1287–1301. doi:10.1007/s00484-015-1108-5

[889] Françon, A., & Forestier, R. (2009). Thermalisme en rhumatologie: indications a partir des recommandations françaises pour la pratique clinique de la Haute Autorité de Santé et européennes de l'European league against rheumatism et de dix-neuf essais cliniques randomisés [Spa therapy in rheumatology. Indications based on the clinical guidelines of the French National Authority for health and the European League Against Rheumatism, and the results of 19 randomized clinical trials]. Bulletin de l'Academie nationale de medecine, 193(6), 1345–1358.

[890] Morer, C., Roques, C. F., Françon, A., Forestier, R., & Maraver, F. (2017). The role of mineral elements and other chemical compounds used in balneology: data from double-blind randomized clinical trials. International journal of biometeorology, 61(12), 2159–2173. https://doi.org/10.1007/s00484-017-1421-2

[891] Karagülle, M., Kardeş, S., Karagülle, O., Dişçi, R., Avcı, A., Durak, İ., & Karagülle, M. Z. (2017). Effect of spa therapy with saline balneotherapy on oxidant/antioxidant status in patients with rheumatoid arthritis: a single-blind randomized controlled trial. International journal of biometeorology, 61(1), 169–180. https://doi.org/10.1007/s00484-016-1201-4

[892] Bender, T., Bariska, J., Vághy, R., Gomez, R., & Imre Kovács (2007). Effect of balneotherapy on the antioxidant system--a controlled pilot study. Archives of medical research, 38(1), 86–89. https://doi.org/10.1016/j.arcmed.2006.08.007

[893] Prandelli, C., Parola, C., Buizza, L., Delbarba, A., Marziano, M., Salvi, V., ... Bosisio, D. (2013). Sulphurous Thermal Water Increases the Release of the Anti-Inflammatory Cytokine IL-10 and Modulates Antioxidant Enzyme Activity. International Journal of Immunopathology and Pharmacology, 26(3), 633–646. doi:10.1177/039463201302600307

[894] Langston, C. (2017). Managing Fluid and Electrolyte Disorders in Kidney Disease. Veterinary Clinics of North America: Small Animal Practice, 47(2), 471–490. doi:10.1016/j.cvsm.2016.09.011

[895] Muhsin, S. A., & Mount, D. B. (2016). Diagnosis and treatment of hypernatremia. Best Practice & Research Clinical Endocrinology & Metabolism, 30(2), 189–203. doi:10.1016/j.beem.2016.02.014

[896] Harvey, K. B., Blumenkrantz, M. J., Levine, S. E., & Blackburn, G. L. (1980). Nutritional assessment and treatment of chronic renal failure. The American Journal of Clinical Nutrition, 33(7), 1586–1597. doi:10.1093/ajcn/33.7.1586

[897] Kaufman, C. E. (1984). Fluid and electrolyte abnormalities in nephrotic syndrome. Postgraduate Medicine, 76(6), 135–143. doi:10.1080/00325481.1984.11698784

[898] Sizykh, T. P., & Panferov, I. V. (1998). Primenenie gidrokarbonatnoĭ magnievo-kal'tsievoĭ mineral'noĭ vody pri nekotorykh zabolevaniakh pochek [The use of magnesium-calcium carbonate mineral water in kidney diseases]. Voprosy kurortologii, fizioterapii, i lechebnoi fizicheskoi kultury, (6), 52–54.

[899] Telina, E. N., Sakhabutdinov, I., Mosikhina, S. S., Anisimova, I. V., & Nizamova, F. A. (1999). Issledovanie éffektivnosti lecheniia sul'fatno-gidrokarbonatnoĭ kal'tsievo-magnievoĭ mineral'noĭ vodoĭ bol'nykh khronicheskim pielonefritom i mochekamennoĭ bolezn'iu [An efficacy study of the treatment of patients with chronic pyelonephritis and urolithiasis using sulfate-bicarbonate calcium-magnesium mineral water]. Voprosy kurortologii, fizioterapii, i lechebnoi fizicheskoi kultury, (4), 26–28.

[900] Benda and Sadílek (2000) 'Natural bicarbonate mineral waters in Spa treatment' Rehabilitace a Fyzikalni Lekarstvi 2000 7:4 (179-193).

[901] Neĭmark, A. I., Davydov, A. V., Bunkov, V. V., Zhiliakova, L. V., & Ukrainskaia, L. M. (2005). Voprosy kurortologii, fizioterapii, i lechebnoi fizicheskoi kultury, (3), 32–34.

[902] Gutenbrunner, C., Gilsdorf, K., & Hildebrandt, G. (1989). Untersuchungen über den Einfluss kalziumhaltiger Mineralwässer auf die Ubersättigung des Harnes mit Kalziumoxalat [The effect of mineral water containing calcium on supersaturation of urine with calcium oxalate]. Der Urologe. Ausg. A, 28(1), 15–19.

[903] Worcester, E. M., & Coe, F. L. (2010). Calcium Kidney Stones. New England Journal of Medicine, 363(10), 954–963. doi:10.1056/nejmcp1001011

[904] Noonan, S. C., & Savage, G. P. (1999). Oxalate content of foods and its effect on humans. Asia Pacific journal of clinical nutrition, 8(1), 64–74.

[905] Heaney, R. P., & Weaver, C. M. (1989). Oxalate: effect on calcium absorbability. The American Journal of Clinical Nutrition, 50(4), 830–832. doi:10.1093/ajcn/50.4.830

[906] Siener, R., Ebert, D., Nicolay, C., & Hesse, A. (2003). Dietary risk factors for hyperoxaluria in calcium oxalate stone formers. Kidney International, 63(3), 1037–1043. doi:10.1046/j.1523-1755.2003.00807.x

[907] Rodgers A. L. (1998). The influence of South African mineral water on reduction of risk of calcium oxalate kidney stone formation. South African medical journal = Suid-Afrikaanse tydskrif vir geneeskunde, 88(4), 448–451.

572

[908] Moss, M., Smith, E., Milner, M., & McCready, J. (2018). Acute ingestion of rosemary water: Evidence of cognitive and cerebrovascular effects in healthy adults. Journal of psychopharmacology (Oxford, England), 32(12), 1319–1329. https://doi.org/10.1177/0269881118798339

[909] Exley, C., Korchazhkina, O., Job, D., Strekopytov, S., Polwart, A., & Crome, P. (2006). Non-invasive therapy to reduce the body burden of aluminium in Alzheimer's disease [JB]. Journal of Alzheimer's Disease, 10(1), 17–24. https://doi.org/10.3233/JAD-2006-10103

[910] Davenward, S., Bentham, P., Wright, J., Crome, P., Job, D., Polwart, A., & Exley, C. (2012). Silicon-Rich Mineral Water as a Non-Invasive Test of the 'Aluminum Hypothesis' in Alzheimer's Disease [JB]. Journal of Alzheimer's Disease, 33(2), 423–430. https://doi.org/10.3233/JAD-2012-121231

[911] Haymes (1991) 'Vitamin and Mineral Supplementation to Athletes', International Journal of Sport Nutrition, 1991, 1, 146-1 69.

[912] Nutrition and Athletic Performance. (2009). Medicine & Science in Sports & Exercise, 41(3), 709–731. doi:10.1249/mss.0b013e31890eb86

[913] Hiller, W. D. B., O'Toole, M. L., Fortess, E. E., Laird, R. H., Imbert, P. C., & Sisk, T. D. (1987). Medical and physiological considerations in triathlons. The American Journal of Sports Medicine, 15(2), 164–167. doi:10.1177/036354658701500212

[914] Nishimuta, M., Kodama, N., Yoshitake, Y., Shimada, M., & Serizawa, N. (2018). Dietary Salt (Sodium Chloride) Requirement and Adverse Effects of Salt Restriction in Humans. Journal of nutritional science and vitaminology, 64(2), 83–89. https://doi.org/10.3177/jnsv.64.83

[915] Galanti et al (2000) 'Effect of high-electrolyte water on restoration of fluid balance after exercise-induced hypohydration', Medicina dello Sport 2000 December;53(4):301-5.

[916] Harris, P. R., Keen, D. A., Constantopoulos, E., Weninger, S. N., Hines, E., Koppinger, M. P., Khalpey, Z. I., & Konhilas, J. P. (2019). Fluid type influences acute hydration and muscle performance recovery in human subjects. Journal of the International Society of Sports Nutrition, 16(1), 15. https://doi.org/10.1186/s12970-019-0282-y

[917] Bergeron, M. F. (2003). Heat cramps: fluid and electrolyte challenges during tennis in the heat. Journal of Science and Medicine in Sport, 6(1), 19–27. doi:10.1016/s1440-2440(03)80005-1

[918] Anastasiou, C. A., Kavouras, S. A., Arnaoutis, G., Gioxari, A., Kollia, M., Botoula, E., & Sidossis, L. S. (2009). Sodium Replacement and Plasma Sodium Drop During Exercise in the Heat When Fluid Intake Matches Fluid Loss. Journal of Athletic Training, 44(2), 117–123. doi:10.4085/1062-6050-44.2.117

[919] Hargreaves, M., Morgan, T. O., Snow, R., & Guerin, M. (1989). Exercise tolerance in the heat on low and normal salt intakes. Clinical Science, 76(5), 553–557. doi:10.1042/cs0760553

[920] Cohn and Emmet (1978) 'The Excretion of Trace Metals in Human Sweat', ANNALS O F CLINICAL AND LABORATORY SCIEN CE, Vol. 8, No. 4, Accessed Online Dec 12 2020: https://citeseerx.ist.psu.edu/viewdoc/download?doi=10.1.1.974.3582&rep=rep1&type=pdf

[921] WALLER, M. F., & HAYMES, E. M. (1996). The effects of heat and exercise on sweat iron loss. Medicine &amp Science in Sports &amp Exercise, 28(2), 197–203. doi:10.1097/00005768-199602000-00007

[922] Armstrong, L. E., Costill, D. L., Fink, W. J., Bassett, D., Hargreaves, M., Nishibata, I., & King, D. S. (1985). Effects of dietary sodium on body and muscle potassium content during heat acclimation. European Journal of Applied Physiology and Occupational Physiology, 54(4), 391–397. doi:10.1007/bf02337183

[923] Hoshi, A., Watanabe, H., Chiba, M., Inaba, Y., Kobayashi, M., Kimura, N., & Ito, T. (2002). Seasonal variation of trace element loss to sweat during exercise in males. Environmental Health and Preventive Medicine, 7(2), 60–63. doi:10.1007/bf02897331

[924] Sato, K., & Dobson, R. L. (1970). Regional and Individual Variations in the Function of the Human Eccrine Sweat Gland. Journal of Investigative Dermatology, 54(6), 443–449. doi:10.1111/1523-1747.ep12259272

[925] Montain et al (2007) 'Sweat Mineral-Element Responses During 7 h of Exercise-Heat Stress', International Journal of Sport Nutrition and Exercise Metabolism, 2007,17.574-582.

[926] Hoshi, A., Watanabe, H., Chiba, M., Inaba, Y., Kobayashi, M., Kimura, N., & Ito, T. (2002). Seasonal variation of trace element loss to sweat during exercise in males. Environmental Health and Preventive Medicine, 7(2), 60–63. doi:10.1007/bf02897331

[927] Omokhodion, F. O., & Howard, J. M. (1994). Trace elements in the sweat of acclimatized persons. Clinica Chimica Acta, 231(1), 23–28. doi:10.1016/0009-8981(94)90250-x

[928] Kuno, Y. (1956) 'Human Perspiration'. Springfield, IL, Charles C Thomas, 1956.

[929] Daly, C and Dill, D.B. (1937) 'Salt economy in humid heat'. Amer. J. Physiol. 118:285-289.

[930] Allan, J. R., & Wilson, C. G. (1971). Influence of acclimatization on sweat sodium concentration. Journal of applied physiology, 30(5), 708–712. https://doi.org/10.1152/jappl.1971.30.5.708

[931] Anatruda and Welt (1953) 'Secretion of electrolytes in thermal sweat'. J. A ppl. Physiol. 5:759-772, 1953.

[932] KAWAHATA A, SAKAMOTO H. Some observations on sweating of the Aino. The Japanese Journal of Physiology. 1951 Nov;2(2):166-169. DOI: 10.2170/jjphysiol.2.166.

[933] Robinson, S., Kincaid, R. K., & Rhamy, R. K. (1950). Effect of Salt Deficiency on the Salt Concentration in Sweat. Journal of Applied Physiology, 3(2), 55–62. doi:10.1152/jappl.1950.3.2.55

[934] Locke, W., Talbot, N. B., Jones, H. S., & Worcester, J. (1951). STUDIES ON THE COMBINED USE OF MEASUREMENTS OF SWEAT ELECTROLYTE COMPOSITION AND RATE OF SWEATING AS AN INDEX OF ADRENAL CORTICAL ACTIVITY 1. Journal of Clinical Investigation, 30(3), 325–337. doi:10.1172/jci102448

[935] Chopra et al (1940) 'On the composition of the sweat of the Indians'. Ind. J. Med. Res. 27:931-935.

[936] Ladell, W. S. S. (1948). The measurement of chloride losses in the sweat. The Journal of Physiology, 107(4), 465–471. doi:10.1113/jphysiol.1948.sp004291

[937] Mickelsen and Keys (1943) 'THE COMPOSITION OF SWEAT, WITH SPECIAL REFERENCE TO THE VITAMINS', J. Biol. Chem. 1943, 149:479-490.

[938] Weiner, J. S., & van Heyningen, R. E. (1952). Observations on Lactate Content of Sweat. Journal of Applied Physiology, 4(9), 734–744. doi:10.1152/jappl.1952.4.9.734

[939] CHINEVERE, T. D., KENEFICK, R. W., CHEUVRONT, S. N., LUKASKI, H. C., & SAWKA, M. N. (2008). Effect of Heat Acclimation on Sweat Minerals. Medicine & Science in Sports & Exercise, 40(5), 886–891. doi:10.1249/mss.0b013e3181641c04

[940] Armstrong, L. E., Hubbard, R. W., Szlyk, P. C., Matthew, W. T., & Sils, I. V. (1985). Voluntary dehydration and electrolyte losses during prolonged exercise in the heat. Aviation, space, and environmental medicine, 56(8), 765–770.

[941] Roberts, M. F., Wenger, C. B., Stolwijk, J. A., & Nadel, E. R. (1977). Skin blood flow and sweating changes following exercise training and heat acclimation. Journal of Applied Physiology, 43(1), 133–137. doi:10.1152/jappl.1977.43.1.133

[942] Tipton, K., Green, N. R., Haymes, E. M., & Waller, M. (1993). Zinc Loss in Sweat of Athletes Exercising in Hot and Neutral Temperatures. International Journal of Sport Nutrition, 3(3), 261–271. doi:10.1123/ijsn.3.3.261

[943] DeRuisseau, K. C., Cheuvront, S. N., Haymes, E. M., & Sharp, R. G. (2002). Sweat Iron and Zinc Losses during Prolonged Exercise. International Journal of Sport Nutrition and Exercise Metabolism, 12(4), 428–437. doi:10.1123/ijsnem.12.4.428

[944] Consolazio, C. F., Matoush, L. O., Nelson, R. A., Hackler, L. R., & Preston, E. E. (1962). Relationship Between Calcium in Sweat, Calcium Balance, and Calcium Requirements. The Journal of Nutrition, 78(1), 78–88. doi:10.1093/jn/78.1.78

[945] Consolazio et al (1964) 'The Trace Mineral Losses in Sweat. Denver, CO: U.S. Army Medical Research and Nutrition Laboratory.

[946] Greenleaf, J. E., Looft-Wilson, R., Wisherd, J. L., Jackson, C. G., Fung, P. P., Ertl, A. C., Barnes, P. R., Jensen, C. D., & Whittam, J. H. (1998). Hypervolemia in men from fluid ingestion at rest and during exercise. Aviation, space, and environmental medicine, 69(4), 374–386.

[947] Sims et al (2007) 'Preexercise sodium loading aids fluid balance and endurance for women exercising in the heat', J Appl Physiol 103: 534–541, 2007. doi:10.1152/japplphysiol.01203.2006.

[948] SIMS, S. T., van VLIET, L., COTTER, J. D., & REHRER, N. J. (2007). Sodium Loading Aids Fluid Balance and Reduces Physiological Strain of Trained Men Exercising in the Heat. Medicine & Science in Sports & Exercise, 39(1), 123–130. doi:10.1249/01.mss.0000241639.97972.4a

[949] Sanders, B., Noakes, T. D., & Dennis, S. C. (2001). Sodium replacement and fluid shifts during prolonged exercise in humans. European Journal of Applied Physiology, 84(5), 419–425. doi:10.1007/s004210000371

[950] Twerenbold et al (2003) 'Effects of different sodium concentrations in replacement fluids during prolonged exercise in women', Br J Sports Med 2003;37:300–303.

[951] Higgins, M. F., Rudkin, B., & Kuo, C. H. (2019). Oral Ingestion of Deep Ocean Minerals Increases High-Intensity Intermittent Running Capacity in Soccer Players after Short-Term Post-Exercise Recovery: A Double-Blind, Placebo-Controlled Crossover Trial. Marine drugs, 17(5), 309. https://doi.org/10.3390/md17050309

[952] Soria, M., González-Haro, C., Esteva, S., Escanero, J. F., & Pina, J. R. (2014). Effect of sulphurous mineral water in haematological and biochemical markers of muscle damage after an endurance exercise in well-trained athletes. Journal of sports sciences, 32(10), 954–962. https://doi.org/10.1080/02640414.2013.868921

[953] Arsenio et al (2006) 'Magnesium and potassium role in muscular performance', Progress in Nutrition 2006 8:1 (11-21).

[954] Laires et al (2014) 'Magnesium status and exercise performance in athletes', Trace Elements and Electrolytes 31(1):13-20, DOI: 10.5414/TEX01304

[955] Halawa, I., Andersson, T., & Tomson, T. (2011). Hyponatremia and risk of seizures: A retrospective cross-sectional study. Epilepsia, no–no. doi:10.1111/j.1528-1167.2010.02939.x

[956] Su and Woo (2012) 'Severe Hyponatremia From Water Intoxication Associated With Preparation for a Urine Flow Study', Journal of Medical Cases, Volume 3, Number 2, April 2012, pages 123-125.

574

[957] Hew-Butler (2018) 'Stay hydrated, but drinking too much water can be deadly, doctors warn.' CBS News, Accessed Online Dec 12 2020: https://www.cbsnews.com/news/stay-hydrated-but-drinking-too-much-water-can-be-deadly-doctors-warn/

[958] McGill University Health Centre. (2018, May 22). Mechanisms of harmful overhydration and brain swelling. ScienceDaily. Retrieved December 12, 2020 from www.sciencedaily.com/releases/2018/05/180522114623.htm

[959] Dreyfuss (2017) 'Every Year, More Athletes Are Injured By Hyponatremia than By Dehydration', M.D. Alert, Accessed Online: https://www.mdalert.com/article/every-year-more-athletes-are-injured-by-hyponatremia-than-by-dehydration

[960] HOFFMAN, M. D., & STUEMPFLE, K. J. (2015). Sodium Supplementation and Exercise-Associated Hyponatremia during Prolonged Exercise. Medicine & Science in Sports & Exercise, 47(9), 1781–1787. doi:10.1249/mss.0000000000000599

[961] Almond, C. S. D., Shin, A. Y., Fortescue, E. B., Mannix, R. C., Wypij, D., Binstadt, B. A., … Greenes, D. S. (2005). Hyponatremia among Runners in the Boston Marathon. New England Journal of Medicine, 352(15), 1550–1556. doi:10.1056/nejmoa043901

[962] Hoorn, E. J., & Zietse, R. (2017). Diagnosis and Treatment of Hyponatremia: Compilation of the Guidelines. Journal of the American Society of Nephrology, 28(5), 1340–1349. doi:10.1681/asn.2016101139

[963] Carr, A. J., Hopkins, W. G., & Gore, C. J. (2011). Effects of Acute Alkalosis and Acidosis on Performance. Sports Medicine, 41(10), 801–814. doi:10.2165/11591440-000000000-00000

[964] Garzon, P., & Eisenberg, M. J. (1998). Variation in the mineral content of commercially available bottled waters: implications for health and disease. The American Journal of Medicine, 105(2), 125–130. doi:10.1016/s0002-9343(98)00189-2

[965] von Wiesenberger A. (1991) 'The Pocket Guide to Bottled Water'. 1st ed. Chicago: Contemporary Books.

[966] Green and Green (1994) 'The Good Water Guide'. London, England: Rosendale Press.

[967] Rosanoff, A. (2013). The high heart health value of drinking-water magnesium. Medical Hypotheses, 81(6), 1063–1065. doi:10.1016/j.mehy.2013.10.003

[968] Stolarz-Skrzypek, K. (2011). Fatal and Nonfatal Outcomes, Incidence of Hypertension, and Blood Pressure Changes in Relation to Urinary Sodium Excretion. JAMA, 305(17), 1777. doi:10.1001/jama.2011.574

[969] Luft, F. C., Zemel, M. B., Sowers, J. A., Fineberg, N. S., & Weinberger, M. H. (1990). Sodium bicarbonate and sodium chloride: effects on blood pressure and electrolyte homeostasis in normal and hypertensive man. Journal of Hypertension, 8(7), 663–670. doi:10.1097/00004872-199007000-00010

[970] Zarse, K., Terao, T., Tian, J., Iwata, N., Ishii, N., & Ristow, M. (2011). Low-dose lithium uptake promotes longevity in humans and metazoans. European Journal of Nutrition, 50(5), 387–389. doi:10.1007/s00394-011-0171-x

[971] Schrauzer, G. N. (2002). Lithium: Occurrence, Dietary Intakes, Nutritional Essentiality. Journal of the American College of Nutrition, 21(1), 14–21. doi:10.1080/07315724.2002.10719188

[972] Andrade Nunes, M., Araujo Viel, T., & Sousa Buck, H. (2013). Microdose Lithium Treatment Stabilized Cognitive Impairment in Patients with Alzheimer's Disease. Current Alzheimer Research, 10(1), 104–107. doi:10.2174/1567205011310010014

[973] Aqua Maestro 'SAN PELLEGRINO', Sparkling Water, Accessed Online Dec 12 2020: https://www.aquamaestro.com/category/sparkling-water/san-pellegrino-water

[974] Rondanelli, M., Miraglia, N., Putignano, P., Peroni, G., Faliva, M. A., Naso, M., … Perna, S. (2020). Short- and Long-Term Effectiveness of Supplementation with Non-Animal Chondroitin Sulphate on Inflammation, Oxidative Stress and Functional Status in Obese Subjects with Moderate Knee Osteoarthritis before and after Physical Stress: A Randomized, Double-Blind, Placebo-Controlled Trial. Antioxidants, 9(12), 1241. doi:10.3390/antiox9121241

[975] Seneff, S., Lauritzen, A., Davidson, R., & Lentz-Marino, L. (2012). Is Endothelial Nitric Oxide Synthase a Moonlighting Protein Whose Day Job is Cholesterol Sulfate Synthesis? Implications for Cholesterol Transport, Diabetes and Cardiovascular Disease. Entropy, 14(12), 2492–2530. doi:10.3390/e14122492

[976] Jez et al (2008) 'Sulfur: A Missing Link between Soils, Crops, and Nutrition', American Society of Agronomy, Inc., Crop Science Society of America, Inc., Soil Science Society of America, Inc., Accessed Online Dec 12 2020: https://portal.sciencesocieties.org/Resources/Files/downloads/pdf/B40720.pdf

[977] Taylor, S. L., Higley, N. A., & Bush, R. K. (1986). Sulfites in Foods: Uses, Analytical Methods, Residues, Fate, Exposure Assessment, Metabolism, Toxicity, and Hypersensitivity. Advances in Food Research, 1–76. doi:10.1016/s0065-2628(08)60347-x

[978] Sapers, G.M. 1993. Browning of foods: control by sulfites, antioxidants, and other means. Food Technol. 47(10): 75–84.

[979] Lester M. R. (1995). Sulfite sensitivity: significance in human health. Journal of the American College of Nutrition, 14(3), 229–232. https://doi.org/10.1080/07315724.1995.10718500

575

[980] Knodel, L.C. 1997. Current Issues in Drug Toxicity; Potential health hazards of sulfites. Toxic Subst. Mech. 16(3): 309–311.

[981] Papazian, R. 1996. Sulfites: Safe for most, dangerous for some. FDA Consumer Magazine. 30(10).

[982] Bohr et al (1904) 'Concerning a Biologically Important Relationship - The Influence of the Carbon Dioxide Content of Blood on its Oxygen Binding', Skand. Arch. Physiol. 16, 401-412 (1904) by Ulf Marquardt for CHEM-342, January 1997, Accessed Online: https://www1.udel.edu/chem/white/C342/Bohr(1904).html

[983] Lee and Levine (1999) 'Acute respiratory alkalosis associated with low minute ventilation in a patient with severe hypothyroidism', Can J Anaesth. 1999 Feb;46(2):185-9.

[984] Woods, Hubert Frank; Cohen, Robert (1976). *Clinical and biochemical aspects of lactic acidosis.* Oxford: Blackwell Scientific

[985] Vander Heiden, M. G., Cantley, L. C., & Thompson, C. B. (2009). Understanding the Warburg effect: the metabolic requirements of cell proliferation. Science (New York, N.Y.), 324(5930), 1029–1033. https://doi.org/10.1126/science.1160809

[986] The Mineral-Calculator 'How many minerals are in your mineral water? It's time to compare.', Accessed Online Dec 12 2020: https://www.mineral-calculator.com/water-faq/

[987] Hamilton (2011) 'Study: Most Plastics Leach Hormone-Like Chemicals', NPR, Accessed Online Dec 12 2020: https://www.npr.org/2011/03/02/134196209/study-most-plastics-leach-hormone-like-chemicals

[988] NIH (2020) 'Endocrine Disruptors', Accessed Online Dec 12 2020: https://www.niehs.nih.gov/health/topics/agents/endocrine/index.cfm

[989] Wozniak, M., & Murias, M. (2008). Ksenoestrogeny: substancje zakłócajace funkcjonowanie układu hormonalnego [Xenoestrogens: endocrine disrupting compounds]. Ginekologia polska, 79(11), 785–790.

[990] Leonard (2018) 'What are the symptoms of high estrogen?', Medical News Today, Accessed Online Dec 12 2020: https://www.medicalnewstoday.com/articles/323280

[991] Stanikova, D., Luck, T., Bae, Y. J., Thiery, J., Ceglarek, U., Engel, C., … Riedel-Heller, S. G. (2018). Increased estrogen level can be associated with depression in males. Psychoneuroendocrinology, 87, 196–203. doi:10.1016/j.psyneuen.2017.10.025

[992] Yang, C. Z., Yaniger, S. I., Jordan, V. C., Klein, D. J., & Bittner, G. D. (2011). Most Plastic Products Release Estrogenic Chemicals: A Potential Health Problem That Can Be Solved. Environmental Health Perspectives, 119(7), 989–996. doi:10.1289/ehp.1003220

[993] Toppari, J., Larsen, J. C., Christiansen, P., Giwercman, A., Grandjean, P., Guillette, L. J., Jr, Jégou, B., Jensen, T. K., Jouannet, P., Keiding, N., Leffers, H., McLachlan, J. A., Meyer, O., Müller, J., Rajpert-De Meyts, E., Scheike, T., Sharpe, R., Sumpter, J., & Skakkebaek, N. E. (1996). Male reproductive health and environmental xenoestrogens. Environmental health perspectives, 104 Suppl 4(Suppl 4), 741–803. https://doi.org/10.1289/ehp.96104s4741

[994] Kucińska, M., & Murias, M. (2013). Kosmetyki jako źródło narazenia na ksenoestrogeny [Cosmetics as source of xenoestrogens exposure]. Przeglad lekarski, 70(8), 647–651.

[995] Detrano, R., Guerci, A. D., Carr, J. J., Bild, D. E., Burke, G., Folsom, A. R., … Kronmal, R. A. (2008). Coronary Calcium as a Predictor of Coronary Events in Four Racial or Ethnic Groups. New England Journal of Medicine, 358(13), 1336–1345. doi:10.1056/nejmoa072100

[996] Li, K., Kaaks, R., Linseisen, J., & Rohrmann, S. (2012). Associations of dietary calcium intake and calcium supplementation with myocardial infarction and stroke risk and overall cardiovascular mortality in the Heidelberg cohort of the European Prospective Investigation into Cancer and Nutrition study (EPIC-Heidelberg). Heart, 98(12), 920–925. doi:10.1136/heartjnl-2011-301345

[997] Xiao, Q., Murphy, R. A., Houston, D. K., Harris, T. B., Chow, W.-H., & Park, Y. (2013). Dietary and Supplemental Calcium Intake and Cardiovascular Disease Mortality. JAMA Internal Medicine, 173(8), 639. doi:10.1001/jamainternmed.2013.3283

[998] Rosanoff, A., Weaver, C. M., & Rude, R. K. (2012). Suboptimal magnesium status in the United States: are the health consequences underestimated? Nutrition Reviews, 70(3), 153–164. doi:10.1111/j.1753-4887.2011.00465.x

[999] DiNicolantonio, J. J., McCarty, M. F., & O'Keefe, J. H. (2017). Decreased magnesium status may mediate the increased cardiovascular risk associated with calcium supplementation. Open Heart, 4(1), e000617. doi:10.1136/openhrt-2017-000617

[1000] Qu et al (2013) 'Magnesium and the Risk of Cardiovascular Events: A Meta-Analysis of Prospective Cohort Studies', PLoS ONE 8(3): e57720. doi:10.1371/journal.pone.0057720

[1001] Del Gobbo, L. C., Imamura, F., Wu, J. H., de Oliveira Otto, M. C., Chiuve, S. E., & Mozaffarian, D. (2013). Circulating and dietary magnesium and risk of cardiovascular disease: a systematic review and meta-analysis of prospective studies. The American Journal of Clinical Nutrition, 98(1), 160–173. doi:10.3945/ajcn.112.053132

[1002] Guasch-Ferré, M., Bulló, M., Estruch, R., Corella, D., Martínez-González, M. A., … Ros, E. (2013). Dietary Magnesium Intake Is Inversely Associated with Mortality in Adults at High Cardiovascular Disease Risk. The Journal of Nutrition, 144(1), 55–60. doi:10.3945/jn.113.183012

[1003] Zhang, W., Iso, H., Ohira, T., Date, C., & Tamakoshi, A. (2012). Associations of dietary magnesium intake with mortality from cardiovascular disease: The JACC study. Atherosclerosis, 221(2), 587–595. doi:10.1016/j.atherosclerosis.2012.01.034

[1004] DiNicolantonio, J. J., O'Keefe, J. H., & Wilson, W. (2018). Subclinical magnesium deficiency: a principal driver of cardiovascular disease and a public health crisis. Open Heart, 5(1), e000668. doi:10.1136/openhrt-2017-000668

[1005] DiNicolantonio, J. J., Liu, J., & O'Keefe, J. H. (2018). Magnesium for the prevention and treatment of cardiovascular disease. Open Heart, 5(2), e000775. doi:10.1136/openhrt-2018-000775

[1006] Hata, A., Doi, Y., Ninomiya, T., Mukai, N., Hirakawa, Y., Hata, J., … Kiyohara, Y. (2013). Magnesium intake decreases Type 2 diabetes risk through the improvement of insulin resistance and inflammation: the Hisayama Study. Diabetic Medicine, 30(12), 1487–1494. doi:10.1111/dme.12250

[1007] Evangelopoulos, A. A., Vallianou, N. G., Panagiotakos, D. B., Georgiou, A., Zacharias, G. A., Alevra, A. N., … Avgerinos, P. C. (2008). An inverse relationship between cumulating components of the metabolic syndrome and serum magnesium levels. Nutrition Research, 28(10), 659–663. doi:10.1016/j.nutres.2008.07.001

[1008] He, K., Song, Y., Belin, R.J. and Chen, Y. (2006), Magnesium Intake and the Metabolic Syndrome: Epidemiologic Evidence to Date. Journal of the CardioMetabolic Syndrome, 1: 351-355. https://doi.org/10.1111/j.1559-4564.2006.05702.x

[1009] McCarty, M. F. (2005). Magnesium may mediate the favorable impact of whole grains on insulin sensitivity by acting as a mild calcium antagonist. Medical Hypotheses, 64(3), 619–627. doi:10.1016/j.mehy.2003.10.034

[1010] Grabarek, Z. (2011). Insights into modulation of calcium signaling by magnesium in calmodulin, troponin C and related EF-hand proteins. Biochimica et Biophysica Acta (BBA) - Molecular Cell Research, 1813(5), 913–921. doi:10.1016/j.bbamcr.2011.01.017

[1011] Iseri, L. T., & French, J. H. (1984). Magnesium: Nature's physiologic calcium blocker. American Heart Journal, 108(1), 188–193. doi:10.1016/0002-8703(84)90572-6

[1012] Wang, L., Manson, J. E., & Sesso, H. D. (2012). Calcium Intake and Risk of Cardiovascular Disease. American Journal of Cardiovascular Drugs, 12(2), 105–116. doi:10.2165/11595400-000000000-00000

[1013] Chan, R., Leung, J., & Woo, J. (2013). A Prospective Cohort Study Examining the Associations of Dietary Calcium Intake with All-Cause and Cardiovascular Mortality in Older Chinese Community-Dwelling People. PLoS ONE, 8(11), e80895. doi:10.1371/journal.pone.0080895

[1014] Anderson, J. J. B., Kruszka, B., Delaney, J. A. C., He, K., Burke, G. L., Alonso, A., … Michos, E. D. (2016). Calcium Intake From Diet and Supplements and the Risk of Coronary Artery Calcification and its Progression Among Older Adults: 10-Year Follow-up of the Multi-Ethnic Study of Atherosclerosis (MESA). Journal of the American Heart Association, 5(10). doi:10.1161/jaha.116.003815

[1015] Samelson, E. J., Booth, S. L., Fox, C. S., Tucker, K. L., Wang, T. J., Hoffmann, U., … Kiel, D. P. (2012). Calcium intake is not associated with increased coronary artery calcification: the Framingham Study. The American Journal of Clinical Nutrition, 96(6), 1274–1280. doi:10.3945/ajcn.112.044230

[1016] Kurnatowska, I., Grzelak, P., Masajtis-Zagajewska, A., Kaczmarska, M., Stefańczyk, L., Vermeer, C., Maresz, K., & Nowicki, M. (2015). Effect of vitamin K2 on progression of atherosclerosis and vascular calcification in nondialyzed patients with chronic kidney disease stages 3-5. Polskie Archiwum Medycyny Wewnetrznej, 125(9), 631–640. https://doi.org/10.20452/pamw.3041

[1017] Riggs, B. L., & Melton, L. J., 3rd (1995). The worldwide problem of osteoporosis: insights afforded by epidemiology. Bone, 17(5 Suppl), 505S–511S. https://doi.org/10.1016/8756-3282(95)00258-4

[1018] Anderson et al (2012) 'Calcium Intakes and Femoral and Lumbar Bone Density of Elderly U.S. Men and Women: National Health and Nutrition Examination Survey 2005–2006 Analysis', The Journal of Clinical Endocrinology & Metabolism, Volume 97, Issue 12, 1 December 2012, Pages 4531–4539, https://doi.org/10.1210/jc.2012-1407

[1019] Warensjo, E., Byberg, L., Melhus, H., Gedeborg, R., Mallmin, H., Wolk, A., & Michaelsson, K. (2011). Dietary calcium intake and risk of fracture and osteoporosis: prospective longitudinal cohort study. BMJ, 342(may24 1), d1473–d1473. doi:10.1136/bmj.d1473

[1020] London, G. M. (2012). Bone-vascular cross-talk. Journal of Nephrology, 25(5), 619–625. doi:10.5301/jn.5000187

[1021] Persy, V., & D'Haese, P. (2009). Vascular calcification and bone disease: the calcification paradox. Trends in molecular medicine, 15(9), 405–416. https://doi.org/10.1016/j.molmed.2009.07.001

[1022] Jensky, N. E., Hyder, J. A., Allison, M. A., Wong, N., Aboyans, V., Blumenthal, R. S., … Criqui, M. H. (2011). The association of bone density and calcified atherosclerosis is stronger in women without dyslipidemia: The multi-ethnic study of atherosclerosis. Journal of Bone and Mineral Research, 26(11), 2702–2709. doi:10.1002/jbmr.469

[1023] Kiel, D. P., Kauppila, L. I., Cupples, L. A., Hannan, M. T., O'Donnell, C. J., & Wilson, P. W. F. (2001). Bone loss and the progression of abdominal aortic calcification over a 25 year period: The Framingham heart study. Calcified Tissue International, 68(5), 271–276. doi:10.1007/bf02390833

577

[1024] Oelzner, P., Lehmann, G., Eidner, T., Franke, S., Müller, A., Wolf, G., & Hein, G. (2006). Hypercalcemia in rheumatoid arthritis: relationship with disease activity and bone metabolism. Rheumatology international, 26(10), 908–915. https://doi.org/10.1007/s00296-005-0095-y

[1025] Orchard, T. S., Larson, J. C., Alghothani, N., Bout-Tabaku, S., Cauley, J. A., Chen, Z., LaCroix, A. Z., Wactawski-Wende, J., & Jackson, R. D. (2014). Magnesium intake, bone mineral density, and fractures: results from the Women's Health Initiative Observational Study. The American journal of clinical nutrition, 99(4), 926–933. https://doi.org/10.3945/ajcn.113.067488

[1026] van Ballegooijen, A. J., Robinson-Cohen, C., Katz, R., Criqui, M., Budoff, M., Li, D., Siscovick, D., Hoofnagle, A., Shea, S. J., Burke, G., de Boer, I. H., & Kestenbaum, B. (2015). Vitamin D metabolites and bone mineral density: The multi-ethnic study of atherosclerosis. Bone, 78, 186–193. https://doi.org/10.1016/j.bone.2015.05.008

[1027] Pearson D. A. (2007). Bone health and osteoporosis: the role of vitamin K and potential antagonism by anticoagulants. Nutrition in clinical practice : official publication of the American Society for Parenteral and Enteral Nutrition, 22(5), 517–544. https://doi.org/10.1177/0115426507022005517

[1028] Vormann (2002) 'Dietary Magnesium: Supply, Requirements and Recommendations - Results From Duplicate and Balance Studies in Man', Journal of Clinical and Basic Cardiology 5(1).

[1029] Canelas, H. M., Assis, L. M. D., & Jorge, F. B. D. (1965). Disorders of magnesium metabolism in epilepsy. Journal of Neurology, Neurosurgery & Psychiatry, 28(4), 378–381. doi:10.1136/jnnp.28.4.378

[1030] Abbott, L. G., & Rude, R. K. (1993). Clinical manifestations of magnesium deficiency. Mineral and electrolyte metabolism, 19(4-5), 314–322.

[1031] Torimitsu et al (2012) '[Role of magnesium in nerve tissue].', Clinical Calcium, 01 Aug 2012, 22(8):1197-1203, PMID: 22846355

[1032] Kielstein, J. T., & David, S. (2012). Magnesium: the "earth cure" of AKI? Nephrology Dialysis Transplantation, 28(4), 785–787. doi:10.1093/ndt/gfs347

[1033] Wacker, W. E. C., & Parisi, A. F. (1968). Magnesium Metabolism. New England Journal of Medicine, 278(12), 658–663. doi:10.1056/nejm196803212781205

[1034] Volpe SL. Magnesium. In: Erdman JW, Macdonald IA, Zeisel SH, eds. Present knowledge in nutrition. 10th ed. Ames, Iowa: John Wiley & Sons, 2012:459–74.

[1035] Vormann, J. (2003). Magnesium: nutrition and metabolism. Molecular Aspects of Medicine, 24(1-3), 27–37. doi:10.1016/s0098-2997(02)00089-4

[1036] Purvis, J.R. and Movahed, A. (1992), Magnesium disorders and cardiovascular diseases. Clin Cardiol, 15: 556-568. https://doi.org/10.1002/clc.4960150804

[1037] Rosanoff A. (2005). '[Magnesium and hypertension]', Clinical calcium, 15(2), 255–260.

[1038] Chipperfield, B., & Chipperfield, J. R. (1977). Magnesium and the heart. American Heart Journal, 93(6), 679–682. doi:10.1016/s0002-8703(77)80061-6

[1039] Sheehan, J. P., & Seelig, M. S. (1984). Interactions of magnesium and potassium in the pathogenesis of cardiovascular disease. Magnesium, 3(4-6), 301–314.

[1040] Altura, B. M., & Altura, B. T. (1984). Interactions of Mg and K on blood vessels--aspects in view of hypertension. Review of present status and new findings. Magnesium, 3(4-6), 175–194.

[1041] Altura, B. M., Altura, B. T., Carella, A., & Turlapaty, P. D. (1981). Hypomagnesemia and vasoconstriction: possible relationship to etiology of sudden death ischemic heart disease and hypertensive vascular diseases. Artery, 9(3), 212–231.

[1042] Madden, J. A., Willems, W. J., Smith, G. A., & Mueller, R. A. (1984). Sodium kinetics and membrane potential in aorta of magnesium-deficient rats. Magnesium, 3(2), 73–80.

[1043] Kharb, S., & Singh, V. (2000). Magnesium deficiency potentiates free radical production associated with myocardial infarction. The Journal of the Association of Physicians of India, 48(5), 484–485.

[1044] Freedman, A. M., Cassidy, M. M., & Weglicki, W. B. (1991). Magnesium-deficient myocardium demonstrates an increased susceptibility to an in vivo oxidative stress. Magnesium research, 4(3-4), 185–189.

[1045] Wiles et al (1996) 'Effect of acute magnesium deficiency (MgD) on aortic endothelial cell (EC) oxidant production', Life Sciences, Volume 60, Issue 3, 6 December 1996, Pages 221-236.

[1046] Kumar, B.P., Shivakumar, K. Depressed antioxidant defense in rat heart in experimental magnesium deficiency implications for the pathogenesis of myocardial lesions. Biol Trace Elem Res 60, 139–144 (1997). https://doi.org/10.1007/BF02783317

[1047] Nazıroğlu, M., Özgül, C., Çiğ, B., Doğan, S., & Uğuz, A. C. (2011). Glutathione modulates Ca(2+) influx and oxidative toxicity through TRPM2 channel in rat dorsal root ganglion neurons. The Journal of membrane biology, 242(3), 109–118. https://doi.org/10.1007/s00232-011-9382-6

[1048] Laurant et al (1999) 'Effect of Magnesium Deficiency on Blood Pressure and Mechanical Properties of Rat Carotid Artery', Hypertension. 1999;33:1105–1110.

[1049] Shibutani, Y., Sakamoto, K., Katsuno, S., Yoshimoto, S., & Matsuura, T. (1988). Serum and erythrocyte magnesium levels in junior high school students: relation to blood pressure and a family history of hypertension. Magnesium, 7(4), 188–194.

[1050] Weglicki and Phillips (1992) 'Pathobiology of magnesium deficiency: a cytokine/neurogenic inflammation hypothesis', American Journal of Physiology-Regulatory, Integrative and Comparative Physiology 1992 263:3, R734-R737

[1051] Ferrè, S., Baldoli, E., Leidi, M., & Maier, J. A. M. (2010). Magnesium deficiency promotes a pro-atherogenic phenotype in cultured human endothelial cells via activation of NFkB. Biochimica et Biophysica Acta (BBA) - Molecular Basis of Disease, 1802(11), 952–958. doi:10.1016/j.bbadis.2010.06.016

[1052] Maier et al (2004) 'Low magnesium promotes endothelial cell dysfunction: implications for atherosclerosis, inflammation and thrombosis', Biochimica et Biophysica Acta (BBA) - Molecular Basis of Disease, Volume 1689, Issue 1, 24 May 2004, Pages 13-21.

[1053] Charles D. Lox, M. Mark Dorsett & R. Moss Hampton (1983) Observations on Clotting Activity During Pre-Eclampsia, Clinical and Experimental Hypertension. Part B: Hypertension in Pregnancy, 2:2, 179-190, DOI: 10.3109/10641958309006078

[1054] Cantón, R., Manzanares, J., Alvarez, E., & Zaragozá, F. (1987). In vitro and in vivo antiaggregant effects of magnesium halogenates. Thrombosis and haemostasis, 58(4), 957–959.

[1055] Herbaczynska-Cedro, K., & Gajkowska, B. (1992). Effect of magnesium on myocardial damage induced by epinephrine. Ultrastructural and cytochemical study. Cardioscience, 3(3), 197–203.

[1056] Freedman, A. M., Atrakchi, A. H., Cassidy, M. M., & Weglicki, W. B. (1990). Magnesium deficiency-induced cardiomyopathy: Protection by vitamin E. Biochemical and Biophysical Research Communications, 170(3), 1102–1106. doi:10.1016/0006-291x(90)90506-i

[1057] Ahmad, A., & Bloom, S. (1989). Sodium pump and calcium channel modulation of Mg-deficiency cardiomyopathy. The American journal of cardiovascular pathology, 2(4), 277–283.

[1058] Wester, P.O. and Dyckner, T. (1986), INTRACELLULAR ELECTROLYTES IN CARDIAC FAILURE. Acta Medica Scandinavica, 219: 33-36. https://doi.org/10.1111/j.0954-6820.1986.tb18112.x

[1059] Altura (1979) 'Sudden-death ischemic heart disease and dietary magnesium intake: Is the target site coronary vascular smooth muscle?', Medical Hypotheses, Volume 5, Issue 8, August 1979, Pages 843-848.

[1060] Khan, A. M., Lubitz, S. A., Sullivan, L. M., Sun, J. X., Levy, D., Vasan, R. S., … Wang, T. J. (2013). Low Serum Magnesium and the Development of Atrial Fibrillation in the Community. Circulation, 127(1), 33–38. doi:10.1161/circulationaha.111.082511

[1061] Parsons RS, Butler T, Sellars EP. The treatment of coronary artery disease with parenteral magnesium sulphate. Med Proc 1959:487.

[1062] el-Hindi HM, Amer HA. Effect of thiamine, magnesium, and sulfate salts on growth, thiamine levels, and serum lipid constituents in rats. J Nutr Sci Vitaminol 1989;35:505–10.

[1063] Altura, B. T., Brust, M., Bloom, S., Barbour, R. L., Stempak, J. G., & Altura, B. M. (1990). Magnesium dietary intake modulates blood lipid levels and atherogenesis. Proceedings of the National Academy of Sciences of the United States of America, 87(5), 1840–1844. https://doi.org/10.1073/pnas.87.5.1840

[1064] Rasmussen, H. S. (1989). Influence of Magnesium Substitution Therapy on Blood Lipid Composition in Patients With Ischemic Heart Disease. Archives of Internal Medicine, 149(5), 1050. doi:10.1001/archinte.1989.00390050052010

[1065] Wang, J., Persuitte, G., Olendzki, B. C., Wedick, N. M., Zhang, Z., Merriam, P. A., Fang, H., Carmody, J., Olendzki, G. F., & Ma, Y. (2013). Dietary magnesium intake improves insulin resistance among non-diabetic individuals with metabolic syndrome participating in a dietary trial. Nutrients, 5(10), 3910–3919. https://doi.org/10.3390/nu5103910

[1066] Humphries, S. (1999). Low dietary magnesium is associated with insulin resistance in a sample of young, nondiabetic black Americans. American Journal of Hypertension, 12(8), 747–756. doi:10.1016/s0895-7061(99)00041-2

[1067] Huerta, M. G., Roemmich, J. N., Kington, M. L., Bovbjerg, V. E., Weltman, A. L., Holmes, V. F., … Nadler, J. L. (2005). Magnesium Deficiency Is Associated With Insulin Resistance in Obese Children. Diabetes Care, 28(5), 1175–1181. doi:10.2337/diacare.28.5.1175

[1068] Rodríguez-Morán, M., Simental Mendía, L. E., Zambrano Galván, G., & Guerrero-Romero, F. (2011). The role of magnesium in type 2 diabetes: a brief based-clinical review. Magnesium research, 24(4), 156–162. https://doi.org/10.1684/mrh.2011.0299

[1069] Hruby, A., O'Donnell, C. J., Jacques, P. F., Meigs, J. B., Hoffmann, U., & McKeown, N. M. (2014). Magnesium Intake Is Inversely Associated With Coronary Artery Calcification. JACC: Cardiovascular Imaging, 7(1), 59–69. doi:10.1016/j.jcmg.2013.10.006

[1070] Maier, J. A. ., Malpuech-Brugère, C., Zimowska, W., Rayssiguier, Y., & Mazur, A. (2004). Low magnesium promotes endothelial cell dysfunction: implications for atherosclerosis, inflammation and thrombosis. Biochimica et Biophysica Acta (BBA) - Molecular Basis of Disease, 1689(1), 13–21. doi:10.1016/j.bbadis.2004.01.002

[1071] HEGGTVEIT, H. A., HERMAN, L., & MISHRA, R. K. (1964). CARDIAC NECROSIS AND CALCIFICATION IN EXPERIMENTAL MAGNESIUM DEFICIENCY. A LIGHT AND ELECTRON MICROSCOPIC STUDY. The American journal of pathology, 45(5), 757–782.

[1072] Battifora, H., Eisenstein, R., Laing, G. H., & McCreary, P. (1966). The kidney in experimental magnesium deprivation. a morphologic and biochemical study. The American journal of pathology, 48(3), 421–437.

[1073] Shechter M. The role of magnesium as antithrombotic therapy. Wien Med Wochenschr 2000;150:343–7.

[1074] Shechter et al (1999) 'Oral magnesium supplementation inhibits platelet-dependent thrombosis in patients with coronary artery disease', Am J Cardiol 1999;84:152–6.

[1075] Pokan, R. (2006). Oral magnesium therapy, exercise heart rate, exercise tolerance, and myocardial function in coronary artery disease patients. British Journal of Sports Medicine, 40(9), 773–778. doi:10.1136/bjsm.2006.027250

[1076] Shechter et al (2000) 'Oral Magnesium Therapy Improves Endothelial Function in Patients With Coronary Artery Disease', Circulation. 2000;102:2353–2358

[1077] Zhang, X., Li, Y., Del Gobbo, L. C., Rosanoff, A., Wang, J., Zhang, W., & Song, Y. (2016). Effects of Magnesium Supplementation on Blood Pressure. Hypertension, 68(2), 324–333. doi:10.1161/hypertensionaha.116.07664

[1078] Kass, L., Weekes, J., & Carpenter, L. (2012). Effect of magnesium supplementation on blood pressure: a meta-analysis. European journal of clinical nutrition, 66(4), 411–418. https://doi.org/10.1038/ejcn.2012.4

[1079] Rosanoff and Plesset (2013) 'Oral magnesium supplements decrease high blood pressure (SBP > 155 mmHg) in hypertensive subjects on anti-hypertensive medications: a targeted meta-analysis', Magnesium Research. 2013;26(3):93-99. doi:10.1684/mrh.2013.0343

[1080] Kass, L., Weekes, J., & Carpenter, L. (2012). Effect of magnesium supplementation on blood pressure: a meta-analysis. European journal of clinical nutrition, 66(4), 411–418. https://doi.org/10.1038/ejcn.2012.4

[1081] Rude, R. K., Singer, F. R., & Gruber, H. E. (2009). Skeletal and hormonal effects of magnesium deficiency. Journal of the American College of Nutrition, 28(2), 131–141. https://doi.org/10.1080/07315724.2009.10719764

[1082] Tucker K. L. (2009). Osteoporosis prevention and nutrition. Current osteoporosis reports, 7(4), 111–117. https://doi.org/10.1007/s11914-009-0020-5

[1083] Mutlu, M., Argun, M., Kilic, E., Saraymen, R., & Yazar, S. (2007). Magnesium, zinc and copper status in osteoporotic, osteopenic and normal post-menopausal women. The Journal of international medical research, 35(5), 692–695. https://doi.org/10.1177/147323000703500514

[1084] Aydin, H., Deyneli, O., Yavuz, D., Gözü, H., Mutlu, N., Kaygusuz, I., & Akalin, S. (2010). Short-term oral magnesium supplementation suppresses bone turnover in postmenopausal osteoporotic women. Biological trace element research, 133(2), 136–143. https://doi.org/10.1007/s12011-009-8416-8

[1085] Waddell, A. L., Board, R. G., Scott, V. D., & Tullett, S. G. (1991). Role of magnesium in egg shell formation in the domestic hen. British poultry science, 32(4), 853–864. https://doi.org/10.1080/00071669108417410

[1086] Durlach (1991) 'Magnesium and extinction of dinosaurs. Was magnesium deficit a major cause?', Magnesium Research, 01 Sep 1991, 4(3-4):201-202.

[1087] Durlach J. (1989). Recommended dietary amounts of magnesium: Mg RDA. Magnesium research, 2(3), 195–203.

[1088] World Health Organization. Calcium and Magnesium in Drinking Water: Public health significance. Geneva: World Health Organization Press; 2009.

[1089] Elin R. J. (2011). Re-evaluation of the concept of chronic, latent, magnesium deficiency. Magnesium research, 24(4), 225–227. https://doi.org/10.1684/mrh.2011.0298

[1090] Marier J. R. (1986). Magnesium content of the food supply in the modern-day world. Magnesium, 5(1), 1–8.

[1091] Wang, J. L., Shaw, N. S., Yeh, H. Y., & Kao, M. D. (2005). Magnesium status and association with diabetes in the Taiwanese elderly. Asia Pacific journal of clinical nutrition, 14(3), 263–269.

[1092] Vormann J, Anke M. Dietary magnesium: supply, requirements and recommendations–results from duplicate and balance studies in man. J Clin Basic Cardiol 2002;5:49–53.

[1093] Touvier, Lioret, Vanrullen, Boclé, Boutron-Ruault, Berta, & Volatier. (2006). Vitamin and Mineral Inadequacy in the French Population: Estimation and Application for the Optimization of Food Fortification. International Journal for Vitamin and Nutrition Research, 76(6), 343–351. doi:10.1024/0300-9831.76.6.343

[1094] Cohen, L., & Kitzes, R. (1981). Infrared spectroscopy and magnesium content of bone mineral in osteoporotic women. Israel journal of medical sciences, 17(12), 1123–1125.

[1095] Nielsen, F. H., Milne, D. B., Gallagher, S., Johnson, L., & Hoverson, B. (2007). Moderate magnesium deprivation results in calcium retention and altered potassium and phosphorus excretion by postmenopausal women. Magnesium research, 20(1), 19–31.

[1096] Tipton IH, Stewart PL, Dickson J. Patterns of elemental excretion in long term balance studies. Health Phys 1969;16:455–62.

[1097] DiNicolantonio JJ, O'Keefe JH, Wilson W. Correction: Subclinical magnesium deficiency: a principal driver of cardiovascular disease and a public health crisis. Open Heart 2018;5.

[1098] Hunt, C. D., & Johnson, L. K. (2006). Magnesium requirements: new estimations for men and women by cross-sectional statistical analyses of metabolic magnesium balance data. The American journal of clinical nutrition, 84(4), 843–852. https://doi.org/10.1093/ajcn/84.4.843

[1099] Nielsen, F. H., & Milne, D. B. (2003). Some magnesium status indicators and oxidative metabolism responses to low-dietary magnesium are affected by dietary copper in postmenopausal women. Nutrition, 19(7-8), 617–626. doi:10.1016/s0899-9007(02)01111-5

[1100] Liebscher, D.-H., & Liebscher, D.-E. (2004). About the Misdiagnosis of Magnesium Deficiency. Journal of the American College of Nutrition, 23(6), 730S–731S. doi:10.1080/07315724.2004.10719416

[1101] Lakshmanan, F. L., Rao, R. B., Kim, W. W., & Kelsay, J. L. (1984). Magnesium intakes, balances, and blood levels of adults consuming self-selected diets. The American Journal of Clinical Nutrition, 40(6), 1380–1389. doi:10.1093/ajcn/40.6.1380

[1102] Spencer, H., Fuller, H., Norris, C., & Williams, D. (1994). Effect of magnesium on the intestinal absorption of calcium in man. Journal of the American College of Nutrition, 13(5), 485–492. doi:10.1080/07315724.1994.10718439

[1103] Nielsen, F. H., Milne, D. B., Klevay, L. M., Gallagher, S., & Johnson, L. (2007). Dietary Magnesium Deficiency Induces Heart Rhythm Changes, Impairs Glucose Tolerance, and Decreases Serum Cholesterol in Post Menopausal Women. Journal of the American College of Nutrition, 26(2), 121–132. doi:10.1080/07315724.2007.10719593

[1104] Wilimzig, C., Latz, R., Vierling, W., Mutschler, E., Trnovec, T., & Nyulassy, S. (1996). Increase in magnesium plasma level after orally administered trimagnesium dicitrate. European Journal of Clinical Pharmacology, 49(4), 317–323. doi:10.1007/bf00226334

[1105] Larsson, S. C., Orsini, N., & Wolk, A. (2012). Dietary magnesium intake and risk of stroke: a meta-analysis of prospective studies. The American journal of clinical nutrition, 95(2), 362–366. https://doi.org/10.3945/ajcn.111.022376

[1106] Larsson, S. C., & Wolk, A. (2007). Magnesium intake and risk of type 2 diabetes: a meta-analysis. Journal of internal medicine, 262(2), 208–214. https://doi.org/10.1111/j.1365-2796.2007.01840.x

[1107] Schulze, M. B., Schulz, M., Heidemann, C., Schienkiewitz, A., Hoffmann, K., & Boeing, H. (2007). Fiber and magnesium intake and incidence of type 2 diabetes: a prospective study and meta-analysis. Archives of internal medicine, 167(9), 956–965. https://doi.org/10.1001/archinte.167.9.956

[1108] Durlach et al (1999) 'Cardiovasoprotective foods and nutrients: Possible importance of magnesium intake', Magnesium research: official organ of the International Society for the Development of Research on Magnesium 12(1):57-61.

[1109] Thomas D. (2007). The mineral depletion of foods available to us as a nation (1940-2002)--a review of the 6th Edition of McCance and Widdowson. Nutrition and health, 19(1-2), 21–55. https://doi.org/10.1177/026010600701900205

[1110] Mayer, A. (1997), "Historical changes in the mineral content of fruits and vegetables", British Food Journal, Vol. 99 No. 6, pp. 207-211. https://doi.org/10.1108/00070709710181540

[1111] Guo, W., Nazim, H., Liang, Z., & Yang, D. (2016). Magnesium deficiency in plants: An urgent problem. The Crop Journal, 4(2), 83–91. doi:10.1016/j.cj.2015.11.003

[1112] Seelig M, Rosanoff A. The Magnesium Factor. New York: Avery; 2003.

[1113] Dean C. The Magnesium Miracle. New York: Ballantine Books; 2007.

[1114] NIH (2020) 'Magnesium: Fact Sheet for Health Professionals', Dietary Supplement Fact Sheets, Accessed Online Jan 26 2021: https://ods.od.nih.gov/factsheets/Magnesium-HealthProfessional/

[1115] Fine, K. D., Santa Ana, C. A., Porter, J. L., & Fordtran, J. S. (1991). Intestinal absorption of magnesium from food and supplements. The Journal of clinical investigation, 88(2), 396–402. https://doi.org/10.1172/JCI115317

[1116] Brink, E. J., & Beynen, A. C. (1992). Nutrition and magnesium absorption: a review. Progress in food & nutrition science, 16(2), 125–162.

[1117] Kelsay, J. L., Behall, K. M., & Prather, E. S. (1978). Effect of fiber from fruits and vegetables on metabolic responses of human subjects I. Bowel transit time, number of defecations, fecal weight, urinary excretions of energy and nitrogen and apparent digestibilities of energy, nitrogen, and fat. The American Journal of Clinical Nutrition, 31(7), 1149–1153. doi:10.1093/ajcn/31.7.1149

[1118] Turnlund, J. R., Betschart, A. A., Liebman, M., Kretsch, M. J., & Sauberlich, H. E. (1992). Vitamin B−6 depletion followed by repletion with animal- or plant-source diets and calcium and magnesium metabolism in young women. The American Journal of Clinical Nutrition, 56(5), 905–910. doi:10.1093/ajcn/56.5.905

[1119] Guillard, O., Piriou, A., Fauconneau, B., Mauco, G., & Mettey, R. (2002). Unexpected toxicity induced by magnesium orotate treatment in congenital hypomagnesemia. Journal of internal medicine, 252(1), 88–90. https://doi.org/10.1046/j.1365-2796.2002.01007.x

[1120] van den Heuvel et al (2009) 'Short-chain fructo-oligosaccharides improve magnesium absorption in adolescent girls with a low calcium intake', Nutrition Research, Volume 29, Issue 4, April 2009, Pages 229-237.

[1121] Bunce, G. E., Sauberlich, H. E., Reeves, P. G., & Oba, T. S. (1965). DIETARY PHOSPHORUS AND MAGNESIUM DEFICIENCY IN THE RAT. The Journal of nutrition, 86, 406–413. https://doi.org/10.1093/jn/86.4.406

[1122] Bunce, G. E., Chiemchaisri, Y., & Phillips, P. H. (1962). The mineral requirements of the dog. IV. Effect of certain dietary and physiologic factors upon the magnesium deficiency syndrome. The Journal of nutrition, 76(1), 23–29. https://doi.org/10.1093/jn/76.1.23

[1123] O'Dell (1960) 'Magnesium requirement and its relation to other dietary constitunents.', Federation Proceedings, 01 Jul 1960, 19:648-654.

[1124] Hodgkinson, A., Marshall, D. H., & Nordin, B. E. C. (1979). Vitamin D and Magnesium Absorption in Man. Clinical Science, 57(1), 121–123. doi:10.1042/cs0570121

[1125] Krejs, G. J., Nicar, M. J., Zerwekh, J. E., Norman, D. A., Kane, M. G., & Pak, C. Y. (1983). Effect of 1,25-dihydroxyvitamin D3 on calcium and magnesium absorption in the healthy human jejunum and ileum. The American journal of medicine, 75(6), 973–976. https://doi.org/10.1016/0002-9343(83)90877-x

[1126] Schmulen, A. C., Lerman, M., Pak, C. Y., Zerwekh, J., Morawski, S., Fordtran, J. S., & Vergne-Marini, P. (1980). Effect of 1,25-(OH)2D3 on jejunal absorption of magnesium in patients with chronic renal disease. The American journal of physiology, 238(4), G349–G352. https://doi.org/10.1152/ajpgi.1980.238.4.G349

[1127] Krejs et al (1983) 'Effect of 1,25-dihydroxyvitamin D3 on calcium and magnesium absorption in the healthy human jejunum and ileum', Am J Med 1983;75:973–6.

[1128] Liu, X., Yao, M., Li, N., Wang, C., Zheng, Y., & Cao, X. (2008). CaMKII promotes TLR-triggered proinflammatory cytokine and type I interferon production by directly binding and activating TAK1 and IRF3 in macrophages. Blood, 112(13), 4961–4970. https://doi.org/10.1182/blood-2008-03-144022

[1129] Grabarek, Z. (2011). Insights into modulation of calcium signaling by magnesium in calmodulin, troponin C and related EF-hand proteins. Biochimica et Biophysica Acta (BBA) - Molecular Cell Research, 1813(5), 913–921. doi:10.1016/j.bbamcr.2011.01.017

[1130] Malmendal, A., Linse, S., Evenäs, J., Forsén, S., & Drakenberg, T. (1999). Battle for the EF-Hands: Magnesium−Calcium Interference in Calmodulin†. Biochemistry, 38(36), 11844–11850. doi:10.1021/bi9909288

[1131] Arayne, M. S., Sultana, N., & Hussain, F. (2005). Interactions between ciprofloxacin and antacids--dissolution and adsorption studies. Drug metabolism and drug interactions, 21(2), 117–129. https://doi.org/10.1515/dmdi.2005.21.2.117

[1132] Dunn, C. J., & Goa, K. L. (2001). Risedronate: a review of its pharmacological properties and clinical use in resorptive bone disease. Drugs, 61(5), 685–712. https://doi.org/10.2165/00003495-200161050-00013

[1133] Wacker, W. E. C., & Parisi, A. F. (1968). Magnesium Metabolism. New England Journal of Medicine, 278(12), 658–663. doi:10.1056/nejm196803212781205

[1134] Smith, R. H. (1959). Calcium and magnesium metabolism in calves. 4. Bone composition in magnesium deficiency and the control of plasma magnesium*. Biochemical Journal, 71(4), 609–614. doi:10.1042/bj0710609

[1135] Rude, R. K., & Gruber, H. E. (2004). Magnesium deficiency and osteoporosis: animal and human observations. The Journal of Nutritional Biochemistry, 15(12), 710–716. doi:10.1016/j.jnutbio.2004.08.001

[1136] Sutton, R. A., & Domrongkitchaiporn, S. (1993). Abnormal renal magnesium handling. Mineral and electrolyte metabolism, 19(4-5), 232–240.

[1137] Neathery, M. W., Crowe, N. A., Miller, W. J., Crowe, C. T., Varnadoe, J. L., & Blackmon, D. M. (1990). Effects of dietary aluminum and phosphorus on magnesium metabolism in dairy calves2. Journal of Animal Science, 68(4), 1133–1138. doi:10.2527/1990.6841133x

[1138] DiNicolantonio, J. J., O'Keefe, J. H., & Wilson, W. (2018). Subclinical magnesium deficiency: a principal driver of cardiovascular disease and a public health crisis. Open Heart, 5(1), e000668. doi:10.1136/openhrt-2017-000668

[1139] Brannan, P. G., Vergne-Marini, P., Pak, C. Y., Hull, A. R., & Fordtran, J. S. (1976). Magnesium absorption in the human small intestine. Results in normal subjects, patients with chronic renal disease, and patients with absorptive hypercalciuria. Journal of Clinical Investigation, 57(6), 1412–1418. doi:10.1172/jci108410

[1140] Bianchetti, M. G., Oetliker, O. H., & Lütschg, J. (1993). Magnesium deficiency in primary distal tubular acidosis. The Journal of Pediatrics, 122(5), 833. doi:10.1016/s0022-3476(06)80045-4

[1141] Lim, P., Dong, S., & Khoo, O. T. (1969). Intracellular Magnesium Depletion in Chronic Renal Failure. New England Journal of Medicine, 280(18), 981–984. doi:10.1056/nejm196905012801803

[1142] Markell MS, Altura BT, Sarn Y, et al. Deficiency of serum ionized magnesium in patients receiving hemodialysis or peritoneal dialysis. Asaio J 1993;39:M801–4.

[1143] Vitale C, Marangella M, Petrarulo M, et al. [Mineral balance during hemodialysis and hemodiafiltration]. Minerva Urol Nefrol 1990;42:173–6.

[1144] Rylander R, Mégevand Y, Lasserre B, et al. Moderate alcohol consumption and urinary excretion of magnesium and calcium. Scand J Clin Lab Invest 2001;61:401–5.

[1145] Tuso PJ, Nortman D. Renal magnesium wasting associated with acetaminophen abuse. Conn Med 1992;56:421–3.

[1146] Fernández-Fernández FJ, Sesma P, Caínzos-Romero T, et al. Intermittent use of pantoprazole and famotidine in severe hypomagnesaemia due to omeprazole. Neth J Med 2010;68:329–30

[1147] Shabajee, N., Lamb, E. J., Sturgess, I., & Sumathipala, R. W. (2008). Omeprazole and refractory hypomagnesaemia. BMJ, 337(jul10 3), a425–a425. doi:10.1136/bmj.39505.738981.be

[1148] Mackay, J. D., & Bladon, P. T. (2010). Hypomagnesaemia due to proton-pump inhibitor therapy: a clinical case series. QJM, 103(6), 387–395. doi:10.1093/qjmed/hcq021

[1149] La, S. A., Lee, J. Y., Kim, D. H., Song, E. L., Park, J. H., & Ju, S. Y. (2015). Low Magnesium Levels in Adults with Metabolic Syndrome: a Meta-Analysis. Biological Trace Element Research, 170(1), 33–42. doi:10.1007/s12011-015-0446-9

[1150] Uğurlu, V., Binay, Ç., Şimşek, E., & Bal, C. (2016). Cellular Trace Element Changes in Type 1 Diabetes Patients. Journal of Clinical Research in Pediatric Endocrinology, 8(2), 180–186. doi:10.4274/jcrpe.2449

[1151] Schnack, C., Bauer, I., Pregant, P., Hopmeier, P., & Schernthaner, G. (1992). Hypomagnesaemia in Type 2 (non-insulin-dependent) diabetes mellitus is not corrected by improvement of long-term metabolic control. Diabetologia, 35(1), 77–79. doi:10.1007/bf00400855

[1152] Booth, C. C., Babouris, N., Hanna, S., & MacIntyre, I. (1963). Incidence of Hypomagnesaemia in Intestinal Malabsorption. BMJ, 2(5350), 141–144. doi:10.1136/bmj.2.5350.141

[1153] Richardson, J. A., & Welt, L. G. (1965). The Hypomagnesemia of Vitamin D Administration. Experimental Biology and Medicine, 118(2), 512–514. doi:10.3181/00379727-118-29891

[1154] Casoni, I., Guglielmini, C., Graziano, L., Reali, M., Mazzotta, D., & Abbasciano, V. (1990). Changes of Magnesium Concentrations in Endurance Athletes. International Journal of Sports Medicine, 11(03), 234–237. doi:10.1055/s-2007-1024798

[1155] Delva, P., Pastori, C., Degan, M., Montesi, G., Brazzarola, P., & Lechi, A. (2000). Intralymphocyte Free Magnesium in Patients With Primary Aldosteronism. Hypertension, 35(1), 113–117. doi:10.1161/01.hyp.35.1.113

[1156] KODAMA, N., NISHIMUTA, M., & SUZUKI, K. (2003). Negative Balance of Calcium and Magnesium under Relatively Low Sodium Intake in Humans. Journal of Nutritional Science and Vitaminology, 49(3), 201–209. doi:10.3177/jnsv.49.201

[1157] Sjögren, A., Florén, C.-H., & Nilsson, A. (1988). Evaluation of Magnesium Status in Crohn's Disease as Assessed by Intracellular Analysis and Intravenous Magnesium Infusion. Scandinavian Journal of Gastroenterology, 23(5), 555–561. doi:10.3109/00365528809093911

[1158] Lipner, A. (1977). Symptomatic magnesium deficiency after small-intestinal bypass for obesity. BMJ, 1(6054), 148–148. doi:10.1136/bmj.1.6054.148

[1159] Mountokalakis TD. Effects of aging, chronic disease, and multiple supplements on magnesium requirements. Magnesium 1987;6:5–11.

[1160] Normén L, Arnaud MJ, Carlsson NG, et al. Small bowel absorption of magnesium and calcium sulphate from a natural mineral water in subjects with ileostomy. Eur J Nutr 2006;45:105–12.

[1161] Oralewska B, Zawadzki J, Jankowska I, et al. Disorders of magnesium homeostasis in the course of liver disease in children. Magnes Res 1996;9:125–8.

[1162] Evans, T. R. J., Harper, C. L., Beveridge, I. G., Wastnage, R., & Mansi, J. L. (1995). A randomised study to determine whether routine intravenous magnesium supplements are necessary in patients receiving cisplatin chemotherapy with continuous infusion 5-fluorouracil. European Journal of Cancer, 31(2), 174–178. doi:10.1016/0959-8049(94)00420-a

[1163] SCHILSKY, R. L. (1979). Hypomagnesemia and Renal Magnesium Wasting in Patients Receiving Cisplatin. Annals of Internal Medicine, 90(6), 929. doi:10.7326/0003-4819-90-6-929

[1164] Lam, M., & Adelstein, D. J. (1986). Hypomagnesemia and Renal Magnesium Wasting in Patients Treated With Cisplatin. American Journal of Kidney Diseases, 8(3), 164–169. doi:10.1016/s0272-6386(86)80020-8

[1165] Bianchetti MG, Kanaka C, Ridolfi-Lüthy A, et al. Chronic renal magnesium loss, hypocalciuria and mild hypokalaemic metabolic alkalosis after cisplatin. Pediatr Nephrol 1990;4:219–22

[1166] Main, A.N., Morgan, R.J., Russell, R.I., Hall, M.J., Mackenzie, J.F., Shenkin, A. and Fell, G.S. (1981), Mg Deficiency in Chronic Inflammatory Bowel Disease and Requirements During Intravenous Nutrition. Journal of Parenteral and Enteral Nutrition, 5: 15-19. https://doi.org/10.1177/014860718100500115

[1167] Revúsová, V., Polakovicová, D., Stefíková, K., & Dzúrik, R. (1991). Pokles magnézia v sére a v krvných lymfocytoch po intravenóznej infúzii glukózy [A decrease in magnesium in the serum and blood lymphocytes after intravenous infusion of glucose]. Casopis lekaru ceskych, 130(16-17), 513–515.

[1168] Djurhuus, M. S., Skøtt, P., Hother-Nielsen, O., Klitgaard, N. A. H., & Beck-Nielsen, H. (1995). Insulin Increases Renal Magnesium Excretion: A Possible Cause of Magnesium Depletion in Hyperinsulinaemic States. Diabetic Medicine, 12(8), 664–669. doi:10.1111/j.1464-5491.1995.tb00566.x

[1169] Hwang, D. L., Yen, C. F., & Nadler, J. L. (1993). Insulin increases intracellular magnesium transport in human platelets. The Journal of Clinical Endocrinology & Metabolism, 76(3), 549–553. doi:10.1210/jcem.76.3.8445010

[1170] Galland L. (1991). Magnesium, stress and neuropsychiatric disorders. Magnesium and trace elements, 10(2-4), 287–301.

[1171] Blasco, L. M., Novo, F., & González-Fernández, C. R. (2012). Chronic Cyclic Nonnephrogenic Magnesium Depletion without Losses. New England Journal of Medicine, 366(19), 1845–1846. doi:10.1056/nejmc1201985

[1172] Seelig M. S. (1990). Increased need for magnesium with the use of combined oestrogen and calcium for osteoporosis treatment. Magnesium research, 3(3), 197–215.

[1173] Kamble TK, Ookalkar DS. Lactational hypomagnesaemia. Lancet 1989;2:155–6.

[1174] DRENICK, E. J., HUNT, I. F., & SWENDSEID, M. E. (1969). Magnesium Depletion During Prolonged Fasting of Obese Males. The Journal of Clinical Endocrinology & Metabolism, 29(10), 1341–1348. doi:10.1210/jcem-29-10-1341

[1175] Nanji AA, Denegri JF. Hypomagnesemia associated with gentamicin therapy. Drug Intell Clin Pharm 1984;18:596–8.

[1176] Zaloga GP, Chernow B, Pock A, et al. Hypomagnesemia is a common complication of aminoglycoside therapy. Surg Gynecol Obstet 1984;158:561–5

[1177] Martin KJ, González EA, Slatopolsky E. Clinical consequences and management of hypomagnesemia. J Am Soc Nephrol 2009;20:2291–5.

[1178] Ohtsuka S, Yamaguchi I. [Magnesium in congestive heart failure]. Clin Calcium 2005;15:181–6.

[1179] Spasov, A. A., Iezhitsa, I. N., Kravchenko, M. S., & Kharitonova, M. V. (2009). Features of Central Neurotransmission in Animals in Conditions of Dietary Magnesium Deficiency and After Its Correction. Neuroscience and Behavioral Physiology, 39(7), 645–653. doi:10.1007/s11055-009-9182-y

[1180] Rylander, R., Remer, T., Berkemeyer, S., & Vormann, J. (2006). Acid-base status affects renal magnesium losses in healthy, elderly persons. The Journal of nutrition, 136(9), 2374–2377. https://doi.org/10.1093/jn/136.9.2374

[1181] Rylander, R., Tallheden, T., & Vormann, J. (2009). Acid-base conditions regulate calcium and magnesium homeostasis. Magnesium Research, 22(4), 262–265. doi:10.1684/mrh.2009.0182

[1182] Papazachariou, I. M., Martinez-Isla, A., Efthimiou, E., Williamson, R. C. ., & Girgis, S. I. (2000). Magnesium deficiency in patients with chronic pancreatitis identified by an intravenous loading test. Clinica Chimica Acta, 302(1-2), 145–154. doi:10.1016/s0009-8981(00)00363-6

[1183] Ryzen E, Rude RK. Low intracellular magnesium in patients with acute pancreatitis and hypocalcemia. West J Med 1990;152:145–8

[1184] Liamis, G., Gianoutsos, C., & Elisaf, M. (2001). Acute Pancreatitis-Induced Hypomagnesemia. Pancreatology, 1(1), 74–76. doi:10.1159/000055796

[1185] Spätling L, Classen HG, Külpmann WR, et al. [Diagnosing magnesium deficiency. Current recommendations of the Society for Magnesium Research]. Fortschr Med Orig 2000;118(Suppl 2):49–53.

[1186] Elin, R. J. (2011). Re-evaluation of the concept of chronic, latent, magnesium deficiency. Magnesium Research, 24(4), 225–227. doi:10.1684/mrh.2011.0298

[1187] Costello, R. B., Elin, R. J., Rosanoff, A., Wallace, T. C., Guerrero-Romero, F., Hruby, A., … Van Horn, L. V. (2016). Perspective: The Case for an Evidence-Based Reference Interval for Serum Magnesium: The Time Has Come. Advances in Nutrition: An International Review Journal, 7(6), 977–993. doi:10.3945/an.116.012765

[1188] Dierck-Hartmut Liebscher & Dierck-Ekkehard Liebscher (2004) About the Misdiagnosis of Magnesium Deficiency, Journal of the American College of Nutrition, 23:6, 730S-731S, DOI: 10.1080/07315724.2004.10719416

[1189] Wang, J. L., Shaw, N. S., Yeh, H. Y., & Kao, M. D. (2005). Magnesium status and association with diabetes in the Taiwanese elderly. Asia Pacific journal of clinical nutrition, 14(3), 263–269.

[1190] Peacock, J. M., Ohira, T., Post, W., Sotoodehnia, N., Rosamond, W., & Folsom, A. R. (2010). Serum magnesium and risk of sudden cardiac death in the Atherosclerosis Risk in Communities (ARIC) Study. American heart journal, 160(3), 464–470. https://doi.org/10.1016/j.ahj.2010.06.012

[1191] Liebscher, D.-H., & Liebscher, D.-E. (2004). About the Misdiagnosis of Magnesium Deficiency. Journal of the American College of Nutrition, 23(6), 730S–731S. doi:10.1080/07315724.2004.10719416

[1192] Costello, R. B., Elin, R. J., Rosanoff, A., Wallace, T. C., Guerrero-Romero, F., Hruby, A., … Van Horn, L. V. (2016). Perspective: The Case for an Evidence-Based Reference Interval for Serum

Magnesium: The Time Has Come. Advances in Nutrition: An International Review Journal, 7(6), 977–993. doi:10.3945/an.116.012765

[1193] Schimatschek and Rempis (2002) 'Prevalence of hypomagnesemia in an unselected German population of 16,000 individuals', Magnesium research: official organ of the International Society for the Development of Research on Magnesium 14(4):283-90.

[1194] Mejía-Rodríguez, F., Shamah-Levy, T., Villalpando, S., García-Guerra, A., & Méndez-Gómez Humarán, I. (2013). Iron, zinc, copper and magnesium deficiencies in Mexican adults from the National Health and Nutrition Survey 2006. Salud Pública de México, 55(3), 275. doi:10.21149/spm.v55i3.7210

[1195] Colli, C. (2014). HAY DEFICIENCIA CRÓNICA LATENTE DE MAGNESIO EN ESTUDIANTES [JB]. NUTRICION HOSPITALARIA, (1), 200–204. https://doi.org/10.3305/nh.2014.30.1.7510

[1196] de Lourdes Lima et al (2006) '[Magnesium deficiency and insulin resistance in patients with type 2 diabetes mellitus]', Arquivos Brasileiros de Endocrinologia & Metabologia 49(6):959-63.

[1197] Whang, R., & Ryder, K. W. (1990). Frequency of hypomagnesemia and hypermagnesemia. Requested vs routine. JAMA, 263(22), 3063–3064.

[1198] Ryzen E. Magnesium homeostasis in critically ill patients. Magnesium 1989;8:201–12.

[1199] Toto and Yucha (1994) 'Magnesium: Homeostasis, imbalances, and therapeutic uses', Critical Care Nursing Clinics of North America, 6(4), http://dx.doi.org/10.1016/S0899-5885(18)30448-9

[1700] Escuela, M. P., Guerra, M., A n, J. M., Mart nez-Vizca no, V., Zapatero, M. D., Garc a-Jal n, A., & Celaya, S. (2004). Total and ionized serum magnesium in critically ill patients. Intensive Care Medicine, 31(1), 151–156. doi:10.1007/s00134-004-2508-x

[1201] Olerich, M. A., & Rude, R. K. (1994). Should we supplement magnesium in critically ill patients?. New horizons (Baltimore, Md.), 2(2), 186–192.

[1202] Whang R. (1987). Routine serum magnesium determination--a continuing unrecognized need. Magnesium, 6(1), 1–4.

[1203] Dabbagh, O. C., Aldawood, A. S., Arabi, Y. M., Lone, N. A., Brits, R., & Pillay, M. (2006). Magnesium supplementation and the potential association with mortality rates among critically ill non-cardiac patients. Saudi medical journal, 27(6), 821–825.

[1204] Abbott, L. G., & Rude, R. K. (1993). Clinical manifestations of magnesium deficiency. Mineral and electrolyte metabolism, 19(4-5), 314–322.

[1205] Touitou, Y., Godard, J. P., Ferment, O., Chastang, C., Proust, J., Bogdan, A., Auzéby, A., & Touitou, C. (1987). Prevalence of magnesium and potassium deficiencies in the elderly. Clinical chemistry, 33(4), 518–523.

[1206] Caddell JL. Magnesium deficiency in man. Del Med J 1968;40:133–8.

[1207] Dørup, I., & Skajaa, K. (1989). Magnesium og langvarig diuretikabehandling [Magnesium and long-term diuretic therapy]. Ugeskrift for laeger, 151(12), 759–763.

[1208] Seelig C. B. (1990). Magnesium deficiency in two hypertensive patient groups. Southern medical journal, 83(7), 739–742. https://doi.org/10.1097/00007611-199007000-00004

[1209] Malini, P. L., Strocchi, E., Valtancoli, G., & Ambrosioni, E. (1990). Angiotensin converting enzyme inhibitors, thiazide diuretics and magnesium balance. A preliminary study. Magnesium research, 3(3), 193–196.

[1210] Hollifield (1986) 'Thiazide treatment of hypertension: Effects of thiazide diuretics on serum potassium, magnesium, and ventricular ectopy', Am J Med 1986;80:8–12.

[1211] Hollifield (1984) 'Potassium and magnesium abnormalities: Diuretics and arrhythmias in hypertension', Am J Med 1984;77:28–32.

[1212] Dyckner and Wester (1987) 'Potassium/magnesium depletion in patients with cardiovascular disease', Am J Med 1987;82:11–17.

[1213] Dyckner and Wester (1979) 'Ventricular extrasystoles and intracellular electrolytes before and after potassium and magnesium infusions in patients on diuretic treatment', American Heart Journal, Volume 97, Issue 1, January 1979, Pages 12-18.

[1214] Dyckner, T. and Wester, P.O. (1981), Relation between Potassium, Magnesium and Cardiac Arrhythmias. Acta Medica Scandinavica, 209: 163-169. https://doi.org/10.1111/j.0954-6820.1981.tb02652.x

[1215] Rasmussen HS, McNair P, Gøransson L, et al. Magnesium deficiency in patients with ischemic heart disease with and without acute myocardial infarction uncovered by an intravenous loading test. Arch Intern Med 1988;148:329–32.

[1216] DiNicolantonio, J. J., O'Keefe, J. H., & Wilson, W. (2018). Subclinical magnesium deficiency: a principal driver of cardiovascular disease and a public health crisis. Open Heart, 5(1), e000668. doi:10.1136/openhrt-2017-000668

[1217] Shils ME. Experimental human magnesium depletion. Medicine 1969;48:61–85.

[1218] De Carvalho, M., Kiernan, M. C., & Swash, M. (2017). Fasciculation in amyotrophic lateral sclerosis: origin and pathophysiological relevance. Journal of Neurology, Neurosurgery & Psychiatry, 88(9), 773–779. doi:10.1136/jnnp-2017-315574

585

[1219] Cieslewicz et al (2012) 'The role of magnesium in cardiac arrhythmias', Journal of Elementology 18(2/2013), DOI: 10.5601/jelem.2013.18.2.11

[1220] Sun-Edelstein, C., & Mauskop, A. (2009). Role of magnesium in the pathogenesis and treatment of migraine. Expert review of neurotherapeutics, 9(3), 369–379. https://doi.org/10.1586/14737175.9.3.369

[1221] Schürks, M., Diener, H. C., & Goadsby, P. (2008). Update on the prophylaxis of migraine. Current treatment options in neurology, 10(1), 20–29. https://doi.org/10.1007/s11940-008-0003-3

[1222] Grobin W. A New Syndrome, Magnesium-Deficiency Tetany. Can Med Assoc J 1960;82:1034–5.

[1223] Jooste, P. L., Wolfswinkel, J. M., Schoeman, J. J., & Strydom, N. B. (1979). Epileptic-type convulsions and magnesium deficiency. Aviation, space, and environmental medicine, 50(7), 734–735.

[1224] Johnson, S. (2001). The multifaceted and widespread pathology of magnesium deficiency. Medical Hypotheses, 56(2), 163–170. doi:10.1054/mehy.2000.1133

[1225] Alloui, A., Begon, S., Chassaing, C., Eschalier, A., Gueux, E., Rayssiguier, Y., & Dubray, C. (2003). Does Mg2+ deficiency induce a long-term sensitization of the central nociceptive pathways? European Journal of Pharmacology, 469(1-3), 65–69. doi:10.1016/s0014-2999(03)01719-9

[1226] Durlach J, Pagès N, Bac P, et al. Headache due to photosensitive magnesium depletion. Magnes Res 2005;18:109–22.

[1227] Cevette, M. J., Barrs, D. M., Patel, A., Conroy, K. P., Sydlowski, S., Noble, B. N., Nelson, G. A., & Stepanek, J. (2011). Phase 2 study examining magnesium-dependent tinnitus. The international tinnitus journal, 16(2), 168–173.

[1228] Cevette, M. J., Vormann, J., & Franz, K. (2003). Magnesium and hearing. Journal of the American Academy of Audiology, 14(4), 202–212.

[1229] RUDE, R. K., OLDHAM, S. B., & SINGER, F. R. (1976). FUNCTIONAL HYPOPARATHYROIDISM AND PARATHYROID HORMONE END-ORGAN RESISTANCE IN HUMAN MAGNESIUM DEFICIENCY. Clinical Endocrinology, 5(3), 209–224. doi:10.1111/j.1365-2265.1976.tb01947.x

[1230] Agarwal, R., Iezhitsa, I. N., Agarwal, P., & Spasov, A. A. (2013). Mechanisms of cataractogenesis in the presence of magnesium deficiency. Magnesium Research, 26(1), 2–8. doi:10.1684/mrh.2013.0336

[1231] Kitliński M, Stepniewski M, Nessler J, et al. Is magnesium deficit in lymphocytes a part of the mitral valve prolapse syndrome? Magnes Res 2004;17:39–45.

[1232] Mccoy, J. H., & Kenney, M. A. (1975). Depressed immune response in the magnesium-deficient rat. The Journal of nutrition, 105(6), 791–797. https://doi.org/10.1093/jn/105.6.791

[1233] Schmitz, C., & Perraud, A.-L. (2017). Magnesium and the Immune Response. Molecular, Genetic, and Nutritional Aspects of Major and Trace Minerals, 319–331. doi:10.1016/b978-0-12-802168-2.00026-9

[1234] Siwek, M., Wróbel, A., Dudek, D., Nowak, G., & Zieba, A. (2005). Udział miedzi i magnezu w patogenezie i terapii zaburzeń afektywnych [The role of copper and magnesium in the pathogenesis and treatment of affective disorders]. Psychiatria polska, 39(5), 911–920.

[1235] Anon. Magnesium deficiency. Br Med J 1967;2:195

[1236] Spisák V. [Magnesium loading test in cardiovascular diseases]. Vnitr Lek 1992;38:337–44.

[1237] Thomas, J., Millot, J.-M., Sebille, S., Delabroise, A.-M., Thomas, E., Manfait, M., & Arnaud, M. J. (2000). Free and total magnesium in lymphocytes of migraine patients — effect of magnesium-rich mineral water intake. Clinica Chimica Acta, 295(1-2), 63–75. doi:10.1016/s0009-8981(00)00186-8

[1238] Kozielec T, Sałacka A, Radomska K, et al. The influence of magnesium supplementation on magnesium and calcium concentrations in hair of children with magnesium shortage. Magnes Res 2001;14:33–8.

[1239] Solarska K, Stepniewski M, Pach J. Concentration of magnesium in hair of inhabitants of down-town Kraków, the protective zone of Steel-Mill "Huta im. Sendzimira" and Tokarnia village. Przegl Lek 1995;52:263–6.

[1240] Witkowski, M., Hubert, J., & Mazur, A. (2011). Methods of assessment of magnesium status in humans: a systematic review. Magnesium research, 24(4), 163–180. https://doi.org/10.1684/mrh.2011.0292

[1241] Caddell JL. Magnesium deficiency in man. Del Med J 1968;40:133–8.

[1242] Gullestad, L., Midtvedt, K., Dolva, L. ø., Norseth, J., & Kjekshus, J. (1994). The magnesium loading test: Reference values in healthy subjects. Scandinavian Journal of Clinical and Laboratory Investigation, 54(1), 23–31. doi:10.3109/00365519409086506

[1243] Gullestad, L., Dolva, L. ø, Waage, A., Falch, D., Fagerthun, H., & Kjekshus, J. (1992). Magnesium deficiency diagnosed by an intravenous loading test. Scandinavian Journal of Clinical and Laboratory Investigation, 52(4), 245–253. doi:10.3109/00365519209088355

[1244] Gullestad, L., Nes, M., Rønneberg, R., Midtvedt, K., Falch, D., & Kjekshus, J. (1994). Magnesium status in healthy free-living elderly Norwegians. Journal of the American College of Nutrition, 13(1), 45–50. doi:10.1080/07315724.1994.10718370

586

[1245] Goto, K., Yasue, H., Okumura, K., Matsuyama, K., Kugiyama, K., Miyagi, H., & Higashi, T. (1990). Magnesium deficiency detected by intravenous loading test in variant angina pectoris. The American Journal of Cardiology, 65(11), 709–712. doi:10.1016/0002-9149(90)91375-g

[1246] Assadi F. Hypomagnesemia: an evidence-based approach to clinical cases. Iran J Kidney Dis 2010;4:13–19.

[1247] Assadi F. (2010). Hypomagnesemia: an evidence-based approach to clinical cases. Iranian journal of kidney diseases, 4(1), 13–19.

[1248] Elisaf, M., Panteli, K., Theodorou, J., & Siamopoulos, K. C. (1997). Fractional excretion of magnesium in normal subjects and in patients with hypomagnesemia. Magnesium research, 10(4), 315–320.

[1249] Nadler, J. L., Malayan, S., Luong, H., Shaw, S., Natarajan, R. D., & Rude, R. K. (1992). Intracellular Free Magnesium Deficiency Plays a Key Role in Increased Platelet Reactivity in Type II Diabetes Mellitus. Diabetes Care, 15(7), 835–841. doi:10.2337/diacare.15.7.835

[1250] DiNicolantonio, J. J., O'Keefe, J. H., & Wilson, W. (2018). Subclinical magnesium deficiency: a principal driver of cardiovascular disease and a public health crisis. Open heart, 5(1), e000668. https://doi.org/10.1136/openhrt-2017-000668

[1251] Bartenstein (2016) 'Magnesium Supplement Guide', Supplement Specs, Accessed Online Feb 04 2021: https://supplementspecs.com/magnesium-supplement-guide/

[1252] Slutsky, I., Abumaria, N., Wu, L. J., Huang, C., Zhang, L., Li, B., Zhao, X., Govindarajan, A., Zhao, M. G., Zhuo, M., Tonegawa, S., & Liu, G. (2010). Enhancement of learning and memory by elevating brain magnesium. Neuron, 65(2), 165–177. https://doi.org/10.1016/j.neuron.2009.12.026

[1253] Liu, G., Weinger, J. G., Lu, Z. L., Xue, F., & Sadeghpour, S. (2016). Efficacy and Safety of MMFS-01, a Synapse Density Enhancer, for Treating Cognitive Impairment in Older Adults: A Randomized, Double-Blind, Placebo-Controlled Trial. Journal of Alzheimer's disease : JAD, 49(4), 971–990. https://doi.org/10.3233/JAD-150538

[1254] Surman, C., Vaudreuil, C., Boland, H., Rhodewalt, L., DiSalvo, M., & Biederman, J. (2020). L-Threonic Acid Magnesium Salt Supplementation in ADHD: An Open-Label Pilot Study. Journal of dietary supplements, 1–13. Advance online publication. https://doi.org/10.1080/19390211.2020.1731044

[1255] Wroolie, T. E., Chen, K., Watson, K. T., Iagaru, A., Sonni, I., Snyder, N., ... Rasgon, N. L. (2017). An 8-week open label trial of l -Threonic Acid Magnesium Salt in patients with mild to moderate dementia. Personalized Medicine in Psychiatry, 4-6, 7–12. doi:10.1016/j.pmip.2017.07.001

[1256] Huang, Y., Huang, X., Zhang, L., Han, F., Pang, K. L., Li, X., & Shen, J. Y. (2018). Magnesium boosts the memory restorative effect of environmental enrichment in Alzheimer's disease mice. CNS neuroscience & therapeutics, 24(1), 70–79. https://doi.org/10.1111/cns.12775

[1257] Blaquiere and Berthon (1987) 'Speciation studies in relation to magnesium bioavailability. Formation of Mg(II) complexes with glutamate, aspartate, glycinate, lactate, pyroglutamate, pyridoxine and citrate, and appraisal of their potential significance towards magnesium gastrointestinal absorption', Inorganica Chimica Acta, Volume 135, Issue 3, March 1987, Pages 179-189.

[1258] Lamontagne C, Sewell JA, Vaillancourt R, Kuhzarani C, (2012) Rapid Resolution of Chronic Back Pain with Magnesium Glycinate in a Pediatric Patient. J Pain Relief 1:101. doi:10.4172/2167-0846.1000101

[1259] Eby, G. A., & Eby, K. L. (2006). Rapid recovery from major depression using magnesium treatment. Medical hypotheses, 67(2), 362–370. https://doi.org/10.1016/j.mehy.2006.01.047

[1260] Schuette, S. A., Lashner, B. A., & Janghorbani, M. (1994). Bioavailability of magnesium diglycinate vs magnesium oxide in patients with ileal resection. JPEN. Journal of parenteral and enteral nutrition, 18(5), 430–435. https://doi.org/10.1177/0148607194018005430

[1261] Porter et al (2010) 'Alternative Medical Interventions Used in the Treatment and Management of Myalgic Encephalomyelitis/Chronic Fatigue Syndrome and Fibromyalgia', The Journal of Alternative and Complementary Medicine Vol. 16, No. 3, https://doi.org/10.1089/acm.2008.0376

[1262] Engen et al (2015) 'Effects of transdermal magnesium chloride on quality of life for patients with fibromyalgia: a feasibility study', Journal of Integrative Medicine, Volume 13, Issue 5, September 2015, Pages 306-313.

[1263] Werbach (2000) 'Nutritional strategies for treating chronic fatigue syndrome', Alternative Medicine Review: a Journal of Clinical Therapeutic 5(2):93-108.

[1264] Uysal, N., Kizildag, S., Yuce, Z., Guvendi, G., Kandis, S., Koc, B., ... Ates, M. (2018). Timeline (Bioavailability) of Magnesium Compounds in Hours: Which Magnesium Compound Works Best? Biological Trace Element Research, 187(1), 128–136. doi:10.1007/s12011-018-1351-9

[1265] Hein J. (2011). Comparison of the efficacy and safety of pantoprazole magnesium and pantoprazole sodium in the treatment of gastro-oesophageal reflux disease: a randomized, double-blind, controlled, multicentre trial. Clinical drug investigation, 31(9), 655–664. https://doi.org/10.2165/11590270-000000000-00000

[1266] Rodríguez-Morán, M., & Guerrero-Romero, F. (2003). Oral magnesium supplementation improves insulin sensitivity and metabolic control in type 2 diabetic subjects: a randomized double-blind controlled trial. Diabetes care, 26(4), 1147–1152. https://doi.org/10.2337/diacare.26.4.1147

[1267] Tarleton et al (2017) 'Role of magnesium supplementation in thetreatment of depression: A randomized clinical trial', PLoS ONE 12(6): e0180067. https://doi.org/10.1371/journal. pone.0180067

[1268] Engen, D. J., McAllister, S. J., Whipple, M. O., Cha, S. S., Dion, L. J., Vincent, A., Bauer, B. A., & Wahner-Roedler, D. L. (2015). Effects of transdermal magnesium chloride on quality of life for patients with fibromyalgia: a feasibility study. Journal of integrative medicine, 13(5), 306–313. https://doi.org/10.1016/S2095-4964(15)60195-9

[1269] Walker, A. F., Marakis, G., Christie, S., & Byng, M. (2003). Mg citrate found more bioavailable than other Mg preparations in a randomised, double-blind study. Magnesium research, 16(3), 183–191.

[1270] Lindberg, J. S., Zobitz, M. M., Poindexter, J. R., & Pak, C. Y. (1990). Magnesium bioavailability from magnesium citrate and magnesium oxide. Journal of the American College of Nutrition, 9(1), 48–55. https://doi.org/10.1080/07315724.1990.10720349

[1271] Schutten, J. C., Joris, P. J., Mensink, R. P., Danel, R. M., Goorman, F., Heiner-Fokkema, M. R., Weersma, R. K., Keyzer, C. A., de Borst, M. H., & Bakker, S. (2019). Effects of magnesium citrate, magnesium oxide and magnesium sulfate supplementation on arterial stiffness in healthy overweight individuals: a study protocol for a randomized controlled trial. Trials, 20(1), 295. https://doi.org/10.1186/s13063-019-3414-4

[1272] Coudray, C., Rambeau, M., Feillet-Coudray, C., Gueux, E., Tressol, J. C., Mazur, A., & Rayssiguier, Y. (2005). Study of magnesium bioavailability from ten organic and inorganic Mg salts in Mg-depleted rats using a stable isotope approach. Magnesium research, 18(4), 215–223.

[1273] Houston, M. (2011), The Role of Magnesium in Hypertension and Cardiovascular Disease. The Journal of Clinical Hypertension, 13: 843-847. https://doi.org/10.1111/j.1751-7176.2011.00538.x

[1274] Azuma J. (1994). Long-term effect of taurine in congestive heart failure: preliminary report. Heart Failure Research with Taurine Group. Advances in experimental medicine and biology, 359, 425–433. https://doi.org/10.1007/978-1-4899-1471-2_46

[1275] McCarty (1996) 'Complementary vascular-protective actions of magnesium and taurine: A rationale for magnesium taurate', Medical Hypotheses, Volume 46, Issue 2, February 1996, Pages 89-100.

[1276] Rouse, D. J., Hirtz, D. G., Thom, E., Varner, M. W., Spong, C. Y., Mercer, B. M., … Roberts, J. M. (2008). A Randomized, Controlled Trial of Magnesium Sulfate for the Prevention of Cerebral Palsy. New England Journal of Medicine, 359(9), 895–905. doi:10.1056/nejmoa0801187

[1277] Gromova, O. A., Torshin, I. Y., Kalacheva, A. G., & Grishina, T. R. (2016). Kardiologiia, 56(3), 73–80. https://doi.org/10.18565/cardio.2016.3.73-80

[1278] Geiss, K. R., Stergiou, N., Jester, Neuenfeld, H. U., & Jester, H. G. (1998). Effects of magnesium orotate on exercise tolerance in patients with coronary heart disease. Cardiovascular drugs and therapy, 12 Suppl 2, 153–156. https://doi.org/10.1023/a:1007796515957

[1279] Classen H. G. (2004). Magnesium orotate--experimental and clinical evidence. Romanian journal of internal medicine = Revue roumaine de medecine interne, 42(3), 491–501.

[1280] Domnitskaia, T. M., D'iachenko, A. V., Kupriianova, O. O., & Domnitskiĭ, M. V. (2005). Kardiologiia, 45(3), 76–81.

[1281] Stepura, O. B., & Martynow, A. I. (2009). Magnesium orotate in severe congestive heart failure (MACH). International journal of cardiology, 134(1), 145–147. https://doi.org/10.1016/j.ijcard.2009.01.047

[1282] Ranade, V. V., & Somberg, J. C. (2001). Bioavailability and pharmacokinetics of magnesium after administration of magnesium salts to humans. American journal of therapeutics, 8(5), 345–357. https://doi.org/10.1097/00045391-200109000-00008

[1283] Ross, J. R., Dargan, P. I., Jones, A. L., & Kostrzewski, A. (2001). A case of hypomagnesaemia due to malabsorption, unresponsive to oral administration of magnesium glycerophosphate, but responsive to oral magnesium oxide supplementation. Gut, 48(6), 857–858. https://doi.org/10.1136/gut.48.6.857

[1284] Garrison et al (2011) 'Magnesium for skeletal muscle cramps', Cochrane Database of Systematic Reviews 2011, Issue 11. Art. No.: CD009402. DOI: 10.1002/14651858.CD009402. Accessed 04 February 2021.

[1285] Schuchardt and Hahn (2017) 'Intestinal Absorption and Factors Influencing Bioavailability of Magnesium- An Update', Current Nutrition & Food Science, Volume 13 , Issue 4 , 2017, DOI : 10.2174/1573401313666170427162740

[1286] Firoz, M., & Graber, M. (2001). Bioavailability of US commercial magnesium preparations. Magnesium research, 14(4), 257–262.

[1287] Van Hook J. W. (1991). Endocrine crises. Hypermagnesemia. Critical care clinics, 7(1), 215–223.

[1288] Toto, K. H., & Yucha, C. B. (1994). Magnesium: homeostasis, imbalances, and therapeutic uses. Critical care nursing clinics of North America, 6(4), 767–783.

[1289] Salem M, Kasinski N, Munoz R, et al. Progressive magnesium deficiency increases mortality from endotoxin challenge: protective effects of acute magnesium replacement therapy. Crit Care Med 1995;23:108–18.

[1290] Musso C. G. (2009). Magnesium metabolism in health and disease. International urology and nephrology, 41(2), 357–362. https://doi.org/10.1007/s11255-009-9548-7

[1291] Ranade, V. V., & Somberg, J. C. (2001). Bioavailability and pharmacokinetics of magnesium after administration of magnesium salts to humans. American journal of therapeutics, 8(5), 345–357. https://doi.org/10.1097/00045391-200109000-00008

[1292] Onishi, S., & Yoshino, S. (2006). Cathartic-induced fatal hypermagnesemia in the elderly. Internal medicine (Tokyo, Japan), 45(4), 207–210. https://doi.org/10.2169/internalmedicine.45.1482

[1293] McGuire, J. K., Kulkarni, M. S., & Baden, H. P. (2000). Fatal hypermagnesemia in a child treated with megavitamin/megamineral therapy. Pediatrics, 105(2), E18. https://doi.org/10.1542/peds.105.2.e18

[1294] Kutsal, E., Aydemir, C., Eldes, N., Demirel, F., Polat, R., Taspnar, O., & Kulah, E. (2007). Severe hypermagnesemia as a result of excessive cathartic ingestion in a child without renal failure. Pediatric emergency care, 23(8), 570–572. https://doi.org/10.1097/PEC.0b013e31812eef1c

[1295] Linus Paulig Institute (2001) 'Calcium', Minerals, Oregon State University, Accessed Online Jan 30 2021: https://lpi.oregonstate.edu/mic/minerals/calcium

[1296] Talmage (1996). 'Foreword'. In Calcium and Phosphorus in Health and Disease; Anderson, J.J.B., Garner, S.C., Eds.; CRC Press: Boca Raton, FL, USA.

[1297] Weaver CM, Heaney RP. Calcium. In: Shils ME, Shike M, Ross AC, Caballero B, Cousins RJ. Modern Nutrition in Health and Disease. 10th ed. Baltimore, MD: Lippincott Williams & Wilkins, 2006:194-210.

[1298] Linus Pauling Institute (2021) 'Calcium', Oregon State University, Accessed Online Feb 01 2021: https://lpi.oregonstate.edu/mic/minerals/calcium

[1299] Haleem, S., Lutchman, L., Mayahi, R., Grice, J. E., & Parker, M. J. (2008). Mortality following hip fracture: trends and geographical variations over the last 40 years. Injury, 39(10), 1157–1163. https://doi.org/10.1016/j.injury.2008.03.022

[1300] Rizzoli, R., Bianchi, M. L., Garabédian, M., McKay, H. A., & Moreno, L. A. (2010). Maximizing bone mineral mass gain during growth for the prevention of fractures in the adolescents and the elderly. Bone, 46(2), 294–305. https://doi.org/10.1016/j.bone.2009.10.005

[1301] Crandall, C. J., Newberry, S. J., Diamant, A., Lim, Y. W., Gellad, W. F., Suttorp, M. J., Motala, A., Ewing, B., Roth, B., Shanman, R., Timmer, M., & Shekelle, P. G. (2012). Treatment To Prevent Fractures in Men and Women With Low Bone Density or Osteoporosis: Update of a 2007 Report. Agency for Healthcare Research and Quality (US).

[1302] Cauley J. A. (2015). Estrogen and bone health in men and women. Steroids, 99(Pt A), 11–15. https://doi.org/10.1016/j.steroids.2014.12.010

[1303] Nie, X., Jin, H., Wen, G., Xu, J., An, J., Liu, X., Xie, R., & Tuo, B. (2020). Estrogen Regulates Duodenal Calcium Absorption Through Differential Role of Estrogen Receptor on Calcium Transport Proteins. Digestive diseases and sciences, 65(12), 3502–3513. https://doi.org/10.1007/s10620-020-06076-x

[1304] Mauras, N., Vieira, N. E., & Yergey, A. L. (1997). Estrogen therapy enhances calcium absorption and retention and diminishes bone turnover in young girls with Turner's syndrome: a calcium kinetic study. Metabolism: clinical and experimental, 46(8), 908–913. https://doi.org/10.1016/s0026-0495(97)90078-0

[1305] Okamura, H., Ishikawa, K., Kudo, Y., Matsuoka, A., Maruyama, H., Emori, H., Yamamura, R., Hayakawa, C., Tani, S., Tsuchiya, K., Shirahata, T., Toyone, T., Nagai, T., & Inagaki, K. (2020). Risk factors predicting osteosarcopenia in postmenopausal women with osteoporosis: A retrospective study. PloS one, 15(8), e0237454. https://doi.org/10.1371/journal.pone.0237454

[1306] Borer K. T. (2005). Physical activity in the prevention and amelioration of osteoporosis in women : interaction of mechanical, hormonal and dietary factors. Sports medicine (Auckland, N.Z.), 35(9), 779–830. https://doi.org/10.2165/00007256-200535090-00004

[1307] Tai, V., Leung, W., Grey, A., Reid, I. R., & Bolland, M. J. (2015). Calcium intake and bone mineral density: systematic review and meta-analysis. BMJ (Clinical research ed.), 351, h4183. https://doi.org/10.1136/bmj.h4183

[1308] Bolland, M. J., Leung, W., Tai, V., Bastin, S., Gamble, G. D., Grey, A., & Reid, I. R. (2015). Calcium intake and risk of fracture: systematic review. BMJ (Clinical research ed.), 351, h4580. https://doi.org/10.1136/bmj.h4580

[1309] Chung, M., Lee, J., Terasawa, T., Lau, J., & Trikalinos, T. A. (2011). Vitamin D with or without calcium supplementation for prevention of cancer and fractures: an updated meta-analysis for the U.S. Preventive Services Task Force. Annals of internal medicine, 155(12), 827–838. https://doi.org/10.7326/0003-4819-155-12-201112200-00005

[1310] Cosman, F., de Beur, S. J., LeBoff, M. S., Lewiecki, E. M., Tanner, B., Randall, S., Lindsay, R., & National Osteoporosis Foundation (2014). Clinician's Guide to Prevention and Treatment of Osteoporosis. Osteoporosis international : a journal established as result of cooperation between the European

589

Foundation for Osteoporosis and the National Osteoporosis Foundation of the USA, 25(10), 2359–2381. https://doi.org/10.1007/s00198-014-2794-2

[1311] Office of the Federal Register, Government Publishing Office. §101.72 Food labeling: health claims: calcium, vitamin D, and osteoporosis. Electronic Code of Federal Regulations, Title 21: Food and Drugs.

[1312] Lind, L., Skarfors, E., Berglund, L., Lithell, H., & Ljunghall, S. (1997). Serum calcium: A new, independent, prospective risk factor for myocardial infarction in middle-aged men followed for 18 years. Journal of Clinical Epidemiology, 50(8), 967–973. doi:10.1016/s0895-4356(97)00104-2

[1313] McKane, W. R., Khosla, S., Egan, K. S., Robins, S. P., Burritt, M. F., & Riggs, B. L. (1996). Role of calcium intake in modulating age-related increases in parathyroid function and bone resorption. The Journal of Clinical Endocrinology & Metabolism, 81(5), 1699–1703. doi:10.1210/jcem.81.5.8626819

[1314] Moe S. M. (2008). Disorders involving calcium, phosphorus, and magnesium. Primary care, 35(2), 215–vi. https://doi.org/10.1016/j.pop.2008.01.007

[1315] Werner, E., Malluche, H. H., Kutschera, J., Hodgson, M., & Schoeppe, W. (1976). Intestinal Calcium Absorption and Whole-body Calcium Retention in Various Stages of Renal Insufficiency. Calcified Tissues 1975, 210–215. doi:10.1007/978-3-662-29272-3_30

[1316] Norman, D. A., Fordtran, J. S., Brinkley, L. J., Zerwekh, J. E., Nicar, M. J., Strowig, S. M., & Pak, C. Y. (1981). Jejunal and ileal adaptation to alterations in dietary calcium: changes in calcium and magnesium absorption and pathogenetic role of parathyroid hormone and 1,25-dihydroxyvitamin D. Journal of Clinical Investigation, 67(6), 1599–1603. doi:10.1172/jci110194

[1317] Kanis, J. A., & Passmore, R. (1989). Calcium supplementation of the diet--I. BMJ, 298(6667), 137–140. doi:10.1136/bmj.298.6667.137

[1318] Bischoff-Ferrari, H. A., Dawson-Hughes, B., Baron, J. A., Burckhardt, P., Li, R., Spiegelman, D., … Willett, W. C. (2007). Calcium intake and hip fracture risk in men and women: a meta-analysis of prospective cohort studies and randomized controlled trials. The American Journal of Clinical Nutrition, 86(6), 1780–1790. doi:10.1093/ajcn/86.5.1780

[1319] Tai, V., Leung, W., Grey, A., Reid, I. R., & Bolland, M. J. (2015). Calcium intake and bone mineral density: systematic review and meta-analysis. BMJ, h4183. doi:10.1136/bmj.h4183

[1320] Bolland, M. J., Leung, W., Tai, V., Bastin, S., Gamble, G. D., Grey, A., & Reid, I. R. (2015). Calcium intake and risk of fracture: systematic review. BMJ, h4580. doi:10.1136/bmj.h4580

[1321] Kärkkäinen, M. U., Lamberg-Allardt, C. J., Ahonen, S., & Välimäki, M. (2001). Does it make a difference how and when you take your calcium? The acute effects of calcium on calcium and bone metabolism. The American Journal of Clinical Nutrition, 74(3), 335–342. doi:10.1093/ajcn/74.3.335

[1322] Berridge, M. J., Lipp, P., & Bootman, M. D. (2000). The versatility and universality of calcium signalling. Nature Reviews Molecular Cell Biology, 1(1), 11–21. doi:10.1038/35036035

[1323] Chalmers, S., & Nicholls, D. G. (2003). The Relationship between Free and Total Calcium Concentrations in the Matrix of Liver and Brain Mitochondria. Journal of Biological Chemistry, 278(21), 19062–19070. doi:10.1074/jbc.m212661200

[1324] Jemmerson, R., Dubinsky, J. M., & Brustovetsky, N. (2005). CytochromecRelease from CNS Mitochondria and Potential for Clinical Intervention in Apoptosis-Mediated CNS Diseases. Antioxidants & Redox Signaling, 7(9-10), 1158–1172. doi:10.1089/ars.2005.7.1158

[1325] Chance, B. (1965). The Energy-linked Reaction of Calcium with Mitochondria. Journal of Biological Chemistry, 240(6), 2729–2748. doi:10.1016/s0021-9258(18)97387-4

[1326] Nicholls, D., & Akerman, K. (1982). Mitochondrial calcium transport. Biochimica et biophysica acta, 683(1), 57–88. https://doi.org/10.1016/0304-4173(82)90013-1

[1327] Puskin, J. S., Gunter, T. E., Gunter, K. K., & Russell, P. R. (1976). Evidence for more than one C2+ion transport mechanism in mitochondria. Biochemistry, 15(17), 3834–3842. doi:10.1021/bi00662a029

[1328] CROMPTON, M., MOSER, R., LUDI, H., & CARAFOLI, E. (1978). The Interrelations between the Transport of Sodium and Calcium in Mitochondria of Various Mammalian Tissues. European Journal of Biochemistry, 82(1), 25–31. doi:10.1111/j.1432-1033.1978.tb11993.x

[1329] CROMPTON, M., & HEID, I. (1978). The Cycling of Calcium, Sodium, and Protons Across the Inner Membrane of Cardiac Mitochondria. European Journal of Biochemistry, 91(2), 599–608. doi:10.1111/j.1432-1033.1978.tb12713.x

[1330] Michelangeli, F., Ogunbayo, O. A., & Wootton, L. L. (2005). A plethora of interacting organellar Ca2+ stores. Current Opinion in Cell Biology, 17(2), 135–140. doi:10.1016/j.ceb.2005.01.005

[1331] Hertz-Picciotto, I., Schramm, M., Watt-Morse, M., Chantala, K., Anderson, J., & Osterloh, J. (2000). Patterns and determinants of blood lead during pregnancy. American journal of epidemiology, 152(9), 829–837. https://doi.org/10.1093/aje/152.9.829

[1332] Ettinger, A. S., Lamadrid-Figueroa, H., Téllez-Rojo, M. M., Mercado-García, A., Peterson, K. E., Schwartz, J., Hu, H., & Hernández-Avila, M. (2009). Effect of calcium supplementation on blood lead levels in pregnancy: a randomized placebo-controlled trial. Environmental health perspectives, 117(1), 26–31. https://doi.org/10.1289/ehp.11868

[1333] Hernandez-Avila, M., Gonzalez-Cossio, T., Hernandez-Avila, J. E., Romieu, I., Peterson, K. E., Aro, A., Palazuelos, E., & Hu, H. (2003). Dietary calcium supplements to lower blood lead levels in lactating women: a randomized placebo-controlled trial. Epidemiology (Cambridge, Mass.), 14(2), 206–212. https://doi.org/10.1097/01.EDE.0000038520.66094.34

[1334] Ettinger, A. S., Téllez-Rojo, M. M., Amarasiriwardena, C., Peterson, K. E., Schwartz, J., Aro, A., Hu, H., & Hernández-Avila, M. (2006). Influence of maternal bone lead burden and calcium intake on levels of lead in breast milk over the course of lactation. American journal of epidemiology, 163(1), 48–56. https://doi.org/10.1093/aje/kwj010

[1335] Muldoon, S. B., Cauley, J. A., Kuller, L. H., Scott, J., & Rohay, J. (1994). Lifestyle and sociodemographic factors as determinants of blood lead levels in elderly women. American journal of epidemiology, 139(6), 599–608. https://doi.org/10.1093/oxfordjournals.aje.a117049

[1336] Roberts H. J. (1983). Potential toxicity due to dolomite and bonemeal. Southern medical journal, 76(5), 556–559. https://doi.org/10.1097/00007611-198305000-00005

[1337] Ross, E. A., Szabo, N. J., & Tebbett, I. R. (2000). Lead content of calcium supplements. JAMA, 284(11), 1425–1429. https://doi.org/10.1001/jama.284.11.1425

[1338] Mindak, W. R., Cheng, J., Canas, B. J., & Bolger, P. M. (2008). Lead in women's and children's vitamins. Journal of agricultural and food chemistry, 56(16), 6892–6896. https://doi.org/10.1021/jf801236w

[1339] Kampman, E., Slattery, M. L., Caan, B., & Potter, J. D. (2000). Calcium, vitamin D, sunshine exposure, dairy products and colon cancer risk (United States). Cancer causes & control : CCC, 11(5), 459–466. https://doi.org/10.1023/a:1008914108739

[1340] Holt, P. R., Atillasoy, E. O., Gilman, J., Guss, J., Moss, S. F., Newmark, H., Fan, K., Yang, K., & Lipkin, M. (1998). Modulation of abnormal colonic epithelial cell proliferation and differentiation by low-fat dairy foods: a randomized controlled trial. JAMA, 280(12), 1074–1079. https://doi.org/10.1001/jama.280.12.1074

[1341] Slattery, M. L., Edwards, S. L., Boucher, K. M., Anderson, K., & Caan, B. J. (1999). Lifestyle and colon cancer: an assessment of factors associated with risk. American journal of epidemiology, 150(8), 869–877. https://doi.org/10.1093/oxfordjournals.aje.a010092

[1342] Bonithon-Kopp, C., Kronborg, O., Giacosa, A., Räth, U., & Faivre, J. (2000). Calcium and fibre supplementation in prevention of colorectal adenoma recurrence: a randomised intervention trial. European Cancer Prevention Organisation Study Group. Lancet (London, England), 356(9238), 1300–1306. https://doi.org/10.1016/s0140-6736(00)02813-0

[1343] Baron, J. A., Beach, M., Mandel, J. S., van Stolk, R. U., Haile, R. W., Sandler, R. S., Rothstein, R., Summers, R. W., Snover, D. C., Beck, G. J., Bond, J. H., & Greenberg, E. R. (1999). Calcium supplements for the prevention of colorectal adenomas. Calcium Polyp Prevention Study Group. The New England journal of medicine, 340(2), 101–107. https://doi.org/10.1056/NEJM199901143400204

[1344] Grau, M. V., Baron, J. A., Sandler, R. S., Wallace, K., Haile, R. W., Church, T. R., Beck, G. J., Summers, R. W., Barry, E. L., Cole, B. F., Snover, D. C., Rothstein, R., & Mandel, J. S. (2007). Prolonged effect of calcium supplementation on risk of colorectal adenomas in a randomized trial. Journal of the National Cancer Institute, 99(2), 129–136. https://doi.org/10.1093/jnci/djk016

[1345] Wu, K., Willett, W. C., Fuchs, C. S., Colditz, G. A., & Giovannucci, E. L. (2002). Calcium intake and risk of colon cancer in women and men. Journal of the National Cancer Institute, 94(6), 437–446. https://doi.org/10.1093/jnci/94.6.437

[1346] Martínez, M. E., & Willett, W. C. (1998). Calcium, vitamin D, and colorectal cancer: a review of the epidemiologic evidence. Cancer epidemiology, biomarkers & prevention : a publication of the American Association for Cancer Research, cosponsored by the American Society of Preventive Oncology, 7(2), 163–168.

[1347] Cascinu, S., Ligi, M., Del Ferro, E., Foglietti, G., Cioccolini, P., Staccioli, M. P., Carnevali, A., Luigi Rocchi, M. B., Alessandroni, P., Giordani, P., Catalano, V., Polizzi, V., Agostinelli, R., Muretto, P., & Catalano, G. (2000). Effects of calcium and vitamin supplementation on colon cell proliferation in colorectal cancer. Cancer investigation, 18(5), 411–416. https://doi.org/10.3109/07357900009032811

[1348] Murphy, N., Norat, T., Ferrari, P., Jenab, M., Bueno-de-Mesquita, B., Skeie, G., Olsen, A., Tjønneland, A., Dahm, C. C., Overvad, K., Boutron-Ruault, M. C., Clavel-Chapelon, F., Nailler, L., Kaaks, R., Teucher, B., Boeing, H., Bergmann, M. M., Trichopoulou, A., Lagiou, P., Trichopoulos, D., … Riboli, E. (2013). Consumption of dairy products and colorectal cancer in the European Prospective Investigation into Cancer and Nutrition (EPIC). PloS one, 8(9), e72715. https://doi.org/10.1371/journal.pone.0072715

[1349] Weingarten, M. A., Zalmanovici, A., & Yaphe, J. (2008). Dietary calcium supplementation for preventing colorectal cancer and adenomatous polyps. The Cochrane database of systematic reviews, (1), CD003548. https://doi.org/10.1002/14651858.CD003548.pub4

[1350] Wactawski-Wende, J., Kotchen, J. M., Anderson, G. L., Assaf, A. R., Brunner, R. L., O'Sullivan, M. J., Margolis, K. L., Ockene, J. K., Phillips, L., Pottern, L., Prentice, R. L., Robbins, J., Rohan, T. E., Sarto, G. E., Sharma, S., Stefanick, M. L., Van Horn, L., Wallace, R. B., Whitlock, E., Bassford, T., … Women's Health Initiative Investigators (2006). Calcium plus vitamin D supplementation and the risk of colorectal cancer. The New England journal of medicine, 354(7), 684–696. https://doi.org/10.1056/NEJMoa055222

591

[1351] Massa, J., Cho, E., Orav, E. J., Willett, W. C., Wu, K., & Giovannucci, E. L. (2014). Total calcium intake and colorectal adenoma in young women. Cancer causes & control : CCC, 25(4), 451–460. https://doi.org/10.1007/s10552-014-0347-9

[1352] Schuurman, A. G., van den Brandt, P. A., Dorant, E., & Goldbohm, R. A. (1999). Animal products, calcium and protein and prostate cancer risk in The Netherlands Cohort Study. British journal of cancer, 80(7), 1107–1113. https://doi.org/10.1038/sj.bjc.6690472

[1353] Kesse, E., Bertrais, S., Astorg, P., Jaouen, A., Arnault, N., Galan, P., & Hercberg, S. (2006). Dairy products, calcium and phosphorus intake, and the risk of prostate cancer: results of the French prospective SU.VI.MAX (Supplémentation en Vitamines et Minéraux Antioxydants) study. The British journal of nutrition, 95(3), 539–545. https://doi.org/10.1079/bjn20051670

[1354] Rodriguez, C., McCullough, M. L., Mondul, A. M., Jacobs, E. J., Fakhrabadi-Shokoohi, D., Giovannucci, E. L., Thun, M. J., & Calle, E. E. (2003). Calcium, dairy products, and risk of prostate cancer in a prospective cohort of United States men. Cancer epidemiology, biomarkers & prevention : a publication of the American Association for Cancer Research, cosponsored by the American Society of Preventive Oncology, 12(7), 597–603.

[1355] Gao, X., LaValley, M. P., & Tucker, K. L. (2005). Prospective studies of dairy product and calcium intakes and prostate cancer risk: a meta-analysis. Journal of the National Cancer Institute, 97(23), 1768–1777. https://doi.org/10.1093/jnci/dji402

[1356] Chan, J. M., & Giovannucci, E. L. (2001). Dairy products, calcium, and vitamin D and risk of prostate cancer. Epidemiologic reviews, 23(1), 87–92. https://doi.org/10.1093/oxfordjournals.epirev.a000800

[1357] Chan, J. M., Giovannucci, E., Andersson, S. O., Yuen, J., Adami, H. O., & Wolk, A. (1998). Dairy products, calcium, phosphorous, vitamin D, and risk of prostate cancer (Sweden). Cancer causes & control : CCC, 9(6), 559–566. https://doi.org/10.1023/a:1008823601897

[1358] Pettersson, A., Kasperzyk, J. L., Kenfield, S. A., Richman, E. L., Chan, J. M., Willett, W. C., Stampfer, M. J., Mucci, L. A., & Giovannucci, E. L. (2012). Milk and dairy consumption among men with prostate cancer and risk of metastases and prostate cancer death. Cancer epidemiology, biomarkers & prevention : a publication of the American Association for Cancer Research, cosponsored by the American Society of Preventive Oncology, 21(3), 428–436. https://doi.org/10.1158/1055-9965.EPI-11-1004

[1359] Aune, D., Navarro Rosenblatt, D. A., Chan, D. S., Vieira, A. R., Vieira, R., Greenwood, D. C., Vatten, L. J., & Norat, T. (2015). Dairy products, calcium, and prostate cancer risk: a systematic review and meta-analysis of cohort studies. The American journal of clinical nutrition, 101(1), 87–117. https://doi.org/10.3945/ajcn.113.067157

[1360] Qin, L. Q., He, K., & Xu, J. Y. (2009). Milk consumption and circulating insulin-like growth factor-I level: a systematic literature review. International journal of food sciences and nutrition, 60 Suppl 7, 330–340. https://doi.org/10.1080/09637480903150114

[1361] Larsson, S. C., Carter, P., Vithayathil, M., Kar, S., Mason, A. M., & Burgess, S. (2020). Insulin-like growth factor-1 and site-specific cancers: A Mendelian randomization study. Cancer medicine, 9(18), 6836–6842. https://doi.org/10.1002/cam4.3345

[1362] Qian, F., & Huo, D. (2020). Circulating Insulin-Like Growth Factor-1 and Risk of Total and 19 Site-Specific Cancers: Cohort Study Analyses from the UK Biobank. Cancer epidemiology, biomarkers & prevention : a publication of the American Association for Cancer Research, cosponsored by the American Society of Preventive Oncology, 29(11), 2332–2342. https://doi.org/10.1158/1055-9965.EPI-20-0743

[1363] Rowlands, M. A., Gunnell, D., Harris, R., Vatten, L. J., Holly, J. M., & Martin, R. M. (2009). Circulating insulin-like growth factor peptides and prostate cancer risk: a systematic review and meta-analysis. International journal of cancer, 124(10), 2416–2429. https://doi.org/10.1002/ijc.24202

[1364] Allen, N. E., Key, T. J., Appleby, P. N., Travis, R. C., Roddam, A. W., Tjønneland, A., Johnsen, N. F., Overvad, K., Linseisen, J., Rohrmann, S., Boeing, H., Pischon, T., Bueno-de-Mesquita, H. B., Kiemeney, L., Tagliabue, G., Palli, D., Vineis, P., Tumino, R., Trichopoulou, A., Kassapa, C., … Riboli, E. (2008). Animal foods, protein, calcium and prostate cancer risk: the European Prospective Investigation into Cancer and Nutrition. British journal of cancer, 98(9), 1574–1581. https://doi.org/10.1038/sj.bjc.6604331

[1365] Huncharek, M., Muscat, J., & Kupelnick, B. (2008). Dairy products, dietary calcium and vitamin D intake as risk factors for prostate cancer: a meta-analysis of 26,769 cases from 45 observational studies. Nutrition and cancer, 60(4), 421–441. https://doi.org/10.1080/01635580801911779

[1366] Zemel, M. B., Richards, J., Milstead, A., & Campbell, P. (2005). Effects of calcium and dairy on body composition and weight loss in African-American adults. Obesity research, 13(7), 1218–1225. https://doi.org/10.1038/oby.2005.144

[1367] Heaney R. P. (2003). Normalizing calcium intake: projected population effects for body weight. The Journal of nutrition, 133(1), 268S–270S. https://doi.org/10.1093/jn/133.1.268S

[1368] Davies, K. M., Heaney, R. P., Recker, R. R., Lappe, J. M., Barger-Lux, M. J., Rafferty, K., & Hinders, S. (2000). Calcium intake and body weight. The Journal of clinical endocrinology and metabolism, 85(12), 4635–4638. https://doi.org/10.1210/jcem.85.12.7063

[1369] Zemel M. B. (2002). Regulation of adiposity and obesity risk by dietary calcium: mechanisms and implications. Journal of the American College of Nutrition, 21(2), 146S–151S. https://doi.org/10.1080/07315724.2002.10719212

[1370] Parikh, S. J., & Yanovski, J. A. (2003). Calcium intake and adiposity. The American journal of clinical nutrition, 77(2), 281–287. https://doi.org/10.1093/ajcn/77.2.281

[1371] Gonzalez, J. T., Rumbold, P. L., & Stevenson, E. J. (2012). Effect of calcium intake on fat oxidation in adults: a meta-analysis of randomized, controlled trials. Obesity reviews : an official journal of the International Association for the Study of Obesity, 13(10), 848–857. https://doi.org/10.1111/j.1467-789X.2012.01013.x

[1372] Christensen, R., Lorenzen, J. K., Svith, C. R., Bartels, E. M., Melanson, E. L., Saris, W. H., Tremblay, A., & Astrup, A. (2009). Effect of calcium from dairy and dietary supplements on faecal fat excretion: a meta-analysis of randomized controlled trials. Obesity reviews : an official journal of the International Association for the Study of Obesity, 10(4), 475–486. https://doi.org/10.1111/j.1467-789X.2009.00599.x

[1373] Jacobsen, R., Lorenzen, J. K., Toubro, S., Krog-Mikkelsen, I., & Astrup, A. (2005). Effect of short-term high dietary calcium intake on 24-h energy expenditure, fat oxidation, and fecal fat excretion. International journal of obesity (2005), 29(3), 292–301. https://doi.org/10.1038/sj.ijo.0802785

[1374] Pathak, K., Soares, M. J., Calton, E. K., Zhao, Y., & Hallett, J. (2014). Vitamin D supplementation and body weight status: a systematic review and meta-analysis of randomized controlled trials. Obesity reviews : an official journal of the International Association for the Study of Obesity, 15(6), 528–537. https://doi.org/10.1111/obr.12162

[1375] Gallagher, J. C., Yalamanchili, V., & Smith, L. M. (2013). The effect of vitamin D supplementation on serum 25(OH)D in thin and obese women. The Journal of steroid biochemistry and molecular biology, 136, 195–200. https://doi.org/10.1016/j.jsbmb.2012.12.003

[1376] Dougkas, A., Reynolds, C. K., Givens, I. D., Elwood, P. C., & Minihane, A. M. (2011). Associations between dairy consumption and body weight: a review of the evidence and underlying mechanisms. Nutrition research reviews, 24(1), 72–95. https://doi.org/10.1017/S095442241000034X

[1377] Zemel, M. B., Thompson, W., Milstead, A., Morris, K., & Campbell, P. (2004). Calcium and dairy acceleration of weight and fat loss during energy restriction in obese adults. Obesity research, 12(4), 582–590. https://doi.org/10.1038/oby.2004.67

[1378] Zemel, M. B., Richards, J., Mathis, S., Milstead, A., Gebhardt, L., & Silva, E. (2005). Dairy augmentation of total and central fat loss in obese subjects. International journal of obesity (2005), 29(4), 391–397. https://doi.org/10.1038/sj.ijo.0802880

[1379] Shi, H., Dirienzo, D., & Zemel, M. B. (2001). Effects of dietary calcium on adipocyte lipid metabolism and body weight regulation in energy-restricted aP2-agouti transgenic mice. FASEB journal : official publication of the Federation of American Societies for Experimental Biology, 15(2), 291–293. https://doi.org/10.1096/fj.00-0584fje

[1380] Heaney, R. P., Davies, K. M., & Barger-Lux, M. J. (2002). Calcium and weight: clinical studies. Journal of the American College of Nutrition, 21(2), 152S–155S. https://doi.org/10.1080/07315724.2002.10719213

[1381] Bortolotti, M., Rudelle, S., Schneiter, P., Vidal, H., Loizon, E., Tappy, L., & Acheson, K. J. (2008). Dairy calcium supplementation in overweight or obese persons: its effect on markers of fat metabolism. The American journal of clinical nutrition, 88(4), 877–885. https://doi.org/10.1093/ajcn/88.4.877

[1382] Yanovski, J. A., Parikh, S. J., Yanoff, L. B., Denkinger, B. I., Calis, K. A., Reynolds, J. C., Sebring, N. G., & McHugh, T. (2009). Effects of calcium supplementation on body weight and adiposity in overweight and obese adults: a randomized trial. Annals of internal medicine, 150(12), 821–W146. https://doi.org/10.7326/0003-4819-150-12-200906160-00005

[1383] Tordoff M. G. (2001). Calcium: taste, intake, and appetite. Physiological reviews, 81(4), 1567–1597. https://doi.org/10.1152/physrev.2001.81.4.1567

[1384] Soares, M. J., Pathak, K., & Calton, E. K. (2014). Calcium and vitamin D in the regulation of energy balance: where do we stand?. International journal of molecular sciences, 15(3), 4938–4945. https://doi.org/10.3390/ijms15034938

[1385] Lutsey, P. L., Alonso, A., Michos, E. D., Loehr, L. R., Astor, B. C., Coresh, J., & Folsom, A. R. (2014). Serum magnesium, phosphorus, and calcium are associated with risk of incident heart failure: the Atherosclerosis Risk in Communities (ARIC) Study. The American journal of clinical nutrition, 100(3), 756–764. https://doi.org/10.3945/ajcn.114.085167

[1386] Foley, R. N., Collins, A. J., Ishani, A., & Kalra, P. A. (2008). Calcium-phosphate levels and cardiovascular disease in community-dwelling adults: the Atherosclerosis Risk in Communities (ARIC) Study. American heart journal, 156(3), 556–563. https://doi.org/10.1016/j.ahj.2008.05.016

[1387] Pentti, K., Tuppurainen, M. T., Honkanen, R., Sandini, L., Kröger, H., Alhava, E., & Saarikoski, S. (2009). Use of calcium supplements and the risk of coronary heart disease in 52-62-year-old women: The Kuopio Osteoporosis Risk Factor and Prevention Study. Maturitas, 63(1), 73–78. https://doi.org/10.1016/j.maturitas.2009.03.006

[1388] Li, K., Kaaks, R., Linseisen, J., & Rohrmann, S. (2012). Associations of dietary calcium intake and calcium supplementation with myocardial infarction and stroke risk and overall cardiovascular mortality in the Heidelberg cohort of the European Prospective Investigation into Cancer and Nutrition study (EPIC-Heidelberg). Heart (British Cardiac Society), 98(12), 920–925. https://doi.org/10.1136/heartjnl-2011-301345

[1389] Bolland, M. J., Barber, P. A., Doughty, R. N., Mason, B., Horne, A., Ames, R., Gamble, G. D., Grey, A., & Reid, I. R. (2008). Vascular events in healthy older women receiving calcium supplementation: randomised controlled trial. BMJ (Clinical research ed.), 336(7638), 262–266. https://doi.org/10.1136/bmj.39440.525752.BE

[1390] Bolland, M. J., Avenell, A., Baron, J. A., Grey, A., MacLennan, G. S., Gamble, G. D., & Reid, I. R. (2010). Effect of calcium supplements on risk of myocardial infarction and cardiovascular events: meta-analysis. BMJ (Clinical research ed.), 341, c3691. https://doi.org/10.1136/bmj.c3691

[1391] Michaëlsson, K., Melhus, H., Warensjö Lemming, E., Wolk, A., & Byberg, L. (2013). Long term calcium intake and rates of all cause and cardiovascular mortality: community based prospective longitudinal cohort study. BMJ (Clinical research ed.), 346, f228. https://doi.org/10.1136/bmj.f228

[1392] Xiao, Q., Murphy, R. A., Houston, D. K., Harris, T. B., Chow, W. H., & Park, Y. (2013). Dietary and supplemental calcium intake and cardiovascular disease mortality: the National Institutes of Health-AARP diet and health study. JAMA internal medicine, 173(8), 639–646. https://doi.org/10.1001/jamainternmed.2013.3283

[1393] Pentti, K., Tuppurainen, M. T., Honkanen, R., Sandini, L., Kröger, H., Alhava, E., & Saarikoski, S. (2009). Use of calcium supplements and the risk of coronary heart disease in 52-62-year-old women: The Kuopio Osteoporosis Risk Factor and Prevention Study. Maturitas, 63(1), 73–78. https://doi.org/10.1016/j.maturitas.2009.03.006

[1394] Bolland, M. J., Grey, A., Avenell, A., Gamble, G. D., & Reid, I. R. (2011). Calcium supplements with or without vitamin D and risk of cardiovascular events: reanalysis of the Women's Health Initiative limited access dataset and meta-analysis. BMJ (Clinical research ed.), 342, d2040. https://doi.org/10.1136/bmj.d2040

[1395] Seely S. (1991). Is calcium excess in western diet a major cause of arterial disease?. International journal of cardiology, 33(2), 191–198. https://doi.org/10.1016/0167-5273(91)90346-q

[1396] Wang, L., Manson, J. E., & Sesso, H. D. (2012). Calcium intake and risk of cardiovascular disease: a review of prospective studies and randomized clinical trials. American journal of cardiovascular drugs : drugs, devices, and other interventions, 12(2), 105–116. https://doi.org/10.2165/11595400-000000000-00000

[1397] Xiao, Q., Murphy, R. A., Houston, D. K., Harris, T. B., Chow, W. H., & Park, Y. (2013). Dietary and supplemental calcium intake and cardiovascular disease mortality: the National Institutes of Health-AARP diet and health study. JAMA internal medicine, 173(8), 639–646. https://doi.org/10.1001/jamainternmed.2013.3283

[1398] Chung, M., Tang, A. M., Fu, Z., Wang, D. D., & Newberry, S. J. (2016). Calcium Intake and Cardiovascular Disease Risk: An Updated Systematic Review and Meta-analysis. Annals of internal medicine, 165(12), 856–866. https://doi.org/10.7326/M16-1165

[1399] Zoccarato, F., & Nicholls, D. G. (1981). Phosphate-independent calcium efflux from liver mitochondria. FEBS Letters, 128(2), 275–277. doi:10.1016/0014-5793(81)80097-x

[1400] REED, K. C., & BYGRAVE, F. L. (1975). A Kinetic Study of Mitochondrial Calcium Transport. European Journal of Biochemistry, 55(3), 497–504. doi:10.1111/j.1432-1033.1975.tb02187.x

[1401] ROSSI, C. S., & LEHNINGER, A. L. (1964). STOICHIOMETRY OF RESPIRATORY STIMULATION, ACCUMULATION OF CA++ AND PHOSPHATE, AND OXIDATIVE PHOSPHORYLATION IN RAT LIVER MITOCHONDRIA. The Journal of biological chemistry, 239, 3971–3980.

[1402] De Oca, A. M., Madueño, J. A., Martinez-Moreno, J. M., Guerrero, F., Muñoz-Castañeda, J., Rodriguez-Ortiz, M. E., … Aguilera-Tejero, E. (2010). High-phosphate-induced calcification is related to SM22α promoter methylation in vascular smooth muscle cells. Journal of Bone and Mineral Research, 25(9), 1996–2005. doi:10.1002/jbmr.93

[1403] Giachelli, C. M., Speer, M. Y., Li, X., Rajachar, R. M., & Yang, H. (2005). Regulation of vascular calcification: roles of phosphate and osteopontin. Circulation research, 96(7), 717–722. https://doi.org/10.1161/01.RES.0000161997.24797.c0

[1404] Ellam, T. J., & Chico, T. J. A. (2012). Phosphate: The new cholesterol? The role of the phosphate axis in non-uremic vascular disease. Atherosclerosis, 220(2), 310–318. doi:10.1016/j.atherosclerosis.2011.09.002

[1405] Medical Xpress (2008) 'High phosphorus linked to coronary calcification in chronic kidney disease', Diseases, Conditions, Syndromes, Accessed Online Jan 22 2021: https://medicalxpress.com/news/2008-12-high-phosphorus-linked-coronary-calcification.html

[1406] Adatorwovor, R., Roggenkamp, K., & Anderson, J. (2015). Intakes of Calcium and Phosphorus and Calculated Calcium-to-Phosphorus Ratios of Older Adults: NHANES 2005–2006 Data. Nutrients, 7(11), 9633–9639. doi:10.3390/nu7115492

[1407] Reid, I. R., Bristow, S. M., & Bolland, M. J. (2015). Cardiovascular Complications of Calcium Supplements. Journal of Cellular Biochemistry, 116(4), 494–501. doi:10.1002/jcb.25028

[1408] Gallagher, J. C., Smith, L. M., & Yalamanchili, V. (2014). Incidence of hypercalciuria and hypercalcemia during vitamin D and calcium supplementation in older women. Menopause, 21(11), 1173–1180. doi:10.1097/gme.0000000000000270

[1409] Mangano, K. M., Walsh, S. J., Insogna, K. L., Kenny, A. M., & Kerstetter, J. E. (2011). Calcium intake in the United States from dietary and supplemental sources across adult age groups: new estimates from the National Health and Nutrition Examination Survey 2003-2006. Journal of the American Dietetic Association, 111(5), 687–695. https://doi.org/10.1016/j.jada.2011.02.014

[1410] Bailey, R. L., Dodd, K. W., Goldman, J. A., Gahche, J. J., Dwyer, J. T., Moshfegh, A. J., ... Picciano, M. F. (2010). Estimation of Total Usual Calcium and Vitamin D Intakes in the United States. The Journal of Nutrition, 140(4), 817–822. doi:10.3945/jn.109.118539

[1411] Leopold, J. A. (2015). Vascular calcification: Mechanisms of vascular smooth muscle cell calcification. Trends in Cardiovascular Medicine, 25(4), 267–274. doi:10.1016/j.tcm.2014.10.021

[1412] McCarty M. F. (2012). Calcium supplementation, renin, and vascular risk. Osteoporosis international : a journal established as result of cooperation between the European Foundation for Osteoporosis and the National Osteoporosis Foundation of the USA, 23(11), 2733–2734. https://doi.org/10.1007/s00198-012-1910-4

[1413] Tomaschitz, A., Pilz, S., Ritz, E., Morganti, A., Grammer, T., Amrein, K., ... Marz, W. (2011). Associations of plasma renin with 10-year cardiovascular mortality, sudden cardiac death, and death due to heart failure. European Heart Journal, 32(21), 2642–2649. doi:10.1093/eurheartj/ehr150

[1414] McCarron, D. A., & Reusser, M. E. (1999). Finding consensus in the dietary calcium-blood pressure debate. Journal of the American College of Nutrition, 18(5 Suppl), 398S–405S. https://doi.org/10.1080/07315724.1999.10718904

[1415] Bucher, H. C., Cook, R. J., Guyatt, G. H., Lang, J. D., Cook, D. J., Hatala, R., & Hunt, D. L. (1996). Effects of dietary calcium supplementation on blood pressure. A meta-analysis of randomized controlled trials. JAMA, 275(13), 1016–1022. https://doi.org/10.1001/jama.1996.03530370054031

[1416] Allender, P. S., Cutler, J. A., Follmann, D., Cappuccio, F. P., Pryer, J., & Elliott, P. (1996). Dietary calcium and blood pressure: a meta-analysis of randomized clinical trials. Annals of internal medicine, 124(9), 825–831. https://doi.org/10.7326/0003-4819-124-9-199605010-00007

[1417] Cappuccio, F. P., Elliott, P., Allender, P. S., Pryer, J., Follman, D. A., & Cutler, J. A. (1995). Epidemiologic association between dietary calcium intake and blood pressure: a meta-analysis of published data. American journal of epidemiology, 142(9), 935–945. https://doi.org/10.1093/oxfordjournals.aje.a117741

[1418] Bucher, H. C., Cook, R. J., Guyatt, G. H., Lang, J. D., Cook, D. J., Hatala, R., & Hunt, D. L. (1996). Effects of dietary calcium supplementation on blood pressure. A meta-analysis of randomized controlled trials. JAMA, 275(13), 1016–1022. https://doi.org/10.1001/jama.1996.03530370054031

[1419] Allender, P. S., Cutler, J. A., Follmann, D., Cappuccio, F. P., Pryer, J., & Elliott, P. (1996). Dietary calcium and blood pressure: a meta-analysis of randomized clinical trials. Annals of internal medicine, 124(9), 825–831. https://doi.org/10.7326/0003-4819-124-9-199605010-00007

[1420] World Health Organization. Guideline: Calcium supplementation in pregnant women. Geneva: World Health Organization, 2013.

[1421] Cudihy, D., & Lee, R. V. (2009). The pathophysiology of pre-eclampsia: current clinical concepts. Journal of obstetrics and gynaecology : the journal of the Institute of Obstetrics and Gynaecology, 29(7), 576–582. https://doi.org/10.1080/01443610903061751

[1422] Hofmeyr, G. J., Lawrie, T. A., Atallah, A. N., Duley, L., & Torloni, M. R. (2014). Calcium supplementation during pregnancy for preventing hypertensive disorders and related problems. The Cochrane database of systematic reviews, (6), CD001059. https://doi.org/10.1002/14651858.CD001059.pub4

[1423] Levine, R. J., Hauth, J. C., Curet, L. B., Sibai, B. M., Catalano, P. M., Morris, C. D., DerSimonian, R., Esterlitz, J. R., Raymond, E. G., Bild, D. E., Clemens, J. D., & Cutler, J. A. (1997). Trial of calcium to prevent preeclampsia. The New England journal of medicine, 337(2), 69–76. https://doi.org/10.1056/NEJM199707103370201

[1424] Kumar, A., Devi, S. G., Batra, S., Singh, C., & Shukla, D. K. (2009). Calcium supplementation for the prevention of pre-eclampsia. International journal of gynaecology and obstetrics: the official organ of the International Federation of Gynaecology and Obstetrics, 104(1), 32–36. https://doi.org/10.1016/j.ijgo.2008.08.027

[1425] Hofmeyr, G. J., Lawrie, T. A., Atallah, A. N., Duley, L., & Torloni, M. R. (2014). Calcium supplementation during pregnancy for preventing hypertensive disorders and related problems. The

Cochrane database of systematic reviews, (6), CD001059. https://doi.org/10.1002/14651858.CD001059.pub4

[1426] Margetts, B. M., Beilin, L. J., Armstrong, B. K., & Vandongen, R. (1985). Vegetarian diet in the treatment of mild hypertension: a randomized controlled trial. Journal of hypertension. Supplement : official journal of the International Society of Hypertension, 3(3), S429–S431.

[1427] Beilin, L. J., Armstrong, B. K., Margetts, B. M., Rouse, I. L., & Vandongen, R. (1987). Vegetarian diet and blood pressure. Nephron, 47 Suppl 1, 37–41. https://doi.org/10.1159/000184551

[1428] Berkow, S. E., & Barnard, N. D. (2005). Blood pressure regulation and vegetarian diets. Nutrition reviews, 63(1), 1–8. https://doi.org/10.1111/j.1753-4887.2005.tb00104.x

[1429] Rouse, I. L., Beilin, L. J., Armstrong, B. K., & Vandongen, R. (1983). Blood-pressure-lowering effect of a vegetarian diet: controlled trial in normotensive subjects. Lancet (London, England), 1(8314-5), 5–10. https://doi.org/10.1016/s0140-6736(83)91557-x

[1430] Appel, L. J., Moore, T. J., Obarzanek, E., Vollmer, W. M., Svetkey, L. P., Sacks, F. M., Bray, G. A., Vogt, T. M., Cutler, J. A., Windhauser, M. M., Lin, P. H., & Karanja, N. (1997). A clinical trial of the effects of dietary patterns on blood pressure. DASH Collaborative Research Group. The New England journal of medicine, 336(16), 1117–1124. https://doi.org/10.1056/NEJM199704173361601

[1431] Miller, G. D., DiRienzo, D. D., Reusser, M. E., & McCarron, D. A. (2000). Benefits of dairy product consumption on blood pressure in humans: a summary of the biomedical literature. Journal of the American College of Nutrition, 19(2 Suppl), 147S–164S. https://doi.org/10.1080/07315724.2000.10718085

[1432] Carafoli, E., Santella, L., Branca, D., & Brini, M. (2001). Generation, Control, and Processing of Cellular Calcium Signals. Critical Reviews in Biochemistry and Molecular Biology, 36(2), 107–260. doi:10.1080/20014091074183

[1433] Smaili, S. S., Hsu, Y.-T., Carvalho, A. C. P., Rosenstock, T. R., Sharpe, J. C., & Youle, R. J. (2003). Mitochondria, calcium and pro-apoptotic proteins as mediators in cell death signaling. Brazilian Journal of Medical and Biological Research, 36(2), 183–190. doi:10.1590/s0100-879x2003000200004

[1434] Duchen, M. R. (2000). Mitochondria and Ca2+in cell physiology and pathophysiology. Cell Calcium, 28(5-6), 339–348. doi:10.1054/ceca.2000.0170

[1435] Brustovetsky, N., Brustovetsky, T., Purl, K. J., Capano, M., Crompton, M., & Dubinsky, J. M. (2003). Increased Susceptibility of Striatal Mitochondria to Calcium-Induced Permeability Transition. The Journal of Neuroscience, 23(12), 4858–4867. doi:10.1523/jneurosci.23-12-04858.2003

[1436] Pandya, J. D., Nukala, V. N., & Sullivan, P. G. (2013). Concentration dependent effect of calcium on brain mitochondrial bioenergetics and oxidative stress parameters. Frontiers in Neuroenergetics, 5. doi:10.3389/fnene.2013.00010

[1437] Starkov, A. A., Polster, B. M., & Fiskum, G. (2002). Regulation of hydrogen peroxide production by brain mitochondria by calcium and Bax. Journal of Neurochemistry, 83(1), 220–228. doi:10.1046/j.1471-4159.2002.01153.x

[1438] Bootman, M. D., Chehab, T., Bultynck, G., Parys, J. B., & Rietdorf, K. (2018). The regulation of autophagy by calcium signals: Do we have a consensus?. Cell calcium, 70, 32–46. https://doi.org/10.1016/j.ceca.2017.08.005

[1439] White, R. J., & Reynolds, I. J. (1997). Mitochondria accumulate Ca2+ following intense glutamate stimulation of cultured rat forebrain neurones. The Journal of physiology, 498 (Pt 1)(Pt 1), 31–47. https://doi.org/10.1113/jphysiol.1997.sp021839

[1440] Thayer, S. A., & Wang, G. J. (1995). Glutamate-induced calcium loads: effects on energy metabolism and neuronal viability. Clinical and experimental pharmacology & physiology, 22(4), 303–304. https://doi.org/10.1111/j.1440-1681.1995.tb02004.x

[1441] Pivovarova, N. B., Nguyen, H. V., Winters, C. A., Brantner, C. A., Smith, C. L., & Andrews, S. B. (2004). Excitotoxic calcium overload in a subpopulation of mitochondria triggers delayed death in hippocampal neurons. The Journal of neuroscience : the official journal of the Society for Neuroscience, 24(24), 5611–5622. https://doi.org/10.1523/JNEUROSCI.0531-04.2004

[1442] Reynolds, I., & Hastings, T. (1995). Glutamate induces the production of reactive oxygen species in cultured forebrain neurons following NMDA receptor activation. The Journal of Neuroscience, 15(5), 3318–3327. doi:10.1523/jneurosci.15-05-03318.1995

[1443] Sengpiel, B., Preis, E., Krieglstein, J., & Prehn, J. H. (1998). NMDA-induced superoxide production and neurotoxicity in cultured rat hippocampal neurons: role of mitochondria. The European journal of neuroscience, 10(5), 1903–1910. https://doi.org/10.1046/j.1460-9568.1998.00202.x

[1444] He, L. M., Chen, L. Y., Lou, X. L., Qu, A. L., Zhou, Z., & Xu, T. (2002). Evaluation of beta-amyloid peptide 25-35 on calcium homeostasis in cultured rat dorsal root ganglion neurons. Brain research, 939(1-2), 65–75. https://doi.org/10.1016/s0006-8993(02)02549-0

[1445] Abramov, A. Y., Canevari, L., & Duchen, M. R. (2003). Changes in Intracellular Calcium and Glutathione in Astrocytes as the Primary Mechanism of Amyloid Neurotoxicity. The Journal of Neuroscience, 23(12), 5088–5095. doi:10.1523/jneurosci.23-12-05088.2003

[1446] Dietary Reference Intakes for Calcium and Vitamin D. (2011). doi:10.17226/13050

[1447] Ross, A. C., Manson, J. E., Abrams, S. A., Aloia, J. F., Brannon, P. M., Clinton, S. K., ... Shapses, S. A. (2011). The 2011 Report on Dietary Reference Intakes for Calcium and Vitamin D from the Institute of Medicine: What Clinicians Need to Know. The Journal of Clinical Endocrinology & Metabolism, 96(1), 53–58. doi:10.1210/jc.2010-2704

[1448] Committee to Review Dietary Reference Intakes for Vitamin D and Calcium, Food and Nutrition Board, Institute of Medicine. Dietary Reference Intakes for Calcium and Vitamin D. Washington, DC: National Academy Press, 2010.

[1449] Hunt, C. D., & Johnson, L. K. (2007). Calcium requirements: new estimations for men and women by cross-sectional statistical analyses of calcium balance data from metabolic studies. The American Journal of Clinical Nutrition, 86(4), 1054–1063. doi:10.1093/ajcn/86.4.1054

[1450] Zhu, K., & Prince, R. L. (2012). Calcium and bone. Clinical biochemistry, 45(12), 936–942. https://doi.org/10.1016/j.clinbiochem.2012.05.006

[1451] Spiegel, D. M., & Brady, K. (2012). Calcium balance in normal individuals and in patients with chronic kidney disease on low- and high-calcium diets. Kidney International, 81(11), 1116–1122. doi:10.1038/ki.2011.490

[1452] Kopple et al (1972) 'METABOLIC STUDIES OF LOW PROTEIN DIETS IN UREMIA, II. CALCIUM, PHOSPHOKUS AND MAGNESIUM', Medicine: November 1973 - Volume 52 - Issue 6 - p 597-607.

[1453] Spiegel, D. M., & Brady, K. (2012). Calcium balance in normal individuals and in patients with chronic kidney disease on low- and high-calcium diets. Kidney International, 81(11), 1116–1122. doi:10.1038/ki.2011.490

[1454] Sarnak, M. J., Levey, A. S., Schoolwerth, A. C., Coresh, J., Culleton, B., Hamm, L. L., ... Wilson, P. W. (2003). Kidney Disease as a Risk Factor for Development of Cardiovascular Disease. Hypertension, 42(5), 1050–1065. doi:10.1161/01.hyp.0000102971.85504.7c

[1455] Chertow, G. M., Burke, S. K., Raggi, P., & for the Treat to Goal Working Group. (2002). Sevelamer attenuates the progression of coronary and aortic calcification in hemodialysis patients. Kidney International, 62(1), 245–252. doi:10.1046/j.1523-1755.2002.00434.x

[1456] Coresh, J., Selvin, E., Stevens, L. A., Manzi, J., Kusek, J. W., Eggers, P., ... Levey, A. S. (2007). Prevalence of Chronic Kidney Disease in the United States. JAMA, 298(17), 2038. doi:10.1001/jama.298.17.2038

[1457] Bailey, R. L., Dodd, K. W., Goldman, J. A., Gahche, J. J., Dwyer, J. T., Moshfegh, A. J., Sempos, C. T., & Picciano, M. F. (2010). Estimation of total usual calcium and vitamin D intakes in the United States. The Journal of nutrition, 140(4), 817–822. https://doi.org/10.3945/jn.109.118539

[1458] Blumberg, J. B., Frei, B. B., Fulgoni, V. L., Weaver, C. M., & Zeisel, S. H. (2017). Impact of Frequency of Multi-Vitamin/Multi-Mineral Supplement Intake on Nutritional Adequacy and Nutrient Deficiencies in U.S. Adults. Nutrients, 9(8), 849. https://doi.org/10.3390/nu9080849

[1459] Ross, A. C., Manson, J. E., Abrams, S. A., Aloia, J. F., Brannon, P. M., Clinton, S. K., Durazo-Arvizu, R. A., Gallagher, J. C., Gallo, R. L., Jones, G., Kovacs, C. S., Mayne, S. T., Rosen, C. J., & Shapses, S. A. (2011). Clarification of DRIs for calcium and vitamin D across age groups. Journal of the American Dietetic Association, 111(10), 1467. https://doi.org/10.1016/j.jada.2011.08.022

[1460] Kit, B. K., Fakhouri, T. H., Park, S., Nielsen, S. J., & Ogden, C. L. (2013). Trends in sugar-sweetened beverage consumption among youth and adults in the United States: 1999-2010. The American journal of clinical nutrition, 98(1), 180–188. https://doi.org/10.3945/ajcn.112.057943

[1461] Calvo M. S. (1993). Dietary phosphorus, calcium metabolism and bone. The Journal of nutrition, 123(9), 1627–1633. https://doi.org/10.1093/jn/123.9.1627

[1462] Li, K., Kaaks, R., Linseisen, J., & Rohrmann, S. (2012). Associations of dietary calcium intake and calcium supplementation with myocardial infarction and stroke risk and overall cardiovascular mortality in the Heidelberg cohort of the European Prospective Investigation into Cancer and Nutrition study (EPIC-Heidelberg). Heart (British Cardiac Society), 98(12), 920–925. https://doi.org/10.1136/heartjnl-2011-301345

[1463] Michaelsson, K., Melhus, H., Warensjo Lemming, E., Wolk, A., & Byberg, L. (2013). Long term calcium intake and rates of all cause and cardiovascular mortality: community based prospective longitudinal cohort study. BMJ, 346(feb12 4), f228–f228. doi:10.1136/bmj.f228

[1464] Wang, X., Chen, H., Ouyang, Y., Liu, J., Zhao, G., Bao, W., & Yan, M. (2014). Dietary calcium intake and mortality risk from cardiovascular disease and all causes: a meta-analysis of prospective cohort studies. BMC Medicine, 12(1). doi:10.1186/s12916-014-0158-6

[1465] Bolland, M. J., Grey, A., Avenell, A., Gamble, G. D., & Reid, I. R. (2011). Calcium supplements with or without vitamin D and risk of cardiovascular events: reanalysis of the Women's Health Initiative limited access dataset and meta-analysis. BMJ, 342(apr19 1), d2040–d2040. doi:10.1136/bmj.d2040

[1466] Curhan, G. C. (1997). Comparison of Dietary Calcium with Supplemental Calcium and Other Nutrients as Factors Affecting the Risk for Kidney Stones in Women. Annals of Internal Medicine, 126(7), 497. doi:10.7326/0003-4819-126-7-199704010-00001

[1467] Karp, H. J., Ketola, M. E., & Lamberg-Allardt, C. J. E. (2009). Acute effects of calcium carbonate, calcium citrate and potassium citrate on markers of calcium and bone metabolism in young women. British Journal of Nutrition, 102(9), 1341–1347. doi:10.1017/s0007114509990195

[1468] Bristow, S. M., Gamble, G. D., Stewart, A., Horne, L., House, M. E., Aati, O., ... Reid, I. R. (2014). Acute and 3-month effects of microcrystalline hydroxyapatite, calcium citrate and calcium carbonate on serum calcium and markers of bone turnover: a randomised controlled trial in postmenopausal women. British Journal of Nutrition, 112(10), 1611–1620. doi:10.1017/s0007114514002785

[1469] Manson, J. E., Allison, M. A., Carr, J. J., Langer, R. D., Cochrane, B. B., Hendrix, S. L., Hsia, J., Hunt, J. R., Lewis, C. E., Margolis, K. L., Robinson, J. G., Rodabough, R. J., Thomas, A. M., & Women's Health Initiative and Women's Health Initiative-Coronary Artery Calcium Study Investigators (2010). Calcium/vitamin D supplementation and coronary artery calcification in the Women's Health Initiative. Menopause (New York, N.Y.), 17(4), 683–691. https://doi.org/10.1097/gme.0b013e3181d683b5

[1470] Seelig M. S. (1990). Increased need for magnesium with the use of combined oestrogen and calcium for osteoporosis treatment. Magnesium research, 3(3), 197–215.

[1471] Dai, Q., Shu, X.-O., Deng, X., Xiang, Y.-B., Li, H., Yang, G., ... Zheng, W. (2013). Modifying effect of calcium/magnesium intake ratio and mortality: a population-based cohort study. BMJ Open, 3(2), e002111. doi:10.1136/bmjopen-2012-002111

[1472] Lakshmanan, F. L., Rao, R. B., Kim, W. W., & Kelsay, J. L. (1984). Magnesium intakes, balances, and blood levels of adults consuming self-selected diets. The American Journal of Clinical Nutrition, 40(6), 1380–1389. doi:10.1093/ajcn/40.6.1380

[1473] Seelig (2012) 'Magnesium Deficiency in the Pathogenesis of Disease: Early Roots of Cardiovascular, Skeletal, and Renal Abnormalities', Springer Science & Business Media.

[1474] Rosanoff, A., Weaver, C. M., & Rude, R. K. (2012). Suboptimal magnesium status in the United States: are the health consequences underestimated? Nutrition Reviews, 70(3), 153–164. doi:10.1111/j.1753-4887.2011.00465.x

[1475] NIH (2020) 'Calcium: Fact Sheet for Health Professionals', Dietary Supplement Fact Sheets, Accessed Online Jan 26 2021: https://ods.od.nih.gov/factsheets/Calcium-HealthProfessional/

[1476] Optimal calcium intake. (1994). NIH consensus statement, 12(4), 1–31.

[1477] Heaney, R. P., Recker, R. R., Stegman, M. R., & Moy, A. J. (1989). Calcium absorption in women: relationships to calcium intake, estrogen status, and age. Journal of bone and mineral research : the official journal of the American Society for Bone and Mineral Research, 4(4), 469–475. https://doi.org/10.1002/jbmr.5650040404

[1478] Committee to Review Dietary Reference Intakes for Vitamin D and Calcium, Food and Nutrition Board, Institute of Medicine. Dietary Reference Intakes for Calcium and Vitamin D. Washington, DC: National Academy Press, 2010.

[1479] Jellin JM, Gregory P, Batz F, Hitchens K. Pharmacist's Letter/Prescriber's Letter Natural Medicines Comprehensive Database. 3rd ed. Stockton, CA: Therapeutic Research Facility, 2000.

[1480] Nordin (1976) 'Calcium, Phosphate, and Magnesium Metabolism'; Churchill Livingstone: Edinburgh, UK; p. 41.

[1481] Lerolle, N., Lantz, B., Paillard, F., Gattegno, B., Flahault, A., Ronco, P., Houillier, P., & Rondeau, E. (2002). Risk factors for nephrolithiasis in patients with familial idiopathic hypercalciuria. The American journal of medicine, 113(2), 99–103. https://doi.org/10.1016/s0002-9343(02)01152-x

[1482] Weaver, C. M., & Heaney, R. P. (1991). Isotopic exchange of ingested calcium between labeled sources. Evidence that ingested calcium does not form a common absorptive pool. Calcified tissue international, 49(4), 244–247. https://doi.org/10.1007/BF02556212

[1483] Hall, W. D., Pettinger, M., Oberman, A., Watts, N. B., Johnson, K. C., Paskett, E. D., Limacher, M. C., & Hays, J. (2001). Risk factors for kidney stones in older women in the southern United States. The American journal of the medical sciences, 322(1), 12–18. https://doi.org/10.1097/00000441-200107000-00003

[1484] Jackson, R. D., LaCroix, A. Z., Gass, M., Wallace, R. B., Robbins, J., Lewis, C. E., Bassford, T., Beresford, S. A., Black, H. R., Blanchette, P., Bonds, D. E., Brunner, R. L., Brzyski, R. G., Caan, B., Cauley, J. A., Chlebowski, R. T., Cummings, S. R., Granek, I., Hays, J., Heiss, G., ... Women's Health Initiative Investigators (2006). Calcium plus vitamin D supplementation and the risk of fractures. The New England journal of medicine, 354(7), 669–683. https://doi.org/10.1056/NEJMoa055218

[1485] Curhan, G. C., Willett, W. C., Knight, E. L., & Stampfer, M. J. (2004). Dietary factors and the risk of incident kidney stones in younger women: Nurses' Health Study II. Archives of internal medicine, 164(8), 885–891. https://doi.org/10.1001/archinte.164.8.885

[1486] Curhan, G. C., Willett, W. C., Rimm, E. B., & Stampfer, M. J. (1993). A prospective study of dietary calcium and other nutrients and the risk of symptomatic kidney stones. The New England journal of medicine, 328(12), 833–838. https://doi.org/10.1056/NEJM199303253281203

[1487] Taylor, E. N., Stampfer, M. J., & Curhan, G. C. (2004). Dietary factors and the risk of incident kidney stones in men: new insights after 14 years of follow-up. Journal of the American Society of Nephrology : JASN, 15(12), 3225–3232. https://doi.org/10.1097/01.ASN.0000146012.44570.20

[1488] Liebman, M., & Chai, W. (1997). Effect of dietary calcium on urinary oxalate excretion after oxalate loads. The American journal of clinical nutrition, 65(5), 1453–1459. https://doi.org/10.1093/ajcn/65.5.1453

[1489] Hess, B., Jost, C., Zipperle, L., Takkinen, R., & Jaeger, P. (1998). High-calcium intake abolishes hyperoxaluria and reduces urinary crystallization during a 20-fold normal oxalate load in humans. Nephrology, dialysis, transplantation : official publication of the European Dialysis and Transplant Association - European Renal Association, 13(9), 2241–2247. https://doi.org/10.1093/ndt/13.9.2241

[1490] Lange, J. N., Wood, K. D., Mufarrij, P. W., Callahan, M. F., Easter, L., Knight, J., Holmes, R. P., & Assimos, D. G. (2012). The impact of dietary calcium and oxalate ratios on stone risk. Urology, 79(6), 1226–1229. https://doi.org/10.1016/j.urology.2012.01.053

[1491] Weaver, C. M., Heaney, R. P., Martin, B. R., & Fitzsimmons, M. L. (1991). Human calcium absorption from whole-wheat products. The Journal of nutrition, 121(11), 1769–1775. https://doi.org/10.1093/jn/121.11.1769

[1492] Heaney R. P. (1996). Bone mass, nutrition, and other lifestyle factors. Nutrition reviews, 54(4 Pt 2), S3–S10. https://doi.org/10.1111/j.1753-4887.1996.tb03891.x

[1493] Weaver, C. M., Proulx, W. R., & Heaney, R. (1999). Choices for achieving adequate dietary calcium with a vegetarian diet. The American journal of clinical nutrition, 70(3 Suppl), 543S–548S. https://doi.org/10.1093/ajcn/70.3.543s

[1494] Meyer, W. J., Transbol, I., Bartter, F. C., & Delea, C. (1976). Control of calcium absorption: Effect of sodium chloride loading and depletion. Metabolism, 25(9), 989–993. doi:10.1016/0026-0495(76)90128-1

[1495] Weaver CM. Calcium. In: Erdman JJ, Macdonald I, Zeisel S, eds. Present Knowledge in Nutrition. 10th ed: John Wiley & Sons, Inc.; 2012:434-446.

[1496] Kanis, J. A., Delmas, P., Burckhardt, P., Cooper, C., & Torgerson, D. (1997). Guidelines for diagnosis and management of osteoporosis. The European Foundation for Osteoporosis and Bone Disease. Osteoporosis international : a journal established as result of cooperation between the European Foundation for Osteoporosis and the National Osteoporosis Foundation of the USA, 7(4), 390–406. https://doi.org/10.1007/BF01623782

[1497] Darling, A. L., Millward, D. J., Torgerson, D. J., Hewitt, C. E., & Lanham-New, S. A. (2009). Dietary protein and bone health: a systematic review and meta-analysis. The American journal of clinical nutrition, 90(6), 1674–1692. https://doi.org/10.3945/ajcn.2009.27799

[1498] Calvez, J., Poupin, N., Chesneau, C., Lassale, C., & Tomé, D. (2012). Protein intake, calcium balance and health consequences. European journal of clinical nutrition, 66(3), 281–295. https://doi.org/10.1038/ejcn.2011.196

[1499] Kerstetter, J. E., O'Brien, K. O., Caseria, D. M., Wall, D. E., & Insogna, K. L. (2005). The impact of dietary protein on calcium absorption and kinetic measures of bone turnover in women. The Journal of clinical endocrinology and metabolism, 90(1), 26–31. https://doi.org/10.1210/jc.2004-0179

[1500] Fenton, T. R., Eliasziw, M., Lyon, A. W., Tough, S. C., & Hanley, D. A. (2008). Meta-analysis of the quantity of calcium excretion associated with the net acid excretion of the modern diet under the acid-ash diet hypothesis. The American journal of clinical nutrition, 88(4), 1159–1166. https://doi.org/10.1093/ajcn/88.4.1159

[1501] Johnson, A. O., Semenya, J. G., Buchowski, M. S., Enwonwu, C. O., & Scrimshaw, N. S. (1993). Correlation of lactose maldigestion, lactose intolerance, and milk intolerance. The American journal of clinical nutrition, 57(3), 399–401. https://doi.org/10.1093/ajcn/57.3.399

[1502] Pribila, B. A., Hertzler, S. R., Martin, B. R., Weaver, C. M., & Savaiano, D. A. (2000). Improved lactose digestion and intolerance among African-American adolescent girls fed a dairy-rich diet. Journal of the American Dietetic Association, 100(5), 524–530. https://doi.org/10.1016/S0002-8223(00)00162-0

[1503] American Dietetic Association, & Dietitians of Canada (2003). Position of the American Dietetic Association and Dietitians of Canada: Vegetarian diets. Journal of the American Dietetic Association, 103(6), 748–765. https://doi.org/10.1053/jada.2003.50142

[1504] Janelle, K. C., & Barr, S. I. (1995). Nutrient intakes and eating behavior scores of vegetarian and nonvegetarian women. Journal of the American Dietetic Association, 95(2), 180–188. https://doi.org/10.1016/s0002-8223(95)00045-3

[1505] Appleby, P., Roddam, A., Allen, N., & Key, T. (2007). Comparative fracture risk in vegetarians and nonvegetarians in EPIC-Oxford. European journal of clinical nutrition, 61(12), 1400–1406. https://doi.org/10.1038/sj.ejcn.1602659

[1506] Reed, J. A., Anderson, J. J., Tylavsky, F. A., & Gallagher, P. N., Jr (1994). Comparative changes in radial-bone density of elderly female lacto-ovovegetarians and omnivores. The American journal of clinical nutrition, 59(5 Suppl), 1197S–1202S. https://doi.org/10.1093/ajcn/59.5.1197S

[1507] Marsh, A. G., Sanchez, T. V., Midkelsen, O., Keiser, J., & Mayor, G. (1980). Cortical bone density of adult lacto-ovo-vegetarian and omnivorous women. Journal of the American Dietetic Association, 76(2), 148–151.

[1508] Massey, L. K., & Whiting, S. J. (1993). Caffeine, urinary calcium, calcium metabolism and bone. The Journal of nutrition, 123(9), 1611–1614. https://doi.org/10.1093/jn/123.9.1611

[1509] Wikoff, D., Welsh, B. T., Henderson, R., Brorby, G. P., Britt, J., Myers, E., Goldberger, J., Lieberman, H. R., O'Brien, C., Peck, J., Tenenbein, M., Weaver, C., Harvey, S., Urban, J., & Doepker, C. (2017). Systematic review of the potential adverse effects of caffeine consumption in healthy adults, pregnant women, adolescents, and children. Food and chemical toxicology : an international journal published for the British Industrial Biological Research Association, 109(Pt 1), 585–648. https://doi.org/10.1016/j.fct.2017.04.002

[1510] Barger-Lux, M. J., Heaney, R. P., & Stegman, M. R. (1990). Effects of moderate caffeine intake on the calcium economy of premenopausal women. The American journal of clinical nutrition, 52(4), 722–725. https://doi.org/10.1093/ajcn/52.4.722

[1511] Barrett-Connor, E., Chang, J. C., & Edelstein, S. L. (1994). Coffee-associated osteoporosis offset by daily milk consumption. The Rancho Bernardo Study. JAMA, 271(4), 280–283. https://doi.org/10.1001/jama.1994.03510280042030

[1512] Heaney, R. P., & Rafferty, K. (2001). Carbonated beverages and urinary calcium excretion. The American journal of clinical nutrition, 74(3), 343–347. https://doi.org/10.1093/ajcn/74.3.343

[1513] Hirsch PE, Peng TC. Effects of alcohol on calcium homeostasis and bone. In: Anderson J, Garner S, eds. Calcium and Phosphorus in Health and Disease. Boca Raton, FL: CRC Press, 1996:289-300.

[1514] Mahabir, S., Baer, D. J., Pfeiffer, R. M., Li, Y., Watkins, B. A., & Taylor, P. R. (2014). Low to moderate alcohol consumption on serum vitamin D and other indicators of bone health in postmenopausal women in a controlled feeding study. European journal of clinical nutrition, 68(11), 1267–1270. https://doi.org/10.1038/ejcn.2014.191

[1515] Breslau N. A. (1994). Calcium, estrogen, and progestin in the treatment of osteoporosis. Rheumatic diseases clinics of North America, 20(3), 691–716.

[1516] Gallagher, J. C., Riggs, B. L., & DeLuca, H. F. (1980). Effect of estrogen on calcium absorption and serum vitamin D metabolites in postmenopausal osteoporosis. The Journal of clinical endocrinology and metabolism, 51(6), 1359–1364. https://doi.org/10.1210/jcem-51-6-1359

[1517] Roberts, J. G., Webber, C. E., & Woolever, C. A. (1986). Estrogen replacement therapy for postmenopausal osteoporosis. Canadian family physician Medecin de famille canadien, 32, 883–891.

[1518] Elders, P. J., Lips, P., Netelenbos, J. C., van Ginkel, F. C., Khoe, E., van der Vijgh, W. J., & van der Stelt, P. F. (1994). Long-term effect of calcium supplementation on bone loss in perimenopausal women. Journal of bone and mineral research : the official journal of the American Society for Bone and Mineral Research, 9(7), 963–970. https://doi.org/10.1002/jbmr.5650090702

[1519] Dawson-Hughes, B., Dallal, G. E., Krall, E. A., Sadowski, L., Sahyoun, N., & Tannenbaum, S. (1990). A controlled trial of the effect of calcium supplementation on bone density in postmenopausal women. The New England journal of medicine, 323(13), 878–883. https://doi.org/10.1056/NEJM199009273231305

[1520] National Institute of Arthritis and Musculoskeletal and Skin Diseases, National Institutes of Health. Osteoporosis Handout on Health. NIH Publication No. 11-5158; 2011.

[1521] North American Menopause Society (2012). The 2012 hormone therapy position statement of: The North American Menopause Society. Menopause (New York, N.Y.), 19(3), 257–271. https://doi.org/10.1097/gme.0b013e31824b970a

[1522] Bendich A. (2000). The potential for dietary supplements to reduce premenstrual syndrome (PMS) symptoms. Journal of the American College of Nutrition, 19(1), 3–12. https://doi.org/10.1080/07315724.2000.10718907

[1523] Bertone-Johnson, E. R., Hankinson, S. E., Bendich, A., Johnson, S. R., Willett, W. C., & Manson, J. E. (2005). Calcium and vitamin D intake and risk of incident premenstrual syndrome. Archives of internal medicine, 165(11), 1246–1252. https://doi.org/10.1001/archinte.165.11.1246

[1524] Thys-Jacobs, S., Starkey, P., Bernstein, D., & Tian, J. (1998). Calcium carbonate and the premenstrual syndrome: effects on premenstrual and menstrual symptoms. Premenstrual Syndrome Study Group. American journal of obstetrics and gynecology, 179(2), 444–452. https://doi.org/10.1016/s0002-9378(98)70377-1

[1525] Shobeiri, F., Araste, F. E., Ebrahimi, R., Jenabi, E., & Nazari, M. (2017). Effect of calcium on premenstrual syndrome: A double-blind randomized clinical trial. Obstetrics & gynecology science, 60(1), 100–105. https://doi.org/10.5468/ogs.2017.60.1.100

[1526] Masoumi, S. Z., Ataollahi, M., & Oshvandi, K. (2016). Effect of Combined Use of Calcium and Vitamin B6 on Premenstrual Syndrome Symptoms: a Randomized Clinical Trial. Journal of caring sciences, 5(1), 67–73. https://doi.org/10.15171/jcs.2016.007

[1527] Alvir, J. M., & Thys-Jacobs, S. (1991). Premenstrual and menstrual symptom clusters and response to calcium treatment. Psychopharmacology bulletin, 27(2), 145–148.

[1528] Thys-Jacobs, S., Ceccarelli, S., Bierman, A., Weisman, H., Cohen, M. A., & Alvir, J. (1989). Calcium supplementation in premenstrual syndrome: a randomized crossover trial. Journal of general internal medicine, 4(3), 183–189. https://doi.org/10.1007/BF02599520

[1529] Drinkwater, B. L., Bruemner, B., & Chesnut, C. H., 3rd (1990). Menstrual history as a determinant of current bone density in young athletes. JAMA, 263(4), 545–548.

[1530] Marcus, R., Cann, C., Madvig, P., Minkoff, J., Goddard, M., Bayer, M., Martin, M., Gaudiani, L., Haskell, W., & Genant, H. (1985). Menstrual function and bone mass in elite women distance runners. Endocrine and metabolic features. Annals of internal medicine, 102(2), 158–163. https://doi.org/10.7326/0003-4819-102-2-158

[1531] Abrams, S. A., Silber, T. J., Esteban, N. V., Vieira, N. E., Stuff, J. E., Meyers, R., Majd, M., & Yergey, A. L. (1993). Mineral balance and bone turnover in adolescents with anorexia nervosa. The Journal of pediatrics, 123(2), 326–331. https://doi.org/10.1016/s0022-3476(05)81714-7

[1532] Nattiv A. (2000). Stress fractures and bone health in track and field athletes. Journal of science and medicine in sport, 3(3), 268–279. https://doi.org/10.1016/s1440-2440(00)80036-5

[1533] Lappe, J., Cullen, D., Haynatzki, G., Recker, R., Ahlf, R., & Thompson, K. (2008). Calcium and vitamin d supplementation decreases incidence of stress fractures in female navy recruits. Journal of bone and mineral research : the official journal of the American Society for Bone and Mineral Research, 23(5), 741–749. https://doi.org/10.1359/jbmr.080102

[1534] Shannon MT, Wilson BA, Stang CL. Health Professionals Drug Guide. Stamford, CT: Appleton and Lange, 2000.

[1535] Peters, M. L., Leonard, M., & Licata, A. A. (2001). Role of alendronate and risedronate in preventing and treating osteoporosis. Cleveland Clinic journal of medicine, 68(11), 945–951. https://doi.org/10.3949/ccjm.68.11.945

[1536] Wood, R. J., & Zheng, J. J. (1997). High dietary calcium intakes reduce zinc absorption and balance in humans. The American journal of clinical nutrition, 65(6), 1803–1809. https://doi.org/10.1093/ajcn/65.6.1803

[1537] Vella, A., Gerber, T. C., Hayes, D. L., & Reeder, G. S. (1999). Digoxin, hypercalcaemia, and cardiac conduction. Postgraduate medical journal, 75(887), 554–556. https://doi.org/10.1136/pgmj.75.887.554

[1538] Lewis, J. R., Zhu, K., & Prince, R. L. (2012). Adverse events from calcium supplementation: relationship to errors in myocardial infarction self-reporting in randomized controlled trials of calcium supplementation. Journal of bone and mineral research : the official journal of the American Society for Bone and Mineral Research, 27(3), 719–722. https://doi.org/10.1002/jbmr.1484

[1539] Straub D. A. (2007). Calcium supplementation in clinical practice: a review of forms, doses, and indications. Nutrition in clinical practice : official publication of the American Society for Parenteral and Enteral Nutrition, 22(3), 286–296. https://doi.org/10.1177/0115426507022003286

[1540] Heaney RP. Phosphorus. In: Erdman JW, Macdonald IA, Zeisel SH, eds. Present Knowledge in Nutrition. 10th ed. Washington, DC: Wiley-Blackwell; 2012:447-58.

[1541] Habibah, T. U., Amlani, D. V., & Brizuela, M. (2020). Hydroxyapatite Dental Material. In StatPearls. StatPearls Publishing.

[1542] Lipmann, D (1944). "Enzymatic Synthesis of Acetyl Phosphate". J Biol Chem. 155: 55–70.

[1543] Garrett, Reginald (1995). Biochemistry. Saunders College.

[1544] Sharma, S., Guthrie, P. H., Chan, S. S., Haq, S., & Taegtmeyer, H. (2007). Glucose phosphorylation is required for insulin-dependent mTOR signalling in the heart. Cardiovascular research, 76(1), 71–80. https://doi.org/10.1016/j.cardiores.2007.05.004

[1545] Hardman G, Perkins S, Ruan Z, Kannan N, Brownridge P, Byrne DP, Eyers PA, Jones AR, Eyers CE (2017). "Extensive non-canonical phosphorylation in human cells revealed using strong-anion exchange-mediated phosphoproteomics". bioRxiv 10.1101/202820

[1546] Fuhs, S. R., & Hunter, T. (2017). pHisphorylation: the emergence of histidine phosphorylation as a reversible regulatory modification. Current opinion in cell biology, 45, 8–16. https://doi.org/10.1016/j.ceb.2016.12.010

[1547] Hruska K. Overview of phosphorus homeostasis. In: Gutierrez OM, Kalantar-Zadeh K, Mehrotra R, eds. Clinical Aspects of Natural and Added Phosphorus in Foods. New York, New York: Springer-Verlag; 2017:11-28.

[1548] de Menezes Filho, H., de Castro, L. C., & Damiani, D. (2006). Hypophosphatemic rickets and osteomalacia. Arquivos brasileiros de endocrinologia e metabologia, 50(4), 802–813. https://doi.org/10.1590/s0004-27302006000400025

[1549] Gattineni, J., & Baum, M. (2012). Genetic disorders of phosphate regulation. Pediatric nephrology (Berlin, Germany), 27(9), 1477–1487. https://doi.org/10.1007/s00467-012-2103-2

[1550] Karpen H. E. (2018). Mineral Homeostasis and Effects on Bone Mineralization in the Preterm Neonate. Clinics in perinatology, 45(1), 129–141. https://doi.org/10.1016/j.clp.2017.11.005

[1551] Abrams S. A. (2007). In utero physiology: role in nutrient delivery and fetal development for calcium, phosphorus, and vitamin D. The American journal of clinical nutrition, 85(2), 604S–607S. https://doi.org/10.1093/ajcn/85.2.604S

[1552] Harding, J. E., Wilson, J., & Brown, J. (2017). Calcium and phosphorus supplementation of human milk for preterm infants. The Cochrane database of systematic reviews, 2(2), CD003310. https://doi.org/10.1002/14651858.CD003310.pub2

[1553] Brunelli and Goldfarb (2007) 'Hypophosphatemia: Clinical Consequences and Management', JASN July 2007, 18 (7) 1999-2003; DOI: https://doi.org/10.1681/ASN.2007020143

[1554] Mehanna, H. M., Moledina, J., & Travis, J. (2008). Refeeding syndrome: what it is, and how to prevent and treat it. BMJ (Clinical research ed.), 336(7659), 1495–1498. https://doi.org/10.1136/bmj.a301

[1555] Camp, M. A., & Allon, M. (1990). Severe hypophosphatemia in hospitalized patients. Mineral and electrolyte metabolism, 16(6), 365–368.

[1556] McCray S, Walker S, Parrish CR. Much ado about refeeding. Practical Gastroenterology2004;XXVIII(12):26-44.

[1557] Parli, S. E., Ruf, K. M., & Magnuson, B. (2014). Pathophysiology, treatment, and prevention of fluid and electrolyte abnormalities during refeeding syndrome. Journal of infusion nursing : the official publication of the Infusion Nurses Society, 37(3), 197–202. https://doi.org/10.1097/NAN.0000000000000038

[1558] Friedli, N., Stanga, Z., Culkin, A., Crook, M., Laviano, A., Sobotka, L., Kressig, R. W., Kondrup, J., Mueller, B., & Schuetz, P. (2018). Management and prevention of refeeding syndrome in medical inpatients: An evidence-based and consensus-supported algorithm. Nutrition (Burbank, Los Angeles County, Calif.), 47, 13–20. https://doi.org/10.1016/j.nut.2017.09.007

[1559] Bazydlo, L. A. L., Needham, M., & Harris, N. S. (2014). Calcium, Magnesium, and Phosphate. Laboratory Medicine, 45(1), e44–e50. doi:10.1309/lmglmz8ciymfnogx

[1560] EFSA Panel on Dietetic Products N, Allergies (2015) 'Scientific Opinion on Dietary Reference Values for phosphorus', EFSA Journal 2015;13:4185.

[1561] Tonelli, M., Sacks, F., Pfeffer, M., Gao, Z., Curhan, G., & Cholesterol And Recurrent Events Trial Investigators (2005). Relation between serum phosphate level and cardiovascular event rate in people with coronary disease. Circulation, 112(17), 2627–2633. https://doi.org/10.1161/CIRCULATIONAHA.105.553198

[1562] Dhingra, R., Sullivan, L. M., Fox, C. S., Wang, T. J., D'Agostino, R. B., Sr, Gaziano, J. M., & Vasan, R. S. (2007). Relations of serum phosphorus and calcium levels to the incidence of cardiovascular disease in the community. Archives of internal medicine, 167(9), 879–885. https://doi.org/10.1001/archinte.167.9.879

[1563] Lopez, F. L., Agarwal, S. K., Grams, M. E., Loehr, L. R., Soliman, E. Z., Lutsey, P. L., Chen, L. Y., Huxley, R. R., & Alonso, A. (2013). Relation of serum phosphorus levels to the incidence of atrial fibrillation (from the Atherosclerosis Risk In Communities [ARIC] study). The American journal of cardiology, 111(6), 857–862. https://doi.org/10.1016/j.amjcard.2012.11.045

[1564] Bai, W., Li, J., & Liu, J. (2016). Serum phosphorus, cardiovascular and all-cause mortality in the general population: A meta-analysis. Clinica chimica acta; international journal of clinical chemistry, 461, 76–82. https://doi.org/10.1016/j.cca.2016.07.020

[1565] Chang, A. R., & Grams, M. E. (2014). Serum phosphorus and mortality in the Third National Health and Nutrition Examination Survey (NHANES III): effect modification by fasting. American journal of kidney diseases : the official journal of the National Kidney Foundation, 64(4), 567–573. https://doi.org/10.1053/j.ajkd.2014.04.028

[1566] Menon, M. C., & Ix, J. H. (2013). Dietary phosphorus, serum phosphorus, and cardiovascular disease. Annals of the New York Academy of Sciences, 1301, 21–26. https://doi.org/10.1111/nyas.12283

[1567] NIH (2020) 'Phosphorus: Fact Sheet for Health Professionals', Dietary Supplement Fact Sheets, Accessed Online Jan 26 2021: https://ods.od.nih.gov/factsheets/Phosphorus-HealthProfessional/

[1568] Institute of Medicine, Food and Nutrition Board. Dietary Reference Intakes for Calcium, Phosphorus, Magnesium, Vitamin D, and Fluoride. Washington, DC: National Academies Press; 1997.

[1569] Institute of Medicine (US) Standing Committee on the Scientific Evaluation of Dietary Reference Intakes. (1997). Dietary Reference Intakes for Calcium, Phosphorus, Magnesium, Vitamin D, and Fluoride. National Academies Press (US).

[1570] Calvo, M. S., & Tucker, K. L. (2013). Is phosphorus intake that exceeds dietary requirements a risk factor in bone health?. Annals of the New York Academy of Sciences, 1301, 29–35. https://doi.org/10.1111/nyas.12300

[1571] Calvo, M. S., & Park, Y. K. (1996). Changing phosphorus content of the U.S. diet: potential for adverse effects on bone. The Journal of nutrition, 126(4 Suppl), 1168S–80S. https://doi.org/10.1093/jn/126.suppl_4.1168S

[1572] USDA (2019) 'What We Eat In America', WWEIA Data Tables, Accessed Online Feb 3 2021: https://www.ars.usda.gov/northeast-area/beltsville-md-bhnrc/beltsville-human-nutrition-research-center/food-surveys-research-group/docs/wweia-data-tables/

[1573] Calvo, M. S., & Uribarri, J. (2013). Public health impact of dietary phosphorus excess on bone and cardiovascular health in the general population. The American journal of clinical nutrition, 98(1), 6–15. https://doi.org/10.3945/ajcn.112.053934

[1574] Yamamoto, K. T., Robinson-Cohen, C., de Oliveira, M. C., Kostina, A., Nettleton, J. A., Ix, J. H., Nguyen, H., Eng, J., Lima, J. A., Siscovick, D. S., Weiss, N. S., & Kestenbaum, B. (2013). Dietary phosphorus is associated with greater left ventricular mass. Kidney international, 83(4), 707–714. https://doi.org/10.1038/ki.2012.303

[1575] Chang, A. R., Lazo, M., Appel, L. J., Gutiérrez, O. M., & Grams, M. E. (2014). High dietary phosphorus intake is associated with all-cause mortality: results from NHANES III. The American journal of clinical nutrition, 99(2), 320–327. https://doi.org/10.3945/ajcn.113.073148

[1576] Malberti F. (2013). Hyperphosphataemia: treatment options. Drugs, 73(7), 673–688. https://doi.org/10.1007/s40265-013-0054-y

[1577] Beloosesky, Y., Grinblat, J., Weiss, A., Grosman, B., Gafter, U., & Chagnac, A. (2003). Electrolyte disorders following oral sodium phosphate administration for bowel cleansing in elderly patients. Archives of internal medicine, 163(7), 803–808. https://doi.org/10.1001/archinte.163.7.803

[1578] Stevens, K. K., Denby, L., Patel, R. K., Mark, P. B., Kettlewell, S., Smith, G. L., Clancy, M. J., Delles, C., & Jardine, A. G. (2017). Deleterious effects of phosphate on vascular and endothelial function via disruption to the nitric oxide pathway. Nephrology, dialysis, transplantation : official publication of the European Dialysis and Transplant Association - European Renal Association, 32(10), 1617–1627. https://doi.org/10.1093/ndt/gfw252

[1579] Shuto, E., Taketani, Y., Tanaka, R., Harada, N., Isshiki, M., Sato, M., Nashiki, K., Amo, K., Yamamoto, H., Higashi, Y., Nakaya, Y., & Takeda, E. (2009). Dietary phosphorus acutely impairs endothelial function. Journal of the American Society of Nephrology : JASN, 20(7), 1504–1512. https://doi.org/10.1681/ASN.2008101106

[1580] Di Marco, G. S., König, M., Stock, C., Wiesinger, A., Hillebrand, U., Reiermann, S., Reuter, S., Amler, S., Köhler, G., Buck, F., Fobker, M., Kümpers, P., Oberleithner, H., Hausberg, M., Lang, D., Pavenstädt, H., & Brand, M. (2013). High phosphate directly affects endothelial function by downregulating annexin II. Kidney international, 83(2), 213–222. https://doi.org/10.1038/ki.2012.300

[1581] Shanahan, C. M., Crouthamel, M. H., Kapustin, A., & Giachelli, C. M. (2011). Arterial calcification in chronic kidney disease: key roles for calcium and phosphate. Circulation research, 109(6), 697–711. https://doi.org/10.1161/CIRCRESAHA.110.234914

[1582] Giachelli C. M. (2003). Vascular calcification: in vitro evidence for the role of inorganic phosphate. Journal of the American Society of Nephrology : JASN, 14(9 Suppl 4), S300–S304. https://doi.org/10.1097/01.asn.0000081663.52165.66

[1583] Giachelli C. M. (2009). The emerging role of phosphate in vascular calcification. Kidney international, 75(9), 890–897. https://doi.org/10.1038/ki.2008.644

[1584] Kemi, V. E., Kärkkäinen, M. U., Rita, H. J., Laaksonen, M. M., Outila, T. A., & Lamberg-Allardt, C. J. (2010). Low calcium:phosphorus ratio in habitual diets affects serum parathyroid hormone concentration and calcium metabolism in healthy women with adequate calcium intake. The British journal of nutrition, 103(4), 561–568. https://doi.org/10.1017/S0007114509992121

[1585] Kemi, V. E., Rita, H. J., Kärkkäinen, M. U., Viljakainen, H. T., Laaksonen, M. M., Outila, T. A., & Lamberg-Allardt, C. J. (2009). Habitual high phosphorus intakes and foods with phosphate additives negatively affect serum parathyroid hormone concentration: a cross-sectional study on healthy premenopausal women. Public Health Nutrition, 12(10), 1885–1892. doi:10.1017/s1368980009004819

[1586] Calvo, M. S., Kumar, R., & Heath, H. (1990). Persistently elevated parathyroid hormone secretion and action in young women after four weeks of ingesting high phosphorus, low calcium diets. The Journal of clinical endocrinology and metabolism, 70(5), 1334–1340. https://doi.org/10.1210/jcem-70-5-1334

[1587] de Boer, I. H., Rue, T. C., & Kestenbaum, B. (2009). Serum phosphorus concentrations in the third National Health and Nutrition Examination Survey (NHANES III). American journal of kidney diseases : the official journal of the National Kidney Foundation, 53(3), 399–407. https://doi.org/10.1053/j.ajkd.2008.07.036

[1588] Lee and Cho (2015) 'Association between phosphorus intake and bone health in the NHANES population', Nutrition Journal volume 14, Article number: 28 (2015)

[1589] Bushinsky, D. A., Parker, W. R., & Asplin, J. R. (2000). Calcium phosphate supersaturation regulates stone formation in genetic hypercalciuric stone-forming rats. Kidney International, 57(2), 550–560. doi:10.1046/j.1523-1755.2000.00875.x

[1590] Chang, A. R., & Anderson, C. (2017). Dietary Phosphorus Intake and the Kidney. Annual review of nutrition, 37, 321–346. https://doi.org/10.1146/annurev-nutr-071816-064607

[1591] Loughrill, E., Wray, D., Christides, T., & Zand, N. (2016). Calcium to phosphorus ratio, essential elements and vitamin D content of infant foods in the UK: Possible implications for bone health. Maternal & Child Nutrition, 13(3), e12368. doi:10.1111/mcn.12368

[1592] Calvo, M. S., Moshfegh, A. J., & Tucker, K. L. (2014). Assessing the health impact of phosphorus in the food supply: issues and considerations. Advances in nutrition (Bethesda, Md.), 5(1), 104–113. https://doi.org/10.3945/an.113.004861

[1593] Kemi, V. E., Kärkkäinen, M. U., Rita, H. J., Laaksonen, M. M., Outila, T. A., & Lamberg-Allardt, C. J. (2010). Low calcium:phosphorus ratio in habitual diets affects serum parathyroid hormone concentration and calcium metabolism in healthy women with adequate calcium intake. The British journal of nutrition, 103(4), 561–568. https://doi.org/10.1017/S0007114509992121

603

[1594] Grimm, M., Müller, A., Hein, G., Fünfstück, R., & Jahreis, G. (2001). High phosphorus intake only slightly affects serum minerals, urinary pyridinium crosslinks and renal function in young women. European journal of clinical nutrition, 55(3), 153–161. https://doi.org/10.1038/sj.ejcn.1601131

[1595] Trautvetter, U., Ditscheid, B., Jahreis, G., & Glei, M. (2018). Habitual Intakes, Food Sources and Excretions of Phosphorus and Calcium in Three German Study Collectives. Nutrients, 10(2), 171. https://doi.org/10.3390/nu10020171

[1596] Brink, E. J., Beynen, A. C., Dekker, P. R., van Beresteijn, E. C., & van der Meer, R. (1992). Interaction of calcium and phosphate decreases ileal magnesium solubility and apparent magnesium absorption in rats. The Journal of nutrition, 122(3), 580–586. https://doi.org/10.1093/jn/122.3.580

[1597] Hardwick, L. L., Jones, M. R., Brautbar, N., & Lee, D. B. (1991). Magnesium absorption: mechanisms and the influence of vitamin D, calcium and phosphate. The Journal of nutrition, 121(1), 13–23. https://doi.org/10.1093/jn/121.1.13

[1598] Uribarri, J., & Calvo, M. S. (2003). Hidden sources of phosphorus in the typical American diet: does it matter in nephrology?. Seminars in dialysis, 16(3), 186–188. https://doi.org/10.1046/j.1525-139x.2003.16037.x

[1599] Seelig (2012) 'Magnesium Deficiency in the Pathogenesis of Disease: Early Roots of Cardiovascular, Skeletal, and Renal Abnormalities', Springer Science & Business Media.

[1600] SELF Nutrition Data (2018) 'Cheese, Cheddar Nutrition Facts and Calories', Accessed Online Jan 26 2021: https://nutritiondata.self.com/facts/dairy-and-egg-products/8/2

[1601] SELF Nutrition Data (2018) 'Seeds, pumpkin and squash seeds, whole, roasted, without salt', Accessed Online Jan 26 2021: https://nutritiondata.self.com/facts/nut-and-seed-products/3141/2

[1602] Spencer, H., Menczel, J., Lewin, I., & Samachson, J. (1965). EFFECT OF HIGH PHOSPHORUS INTAKE ON CALCIUM AND PHOSPHORUS METABOLISM IN MAN. The Journal of nutrition, 86, 125–132. https://doi.org/10.1093/jn/86.2.125

[1603] Farquharson, R. F., Salter, W. T., & Aub, J. C. (1931). STUDIES OF CALCIUM AND PHOSPHORUS METABOLISM: XIII. The Effect of Ingestion of Phosphates on the Excretion of Calcium. The Journal of clinical investigation, 10(2), 251–269. https://doi.org/10.1172/JCI100348

[1604] McClure, S. T., Chang, A. R., Selvin, E., Rebholz, C. M., & Appel, L. J. (2017). Dietary Sources of Phosphorus among Adults in the United States: Results from NHANES 2001-2014. Nutrients, 9(2), 95. https://doi.org/10.3390/nu9020095

[1605] Moshfegh AJ, Kovalchik AF, Clemens JC. Phosphorus Intake of Americans: What We Eat in American, NHANES 2011-2012. Food Surveys Research Group Dietary Data Brief No. 15. 2016.

[1606] Foment S, Nelson S. Calcium, phosphorus, magnesium, and sulfur. In: Foment S, editor. Nutrition of Normal Infants. St. Louis, MO: Mosby-Year Book, Inc; 1993. pp. 192–216.

[1607] Venkataraman, P. S., Tsang, R. C., Greer, F. R., Noguchi, A., Laskarzewski, P., & Steichen, J. J. (1985). Late infantile tetany and secondary hyperparathyroidism in infants fed humanized cow milk formula. Longitudinal follow-up. American journal of diseases of children (1960), 139(7), 664–668. https://doi.org/10.1001/archpedi.1985.02140090026018

[1608] Specker, B. L., Tsang, R. C., Ho, M. L., Landi, T. M., & Gratton, T. L. (1991). Low serum calcium and high parathyroid hormone levels in neonates fed 'humanized' cow's milk-based formula. American journal of diseases of children (1960), 145(8), 941–945. https://doi.org/10.1001/archpedi.1991.02160080119033

[1609] Gutiérrez, O. M., Luzuriaga-McPherson, A., Lin, Y., Gilbert, L. C., Ha, S. W., & Beck, G. R., Jr (2015). Impact of Phosphorus-Based Food Additives on Bone and Mineral Metabolism. The Journal of clinical endocrinology and metabolism, 100(11), 4264–4271. https://doi.org/10.1210/jc.2015-2279

[1610] Calvo, M. S., & Uribarri, J. (2013). Contributions to total phosphorus intake: all sources considered. Seminars in dialysis, 26(1), 54–61. https://doi.org/10.1111/sdi.12042

[1611] Calvo, M. S., & Park, Y. K. (1996). Changing phosphorus content of the U.S. diet: potential for adverse effects on bone. The Journal of nutrition, 126(4 Suppl), 1168S–80S. https://doi.org/10.1093/jn/126.suppl_4.1168S

[1612] León, J. B., Sullivan, C. M., & Sehgal, A. R. (2013). The prevalence of phosphorus-containing food additives in top-selling foods in grocery stores. Journal of renal nutrition : the official journal of the Council on Renal Nutrition of the National Kidney Foundation, 23(4), 265–270.e2. https://doi.org/10.1053/j.jrn.2012.12.003

[1613] Carrigan, A., Klinger, A., Choquette, S. S., Luzuriaga-McPherson, A., Bell, E. K., Darnell, B., & Gutiérrez, O. M. (2014). Contribution of food additives to sodium and phosphorus content of diets rich in processed foods. Journal of renal nutrition : the official journal of the Council on Renal Nutrition of the National Kidney Foundation, 24(1), 13–19e1. https://doi.org/10.1053/j.jrn.2013.09.003

[1614] Itkonen ST, Karp HJ, Lamberg-Allardt CJ. Bioavailability of phosphorus. In: Uribarri J, Calvo MS, eds. Dietary Phosphorus: Health, Nutrition, and Regulatory Aspects. Boca Raton, Florida: CRC Press; 2018:221-33.

604

[1615] American Kidney Fund (2019) 'Phosphorus food guide', Guides to help you cook and shop, Accessed Online Feb 04 2021: http://kitchen.kidneyfund.org/wp-content/uploads/2019/09/Phosphorus_Guide_090419.pdf

[1616] NIH (2020) 'Phosphorus: Fact Sheet for Health Professionals', Dietary Supplement Fact Sheets, Accessed Online Jan 26 2021: https://ods.od.nih.gov/factsheets/Phosphorus-HealthProfessional/

[1617] Calvo, M. S., Moshfegh, A. J., & Tucker, K. L. (2014). Assessing the health impact of phosphorus in the food supply: issues and considerations. Advances in nutrition (Bethesda, Md.), 5(1), 104–113. https://doi.org/10.3945/an.113.004861

[1618] Uribarri, J., & Calvo, M. S. (2003). Hidden sources of phosphorus in the typical American diet: does it matter in nephrology?. Seminars in dialysis, 16(3), 186–188. https://doi.org/10.1046/j.1525-139x.2003.16037.x

[1619] Scanni, R., vonRotz, M., Jehle, S., Hulter, H. N., & Krapf, R. (2014). The human response to acute enteral and parenteral phosphate loads. Journal of the American Society of Nephrology : JASN, 25(12), 2730–2739. https://doi.org/10.1681/ASN.2013101076

[1620] Karp, H., Ekholm, P., Kemi, V., Hirvonen, T., & Lamberg-Allardt, C. (2012). Differences among total and in vitro digestible phosphorus content of meat and milk products. Journal of renal nutrition : the official journal of the Council on Renal Nutrition of the National Kidney Foundation, 22(3), 344–349. https://doi.org/10.1053/j.jrn.2011.07.004

[1621] Taylor, T. G., & Coleman, J. W. (1979). A comparative study of the absorption of calcium and the availability of phytate-phosphorus in the golden hamster (Mesocricetus auratus) and the laboratory rat. The British journal of nutrition, 42(1), 113–119. https://doi.org/10.1079/bjn19790095

[1622] Heaney, R. P., & Nordin, B. E. (2002). Calcium effects on phosphorus absorption: implications for the prevention and co-therapy of osteoporosis. Journal of the American College of Nutrition, 21(3), 239–244. https://doi.org/10.1080/07315724.2002.10719216

[1623] de Fornasari, M. L., & Dos Santos Sens, Y. A. (2017). Replacing Phosphorus-Containing Food Additives With Foods Without Additives Reduces Phosphatemia in End-Stage Renal Disease Patients: A Randomized Clinical Trial. Journal of renal nutrition : the official journal of the Council on Renal Nutrition of the National Kidney Foundation, 27(2), 97–105. https://doi.org/10.1053/j.jrn.2016.08.009

[1624] Calvo, M. S., Sherman, R. A., & Uribarri, J. (2019). Dietary Phosphate and the Forgotten Kidney Patient: A Critical Need for FDA Regulatory Action. American journal of kidney diseases : the official journal of the National Kidney Foundation, 73(4), 542–551. https://doi.org/10.1053/j.ajkd.2018.11.004

[1625] Liu, Z., Su, G., Guo, X., Wu, Y., Liu, X., Zou, C., Zhang, L., Yang, Q., Xu, Y., & Ma, W. (2015). Dietary interventions for mineral and bone disorder in people with chronic kidney disease. The Cochrane database of systematic reviews, (9), CD010350. https://doi.org/10.1002/14651858.CD010350.pub2

[1626] Moore, L. W., Nolte, J. V., Gaber, A. O., & Suki, W. N. (2015). Association of dietary phosphate and serum phosphorus concentration by levels of kidney function. The American journal of clinical nutrition, 102(2), 444–453. https://doi.org/10.3945/ajcn.114.102715

[1627] Moe, S., Drüeke, T., Cunningham, J., Goodman, W., Martin, K., Olgaard, K., Ott, S., Sprague, S., Lameire, N., Eknoyan, G., & Kidney Disease: Improving Global Outcomes (KDIGO) (2006). Definition, evaluation, and classification of renal osteodystrophy: a position statement from Kidney Disease: Improving Global Outcomes (KDIGO). Kidney international, 69(11), 1945–1953. https://doi.org/10.1038/sj.ki.5000414

[1628] Moe, S., Drüeke, T., Cunningham, J., Goodman, W., Martin, K., Olgaard, K., Ott, S., Sprague, S., Lameire, N., Eknoyan, G., & Kidney Disease: Improving Global Outcomes (KDIGO) (2006). Definition, evaluation, and classification of renal osteodystrophy: a position statement from Kidney Disease: Improving Global Outcomes (KDIGO). Kidney international, 69(11), 1945–1953. https://doi.org/10.1038/sj.ki.5000414

[1629] Palmer, S. C., Hayen, A., Macaskill, P., Pellegrini, F., Craig, J. C., Elder, G. J., & Strippoli, G. F. (2011). Serum levels of phosphorus, parathyroid hormone, and calcium and risks of death and cardiovascular disease in individuals with chronic kidney disease: a systematic review and meta-analysis. JAMA, 305(11), 1119–1127. https://doi.org/10.1001/jama.2011.308

[1630] Cheungpasitporn, W., Thongprayoon, C., Mao, M. A., Kittanamongkolchai, W., Sakhuja, A., & Erickson, S. B. (2018). Admission serum phosphate levels predict hospital mortality. Hospital practice (1995), 46(3), 121–127. https://doi.org/10.1080/21548331.2018.1483172

[1631] Da, J., Xie, X., Wolf, M., Disthabanchong, S., Wang, J., Zha, Y., Lv, J., Zhang, L., & Wang, H. (2015). Serum Phosphorus and Progression of CKD and Mortality: A Meta-analysis of Cohort Studies. American journal of kidney diseases : the official journal of the National Kidney Foundation, 66(2), 258–265. https://doi.org/10.1053/j.ajkd.2015.01.009

[1632] Hou, Y., Li, X., Sun, L., Qu, Z., Jiang, L., & Du, Y. (2017). Phosphorus and mortality risk in end-stage renal disease: A meta-analysis. Clinica chimica acta; international journal of clinical chemistry, 474, 108–113. https://doi.org/10.1016/j.cca.2017.09.005

[1633] Selamet, U., Tighiouart, H., Sarnak, M. J., Beck, G., Levey, A. S., Block, G., & Ix, J. H. (2016). Relationship of dietary phosphate intake with risk of end-stage renal disease and mortality in chronic

605

kidney disease stages 3-5: The Modification of Diet in Renal Disease Study. Kidney international, 89(1), 176–184. https://doi.org/10.1038/ki.2015.284

[1634] Murtaugh, M. A., Filipowicz, R., Baird, B. C., Wei, G., Greene, T., & Beddhu, S. (2012). Dietary phosphorus intake and mortality in moderate chronic kidney disease: NHANES III. Nephrology, dialysis, transplantation : official publication of the European Dialysis and Transplant Association - European Renal Association, 27(3), 990–996. https://doi.org/10.1093/ndt/gfr367

[1635] Erratum: Kidney Disease: Improving Global Outcomes (KDIGO) CKD-MBD Update Work Group. KDIGO 2017 Clinical Practice Guideline Update for the Diagnosis, Evaluation, Prevention, and Treatment of Chronic Kidney Disease-Mineral and Bone Disorder (CKD-MBD). Kidney Int Suppl. 2017;7:1-59. (2017). Kidney international supplements, 7(3), e1. https://doi.org/10.1016/j.kisu.2017.10.001

[1636] Shinaberger, C. S., Greenland, S., Kopple, J. D., Van Wyck, D., Mehrotra, R., Kovesdy, C. P., & Kalantar-Zadeh, K. (2008). Is controlling phosphorus by decreasing dietary protein intake beneficial or harmful in persons with chronic kidney disease?. The American journal of clinical nutrition, 88(6), 1511–1518. https://doi.org/10.3945/ajcn.2008.26665

[1637] Chines, A., & Pacifici, R. (1990). Antacid and sucralfate-induced hypophosphatemic osteomalacia: a case report and review of the literature. Calcified tissue international, 47(5), 291–295. https://doi.org/10.1007/BF02555911

[1638] Ruospo, M., Palmer, S. C., Natale, P., Craig, J. C., Vecchio, M., Elder, G. J., & Strippoli, G. F. (2018). Phosphate binders for preventing and treating chronic kidney disease-mineral and bone disorder (CKD-MBD). The Cochrane database of systematic reviews, 8(8), CD006023. https://doi.org/10.1002/14651858.CD006023.pub3

[1639] Casais, M. N., Rosa-Diez, G., Pérez, S., Mansilla, E. N., Bravo, S., & Bonofiglio, F. C. (2009). Hyperphosphatemia after sodium phosphate laxatives in low risk patients: prospective study. World journal of gastroenterology, 15(47), 5960–5965. https://doi.org/10.3748/wjg.15.5960

[1640] US FDA (2016) 'FDA Drug Safety Communication: FDA warns of possible harm from exceeding recommended dose of over-the-counter sodium phosphate products to treat constipation', Drug Safety and Availability, Accessed Online Feb 3 2021: https://www.fda.gov/drugs/drug-safety-and-availability/fda-drug-safety-communication-fda-warns-possible-harm-exceeding-recommended-dose-over-counter-sodium

[1641] Vest K.E., Hashemi H.F., Cobine P.A. (2013) The Copper Metallome in Eukaryotic Cells. In: Banci L. (eds) Metallomics and the Cell. Metal Ions in Life Sciences, vol 12. Springer, Dordrecht. https://doi.org/10.1007/978-94-007-5561-1_13

[1642] FRIEDEN (1962) ' The copper complex of nature, in Horizons in Biochemistry. Academic Press, New York.

[1643] Decker, H., & Terwilliger, N. (2000). Cops and robbers: putative evolution of copper oxygen-binding proteins. The Journal of experimental biology, 203(Pt 12), 1777–1782.

[1644] Sommer, A. L. (1931). COPPER AS AN ESSENTIAL FOR PLANT GROWTH. Plant Physiology, 6(2), 339–345. doi:10.1104/pp.6.2.339

[1645] VPIOGRAWV (1953) 'The Elementary Chemical Composition of Marine Organisms.' Sears Foundation for Marine Research, Memoir No. 2, Yale University, New Haven.

[1646] SCHENBERG and SERNLIEB (1960) Copper metabolism, Pharmacol. Rev. 12,355.

[1647] STEWARD, F. C. (Editor) (1963) Plant Physiology, A Treatise, Vol. III. Academic Press, New York.

[1648] Linder (1991) ' The Biochemistry of Copper', Plenum Press, New York.

[1649] Copper Development Association Inc. 'Copper in Human Health', Accessed Online: https://www.copper.org/consumers/health/cu_health_uk.html

[1650] Kelley et al (1995) 'Effects of low-copper diets on human immune response', The American Journal of Clinical Nutrition, Volume 62, Issue 2, August 1995, Pages 412–416, https://doi.org/10.1093/ajcn/62.2.412

[1651] Klevay L. M. (2011). Is the Western diet adequate in copper?. Journal of trace elements in medicine and biology : organ of the Society for Minerals and Trace Elements (GMS), 25(4), 204–212. https://doi.org/10.1016/j.jtemb.2011.08.146

[1652] Chambers, A., Krewski, D., Birkett, N., Plunkett, L., Hertzberg, R., Danzeisen, R., Aggett, P. J., Starr, T. B., Baker, S., Dourson, M., Jones, P., Keen, C. L., Meek, B., Schoeny, R., & Slob, W. (2010). An exposure-response curve for copper excess and deficiency. Journal of toxicology and environmental health. Part B, Critical reviews, 13(7-8), 546–578. https://doi.org/10.1080/10937404.2010.538657

[1653] Schroeder, H. A., Nason, A. P., Tipton, I. H., & Balassa, J. J. (1966). Essential trace metals in man: Copper. Journal of Chronic Diseases, 19(9), 1007–1034. doi:10.1016/0021-9681(66)90033-6

[1654] Merriam-Webster. (n.d.). Copper. In Merriam-Webster.com dictionary. Retrieved December 3, 2020, from https://www.merriam-webster.com/dictionary/copper

[1655] Scheiber, I., Dringen, R., & Mercer, J. F. (2013). Copper: effects of deficiency and overload. Metal ions in life sciences, 13, 359–387. https://doi.org/10.1007/978-94-007-7500-8_11

[1656] Angelé-Martínez, C., Nguyen, K. V., Ameer, F. S., Anker, J. N., & Brumaghim, J. L. (2017). Reactive oxygen species generation by copper(II) oxide nanoparticles determined by DNA damage assays and EPR spectroscopy. Nanotoxicology, 11(2), 278–288. https://doi.org/10.1080/17435390.2017.1293750

[1657] Lazarchick J. (2012). Update on anemia and neutropenia in copper deficiency. Current opinion in hematology, 19(1), 58–60. https://doi.org/10.1097/MOH.0b013e32834da9d2

[1658] DiNicolantonio JJ, Mangan D, O'Keefe JHCopper deficiency may be a leading cause of ischaemic heart diseaseOpen Heart 2018;5:e000784. doi: 10.1136/openhrt-2018-000784

[1659] Breasted (1930) 'The Edwin Smith Surgical Papyrus', Chicago: The University of Chicago Press, 1930, Oriental Institute Publications 3, ISBN 978-0-918986-73-3

[1660] Dollwet, H.H.A. and Sorenson, J.R.J. (2001) Historic Uses of Copper Compounds in Medicine. Trace Elements in Medicine. 2nd Edition, The Humana Press Inc., Arkansas, 80-87.

[1661] Joachim (1880) 'Papyros Ebers: das alteste Buch uber Heilkunde.' Druck und Verlag von Georg Reimer, Berlin.

[1662] Dollwet, H.H.A. and Sorenson, J.R.J. (2001) Historic Uses of Copper Compounds in Medicine. Trace Elements in Medicine. 2nd Edition, The Humana Press Inc., Arkansas, 80-87.

[1663] Majno (1975) 'The Healing Hand. Man and Wound in the Ancient World', Harvard University Press, Cambridge, ISBN 0674383311, 9780674383319

[1664] Gunther (1934) 'The Greek Herbal of Dioscorides' Nature 133, 231–233. https://doi.org/10.1038/133231a0

[1665] Arendsen, L. P., Thakar, R., & Sultan, A. H. (2019). The Use of Copper as an Antimicrobial Agent in Health Care, Including Obstetrics and Gynecology. Clinical Microbiology Reviews, 32(4). doi:10.1128/cmr.00125-18

[1666] St. Clair, Kassia (2016). The Secret Lives of Colour. London: John Murray. p. 215. ISBN 9781473630819.

[1667] Dollwet, H.H.A. and Sorenson, J.R.J. (2001) Historic Uses of Copper Compounds in Medicine. Trace Elements in Medicine. 2nd Edition, The Humana Press Inc., Arkansas, 80-87.

[1668] Dollwet, H.H.A. and Sorenson, J.R.J. (2001) Historic Uses of Copper Compounds in Medicine. Trace Elements in Medicine. 2nd Edition, The Humana Press Inc., Arkansas, 80-87.

[1669] Wilks, S. A., Michels, H., & Keevil, C. W. (2005). The survival of Escherichia coli O157 on a range of metal surfaces. International journal of food microbiology, 105(3), 445–454. https://doi.org/10.1016/j.ijfoodmicro.2005.04.021

[1670] Avakian, Z. A., & Rabotnova, I. L. (1966). Ob opredelenii kontsentratsiï medi, toksichnykh dlia mikroorganizmov [On determination of copper concentrations toxic to microorganisms]. Mikrobiologiia, 35(5), 805–811.

[1671] Colobert, L (1962). "Sensitivity of poliomyelitis virus to catalytic systems generating free hydroxyl radicals". Revue de Pathologie Generale et de Physiologie Clinique. 62: 551–5. PMID 14041393.

[1672] Robert B. Thurman, Charles P. Gerba & Gabriel Bitton (1989) The molecular mechanisms of copper and silver ion disinfection of bacteria and viruses, Critical Reviews in Environmental Control, 18:4, 295-315, DOI: 10.1080/10643388909388351

[1673] Spencer (1935) 'Celsus On Medicine, Volume I', Books 1–4, Loeb Classical Library 292, Harvard University Press, ISBN 9780674993228

[1674] Rackham (1950) 'Pliny, Natural History, Volume V: Books 17-19', Loeb Classical Library 371, Harvard University Press, Cambridge.

[1675] Dollwet, H.H.A. and Sorenson, J.R.J. (2001) Historic Uses of Copper Compounds in Medicine. Trace Elements in Medicine. 2nd Edition, The Humana Press Inc., Arkansas, 80-87.

[1676] Dollwet, H.H.A. and Sorenson, J.R.J. (2001) Historic Uses of Copper Compounds in Medicine. Trace Elements in Medicine. 2nd Edition, The Humana Press Inc., Arkansas, 80-87.

[1677] Emmart (1940) 'The Badianus Manuscript (Codex Barberini Latin 241): An Aztec Herbal of 1552'. Baltimore: Johns Hopkins University Press.

[1678] Kobert (1895) 'Ueber den jetzigen Stand der Frage nach den pharmakologischen Wirkungen des Kupfers'. Deutsche Med Wochen 5, 42-45.

[1679] Wise (1845) 'Commentary on the Hindu system of medicine', London, Smith, Elder and Co.

[1680] Harawi (1893) 'Die phannakologischen Crundsatze (Liberfundamentorum phannacologiae)', In: Kobert R (ed) 'Historische Studien aus dem phannakologischen Institute der Kaiserlichen Universitat Dorpat'. Verlag von Tausch und Grosse, Halle a. S.

[1681] Burq (1853) 'Métallothérapie : nouveau traitement par les applications metalliques : abrégé historique, théorique et pratique', Paris : Rignoux, imprimeur de la Faculte de Medecine.

[1682] Spiro (1925) 'Einige Ergebnisse über Vorkommen und Wirkung der weniger verbreiteten Elemente'. Ergebnisse der Physiologie 24, 474–516 (1925). https://doi.org/10.1007/BF02321466

[1683] Bergmann (1969) 'Nomadische Streifereien unter den Kalmücken in den Jahren 1802 und 1803'. Riga 1804/5, Anthropological Publications, Oosterhout.

[1684] Burq (1871) 'Metallotherapie. Traitement des Maladies Nerveuses', Paris: G. Baillière, 1 vol. (122 p.) ; In-16.

[1685] Dollwet, H.H.A. and Sorenson, J.R.J. (2001) Historic Uses of Copper Compounds in Medicine. Trace Elements in Medicine. 2nd Edition, The Humana Press Inc., Arkansas, 80-87.

[1686] Walusinski O. (2018). The Scientific Illusion of Victor Burq (1822-1884). European neurology, 79(3-4), 135–149. https://doi.org/10.1159/000487667

[1687] Dollwet, H.H.A. and Sorenson, J.R.J. (2001) Historic Uses of Copper Compounds in Medicine. Trace Elements in Medicine. 2nd Edition, The Humana Press Inc., Arkansas, 80-87.

[1688] Burq (1871) 'Metallotherapie. Traitement des Maladies Nerveuses', Paris: G. Baillière, 1 vol. (122 p.) ; In-16.

[1689] Kobert (1895) 'Ueber den jetzigen Stand der Frage nach den pharmakologischen Wirkungen des Kupfers'. Deutsche Med Wochen 5, 42-45.

[1690] Schulz (1890) 'Arseniksaures Kupfer bei akuten Erkrankungen des Darmes'. Therapeutische Monatshefte 4: 307.

[1691] Von Linden (1935) 'Das Kupfer in seiner Biologischen und therapeutischen Bedeutung'. Schweizerische Medizinische Wochenschrift. 29: 660.

[1692] Srivastava (1953) 'History of Indian Pharmacy'. Banaras Hindu Press, Banaras.

[1693] Wise (1845) 'Commentary on the Hindu system of medicine', London, Smith, Elder and Co.

[1694] Dollwet, H.H.A. and Sorenson, J.R.J. (2001) Historic Uses of Copper Compounds in Medicine. Trace Elements in Medicine. 2nd Edition, The Humana Press Inc., Arkansas, 80-87.

[1695] Köchlin (1837) 'Von den Wirkungen der gebrauchlichen Metalle auf den menschlichen Organismum iiberhaupt und als Heilmittel und dem Kupfersalmiak-Liquor und anderen Kupferpraparaten als soIehe insbesondere'. Medic. Chirurg, Ztg. 1818 S. Hohr, Zurich, vol II.

[1696] Köchlin (1837) 'Von den Wirkungen der gebrauchlichen Metalle auf den menschlichen Organismum iiberhaupt und als Heilmittel und dem Kupfersalmiak-Liquor und anderen Kupferpraparaten als soIehe insbesondere'. Medic. Chirurg, Ztg. 1818 S. Hohr, Zurich, vol II.

[1697] Hignett (1952) 'Some nutritional factors affecting herd fertility in cattle in Britain'. IInd International Congress of Physiology and Pathology of Animal Reproduction. Copenhagen 2: 75.

[1698] Millon (1848) 'De la présence normale de plusiers métaux dans le sang de l'homme, et de l'analyse des sels fixes contenus dans ce liquide'. Comptes Rend de l'Acad des Sci à Paris 26, 41–43.

[1699] Melsens. (1848) 'De l'absence du cuivre et du plomb dans le sang'. Annales de Chim et de Phys 23, 358–371.

[1700] Béchamp (1859) 'Sur les metaux qui peuvent exister dans le sang ou les viscères, et spécialement sur le cuivre dit physiologique'. Montpellier Méd 3, 311–339.

[1701] Fox P. L. (2003). The copper-iron chronicles: the story of an intimate relationship. Biometals : an international journal on the role of metal ions in biology, biochemistry, and medicine, 16(1), 9–40. https://doi.org/10.1023/a:1020799512190

[1702] Schulz (1920) 'Vorlesungen über Wirkung und Anwendung der unorganischen Arzneistoffe für Aerzte und Studierende : Unveränderter Neudruck mit einer Ergänzung "XXIII. Vorlesung', Leipzig : Thieme.

[1703] Rademacher (1848) 'Rechtfertigung der von den Gelehrten misskannten: verstandesrechten Erfahrungsheillehre der alten scheidekünstigen Geheimärzte und treue Mittheilung des Ergebnisses einer 25 Jährigen Erprobung dieser Lehre am Krankenbette', Berlin : G. Reimer.

[1704] Dollwet, H.H.A. and Sorenson, J.R.J. (2001) Historic Uses of Copper Compounds in Medicine. Trace Elements in Medicine. 2nd Edition, The Humana Press Inc., Arkansas, 80-87.

[1705] Keen, C. L., Lönnerdal, B., & Hurley, L. S. (1982). Teratogenic Effects of Copper Deficiency and Excess. Inflammatory Diseases and Copper, 109–121. doi:10.1007/978-1-4612-5829-2_11

[1706] Dollwet, H.H.A. and Sorenson, J.R.J. (2001) Historic Uses of Copper Compounds in Medicine. Trace Elements in Medicine. 2nd Edition, The Humana Press Inc., Arkansas, 80-87.

[1707] Luton (1885) 'De l'acetate de cuivre en therapeutique'. Union Medicale et Scientifique du Nord-Est. 9: 317.

[1708] Luton (1886) 'Tuberculose et sels de cuivre'. ibid 10: 77.

[1709] Luton (1887) 'Tuberculose et sels (phosphate) de cuivre'. ibid. 11:33.

[1710] Dollwet, H.H.A. and Sorenson, J.R.J. (2001) Historic Uses of Copper Compounds in Medicine. Trace Elements in Medicine. 2nd Edition, The Humana Press Inc., Arkansas, 80-87.

[1711] von Linden (1920) 'Die entwicklungshemmende Wirkung von Kupfersalzen auf Krankheit erregende Bakterien'. Centralblatt fiir Bakteriologie, Parasitenkunde und Infektionskrankheiten. 85: 136.

[1712] Sorgo-Alland (1913) 'Erfahrungen mit dem Finklerschen Heilverfahren bei Lungenphthise. Gesellschaft Deutscher Naturforscher und Arzte'. Verhandlungen der Ges. Deut. Naturf Arzte. Springer Verlag, Berlin, New York.

[1713] Ritter (1937) 'Bemerkungen zur Behandlung mit Gold, Kupfer und Jodsilber'. Beitrage zur Klinik der Tuberkulose und spezifischen Tuberkulose-Forschung. 89: 652.

[1714] Tücher and Ranzenhofer (1940) 'Cuprion, ein neuartiges Schwermetallsalz zur Behandlung der Tuberkulose'. Wiener Medizinische Wochenschrift. 90: 115

[1715] Goraletoski (1940) 'Das Kupfer in der Behandlung der Lungentuberkulose'. Zeitschrift fiir Tuberkulose. 84: 313

[1716] Dollwet, H.H.A. and Sorenson, J.R.J. (2001) Historic Uses of Copper Compounds in Medicine. Trace Elements in Medicine. 2nd Edition, The Humana Press Inc., Arkansas, 80-87.

[1717] Dollwet, H.H.A. and Sorenson, J.R.J. (2001) Historic Uses of Copper Compounds in Medicine. Trace Elements in Medicine. 2nd Edition, The Humana Press Inc., Arkansas, 80-87.

[1718] Sorenson (1979) 'Therapeutic Uses of Copper'. In: Nriagu JO (ed) Copper in the Environment, Part II: Health Effects. John Wiley and Sons, New York p 83.
Wiley and Sons, New York p 83

[1719] Sorenson et al (1979) 'Anticonvulsant Activity of Some Copper Complexes'. In: Hemphill DD (ed) Trace Substances in Environmental Health. University of Missouri Press, Columbia, vol XIII, p 360.

[1720] Sorenson et al (1980) 'Anticonvulsant Copper Complexes'. In: Hemphill DO (ed) Trace Substances in Environmental Health. University of Missouri Press, Columbia, vol XIV p 252.

[1721] Sorenson et al (1983) 'Copper Complexes: A Physiological Approach to the Treatment of "Inflammatory Diseases"'. Inorg. Chim. Acta. 79: 45.

[1722] Strauss (1912) 'Epitheliobehandlung mit Kupfersalzen (Kupferlezithin)'. Deutsche Medizinische Wochenschrift. 38: 2122.

[1723] Gelarie, A. J. (1913). THE INFLUENCE OF COPPER UPON THE GROWTH OF MOUSE CARCINOMA. BMJ, 2(2744), 222–223. doi:10.1136/bmj.2.2744.222

[1724] Moullin (1918) 'Colloid copper and cancer'. British Medical J. 1: 427.

[1725] Sugiura and Benedict (1922) 'The Influence of Inorganic Salts Upon Tumor Growth in Albino Rats', Cancer Research, October 1922, Volume 7, Issue 4, DOI: 10.1158/jcr.1922.329

[1726] De Nabias (1930) 'Quelques indications de l'emploi des injections de cuivre colloidal dans la therapeutique des cancers'. Bulletin de l'Association Francaise pour l'Etude du Cancer. 19: 343.

[1727] Voisin (1959) 'Soil, Grass and Cancer'. Philosophical Library Inc., New York.

[1728] Kobert (1895) 'Ueber den jetzigen Stand der Frage nach den pharmakologischen Wirkungen des Kupfers'. Deutsche Med Wochen 5, 42-45.

[1729] Heitmeyer and Sueoe (1938) 'Der Eisen-Kupferantogonismus im Blutplasma beim Infektionsgeschehen'. Klinische Wochenschrift. 17: 925.

[1730] Fenz (1941) 'Kupfer, ein neues Mittel gegen chronischen und subakuten Gelenkrheumatismus'. Mtinchner Medizinische Wochenschrift. 88: 1101.

[1731] Forestier (1944) 'Les sels organiques de cuivre dans le traitement des rhumatismes chroniques'. Bulletin de l'Academie Nationale de Medecine, 128: 22.

[1732] Forestier and Certonciny (1946) 'Le traitement des rhumatismes chroniques par les sels organiques de cuivre'. La Presse Medicale, 64: 884.

[1733] Forestier et al (1948) 'La cuprotherapie intra-museulaire dans le rhumatismes chroniques inflammatoires'. La Presse Medicale, 29: 351.

[1734] Forestier (1949) 'Comparative Results of Copper Salts and Gold Salts in Rheumatoid Arthritis'. Ann. Rheum. Dis. 8: 132.

[1735] Garber-Duuernay and Van Moorleghem (1950) 'Le Morrhuate de Cuivre dans la Therapeutique des Polyarthrites Chroniques'. Lyon Medicale. 183: 113.

[1736] Hangarter W. (1980). Kupfersalizylat bei rheumatoider Arthritis und Rheuma-ähnlichen degenerativen Erkrankungen [Copper salicylate in rheumatoid arthritis and rheumatism--like degenerative diseases]. Die Medizinische Welt, 31(45), 1625–1628.

[1737] Hangarter and Lubke (1952) 'Dber die Behandlung rheumatischer Erkrankungen mit einer Kupfer-Natrium-Salizylat-Komplexverbindung (Pennalon)'. Deutsche Medizinische Wochenschrift. 77: 870.

[1738] Dollwet, H.H.A. and Sorenson, J.R.J. (2001) Historic Uses of Copper Compounds in Medicine. Trace Elements in Medicine. 2nd Edition, The Humana Press Inc., Arkansas, 80-87.

[1739] Loudon, I. S. (1980). Chlorosis, anaemia, and anorexia nervosa. BMJ, 281(6256), 1669–1675. doi:10.1136/bmj.281.6256.1669

[1740] McLean, E., Cogswell, M., Egli, I., Wojdyla, D., & de Benoist, B. (2008). Worldwide prevalence of anaemia, WHO Vitamin and Mineral Nutrition Information System, 1993–2005. Public Health Nutrition, 12(04), 444. doi:10.1017/s1368980008002401

[1741] de Benoist B et al., eds. (2008) 'Worldwide prevalence of anaemia 1993-2005'. WHO Global Database on Anaemia Geneva, World Health Organization. Accessed Online Dec 5 2020: https://www.who.int/vmnis/anaemia/prevalence/summary/anaemia_data_status_t2/en/

[1742] Rodak et al (2011) 'Hematology: Clinical Principles and Applications', Saunders; 4th edition (March 4, 2011), ISBN-13 : 978-1437706925

[1743] World Health Organization (2011) 'Haemoglobin concentrations for the diagnosis of anaemia and assessment of severity', Vitamin and Mineral Nutrition Information System, Accessed Online Dec 5th 2020: https://www.who.int/vmnis/indicators/haemoglobin.pdf

[1744] Barrell (2020) 'What's to know about hemoglobin levels?', Medical News Today, Accessed Online Dec 8 2020: https://www.medicalnewstoday.com/articles/318050

[1745] Bager P. (2014). Fatigue and acute/chronic anaemia. Danish medical journal, 61(4), B4824.

[1746] Kalantri, A., Karambelkar, M., Joshi, R., Kalantri, S., & Jajoo, U. (2010). Accuracy and reliability of pallor for detecting anaemia: a hospital-based diagnostic accuracy study. PloS one, 5(1), e8545. https://doi.org/10.1371/journal.pone.0008545

[1747] Tansarli, G. S., Karageorgopoulos, D. E., Kapaskelis, A., Gkegkes, I., & Falagas, M. E. (2013). Iron deficiency and susceptibility to infections: evaluation of the clinical evidence. European journal of clinical microbiology & infectious diseases : official publication of the European Society of Clinical Microbiology, 32(10), 1253–1258. https://doi.org/10.1007/s10096-013-1877-x

[1748] Silva-Gomes, S., Vale-Costa, S., Appelberg, R., & Gomes, M. S. (2013). Iron in intracellular infection: to provide or to deprive?. Frontiers in cellular and infection microbiology, 3, 96. https://doi.org/10.3389/fcimb.2013.00096

[1749] Robb-Smith (1933) 'The history of the hedgehog's rosary'. St Bartholomew's Hosp J 40, 149–152, 166–168, 211–216, 238–240; 41, 13–15.

[1750] Liégeois (1900) 'Fer, arsenic ou cuivre dans la chlorose'. J des Praticiens, 615.

[1751] Reynolds, L. G., & Klein, M. (1985). Iron poisoning--a preventable hazard of childhood. South African medical journal = Suid-Afrikaanse tydskrif vir geneeskunde, 67(17), 680–683.

[1752] Chang, T. P., & Rangan, C. (2011). Iron poisoning: a literature-based review of epidemiology, diagnosis, and management. Pediatric emergency care, 27(10), 978–985. https://doi.org/10.1097/PEC.0b013e3182302604

[1753] Manoguerra, A. S., Erdman, A. R., Booze, L. L., Christianson, G., Wax, P. M., Scharman, E. J., Woolf, A. D., Chyka, P. A., Keyes, D. C., Olson, K. R., Caravati, E. M., & Troutman, W. G. (2005). Iron ingestion: an evidence-based consensus guideline for out-of-hospital management. Clinical toxicology (Philadelphia, Pa.), 43(6), 553–570. https://doi.org/10.1081/clt-200068842

[1754] BRUBAKER, C., & STURGEON, P. (1956). Copper deficiency in infants; a syndrome characterized by hypocupremia, iron deficiency anemia, and hypoproteinemia. A.M.A. journal of diseases of children, 92(3), 254–265.

[1755] Olivares, M., Araya, M., Pizarro, F., & Letelier, A. (2006). Erythrocyte CuZn Superoxide Dismutase Activity Is Decreased in Iron-Deficiency Anemia. Biological Trace Element Research, 112(3), 213–220. doi:10.1385/bter:112:3:213

[1756] Pécholier and Saintpierre (1864) 'Étude sur L'hygiène des ouvriers employés a la fabrication du verdet'. Montpellier Méd 12, 97–127.

[1757] Mendini (1862) 'Di un rimedio per l'amenorrea et di altro per la sordita ipostenica'. Gazz Med Ital Prov Venete 5, 36–37.

[1758] Levi and Barduzzi (1877b) 'Di alcune applicazioni terapeutiche poco note del solfato di rame. Ricerche sperimentali e cliniche'. Parte seconda. Giorn di Anat Fisiol e Patol degli Animali 9, 337–352.

[1759] Rock et al (2000) 'The effect of copper supplementation on red blood cell oxidizability and plasma antioxidants in middle-aged healthy volunteers', Free Radical Biology and Medicine, Volume 28, Issue 3, 1 February 2000, Pages 324-329.

[1760] Chevallier and Boys de Loury (1848) 'Memoire sur les ouvriers qui travaillent le cuivre et ses alliages'. Ann d'Hygiène Pub et de Méd Lég 43, 369.

[1761] Pécholier and Saintpierre (1864) '*Étude sur L'hygiène des ouvriers employés a la fabrication du verdet*'. Montpellier Méd 12, 97–127.

[1762] Liégeois (1891) 'Fer et chlorose. Remarques pratiques sur le choix et le mode d'administration des meilleures preparations ferrugineuses'. Rev Méd de l'Est 23, 545–554.

[1763] Hare (1892) 'The treatment of anaemia by copper and arsenic'. Therapeut Gaz 16, 30–31.

[1764] Cervello and Barabini (1894) 'Sul potere ematogeno dei metallic pesanti. Palermo: Tipografia editrice Tempo.

[1765] Von Linden (1935) 'Das Kupfer in seiner Biologischen und therapeutischen Bedeutung'. Schweizerische Medizinische Wochenschrift. 29: 660.

[1766] Hart, E. B., Steenbock, H., Waddell, J. and Elvehjem, C. A. (1928). Iron in nutrition. VII. Copper as a supplement to iron for hemoglobin building in the rat. J. Biol. Chem. 77, 797-812.

[1767] Pécholier and Saintpierre (1864) '*Étude sur L'hygiène des ouvriers employés a la fabrication du verdet*'. Montpellier Méd 12, 97–127.

[1768] Hart, E. B.; Steenbock, H.; Waddell, J. (1928). "Iron nutrition. VII: Copper is a supplement to iron for hemoglobin building in the rat". The Journal of Biological Chemistry. 77: 797–833.

[1769] Hart, E. B.; Steenbock, H.; Waddell, J. (1928). "Iron nutrition. VII: Copper is a supplement to iron for hemoglobin building in the rat". The Journal of Biological Chemistry. 77: 797–833.

[1770] Matak P, Zumerle S, Mastrogiannaki M, El Balkhi S, Delga S, Mathieu JRR, et al. (2013) Copper Deficiency Leads to Anemia, Duodenal Hypoxia, Upregulation of HIF-2α and Altered Expression of Iron Absorption Genes in Mice. PLoS ONE 8(3): e59538. https://doi.org/10.1371/journal.pone.0059538

[1771] Istvan Molnar, Dora Il'yasova, Anastasia Ivanova, Mary A. Knovich; The Association between Serum Copper and Anemia in the Adult NHANES II Population.. Blood 2005; 106 (11): 3766. doi: https://doi.org/10.1182/blood.V106.11.3766.3766

[1772] Mills E. S. (1930). THE TREATMENT OF IDIOPATHIC (HYPOCHROMIC) ANAEMIA WITH IRON AND COPPER. Canadian Medical Association journal, 22(2), 175–178.

[1773] McHargue et al (1928) 'THE RELATION OF COPPER TO THE HEMOGLOBIN CONTENT OF RAT BLOOD: PRELIMINARY REPORT', J. Biol. Chem. 1928, 78:637-641.

[1774] Elvehjem et al (1932) 'THE NECESSITY OF COPPER AS A SUPPLEMENT TO IRON FOR HEMOGLOBIN FORMATION IN THE PIG', J. Biol. Chem. 1932, 95:363-370.

[1775] ELVEHJEM et al (1938) 'ANEMIA STUDIES WITH DOGS', J. Biol. Chem. 1938, 126:155-173.

[1776] Elvehjem et al (1929) 'THE RELATION OF IRON AND COPPER TO HEMOGLOBIN SYNTHESIS IN THE CHICK'. J. Biol. Chem. 1929, 84:131-141.

[1777] Elvehjem et al (1929) 'IS COPPER A CONSTITUENT OF THE HEMOGLOBIN MOLECULE? THE DISTRIBUTION OF COPPER IN BLOOD', J. Biol. Chem. 1929, 83:21-25.

[1778] Higuchi, T., Matsukawa, Y., Okada, K., Oikawa, O., Yamazaki, T., Ohnishi, Y., … Matsumoto, K. (2006). Correction of Copper Deficiency Improves Erythropoietin Unresponsiveness in Hemodialysis Patients with Anemia. Internal Medicine, 45(5), 271–273. doi:10.2169/internalmedicine.45.1541

[1779] Cook SF, Spilles NM. 1931 Some factors regulating the utilization of splenic iron. Am J Physiol 98, 626-635.

[1780] Broderius, M., Mostad, E., & Prohaska, J. R. (2012). Suppressed hepcidin expression correlates with hypotransferrinemia in copper-deficient rat pups but not dams. Genes & Nutrition, 7(3), 405–414. doi:10.1007/s12263-012-0293-7

[1781] Jenkitkasemwong, S., Broderius, M., Nam, H., Prohaska, J. R., & Knutson, M. D. (2010). Anemic copper-deficient rats, but not mice, display low hepcidin expression and high ferroportin levels. The Journal of nutrition, 140(4), 723–730. https://doi.org/10.3945/jn.109.117077

[1782] Chen, H., Huang, G., Su, T., Gao, H., Attieh, Z. K., McKie, A. T., … Vulpe, C. D. (2006). Decreased Hephaestin Activity in the Intestine of Copper-Deficient Mice Causes Systemic Iron Deficiency. The Journal of Nutrition, 136(5), 1236–1241. doi:10.1093/jn/136.5.1236

[1783] CHASE, M. S., GUBLER, C. J., CARTWRIGHT, G. E., & WINTROBE, M. M. (1952). Studies on copper metabolism. IV. The influence of copper on the absorption of iron. The Journal of biological chemistry, 199(2), 757–763.

[1784] Bing et al (1934) 'Studies in the nutritional anemia of the rat. X. Hemoglobin production and iron and copper metabolism with milk of low copper content. J Biol Chem 105, 343–354.

[1785] Matak, P., Zumerle, S., Mastrogiannaki, M., El Balkhi, S., Delga, S., Mathieu, J. R. R., … Peyssonnaux, C. (2013). Copper Deficiency Leads to Anemia, Duodenal Hypoxia, Upregulation of HIF-2α and Altered Expression of Iron Absorption Genes in Mice. PLoS ONE, 8(3), e59538. doi:10.1371/journal.pone.0059538

[1786] Josephs H. 1931 Treatment of anaemia of infancy with iron and copper. Bull Johns Hopkins Hosp 49, 246-258.

[1787] LEWIS, M. S. (1931). IRON AND COPPER IN THE TREATMENT OF ANEMIA IN CHILDREN. JAMA: The Journal of the American Medical Association, 96(14), 1135. doi:10.1001/jama.1931.02720400033010

[1788] Elvehjem et al (1935) 'EFFECT OF IRON AND COPPER THERAPY ON HEMOGLOBIN CONTENT OF THE BLOOD OF INFANTS', Am J Dis Child. 1935;50(1):28-35. doi:10.1001/archpedi.1935.01970070037003

[1789] Hutchinson (1938) 'THE ROLE OF COPPER IN IRON-DEFICIENCY ANAEMIA IN INFANCY', QJM: An International Journal of Medicine, Volume 7, Issue 3, July 1938, Pages 397–419, https://doi.org/10.1093/oxfordjournals.qjmed.a068595

[1790] Lazarchick, J. (2012). Update on anemia and neutropenia in copper deficiency. Current Opinion in Hematology, 19(1), 58–60. doi:10.1097/moh.0b013e32834da9d2

[1791] GUBLER, C. J., LAHEY, M. E., CHASE, M. S., CARTWRIGHT, G. E., & WINTROBE, M. M. (1952). Studies on copper metabolism. III. The metabolism of iron in copper deficient swine. Blood, 7(11), 1075–1092.

[1792] LAHEY, M. E., GUBLER, C. J., CHASE, M. S., CARTWRIGHT, G. E., & WINTROBE, M. M. (1952). Studies on copper metabolism. II. Hematologic manifestations of copper deficiency in swine. Blood, 7(11), 1053–1074.

[1793] Cherukuri et al (2005) 'Unexpected role of ceruloplasmin in intestinal iron absorption', Cell Metabolism, VOLUME 2, ISSUE 5, P309-319, DOI:https://doi.org/10.1016/j.cmet.2005.10.003

[1794] Holmberg CG, Laurell CB (1948). "Investigations in serum copper. II. Isolation of the Copper containing protein, and a description of its properties". Acta Chem Scand. 2: 550–56. doi:10.3891/acta.chem.scand.02-0550.

[1795] Song, D., & Dunaief, J. L. (2013). Retinal iron homeostasis in health and disease. Frontiers in aging neuroscience, 5, 24. https://doi.org/10.3389/fnagi.2013.00024

[1796] Curzon, G. (1961). Some properties of coupled iron–caeruloplasmin oxidation systems. Biochemical Journal, 79(3), 656–663. doi:10.1042/bj0790656

611

[1797] Osaki S. (1966). Kinetic studies of ferrous ion oxidation with crystalline human ferroxidase (ceruloplasmin). The Journal of biological chemistry, 241(21), 5053–5059.

[1798] Fox P. L. (2003). The copper-iron chronicles: the story of an intimate relationship. Biometals : an international journal on the role of metal ions in biology, biochemistry, and medicine, 16(1), 9–40. https://doi.org/10.1023/a:1020799512190

[1799] Osaki, S., Johnson, D. A., & Frieden, E. (1971). The mobilization of iron from the perfused mammalian liver by a serum copper enzyme, ferroxidase I. The Journal of biological chemistry, 246(9), 3018–3023.

[1800] Fox P. L. (2003). The copper-iron chronicles: the story of an intimate relationship. Biometals : an international journal on the role of metal ions in biology, biochemistry, and medicine, 16(1), 9–40. https://doi.org/10.1023/a:1020799512190

[1801] O'Reilly et al (1968) 'Iron metabolism in Wilson's disease, Kinetic studies with iron', Neurology Jul 1968, 18 (7) 634; DOI: 10.1212/WNL.18.7.634

[1802] Roeser, H. P., Lee, G. R., Nacht, S., & Cartwright, G. E. (1970). The role of ceruloplasmin in iron metabolism. Journal of Clinical Investigation, 49(12), 2408–2417. doi:10.1172/jci106460

[1803] Osaki, S., Johnson, D. A., & Frieden, E. (1971). The mobilization of iron from the perfused mammalian liver by a serum copper enzyme, ferroxidase I. The Journal of biological chemistry, 246(9), 3018–3023.

[1804] Osaki, S., Johnson, D. A., & Frieden, E. (1971). The mobilization of iron from the perfused mammalian liver by a serum copper enzyme, ferroxidase I. The Journal of biological chemistry, 246(9), 3018–3023.

[1805] Patel, B. N., & David, S. (1997). A Novel Glycosylphosphatidylinositol-anchored Form of Ceruloplasmin Is Expressed by Mammalian Astrocytes. Journal of Biological Chemistry, 272(32), 20185–20190. doi:10.1074/jbc.272.32.20185

[1806] Osaki, S., & Johnson, D. A. (1969). Mobilization of liver iron by ferroxidase (ceruloplasmin). The Journal of biological chemistry, 244(20), 5757–5758.

[1807] Evans and Abraham (1973) 'Anemia, Iron Storage and Ceruloplasmin in Copper Nutrition in the Growing Rat', The Journal of Nutrition, Volume 103, Issue 2, February 1973, Pages 196–201, https://doi.org/10.1093/jn/103.2.196

[1808] Chen, H., Huang, G., Su, T., Gao, H., Attieh, Z. K., McKie, A. T., … Vulpe, C. D. (2006). Decreased Hephaestin Activity in the Intestine of Copper-Deficient Mice Causes Systemic Iron Deficiency. The Journal of Nutrition, 136(5), 1236–1241. doi:10.1093/jn/136.5.1236

[1809] Collins, J. F., Prohaska, J. R., & Knutson, M. D. (2010). Metabolic crossroads of iron and copper. Nutrition Reviews, 68(3), 133–147. doi:10.1111/j.1753-4887.2010.00271.x

[1810] Miyajima, H., Nishimura, Y., Mimguchi, K., Sakamoto, M., Shimizu, T., & Honda, N. (1987). Familial apoceruloplasmin deficiency associated with blepharospasm and retinal degeneration. Neurology, 37(5), 761–761. doi:10.1212/wnl.37.5.761

[1811] Morita, H., Ikeda, S.-I., Yamamoto, K., Morita, S., Yoshida, K., Nomoto, S., … Yanagisawa, N. (1995). Hereditary ceruloplasmin deficiency with hemosiderosis: A clinicopathological study of a japanese family. Annals of Neurology, 37(5), 646–656. doi:10.1002/ana.410370515

[1812] Hereditary caeruloplasmin deficiency, dementia and diabetes mellitus. (1994). QJM: An International Journal of Medicine. doi:10.1093/oxfordjournals.qjmed.a068881

[1813] Harris, Z. L., Durley, A. P., Man, T. K., & Gitlin, J. D. (1999). Targeted gene disruption reveals an essential role for ceruloplasmin in cellular iron efflux. Proceedings of the National Academy of Sciences, 96(19), 10812–10817. doi:10.1073/pnas.96.19.10812

[1814] Broderius, M., Mostad, E., Wendroth, K., & Prohaska, J. R. (2010). Levels of plasma ceruloplasmin protein are markedly lower following dietary copper deficiency in rodents. Comparative Biochemistry and Physiology Part C: Toxicology & Pharmacology, 151(4), 473–479. doi:10.1016/j.cbpc.2010.02.005

[1815] Thackeray, E. W., Sanderson, S. O., Fox, J. C., & Kumar, N. (2011). Hepatic Iron Overload or Cirrhosis May Occur in Acquired Copper Deficiency and is Likely Mediated by Hypoceruloplasminemia. Journal of Clinical Gastroenterology, 45(2), 153–158. doi:10.1097/mcg.0b013e3181dc25f7

[1816] Kono, S. (2013). Aceruloplasminemia. Metal Related Neurodegenerative Disease, 125–151. doi:10.1016/b978-0-12-410502-7.00007-7

[1817] Aigner, E., Theurl, I., Haufe, H., Seifert, M., Hohla, F., Scharinger, L., … Datz, C. (2008). Copper Availability Contributes to Iron Perturbations in Human Nonalcoholic Fatty Liver Disease. Gastroenterology, 135(2), 680–688.e1. doi:10.1053/j.gastro.2008.04.007

[1818] Torti, S. V., & Torti, F. M. (2013). Iron and cancer: more ore to be mined. Nature reviews. Cancer, 13(5), 342–355. https://doi.org/10.1038/nrc3495

[1819] Fleming, R. E., & Ponka, P. (2012). Iron overload in human disease. The New England journal of medicine, 366(4), 348–359. https://doi.org/10.1056/NEJMra1004967

[1820] Qiao, L., & Feng, Y. (2013). Intakes of heme iron and zinc and colorectal cancer incidence: a meta-analysis of prospective studies. Cancer causes & control : CCC, 24(6), 1175–1183. https://doi.org/10.1007/s10552-013-0197-x

[1821] Atamna, H. (2004). Heme, iron, and the mitochondrial decay of ageing. Ageing Research Reviews, 3(3), 303–318. doi:10.1016/j.arr.2004.02.002

[1822] Klevay, L. M. (2001). Iron overload can induce mild copper deficiency. Journal of Trace Elements in Medicine and Biology, 14(4), 237–240. doi:10.1016/s0946-672x(01)80009-2

[1823] Nittis T, Gitlin JD. Role of copper in the proteosomemediated degradation of the multicopper oxidase hephaestin. J Biol Chem. 2004;279:25696–25702.

[1824] Höhn, A., Jung, T., Grimm, S., & Grune, T. (2010). Lipofuscin-bound iron is a major intracellular source of oxidants: Role in senescent cells. Free Radical Biology and Medicine, 48(8), 1100–1108. doi:10.1016/j.freeradbiomed.2010.01.030

[1825] Williams, D. M., Loukopoulos, D., Lee, G. R., & Cartwright, G. E. (1976). Role of copper in mitochondrial iron metabolism. Blood, 48(1), 77–85.

[1826] Williams, D. M., Barbuto, A. J., Atkin, C. L., & Lee, G. R. (1978). Evidence for an iron carrier substance in copper-deficient mitochondria. Progress in clinical and biological research, 21, 539–549.

[1827] Bush, J. A., Jensen, W. N., Athens, J. W., Ashenbrucker, H., Cartwright, G. E., & Wintrobe, M. M. (1956). STUDIES ON COPPER METABOLISM. XIX. Journal of Experimental Medicine, 103(5), 701–712. doi:10.1084/jem.103.5.701

[1828] Reeves, P. G., & DeMars, L. C. S. (2006). Signs of iron deficiency in copper-deficient rats are not affected by iron supplements administered by diet or by injection. The Journal of Nutritional Biochemistry, 17(9), 635–642. doi:10.1016/j.jnutbio.2006.04.004

[1829] Sarata and Suzuki (1934) 'Studies in the biochemistry of copper. V. Effect of rapid loss of blood upon the copper content of blood'. Jap J Med Sci II, Biochem 2, 341–354.

[1830] Sachs, A. (1937). The effect of bleeding ulcers and hemorrhagic anemia upon whole blood copper and iron. American Journal of Digestive Diseases and Nutrition, 4(12), 803–804. doi:10.1007/bf03003043

[1831] CARTWRIGHT, G. E., & HUGULEY, C. M., Jr (1948). Studies on free erythrocyte protoporphyrin, plasma iron and plasma copper in normal and anemic subjects. Blood, 3(5), 501–525.

[1832] Lahey, M. E., Gubler, C. J., Cartwright, G. E., & Wintrobe, M. M. (1953). STUDIES ON COPPER METABOLISM. VII. BLOOD COPPER IN PREGNANCY AND VARIOUS PATHOLOGIC STATES 1. Journal of Clinical Investigation, 32(4), 329–339. doi:10.1172/jci102743

[1833] Klevay, L. M. (2000). Cardiovascular Disease from Copper Deficiency—A History. The Journal of Nutrition, 130(2), 489S–492S. doi:10.1093/jn/130.2.489s

[1834] Klevay (2000), 'Dietary copper and risk of coronary heart disease', The American Journal of Clinical Nutrition, Volume 71, Issue 5, May 2000, Pages 1213–1214, https://doi.org/10.1093/ajcn/71.5.1213

[1835] Klevay (2015) 'Copper, Coronary Heart Disease, and Dehydroepiandrosterone', J Am Coll Cardiol. 2015 May, 65 (19) 2151–2152.

[1836] Russo, C., Olivieri, O., Girelli, D., Faccini, G., Zenari, M. L., Lombardi, S., & Corrocher, R. (1998). Anti-oxidant status and lipid peroxidation in patients with essential hypertension. Journal of hypertension, 16(9), 1267–1271. https://doi.org/10.1097/00004872-199816090-00007

[1837] Reiser, S., Smith, J. C., Jr, Mertz, W., Holbrook, J. T., Scholfield, D. J., Powell, A. S., Canfield, W. K., & Canary, J. J. (1985). Indices of copper status in humans consuming a typical American diet containing either fructose or starch. The American journal of clinical nutrition, 42(2), 242–251. https://doi.org/10.1093/ajcn/42.2.242

[1838] Saldivar, V. A., Dick, M., Rosenthal, A., Vawter, G. F., Weymouth, R. E., Calder, A. L., … Van Praagh, R. (1974). Generalized arterial disease with angina pectoris in an adolescent girl. The American Journal of Cardiology, 34(3), 376–381. doi:10.1016/0002-9149(74)90043-5

[1839] Wester, P. O. (1971). Trace elements in the coronary arteries in the presence and absence of atherosclerosis. Atherosclerosis, 13(3), 395–412. doi:10.1016/0021-9150(71)90082-7

[1840] Waisman, J., Cancilla, P. A., & Coulson, W. F. (1969). Cardiovascular studies on copper-deficient swine. 13. The effect of chronic copper deficiency on the cardiovascular system of miniature pigs. Laboratory investigation; a journal of technical methods and pathology, 21(6), 548–554.

[1841] Klevay, L. M. (2011). Is the Western diet adequate in copper? Journal of Trace Elements in Medicine and Biology, 25(4), 204–212. doi:10.1016/j.jtemb.2011.08.146

[1842] Klevay, L. M. (2007). Copper Deficiency, Lead, and Paraoxonase. Environmental Health Perspectives, 115(7). doi:10.1289/ehp.10151

[1843] Klevay, L. M. (2016). IHD from copper deficiency: a unified theory. Nutrition Research Reviews, 29(2), 172–179. doi:10.1017/s0954422416000093

[1844] Kirk (1969) 'Enzymes of the Arterial Wall', Academic Press, New York and London.

[1845] Kreuter, K., Lee, J., Mukai, D., Mahon, S., Waddington, T., Armstrong, J., … Brenner, M. (2005). DIFFUSE OPTICAL SPECTROSCOPY MONITORING OF CYANIDE TOXICITY AND TREATMENT USING HYDROXOCOBALAMIN IN AN ANIMAL MODEL. Chest, 128(4), 301S. doi:10.1378/chest.128.4_meetingabstracts.301s-a

[1846] BAJUSZ, E., & JASMIN, G. (1964). HISTOCHEMICAL STUDIES ON THE MYOCARDIUM FOLLOWING EXPERIMENTAL INTERFERENCE WITH CORONARY CIRCULATION IN THE RAT. I. OCCLUSION OF CORONARY ARTERY. Acta histochemica, 18, 222–237.

[1847] REDETZKI, H., RUSKIN, A., NOWINSKI, W., SINCLAIR, J. G., ROSENTHAL, P., & RUSKIN, B. (1958). Changes in enzyme activity (glutamic oxaloacetic transaminase, lactic dehydrogenase, cytochrome c, and cytochrome oxidase) in serum and heart muscle after experimental myocardial infarction in the dog. Texas reports on biology and medicine, 16(1), 101–115.

[1848] Adelstein, S. J., Coombs, T. L., & Vallee, B. L. (1956). Metalloenzymes and Myocardial Infarction. New England Journal of Medicine, 255(3), 105–109. doi:10.1056/nejm195607192550301

[1849] VALLEE B. L. (1952). The time course of serum copper concentrations of patients with myocardial infarctions. I. Metabolism: clinical and experimental, 1(5), 420–434.

[1850] HANSON, A., & BIORCK, G. (1957). Glutamic-oxalacetic transaminase in the diagnosis of myocardial infarction. II. Comparison of serum transaminase activity with determinations of serum aldolase, cholesterol, alpha2-globulin, iron, copper and lactic dehydrogenase. Acta medica Scandinavica, 157(6), 493–502.

[1851] Kanabrocki, E. L., Fields, T., Decker, C. F., Case, L. F., Miller, E. B., Kaplan, E., & Oester, Y. T. (1964). Neutron activation studies of biological fluids: Manganese and copper. The International Journal of Applied Radiation and Isotopes, 15(4), 175–190. doi:10.1016/0020-708x(64)90064-x

[1852] HANSON, A., & BIORCK, G. (1957). Glutamic-oxalacetic transaminase in the diagnosis of myocardial infarction. II. Comparison of serum transaminase activity with determinations of serum aldolase, cholesterol, alpha2-globulin, iron, copper and lactic dehydrogenase. Acta medica Scandinavica, 157(6), 493–502.

[1853] Schroeder, H. A., Nason, A. P., Tipton, I. H., & Balassa, J. J. (1966). Essential trace metals in man: copper. Journal of chronic diseases, 19(9), 1007–1034. https://doi.org/10.1016/0021-9681(66)90033-6

[1854] Oladunni Taylor, G., & Olufemi Williams, A. (1974). Lipid and trace metal content in coronary arteries of Nigerian Africans. Experimental and Molecular Pathology, 21(3), 371–380. doi:10.1016/0014-4800(74)90103-8

[1855] TAYLOR, G. O., WILLIAMS, A. O., RESCH, J. A., BARBER, J. B., JACKSON, M. A., & PAULISSEN, G. A. (1975). Trace Metal Content of Cerebral Vessels in American Blacks, Caucasians and Nigerian Africans. Stroke, 6(6), 684–690. doi:10.1161/01.str.6.6.684

[1856] Sullivan, JL (1981) Iron and the sex difference in heart disease risk. Lancet i, 1293–1294.

[1857] Kaluza, J., Larsson, S. C., Håkansson, N., & Wolk, A. (2014). Heme iron intake and acute myocardial infarction: a prospective study of men. International journal of cardiology, 172(1), 155–160. https://doi.org/10.1016/j.ijcard.2013.12.176

[1858] Klevay, L. M. (2001). Iron overload can induce mild copper deficiency. Journal of Trace Elements in Medicine and Biology, 14(4), 237–240. doi:10.1016/s0946-672x(01)80009-2

[1859] Harris, E. D., Rayton, J. K., Balthrop, J. E., DiSilvestro, R. A., & Garcia-de-Quevedo, M. (1980). Copper and the synthesis of elastin and collagen. Ciba Foundation symposium, 79, 163–182. https://doi.org/10.1002/9780470720622.ch9

[1860] Rucker, R. B., Kosonen, T., Clegg, M. S., Mitchell, A. E., Rucker, B. R., Uriu-Hare, J. Y., & Keen, C. L. (1998). Copper, lysyl oxidase, and extracellular matrix protein cross-linking. The American Journal of Clinical Nutrition, 67(5), 996S–1002S. doi:10.1093/ajcn/67.5.996s

[1861] Klevay, LM (2006) How dietary deficiency, genes and a toxin can cooperate to produce arteriosclerosis and ischaemic heart disease. Cell Mol Biol 52, 11–15.

[1862] Klevay L. M. (2004). Ischemic heart disease as deficiency disease. Cellular and molecular biology (Noisy-le-Grand, France), 50(8), 877–884.

[1863] Clarke et al (2002) 'Homocysteine and Risk of Ischemic Heart Disease and Stroke: A Meta-Analysis', JAMA. 2002;288(16):2015–2022. doi:10.1001/jama.288.16.2015

[1864] Barter and Rye (2006) 'Homocysteine and Cardiovascular Disease: Is HDL the Link?', Circulation Research. 2006;99:565–566, DOI: https://doi.org/10.1161/01.RES.0000243583.39694.1f

[1865] Linnebank, M., Lutz, H., Jarre, E., Vielhaber, S., Noelker, C., Struys, E., Jakobs, C., Klockgether, T., Evert, B. O., Kunz, W. S., & Wüllner, U. (2006). Binding of copper is a mechanism of homocysteine toxicity leading to COX deficiency and apoptosis in primary neurons, PC12 and SHSY-5Y cells. Neurobiology of disease, 23(3), 725–730. https://doi.org/10.1016/j.nbd.2006.06.010

[1866] Hughes, W. M., Jr, Rodriguez, W. E., Rosenberger, D., Chen, J., Sen, U., Tyagi, N., Moshal, K. S., Vacek, T., Kang, Y. J., & Tyagi, S. C. (2008). Role of copper and homocysteine in pressure overload heart failure. Cardiovascular toxicology, 8(3), 137–144. https://doi.org/10.1007/s12012-008-9021-3

[1867] Urso, E., & Maffia, M. (2015). Behind the Link between Copper and Angiogenesis: Established Mechanisms and an Overview on the Role of Vascular Copper Transport Systems. Journal of vascular research, 52(3), 172–196. https://doi.org/10.1159/000438485

[1868] Demura, Y., Ameshima, S., Ishizaki, T., Okamura, S., Miyamori, I., & Matsukawa, S. (1998). The Activation of eNOS by Copper Ion (Cu2) in Human Pulmonary Arterial Endothelial Cells (HPAEC). Free Radical Biology and Medicine, 25(3), 314–320. doi:10.1016/s0891-5849(98)00056-2

[1869] Demura, Y., Ishizaki, T., Ameshima, S., Okamura, S., Hayashi, T., Matsukawa, S., & Miyamori, I. (1998). The activation of nitric oxide synthase by copper ion is mediated by intracellular Ca2+

614

mobilization in human pulmonary arterial endothelial cells. British Journal of Pharmacology, 125(6), 1180–1187. doi:10.1038/sj.bjp.0702197

[1870] Ma, J., Xie, Y., Zhou, Y., Wang, D., Cao, L., Zhou, M., … Chen, W. (2020). Urinary copper, systemic inflammation, and blood lipid profiles: Wuhan-Zhuhai cohort study. Environmental Pollution, 267, 115647. doi:10.1016/j.envpol.2020.115647

[1871] PEDRERO, E., Jr, & KOZELKA, F. L. (1951). Effect of various pathological conditions on the copper content of human tissues. A.M.A. archives of pathology, 52(5), 447–454.

[1872] Zhang, S., Xu, H., Liu, H., Amarsingh, G., & Cooper, G. J. S. (2013). P4.27 DIABETES-EVOKED PATHOGENIC CHANGES ASSOCIATED WITH ALTERED COPPER UPTAKE/TRANSPORT PATHWAYS IN THE AORTA OF STZ-DIABETIC RATS: EFFECTS OF TREATMENT BY CU(II)-SELECTIVE CHELATION. Artery Research, 7(3-4), 143. doi:10.1016/j.artres.2013.10.145

[1873] M, S., & DR, M. (2014). Inflammation and Diabetes. Interdisciplinary Journal of Microinflammation, 01(01). doi:10.4172/ijm.1000110

[1874] Washington University in St. Louis. (2016, November 2). Cause of inflammation in diabetes identified. ScienceDaily. Retrieved December 6, 2020 from www.sciencedaily.com/releases/2016/11/161102080309.htm

[1875] Wolf, M., Sauk, J., Shah, A., Vossen Smirnakis, K., Jimenez-Kimble, R., Ecker, J. L., & Thadhani, R. (2003). Inflammation and Glucose Intolerance: A prospective study of gestational diabetes mellitus. Diabetes Care, 27(1), 21–27. doi:10.2337/diacare.27.1.21

[1876] Vyden, J. K., Thorner, J., Nagasawa, K., Takano, T., Groseth-Dittrich, M. F., Perlow, R., & Swan, H. J. (1975). Metabolic and cardiovascular abnormalities in patients with peripheral arterial disease. American heart journal, 90(6), 703–708. https://doi.org/10.1016/0002-8703(75)90459-7

[1877] Niedermeier, W., Creitz, E. E., & Holley, H. L. (1962). Trace metal composition of synovial fluid from patients with rheumatoid arthritis. Arthritis & Rheumatism, 5(5), 439–444. doi:10.1002/art.1780050502

[1878] Saltman, P. D., & Strause, L. G. (1993). The role of trace minerals in osteoporosis. Journal of the American College of Nutrition, 12(4), 384–389. doi:10.1080/07315724.1993.10718327

[1879] Carty H. (1988). Brittle or battered. Archives of disease in childhood, 63(4), 350–352. https://doi.org/10.1136/adc.63.4.350

[1880] Chapman S. (1987). Child abuse or copper deficiency? A radiological view. British medical journal (Clinical research ed.), 294(6584), 1370. https://doi.org/10.1136/bmj.294.6584.1370

[1881] Jonas, J., Burns, J., Abel, E. W., Cresswell, M. J., Strain, J. J., & Paterson, C. R. (1993). Impaired Mechanical Strength of Bone in Experimental Copper Deficiency. Annals of Nutrition and Metabolism, 37(5), 245–252. doi:10.1159/000177774

[1882] Opsahl, W., Zeronian, H., Ellison, M., Lewis, D., Rucker, R. B., & Riggins, R. S. (1982). Role of Copper in Collagen Cross-linking and Its Influence on Selected Mechanical Properties of Chick Bone and Tendon. The Journal of Nutrition, 112(4), 708–716. doi:10.1093/jn/112.4.708

[1883] Marquardt, M. L., Done, S. L., Sandrock, M., Berdon, W. E., & Feldman, K. W. (2012). Copper Deficiency Presenting as Metabolic Bone Disease in Extremely Low Birth Weight, Short-Gut Infants. PEDIATRICS, 130(3), e695–e698. doi:10.1542/peds.2011-1295

[1884] Medeiros D. M. (2016). Copper, iron, and selenium dietary deficiencies negatively impact skeletal integrity: A review. Experimental biology and medicine (Maywood, N.J.), 241(12), 1316–1322. https://doi.org/10.1177/1535370216648805

[1885] Zheng, J., Mao, X., Ling, J., He, Q., & Quan, J. (2014). Low Serum Levels of Zinc, Copper, and Iron as Risk Factors for Osteoporosis: a Meta-analysis. Biological Trace Element Research, 160(1), 15–23. doi:10.1007/s12011-014-0031-7

[1886] Strain, J. J. (1988). A reassessment of diet and osteoporosis — Possible role for copper. Medical Hypotheses, 27(4), 333–338. doi:10.1016/0306-9877(88)90016-3

[1887] Menczel, J., Reshef, A., Schwartz, A., Guggenheim, K., Hegsted, D. M., & Stare, F. J. (1971). Aortic calcification in Israel. An epidemiological study. Archives of environmental health, 22(6), 667–671. https://doi.org/10.1080/00039896.1971.10665921

[1888] Cox, J. M., Gideon, D., & Rogers, F. J. (1983). Incidence of osteophytic lipping of the thoracic spine in coronary heart disease: results of a pilot study. The Journal of the American Osteopathic Association, 82(11), 837–838.

[1889] BAXTER, J. H., VAN WYK, J. J., & FOLLIS, R. H., Jr (1953). A bone disorder associated with copper deficiency. II. Histological and chemical studies on the bones. Bulletin of the Johns Hopkins Hospital, 93(1), 25–39.

[1890] Riggs (1992) 'Osteoporosis. In Wyngaarden JB', in Smith LH Jr, Bennett JC (eds): "Cecil Textbook of Medicine," 19th ed. Philadelphia: W.B. Saunders Company, pp 1426-1431.

[1891] Rosenberg A. E. (1991). The pathology of metabolic bone disease. Radiologic clinics of North America, 29(1), 19–36.

[1892] Gillespie, T., 3rd, & Gillespie, M. P. (1991). Osteoporosis. Radiologic clinics of North America, 29(1), 77–84.

[1893] Strause, L., Saltman, P., Smith, K. T., Bracker, M., & Andon, M. B. (1994). Spinal Bone Loss in Postmenopausal Women Supplemented with Calcium and Trace Minerals. The Journal of Nutrition, 124(7), 1060–1064. doi:10.1093/jn/124.7.1060

[1894] Cox, J. M., Gideon, D., & Rogers, F. J. (1983). Incidence of osteophytic lipping of the thoracic spine in coronary heart disease: results of a pilot study. The Journal of the American Osteopathic Association, 82(11), 837–838.

[1895] Milachowski, K.A. Investigation of ischaemic necrosis of the femoral head with trace elements. International Orthopaedics 12, 323–330 (1988). https://doi.org/10.1007/BF00317832

[1896] Qu, X., He, Z., Qiao, H., Zhai, Z., Mao, Z., Yu, Z., & Dai, K. (2018). Serum copper levels are associated with bone mineral density and total fracture. Journal of Orthopaedic Translation, 14, 34–44. doi:10.1016/j.jot.2018.05.001

[1897] Howard et al (1992) 'Low serum copper, a risk factor additional to low dietary calcium in postmenopausal bone loss', The Journal of Trace Elements in Experimental Medicine 5(1):23-31.

[1898] Altobelli, G. G., Van Noorden, S., Balato, A., & Cimini, V. (2020). Copper/Zinc Superoxide Dismutase in Human Skin: Current Knowledge. Frontiers in Medicine, 7. doi:10.3389/fmed.2020.00183

[1899] Murphy, M. P., Echtay, K. S., Blaikie, F. H., Asin-Cayuela, J., Cochemé, H. M., Green, K., … Brand, M. D. (2003). Superoxide Activates Uncoupling Proteins by Generating Carbon-centered Radicals and Initiating Lipid Peroxidation. Journal of Biological Chemistry, 278(49), 48534–48545. doi:10.1074/jbc.m308529200

[1900] McCormick, M. L., Gavrila, D., & Weintraub, N. L. (2007). Role of Oxidative Stress in the Pathogenesis of Abdominal Aortic Aneurysms. Arteriosclerosis, Thrombosis, and Vascular Biology, 27(3), 461–469. doi:10.1161/01.atv.0000257552.94483.14

[1901] Rocha, M., Apostolova, N., Hernandez-Mijares, A., Herance, R., & Victor, V. M. (2010). Oxidative stress and endothelial dysfunction in cardiovascular disease: mitochondria-targeted therapeutics. Current medicinal chemistry, 17(32), 3827–3841. https://doi.org/10.2174/092986710793205444

[1902] Auger, C., Pollet, B., Marx, C., Benchabane, D., & Schini-Kerth, V. B. (2014). 0179: Polyphenol-rich blackcurrant juice induces NO-mediated relaxation in porcine coronary artery rings via a copper- and iron-dependent redox-sensitive activation of the Src/PI3-kinase/Akt/eNOS pathway. Archives of Cardiovascular Diseases Supplements, 6, 17. doi:10.1016/s1878-6480(14)71309-6

[1903] Davis, C. D. (2003). Low Dietary Copper Increases Fecal Free Radical Production, Fecal Water Alkaline Phosphatase Activity and Cytotoxicity in Healthy Men. The Journal of Nutrition, 133(2), 522–527. doi:10.1093/jn/133.2.522

[1904] Granger, D. N., & Kvietys, P. R. (2015). Reperfusion injury and reactive oxygen species: The evolution of a concept. Redox biology, 6, 524–551. https://doi.org/10.1016/j.redox.2015.08.020

[1905] Sudhahar, V., Urao, N., Oshikawa, J., McKinney, R. D., Llanos, R. M., Mercer, J. F., Ushio-Fukai, M., & Fukai, T. (2013). Copper transporter ATP7A protects against endothelial dysfunction in type 1 diabetic mice by regulating extracellular superoxide dismutase. Diabetes, 62(11), 3839–3850. https://doi.org/10.2337/db12-1228

[1906] Malinowska, K., Morawiec-Sztandera, A., Majsterek, I., & Kaczmarczyk, D. (2016). Effect of copper(II) the activity of glutathione peroxidase in patients with head and neck cancer. Otolaryngologia polska = The Polish otolaryngology, 70(6), 20–25. https://doi.org/10.5604/01.3001.0009.3735

[1907] Jenkinson, S. G., Lawrence, R. A., Burk, R. F., & Williams, D. M. (1982). Effects of copper deficiency on the activity of the selenoenzyme glutathione peroxidase and on excretion and tissue retention of 75SeO3(2-). The Journal of nutrition, 112(1), 197–204. https://doi.org/10.1093/jn/112.1.197

[1908] ARAYA, M., PIZARRO, F., OLIVARES, M., ARREDONDO, M., GONZÁLEZ, M., & MÉNDEZ, M. (2006). Understanding copper homeostasis in humans and copper effects on health. Biological Research, 39(1). doi:10.4067/s0716-97602006000100020

[1909] Freedman et al (1989) 'The Role of Glutathione in Copper Metabolism and Toxicity', THE JOURNAL OF BIOLOGICAL CHEMISTRY, Vol. 264, No. 10, Issue of April 5, pp. 5598-5605.

[1910] Bustos, R. I., Jensen, E. L., Ruiz, L. M., Rivera, S., Ruiz, S., Simon, F., … Elorza, A. A. (2013). Copper deficiency alters cell bioenergetics and induces mitochondrial fusion through up-regulation of MFN2 and OPA1 in erythropoietic cells. Biochemical and Biophysical Research Communications, 437(3), 426–432. doi:10.1016/j.bbrc.2013.06.095

[1911] van der Mijn, J. C., Kuiper, M. J., Siegert, C., Wassenaar, A. E., van Noesel, C., & Ogilvie, A. C. (2017). Lactic Acidosis in Prostate Cancer: Consider the Warburg Effect. Case reports in oncology, 10(3), 1085–1091. https://doi.org/10.1159/000485242

[1912] Yang (2016) 'Copper is Key in Burning Fat', News Center, (510) 486-4575 • June 6, 2016.

[1913] DOE/Lawrence Berkeley National Laboratory. (2016, June 6). Copper is key in burning fat: Scientist says results could provide new target for obesity research. ScienceDaily. Retrieved December 5, 2020 from www.sciencedaily.com/releases/2016/06/160606200439.htm

[1914] Berardi (2020) 'How to fix a broken diet: 3 ways to get your eating on track.', Precision Nutrition, Accessed Online Nov 11 2020: https://www.precisionnutrition.com/fix-a-broken-diet

[1915] Klevay, L. M. (1998). Lack of a Recommended Dietary Allowance for Copper may be Hazardous to Your Health. Journal of the American College of Nutrition, 17(4), 322–326. doi:10.1080/07315724.1998.10718769

[1916] Friedman, S., & Kaufman, S. (1965). 3,4-dihydroxyphenylethylamine beta-hydroxylase. Physical properties, copper content, and role of copper in the catalytic acttivity. The Journal of biological chemistry, 240(12), 4763–4773.

[1917] Feng, W., Ye, F., Xue, W., Zhou, Z., & Kang, Y. J. (2009). Copper regulation of hypoxia-inducible factor-1 activity. Molecular pharmacology, 75(1), 174–182. https://doi.org/10.1124/mol.108.051516

[1918] Rochlani, Y., Pothineni, N. V., Kovelamudi, S., & Mehta, J. L. (2017). Metabolic syndrome: pathophysiology, management, and modulation by natural compounds. Therapeutic Advances in Cardiovascular Disease, 11(8), 215–225. doi:10.1177/1753944717711379

[1919] Grundy, S. M., Hansen, B., Smith, S. C., Cleeman, J. I., & Kahn, R. A. (2004). Clinical Management of Metabolic Syndrome. Arteriosclerosis, Thrombosis, and Vascular Biology, 24(2). doi:10.1161/01.atv.0000112379.88385.67

[1920] Mottillo, S., Filion, K. B., Genest, J., Joseph, L., Pilote, L., Poirier, P., … Eisenberg, M. J. (2010). The Metabolic Syndrome and Cardiovascular Risk. Journal of the American College of Cardiology, 56(14), 1113–1132. doi:10.1016/j.jacc.2010.05.034

[1921] Fields, M., Ferretti, R. J., Smith, J. C., Jr, & Reiser, S. (1983). Effect of copper deficiency on metabolism and mortality in rats fed sucrose or starch diets. The Journal of nutrition, 113(7), 1335–1345. https://doi.org/10.1093/jn/113.7.1335

[1922] Reiser, S., Ferretti, R. J., Fields, M., & Smith, J. C. (1983). Role of dietary fructose in the enhancement of mortality and biochemical changes associated with copper deficiency in rats. The American Journal of Clinical Nutrition, 38(2), 214–222. doi:10.1093/ajcn/38.2.214

[1923] Hassel, C. A., Marchello, J. A., & Lei, K. Y. (1983). Impaired glucose tolerance in copper-deficient rats. The Journal of nutrition, 113(5), 1081–1083. https://doi.org/10.1093/jn/113.5.1081

[1924] Medeiros, D., Pellum, L. & Brown, B. (1983) Serum lipids and glucose as associated with hemoglobin levels and copper and zinc intake in young adults. Life Sci. 32, 1897-1904.

[1925] Nagisa, Y., Kato, K., Watanabe, K., Murakoshi, H., Odaka, H., Yoshikawa, K. and Sugiyama, Y. (2003), Changes in glycated haemoglobin levels in diabetic rats measured with an automatic affinity HPLC. Clinical and Experimental Pharmacology and Physiology, 30: 752-758. https://doi.org/10.1046/j.1440-1681.2003.03902.x

[1926] Beck-Nielsen, H., Pederson, O. & Lindskov, H. O. (1980) Impaired cellular insulin binding and insulin sensitivity induced by high-fructose feeding in normal subjects. Am. J. Clin. Nutr. 33, 273-278.

[1927] Takahashi, Y., Miyajima, H., Shirabe, S., Nagataki, S., Suenaga, A., & Gitlin, J. D. (1996). Characterization of a nonsense mutation in the ceruloplasmin gene resulting in diabetes and neurodegenerative disease. Human molecular genetics, 5(1), 81–84. https://doi.org/10.1093/hmg/5.1.81

[1928] Uriu-Adams, J. Y., & Keen, C. L. (2005). Copper, oxidative stress, and human health. Molecular aspects of medicine, 26(4-5), 268–298. https://doi.org/10.1016/j.mam.2005.07.015

[1929] L., J., & Lutsenko, S. (2013). The Role of Copper as a Modifier of Lipid Metabolism. Lipid Metabolism. doi:10.5772/51819

[1930] Kaya, A., Altıner, A., & Özpınar, A. (2006). Effect of Copper Deficiency on Blood Lipid Profile and Haematological Parameters in Broilers. Journal of Veterinary Medicine Series A, 53(8), 399–404. doi:10.1111/j.1439-0442.2006.00835.x

[1931] Klevay, LM, Inman, L, Johnson, LK, et al. (1984) Increased cholesterol in plasma in a young man during experimental copper depletion. Metabolism 33, 1112–1118.

[1932] Alarcón-Corredor, O. M., Guerrero, Y., Ramírez de Fernández, M., D'Jesús, I., Burguera, M., Burguera, J. L., Di Bernardo, M. L., García, M. Y., & Alarcón, A. O. (2004). Efecto de la suplementación oral con cobre en el perfil lipídico de pacientes Venezolanos hiperlipémicos [Effect of copper supplementation on lipid profile of Venezuelan hyperlipemic patients]. Archivos latinoamericanos de nutricion, 54(4), 413–418.

[1933] Klevay, LM (2000) Trace element and mineral nutrition in disease: ischemic heart disease. In Clinical Nutrition of the Essential Trace Elements and Minerals: The Guide for Health Professionals, 1st ed., pp. 251–271 [JD Bogden and LM Klevay, editors]. Totowa, NJ: Humana Press Inc.

[1934] Harold et al (1977) 'Influence of dietary copper and zinc on rat lipid metabolism', Journal of Agricultural and Food Chemistry 1977 25 (5), 1105-1109.

[1935] Valsala, P., & Kurup, P. A. (1987). Investigations on the mechanism of hypercholesterolemia observed in copper deficiency in rats. Journal of Biosciences, 12(2), 137–142. doi:10.1007/bf02702965

[1936] Wilson, J., Kim, S., Allen, K. G., Baillie, R., & Clarke, S. D. (1997). Hepatic fatty acid synthase gene transcription is induced by a dietary copper deficiency. The American journal of physiology, 272(6 Pt 1), E1124–E1129. https://doi.org/10.1152/ajpendo.1997.272.6.E1124

[1937] Lukaski et al (1995) 'Body temperature and thyroid hormone metabolism of copper-deficient rats', The Journal of Nutritional Biochemistry, Volume 6, Issue 8, August 1995, Pages 445-451. https://doi.org/10.1016/0955-2863(95)00062-5

[1938] Blasig et al (2016) 'Positive correlation of thyroid hormones and serum copper in children with congenital hypothyroidism', Journal of Trace Elements in Medicine and Biology, Volume 37, September 2016, Pages 90-95, https://doi.org/10.1016/j.jtemb.2016.05.007

[1939] Rasic-Milutinovic, Z., Jovanovic, D., Bogdanovic, G., Trifunovic, J., & Mutic, J. (2017). Potential Influence of Selenium, Copper, Zinc and Cadmium on L-Thyroxine Substitution in Patients with Hashimoto Thyroiditis and Hypothyroidism. Experimental and clinical endocrinology & diabetes : official journal, German Society of Endocrinology [and] German Diabetes Association, 125(2), 79–85. https://doi.org/10.1055/s-0042-116070

[1940] Aihara, K., Nishi, Y., Hatano, S., Kihara, M., Yoshimitsu, K., Takeichi, N., Ito, T., Ezaki, H., & Usui, T. (1984). Zinc, copper, manganese, and selenium metabolism in thyroid disease. The American journal of clinical nutrition, 40(1), 26–35. https://doi.org/10.1093/ajcn/40.1.26

[1941] Bastian, T. W., Prohaska, J. R., Georgieff, M. K., & Anderson, G. W. (2010). Perinatal iron and copper deficiencies alter neonatal rat circulating and brain thyroid hormone concentrations. Endocrinology, 151(8), 4055–4065. https://doi.org/10.1210/en.2010-0252

[1942] Olin, K. L., Walter, R. M., & Keen, C. L. (1994). Copper deficiency affects selenoglutathione peroxidase and selenodeiodinase activities and antioxidant defense in weanling rats. The American journal of clinical nutrition, 59(3), 654–658. https://doi.org/10.1093/ajcn/59.3.654

[1943] Jain R. B. (2014). Thyroid function and serum copper, selenium, and zinc in general U.S. population. Biological trace element research, 159(1-3), 87–98. https://doi.org/10.1007/s12011-014-9992-9

[1944] Mittag, J., Behrends, T., Nordström, K., Anselmo, J., Vennström, B., & Schomburg, L. (2012). Serum copper as a novel biomarker for resistance to thyroid hormone. Biochemical Journal, 443(1), 103–109. doi:10.1042/bj20111817

[1945] Arora et al (2018) 'Study of Trace Elements in Patients of Hypothyroidism with Special Reference to Zinc and Copper', Biomed J Sci & Tech Res, 6(2)-2018. BJSTR. MS.ID.001336. DOI: 10.26717/BJSTR.2018.06.001336.

[1946] Kinsella, J., & Sacktor, B. (1985). Thyroid hormones increase Na+-H+ exchange activity in renal brush border membranes. Proceedings of the National Academy of Sciences, 82(11), 3606–3610. doi:10.1073/pnas.82.11.3606

[1947] Bizhanova, A., & Kopp, P. (2009). The Sodium-Iodide Symporter NIS and Pendrin in Iodide Homeostasis of the Thyroid. Endocrinology, 150(3), 1084–1090. doi:10.1210/en.2008-1437

[1948] Ravera, S., Reyna-Neyra, A., Ferrandino, G., Amzel, L. M., & Carrasco, N. (2017). The Sodium/Iodide Symporter (NIS): Molecular Physiology and Preclinical and Clinical Applications. Annual Review of Physiology, 79(1), 261–289. doi:10.1146/annurev-physiol-022516-034125

[1949] Nicola, J. P., Carrasco, N., & Mario Amzel, L. (2014). Physiological sodium concentrations enhance the iodide affinity of the Na+/I− symporter. Nature Communications, 5(1). doi:10.1038/ncomms4948

[1950] Sakamaki, Y., Goto, K., Watanabe, Y., Takata, T., Yamazaki, H., Imai, N., … Narita, I. (2014). Nephrotic Syndrome and End-stage Kidney Disease Accompanied by Bicytopenia due to Copper Deficiency. Internal Medicine, 53(18), 2101–2106. doi:10.2169/internalmedicine.53.2338

[1951] Sakamaki, Y., Goto, K., Watanabe, Y., Takata, T., Yamazaki, H., Imai, N., … Narita, I. (2014). Nephrotic Syndrome and End-stage Kidney Disease Accompanied by Bicytopenia due to Copper Deficiency. Internal Medicine, 53(18), 2101–2106. doi:10.2169/internalmedicine.53.2338

[1952] Emenaker, N. J., DiSilvestro, R. A., Nahman, N. S., Jr, & Percival, S. (1996). Copper-related blood indexes in kidney dialysis patients. The American journal of clinical nutrition, 64(5), 757–760. https://doi.org/10.1093/ajcn/64.5.757

[1953] Brown, E. A., Sampson, B., Muller, B. R., & Curtis, J. R. (1984). Urinary iron loss in the nephrotic syndrome--an unusual cause of iron deficiency with a note on urinary copper losses. Postgraduate Medical Journal, 60(700), 125–128. doi:10.1136/pgmj.60.700.125

[1954] MARKOWITZ, H., GUBLER, C. J., MAHONEY, J. P., CARTWRIGHT, G. E., & WINTROBE, M. M. (1955). Studies on copper metabolism. XIV. Copper, ceruloplasmin and oxidase activity in sera of normal human subjects, pregnant women, and patients with infection, hepatolenticular degeneration and the nephrotic syndrome. The Journal of clinical investigation, 34(10), 1498–1508. https://doi.org/10.1172/JCI103201

[1955] Tvrda, E., Peer, R., Sikka, S. C., & Agarwal, A. (2014). Iron and copper in male reproduction: a double-edged sword. Journal of Assisted Reproduction and Genetics, 32(1), 3–16. doi:10.1007/s10815-014-0344-7

[1956] Tvrda, E., Peer, R., Sikka, S. C., & Agarwal, A. (2014). Iron and copper in male reproduction: a double-edged sword. Journal of Assisted Reproduction and Genetics, 32(1), 3–16. doi:10.1007/s10815-014-0344-7

[1957] Tvrda, E., Peer, R., Sikka, S. C., & Agarwal, A. (2014). Iron and copper in male reproduction: a double-edged sword. Journal of Assisted Reproduction and Genetics, 32(1), 3–16. doi:10.1007/s10815-014-0344-7

[1958] Muñoz, C., Rios, E., Olivos, J., Brunser, O., & Olivares, M. (2007). Iron, copper and immunocompetence. British Journal of Nutrition, 98(S1), S24–S28. doi:10.1017/s0007114507833046

618

[1959] Prohaska, J. R., Downing, S. W., & Lukasewycz, O. A. (1983). Chronic Dietary Copper Deficiency Alters Biochemical and Morphological Properties of Mouse Lymphoid Tissues. The Journal of Nutrition, 113(8), 1583–1590. doi:10.1093/jn/113.8.1583

[1960] Tong et al (1996) 'The effects of copper deficiency on human lymphoid and myeloid cells: An in vitro model', British Journal Of Nutrition 75(1):97-108, DOI: 10.1079/BJN19960113

[1961] Muñoz, C., Rios, E., Olivos, J., Brunser, O., & Olivares, M. (2007). Iron, copper and immunocompetence. British Journal of Nutrition, 98(S1), S24–S28. doi:10.1017/s0007114507833046

[1962] Arredondo, M., & Núñez, M. T. (2005). Iron and copper metabolism. Molecular Aspects of Medicine, 26(4-5), 313–327. doi:10.1016/j.mam.2005.07.010

[1963] Horn, D., & Barrientos, A. (2008). Mitochondrial copper metabolism and delivery to cytochrome c oxidase. IUBMB life, 60(7), 421–429. https://doi.org/10.1002/iub.50

[1964] Blumberg, W. E., Peisach, J., Eisenberger, P., & Fee, J. A. (1978). Superoxide dismutase, a study of the electronic properties of the copper and zinc by X-ray absorption spectroscopy. Biochemistry, 17(10), 1842–1846. https://doi.org/10.1021/bi00603a006

[1965] Chen, Y., Saari, J. T., & Kang, Y. J. (1994). Weak antioxidant defenses make the heart a target for damage in copper-deficient rats. Free radical biology & medicine, 17(6), 529–536. https://doi.org/10.1016/0891-5849(94)90092-2

[1966] Petris, M. J., Strausak, D., & Mercer, J. F. (2000). The Menkes copper transporter is required for the activation of tyrosinase. Human molecular genetics, 9(19), 2845–2851. https://doi.org/10.1093/hmg/9.19.2845

[1967] Vendelboe et al (2016) 'The crystal structure of human dopamine β-hydroxylase at 2.9 Å resolution', Science Advances 08 Apr 2016: Vol. 2, no. 4, e1500980, DOI: 10.1126/sciadv.1500980.

[1968] Bousquet-Moore, D., Mains, R. E., & Eipper, B. A. (2010). Peptidylglycine α-amidating monooxygenase and copper: A gene-nutrient interaction critical to nervous system function. Journal of Neuroscience Research, 88(12), 2535–2545. doi:10.1002/jnr.22404

[1969] El Meskini, R., Culotta, V. C., Mains, R. E., & Eipper, B. A. (2003). Supplying Copper to the Cuproenzyme Peptidylglycine α-Amidating Monooxygenase. Journal of Biological Chemistry, 278(14), 12278–12284. doi:10.1074/jbc.m211413200

[1970] Werman et al (1997) 'Dietary copper intake influences skin lysyl oxidase in young men', The Journal of Nutritional Biochemistry, Volume 8, Issue 4, April 1997, Pages 201-204.

[1971] Lin, W., Xu, L., & Li, G. (2020). Molecular Insights Into Lysyl Oxidases in Cartilage Regeneration and Rejuvenation. Frontiers in Bioengineering and Biotechnology, 8. doi:10.3389/fbioe.2020.00359

[1972] Fife, R. S., Kluve-Beckerman, B., Houser, D. S., Proctor, C., Liepnieks, J., Masuda, I., McCarty, D. J., & Ryan, L. M. (1993). Evidence that a 550,000-dalton cartilage matrix glycoprotein is a chondrocyte membrane-associated protein closely related to ceruloplasmin. The Journal of biological chemistry, 268(6), 4407–4411.

[1973] FIFE, R., MOODY, S., HOUSER, D., & PROCTOR, C. (1994). Studies of copper transport in cultured bovine chondrocytes☆. Biochimica et Biophysica Acta (BBA) - General Subjects, 1201(1), 19–22. doi:10.1016/0304-4165(94)90145-7

[1974] Shi, Y., Hu, X., Cheng, J., Zhang, X., Zhao, F., Shi, W., … Ao, Y. (2019). A small molecule promotes cartilage extracellular matrix generation and inhibits osteoarthritis development. Nature Communications, 10(1). doi:10.1038/s41467-019-09839-x

[1975] Sandler (1987) 'MONOAMINE OXIDASE AND COPPER', VOLUME 329, ISSUE 8540, P1034, MAY 02, 1987, DOI:https://doi.org/10.1016/S0140-6736(87)92303-8

[1976] Jalkanen, S., & Salmi, M. (2001). Cell surface monoamine oxidases: enzymes in search of a function. The EMBO journal, 20(15), 3893–3901. https://doi.org/10.1093/emboj/20.15.3893

[1977] Sorenson (2012) 'Inflammatory Diseases and Copper: The Metabolic and Therapeutic Roles of Copper and Other Essential Metalloelements in Humans', Springer Science & Business Media, Dec 6, 2012.

[1978] Chang, T.-S. (2009). An Updated Review of Tyrosinase Inhibitors. International Journal of Molecular Sciences, 10(6), 2440–2475. doi:10.3390/ijms10062440

[1979] Bourre, J. M., Cloez, I., Galliot, M., Buisine, A., Dumont, O., Piciotti, M., … Bourdon, R. (1987). Occurrence of manganese, copper and zinc in myelin. Alterations in the peripheral nervous system of dysmyelinating trembler mutant are at variance with brain mutants (quaking and shiverer). Neurochemistry International, 10(3), 281–286. doi:10.1016/0197-0186(87)90101-x

[1980] Sant-Rayn Pasricha, Hal Drakesmith, James Black, David Hipgrave, Beverley-Ann Biggs; Control of iron deficiency anemia in low- and middle-income countries. Blood 2013; 121 (14): 2607–2617. doi: https://doi.org/10.1182/blood-2012-09-453522

[1981] De Benoist et al (2008) 'Worldwide prevalence of anaemia 1993-2005; WHO Global Database of anaemia', CDC Stacks, Accessed Online Dec 14 2020: https://stacks.cdc.gov/view/cdc/5351

[1982] Halfdanarson, T. R., Kumar, N., Li, C.-Y., Phyliky, R. L., & Hogan, W. J. (2008). Hematological manifestations of copper deficiency: a retrospective review. European Journal of Haematology, 80(6), 523–531. doi:10.1111/j.1600-0609.2008.01050.x

619

[1983] Gletsu-Miller, N., Broderius, M., Frediani, J. K., Zhao, V. M., Griffith, D. P., Davis, S. S., Jr, Sweeney, J. F., Lin, E., Prohaska, J. R., & Ziegler, T. R. (2012). Incidence and prevalence of copper deficiency following roux-en-y gastric bypass surgery. International journal of obesity (2005), 36(3), 328–335. https://doi.org/10.1038/ijo.2011.159

[1984] Griffith, D. P., Liff, D. A., Ziegler, T. R., Esper, G. J., & Winton, E. F. (2009). Acquired Copper Deficiency: A Potentially Serious and Preventable Complication Following Gastric Bypass Surgery. Obesity, 17(4), 827–831. doi:10.1038/oby.2008.614

[1985] Chan, L. N., & Mike, L. A. (2014). The science and practice of micronutrient supplementations in nutritional anemia: an evidence-based review. JPEN. Journal of parenteral and enteral nutrition, 38(6), 656–672. https://doi.org/10.1177/0148607114533726

[1986] F. S. Robscheit-Robbins, G. H. Whipple; COPPER AND COBALT RELATED HEMOGLOBIN PRODUCTION IN EXPERIMENTAL ANEMIA . J Exp Med 1 May 1942; 75 (5): 481–487. doi: https://doi.org/10.1084/jem.75.5.481

[1987] G. E. CARTWRIGHT, M. M. WINTROBE, The Question of Copper Deficiency in Man, The American Journal of Clinical Nutrition, Volume 15, Issue 2, August 1964, Pages 94–110, https://doi.org/10.1093/ajcn/15.2.94

[1988] Butterworth, C. E., Gubler, C. J., Cartwright, G. E., & Wintrobe, M. M. (1958). Studies on Copper Metabolism. XXVI. Plasma Copper in Patients with Tropical Sprue. Experimental Biology and Medicine, 98(3), 594–597. doi:10.3181/00379727-98-24117

[1989] Vulpe, C. D., Kuo, Y. M., Murphy, T. L., Cowley, L., Askwith, C., Libina, N., Gitschier, J., & Anderson, G. J. (1999). Hephaestin, a ceruloplasmin homologue implicated in intestinal iron transport, is defective in the sla mouse. Nature genetics, 21(2), 195–199. https://doi.org/10.1038/5979

[1990] Joseph R. Prohaska, Impact of Copper Limitation on Expression and Function of Multicopper Oxidases (Ferroxidases), Advances in Nutrition, Volume 2, Issue 2, 01 March 2011, Pages 89–95, https://doi.org/10.3945/an.110.000208

[1991] Watts (1989) 'The Nutritional Relationships of Copper', Journal of Orthomolecular Medicine, Vol. 4, No. 2, Accessed Online Nov 4 2020: http://traceelements.com/Docs/The%20Nutritional%20Relationships%20of%20Copper.pdf

[1992] Klevay, L. M. (2001). Iron overload can induce mild copper deficiency. Journal of Trace Elements in Medicine and Biology, 14(4), 237–240. doi:10.1016/s0946-672x(01)80009-2

[1993] Fields, M., Lewis, C. G., Lure, M. D., Burns, W. A., & Antholine, W. E. (1991). The severity of copper deficiency can be ameliorated by deferoxamine. Metabolism, 40(1), 105–109. doi:10.1016/0026-0495(91)90200-g

[1994] Gerrior, S., Bente, L., & Hiza, H. (2004). Nutrient Content of the U.S. Food Supply, 1909-2000. (Home Economics Research Report No. 56). U.S. Department of Agriculture, Center for Nutrition Policy and Promotion.

[1995] Altunoğlu, E., Müderrisoğlu, C., Erdenen, F., Ülgen, E., & Ar, M. C. (2014). The Impact of Obesity and Insulin Resistance on Iron and Red Blood Cell Parameters: A Single Center, Cross-Sectional Study. Turkish Journal of Hematology, 31(1), 61–67. doi:10.4274/tjh.2012.0187

[1996] Fernandez-Real, J. M., Lopez-Bermejo, A., & Ricart, W. (2002). Cross-Talk Between Iron Metabolism and Diabetes. Diabetes, 51(8), 2348–2354. doi:10.2337/diabetes.51.8.2348

[1997] Fox P. L. (2003). The copper-iron chronicles: the story of an intimate relationship. Biometals : an international journal on the role of metal ions in biology, biochemistry, and medicine, 16(1), 9–40. https://doi.org/10.1023/a:1020799512190

[1998] CORDANO, A., BAERTL, J. M., & GRAHAM, G. G. (1964). COPPER DEFICIENCY IN INFANCY. Pediatrics, 34, 324–336.

[1999] CORDANO, A., BAERTL, J. M., & GRAHAM, G. G. (1964). COPPER DEFICIENCY IN INFANCY. Pediatrics, 34, 324–336.

[2000] Graham, G. G., & Cordano, A. (1969). Copper depletion and deficiency in the malnourished infant. The Johns Hopkins medical journal, 124(3), 139–150.

[2001] Levy, Y., Zeharia, A., Grunebaum, M., Nitzan, M., & Steinherz, R. (1985). Copper deficiency in infants fed cow milk. The Journal of Pediatrics, 106(5), 786–788. doi:10.1016/s0022-3476(85)80356-5

[2002] Dörner, K., Dziadzka, S., Höhn, A., Sievers, E., Oldigs, H.-D., Schulz-Lell, G., & Schaub, J. (1989). Longitudinal manganese and copper balances in young infants and preterm infants fed on breast-milk and adapted cow's milkformulas. British Journal of Nutrition, 61(3), 559–572. doi:10.1079/bjn19890143

[2003] World Health Organization and Food and Agricultural Organization (2016) 'Guidelines on food fortification with micronutrients', Edited by Lindsay Allen, Bruno de Benoist, Omar Dary and Richard Hurrell, Accessed Online Dec 5 2020: https://www.who.int/nutrition/publications/guide_food_fortification_micronutrients.pdf

[2004] Food and Agricultural Organization of the United Nations 'Micronutrient Fortification of Food: Technology and Quality Control', Accessed Online Dec 5 2020: http://www.fao.org/3/W2840E/w2840e0b.htm

[2005] Moon and Weinberg (2008) 'Iron: The Most Toxic Metal', George Ohsawa Macrobiotic Foundation.

[2006] Elwood (1977), 'The Enrichment Dabate', Nutrition Today: July-August 1977 - p 18-24..

[2007] LEWIS, M. S. (1931). IRON AND COPPER IN THE TREATMENT OF ANEMIA IN CHILDREN. JAMA: The Journal of the American Medical Association, 96(14), 1135. doi:10.1001/jama.1931.02720400033010

[2008] Arredondo, M., & Núñez, M. T. (2005). Iron and copper metabolism. Molecular Aspects of Medicine, 26(4-5), 313–327. doi:10.1016/j.mam.2005.07.010

[2009] National Research Council (US) Subcommittee on the Tenth Edition of the Recommended Dietary Allowances. (1989). Recommended Dietary Allowances: 10th Edition. National Academies Press (US).

[2010] Institute of Medicine (US) Panel on Micronutrients. (2001). Dietary Reference Intakes for Vitamin A, Vitamin K, Arsenic, Boron, Chromium, Copper, Iodine, Iron, Manganese, Molybdenum, Nickel, Silicon, Vanadium, and Zinc. National Academies Press (US).

[2011] Chambers, A., Krewski, D., Birkett, N., Plunkett, L., Hertzberg, R., Danzeisen, R., Aggett, P. J., Starr, T. B., Baker, S., Dourson, M., Jones, P., Keen, C. L., Meek, B., Schoeny, R., & Slob, W. (2010). An exposure-response curve for copper excess and deficiency. Journal of toxicology and environmental health. Part B, Critical reviews, 13(7-8), 546–578. https://doi.org/10.1080/10937404.2010.538657

[2012] National Research Council (1989). 'Recommended dietary allowances.' 10th ed. Washington, DC: National Academy Press.

[2013] Anon (1994) 'How Should the Recommended Dietary Allowances be Revised?', Washington, DC: National Academy Press, pp vii,2,3,11.

[2014] Harvey et al (2003) 'Adaptive response in men fed low- and high-copper diets', British Journal of Nutrition, Volume 90, Issue 1, 1 July 2003, Pages 161-168.

[2015] J R Turnlund, Human whole-body copper metabolism, The American Journal of Clinical Nutrition, Volume 67, Issue 5, May 1998, Pages 960S–964S, https://doi.org/10.1093/ajcn/67.5.960S

[2016] Bost et al (2016) 'Dietary copper and human health: Current evidence and unresolved issues', Journal of Trace Elements in Medicine and Biology, Volume 35, May 2016, Pages 107-115, https://doi.org/10.1016/j.jtemb.2016.02.006

[2017] Milne (1998) 'Copper intake and assessment of copper status', The American Journal of Clinical Nutrition, Volume 67, Issue 5, May 1998, Pages 1041S–1045S, https://doi.org/10.1093/ajcn/67.5.1041S.

[2018] Milne and Nielsen (1996) 'Effects of a diet low in copper on copper-status indicators in postmenopausal women', American Journal of Clinical Nutrition 63(3):358-64, DOI: 10.1093/ajcn/63.3.358.

[2019] Milne et al (1990) 'Effect of copper intake on balance, absorption, and status indices of copper in men', Nutrition Research, Volume 10, Issue 9, September 1990, Pages 975-986, https://doi.org/10.1016/S0271-5317(05)80039-9

[2020] Reiser, S., Smith, J. C., Jr, Mertz, W., Holbrook, J. T., Scholfield, D. J., Powell, A. S., Canfield, W. K., & Canary, J. J. (1985). Indices of copper status in humans consuming a typical American diet containing either fructose or starch. The American journal of clinical nutrition, 42(2), 242–251. https://doi.org/10.1093/ajcn/42.2.242

[2021] Klevay, L. M., Inman, L., Johnson, L. K., Lawler, M., Mahalko, J. R., Milne, D. B., Lukaski, H. C., Bolonchuk, W., & Sandstead, H. H. (1984). Increased cholesterol in plasma in a young man during experimental copper depletion. Metabolism: clinical and experimental, 33(12), 1112–1118. https://doi.org/10.1016/0026-0495(84)90096-9

[2022] U.S. Department of Agriculture, Agricultural Research Service (2007) Continuing Survey of Food Intakes by Individuals 1994-96, 1998 and Diet and Health Knowledge Survey 1994-96, Food Surveys Research Group, Beltsville, MD

[2023] Klevay L. M. (2011). Is the Western diet adequate in copper?. Journal of trace elements in medicine and biology : organ of the Society for Minerals and Trace Elements (GMS), 25(4), 204–212. https://doi.org/10.1016/j.jtemb.2011.08.146

[2024] Knovich, M. A., Il'yasova, D., Ivanova, A., & Molnár, I. (2008). The association between serum copper and anaemia in the adult Second National Health and Nutrition Examination Survey (NHANES II) population. The British journal of nutrition, 99(6), 1226–1229. https://doi.org/10.1017/s0007114507864828

[2025] Klevay, L. M. (1998) Lack of a recommended dietary allowance for copper may be hazardous to your health. J. Am. Coll. Nutr.17:322–326.

[2026] Leslie M. Klevay, Denis M. Medeiros, Deliberations and Evaluations of the Approaches, Endpoints and Paradigms for Dietary Recommendations about Copper, The Journal of Nutrition, Volume 126, Issue suppl_9, September 1996, Pages 2419S–2426S, https://doi.org/10.1093/jn/126.suppl_9.2419S

[2027] Klevay, LM (1990) Ischemic heart disease: toward a unified theory. In Role of Copper in Lipid Metabolism, 1st ed., pp. 233–267 [KY Lei and TP Carr, editors]. Boca Raton, FL: CRC Press.

[2028] Klevay (1993) 'Copper in the western diet (Belgium, Canada, UK and USA)'. In Anke M, Meissner D, Mills CF (eds): "Proc. 8th Int. Symposium on Trace Elements in Man and Animals." Gersdorf, Germany: Verlag Media Tourishk, pp 207–210.

[2029] Klevay, L. M., Reck, S. J., & Barcome, D. F. (1979). Evidence of dietary copper and zinc deficiencies. JAMA, 241(18), 1916–1918. https://doi.org/10.1001/jama.1979.03290440038025

[2030] Kashian and Fathiavand (2015) 'Estimated daily intake of Fe, Cu, Ca and Zn through common cereals in Tehran, Iran', Food Chemistry, Volume 176, 1 June 2015, Pages 193-196.

[2031] Đermanović, M., Miletić, I. & Pavlović, Z. A Comparative Analysis of the Contents Of Iron, Zinc, Copper, Manganese, and Calcium in the Collective Diet Of Preschool Children in the Northwestern Region of Bosnia. Biol Trace Elem Res 175, 27–32 (2017). https://doi.org/10.1007/s12011-016-0755-7

[2032] Reiser et al (1987) 'Effect of copper intake on blood cholesterol and its lipoprotein distribution in men', Nutr. Rep. Int., 36 (1987), pp. 641-649.

[2033] Klevay, L. M., Inman, L., Johnson, L. K., Lawler, M., Mahalko, J. R., Milne, D. B., Lukaski, H. C., Bolonchuk, W., & Sandstead, H. H. (1984). Increased cholesterol in plasma in a young man during experimental copper depletion. Metabolism: clinical and experimental, 33(12), 1112–1118. https://doi.org/10.1016/0026-0495(84)90096-9

[2034] Reiser, S., Smith, J. C., Jr, Mertz, W., Holbrook, J. T., Scholfield, D. J., Powell, A. S., Canfield, W. K., & Canary, J. J. (1985). Indices of copper status in humans consuming a typical American diet containing either fructose or starch. The American journal of clinical nutrition, 42(2), 242–251. https://doi.org/10.1093/ajcn/42.2.242

[2035] Klevay LM, Canfield WK, Gallagher SK, Henriksen LK, Lukaski HC, Bolonchuk W, Johnson LK, Milne DB. Decreased glucose tolerance in two men during experimental copper depletion. Nutr Rep Int. 1986;33:371–382.

[2036] Lukaski, H.C., Klevay, L.M. & Milne, D.B. Effects of dietary copper on human autonomic cardiovascular function. Europ. J. Appl. Physiol. 58, 74–80 (1988). https://doi.org/10.1007/BF00636606

[2037] Willis et al (2005) 'Zinc-Induced Copper Deficiency: A Report of Three Cases Initially Recognized on Bone Marrow Examination', American Journal of Clinical Pathology, Volume 123, Issue 1, January 2005, Pages 125–131, https://doi.org/10.1309/V6GVYW2QTYD5C5PJ.

[2038] Chan and Mike (2014) 'The Science and Practice of Micronutrient Supplementations in Nutritional Anemia: An Evidence-Based Review', Journal of Parenteral and Enteral Nutrition 38(6), DOI: 10.1177/0148607114533726

[2039] Klevay et al (1995) 'The copper requirement of women losing weight exceeds 1.23 mg/day'. Am J Clin Nutr 61:909–909.

[2040] Błażewicz, A., Klatka, M., Astel, A. et al. Differences in Trace Metal Concentrations (Co, Cu, Fe, Mn, Zn, Cd, and Ni) in Whole Blood, Plasma, and Urine of Obese and Nonobese Children. Biol Trace Elem Res 155, 190–200 (2013). https://doi.org/10.1007/s12011-013-9783-8

[2041] Pinhas-Hamiel, O., Newfield, R., Koren, I. et al. Greater prevalence of iron deficiency in overweight and obese children and adolescents. Int J Obes 27, 416–418 (2003). https://doi.org/10.1038/sj.ijo.0802224

[2042] Ebesh, O., Barone, A., Harper, R. G., & Wapnir, R. A. (1999). Combined effect of high-fat diet and copper deficiency during gestation on fetal copper status in the rat. Biological trace element research, 67(2), 139–150. https://doi.org/10.1007/BF02784069

[2043] Jacob, R. A., Sandstead, H. H., Munoz, J. M., Klevay, L. M., & Milne, D. B. (1981). Whole body surface loss of trace metals in normal males. The American Journal of Clinical Nutrition, 34(7), 1379–1383. doi:10.1093/ajcn/34.7.1379

[2044] Cohn, J. R., & Emmett, E. A. (1978). The excretion of trace metals in human sweat. Annals of clinical and laboratory science, 8(4), 270–275.

[2045] CARTWRIGHT, G. E., GUBLER, C. J., & WINTROBE, M. M. (1954). Studies on copper metabolism. XI. Copper and iron metabolism in the nephrotic syndrome. The Journal of clinical investigation, 33(4), 685–698. https://doi.org/10.1172/JCI102939

[2046] Wapnir, R. A., & Devas, G. (1995). Copper deficiency: interaction with high-fructose and high-fat diets in rats. The American journal of clinical nutrition, 61(1), 105–110. https://doi.org/10.1093/ajcn/61.1.105

[2047] Song, M., Schuschke, D. A., Zhou, Z., Chen, T., Pierce, W. M., Wang, R., … McClain, C. J. (2012). High fructose feeding induces copper deficiency in Sprague–Dawley rats: A novel mechanism for obesity related fatty liver. Journal of Hepatology, 56(2), 433–440. doi:10.1016/j.jhep.2011.05.030

[2048] DiNicolantonio JJ, Mangan D, O'Keefe JH. The fructose–copper connection: Added sugars induce fatty liver and insulin resistance via copper deficiency. J. insul. resist. 2018;3(1), a43. https://doi.org/10.4102/jir.v3i1.43

[2049] Fields, M., Ferretti, R. J., Smith, J. C., & Reiser, S. (1984). The interaction of type of dietary carbohydrates with copper deficiency. The American Journal of Clinical Nutrition, 39(2), 289–295. doi:10.1093/ajcn/39.2.289

[2050] Reiser, S., Smith, J. C., Jr, Mertz, W., Holbrook, J. T., Scholfield, D. J., Powell, A. S., Canfield, W. K., & Canary, J. J. (1985). Indices of copper status in humans consuming a typical American diet containing either fructose or starch. The American journal of clinical nutrition, 42(2), 242–251. https://doi.org/10.1093/ajcn/42.2.242

[2051] Ito, S., Fujita, H., Narita, T., Yaginuma, T., Kawarada, Y., Kawagoe, M., & Sugiyama, T. (2001). Urinary copper excretion in type 2 diabetic patients with nephropathy. Nephron, 88(4), 307–312. https://doi.org/10.1159/000046013

[2052] Moon, P.-G., Lee, J.-E., You, S., Kim, T.-K., Cho, J.-H., Kim, I.-S., Kwon, T.-H., Kim, C.-D., Park, S.-H., Hwang, D., Kim, Y.-L. and Baek, M.-C. (2011), Proteomic analysis of urinary exosomes from patients of early IgA nephropathy and thin basement membrane nephropathy. Proteomics, 11: 2459-2475. https://doi.org/10.1002/pmic.201000443

[2053] Hacibekiroglu, T., Basturk, A., Akinci, S., Bakanay, S. M., Ulas, T., Guney, T., & Dilek, I. (2015). Evaluation of serum levels of zinc, copper, and Helicobacter pylori IgG and IgA in iron deficiency anemia cases. European review for medical and pharmacological sciences, 19(24), 4835–4840.

[2054] Berger et al (1992) 'Cutaneous copper and zinc losses in burns', Burns, Volume 18, Issue 5, October 1992, Pages 373-380, https://doi.org/10.1016/0305-4179(92)90035-S

[2055] Goyens, P., Brasseur, D., & Cadranel, S. (1985). Copper deficiency in infants with active celiac disease. Journal of pediatric gastroenterology and nutrition, 4(4), 677–680. https://doi.org/10.1097/00005176-198508000-00033

[2056] BRAGA, C. B. M., FERREIRA, I. M. de L., MARCHINI, J. S., & CUNHA, S. F. de C. da. (2015). COPPER AND MAGNESIUM DEFICIENCIES IN PATIENTS WITH SHORT BOWEL SYNDROME RECEIVING PARENTERAL NUTRITION OR ORAL FEEDING. Arquivos de Gastroenterologia, 52(2), 94–99. doi:10.1590/s0004-28032015000200004

[2057] Hujoel, I.A. (2020), Nutritional status in irritable bowel syndrome: A North American population-based study. JGH Open, 4: 656-662. https://doi.org/10.1002/jgh3.12311

[2058] Hoyle, G. S., Schwartz, R. P., & Auringer, S. T. (1999). Pseudoscurvy caused by copper deficiency. The Journal of pediatrics, 134(3), 379. https://doi.org/10.1016/s0022-3476(99)70470-1

[2059] Rapoport, Y., & Lavin, P. J. (2016). Nutritional Optic Neuropathy Caused by Copper Deficiency After Bariatric Surgery. Journal of neuro-ophthalmology : the official journal of the North American Neuro-Ophthalmology Society, 36(2), 178–181. https://doi.org/10.1097/WNO.0000000000000333

[2060] Stec, J., Podracká, L., Pavkovceková, O., & Kollár, J. (1990). Zinc and copper metabolism in nephrotic syndrome. Nephron, 56(2), 186–187. https://doi.org/10.1159/000186130

[2061] Moore, R. J., Hall, C. B., Carlson, E. C., Lukaski, H. C., & Klevay, L. M. (1989). Acute renal failure and fluid retention and kidney damage in copper-deficient rats fed a high-NaCl diet. The Journal of laboratory and clinical medicine, 113(4), 516–524.

[2062] Moss H. E. (2016). Bariatric Surgery and the Neuro-Ophthalmologist. Journal of neuro-ophthalmology : the official journal of the North American Neuro-Ophthalmology Society, 36(1), 78–84. https://doi.org/10.1097/WNO.0000000000000332

[2063] Goodman J. C. (2015). Neurological Complications of Bariatric Surgery. Current neurology and neuroscience reports, 15(12), 79. https://doi.org/10.1007/s11910-015-0597-2

[2064] Dalal et al (2015) 'Copper deficiency mimicking myelodysplastic syndrome', Clinical Case Reports 2015; 3(5): 325– 327.

[2065] Takikita, S., Takano, T., Narita, T., & Maruo, Y. (2015). Increased apoptosis and hypomyelination in cerebral white matter of macular mutant mouse brain. Molecular genetics and metabolism reports, 4, 25–29. https://doi.org/10.1016/j.ymgmr.2015.05.005

[2066] Mittal, S. O., & Machado, D. G. (2014). Hypocupremia: a possible association with late cortical cerebellar atrophy. Tremor and other hyperkinetic movements (New York, N.Y.), 4, 202. https://doi.org/10.7916/D8G44NHV

[2067] Shi, Y., Ivannikov, M. V., Walsh, M. E., Liu, Y., Zhang, Y., Jaramillo, C. A., Macleod, G. T., & Van Remmen, H. (2014). The lack of CuZnSOD leads to impaired neurotransmitter release, neuromuscular junction destabilization and reduced muscle strength in mice. PloS one, 9(6), e100834. https://doi.org/10.1371/journal.pone.0100834

[2068] Prohaska, J. R., & Heller, L. J. (1982). Mechanical properties of the copper-deficient rat heart. The Journal of nutrition, 112(11), 2142–2150. https://doi.org/10.1093/jn/112.11.2142

[2069] Li, Y., Wang, L., Schuschke, D. A., Zhou, Z., Saari, J. T., & Kang, Y. J. (2005). Marginal dietary copper restriction induces cardiomyopathy in rats. The Journal of nutrition, 135(9), 2130–2136. https://doi.org/10.1093/jn/135.9.2130

[2070] Dudakova et al (2015) 'Is copper imbalance an environmental factor influencing keratoconus development?', Medical Hypotheses, Volume 84, Issue 5, May 2015, Pages 518-524.

[2071] Yu, L., Liou, I.W., Biggins, S.W., Yeh, M., Jalikis, F., Chan, L.-N. and Burkhead, J. (2019), Copper Deficiency in Liver Diseases: A Case Series and Pathophysiological Considerations. Hepatol Commun, 3: 1159-1165. https://doi.org/10.1002/hep4.1393

[2072] Song, M., Zhou, Z., Chen, T., Zhang, J., & McClain, C. J. (2011). Copper deficiency exacerbates bile duct ligation-induced liver injury and fibrosis in rats. The Journal of pharmacology and experimental therapeutics, 339(1), 298–306. https://doi.org/10.1124/jpet.111.184325

623

[2073] Sakiyama, H., Fujiwara, N., Yoneoka, Y., Yoshihara, D., Eguchi, H., & Suzuki, K. (2016). Cu,Zn-SOD deficiency induces the accumulation of hepatic collagen. Free radical research, 50(6), 666–677. https://doi.org/10.3109/10715762.2016.1164856

[2074] Jung, K. H., Chu, K., Lee, S. T., Shin, Y. W., Lee, K. J., Park, D. K., Yoo, J. S., Kim, S., Kim, M., Lee, S. K., & Roh, J. K. (2016). Experimental Induction of Cerebral Aneurysms by Developmental Low Copper Diet. Journal of neuropathology and experimental neurology, 75(5), 455–463. https://doi.org/10.1093/jnen/nlw020

[2075] Jung, K. H., Chu, K., Lee, S. T., Shin, Y. W., Lee, K. J., Park, D. K., Yoo, J. S., Kim, S., Kim, M., Lee, S. K., & Roh, J. K. (2016). Experimental Induction of Cerebral Aneurysms by Developmental Low Copper Diet. Journal of neuropathology and experimental neurology, 75(5), 455–463. https://doi.org/10.1093/jnen/nlw020

[2076] Amorós, R., Murcia, M., González, L., Soler-Blasco, R., Rebagliato, M., Iñiguez, C., Carrasco, P., Vioque, J., Broberg, K., Levi, M., Lopez-Espinosa, M. J., Ballester, F., & Llop, S. (2019). Maternal copper status and neuropsychological development in infants and preschool children. International journal of hygiene and environmental health, 222(3), 503–512. https://doi.org/10.1016/j.ijheh.2019.01.007

[2077] Gambling, L., Kennedy, C., & McArdle, H. J. (2011). Iron and copper in fetal development. Seminars in cell & developmental biology, 22(6), 637–644. https://doi.org/10.1016/j.semcdb.2011.08.011

[2078] Duncan, A., Talwar, D., & Morrison, I. (2016). The predictive value of low plasma copper and high plasma zinc in detecting zinc-induced copper deficiency. Annals of clinical biochemistry, 53(Pt 5), 575–579. https://doi.org/10.1177/0004563215620821

[2079] Merza, H., Sood, N., & Sood, R. (2015). Idiopathic hyperzincemia with associated copper deficiency anemia: a diagnostic dilemma. Clinical Case Reports, 3(10), 819–822. doi:10.1002/ccr3.344

[2080] Prasad, R., Hawthorne, B., Durai, D., & McDowell, I. (2015). Zinc in denture adhesive: a rare cause of copper deficiency in a patient on home parenteral nutrition: Figure 1. BMJ Case Reports, bcr2015211390. doi:10.1136/bcr-2015-211390

[2081] Sierpinska, T., Konstantynowicz, J., Orywal, K., Golebiewska, M., & Szmitkowski, M. (2014). Copper deficit as a potential pathogenic factor of reduced bone mineral density and severe tooth wear. Osteoporosis international : a journal established as result of cooperation between the European Foundation for Osteoporosis and the National Osteoporosis Foundation of the USA, 25(2), 447–454. https://doi.org/10.1007/s00198-013-2410-x

[2082] Plantone, D., Renna, R., Primiano, G., Shukralla, A., & Koudriavtseva, T. (2015). PPIs as possible risk factor for copper deficiency myelopathy. Journal of the neurological sciences, 349(1-2), 258–259. https://doi.org/10.1016/j.jns.2015.01.009

[2083] Eife, R., Weiss, M., Müller-Höcker, M., Lang, T., Barros, V., Sigmund, B., Thanner, F., Welling, P., Lange, H., Wolf, W., Rodeck, B., Kittel, J., Schramel, P., & Reiter, K. (1999). Chronic poisoning by copper in tap water: II. Copper intoxications with predominantly systemic symptoms. European journal of medical research, 4(6), 224–228.

[2084] O'Donohue, J., Reid, M., Varghese, A., Portmann, B., & Williams, R. (1999). A case of adult chronic copper self-intoxication resulting in cirrhosis. European journal of medical research, 4(6), 252.

[2085] Ware (2017) 'Health benefits and risks of copper', Medical News Today, Accessed Online Dec 9 2020: https://www.medicalnewstoday.com/articles/288165

[2086] Pratt et al (1985) 'Lack of effects of copper gluconate supplementation', The American Journal of Clinical Nutrition, Volume 42, Issue 4, October 1985, Pages 681–682, https://doi.org/10.1093/ajcn/42.4.681.

[2087] O'Donohue, JW, Reid, MA, Varghese, A et al. (1993) 'Micronodular cirrhosis and acute liver failure due to chronic copper self-intoxication'. Eur J Gastroenterol 5, 561–562.

[2088] Turnlund et al (2005) 'Long-term high copper intake: effects on copper absorption, retention, and homeostasis in men', Am J Clin Nutr 2005;81:822– 8.

[2089] Turnlund, J. R., Keyes, W. R., Anderson, H. L., & Acord, L. L. (1989). Copper absorption and retention in young men at three levels of dietary copper by use of the stable isotope 65Cu. The American Journal of Clinical Nutrition, 49(5), 870–878. doi:10.1093/ajcn/49.5.870

[2090] Turnlund, J. R., Keyes, W. R., Peiffer, G. L., & Scott, K. C. (1998). Copper absorption, excretion, and retention by young men consuming low dietary copper determined by using the stable isotope 65Cu. The American journal of clinical nutrition, 67(6), 1219–1225. https://doi.org/10.1093/ajcn/67.6.1219

[2091] Harvey, L. J., Majsak-Newman, G., Dainty, J. R., Lewis, D. J., Langford, N. J., Crews, H. M., & Fairweather-Tait, S. J. (2003). Adaptive responses in men fed low- and high-copper diets. The British journal of nutrition, 90(1), 161–168. https://doi.org/10.1079/bjn2003887

[2092] Cashman, K., Baker, A., Ginty, F., Flynn, A., Strain, J., Bonham, M., … Sandström, B. (2001). No effect of copper supplementation on biochemical markers of bone metabolism in healthy young adult females despite apparently improved copper status. European Journal of Clinical Nutrition, 55(7), 525–531. doi:10.1038/sj.ejcn.1601177

[2093] Schroeder et al (1966) 'Essential trace metals in man: Copper', Journal of Chronic Diseases, Volume 19, Issue 9, September 1966, Pages 1007-1034.

[2094] Underwood (1962) 'Trace Elements in Human and Animal Nutrition 2nd Edn. Academic Press, New York.

[2095] Eife, R., Weiss, M., Barros, V., Sigmund, B., Goriup, U., Komb, D., Wolf, W., Kittel, J., Schramel, P., & Reiter, K. (1999). Chronic poisoning by copper in tap water: I. Copper intoxications with predominantly gastrointestinal symptoms. European journal of medical research, 4(6), 219–223.

[2096] (1965). Copper Deficiency in Malnourished Infants. Nutrition Reviews, 23(6)

[2097] Fujita, M., Itakura, T., Takagi, Y., & Okada, A. (1989). Copper deficiency during total parenteral nutrition: clinical analysis of three cases. JPEN. Journal of parenteral and enteral nutrition, 13(4), 421–425. https://doi.org/10.1177/0148607189013004421

[2098] Hassan et al (2000) 'Zinc-induced copper deficiency in a coin swallower', The American Journal of Gastroenterology, Volume 95, Issue 10, October 2000, Pages 2975-2977. https://doi.org/10.1016/S0002-9270(00)01128-X

[2099] Gyorffy, E. J., & Chan, H. (1992). Copper deficiency and microcytic anemia resulting from prolonged ingestion of over-the-counter zinc. The American journal of gastroenterology, 87(8), 1054–1055.

[2100] Naveh, Y., Hazani, A., & Berant, M. (1981). Copper deficiency with cow's milk diet. Pediatrics, 68(3), 397–400.

[2101] Karan, S., & Pathak, A. (1975). Systemic bone disease associated with low serum copper levels in preterm low-birth weight twin infants. Indian pediatrics, 12(9), 903–906.

[2102] Kawada, E., Moridaira, K., Itoh, K., Hoshino, A., Tamura, J., & Morita, T. (2006). In long-term bedridden elderly patients with dietary copper deficiency, biochemical markers of bone resorption are increased with copper supplementation during 12 weeks. Annals of nutrition & metabolism, 50(5), 420–424. https://doi.org/10.1159/000094633

[2103] Cordano, A., & Grahma, G. G. (1966). Copper deficiency complicating severe chronic intestinal malabsorption. Pediatrics, 38(4), 596–604.

[2104] Danks (1988) 'Copper Deficiency in Humans', Annual Review of Nutrition, Volume 8, Danks, pp 235-257.

[2105] Williams D. M. (1983). Copper deficiency in humans. Seminars in hematology, 20(2), 118–128.

[2106] Knobeloch, L., Schubert, C., Hayes, J., Clark, J., Fitzgerald, C., & Fraundorff, A. (1998). Gastrointestinal upsets and new copper plumbing--is there a connection?. WMJ : official publication of the State Medical Society of Wisconsin, 97(1), 49–53.

[2107] Oon and Yap (2006) 'Acute copper toxicity following copper glycinate injection', Internal Medicine Journal 36(11):741-3, DOI: 10.1111/j.1445-5994.2006.01195.x

[2108] Olivares, M., & Uauy, R. (1996). Copper as an essential nutrient. The American Journal of Clinical Nutrition, 63(5), 791S–796S. doi:10.1093/ajcn/63.5.791

[2109] Medeiros, D.M. Perspectives on the Role and Relevance of Copper in Cardiac Disease. Biol Trace Elem Res 176, 10–19 (2017). https://doi.org/10.1007/s12011-016-0807-z

[2110] Nargund, S., Qiu, J., & Goudar, C. T. (2015). Elucidating the role of copper in CHO cell energy metabolism using (13)C metabolic flux analysis. Biotechnology progress, 31(5), 1179–1186. https://doi.org/10.1002/btpr.2131

[2111] Chan et al (2014) 'The Science and Practice of Micronutrient Supplementations in Nutritional Anemia: An Evidence-Based Review', Journal of Parenteral and Enteral Nutrition 38(6), DOI: 10.1177/0148607114533726.

[2112] Bo, S., Durazzo, M., Gambino, R., Berutti, C., Milanesio, N., Caropreso, A., … Pagano, G. (2008). Associations of Dietary and Serum Copper with Inflammation, Oxidative Stress, and Metabolic Variables in Adults. The Journal of Nutrition, 138(2), 305–310. doi:10.1093/jn/138.2.305

[2113] Mirastschijski, U., Martin, A., Jorgensen, L. N., Sampson, B., & Ågren, M. S. (2013). Zinc, Copper, and Selenium Tissue Levels and Their Relation to Subcutaneous Abscess, Minor Surgery, and Wound Healing in Humans. Biological Trace Element Research, 153(1-3), 76–83. doi:10.1007/s12011-013-9658-z

[2114] Malek, F., Jiresova, E., Dohnalova, A., Koprivova, H., & Spacek, R. (2006). Serum copper as a marker of inflammation in prediction of short term outcome in high risk patients with chronic heart failure. International journal of cardiology, 113(2), e51–e53. https://doi.org/10.1016/j.ijcard.2006.05.022

[2115] Bui, V.Q., Stein, A.D., DiGirolamo, A.M. et al. Associations between Serum C-reactive Protein and Serum Zinc, Ferritin, and Copper in Guatemalan School Children. Biol Trace Elem Res 148, 154–160 (2012). https://doi.org/10.1007/s12011-012-9358-0

[2116] Klevay L. M. (2016). Improving accuracy of normal serum copper. Journal of trace elements in medicine and biology : organ of the Society for Minerals and Trace Elements (GMS), 34, 38. https://doi.org/10.1016/j.jtemb.2015.10.005

[2117] Mielcarz, G., Howard, A. N., Mielcarz, B., Williams, N. R., Rajput-Williams, J., Nigdigar, S. V., & Stone, D. L. (2001). Leucocyte copper, a marker of copper body status is low in coronary artery disease. Journal of Trace Elements in Medicine and Biology, 15(1), 31–35. doi:10.1016/s0946-672x(01)80023-7

[2118] KINSMAN, G. D., HOWARD, A. N., STONE, D. L., & MULLINS, P. A. (1990). Studies in copper status and atherosclerosis. Biochemical Society Transactions, 18(6), 1186–1188. doi:10.1042/bst0181186

[2119] Fletcher, D. J. (1982). Hair analysis. Postgraduate Medicine, 72(5), 79–88. doi:10.1080/00325481.1982.11716248

[2120] HAMMER, D. I., FINKLEA, J. F., HENDRICKS, R. H., SHY, C. M., & HORTON, R. J. M. (1971). HAIR TRACE METAL LEVELS AND ENVIRONMENTAL EXPOSURE. American Journal of Epidemiology, 93(2), 84–92. doi:10.1093/oxfordjournals.aje.a121238

[2121] Dittmer, K. E., Hitchcock, B., McDougall, S., & Hunnam, J. C. (2016). Pathophysiology of humeral fractures in a sample of dairy heifers. New Zealand veterinary journal, 64(4), 230–237. https://doi.org/10.1080/00480169.2016.1171173

[2122] Mao, S., Zhang, A., & Huang, S. (2014). Meta-analysis of Zn, Cu and Fe in the hair of Chinese children with recurrent respiratory tract infection. Scandinavian journal of clinical and laboratory investigation, 74(7), 561–567. https://doi.org/10.3109/00365513.2014.921323

[2123] Halfdanarson, T. R., Kumar, N., Li, C.-Y., Phyliky, R. L., & Hogan, W. J. (2008). Hematological manifestations of copper deficiency: a retrospective review. European Journal of Haematology, 80(6), 523–531. doi:10.1111/j.1600-0609.2008.01050.x

[2124] Gabreyes, A. A., Abbasi, H. N., Forbes, K. P., McQuaker, G., Duncan, A., & Morrison, I. (2013). Hypocupremia associated cytopenia and myelopathy: a national retrospective review. European journal of haematology, 90(1), 1–9. https://doi.org/10.1111/ejh.12020

[2125] Harvey, L., & McArdle, H. (2008). Biomarkers of copper status: A brief update. British Journal of Nutrition, 99(S3), S10-S13. doi:10.1017/S0007114508006806

[2126] Manson, P., & Zlotkin, S. (1985). Hair analysis--a critical review. Canadian Medical Association journal, 133(3), 186–188.

[2127] Afridi et al (2013) 'Distribution of Copper, Iron, and Zinc in Biological Samples of Pakistani Hypertensive Patients and Referent Subjects of Different Age Groups', Clinical Laboratory 59(9-10):959-67, DOI: 10.7754/Clin.Lab.2012.120704

[2128] Laker M. (1982). On determining trace element levels in man: the uses of blood and hair. Lancet (London, England), 2(8292), 260–262. https://doi.org/10.1016/s0140-6736(82)90336-1

[2129] Aggett, P. J., & Harries, J. T. (1979). Current status of zinc in health and disease states. Archives of Disease in Childhood, 54(12), 909–917. doi:10.1136/adc.54.12.909

[2130] Wilhelm, M., Ohnesorge, F. K., Lombeck, I., & Hafner, D. (1989). Uptake of Aluminum, Cadmium, Copper, Lead, and Zinc by Human Scalp Hair and Elution of the Adsorbed Metals. Journal of Analytical Toxicology, 13(1), 17–21. doi:10.1093/jat/13.1.17

[2131] McNeill et al (2008) 'The Neurological Presentation of Ceruloplasmin Gene Mutations', European Neurology 60(4):200-205, DOI: 10.1159/000148691

[2132] Oakes et al (2008) 'Acute inflammatory response does not affect erythrocyte concentrations of copper, zinc and selenium', Clinical Nutrition, Volume 27, Issue 1, February 2008, Pages 115-120.

[2133] Jardim-Botelho and Gurgel (2015) 'Micronutrient deficiencies in normal and overweight infants in a low socio-economic population in north-east Brazil', Paediatrics and International Child Health 36(3):2046905515Y0000000035

[2134] Institute of Medicine (2001) 'Food and Nutrition Board. Dietary Reference Intakes for Vitamin A, Vitamin K, Arsenic, Boron, Chromium, Copper, Iodine, Iron, Manganese, Molybdenum, Nickel, Silicon, Vanadium, and Zinc : a Report of the Panel on Micronutrients', Washington, DC: National Academy Press.

[2135] Leonard (2018) 'What to know about ferritin blood tests for anemia', Medical News Today, Accessed Online Dec 9 2020 https://www.medicalnewstoday.com/articles/323713

[2136] Camaschella C. (2015). Iron-deficiency anemia. The New England journal of medicine, 372(19), 1832–1843. https://doi.org/10.1056/NEJMra1401038

[2137] Reynolds, L. G., & Klein, M. (1985). Iron poisoning--a preventable hazard of childhood. South African medical journal = Suid-Afrikaanse tydskrif vir geneeskunde, 67(17), 680–683.

[2138] Chang, T. P., & Rangan, C. (2011). Iron poisoning: a literature-based review of epidemiology, diagnosis, and management. Pediatric emergency care, 27(10), 978–985. https://doi.org/10.1097/PEC.0b013e3182302604

[2139] Manoguerra, A. S., Erdman, A. R., Booze, L. L., Christianson, G., Wax, P. M., Scharman, E. J., Woolf, A. D., Chyka, P. A., Keyes, D. C., Olson, K. R., Caravati, E. M., & Troutman, W. G. (2005). Iron ingestion: an evidence-based consensus guideline for out-of-hospital management. Clinical toxicology (Philadelphia, Pa.), 43(6), 553–570. https://doi.org/10.1081/clt-200068842

[2140] Pietrangelo A. (2010). Hereditary hemochromatosis: pathogenesis, diagnosis, and treatment. Gastroenterology, 139(2), 393–408.e4082. https://doi.org/10.1053/j.gastro.2010.06.013

[2141] Gordeuk V. R. (2002). African iron overload. Seminars in hematology, 39(4), 263–269. https://doi.org/10.1053/shem.2002.35636

[2142] NIH (2020) 'Iron: Fact Sheet for Health Professionals', Dietary Supplement Fact Sheets, Accessed Online Dec 9 2020: https://ods.od.nih.gov/factsheets/Iron-HealthProfessional/

[2143] Valenzuela, C., de Romaña, D. L., Olivares, M., Morales, M. S., & Pizarro, F. (2009). Total iron and heme iron content and their distribution in beef meat and viscera. Biological trace element research, 132(1-3), 103–111. https://doi.org/10.1007/s12011-009-8400-3

[2144] NIH (2020) 'Copper: Fact Sheet for Health Professionals', Dietary Supplement Fact Sheets, Accessed Online Dec 9 2020: https://ods.od.nih.gov/factsheets/Copper-HealthProfessional/

[2145] Lurie et al (1989) 'The copper content of foods based on a critical evaluation of published analytical data'. J Food Comp Anal 2:298–316.

[2146] SELF Nutrition Data (2018) 'Foods highest in Copper', Accessed Online Dec 9 2020: https://nutritiondata.self.com/foods-000125000000000000000-w.html

[2147] Klevay, L. M., & Wildman, R. E. C. (2002). Meat diets and fragile bones: Inferences about osteoporosis. Journal of Trace Elements in Medicine and Biology, 16(3), 149–154. doi:10.1016/s0946-672x(02)80017-7

[2148] Brzozowska A. (1989). Interakcje zelaza, cynku i miedzi w organizmie zwierzat i człowieka [Interaction of iron, zinc and copper in the body of animals and humans]. Roczniki Panstwowego Zakladu Higieny, 40(4-6), 302–312.

[2149] Wan, Q., Yang, B. S., & Kato, N. (1996). Feeding of excessive cystine and cysteine enhances defects of dietary copper deficiency in rats by differential mechanisms involving altered iron status. Journal of nutritional science and vitaminology, 42(3), 185–193. https://doi.org/10.3177/jnsv.42.185

[2150] Whitbread (2020) 'Top 10 Foods Highest in Cystine (Cysteine)', My Food Data, USDA Nutrition Data, Accessed Online Dec 10 2020: https://www.myfooddata.com/articles/high-cystine-foods.php

[2151] WILLIAMS, P. (2007). Nutritional composition of red meat. Nutrition & Dietetics, 64(s4 The Role of), S113–S119. doi:10.1111/j.1747-0080.2007.00197.x

[2152] Foster, M., & Samman, S. (2015). Vegetarian diets across the lifecycle: impact on zinc intake and status. Advances in food and nutrition research, 74, 93–131. https://doi.org/10.1016/bs.afnr.2014.11.003

[2153] Hunt, J. R., & Vanderpool, R. A. (2001). Apparent copper absorption from a vegetarian diet. The American Journal of Clinical Nutrition, 74(6), 803–807. doi:10.1093/ajcn/74.6.803

[2154] Lee, D.-Y., Schroeder, J., & Gordon, D. T. (1988). Enhancement of Cu Bioavailability in the Rat by Phytic Acid. The Journal of Nutrition, 118(6), 712–717. doi:10.1093/jn/118.6.712

[2155] Abdulla et al (1981) 'Nutrient intake and health status of vegans. Chemical analyses of diets using the duplicate portion sampling technique', American Journal of Clinical Nutrition, Volume 34, Issue 11, 1981, Pages 2464-2477.

[2156] Donovan and Gibson (1996) 'Dietary intakes of adolescent females consuming vegetarian, semi-vegetarian, and omnivorous diets', Journal of Adolescent Health, Volume 18, Issue 4, April 1996, Pages 292-300. https://doi.org/10.1016/1054-139X(95)00133-D

[2157] Janet R Hunt, Richard A Vanderpool, Apparent copper absorption from a vegetarian diet, The American Journal of Clinical Nutrition, Volume 74, Issue 6, December 2001, Pages 803–807, https://doi.org/10.1093/ajcn/74.6.803

[2158] Behall, K. M., Scholfield, D. J., Lee, K., Powell, A. S., & Moser, P. B. (1987). Mineral balance in adult men: effect of four refined fibers. The American journal of clinical nutrition, 46(2), 307–314. https://doi.org/10.1093/ajcn/46.2.307

[2159] Saari, J. T., Reeves, P. G., Johnson, W. T., & Johnson, L. K. (2006). Pinto beans are a source of highly bioavailable copper in rats. The Journal of nutrition, 136(12), 2999–3004. https://doi.org/10.1093/jn/136.12.2999

[2160] Ducros, V., Arnaud, J., Tahiri, M., Coudray, C., Bornet, F., Bouteloup-Demange, C., Brouns, F., Rayssiguier, Y., & Roussel, A. M. (2005). Influence of short-chain fructo-oligosaccharides (sc-FOS) on absorption of Cu, Zn, and Se in healthy postmenopausal women. Journal of the American College of Nutrition, 24(1), 30–37. https://doi.org/10.1080/07315724.2005.10719440

[2161] Lönnerdal, B., Bell, J. G., & Keen, C. L. (1985). Copper absorption from human milk, cow's milk, and infant formulas using a suckling rat model. The American journal of clinical nutrition, 42(5), 836–844. https://doi.org/10.1093/ajcn/42.5.836

[2162] Davis, P. N., Norris, L. C., & Kratzer, F. H. (1962). Interference of soybean proteins with the utilization of trace minerals. The Journal of nutrition, 77(2), 217–223. https://doi.org/10.1093/jn/77.2.217

[2163] De Romaña, D. L., Olivares, M., Uauy, R., & Araya, M. (2011). Risks and benefits of copper in light of new insights of copper homeostasis. Journal of Trace Elements in Medicine and Biology, 25(1), 3–13. doi:10.1016/j.jtemb.2010.11.004

[2164] Klevay L. M. (1975). Coronary heart disease: the zinc/copper hypothesis. The American journal of clinical nutrition, 28(7), 764–774. https://doi.org/10.1093/ajcn/28.7.764

[2165] Klevay, L. M., & Hyg, S. D. (1973). Hypercholesterolemia in rats produced by an increase in the ratio of zinc to copper ingested. The American Journal of Clinical Nutrition, 26(10), 1060–1068. doi:10.1093/ajcn/26.10.1060

[2166] Neggers, Y. H., Bindon, J. R., & Dressler, W. W. (2001). The relationship between zinc and copper status and lipid levels in African-Americans. Biological trace element research, 79(1), 1–13. https://doi.org/10.1385/BTER:79:1:01

627

[2167] Lutfi, M. F., Elhakeem, R. F., Khogaly, R. S., Abdrabo, A. A., Ali, A. B., Gasim, G. I., & Adam, I. (2015). Zinc and copper levels are not correlated with angiographically-defined coronary artery disease in sudanese patients. Frontiers in Physiology, 6. doi:10.3389/fphys.2015.00191

[2168] Mielcarz, G., Howard, A. N., Mielcarz, B., Williams, N. R., Rajput-Williams, J., Nigdigar, S. V., & Stone, D. L. (2001). Leucocyte copper, a marker of copper body status is low in coronary artery disease. Journal of Trace Elements in Medicine and Biology, 15(1), 31–35. doi:10.1016/s0946-672x(01)80023-7

[2169] KINSMAN, G. D., HOWARD, A. N., STONE, D. L., & MULLINS, P. A. (1990). Studies in copper status and atherosclerosis. Biochemical Society Transactions, 18(6), 1186–1188. doi:10.1042/bst0181186

[2170] Ghayour-Mobarhan, M., Shapouri-Moghaddam, A., Azimi-Nezhad, M., Esmaeili, H., Parizadeh, S. M., Safarian, M., Kazemi-Bajestani, S. M., Khodaei, G. H., Hosseini, S. J., Parizadeh, S. M., & Ferns, G. A. (2009). The relationship between established coronary risk factors and serum copper and zinc concentrations in a large Persian cohort. Journal of trace elements in medicine and biology : organ of the Society for Minerals and Trace Elements (GMS), 23(3), 167–175. https://doi.org/10.1016/j.jtemb.2009.03.006

[2171] Singh, R. B., Niaz, M. A., Rastogi, S. S., Bajaj, S., Gaoli, Z., & Shoumin, Z. (1998). Current zinc intake and risk of diabetes and coronary artery disease and factors associated with insulin resistance in rural and urban populations of North India. Journal of the American College of Nutrition, 17(6), 564–570. https://doi.org/10.1080/07315724.1998.10718804

[2172] Reunanen, A., Knekt, P., Marniemi, J., Mäki, J., Maatela, J., & Aromaa, A. (1996). Serum calcium, magnesium, copper and zinc and risk of cardiovascular death. European journal of clinical nutrition, 50(7), 431–437.

[2173] Olusi, S., Al-Awadhi, A., Abiaka, C., Abraham, M., & George, S. (2003). Serum copper levels and not zinc are positively associated with serum leptin concentrations in the healthy adult population. Biological trace element research, 91(2), 137–144. https://doi.org/10.1385/BTER:91:2:137

[2174] Yuzbasiyan-Gurkan, V., Grider, A., Nostrant, T., Cousins, R. J., & Brewer, G. J. (1992). Treatment of Wilson's disease with zinc: X. Intestinal metallothionein induction. The Journal of laboratory and clinical medicine, 120(3), 380–386.

[2175] Fox P. L. (2003). The copper-iron chronicles: the story of an intimate relationship. Biometals : an international journal on the role of metal ions in biology, biochemistry, and medicine, 16(1), 9–40. https://doi.org/10.1023/a:1020799512190

[2176] Duncan, A., Yacoubian, C., Watson, N., & Morrison, I. (2015). The risk of copper deficiency in patients prescribed zinc supplements. Journal of Clinical Pathology, 68(9), 723–725. doi:10.1136/jclinpath-2014-202837

[2177] Duncan, A., Gallacher, G., & Willox, L. (2016). The role of the clinical biochemist in detection of zinc-induced copper deficiency. Annals of Clinical Biochemistry, 53(2), 298–301. doi:10.1177/0004563215595429

[2178] Yadrick, M. K., Kenney, M. A., & Winterfeldt, E. A. (1989). Iron, copper, and zinc status: response to supplementation with zinc or zinc and iron in adult females. The American Journal of Clinical Nutrition, 49(1), 145–150. doi:10.1093/ajcn/49.1.145

[2179] Klevay et al (1994) 'Decreased high density lipoprotein cholesterol and apoprotein A-I in plasma and ultrastructural pathology in cardiac muscle of young pigs fed a diet high in zinc', Nutrition Research, Volume 14, Issue 8, August 1994, Pages 1227-1239. https://doi.org/10.1016/S0271-5317(05)80249-0

[2180] Iskandar, M., Swist, E., Trick, K. D., Wang, B., L'Abbé, M. R., & Bertinato, J. (2005). Copper Chaperone for Cu/Zn Superoxide Dismutase is a sensitive biomarker of mild copper deficiency induced by moderately high intakes of zinc. Nutrition Journal, 4(1). doi:10.1186/1475-2891-4-35

[2181] Fischer, P. W., Giroux, A., & L'Abbé, M. R. (1984). Effect of zinc supplementation on copper status in adult man. The American Journal of Clinical Nutrition, 40(4), 743–746. doi:10.1093/ajcn/40.4.743

[2182] Yadrick, M. K., Kenney, M. A., & Winterfeldt, E. A. (1989). Iron, copper, and zinc status: response to supplementation with zinc or zinc and iron in adult females. The American Journal of Clinical Nutrition, 49(1), 145–150. doi:10.1093/ajcn/49.1.145

[2183] Uriu-Adams, J. Y., & Keen, C. L. (2005). Copper, oxidative stress, and human health. Molecular Aspects of Medicine, 26(4-5), 268–298. doi:10.1016/j.mam.2005.07.015

[2184] Goodwin, J. S., Hunt, W. C., Hooper, P., & Garry, P. J. (1985). Relationship between zinc intake, physical activity, and blood levels of high-density lipoprotein cholesterol in a healthy elderly population. Metabolism: clinical and experimental, 34(6), 519–523. https://doi.org/10.1016/0026-0495(85)90187-8

[2185] Institute of Medicine (2002) 'Zinc. Dietary reference intakes: vitamin A, vitamin K, arsenic, boron, chromium, copper, iodine, iron, manganese, molybdenum, nickel, silicon, vanadium, and zinc. Food and Nutrition Board. National Academy Press, Washington, DC, pp. 442–501.

[2186] Sandstead H. H. (1995). Requirements and toxicity of essential trace elements, illustrated by zinc and copper. The American journal of clinical nutrition, 61(3 Suppl), 621S–624S. https://doi.org/10.1093/ajcn/61.3.621S

628

[2187] Prasad et al (2000) 'Duration of Symptoms and Plasma Cytokine Levels in Patients with the Common Cold Treated with Zinc Acetate A Randomized, Double-Blind, Placebo-Controlled Trial', Annals of Internal Medicine 133(4):245-52.

[2188] Rowin, J. (2005). Copper deficiency myeloneuropathy and pancytopenia secondary to overuse of zinc supplementation. Journal of Neurology, Neurosurgery & Psychiatry, 76(5), 750–751. doi:10.1136/jnnp.2004.046987

[2189] Hedera, P., Fink, J. K., Bockenstedt, P. L., & Brewer, G. J. (2003). Myelopolyneuropathy and pancytopenia due to copper deficiency and high zinc levels of unknown origin: further support for existence of a new zinc overload syndrome. Archives of neurology, 60(9), 1303–1306. https://doi.org/10.1001/archneur.60.9.1303

[2190] Kumar et al (2004) 'Copper deficiency myelopathy produces a clinical picture like subacute combined degeneration', Neurology, July 13, 2004; 63 (1), DOI: https://doi.org/10.1212/01.WNL.0000132644.52613.FA

[2191] Tan, J. C., Burns, D. L., & Jones, H. R. (2006). Severe ataxia, myelopathy, and peripheral neuropathy due to acquired copper deficiency in a patient with history of gastrectomy. JPEN. Journal of parenteral and enteral nutrition, 30(5), 446–450. https://doi.org/10.1177/0148607106030005446

[2192] Nations, S. P., Boyer, P. J., Love, L. A., Burritt, M. F., Butz, J. A., Wolfe, G. I., Hynan, L. S., Reisch, J., & Trivedi, J. R. (2008). Denture cream: an unusual source of excess zinc, leading to hypocupremia and neurologic disease. Neurology, 71(9), 639–643. https://doi.org/10.1212/01.wnl.0000312375.79881.94

[2193] Hedera, P., Peltier, A., Fink, J. K., Wilcock, S., London, Z., & Brewer, G. J. (2009). Myelopolyneuropathy and pancytopenia due to copper deficiency and high zinc levels of unknown origin II. The denture cream is a primary source of excessive zinc. Neurotoxicology, 30(6), 996–999. https://doi.org/10.1016/j.neuro.2009.08.008

[2194] Shah NB, Gounaris MC, Holeva KT, inventors. Richarson-Vicks, Inc, assignee. Denture stabilizing zinc and strontium salts of AVE/MA copolymer. 4758630. US patent. 1988 Jul 19.

[2195] Wapnir (1998) 'Copper absorption and bioavailability', The American Journal of Clinical Nutrition, Volume 67, Issue 5, May 1998, Pages 1054S–1060S, https://doi.org/10.1093/ajcn/67.5.1054S

[2196] Nikolić, M., Nikić, D., & Petrović, B. (2008). Fruit and vegetable intake and the risk for developing coronary heart disease. Central European journal of public health, 16(1), 17–20.

[2197] Dauchet et al (2006) 'Fruit and Vegetable Consumption and Risk of Coronary Heart Disease: A Meta-Analysis of Cohort Studies ', The Journal of Nutrition, Volume 136, Issue 10, October 2006, Pages 2588–2593, https://doi.org/10.1093/jn/136.10.2588

[2198] Joshipura, K. J., Hu, F. B., Manson, J. E., Stampfer, M. J., Rimm, E. B., Speizer, F. E., Colditz, G., Ascherio, A., Rosner, B., Spiegelman, D., & Willett, W. C. (2001). The effect of fruit and vegetable intake on risk for coronary heart disease. Annals of internal medicine, 134(12), 1106–1114. https://doi.org/10.7326/0003-4819-134-12-200106190-00010

[2199] Klevay, L. M., 1975a, The ratio of zinc to copper of diets in the United States, Nutr. Rep. Int 11: 237.

[2200] Shamah-Levy, T., Villalpando, S., Jáuregui, A., & Rivera, J. A. (2012). Overview of the nutritional status of selected micronutrients in Mexican children in 2006. Salud publica de Mexico, 54(2), 146–151.

[2201] Cruz-Góngora et al (2012) 'Anemia and Iron, Zinc, Copper and Magnesium deficiency in Mexican adolescents: National Health and Nutrition Survey 2006', Salud publica de Mexico 54(2):135-45, DOI: 10.1590/S0036-36342012000200009

[2202] Barquera et al (2006) 'Energy and nutrient consumption in adults: analysis of the Mexican National Health and Nutrition Survey 2006', Salud Publica Mex 2009;51 Suppl 4:S562-573.

[2203] Bellof, G., Most, E., & Pallauf, J. (2007). Concentration of copper, iron, manganese and zinc in muscle, fat and bone tissue of lambs of the breed German Merino Landsheep in the course of the growing period and different feeding intensities. Journal of Animal Physiology and Animal Nutrition, 91(3-4), 100–108. doi:10.1111/j.1439-0396.2006.00648.x

[2204] WILLIAMS, P. (2007). Nutritional composition of red meat. Nutrition & Dietetics, 64(s4 The Role of), S113–S119. doi:10.1111/j.1747-0080.2007.00197.x

[2205] Bellof, G., Most, E., & Pallauf, J. (2007). Concentration of copper, iron, manganese and zinc in muscle, fat and bone tissue of lambs of the breed German Merino Landsheep in the course of the growing period and different feeding intensities. Journal of Animal Physiology and Animal Nutrition, 91(3-4), 100–108. doi:10.1111/j.1439-0396.2006.00648.x

[2206] SELF Nutrition Data (2018) 'Beef, variety meats and by-products, liver, cooked, pan-fried', Beef Products, Accessed Online Dec 10 2020: https://nutritiondata.self.com/facts/beef-products/3470/2

[2207] Jacob RA, Baesler LG, Klevay LM, Lee DE, and Wherry PL (1977) HyperchoLesterolemia in mice with meat anemia. Nutr. Rep. Int. 16:73-79

[2208] Fuhrman, J., Sarter, B., Glaser, D., & Acocella, S. (2010). Changing perceptions of hunger on a high nutrient density diet. Nutrition Journal, 9(1). doi:10.1186/1475-2891-9-51

[2209] Sandstead H. H. (1973). Zinc nutrition in the United States. The American journal of clinical nutrition, 26(11), 1251–1260. https://doi.org/10.1093/ajcn/26.11.1251

[2210] U.S. Department of Agriculture (2019), 'Agricultural Research Service'. Food Data Central.

629

[2211] NIH (2020) 'Zinc: Fact Sheet for Health Professionals', Dietary Supplement Fact Sheets, Accessed Online Dec 10 2020: https://ods.od.nih.gov/factsheets/Zinc-HealthProfessional/

[2212] Whitbread (2020) 'Top 10 Foods Highest in Zinc', My Food Data, Accessed Online Dec 10 2020: https://www.myfooddata.com/articles/high-zinc-foods.php

[2213] Klevay (1974) 'The ratio of zinc to copper in milk and mortality due to coronary heart disease: An association', in Trace Substances in Environmental Health VIII. D.D. Hemphill, ed. University of Missouri Press, Columbia, pp. 9–14.

[2214] Klevay, L. M. (1975). The ratio of zinc to copper of diets in the United States. Nutrition reports international, 11, 237.

[2215] Klevay, L. M. (1972). Coronary heart disease: the zinc/copper hypothesis. The American Journal of Clinical Nutrition, 28(7), 764–774. doi:10.1093/ajcn/28.7.764

[2216] Macfarlane (2017) 'Understanding Cronometer's Nutrient Ratios – Zinc/Copper', Cronometer, Nutrition, Accessed Online Dec 10 2020: https://cronometer.com/blog/nutrient-ratios-zinccopper/

[2217] Prather (2001) 'Valentine's Day Lovers Delight: Chocolate Is Rich in Dietary Copper!', Copper Development Association Inc., Accessed Online Nov 4 2020: https://www.copper.org/about/pressreleases/2001/ValentinesDay.html

[2218] Tokuda, Y., Kashima, M., Kayo, M., Nakazato, N., & Stein, G. H. (2006). Cocoa supplementation for copper deficiency associated with tube feeding nutrition. Internal medicine (Tokyo, Japan), 45(19), 1079–1085. https://doi.org/10.2169/internalmedicine.45.1525

[2219] Copper Development Association Inc. (2001) 'Valentine's Day Lovers Delight: Chocolate Is Rich in Dietary Copper!', 2001 Press Releases, Accessed Online Dec 10 2020: https://www.copper.org/about/pressreleases/2001/ValentinesDay.html

[2220] Arthington, J. D., Corah, L. R., & Blecha, F. (1996). The effect of molybdenum-induced copper deficiency on acute-phase protein concentrations, superoxide dismutase activity, leukocyte numbers, and lymphocyte proliferation in beef heifers inoculated with bovine herpesvirus-1. Journal of animal science, 74(1), 211–217. https://doi.org/10.2527/1996.741211x

[2221] Flores et al (2011) 'Trace elements status in diabetes mellitus type 2: Possible role of the interaction between molybdenum and copper in the progress of typical complications', Diabetes Research and Clinical Practice, Volume 91, Issue 3, March 2011, Pages 333-341.

[2222] Frank et al (2002) 'Myocardial cytochrome c oxidase activity in Swedish moose (Alces alces L.) affected by molybdenosis', Science of The Total Environment, Volume 290, Issues 1–3, 6 May 2002, Pages 121-129.

[2223] Frank et al (2000) 'A syndrome of molybdenosis, copper deficiency, and type 2 diabetes in the moose population of south-west Sweden', Science of The Total Environment, Volume 249, Issues 1–3, 17 April 2000, Pages 123-131, https://doi.org/10.1016/S0048-9697(99)00516-1

[2224] Frank (1998) ''Mysterious' moose disease in Sweden. Similarities to copper deficiency and/or molybdenosis in cattle and sheep. Biochemical background of clinical signs and organ lesions', Science of The Total Environment, Volume 209, Issue 1, 8 January 1998, Pages 17-26. https://doi.org/10.1016/S0048-9697(97)00303-3

[2225] Frank A. (2004). A review of the "mysterious" wasting disease in Swedish moose (Alces alces L.) related to molybdenosis and disturbances in copper metabolism. Biological trace element research, 102(1-3), 143–159. https://doi.org/10.1385/BTER:102:1-3:143

[2226] Yu, L., Liou, I.W., Biggins, S.W., Yeh, M., Jalikis, F., Chan, L.-N. and Burkhead, J. (2019), Copper Deficiency in Liver Diseases: A Case Series and Pathophysiological Considerations. Hepatol Commun, 3: 1159-1165. https://doi.org/10.1002/hep4.1393

[2227] Song, M., Zhou, Z., Chen, T., Zhang, J., & McClain, C. J. (2011). Copper deficiency exacerbates bile duct ligation-induced liver injury and fibrosis in rats. The Journal of pharmacology and experimental therapeutics, 339(1), 298–306. https://doi.org/10.1124/jpet.111.184325

[2228] Ackerman, Z., Skarzinski, G., Grozovski, M., Oron-Herman, M., & Sela, B. A. (2014). Effects of antihypertensive and triglyceride-lowering agents on hepatic copper concentrations in rats with fatty liver disease. Basic & clinical pharmacology & toxicology, 115(6), 545–551. https://doi.org/10.1111/bcpt.12283

[2229] Goyens, P., Brasseur, D., & Cadranel, S. (1985). Copper deficiency in infants with active celiac disease. Journal of pediatric gastroenterology and nutrition, 4(4), 677–680. https://doi.org/10.1097/00005176-198508000-00033

[2230] BRAGA, C. B. M., FERREIRA, I. M. de L., MARCHINI, J. S., & CUNHA, S. F. de C. da. (2015). COPPER AND MAGNESIUM DEFICIENCIES IN PATIENTS WITH SHORT BOWEL SYNDROME RECEIVING PARENTERAL NUTRITION OR ORAL FEEDING. Arquivos de Gastroenterologia, 52(2), 94–99. doi:10.1590/s0004-28032015000200004

[2231] Hujoel, I.A. (2020), Nutritional status in irritable bowel syndrome: A North American population-based study. JGH Open, 4: 656-662. https://doi.org/10.1002/jgh3.12311

630

[2232] Goyens, P., Brasseur, D., & Cadranel, S. (1985). Copper deficiency in infants with active celiac disease. Journal of pediatric gastroenterology and nutrition, 4(4), 677–680. https://doi.org/10.1097/00005176-198508000-00033

[2233] Halfdanarson, T. R., Litzow, M. R., & Murray, J. A. (2007). Hematologic manifestations of celiac disease. Blood, 109(2), 412–421. https://doi.org/10.1182/blood-2006-07-031104

[2234] Halfdanarson, T. R., Kumar, N., Hogan, W. J., & Murray, J. A. (2009). Copper deficiency in celiac disease. Journal of clinical gastroenterology, 43(2), 162–164. https://doi.org/10.1097/MCG.0b013e3181354294

[2235] Chhetri, S. K., Mills, R. J., Shaunak, S., & Emsley, H. C. (2014). Copper deficiency. BMJ (Clinical research ed.), 348, g3691. https://doi.org/10.1136/bmj.g3691

[2236] Livingston, E. H. (2010). The incidence of bariatric surgery has plateaued in the U.S. The American Journal of Surgery, 200(3), 378–385. doi:10.1016/j.amjsurg.2009.11.007

[2237] Institute of Medicine, Food and Nutrition Board. Dietary Reference Intakes for Vitamin A, Vitamin K, Arsenic, Boron, Chromium, Copper, Iodine, Iron, Manganese, Molybdenum, Nickel, Silicon, Vanadium, and Zinc. Washington, DC: National Academies Press; 2001.

[2238] Wapnir R. A. (1998). Copper absorption and bioavailability. The American journal of clinical nutrition, 67(5 Suppl), 1054S–1060S. https://doi.org/10.1093/ajcn/67.5.1054S

[2239] Wapnir (1998) 'Copper absorption and bioavailability', Am J Clin Nutr 1998;67(suppl):1054S–60S.

[2240] Wapnir R. A. (1998). Copper absorption and bioavailability. The American journal of clinical nutrition, 67(5 Suppl), 1054S–1060S. https://doi.org/10.1093/ajcn/67.5.1054S

[2241] Crisponi et al (2010) 'Copper-related diseases: From chemistry to molecular pathology', Coordination Chemistry Reviews 254(17-18):876, DOI: 10.1016/j.ccr.2009.12.018

[2242] Johnson, R. J., Rivard, C., Lanaspa, M. A., Otabachian-Smith, S., Ishimoto, T., Cicerchi, C., ... Hess, T. (2013). Fructokinase, Fructans, Intestinal Permeability, and Metabolic Syndrome: An Equine Connection? Journal of Equine Veterinary Science, 33(2), 120–126. doi:10.1016/j.jevs.2012.05.004

[2243] Andres-Hernando, A., Orlicky, D. J., Kuwabara, M., Ishimoto, T., Nakagawa, T., Johnson, R. J., & Lanaspa, M. A. (2020). Deletion of Fructokinase in the Liver or in the Intestine Reveals Differential Effects on Sugar-Induced Metabolic Dysfunction. Cell Metabolism, 32(1), 117–127.e3. doi:10.1016/j.cmet.2020.05.012

[2244] Wang, X., Flores, S. R., Ha, J.-H., Doguer, C., Woloshun, R. R., Xiang, P., ... Collins, J. F. (2018). Intestinal DMT1 Is Essential for Optimal Assimilation of Dietary Copper in Male and Female Mice with Iron-Deficiency Anemia. The Journal of Nutrition, 148(8), 1244–1252. doi:10.1093/jn/nxy111

[2245] Joseph R Prohaska, Role of copper transporters in copper homeostasis, The American Journal of Clinical Nutrition, Volume 88, Issue 3, September 2008, Pages 826S–829S, https://doi.org/10.1093/ajcn/88.3.826S

[2246] Skjørringe, T., Burkhart, A., Johnsen, K. B., & Moos, T. (2015). Divalent metal transporter 1 (DMT1) in the brain: implications for a role in iron transport at the blood-brain barrier, and neuronal and glial pathology. Frontiers in Molecular Neuroscience, 8. doi:10.3389/fnmol.2015.00019

[2247] J.J. Ravia, R.M. Stephen, F.K. Ghishan, J.F. Collins, J. Biol. Chem. 280 (2005) 36221.

[2248] Espinoza, A., Le Blanc, S., Olivares, M., Pizarro, F., Ruz, M., & Arredondo, M. (2011). Iron, Copper, and Zinc Transport: Inhibition of Divalent Metal Transporter 1 (DMT1) and Human Copper Transporter 1 (hCTR1) by shRNA. Biological Trace Element Research, 146(2), 281–286. doi:10.1007/s12011-011-9243-2

[2249] Wapnir, R. A. (1991). Copper-Sodium Linkage during Intestinal Absorption: Inhibition by Amiloride. Experimental Biology and Medicine, 196(4), 410–414. doi:10.3181/00379727-196-43208

[2250] Wapnir, R. A., & Stiel, L. (1987). Intestinal absorption of copper: effect of sodium. Proceedings of the Society for Experimental Biology and Medicine. Society for Experimental Biology and Medicine (New York, N.Y.), 185(3), 277–282. https://doi.org/10.3181/00379727-185-42545

[2251] Fields, M., Ferretti, R. J., Reiser, S., & Smith, J. C. (1984). The Severity of Copper Deficiency in Rats is Determined by the Type of Dietary Carbohydrate. Experimental Biology and Medicine, 175(4), 530–537. doi:10.3181/00379727-175-41832

[2252] Reiser, S., Ferretti, R. J., Fields, M., & Smith, J. C. (1983). Role of dietary fructose in the enhancement of mortality and biochemical changes associated with copper deficiency in rats. The American Journal of Clinical Nutrition, 38(2), 214–222. doi:10.1093/ajcn/38.2.214

[2253] Lee, J., Peña, M. M. O., Nose, Y., & Thiele, D. J. (2001). Biochemical Characterization of the Human Copper Transporter Ctr1. Journal of Biological Chemistry, 277(6), 4380–4387. doi:10.1074/jbc.m104728200

[2254] Plantone et al (2015) 'PPIs as possible risk factor for copper deficiency myelopathy', Journal of the Neurological Sciences 349(1-2), DOI: 10.1016/j.jns.2015.01.009

[2255] Gollan, J. L. (1975). Studies on the Nature of Complexes Formed by Copper with Human Alimentary Secretions and Their Influence on Copper Absorption in the Rat. Clinical Science, 49(3), 237–245. doi:10.1042/cs0490237

631

[2256] Plantone et al (2015) 'PPIs as possible risk factor for copper deficiency myelopathy', Journal of the Neurological Sciences 349(1-2), DOI: 10.1016/j.jns.2015.01.009

[2257] Harris, E. D., & Percival, S. S. (1991). A role for ascorbic acid in copper transport. The American journal of clinical nutrition, 54(6 Suppl), 1193S–1197S. https://doi.org/10.1093/ajcn/54.6.1193s

[2258] Davies, J. D., & Newson, J. (1974). Ascorbic acid and cholesterol levels in pastoral peoples in Kenya. The American journal of clinical nutrition, 27(10), 1039–1042. https://doi.org/10.1093/ajcn/27.8.1039

[2259] Milne, D. B., & Omaye, S. T. (1980). Effect of vitamin C on copper and iron metabolism in the guinea pig. International journal for vitamin and nutrition research. Internationale Zeitschrift fur Vitamin- und Ernahrungsforschung. Journal international de vitaminologie et de nutrition, 50(3), 301–308.

[2260] Hallberg, L., Brune, M., & Rossander, L. (1989). The role of vitamin C in iron absorption. International journal for vitamin and nutrition research. Supplement = Internationale Zeitschrift fur Vitamin- und Ernahrungsforschung. Supplement, 30, 103–108.

[2261] Cinar, M., Yildirim, E., Yigit, A. A., Yalcinkaya, I., Duru, O., Kisa, U., & Atmaca, N. (2014). Effects of Dietary Supplementation with Vitamin C and Vitamin E and Their Combination on Growth Performance, Some Biochemical Parameters, and Oxidative Stress Induced by Copper Toxicity in Broilers. Biological Trace Element Research, 158(2), 186–196. doi:10.1007/s12011-014-9926-6

[2262] Rifici, V. A., & Khachadurian, A. K. (1996). Effects of dietary vitamin C and E supplementation on the copper mediated oxidation of HDL and on HDL mediated cholesterol efflux. Atherosclerosis, 127(1), 19–26. doi:10.1016/s0021-9150(96)05928-x

[2263] Kaplan, J. H., & Lutsenko, S. (2009). Copper Transport in Mammalian Cells: Special Care for a Metal with Special Needs. Journal of Biological Chemistry, 284(38), 25461–25465. doi:10.1074/jbc.r109.031286

[2264] Feng et al (2000) 'Thyroid Hormone Regulation of Hepatic Genes in Vivo Detected by Complementary DNA Microarray', Molecular Endocrinology, Volume 14, Issue 7, 1 July 2000, Pages 947–955, https://doi.org/10.1210/mend.14.7.0470

[2265] Flores-Morales et al (2002) 'Patterns of Liver Gene Expression Governed by TRβ', Molecular Endocrinology, Volume 16, Issue 6, 1 June 2002, Pages 1257–1268, https://doi.org/10.1210/mend.16.6.0846

[2266] Arora et al (2018) 'Study of Trace Elements in Patients of Hypothyroidism with Special Reference to Zinc and Copper', Biomed J Sci&Tech Res 6(2)-2018. BJSTR. MS.ID.001336. DOI: 10.26717/BJSTR.2018.06.001336.

[2267] Mittag, J., Behrends, T., Nordström, K., Anselmo, J., Vennström, B., & Schomburg, L. (2012). Serum copper as a novel biomarker for resistance to thyroid hormone. Biochemical Journal, 443(1), 103–109. doi:10.1042/bj20111817

[2268] Camakaris et al (1999) 'Molecular Mechanisms of Copper Homeostasis', Biochemical and Biophysical Research Communications, Volume 261, Issue 2, 2 August 1999, Pages 225-232.

[2269] Turnlund, J. R., Keen, C. L., & Smith, R. G. (1990). Copper status and urinary and salivary copper in young men at three levels of dietary copper. The American journal of clinical nutrition, 51(4), 658–664. https://doi.org/10.1093/ajcn/51.4.658

[2270] Bonham and O'Connor (2000) 'Response of putative indices of copper status to copper supplementation in human subjects', British Journal Of Nutrition 84(2):151-6, DOI: 10.1017/S0007114500001379

[2271] Berghe and Klomp (2009) 'New developments in the regulation of intestinal copper absorption', Nutrition Reviews, Volume 67, Issue 11, 1 November 2009, Pages 658–672, https://doi.org/10.1111/j.1753-4887.2009.00250.x

[2272] Ala, A., Walker, A. P., Ashkan, K., Dooley, J. S., & Schilsky, M. L. (2007). Wilson's disease. Lancet (London, England), 369(9559), 397–408. https://doi.org/10.1016/S0140-6736(07)60196-2

[2273] Brewer, G. J., Dick, R. D., Johnson, V., Wang, Y., Yuzbasiyan-Gurkan, V., Kluin, K., Fink, J. K., & Aisen, A. (1994). Treatment of Wilson's disease with ammonium tetrathiomolybdate. I. Initial therapy in 17 neurologically affected patients. Archives of neurology, 51(6), 545–554. https://doi.org/10.1001/archneur.1994.00540180023009

[2274] Walshe, J. M. (1956). WILSON'S DISEASE. The Lancet, 267(6906), 25–26. doi:10.1016/s0140-6736(56)91859-1

[2275] Brewer, G. J. (1994). Treatment of Wilson's Disease With Ammonium Tetrathiomolybdate. Archives of Neurology, 51(6), 545. doi:10.1001/archneur.1994.00540180023009

[2276] Brewer, G. J., Yuzbasiyan-Gurkan, V., & Johnson, V. (1991). Treatment of Wilson's disease with zinc. IX: Response of serum lipids. The Journal of laboratory and clinical medicine, 118(5), 466–470.

[2277] Danks DM . Disorders of copper transport. In: Scriver CR Beaudet AL Sly WM Valle D, eds. The Metabolic and Molecular Basis of Inherited Disease. New York: McGraw-Hill; 1995:2211–2235.

[2278] Tønnesen, T., Kleijer, W. J., & Horn, N. (1991). Incidence of Menkes disease. Human genetics, 86(4), 408–410. https://doi.org/10.1007/BF00201846

[2279] Danks D. M. (1988). The mild form of Menkes disease: progress report on the original case. American journal of medical genetics, 30(3), 859–864. https://doi.org/10.1002/ajmg.1320300325

[2280] Sarkar, B., Lingertat-Walsh, K., & Clarke, J. T. (1993). Copper-histidine therapy for Menkes disease. The Journal of pediatrics, 123(5), 828–830. https://doi.org/10.1016/s0022-3476(05)80870-4

[2281] Brem, S. S., Zagzag, D., Tsanaclis, A. M., Gately, S., Elkouby, M. P., & Brien, S. E. (1990). Inhibition of angiogenesis and tumor growth in the brain. Suppression of endothelial cell turnover by penicillamine and the depletion of copper, an angiogenic cofactor. The American journal of pathology, 137(5), 1121–1142.

[2282] Lowndes, S. A., & Harris, A. L. (2004). Copper chelation as an antiangiogenic therapy. Oncology research, 14(11-12), 529–539. https://doi.org/10.3727/0965040042707952

[2283] Sen, C. K., Khanna, S., Venojarvi, M., Trikha, P., Ellison, E. C., Hunt, T. K., & Roy, S. (2002). Copper-induced vascular endothelial growth factor expression and wound healing. American journal of physiology. Heart and circulatory physiology, 282(5), H1821–H1827. https://doi.org/10.1152/ajpheart.01015.2001

[2284] Lugano, R., Ramachandran, M. & Dimberg, A. Tumor angiogenesis: causes, consequences, challenges and opportunities. Cell. Mol. Life Sci. 77, 1745–1770 (2020). https://doi.org/10.1007/s00018-019-03351-7

[2285] Harris, E.D., 2004. A requirement for copper in angiogenesis. Nutr. Rev. 62, 60–64.

[2286] Goodman, V. L., Brewer, G. J., & Merajver, S. D. (2004). Copper deficiency as an anti-cancer strategy. Endocrine-related cancer, 11(2), 255–263. https://doi.org/10.1677/erc.0.0110255

[2287] Cooper, G. J., Chan, Y. K., Dissanayake, A. M., Leahy, F. E., Keogh, G. F., Frampton, C. M., Gamble, G. D., Brunton, D. H., Baker, J. R., & Poppitt, S. D. (2005). Demonstration of a hyperglycemia-driven pathogenic abnormality of copper homeostasis in diabetes and its reversibility by selective chelation: quantitative comparisons between the biology of copper and eight other nutritionally essential elements in normal and diabetic individuals. Diabetes, 54(5), 1468–1476. https://doi.org/10.2337/diabetes.54.5.1468

[2288] Samsel, A., & Seneff, S. (2013). Glyphosate, pathways to modern diseases II: Celiac sprue and gluten intolerance. Interdisciplinary toxicology, 6(4), 159–184. https://doi.org/10.2478/intox-2013-0026

[2289] Leino et al (2020) 'Classification of the glyphosate target enzyme (5-enolpyruvylshikimate-3-phosphate synthase) for assessing sensitivity of organisms to the herbicide', Journal of Hazardous Materials, Available online 14 November 2020, 124556, https://doi.org/10.1016/j.jhazmat.2020.124556

[2290] Motekaitis RJ, Martell AE. Metal chelate formation by N-phosphono- methylglycine and related ligands. J Coord Chem. 1985;14:139–149.

[2291] Madsen HEL, Christensen HH, Gottlieb-Petersen C. Stability constants of copper(II), zinc, manganese(II), calcium, and magnesium complexes of N-(phosphonomethyl)glycine (glyphosate) Acta Chem Scand. 1978;32:79–83.

[2292] Undabeytia, T., Morillo, E., & Maqueda, C. (2002). FTIR study of glyphosate-copper complexes. Journal of agricultural and food chemistry, 50(7), 1918–1921. https://doi.org/10.1021/jf010988w

[2293] Cakmak, I., Yazici, A., Tutus, Y., & Ozturk, L. (2009). Glyphosate reduced seed and leaf concentrations of calcium, manganese, magnesium, and iron in non-glyphosate resistant soybean. European Journal of Agronomy, 31(3), 114–119. doi:10.1016/j.eja.2009.07.001

[2294] Mehta, S. W., & Eikum, R. (1989). Effect of Estrogen on Serum and Tissue Levels of Copper and Zinc. Copper Bioavailability and Metabolism, 155–162. doi:10.1007/978-1-4613-0537-8_13

[2295] King J. C. (1987). Do women using oral contraceptive agents require extra zinc?. The Journal of nutrition, 117(1), 217–219. https://doi.org/10.1093/jn/117.1.217

[2296] Solomons N. W. (1998). Mild human zinc deficiency produces an imbalance between cell-mediated and humoral immunity. Nutrition reviews, 56(1 Pt 1), 27–28. https://doi.org/10.1111/j.1753-4887.1998.tb01656.x

[2297] Pisano, M., & Hilas, O. (2016). Zinc and Taste Disturbances in Older Adults: A Review of the Literature. The Consultant pharmacist : the journal of the American Society of Consultant Pharmacists, 31(5), 267–270. https://doi.org/10.4140/TCP.n.2016.267

[2298] Sandstead H. H. (1994). Understanding zinc: recent observations and interpretations. The Journal of laboratory and clinical medicine, 124(3), 322–327.

[2299] Prasad A. S. (1995). Zinc: an overview. Nutrition (Burbank, Los Angeles County, Calif.), 11(1 Suppl), 93–99.

[2300] SIMMER, K., & THOMPSON, R. P. H. (1985). Zinc in the Fetus and Newborn. Acta Paediatrica, 74(s319), 158–163. doi:10.1111/j.1651-2227.1985.tb10126.x

[2301] Taylor, G. A., & Blackshear, P. J. (1995). Zinc inhibits turnover of labile mRNAs in intact cells. Journal of Cellular Physiology, 162(3), 378–387. doi:10.1002/jcp.1041620310

[2302] Wu, F. Y. H., & Wu, C. W. (1987). Zinc in DNA Replication and Transcription. Annual Review of Nutrition, 7(1), 251–272. doi:10.1146/annurev.nu.07.070187.001343

[2303] Sandstead, H. H., & Rinaldi, R. A. (1969). Impairment of deoxyribonucleic acid synthesis by dietary zinc deficiency in the rat. Journal of cellular physiology, 73(1), 81–83. https://doi.org/10.1002/jcp.1040730111

[2304] Chesters JK (1992) Trace elements–gene interactions. Nutrition Reviews 50, 217–223.

[2305] Umezawa, K., Nakazawa, K., Uchihata, Y., & Otsuka, M. (1999). Screening for inducers of apoptosis in apoptosis-resistant human carcinoma cells. Advances in Enzyme Regulation, 39(1), 145–156. doi:10.1016/s0065-2571(98)00022-3

[2306] Jiang et al (1995) 'Lack of Ca2+ involvement in thymocyte apoptosis induced by chelation of intracellular Zn2+', Laboratory Investigation 73(1):111-7.

[2307] Zalewski PD & Forbes IJ (1993) 'Intracellular zinc and the regulation of apoptosis'. In Programmed Cell Death: The Cellular and Molecular Biology of Apoptosis, pp. 73–85 [M Laviri and D Watters, editors]. Melbourne: Harword Academic Press

[2308] Ploysangam, A., Falciglia, G. A., & Brehm, B. J. (1997). Effect of marginal zinc deficiency on human growth and development. Journal of tropical pediatrics, 43(4), 192–198. https://doi.org/10.1093/tropej/43.4.192

[2309] Prasad A. S. (2004). Zinc deficiency: its characterization and treatment. Metal ions in biological systems, 41, 103–137.

[2310] Hambidge KM, 'Mild zinc deficiency in human subjects'. In: Mills CF, ed. Zinc in Human Biology. New York, NY: Springer-Verlag, 1989:281-96.

[2311] Favier AE (1992) The role of zinc in reproduction. Hormonal mechanisms. Biological Trace Element Research 32, 363–382.

[2312] JAMESON, S. (1993). Zinc Status in Pregnancy: The Effect of Zinc Therapy on Perinatal Mortality, Prematurity, and Placental Ablation. Annals of the New York Academy of Sciences, 678(1 Maternal Nutr), 178–192. doi:10.1111/j.1749-6632.1993.tb26121.x

[2313] PRASAD, A. S. (1963). Biochemical Studies on Dwarfism,Hypogonadism, and Anemia. Archives of Internal Medicine, 111(4), 407. doi:10.1001/archinte.1963.03620280007003

[2314] Sandstead, H. H., Prasad, A. S., Schulert, A. R., Farid, Z., Miale, A., Jr, Bassilly, S., & Darby, W. J. (1967). Human zinc deficiency, endocrine manifestations and response to treatment. The American journal of clinical nutrition, 20(5), 422–442. https://doi.org/10.1093/ajcn/20.5.422

[2315] Prasad A. S. (2012). Discovery of human zinc deficiency: 50 years later. Journal of trace elements in medicine and biology : organ of the Society for Minerals and Trace Elements (GMS), 26(2-3), 66–69. https://doi.org/10.1016/j.jtemb.2012.04.004

[2316] Brown, K. H., Wuehler, S. E., & Peerson, J. M. (2001). The Importance of Zinc in Human Nutrition and Estimation of the Global Prevalence of Zinc Deficiency. Food and Nutrition Bulletin, 22(2), 113–125. https://doi.org/10.1177/156482650102200201

[2317] Rivera, J. A., Ruel, M. T., Santizo, M. C., Lönnerdal, B., & Brown, K. H. (1998). Zinc Supplementation Improves the Growth of Stunted Rural Guatemalan Infants. The Journal of Nutrition, 128(3), 556–562. doi:10.1093/jn/128.3.556

[2318] Darnton-Hill (2013) 'Zinc supplementation and growth in children: Biological, behavioural and contextual rationale', e-Library of Evidence for Nutrition Actions (eLENA), World Health Organization, Accessed Online Dec 19 2020: https://www.who.int/elena/bbc/zinc_stunting/en/

[2319] Lehto, R. S. (1968). "Zinc". In Clifford A. Hampel (ed.). The Encyclopedia of the Chemical Elements. New York: Reinhold Book Corporation. pp. 822–830. ISBN 978-0-442-15598-8. LCCN 68-29938.

[2320] Thornton, C. P. (2007). Of brass and bronze in prehistoric Southwest Asia (PDF). Papers and Lectures Online. Archetype Publications. ISBN 978-1-904982-19-7.

[2321] Greenwood, N. N.; Earnshaw, A. (1997). Chemistry of the Elements (2nd ed.). Oxford: Butterworth-Heinemann, p 1201. ISBN 978-0-7506-3365-9.

[2322] Craddock (1978) 'The composition of the copper alloys used by the Greek, Etruscan and Roman civilizations: 3. The Origins and Early Use of Brass', Journal of Archaeological Science, Volume 5, Issue 1, March 1978, Pages 1-16, https://doi.org/10.1016/0305-4403(78)90015-8

[2323] Giachi, G., Pallecchi, P., Romualdi, A., Ribechini, E., Lucejko, J. J., Colombini, M. P., & Mariotti Lippi, M. (2013). Ingredients of a 2,000-y-old medicine revealed by chemical, mineralogical, and botanical investigations. Proceedings of the National Academy of Sciences of the United States of America, 110(4), 1193–1196. https://doi.org/10.1073/pnas.1216776110

[2324] P. T. Craddock, L. K. Gurjar & K. T. M. Hegde (1983) Zinc production in medieval India, World Archaeology, 15:2, 211-217, DOI: 10.1080/00438243.1983.9979899

[2325] Gandhi (2000) 'Ancient mining and metallurgy in Rajasthan', chapter 2 in Crustal Evolution and Metallogeny in the Northwestern Indian Shield: A Festschrift for Asoke Mookherjee, M. Deb, ed., Alpha Science Int'l Ltd., p. 46, ISBN 1-84265-001-7.

[2326] Habashi (2015) 'Discovering the 8th Metal: A History of Zinc', International Zinc Association (IZA), www.zincworld.org, Accessed Online Nov 10 2020: https://web.archive.org/web/20150606210821/http://www.zinc.org/general/ZP-Discovering_the_8th_Metal1.pdf

[2327] Gerhartz, Wolfgang; et al. (1996). Ullmann's Encyclopedia of Industrial Chemistry (5th ed.). VHC. p. 509.

[2328] Arny, Henry Vinecome (1917). Principles of Pharmacy (2nd ed.). W. B. Saunders company. p. 483.

[2329] Raulin J (1869) '*Etudes chimique sur la vegetation (Chemical studies on plants)*'. Annales des Sciences Naturelles Botanique et Biologie Vegetale 11, 293–299.

[2330] TODD, W. R., ELVEHJEM, C. A., & HART, E. B. (2009). ZINC IN THE NUTRITION OF THE RAT. Nutrition Reviews, 38(4), 151–154. doi:10.1111/j.1753-4887.1980.tb05879.x

[2331] Vallee, B. L., Wacker, W. E. C., Bartholomay, A. F., & Hoch, F. L. (1957). Zinc Metabolism in Hepatic Dysfunction. New England Journal of Medicine, 257(22), 1055–1065. doi:10.1056/nejm195711282572201

[2332] Prasad, A. S., Halsted, J. A., & Nadimi, M. (1961). Syndrome of iron deficiency anemia, hepatosplenomegaly, hypogonadism, dwarfism and geophagia. The American Journal of Medicine, 31(4), 532–546. doi:10.1016/0002-9343(61)90137-1

[2333] Hoekstra W. G. (1969). Skeletal and skin lesions of zinc-deficiency chickens and swine. Possible relationship to "connective tissue diseases" of man. The American journal of clinical nutrition, 22(9), 1268–1277. https://doi.org/10.1093/ajcn/22.9.1268

[2334] Hurley, L. S., Gowan, J., & Milhaud, G. (1969). Calcium metabolism in manganese-deficient and zinc-deficient rats. Proceedings of the Society for Experimental Biology and Medicine. Society for Experimental Biology and Medicine (New York, N.Y.), 130(3), 856–860. https://doi.org/10.3181/00379727-130-33672

[2335] Fernandez-Madrid, F., Prasad, A. S., & Oberleas, D. (1971). Effect of zinc deficiency on collagen metabolism. The Journal of laboratory and clinical medicine, 78(5), 853.

[2336] Kjaer, M., Frederiksen, A. K. S., Nissen, N. I., Willumsen, N., van Hall, G., Jorgensen, L. N., … Ågren, M. S. (2020). Multinutrient Supplementation Increases Collagen Synthesis during Early Wound Repair in a Randomized Controlled Trial in Patients with Inguinal Hernia. The Journal of Nutrition, 150(4), 792–799. doi:10.1093/jn/nxz324

[2337] Cohen C. (1968). Zinc sulphate and bedsores. British medical journal, 2(5604), 561. https://doi.org/10.1136/bmj.2.5604.561-b

[2338] Pories, W. J., Henzel, J. H., Rob, C. G., & Strain, W. H. (1967). Acceleration of healing with zinc sulfate. Annals of surgery, 165(3), 432–436. https://doi.org/10.1097/00000658-196703000-00015

[2339] Brodribb and Ricketts (1972) 'The effect of zinc in the healing of burns', Injury, Volume 3, Issue 1, 1972, Pages 25-29, https://doi.org/10.1016/S0020-1383(71)80132-8

[2340] Sandstead, H. H., & Shepard, G. H. (1968). The effect of zinc deficiency on the tensile strength of healing surgical incisions in the integument of the rat. Proceedings of the Society for Experimental Biology and Medicine. Society for Experimental Biology and Medicine (New York, N.Y.), 128(3), 687–689. https://doi.org/10.3181/00379727-128-33100

[2341] Sandstead, H. H., Lanier, V. C., Jr, Shephard, G. H., & Gillespie, D. D. (1970). Zinc and wound healing. Effects of zinc deficiency and zinc supplementation. The American journal of clinical nutrition, 23(5), 514–519. https://doi.org/10.1093/ajcn/23.5.514

[2342] Latafat Husain, S. (1969). ORAL ZINC SULPHATE IN LEG ULCERS. The Lancet, 293(7605), 1069–1071. doi:10.1016/s0140-6736(69)91706-1

[2343] Momen-Heravi, M., Barahimi, E., Razzaghi, R., Bahmani, F., Gilasi, H. R., & Asemi, Z. (2017). The effects of zinc supplementation on wound healing and metabolic status in patients with diabetic foot ulcer: A randomized, double-blind, placebo-controlled trial. Wound Repair and Regeneration, 25(3), 512–520. doi:10.1111/wrr.12537

[2344] Greaves, M. W., & Skillen, A. W. (1970). Effects of long-continued ingestion of zinc sulphate in patients with venous leg ulceration. Lancet (London, England), 2(7679), 889–891. https://doi.org/10.1016/s0140-6736(70)92066-0

[2345] Serjeant, G., Galloway, R., & Gueri, M. (1970). ORAL ZINC SULPHATE IN SICKLE-CELL ULCERS. The Lancet, 296(7679), 891–893. doi:10.1016/s0140-6736(70)92067-2

[2346] Nakamura, H., Sekiguchi, A., Ogawa, Y., Kawamura, T., Akai, R., Iwawaki, T., … Motegi, S. (2019). Zinc deficiency exacerbates pressure ulcers by increasing oxidative stress and ATP in the skin. Journal of Dermatological Science, 95(2), 62–69. doi:10.1016/j.jdermsci.2019.07.004

[2347] Han, B., Fang, W. H., Zhao, S., Yang, Z., & Hoang, B. X. (2020). Zinc sulfide nanoparticles improve skin regeneration. Nanomedicine: Nanotechnology, Biology and Medicine, 29, 102263. doi:10.1016/j.nano.2020.102263

[2348] STRAIN, W. H., HUEGIN, F., LANKAU, C. A., Jr, BERLINER, W. P., MCEVOY, R. K., & PORIES, W. J. (1964). ZINC-65 RETENTION BY AORTIC TISSUE OF RATS. The International journal of applied radiation and isotopes, 15, 231–237. https://doi.org/10.1016/0020-708x(64)90069-9

[2349] Hermann, J., Arquitt, A., & Hanson, C. (1993). Relationships between dietary minerals and plasma lipids and glucose among older adults. Journal of nutrition for the elderly, 12(3), 1–14. https://doi.org/10.1300/j052v12n03_01

[2350] Ripa, S., & Ripa, R. (1994). Zinco ed aterosclerosi [Zinc and atherosclerosis]. Minerva medica, 85(12), 647–654.

[2351] Wilkins, G. M., & Leake, D. S. (1994). The oxidation of low density lipoprotein by cells or iron is inhibited by zinc. FEBS letters, 341(2-3), 259–262. https://doi.org/10.1016/0014-5793(94)80468-0

[2352] Hughes, S., & Samman, S. (2006). The effect of zinc supplementation in humans on plasma lipids, antioxidant status and thrombogenesis. Journal of the American College of Nutrition, 25(4), 285–291. https://doi.org/10.1080/07315724.2006.10719537

[2353] Giacconi, R., Caruso, C., Malavolta, M., Lio, D., Balistreri, C. R., Scola, L., Candore, G., Muti, E., & Mocchegiani, E. (2008). Pro-inflammatory genetic background and zinc status in old atherosclerotic subjects. Ageing research reviews, 7(4), 306–318. https://doi.org/10.1016/j.arr.2008.06.001

[2354] Wang, J., Song, Y., Elsherif, L., Song, Z., Zhou, G., Prabhu, S. D., ... Cai, L. (2006). Cardiac Metallothionein Induction Plays the Major Role in the Prevention of Diabetic Cardiomyopathy by Zinc Supplementation. Circulation, 113(4), 544–554. doi:10.1161/circulationaha.105.537894

[2355] Kang, Y. J. (1999). The Antioxidant Function of Metallothionein in the Heart (44451). Proceedings of the Society for Experimental Biology and Medicine, 222(3), 263–273. https://doi.org/10.1177/153537029922200309

[2356] Kang et al (2015) 'Reduced metallothionein expression induced by Zinc deficiency results in apoptosis in hepatic stellate cell line LX-2', Int J Clin Exp Med 2015;8(11):20603-20609.

[2357] Kang et al (1997) 'Overexpression of Metallothionein in the Heart of Transgenic Mice Suppresses Doxorubicin Cardiotoxicity', J. Clin. Invest, Volume 100, Number 6, September 1997, 1501–1506.

[2358] Wang, L., Zhou, Z., Saari, J. T., & Kang, Y. J. (2005). Alcohol-Induced Myocardial Fibrosis in Metallothionein-Null Mice. The American Journal of Pathology, 167(2), 337–344. doi:10.1016/s0002-9440(10)62979-3

[2359] Mocchegiani, E., Malavolta, M., Muti, E., Costarelli, L., Cipriano, C., Piacenza, F., Tesei, S., Giacconi, R., & Lattanzio, F. (2008). Zinc, metallothioneins and longevity: interrelationships with niacin and selenium. Current pharmaceutical design, 14(26), 2719–2732. https://doi.org/10.2174/138161208786264188

[2360] Vasto, S., Mocchegiani, E., Malavolta, M., Cuppari, I., Listì, F., Nuzzo, D., Ditta, V., Candore, G., & Caruso, C. (2007). Zinc and inflammatory/immune response in aging. Annals of the New York Academy of Sciences, 1100, 111–122. https://doi.org/10.1196/annals.1395.009

[2361] Barbato, J. C., Catanescu, O., Murray, K., DiBello, P. M., & Jacobsen, D. W. (2007). Targeting of Metallothionein by L-Homocysteine. Arteriosclerosis, Thrombosis, and Vascular Biology, 27(1), 49–54. doi:10.1161/01.atv.0000251536.49581.8a

[2362] Colgan, S. M., & Austin, R. C. (2007). Homocysteinylation of Metallothionein Impairs Intracellular Redox Homeostasis. Arteriosclerosis, Thrombosis, and Vascular Biology, 27(1), 8–11. doi:10.1161/01.atv.0000254151.00086.26

[2363] Stadler, N., Stanley, N., Heeneman, S., Vacata, V., Daemen, M. J., Bannon, P. G., Waltenberger, J., & Davies, M. J. (2008). Accumulation of zinc in human atherosclerotic lesions correlates with calcium levels but does not protect against protein oxidation. Arteriosclerosis, thrombosis, and vascular biology, 28(5), 1024–1030. https://doi.org/10.1161/ATVBAHA.108.162735

[2364] Lee, R. T., & Libby, P. (1997). The Unstable Atheroma. Arteriosclerosis, Thrombosis, and Vascular Biology, 17(10), 1859–1867. doi:10.1161/01.atv.17.10.1859

[2365] Bittencourt, M. S., & Cerci, R. J. (2015). Statin effects on atherosclerotic plaques: regression or healing?. BMC medicine, 13, 260. https://doi.org/10.1186/s12916-015-0499-9

[2366] Leonhardt, W., Kurktschiev, T., Meissner, D., Lattke, P., Abletshauser, C., Weidinger, G., Jaross, W., & Hanefeld, M. (1997). Effects of fluvastatin therapy on lipids, antioxidants, oxidation of low density lipoproteins and trace metals. European journal of clinical pharmacology, 53(1), 65–69. https://doi.org/10.1007/s002280050338

[2367] Leone, N., Courbon, D., Ducimetiere, P., & Zureik, M. (2006). Zinc, copper, and magnesium and risks for all-cause, cancer, and cardiovascular mortality. Epidemiology (Cambridge, Mass.), 17(3), 308–314. https://doi.org/10.1097/01.ede.0000209454.41466.b7

[2368] Giannoglou, G. D., Konstantinou, D. M., Kovatsi, L., Chatzizisis, Y. S., & Mikhailidis, D. P. (2010). Association of reduced zinc status with angiographically severe coronary atherosclerosis: a pilot study. Angiology, 61(5), 449–455. https://doi.org/10.1177/0003319710366702

[2369] VOLKOV N. F. (1963). COBALT, MANGANESE AND ZINC CONTENT IN THE BLOOD OF ATHEROSCLEROSIS PATIENTS. Federation proceedings. Translation supplement; selected translations from medical-related science, 22, 897–899.

[2370] ULMER, D. D., VALLEE, B. L., & WACKER, W. E. (1956). Metalloenzymes and myocardial infarction. II. Malic and lactic dehydrogenase activities and zinc concentrations in serum. The New England journal of medicine, 255(10), 450–456.

[2371] Nakashima, A. S., & Dyck, R. H. (2009). Zinc and cortical plasticity. Brain research reviews, 59(2), 347–373. https://doi.org/10.1016/j.brainresrev.2008.10.003

[2372] Prakash, A., Bharti, K., & Majeed, A. B. (2015). Zinc: indications in brain disorders. Fundamental & clinical pharmacology, 29(2), 131–149. https://doi.org/10.1111/fcp.12110

[2373] Ronaghy, H., Fox, M. R., Garnsm, Israel, H., Harp, A., Moe, P. G., & Halsted, J. A. (1969). Controlled zinc supplementation for malnourished school boys: a pilot experiment. The American journal of clinical nutrition, 22(10), 1279–1289. https://doi.org/10.1093/ajcn/22.10.1279

636

[2374] Cherasse, Y., & Urade, Y. (2017). Dietary Zinc Acts as a Sleep Modulator. International journal of molecular sciences, 18(11), 2334. https://doi.org/10.3390/ijms18112334

[2375] Bitanihirwe, B. K., & Cunningham, M. G. (2009). Zinc: the brain's dark horse. Synapse (New York, N.Y.), 63(11), 1029–1049. https://doi.org/10.1002/syn.20683

[2376] Tyszka-Czochara, M., Grzywacz, A., Gdula-Argasińska, J., Librowski, T., Wiliński, B., & Opoka, W. (2014). The role of zinc in the pathogenesis and treatment of central nervous system (CNS) diseases. Implications of zinc homeostasis for proper CNS function. Acta poloniae pharmaceutica, 71(3), 369–377.

[2377] Quarterman J. (1972). The effect of zinc deficiency on the activity of the adrenal glands. The Proceedings of the Nutrition Society, 31(2), 74A–75A.

[2378] Chen, S. M., Kuo, C. D., Ho, L. T., & Liao, J. F. (2005). Effect of hypothyroidism on intestinal zinc absorption and renal zinc disposal in five-sixths nephrectomized rats. The Japanese journal of physiology, 55(4), 211–219. https://doi.org/10.2170/jjphysiol.R2124

[2379] Freake, H. C., Govoni, K. E., Guda, K., Huang, C., & Zinn, S. A. (2001). Actions and interactions of thyroid hormone and zinc status in growing rats. The Journal of nutrition, 131(4), 1135–1141. https://doi.org/10.1093/jn/131.4.1135

[2380] Binitha, M., Sarita, S., & Betsy, A. (2013). Zinc deficiency associated with hypothyroidism: An overlooked cause of severe alopecia. International Journal of Trichology, 5(1), 40. doi:10.4103/0974-7753.114714

[2381] Napolitano G, Palka G, Lio S, et al. Is zinc deficiency a cause of subclinical hypothyroidism in Down syndrome? Annales de Genetique. 1990 ;33(1):9-15.

[2382] Bucci, I., Napolitano, G., Giuliani, C., Lio, S., Minnucci, A., Giacomo, F. D., ... Monaco, F. (1999). Zinc sulfate supplementation improves thyroid function in hypozincemic down children. Biological Trace Element Research, 67(3), 257–268. doi:10.1007/bf02784425

[2383] Wijesekara, N., Chimienti, F., & Wheeler, M. B. (2009). Zinc, a regulator of islet function and glucose homeostasis. Diabetes, obesity & metabolism, 11 Suppl 4, 202–214. https://doi.org/10.1111/j.1463-1326.2009.01110.x

[2384] Zheng, Y., Li, X.-K., Wang, Y., & Cai, L. (2008). The Role of Zinc, Copper and Iron in the Pathogenesis of Diabetes and Diabetic Complications: Therapeutic Effects by Chelators. Hemoglobin, 32(1-2), 135–145. doi:10.1080/03630260701727077

[2385] Maruthur, N. M., Clark, J. M., Fu, M., Linda Kao, W. H., & Shuldiner, A. R. (2014). Effect of zinc supplementation on insulin secretion: interaction between zinc and SLC30A8 genotype in Old Order Amish. Diabetologia, 58(2), 295–303. doi:10.1007/s00125-014-3419-1

[2386] Quarterman J. (1969). The effect of zinc on the uptake of glucose by adipose tissue. Biochimica et biophysica acta, 177(3), 644–646. https://doi.org/10.1016/0304-4165(69)90331-6

[2387] Aksoy M. (1972). Carbohydrate metabolism in severe and longstanding iron-deficiency anemia due to dietary and zinc deficiencies. The American journal of clinical nutrition, 25(3), 262–263. https://doi.org/10.1093/ajcn/25.3.262

[2388] Mills, C. F., Quarterman, J., Chesters, J. K., Williams, R. B., & Dalgarno, A. C. (1969). Metabolic role of zinc. The American journal of clinical nutrition, 22(9), 1240–1249. https://doi.org/10.1093/ajcn/22.9.1240

[2389] Hendricks, D. G., & Mahoney, A. W. (1972). Glucose tolerance in zinc-deficient rats. The Journal of nutrition, 102(8), 1079–1084. https://doi.org/10.1093/jn/102.8.1079

[2390] Jayawardena, R., Ranasinghe, P., Galappatthy, P., Malkanthi, R., Constantine, G., & Katulanda, P. (2012). Effects of zinc supplementation on diabetes mellitus: a systematic review and meta-analysis. Diabetology & metabolic syndrome, 4(1), 13. https://doi.org/10.1186/1758-5996-4-13

[2391] Shidfar, F., Aghasi, M., Vafa, M., Heydari, I., Hosseini, S., & Shidfar, S. (2010). Effects of combination of zinc and vitamin A supplementation on serum fasting blood sugar, insulin, apoprotein B and apoprotein A-I in patients with type I diabetes. International journal of food sciences and nutrition, 61(2), 182–191. https://doi.org/10.3109/09637480903334171

[2392] Mills, C. F., Quarterman, J., Williams, R. B., & Dalgarno, A. C. (1967). The effects of zinc deficiency on pancreatic carboxypeptidase activity and protein digestion and absorption in the rat. The Biochemical journal, 102(3), 712–718. https://doi.org/10.1042/bj1020712

[2393] Polastri, L., Galbiati, F., Folli, F., & Davalli, A. M. (2002). Effects of carboxypeptidase E overexpression on insulin mRNA levels, regulated insulin secretion, and proinsulin processing of pituitary GH3 cells transfected with a furin-cleavable human proinsulin cDNA. Cell transplantation, 11(8), 803–811.

[2394] Huber, A. M., & Gershoff, S. N. (1973). Effect of zinc deficiency in rats on insulin release from the pancreas. The Journal of nutrition, 103(12), 1739–1744. https://doi.org/10.1093/jn/103.12.1739

[2395] Quarterman, J., Mills, C. F., & Humphries, W. R. (1966). The reduced secretion of, and sensitivity to insulin in zinc-deficient rats. Biochemical and Biophysical Research Communications, 25(3), 354–358. doi:10.1016/0006-291x(66)90785-6

[2396] Hashemipour, M., Kelishadi, R., Shapouri, J., Sarrafzadegan, N., Amini, M., Tavakoli, N., Movahedian-Attar, A., Mirmoghtadaee, P., & Poursafa, P. (2009). Effect of zinc supplementation on

637

insulin resistance and components of the metabolic syndrome in prepubertal obese children. Hormones (Athens, Greece), 8(4), 279–285. https://doi.org/10.14310/horm.2002.1244

[2397] Sjöblom, B., Polentarutti, M., & Djinovic-Carugo, K. (2009). Structural study of X-ray induced activation of carbonic anhydrase. Proceedings of the National Academy of Sciences of the United States of America, 106(26), 10609–10613. https://doi.org/10.1073/pnas.0904184106

[2398] Campbell, W. W., & Anderson, R. A. (1987). Effects of aerobic exercise and training on the trace minerals chromium, zinc and copper. Sports medicine (Auckland, N.Z.), 4(1), 9–18. https://doi.org/10.2165/00007256-198704010-00002

[2399] Prasad, A. S., Oberleas, D., Wolf, P., Horwitz, J. P., Collins, R., & Vazquez, J. M. (1967). Studies on Zinc Deficiency: Changes in Trace Elements and Enzyme Activities in Tissues of Zinc-deficient Rats *. Journal of Clinical Investigation, 46(4), 549–557. doi:10.1172/jci105556

[2400] Prasad A. S. (2013). Discovery of human zinc deficiency: its impact on human health and disease. Advances in nutrition (Bethesda, Md.), 4(2), 176–190. https://doi.org/10.3945/an.112.003210

[2401] Zemel, B. S., Kawchak, D. A., Fung, E. B., Ohene-Frempong, K., & Stallings, V. A. (2002). Effect of zinc supplementation on growth and body composition in children with sickle cell disease. The American journal of clinical nutrition, 75(2), 300–307. https://doi.org/10.1093/ajcn/75.2.300

[2402] Abdollahi, M., Ajami, M., Abdollahi, Z., Kalantari, N., Houshiarrad, A., Fozouni, F., Fallahrokni, A., & Mazandarani, F. S. (2019). Zinc supplementation is an effective and feasible strategy to prevent growth retardation in 6 to 24 month children: A pragmatic double blind, randomized trial. Heliyon, 5(11), e02581. https://doi.org/10.1016/j.heliyon.2019.e02581

[2403] Baer et al (1978) 'Acne in Zinc Deficiency', Arch Dermatol. 1978;114(7):1093. doi:10.1001/archderm.1978.01640190071030

[2404] Gray, N. A., Dhana, A., Stein, D. J., & Khumalo, N. P. (2019). Zinc and atopic dermatitis: a systematic review and meta-analysis. Journal of the European Academy of Dermatology and Venereology : JEADV, 33(6), 1042–1050. https://doi.org/10.1111/jdv.15524

[2405] Lei, L., Su, J., Chen, J., Chen, W., Chen, X., & Peng, C. (2019). Abnormal Serum Copper and Zinc Levels in Patients with Psoriasis: A Meta-Analysis. Indian journal of dermatology, 64(3), 224–230. https://doi.org/10.4103/ijd.IJD_475_18

[2406] DAVID, T. J., WELLS, F. E., SHARPE, T. C., & GIBBS, A. C. C. (1984). Low serum zinc in children with atopic eczema. British Journal of Dermatology, 111(5), 597–601. doi:10.1111/j.1365-2133.1984.tb06630.x

[2407] Ikeda, M., Ikui, A., Komiyama, A., Kobayashi, D., & Tanaka, M. (2008). Causative factors of taste disorders in the elderly, and therapeutic effects of zinc. The Journal of laryngology and otology, 122(2), 155–160. https://doi.org/10.1017/S0022215107008833

[2408] McDaid, O., Stewart-Knox, B., Parr, H., & Simpson, E. (2007). Dietary zinc intake and sex differences in taste acuity in healthy young adults. Journal of human nutrition and dietetics : the official journal of the British Dietetic Association, 20(2), 103–110. https://doi.org/10.1111/j.1365-277X.2007.00756.x

[2409] Suzuki, H., Asakawa, A., Li, J. B., Tsai, M., Amitani, H., Ohinata, K., Komai, M., & Inui, A. (2011). Zinc as an appetite stimulator - the possible role of zinc in the progression of diseases such as cachexia and sarcopenia. Recent patents on food, nutrition & agriculture, 3(3), 226–231. https://doi.org/10.2174/2212798411103030226

[2410] Christian, P., Khatry, S. K., Yamini, S., Stallings, R., LeClerq, S. C., Shrestha, S. R., Pradhan, E. K., & West, K. P., Jr (2001). Zinc supplementation might potentiate the effect of vitamin A in restoring night vision in pregnant Nepalese women. The American journal of clinical nutrition, 73(6), 1045–1051. https://doi.org/10.1093/ajcn/73.6.1045

[2411] Shankar, A. H., & Prasad, A. S. (1998). Zinc and immune function: the biological basis of altered resistance to infection. The American journal of clinical nutrition, 68(2 Suppl), 447S–463S. https://doi.org/10.1093/ajcn/68.2.447S

[2412] Lassi, Z. S., Moin, A., & Bhutta, Z. A. (2016). Zinc supplementation for the prevention of pneumonia in children aged 2 months to 59 months. The Cochrane database of systematic reviews, 12(12), CD005978. https://doi.org/10.1002/14651858.CD005978.pub3

[2413] Black, R. E., & Sazawal, S. (2001). Zinc and childhood infectious disease morbidity and mortality. The British journal of nutrition, 85 Suppl 2, S125–S129. https://doi.org/10.1079/bjn2000304

[2414] Young, G. P., Mortimer, E. K., Gopalsamy, G. L., Alpers, D. H., Binder, H. J., Manary, M. J., Ramakrishna, B. S., Brown, I. L., & Brewer, T. G. (2014). Zinc deficiency in children with environmental enteropathy-development of new strategies: report from an expert workshop. The American journal of clinical nutrition, 100(4), 1198–1207. https://doi.org/10.3945/ajcn.113.075036

[2415] Takeda A. (2000). Movement of zinc and its functional significance in the brain. Brain research. Brain research reviews, 34(3), 137–148. https://doi.org/10.1016/s0165-0173(00)00044-8

[2416] Anbari-Nogyni, Z., Bidaki, R., Madadizadeh, F., Sangsefidi, Z. S., Fallahzadeh, H., Karimi-Nazari, E., & Nadjarzadeh, A. (2020). Relationship of zinc status with depression and anxiety among elderly population. Clinical nutrition ESPEN, 37, 233–239. https://doi.org/10.1016/j.clnesp.2020.02.008

[2417] Grønli, O., Kvamme, J. M., Friborg, O., & Wynn, R. (2013). Zinc Deficiency Is Common in Several Psychiatric Disorders. PLoS ONE, 8(12), e82793. doi:10.1371/journal.pone.0082793

[2418] Dodig-Curković, K., Dovhanj, J., Curković, M., Dodig-Radić, J., & Degmecić, D. (2009). Uloga cinka u lijecenju hiperaktivnog poremećaja u djece [The role of zinc in the treatment of hyperactivity disorder in children]. Acta medica Croatica : casopis Hrvatske akademije medicinskih znanosti, 63(4), 307–313.

[2419] Swardfager, W., Herrmann, N., Mazereeuw, G., Goldberger, K., Harimoto, T., & Lanctôt, K. L. (2013). Zinc in depression: a meta-analysis. Biological psychiatry, 74(12), 872–878. https://doi.org/10.1016/j.biopsych.2013.05.008

[2420] Petrilli, M. A., Kranz, T. M., Kleinhaus, K., Joe, P., Getz, M., Johnson, P., Chao, M. V., & Malaspina, D. (2017). The Emerging Role for Zinc in Depression and Psychosis. Frontiers in pharmacology, 8, 414. https://doi.org/10.3389/fphar.2017.00414

[2421] Maret W. (2003). Cellular zinc and redox states converge in the metallothionein/thionein pair. The Journal of nutrition, 133(5 Suppl 1), 1460S–2S. https://doi.org/10.1093/jn/133.5.1460S

[2422] Severo, J. S., Morais, J., de Freitas, T., Andrade, A., Feitosa, M. M., Fontenelle, L. C., de Oliveira, A., Cruz, K., & do Nascimento Marreiro, D. (2019). The Role of Zinc in Thyroid Hormones Metabolism. International journal for vitamin and nutrition research. Internationale Zeitschrift fur Vitamin- und Ernahrungsforschung. Journal international de vitaminologie et de nutrition, 89(1-2), 80–88. https://doi.org/10.1024/0300-9831/a000262

[2423] Jalali, G. R., Roozbeh, J., Mohammadzadeh, A., Sharifian, M., Sagheb, M. M., Hamidian Jahromi, A., Shabani, S., Ghaffarpasand, F., & Afshariani, R. (2010). Impact of oral zinc therapy on the level of sex hormones in male patients on hemodialysis. Renal failure, 32(4), 417–419. https://doi.org/10.3109/08860221003706958

[2424] Baltaci, A. K., Mogulkoc, R., & Baltaci, S. B. (2019). Review: The role of zinc in the endocrine system. Pakistan journal of pharmaceutical sciences, 32(1), 231–239.

[2425] Maruthur, N. M., Clark, J. M., Fu, M., Linda Kao, W. H., & Shuldiner, A. R. (2015). Effect of zinc supplementation on insulin secretion: interaction between zinc and SLC30A8 genotype in Old Order Amish. Diabetologia, 58(2), 295–303. https://doi.org/10.1007/s00125-014-3419-1

[2426] Scholze, P., Nørregaard, L., Singer, E. A., Freissmuth, M., Gether, U., & Sitte, H. H. (2002). The role of zinc ions in reverse transport mediated by monoamine transporters. The Journal of biological chemistry, 277(24), 21505–21513. https://doi.org/10.1074/jbc.M112265200

[2427] Liuzzi, J. P., & Pazos, R. (2020). Interplay Between Autophagy and Zinc. Journal of Trace Elements in Medicine and Biology, 62, 126636. doi:10.1016/j.jtemb.2020.126636

[2428] Popp, L., & Segatori, L. (2019). Zinc Oxide Particles Induce Activation of the Lysosome–Autophagy System. ACS Omega, 4(1), 573–581. doi:10.1021/acsomega.8b01497

[2429] WILLIAMS, R. J. P. (1960). Binding of Zinc in Carboxypeptidase. Nature, 188(4747), 322–322. doi:10.1038/188322a0

[2430] Göktuğ Kadıoğlu, B., Nalçakan, A., & Dilek, E. (2020). Relationship between zinc content and carbonic anhydrase activity in blood of anemic pregnant women in Turkey. Journal of Obstetrics and Gynaecology Research, 46(12), 2612–2617. doi:10.1111/jog.14506

[2431] McCall, K. A., Huang, C., & Fierke, C. A. (2000). Function and Mechanism of Zinc Metalloenzymes. The Journal of Nutrition, 130(5), 1437S–1446S. doi:10.1093/jn/130.5.1437s

[2432] Shankar, A. H., & Prasad, A. S. (1998). Zinc and immune function: the biological basis of altered resistance to infection. The American journal of clinical nutrition, 68(2 Suppl), 447S–463S. https://doi.org/10.1093/ajcn/68.2.447S

[2433] Gao, H., Dai, W., Zhao, L., Min, J., & Wang, F. (2018). The Role of Zinc and Zinc Homeostasis in Macrophage Function. Journal of Immunology Research, 2018, 1–11. doi:10.1155/2018/6872621

[2434] Ruz, M., Cavan, K. R., Bettger, W. J., & Gibson, R. S. (1992). Erythrocytes, erythrocyte membranes, neutrophils and platelets as biopsy materials for the assessment of zinc status in humans. British Journal of Nutrition, 68(2), 515–527. doi:10.1079/bjn19920109

[2435] Rolles, B., Maywald, M., & Rink, L. (2018). Influence of zinc deficiency and supplementation on NK cell cytotoxicity. Journal of Functional Foods, 48, 322–328. doi:10.1016/j.jff.2018.07.027

[2436] Bozalioğlu, S., Özkan, Y., Turan, M., & Şimşek, B. (2005). Prevalence of zinc deficiency and immune response in short-term hemodialysis. Journal of Trace Elements in Medicine and Biology, 18(3), 243–249. doi:10.1016/j.jtemb.2005.01.003

[2437] Beck, F. W., Prasad, A. S., Kaplan, J., Fitzgerald, J. T., & Brewer, G. J. (1997). Changes in cytokine production and T cell subpopulations in experimentally induced zinc-deficient humans. The American journal of physiology, 272(6 Pt 1), E1002–E1007. https://doi.org/10.1152/ajpendo.1997.272.6.E1002

[2438] Prasad A. S. (2000). Effects of zinc deficiency on Th1 and Th2 cytokine shifts. The Journal of infectious diseases, 182 Suppl 1, S62–S68. https://doi.org/10.1086/315916

[2439] Rolles, B., Maywald, M., & Rink, L. (2018). Influence of zinc deficiency and supplementation on NK cell cytotoxicity. Journal of Functional Foods, 48, 322–328. doi:10.1016/j.jff.2018.07.027

[2440] Beach RS, Gershwin ME, Hurley LS. Gestational zinc deprivation in mice: persistence of immunodeficiency for three generations. Science 1982;218:469–71.

639

[2441] Vruwink K, Gershwin ME, Keen CL. Effects of gestational zinc deficiency in mice on growth and immune function. J Nutr Immunol 1993;2:25–41.

[2442] Bach, J.-F. (1981). The multi-faceted zinc dependency of the immune system. Immunology Today, 2(11), 225–227. doi:10.1016/0167-5699(81)90052-9

[2443] Bach, JF (1983) Thymulin (FTS-Zn). Clinics in Immunology and Allergy 3, 133–150.

[2444] Dardenne, M., Savino, W., Wade, S., Kaiserlian, D., Lemonnier, D., & Bach, J. F. (1984). In vivo and in vitro studies of thymulin in marginally zinc-deficient mice. European journal of immunology, 14(5), 454–458. https://doi.org/10.1002/eji.1830140513

[2445] Saha, A. R., Hadden, E. M., & Hadden, J. W. (1995). Zinc induces thymulin secretion from human thymic epithelial cells In vitro and augments splenocyte and thymocyte responses In vivo. International Journal of Immunopharmacology, 17(9), 729–733. doi:10.1016/0192-0561(95)00061-6

[2446] Simkin, P. (1976). ORAL ZINC SULPHATE IN RHEUMATOID ARTHRITIS. The Lancet, 308(7985), 539–542. doi:10.1016/s0140-6736(76)91793-1

[2447] Coto, J. A., Hadden, E. M., Sauro, M., Zorn, N., & Hadden, J. W. (1992). Interleukin 1 regulates secretion of zinc-thymulin by human thymic epithelial cells and its action on T-lymphocyte proliferation and nuclear protein kinase C. Proceedings of the National Academy of Sciences, 89(16), 7752–7756. doi:10.1073/pnas.89.16.7752

[2448] Kido, T., Ishiwata, K., Suka, M., & Yanagisawa, H. (2019). Inflammatory response under zinc deficiency is exacerbated by dysfunction of the T helper type 2 lymphocyte-M2 macrophage pathway. Immunology, 156(4), 356–372. https://doi.org/10.1111/imm.13033

[2449] Mercalli, M. E., Seri, S., Aquilio, E., Cramarossa, L., Gobbo, V. D., Accinni, L., & Toniette, G. (1984). Zinc deficiency and thymus ultrastructure in rats. Nutrition Research, 4(4), 665–671. doi:10.1016/s0271-5317(84)80040-8

[2450] Mocchegiani, E., Santarelli, L., Muzzioli, M., & Fabris, N. (1995). Reversibility of the thymic involution and of age-related peripheral immune dysfunctions by zinc supplementation in old mice. International Journal of Immunopharmacology, 17(9), 703–718. doi:10.1016/0192-0561(95)00059-b

[2451] Rajagopalan, S., Winter, C. C., Wagtmann, N., & Long, E. O. (1995). The Ig-related killer cell inhibitory receptor binds zinc and requires zinc for recognition of HLA-C on target cells. Journal of immunology (Baltimore, Md. : 1950), 155(9), 4143–4146.

[2452] Allen, J. I., Perri, R. T., McClain, C. J., & Kay, N. E. (1983). Alterations in human natural killer cell activity and monocyte cytotoxicity induced by zinc deficiency. The Journal of laboratory and clinical medicine, 102(4), 577–589.

[2453] Keen, C. L., & Gershwin, M. E. (1990). Zinc Deficiency and Immune Function. Annual Review of Nutrition, 10(1), 415–431. doi:10.1146/annurev.nu.10.070190.002215

[2454] Kirchner, H., & Rühl, H. (1970). Stimulation of human peripheral lymphocytes by Zn2+ in vitro. Experimental Cell Research, 61(1), 229–230. doi:10.1016/0014-4827(70)90284-3

[2455] Rühl, H., Kirchner, H., & Bochert, G. (1971). Kinetics of the Zn 2+ - stimulation of human peripheral lmphocytes in vitro. Proceedings of the Society for Experimental Biology and Medicine. Society for Experimental Biology and Medicine (New York, N.Y.), 137(3), 1089–1092.

[2456] Berger, N. A., & Skinner, S. A. M. (1974). CHARACTERIZATION OF LYMPHOCYTE TRANSFORMATION INDUCED BY ZINC IONS. Journal of Cell Biology, 61(1), 45–55. doi:10.1083/jcb.61.1.45

[2457] Salas, M., & Kirchner, H. (1987). Induction of interferon-γ in human leukocyte cultures stimulated by Zn2+. Clinical Immunology and Immunopathology, 45(1), 139–142. doi:10.1016/0090-1229(87)90120-6

[2458] Scuderi, P. (1990). Differential effects of copper and zinc on human peripheral blood monocyte cytokine secretion. Cellular Immunology, 126(2), 391–405. doi:10.1016/0008-8749(90)90330-t

[2459] Driessen, C., Hirv, K., Rink, L., & Kirchner, H. (1994). Induction of cytokines by zinc ions in human peripheral blood mononuclear cells and separated monocytes. Lymphokine and cytokine research, 13(1), 15–20.

[2460] Brooks, W. A., Santosham, M., Naheed, A., Goswami, D., Wahed, M. A., Diener-West, M., Faruque, A. S., & Black, R. E. (2005). Effect of weekly zinc supplements on incidence of pneumonia and diarrhoea in children younger than 2 years in an urban, low-income population in Bangladesh: randomised controlled trial. Lancet (London, England), 366(9490), 999–1004. https://doi.org/10.1016/S0140-6736(05)67109-7

[2461] Bahl, R., Bhandari, N., Hambidge, K. M., & Bhan, M. K. (1998). Plasma zinc as a predictor of diarrheal and respiratory morbidity in children in an urban slum setting. The American journal of clinical nutrition, 68(2 Suppl), 414S–417S. https://doi.org/10.1093/ajcn/68.2.414S

[2462] Meydani, S. N., Barnett, J. B., Dallal, G. E., Fine, B. C., Jacques, P. F., Leka, L. S., & Hamer, D. H. (2007). Serum zinc and pneumonia in nursing home elderly. The American journal of clinical nutrition, 86(4), 1167–1173. https://doi.org/10.1093/ajcn/86.4.1167

[2463] Black, R. E. (2003). Zinc Deficiency, Infectious Disease and Mortality in the Developing World. The Journal of Nutrition, 133(5), 1485S–1489S. doi:10.1093/jn/133.5.1485s

[2464] Lukacik, M., Thomas, R. L., & Aranda, J. V. (2008). A meta-analysis of the effects of oral zinc in the treatment of acute and persistent diarrhea. Pediatrics, 121(2), 326–336. https://doi.org/10.1542/peds.2007-0921

[2465] Bhutta, Z. A., Bird, S. M., Black, R. E., Brown, K. H., Gardner, J. M., Hidayat, A., Khatun, F., Martorell, R., Ninh, N. X., Penny, M. E., Rosado, J. L., Roy, S. K., Ruel, M., Sazawal, S., & Shankar, A. (2000). Therapeutic effects of oral zinc in acute and persistent diarrhea in children in developing countries: pooled analysis of randomized controlled trials. The American journal of clinical nutrition, 72(6), 1516–1522. https://doi.org/10.1093/ajcn/72.6.1516

[2466] Black R. E. (1998). Therapeutic and preventive effects of zinc on serious childhood infectious diseases in developing countries. The American journal of clinical nutrition, 68(2 Suppl), 476S–479S. https://doi.org/10.1093/ajcn/68.2.476S

[2467] Himoto, T., Hosomi, N., Nakai, S., Deguchi, A., Kinekawa, F., Matsuki, M., … Kuriyama, S. (2007). Efficacy of zinc administration in patients with hepatitis C virus-related chronic liver disease. Scandinavian Journal of Gastroenterology, 42(9), 1078–1087. doi:10.1080/00365520701272409

[2468] Sanna, A., Firinu, D., Zavattari, P., & Valera, P. (2018). Zinc Status and Autoimmunity: A Systematic Review and Meta-Analysis. Nutrients, 10(1), 68. doi:10.3390/nu10010068

[2469] Jothimani, D., Kailasam, E., Danielraj, S., Nallathambi, B., Ramachandran, H., Sekar, P., Manoharan, S., Ramani, V., Narasimhan, G., Kaliamoorthy, I., & Rela, M. (2020). COVID-19: Poor outcomes in patients with zinc deficiency. International journal of infectious diseases : IJID : official publication of the International Society for Infectious Diseases, 100, 343–349. https://doi.org/10.1016/j.ijid.2020.09.014

[2470] Te Velthuis et al (2010). Zn2+ Inhibits Coronavirus and Arterivirus RNA Polymerase Activity In Vitro and Zinc Ionophores Block the Replication of These Viruses in Cell Culture. PLoS Pathogens, 6(11), e1001176. doi:10.1371/journal.ppat.1001176

[2471] Hulisz D. (2004). Efficacy of zinc against common cold viruses: an overview. Journal of the American Pharmacists Association : JAPhA, 44(5), 594–603. https://doi.org/10.1331/1544-3191.44.5.594.hulisz

[2472] Allan, G. & Arroll, B. (2014). Prevention and treatment of the common cold: making sense of the evidence. CMAJ 186 (3): 190–199.

[2473] Prasad, A. S., Beck, F. W., Bao, B., Snell, D., & Fitzgerald, J. T. (2008). Duration and severity of symptoms and levels of plasma interleukin-1 receptor antagonist, soluble tumor necrosis factor receptor, and adhesion molecules in patients with common cold treated with zinc acetate. The Journal of infectious diseases, 197(6), 795–802. https://doi.org/10.1086/528803

[2474] Turner, R. B., & Cetnarowski, W. E. (2000). Effect of treatment with zinc gluconate or zinc acetate on experimental and natural colds. Clinical infectious diseases : an official publication of the Infectious Diseases Society of America, 31(5), 1202–1208. https://doi.org/10.1086/317437

[2475] Eby, G. A., & Halcomb, W. W. (2006). Ineffectiveness of zinc gluconate nasal spray and zinc orotate lozenges in common-cold treatment: a double-blind, placebo-controlled clinical trial. Alternative therapies in health and medicine, 12(1), 34–38.

[2476] Caruso, T. J., Prober, C. G., & Gwaltney, J. M., Jr (2007). Treatment of naturally acquired common colds with zinc: a structured review. Clinical infectious diseases : an official publication of the Infectious Diseases Society of America, 45(5), 569–574. https://doi.org/10.1086/520031

[2477] Hemilä, H. & Chalker, E. (2017). Zinc for preventing and treating the common cold. Cochrane Database of Systematic Reviews 2017 (9): CD012808.

[2478] Sohnle, P. G., Collins-Lech, C., & Wiessner, J. H. (1991). The Zinc-Reversible Antimicrobial Activity of Neutrophil Lysates and Abscess Fluid Supernatants. Journal of Infectious Diseases, 164(1), 137–142. doi:10.1093/infdis/164.1.137

[2479] Miyasaki, K. T., Bodeau, A. L., Murthy, A. R. K., & Lehrer, R. I. (1993). In vitro Antimicrobial Activity of the Human Neutrophil Cytosolic S-100 Protein Complex, Calprotectin, Against Capnocytophaga sputigena. Journal of Dental Research, 72(2), 517–523. doi:10.1177/00220345930720020801

[2480] CLOHESSY, P. A., & GOLDEN, B. E. (1995). Calprotectin-Mediated Zinc Chelation as a Biostatic Mechanism in Host Defence. Scandinavian Journal of Immunology, 42(5), 551–556. doi:10.1111/j.1365-3083.1995.tb03695.x

[2481] Klosterhalfen, B., Töns, C., Hauptmann, S., Tietze, L., Offner, F. A., Küpper, W., & Kirkpatrick, C. J. (1996). Influence of heat shock protein 70 and metallothionein induction by Zinc-Bis-(DL-Hydrogenaspartate) on the release of inflammatory mediators in a porcine model of recurrent endotoxemia. Biochemical Pharmacology, 52(8), 1201–1210. doi:10.1016/0006-2952(96)00469-8

[2482] Wellinghausen N, Schromm AB, Seydel U, Brandenburg K, Luhm J, Kirchner H & Rink L (1996) Zinc enhances lipopolysaccharide-induced monokine secretion by a fluidity change of lipopolysaccharide. Journal of Immunology 157, 3139–3145.

[2483] Porter, K. G., Mcmaster, D., Elmes, M. E., & Love, A. H. G. (1977). ANÆMIA AND LOW SERUM-COPPER DURING ZINC THERAPY. The Lancet, 310(8041), 774. doi:10.1016/s0140-6736(77)90295-1

[2484] Provinciali M, Montenovo A, Di-Stefano G, Colombo M, Daghetta L, Cairati M, Veroni C, Cassino R, Della-Torre F & Fabris N (1998) Effect of zinc or zinc plus arginine supplementation on antibody titre and lymphocyte subsets after influenza vaccination in elderly subjects: a randomized controlled trial. Age and Ageing 27, 715–722.

[2485] Reinhold, D., Ansorge, S., & Grüngreiff, K. (1999). Immunobiology of zinc and zinc therapy. Immunology Today, 20(2), 102. doi:10.1016/s0167-5699(98)01400-5

[2486] Sandstead, H. H., Henriksen, L. K., Greger, J. L., Prasad, A. S., & Good, R. A. (1982). Zinc nutriture in the elderly in relation to taste acuity, immune response, and wound healing. The American Journal of Clinical Nutrition, 36(5), 1046–1059. doi:10.1093/ajcn/36.5.1046

[2487] Prasad, A. S., Beck, F. W., Bao, B., Fitzgerald, J. T., Snell, D. C., Steinberg, J. D., & Cardozo, L. J. (2007). Zinc supplementation decreases incidence of infections in the elderly: effect of zinc on generation of cytokines and oxidative stress. The American Journal of Clinical Nutrition, 85(3), 837–844. doi:10.1093/ajcn/85.3.837

[2488] Scott, B. J., & Bradwell, A. R. (1983). Identification of the serum binding proteins for iron, zinc, cadmium, nickel, and calcium. Clinical chemistry, 29(4), 629–633.

[2489] Wastney, M. E., Aamodt, R. L., Rumble, W. F., & Henkin, R. I. (1986). Kinetic analysis of zinc metabolism and its regulation in normal humans. The American journal of physiology, 251(2 Pt 2), R398–R408. https://doi.org/10.1152/ajpregu.1986.251.2.R398

[2490] Mills CF (1989) Zinc in Human Biology. Human Nutrition Reviews. London: Springer Verlag.

[2491] Favier A & Favier M (1990) 'Consequences des deficits en zinc durant la grossesse pour la mère et le nouveau-né (Consequences of zinc deficits during pregnancy for the mother and newborn)'. Revue Française de Gynecologie et d'Obstetrique 85, 13–27.

[2492] Institute of Medicine (2002) 'Zinc. Dietary reference intakes: vitamin A, vitamin K, arsenic, boron, chromium, copper, iodine, iron, manganese, molybdenum, nickel, silicon, vanadium, and zinc. Food and Nutrition Board. National Academy Press, Washington, DC, pp. 442–501.

[2493] Sadler, P. J. (1982). Trace Elements in Human and Animal Nutrition. Biochemical Education, 10(1), 36. doi:10.1016/0307-4412(82)90035-8

[2494] Cotton, P. A., Subar, A. F., Friday, J. E., & Cook, A. (2004). Dietary sources of nutrients among US adults, 1994 to 1996. Journal of the American Dietetic Association, 104(6), 921–930. https://doi.org/10.1016/j.jada.2004.03.019

[2495] Ma, J., & Betts, N. M. (2000). Zinc and copper intakes and their major food sources for older adults in the 1994-96 continuing survey of food intakes by individuals (CSFII). The Journal of nutrition, 130(11), 2838–2843. https://doi.org/10.1093/jn/130.11.2838

[2496] Alaimo K, McDowell MA, Briefel RR, et al. Dietary intake of vitamins, minerals, and fiber of persons ages 2 months and over in the United States: Third National Health and Nutrition Examination Survey, Phase 1, 1986-91. Advance data from vital and health statistics no 258external link disclaimer. Hyattsville, Maryland: National Center for Health Statistics. 1994.

[2497] Alaimo K, McDowell MA, Briefel RR, et al. Dietary intake of vitamins, minerals, and fiber of persons ages 2 months and over in the United States: Third National Health and Nutrition Examination Survey, Phase 1, 1986-91. Advance data from vital and health statistics no 258external link disclaimer. Hyattsville, Maryland: National Center for Health Statistics. 1994.

[2498] Ribar DS, Hamrick KS. Dynamics of Poverty and Food Sufficiency. Food Assistance and Nutrition Report Number 36, 2003. Washington, DC: U.S. Department of Agriculture, Economic Research Service. [http://www.ers.usda.gov/publications/fanrr36/fanrr36.pdfexternal link disclaimer]

[2499] Dixon LB, Winkleby MA, Radimer KL. Dietary intakes and serum nutrients differ between adults from food-insufficient and food-sufficient families: Third National Health and Nutrition Examination Survey, 1988-1994. J Nutr 2001;131:1232-46.

[2500] Henderson L, Irving K, Gregory J, Bates C, Prentice A, Perks J, et al. The National Diet and Nutrition Survey: adults aged 19 to 64 years. Vitamin and mineral intake and urinary analytes. 1st ed. Norwich: Her Majesty's Stationery Office; 2003.

[2501] Thane CW, Bates CJ, Prentice A. Zinc and vitamin A intake and status in a national sample of British young people aged 4–18 y. Eur J Clin Nutr 2004;58: 363–75

[2502] Milne et al (1987) 'Ethanol metabolism in postmenopausal women fed a diet marginal in zinc', The American Journal of Clinical Nutrition, Volume 46, Issue 4, October 1987, Pages 688–693, https://doi.org/10.1093/ajcn/46.4.688

[2503] Penland, J.G. Cognitive performance affects low zinc (Zn) intakes in healthy adult men (abstract). FASEB J 1991; 5: A938.

[2504] Sandstead, H. H., & Smith, J. C., Jr (1996). Deliberations and evaluations of approaches, endpoints and paradigms for determining zinc dietary recommendations. The Journal of nutrition, 126(9 Suppl), 2410S–2418S. https://doi.org/10.1093/jn/126.suppl_9.2410S

[2505] Gibson R. Zinc nutrition in developing countries. Nutr Res Rev 1994;7:151–73.

[2506] Walsh, C. T., Sandstead, H. H., Prasad, A. S., Newberne, P. M., & Fraker, P. J. (1994). Zinc: health effects and research priorities for the 1990s. Environmental Health Perspectives, 102(suppl 2), 5–46. doi:10.1289/ehp.941025

[2507] Yokoi, K., Egger, N. G., Ramanujam, V. M., Alcock, N. W., Dayal, H. H., Penland, J. G., & Sandstead, H. H. (2003). Association between plasma zinc concentration and zinc kinetic parameters in premenopausal women. American journal of physiology. Endocrinology and metabolism, 285(5), E1010–E1020. https://doi.org/10.1152/ajpendo.00533.2002

[2508] Yokoi, K., Alcock, N. W., & Sandstead, H. H. (1994). Iron and zinc nutriture of premenopausal women: associations of diet with serum ferritin and plasma zinc disappearance and of serum ferritin with plasma zinc and plasma zinc disappearance. The Journal of laboratory and clinical medicine, 124(6), 852–861.

[2509] Milne, D. B., Canfield, W. K., Mahalko, J. R., & Sandstead, H. H. (1983). Effect of dietary zinc on whole body surface loss of zinc: impact on estimation of zinc retention by balance method. The American Journal of Clinical Nutrition, 38(2), 181–186. doi:10.1093/ajcn/38.2.181

[2510] Gibson R. S. (1994). Content and bioavailability of trace elements in vegetarian diets. The American journal of clinical nutrition, 59(5 Suppl), 1223S–1232S. https://doi.org/10.1093/ajcn/59.5.1223S

[2511] TRIBBLE, H. M., & SCOULAR, F. I. (1954). The Journal of nutrition, 52(2), 209–216. https://doi.org/10.1093/jn/52.2.209

[2512] Gallaher DD, Johnson PE, Hunt JR, Lykken GI, Marchello MJ. Bioavailability in humans of zinc from beef: intrinsic vs. extrinsic labels. Am J Clin Nutr 1988;48:350–4.

[2513] TRIBBLE, H. M., & SCOULAR, F. I. (1954). The Journal of nutrition, 52(2), 209–216. https://doi.org/10.1093/jn/52.2.209

[2514] Hambidge, K. M., Hambidge, C., Jacobs, M., & Baum, J. D. (1972). Low levels of zinc in hair, anorexia, poor growth, and hypogeusia in children. Pediatric research, 6(12), 868–874. https://doi.org/10.1203/00006450-197212000-00003

[2515] Henkin, R. I., 'Newer aspects of copper and zinc metabolism', in Newer Trace Elements in Nutrition, edited by W. Mertz and W. E. Cornatzer, Marcel Dekker, New York, 1971, pp. 297-308.

[2516] Henkin, R. I. (1971). Idiopathic Hypogeusia With Dysgeusia, Hyposmia, and Dysosmia. JAMA, 217(4), 434. doi:10.1001/jama.1971.03190040028006

[2517] Gibson, R. S., Raboy, V., & King, J. C. (2018). Implications of phytate in plant-based foods for iron and zinc bioavailability, setting dietary requirements, and formulating programs and policies. Nutrition reviews, 76(11), 793–804. https://doi.org/10.1093/nutrit/nuy028

[2518] O'Deli, B. L., & Savage, J. E. (1960). Effect of Phytic Acid on Zinc Availability. Experimental Biology and Medicine, 103(2), 304–306. doi:10.3181/00379727-103-25498

[2519] Jung, S. K., Kim, M. K., Lee, Y. H., Shin, D. H., Shin, M. H., Chun, B. Y., & Choi, B. Y. (2013). Lower zinc bioavailability may be related to higher risk of subclinical atherosclerosis in Korean adults. PloS one, 8(11), e80115. https://doi.org/10.1371/journal.pone.0080115

[2520] O'Dell B. L. (1969). Effect of dietary components upon zinc vailability. A review with original data. The American journal of clinical nutrition, 22(10), 1315–1322. https://doi.org/10.1093/ajcn/22.10.1315

[2521] O'Dell, B. L., Burpo, C. E., & Savage, J. E. (1972). Evaluation of zinc availability in foodstuffs of plant and animal origin. The Journal of nutrition, 102(5), 653–660. https://doi.org/10.1093/jn/102.5.653

[2522] Reinhold, J. G., Nasr, K., Lahimgarzadeh, A., & Hedayati, H. (1973). Effects of purified phytate and phytate-rich bread upon metabolism of zinc, calcium, phosphorus, and nitrogen in man. Lancet (London, England), 1(7798), 283–288. https://doi.org/10.1016/s0140-6736(73)91538-9

[2523] Reinhold J. G. (1971). High phytate content of rural Iranian bread: a possible cause of human zinc deficiency. The American journal of clinical nutrition, 24(10), 1204–1206. https://doi.org/10.1093/ajcn/24.10.1204

[2524] Loladze, I. (2014). Hidden shift of the ionome of plants exposed to elevated CO2 depletes minerals at the base of human nutrition. eLife, 3. doi:10.7554/elife.02245

[2525] Myers, S. S., Zanobetti, A., Kloog, I., Huybers, P., Leakey, A. D., Bloom, A. J., Carlisle, E., Dietterich, L. H., Fitzgerald, G., Hasegawa, T., Holbrook, N. M., Nelson, R. L., Ottman, M. J., Raboy, V., Sakai, H., Sartor, K. A., Schwartz, J., Seneweera, S., Tausz, M., & Usui, Y. (2014). Increasing CO2 threatens human nutrition. Nature, 510(7503), 139–142. https://doi.org/10.1038/nature13179

[2526] Prasad et al (1963) 'Zinc and Iron Deficiencies in Male Subjects with Dwarfism and Hypogonadism but Without Ancylostomiasis, Schistosomiasis or Severe Anemia', American Journal of Clinical Nutrition 12:437-44, DOI: 10.1093/ajcn/12.6.437

[2527] Prasad AS. Discovery of human zinc deficiency and marginal deficiency of zinc. In: Tomita H, ed. Modern nutrition in health and disease. Tokyo: Springer-Verlag, 1990:3–14.

[2528] Milne, D. B., Canfield, W. K., Mahalko, J. R., & Sandstead, H. H. (1984). Effect of oral folic acid supplements on zinc, copper, and iron absorption and excretion. The American journal of clinical nutrition, 39(4), 535–539. https://doi.org/10.1093/ajcn/39.4.535

643

[2529] Sreenivasulu, K., Raghu, P., & Nair, K. M. (2010). Polyphenol-rich beverages enhance zinc uptake and metallothionein expression in Caco-2 cells. Journal of food science, 75(4), H123–H128. https://doi.org/10.1111/j.1750-3841.2010.01582.x

[2530] Oberleas, D., Muhrer, M. E., & O'Dell, B. L. (1966). Dietary metal-complexing agents and zinc availability in the rat. The Journal of nutrition, 90(1), 56–62. https://doi.org/10.1093/jn/90.1.56

[2531] Ferguson, E. L., Gibson, R. S., Thompson, L. U., & Ounpuu, S. (1989). Dietary calcium, phytate, and zinc intakes and the calcium, phytate, and zinc molar ratios of the diets of a selected group of East African children. The American journal of clinical nutrition, 50(6), 1450–1456. https://doi.org/10.1093/ajcn/50.6.1450

[2532] ROBERTSON, B. T., & BURNS, M. J. (1963). ZINC METABOLISM AND THE ZINC-DEFICIENCY SYNDROME IN THE DOG. American journal of veterinary research, 24, 997–1002.

[2533] ZINC DEFICIENCY and dietary calcium in swine. (1957). Nutrition reviews, 15(11), 334–336. https://doi.org/10.1111/j.1753-4887.1957.tb00432.x

[2534] ZINC DEFICIENCY IN PIGS. (1955). Nutrition Reviews, 13(10), 303–304. doi:10.1111/j.1753-4887.1955.tb03353.x

[2535] Valberg, L. S., Flanagan, P. R., & Chamberlain, M. J. (1984). Effects of iron, tin, and copper on zinc absorption in humans. The American Journal of Clinical Nutrition, 40(3), 536–541. doi:10.1093/ajcn/40.3.536

[2536] Solomons N. W. (1986). Competitive interaction of iron and zinc in the diet: consequences for human nutrition. The Journal of nutrition, 116(6), 927–935. https://doi.org/10.1093/jn/116.6.927

[2537] Solomons, N. W., & Jacob, R. A. (1981). Studies on the bioavailability of zinc in humans: effects of heme and nonheme iron on the absorption of zinc. The American journal of clinical nutrition, 34(4), 475–482. https://doi.org/10.1093/ajcn/34.4.475

[2538] Meadows, N. J., Grainger, S. L., Ruse, W., Keeling, P. W., & Thompson, R. P. (1983). Oral iron and the bioavailability of zinc. BMJ, 287(6398), 1013–1014. doi:10.1136/bmj.287.6398.1013

[2539] Whittaker, P. (1998). Iron and zinc interactions in humans. The American Journal of Clinical Nutrition, 68(2), 442S–446S. doi:10.1093/ajcn/68.2.442s

[2540] Solomons, N. W., Pineda, O., Viteri, F., & Sandstead, H. H. (1983). Studies on the Bioavailability of Zinc in Humans: Mechanism of the Intestinal Interaction of Nonheme Iron and Zinc. The Journal of Nutrition, 113(2), 337–349. doi:10.1093/jn/113.2.337

[2541] Crofton et al (1989) 'Inorganic zinc and the intestinal absorption of ferrous iron', American Journal of Clinical Nutrition 50(1):141-4, DOI: 10.1093/ajcn/50.1.141

[2542] National Academy of Sciences. 1987 poundage and technical effects update of substances added to food. Springfield, VA: Department of Commerce, National Technical Information Service, 1989.

[2543] Lomaestro, B. M., & Bailie, G. R. (1995). Absorption interactions with fluoroquinolones. 1995 update. Drug safety, 12(5), 314–333. https://doi.org/10.2165/00002018-199512050-00004

[2544] Penttilä, O., Hurme, H., & Neuvonen, P. J. (1975). Effect of zinc sulphate on the absorption of tetracycline and doxycycline in man. European journal of clinical pharmacology, 9(2-3), 131–134. https://doi.org/10.1007/BF00614009

[2545] Brewer, G. J., Yuzbasiyan-Gurkan, V., Johnson, V., Dick, R. D., & Wang, Y. (1993). Treatment of Wilson's disease with zinc: XI. Interaction with other anticopper agents. Journal of the American College of Nutrition, 12(1), 26–30. https://doi.org/10.1080/07315724.1993.10718278

[2546] Wester P. O. (1980). Urinary zinc excretion during treatment with different diuretics. Acta medica Scandinavica, 208(3), 209–212. https://doi.org/10.1111/j.0954-6820.1980.tb01179.x

[2547] Golik, A., Modai, D., Averbukh, Z., Sheffy, M., Shamis, A., Cohen, N., Shaked, U., & Dolev, E. (1990). Zinc metabolism in patients treated with captopril versus enalapril. Metabolism: clinical and experimental, 39(7), 665–667. https://doi.org/10.1016/0026-0495(90)90098-w

[2548] Joshaghani, H., Amiriani, T., Vaghari, G., Besharat, S., Molana, A., Badeleh, M., & Roshandel, G. (2012). Effects of omeprazole consumption on serum levels of trace elements. Journal of trace elements in medicine and biology : organ of the Society for Minerals and Trace Elements (GMS), 26(4), 234–237. https://doi.org/10.1016/j.jtemb.2012.02.002

[2549] Cakman, I., Rohwer, J., Schütz, R.-M., Kirchner, H., & Rink, L. (1996). Dysregulation between TH1 and TH2 T cell subpopulations in the elderly. Mechanisms of Ageing and Development, 87(3), 197–209. doi:10.1016/0047-6374(96)01708-3

[2550] Hambidge, K. M. (1989). Mild Zinc Deficiency in Human Subjects. Zinc in Human Biology, 281–296. doi:10.1007/978-1-4471-3879-2_18

[2551] Bistrian, B. R. (2006). Modern Nutrition in Health and Disease (Tenth Edition). Critical Care Medicine, 34(9), 2514. doi:10.1097/01.ccm.0000236502.51400.9f

[2552] Klaiman, A. P., Victery, W., Kluger, M. J., & Vander, A. J. (1981). Urinary Excretion of Zinc and Iron following Acute Injection of Dead Bacteria in Dog. Experimental Biology and Medicine, 167(2), 165–171. doi:10.3181/00379727-167-41143

[2553] Weiss, G., Widner, B., Zoller, H., & Fuchs, D. (1998). The immunobiology of zinc and the kidney. Immunology Today, 19(4), 193–194. doi:10.1016/s0167-5699(97)01221-8

[2554] Evans (1982) 'Dietary supplementation with essential metal picolinates', United States Patent No 4,315,927. Accessed Online Jan 11 2021: https://patents.google.com/patent/US4315927A/en

[2555] Evans G. W. (1980). Normal and abnormal zinc absorption in man and animals: the tryptophan connection. Nutrition reviews, 38(4), 137–141. https://doi.org/10.1111/j.1753-4887.1980.tb05874.x

[2556] McClain C. J. (1985). Zinc metabolism in malabsorption syndromes. Journal of the American College of Nutrition, 4(1), 49–64. https://doi.org/10.1080/07315724.1985.10720066

[2557] Vasseur, P., Dugelay, E., Benamouzig, R., Savoye, G., Hercberg, S., Touvier, M., Hugot, J. P., Julia, C., Lan, A., & Buscail, C. (2020). Dietary Zinc Intake and Inflammatory Bowel Disease in the French NutriNet-Santé Cohort. The American journal of gastroenterology, 115(8), 1293–1297. https://doi.org/10.14309/ajg.0000000000000688

[2558] Solomons, N. W., Rosenberg, I. H., Sandstead, H. H., & Vo-Khactu, K. P. (1977). Zinc deficiency in Crohn's disease. Digestion, 16(1-2), 87–95. https://doi.org/10.1159/000198059

[2559] Prasad A. S. (1997). Malnutrition in sickle cell disease patients. The American journal of clinical nutrition, 66(2), 423–424. https://doi.org/10.1093/ajcn/66.2.423

[2560] Dhingra et al (2020) 'Lower-Dose Zinc for Childhood Diarrhea — A Randomized, Multicenter Trial', N Engl J Med 2020; 383:1231-1241, DOI: 10.1056/NEJMoa1915905

[2561] Hoque and Binder (2006) 'Zinc in the Treatment of Acute Diarrhea: Current Status and Assessment', Gastroenterology, SPECIAL REPORT AND REVIEW| VOLUME 130, ISSUE 7, P2201-2205, JUNE 01, 2006, DOI:https://doi.org/10.1053/j.gastro.2006.02.062

[2562] STRONG, E. K. Effects of Hookworm on the Mental and Physical Development of Children. Publ. no. 3. Internatl. Health Comm., Rockefeller Found., 1916, 121 pp.

[2563] AITE and Neilson. (1919) 'A study of the effects of hookworm infection upon the mental development of North Queensland school children', Med. J. Australia 1: 1, 1919.

[2564] Vallee BL, Wacker WEC, Bartholomay AF, Robin ED. Zinc metabolism in hepatic dysfunction. NE J Med 1956;255:403–8.

[2565] Sullivan, J. F., & Lankford, H. G. (1962). Urinary excretion of zinc in alcoholism and postalcoholic cirrhosis. The American journal of clinical nutrition, 10, 153–157. https://doi.org/10.1093/ajcn/10.2.153

[2566] McClain, C. J., Antonow, D. R., Cohen, D. A., & Shedlofsky, S. I. (1986). Zinc Metabolism in Alcoholic Liver Disease. Alcoholism: Clinical and Experimental Research, 10(6), 582–589. doi:10.1111/j.1530-0277.1986.tb05149.x

[2567] Powanda M. C. (1980). Host metabolic alterations during inflammatory stress as related to nutritional status. American journal of veterinary research, 41(11), 1905–1911.

[2568] PRASAD, A. S., SANDSTEAD, H. H., SCHULERT, A. R., & EL-ROOBY, A. S. (1963). URINARY EXCRETION OF ZINC IN PATIENTS WITH THE SYNDROME OF ANEMIA, HEPATOSPLENOMEGALY, DWARFISM, AND HYPOGONADISM. The Journal of laboratory and clinical medicine, 62, 591–599.

[2569] El-Safty, I. A., Gadallah, M., Shafik, A., & Shouman, A. E. (2002). Effect of mercury vapour exposure on urinary excretion of calcium, zinc and copper: relationship to alterations in functional and structural integrity of the kidney. Toxicology and industrial health, 18(8), 377–388. https://doi.org/10.1191/0748233702th160oa

[2570] Funk, A. E., Day, F. A., & Brady, F. O. (1987). Displacement of zinc and copper from copper-induced metallothionein by cadmium and by mercury: in vivo and ex vivo studies. Comparative biochemistry and physiology. C, Comparative pharmacology and toxicology, 86(1), 1–6. https://doi.org/10.1016/0742-8413(87)90133-2

[2571] Ziegler, E. E., Serfass, R. E., Nelson, S. E., Figueroa-Colón, R., Edwards, B. B., Houk, R. S., & Thompson, J. J. (1989). Effect of Low Zinc Intake on Absorption and Excretion of Zinc by Infants Studied with 70Zn as Extrinsic Tag. The Journal of Nutrition, 119(11), 1647–1653. doi:10.1093/jn/119.11.1647

[2572] German Society of Nutrition (1995) 'Ausschuß Nahrungsbedarf der DGE Zufuhrempfehlungen und Nährstoffbedarf. Teil II: Vergleich der Vorschläge von SCF/EC mit den Empfehlungen der DGE (Dietary requirements committee of DGE recommended intakes and nutrient requirements. Part 2. Comparison of proposals of SCF/EC with the recommendations of DGE)'. Ernährungsumschau 42, 4–10.

[2573] Prasad A. S. (1996). Zinc deficiency in women, infants and children. Journal of the American College of Nutrition, 15(2), 113–120. https://doi.org/10.1080/07315724.1996.10718575

[2574] Sallé, A., Demarsy, D., Poirier, A. L., Lelièvre, B., Topart, P., Guilloteau, G., Bécouarn, G., & Rohmer, V. (2010). Zinc deficiency: a frequent and underestimated complication after bariatric surgery. Obesity surgery, 20(12), 1660–1670. https://doi.org/10.1007/s11695-010-0237-5

[2575] Marreiro, D. N., Geloneze, B., Tambascia, M. A., Lerário, A. C., Halpern, A., & Cozzolino, S. M. (2006). Effect of zinc supplementation on serum leptin levels and insulin resistance of obese women. Biological trace element research, 112(2), 109–118. https://doi.org/10.1385/bter:112:2:109

[2576] Bouglé, D. L., Bureau, F., & Laroche, D. (2009). Trace element status in obese children: Relationship with metabolic risk factors. e-SPEN, the European e-Journal of Clinical Nutrition and Metabolism, 4(2), e98–e100. doi:10.1016/j.eclnm.2009.01.012

645

[2577] Marreiro, D. N., Fisberg, M., & Cozzolino, S. M. (2002). Zinc nutritional status in obese children and adolescents. Biological trace element research, 86(2), 107–122. https://doi.org/10.1385/bter:86:2:107

[2578] Konukoglu, D., Turhan, M. S., Ercan, M., & Serin, O. (2004). Relationship between plasma leptin and zinc levels and the effect of insulin and oxidative stress on leptin levels in obese diabetic patients. The Journal of nutritional biochemistry, 15(12), 757–760. https://doi.org/10.1016/j.jnutbio.2004.07.007

[2579] Chu et al (2018) 'Zinc status at baseline is not related to acute changes in serum zinc concentration following bouts of running or cycling', Journal of Trace Elements in Medicine and Biology, Volume 50, December 2018, Pages 105-110. https://doi.org/10.1016/j.jtemb.2018.06.004

[2580] Sandstead, H. H., Prasad, A. S., Schulert, A. R., Farid, Z., Miale, A., Jr, Bassilly, S., & Darby, W. J. (1967). Human zinc deficiency, endocrine manifestations and response to treatment. The American journal of clinical nutrition, 20(5), 422–442. https://doi.org/10.1093/ajcn/20.5.422

[2581] PRASAD, A. S., SCHULERT, A. R., SANDSTEAD, H. H., MIALE, A., Jr, & FARID, Z. (1963). Zinc, iron, and nitrogen content of sweat in normal and deficient subjects. The Journal of laboratory and clinical medicine, 62, 84–89.

[2582] National Research Council (US) Subcommittee on the Tenth Edition of the Recommended Dietary Allowances. (1989). Recommended Dietary Allowances: 10th Edition. National Academies Press (US).

[2583] Mittermeier, L., Demirkhanyan, L., Stadlbauer, B., Breit, A., Recordati, C., Hilgendorff, A., Matsushita, M., Braun, A., Simmons, D. G., Zakharian, E., Gudermann, T., & Chubanov, V. (2019). TRPM7 is the central gatekeeper of intestinal mineral absorption essential for postnatal survival. Proceedings of the National Academy of Sciences of the United States of America, 116(10), 4706–4715. https://doi.org/10.1073/pnas.1810633116

[2584] Kasana, S., Din, J., & Maret, W. (2015). Genetic causes and gene–nutrient interactions in mammalian zinc deficiencies: acrodermatitis enteropathica and transient neonatal zinc deficiency as examples. Journal of trace elements in medicine and biology : organ of the Society for Minerals and Trace Elements (GMS), 29, 47–62. https://doi.org/10.1016/j.jtemb.2014.10.003

[2585] BROWN, M. A., THOM, J. V., ORTH, G. L., COVA, P., & JUAREZ, J. (1964). FOOD POISONING INVOLVING ZINC CONTAMINATION. Archives of environmental health, 8, 657–660. https://doi.org/10.1080/00039896.1964.10663736

[2586] Lewis, M. R., & Kokan, L. (1998). Zinc gluconate: acute ingestion. Journal of toxicology. Clinical toxicology, 36(1-2), 99–101. https://doi.org/10.3109/15563659809162595

[2587] Hooper, P. L., Visconti, L., Garry, P. J., & Johnson, G. E. (1980). Zinc lowers high-density lipoprotein-cholesterol levels. JAMA, 244(17), 1960–1961.

[2588] Johnson, A. R., Munoz, A., Gottlieb, J. L., & Jarrard, D. F. (2007). High dose zinc increases hospital admissions due to genitourinary complications. The Journal of urology, 177(2), 639–643. https://doi.org/10.1016/j.juro.2006.09.047

[2589] Chandra R. K. (1984). Excessive intake of zinc impairs immune responses. JAMA, 252(11), 1443–1446.

[2590] Faber, C., Gabriel, P., Ibs, K. H., & Rink, L. (2004). Zinc in pharmacological doses suppresses allogeneic reaction without affecting the antigenic response. Bone marrow transplantation, 33(12), 1241–1246. https://doi.org/10.1038/sj.bmt.1704509

[2591] Goodwin, J. S., Hunt, W. C., Hooper, P., & Garry, P. J. (1985). Relationship between zinc intake, physical activity, and blood levels of high-density lipoprotein cholesterol in a healthy elderly population. Metabolism: clinical and experimental, 34(6), 519–523. https://doi.org/10.1016/0026-0495(85)90187-8

[2592] Jafek, B. W., Linschoten, M. R., & Murrow, B. W. (2004). Anosmia after intranasal zinc gluconate use. American journal of rhinology, 18(3), 137–141.

[2593] Alexander, T. H., & Davidson, T. M. (2006). Intranasal Zinc and Anosmia: The Zinc-Induced Anosmia Syndrome. The Laryngoscope, 116(2), 217–220. doi:10.1097/01.mlg.0000191549.17796.13

[2594] U.S. Food and Drug Administration. Warnings on Three Zicam Intranasal Zinc Products. [http://www.fda.gov/ForConsumers/ConsumerUpdates/ucm166931.htmexternal link disclaimer]

[2595] Uriu-Adams, J. Y., & Keen, C. L. (2005). Copper, oxidative stress, and human health. Molecular Aspects of Medicine, 26(4-5), 268–298. doi:10.1016/j.mam.2005.07.015

[2596] Domingo JL, Llobet JM, Paternain JL, Corbella J. Acute zinc intoxication: comparison of the antidotal efficacy of several chelating agents. Veterinary and Human Toxicology. 1988 Jun;30(3):224-228.

[2597] Newberne, P. M., Schrager, T. F., & Broitman, S. (1997). Esophageal carcinogenesis in the rat: zinc deficiency and alcohol effects on tumor induction. Pathobiology : journal of immunopathology, molecular and cellular biology, 65(1), 39–45. https://doi.org/10.1159/000164101

[2598] Leitzmann, M. F., Stampfer, M. J., Wu, K., Colditz, G. A., Willett, W. C., & Giovannucci, E. L. (2003). Zinc supplement use and risk of prostate cancer. Journal of the National Cancer Institute, 95(13), 1004–1007. https://doi.org/10.1093/jnci/95.13.1004

[2599] Stewart, A. K., & Magee, A. C. (1964). Effect of Zinc Toxicity on Calcium, Phosphorus and Magnesium Metabolism of Young Rats. The Journal of Nutrition, 82(2), 287–295. doi:10.1093/jn/82.2.287

[2600] Prasad, A. S., & Cossack, Z. T. (1982). Neutrophil zinc: an indicator of zinc status in man. Transactions of the Association of American Physicians, 95, 165–176.

[2601] Prasad, A. S., Fitzgerald, J. T., Hess, J. W., Kaplan, J., Pelen, F., & Dardenne, M. (1993). Zinc deficiency in elderly patients. Nutrition (Burbank, Los Angeles County, Calif.), 9(3), 218–224.

[2602] Beck FWJ, Prasad AS, Kaplan J, Fitzgerald JT, Brewer GJ. Changes in cytokine production and T cell subpopulations in experimentally induced zinc-deficient humans. Am J Physiol 1997;272:E1002–7.

[2603] Lewis et al (1957) 'RESTRICTED CALCIUM FEEDING VERSUS ZINC SUPPLEMENTATION FOR THE CONTROL OF PARAKERATOSIS IN SWINE', Journal of Animal Science, Volume 16, Issue 3, August 1957, Pages 578–588, https://doi.org/10.2527/1957.163578x

[2604] Macapinlac et al (1967) 'Production of Zinc Deficiency in the Squirrel Monkey (Saimiri sciureus)', The Journal of Nutrition, Volume 93, Issue 4, December 1967, Pages 499–510, https://doi.org/10.1093/jn/93.4.499

[2605] Miller et al (1965) 'Factors Affecting Zinc Content of Bovine Hair', Journal of Dairy Science, Volume 48, Issue 8, August 1965, Pages 1091-1095, https://doi.org/10.3168/jds.S0022-0302(65)88397-7

[2606] McBean, L. D., Mahloudji, M., Reinhold, J. G., & Halsted, J. A. (1971). Correlation of zinc concentrations in human plasma and hair. The American journal of clinical nutrition, 24(5), 506–509. https://doi.org/10.1093/ajcn/24.5.506

[2607] Strain, W. H., Steadman, L. T., Lankau, C. A., Jr, Berliner, W. P., & Pories, W. J. (1966). Analysis of zinc levels in hair for the diagnosis of zinc deficiency in man. The Journal of laboratory and clinical medicine, 68(2), 244–249.

[2608] Prasad (1966) 'Metabolism of zinc and its deficiency in human subjects'. Springield Thomas, p 250.

[2609] PRASAD, A. S., OBERLEAS, D., WOLF, P., HORWITZ, J. P., MILLER, E. R., & LUECKE, R. W. (1969). Changes in Trace Elements and Enzyme Activities in Tissues of Zinc-Deficient Pigs. The American Journal of Clinical Nutrition, 22(5), 628–637. doi:10.1093/ajcn/22.5.628

[2610] Prasad, A. S., Rabbani, P., Abbasii, A., Bowersox, E., & Fox, M. R. (1978). Experimental zinc deficiency in humans. Annals of internal medicine, 89(4), 483–490. https://doi.org/10.7326/0003-4819-89-4-483

[2611] Maret, W., & Sandstead, H. H. (2006). Zinc requirements and the risks and benefits of zinc supplementation. Journal of trace elements in medicine and biology : organ of the Society for Minerals and Trace Elements (GMS), 20(1), 3–18. https://doi.org/10.1016/j.jtemb.2006.01.006

[2612] Lukaski, H. C., Bolonchuk, W. W., Klevay, L. M., Milne, D. B., & Sandstead, H. H. (1984). Changes in plasma zinc content after exercise in men fed a low-zinc diet. The American journal of physiology, 247(1 Pt 1), E88–E93. https://doi.org/10.1152/ajpendo.1984.247.1.E88

[2613] Prasad, A. S., Oberleas, D., & Halsted, J. A. (1965). Determination of zinc in biological fluids by atomic absorption spectrophotometry in normal and cirrhotic subjects. The Journal of laboratory and clinical medicine, 66(3), 508–516.

[2614] Hackley, B. M., Smith, J. C., & Halsted, J. A. (1968). A simplified method for plasma zinc determination by atomic absorption spectrophotometry. Clinical chemistry, 14(1), 1–5.

[2615] Hovmark A. (1977). An in vitro study of depressed cell-mediated immunity and of T and B lymphocytes in atopic dermatitis. Acta dermato-venereologica, 57(3), 237–242.

[2616] Kempson, I. M., Skinner, W. M., & Kirkbride, K. P. (2007). The occurrence and incorporation of copper and zinc in hair and their potential role as bioindicators: a review. Journal of toxicology and environmental health. Part B, Critical reviews, 10(8), 611–622. https://doi.org/10.1080/10937400701389917

[2617] Yuzbasiyan-Gurkan, V., Grider, A., Nostrant, T., Cousins, R. J., & Brewer, G. J. (1992). Treatment of Wilson's disease with zinc: X. Intestinal metallothionein induction. The Journal of laboratory and clinical medicine, 120(3), 380–386.

[2618] Klevay, L. M., & Hyg., S. D. (1973). Hypercholesterolemia in rats produced by an increase in the ratio of zinc to copper ingested. The American Journal of Clinical Nutrition, 26(10), 1060–1068. doi:10.1093/ajcn/26.10.1060

[2619] Troost et al (2003) 'Iron supplements inhibit zinc but not copper absorption in vivo in ileostomy subjects', The American Journal of Clinical Nutrition, Volume 78, Issue 5, November 2003, Pages 1018–1023, https://doi.org/10.1093/ajcn/78.5.1018

[2620] Lönnerdal B. (2000). Dietary factors influencing zinc absorption. The Journal of nutrition, 130(5S Suppl), 1378S–83S. https://doi.org/10.1093/jn/130.5.1378S

[2621] Layman, D. K., Anthony, T. G., Rasmussen, B. B., Adams, S. H., Lynch, C. J., Brinkworth, G. D., & Davis, T. A. (2015). Defining meal requirements for protein to optimize metabolic roles of amino acids. The American journal of clinical nutrition, 101(6), 1330S–1338S. https://doi.org/10.3945/ajcn.114.084053

[2622] Bosse, J. D., & Dixon, B. M. (2012). Dietary protein to maximize resistance training: a review and examination of protein spread and change theories. Journal of the International Society of Sports Nutrition, 9(1), 42. https://doi.org/10.1186/1550-2783-9-42

647

[2623] Wycherley, T. P., Moran, L. J., Clifton, P. M., Noakes, M., & Brinkworth, G. D. (2012). Effects of energy-restricted high-protein, low-fat compared with standard-protein, low-fat diets: a meta-analysis of randomized controlled trials. The American journal of clinical nutrition, 96(6), 1281–1298. https://doi.org/10.3945/ajcn.112.044321

[2624] Blom, W. A., Lluch, A., Stafleu, A., Vinoy, S., Holst, J. J., Schaafsma, G., & Hendriks, H. F. (2006). Effect of a high-protein breakfast on the postprandial ghrelin response. The American journal of clinical nutrition, 83(2), 211–220. https://doi.org/10.1093/ajcn/83.2.211

[2625] Lejeune, M. P., Westerterp, K. R., Adam, T. C., Luscombe-Marsh, N. D., & Westerterp-Plantenga, M. S. (2006). Ghrelin and glucagon-like peptide 1 concentrations, 24-h satiety, and energy and substrate metabolism during a high-protein diet and measured in a respiration chamber. The American journal of clinical nutrition, 83(1), 89–94. https://doi.org/10.1093/ajcn/83.1.89

[2626] Wycherley, T. P., Moran, L. J., Clifton, P. M., Noakes, M., & Brinkworth, G. D. (2012). Effects of energy-restricted high-protein, low-fat compared with standard-protein, low-fat diets: a meta-analysis of randomized controlled trials. The American journal of clinical nutrition, 96(6), 1281–1298. https://doi.org/10.3945/ajcn.112.044321

[2627] Bonjour J. P. (2005). Dietary protein: an essential nutrient for bone health. Journal of the American College of Nutrition, 24(6 Suppl), 526S–36S. https://doi.org/10.1080/07315724.2005.10719501

[2628] Kerstetter, J. E., Kenny, A. M., & Insogna, K. L. (2011). Dietary protein and skeletal health: a review of recent human research. Current opinion in lipidology, 22(1), 16–20. https://doi.org/10.1097/MOL.0b013e3283419441

[2629] Morton, R. W., Murphy, K. T., McKellar, S. R., Schoenfeld, B. J., Henselmans, M., Helms, E., ... Phillips, S. M. (2017). A systematic review, meta-analysis and meta-regression of the effect of protein supplementation on resistance training-induced gains in muscle mass and strength in healthy adults. British Journal of Sports Medicine, 52(6), 376–384. doi:10.1136/bjsports-2017-097608

[2630] Moeller, L. C., & Broecker-Preuss, M. (2011). Transcriptional regulation by nonclassical action of thyroid hormone. Thyroid research, 4 Suppl 1(Suppl 1), S6. https://doi.org/10.1186/1756-6614-4-S1-S6

[2631] Yen P. M. (2001). Physiological and molecular basis of thyroid hormone action. Physiological reviews, 81(3), 1097–1142. https://doi.org/10.1152/physrev.2001.81.3.1097

[2632] Venturi (2015) 'Iodine, PUFAs and Iodolipids in Health and Diseases: An Evolutionary Perspective', Human Evolution. 29 (1–3): 185–205. ISSN 0393-9375.

[2633] Cocchi and Venturi (2000) 'Iodide, antioxidant function and omega-6 and omega-3 fatty acids: A new hypothesis of biochemical cooperation?', Progress in Nutrition 2:15-19.

[2634] Mehran, L., Amouzegar, A., Rahimabad, P. K., Tohidi, M., Tahmasebinejad, Z., & Azizi, F. (2017). Thyroid Function and Metabolic Syndrome: A Population-Based Thyroid Study. Hormone and metabolic research = Hormon- und Stoffwechselforschung = Hormones et metabolisme, 49(3), 192–200. https://doi.org/10.1055/s-0042-117279

[2635] Cappola, A. R., Desai, A. S., Medici, M., Cooper, L. S., Egan, D., Sopko, G., ... Wassner, A. J. (2019). Thyroid and Cardiovascular Disease. Circulation, 139(25), 2892–2909. doi:10.1161/circulationaha.118.036859

[2636] Laurberg, P., Knudsen, N., Andersen, S., Carlé, A., Pedersen, I. B., & Karmisholt, J. (2012). Thyroid Function and Obesity. European Thyroid Journal, 1(3), 159–167. doi:10.1159/000342994

[2637] Samuels, M. H. (2014). Psychiatric and cognitive manifestations of hypothyroidism. Current Opinion in Endocrinology & Diabetes and Obesity, 21(5), 377–383. doi:10.1097/med.0000000000000089

[2638] Bennett, W. E., & Heuckeroth, R. O. (2012). Hypothyroidism Is a Rare Cause of Isolated Constipation. Journal of Pediatric Gastroenterology and Nutrition, 54(2), 285–287. doi:10.1097/mpg.0b013e318239714f

[2639] (2013). International Journal of Geriatric Psychiatry, 28(2). doi:10.1002/gps.v28.2

[2640] Harvey, C. B., & Williams, G. R. (2002). Mechanism of thyroid hormone action. Thyroid : official journal of the American Thyroid Association, 12(6), 441–446. https://doi.org/10.1089/105072502760143791

[2641] Brent G. A. (2000). Tissue-specific actions of thyroid hormone: insights from animal models. Reviews in endocrine & metabolic disorders, 1(1-2), 27–33. https://doi.org/10.1023/a:1010056202122

[2642] ROBBINS, J., & RALL, J. E. (1960). Proteins associated with the thyroid hormones. Physiological reviews, 40, 415–489. https://doi.org/10.1152/physrev.1960.40.3.415

[2643] ROBBINS, J., & RALL, J. E. (1957). The interaction of thyroid hormones and protein in biological fluids. Recent progress in hormone research, 13, 161–208.

[2644] INGBAR, S. H., & FREINKEL, N. (1960). Regulation of the peripheral metabolism of the thyroid hormones. Recent progress in hormone research, 16, 353–403.

[2645] Rao, G. S., Eckel, J., Rao, M. L., & Breuer, H. (1976). Uptake of thyroid hormone by isolated rat liver cells. Biochemical and biophysical research communications, 73(1), 98–104. https://doi.org/10.1016/0006-291x(76)90502-7

[2646] Zonefrati, R., Rotella, C. M., Toccafondi, R. S., & Arcangeli, P. (1983). Thyroid hormone receptors in human cultured fibroblasts: evidence for cellular T4 transport and nuclear T3 binding. Hormone and metabolic research = Hormon- und Stoffwechselforschung = Hormones et metabolisme, 15(3), 151–154. https://doi.org/10.1055/s-2007-1018654

[2647] Mitchell, A. M., Manley, S. W., & Mortimer, R. H. (1992). Uptake of L-tri-iodothyronine by human cultured trophoblast cells. The Journal of endocrinology, 133(3), 483–486. https://doi.org/10.1677/joe.0.1330483

[2648] Krenning, E. P., Docter, R., Bernard, H. F., Visser, T. J., & Hennemann, G. (1978). Active transport of triiodothyronine (T3) into isolated rat liver cells. FEBS letters, 91(1), 113–116. https://doi.org/10.1016/0014-5793(78)80029-5

[2649] Hennemann, G., Docter, R., Friesema, E. C. H., de Jong, M., Krenning, E. P., & Visser, T. J. (2001). Plasma Membrane Transport of Thyroid Hormones and Its Role inThyroid Hormone Metabolism and Bioavailability. Endocrine Reviews, 22(4), 451–476. doi:10.1210/edrv.22.4.0435

[2650] Krenning, E., Docter, R., Bernard, B., Visser, T., & Hennemann, G. (1981). Characteristics of active transport of thyroid hormone into rat hepatocytes. Biochimica et biophysica acta, 676(3), 314–320. https://doi.org/10.1016/0304-4165(81)90165-3

[2651] Centanni, M., & Robbins, J. (1987). Role of sodium in thyroid hormone uptake by rat skeletal muscle. The Journal of clinical investigation, 80(4), 1068–1072. https://doi.org/10.1172/JCI113162

[2652] de Jong, M., Visser, T. J., Bernard, B. F., Docter, R., Vos, R. A., Hennemann, G., & Krenning, E. P. (1993). Transport and metabolism of iodothyronines in cultured human hepatocytes. The Journal of clinical endocrinology and metabolism, 77(1), 139–143. https://doi.org/10.1210/jcem.77.1.8392080

[2653] Krenning, E., Docter, R., Bernard, B., Visser, T., & Hennemann, G. (1980). Regulation of the active transport of 3,3',5-triiodothyronine (T3) into primary cultured rat hepatocytes by ATP. FEBS letters, 119(2), 279–282. https://doi.org/10.1016/0014-5793(80)80271-7

[2654] Osty, J., Valensi, P., Samson, M., Francon, J., & Blondeau, J. P. (1990). Transport of thyroid hormones by human erythrocytes: kinetic characterization in adults and newborns. The Journal of clinical endocrinology and metabolism, 71(6), 1589–1595. https://doi.org/10.1210/jcem-71-6-1589

[2655] Dai, G., Levy, O., & Carrasco, N. (1996). Cloning and characterization of the thyroid iodide transporter. Nature, 379(6564), 458–460. https://doi.org/10.1038/379458a0

[2656] Krenning, E. P., Docter, R., Bernard, H. F., Visser, T. J., & Hennemann, G. (1979). The essential role of albumin in the active transport of thyroid hormones into primary cultured rat hepatocytes. FEBS letters, 107(1), 227–230. https://doi.org/10.1016/0014-5793(79)80501-3

[2657] Sellitti, D. F., & Suzuki, K. (2014). Intrinsic Regulation of Thyroid Function by Thyroglobulin. Thyroid, 24(4), 625–638. doi:10.1089/thy.2013.0344

[2658] Arriagada, A. A., Albornoz, E., Opazo, M. C., Becerra, A., Vidal, G., Fardella, C., … Riedel, C. A. (2015). Excess Iodide Induces an Acute Inhibition of the Sodium/Iodide Symporter in Thyroid Male Rat Cells by Increasing Reactive Oxygen Species. Endocrinology, 156(4), 1540–1551. doi:10.1210/en.2014-1371

[2659] Milanesi and Brent (2017) 'Chapter 12 - Iodine and Thyroid Hormone Synthesis, Metabolism, and Action', Molecular, Genetic, and Nutritional Aspects of Major and Trace Minerals, Pages 143-150, DOI: https://doi.org/10.1016/B978-0-12-802168-2.00012-9

[2660] Knudsen, N., Laurberg, P., Perrild, H., Bülow, I., Ovesen, L., & Jørgensen, T. (2002). Risk factors for goiter and thyroid nodules. Thyroid : official journal of the American Thyroid Association, 12(10), 879–888. https://doi.org/10.1089/105072502761016502

[2661] Greenwood and Earshaw (1997) 'Chemistry of the Elements: 2nd Edition', Butterworth-Heinemann, pp. 795–796.

[2662] Swain, Patricia A. (2005). "Bernard Courtois (1777–1838) famed for discovering iodine (1811), and his life in Paris from 1798". Bulletin for the History of Chemistry. 30 (2): 103.

[2663] Gay-Lussac, J. (1813). "Sur un nouvel acide formé avec la substance découverte par M. Courtois". Annales de Chimie. 88: 311.

[2664] Patwardhan, N., & Kelkar, U. (2011). Disinfection, sterilization and operation theater guidelines for dermatosurgical practitioners in India. Indian journal of dermatology, venereology and leprology, 77(1), 83–93. https://doi.org/10.4103/0378-6323.74965

[2665] Venturi (2015) 'Iodine, PUFAs and Iodolipids in Health and Diseases: An Evolutionary Perspective', Human Evolution. 29 (1–3): 185–205. ISSN 0393-9375.

[2666] Cocchi and Venturi (2000) 'Iodide, antioxidant function and omega-6 and omega-3 fatty acids: A new hypothesis of biochemical cooperation?', Progress in Nutrition 2:15-19.

[2667] Cocchi and Venturi (2000) 'Iodide, antioxidant function and omega-6 and omega-3 fatty acids: A new hypothesis of biochemical cooperation?', Progress in Nutrition 2:15-19.

[2668] Zoeller, R. T., Tan, S. W., & Tyl, R. W. (2007). General background on the hypothalamic-pituitary-thyroid (HPT) axis. Critical reviews in toxicology, 37(1-2), 11–53. https://doi.org/10.1080/10408440601123446

[2669] Hennemann (1986) Thyroid hormone deiodination in healthy men. In: Hennemann G, ed. Thyroid hormone metabolism. New York: Marcel Dekker; 277–296

[2670] Visser TJ (1990) Importance of deiodination and conjugation in the hepatic metabolism of thyroid hormone. In: Greer MA, ed. The thyroid gland. New York: Raven Press; 255–283

[2671] Visser, T. J., Kaptein, E., Terpstra, O. T., & Krenning, E. P. (1988). Deiodination of thyroid hormone by human liver. The Journal of clinical endocrinology and metabolism, 67(1), 17–24. https://doi.org/10.1210/jcem-67-1-17

[2672] Larsen PR 1997 An update on thyroxine activation in humans. Thyroid Int 4:8–14.

[2673] Cocchi and Venturi (2000) 'Iodide, antioxidant function and omega-6 and omega-3 fatty acids: A new hypothesis of biochemical cooperation?', Progress in Nutrition 2:15-19.

[2674] Dohán, O., De la Vieja, A., Paroder, V., Riedel, C., Artani, M., Reed, M., Ginter, C. S., & Carrasco, N. (2003). The sodium/iodide Symporter (NIS): characterization, regulation, and medical significance. Endocrine reviews, 24(1), 48–77. https://doi.org/10.1210/er.2001-0029

[2675] Eskandari, S., Loo, D. D. F., Dai, G., Levy, O., Wright, E. M., & Carrasco, N. (1997). Thyroid Na+/I−Symporter. Journal of Biological Chemistry, 272(43), 27230–27238. doi:10.1074/jbc.272.43.27230

[2676] Zimmermann, M. B., Jooste, P. L., & Pandav, C. S. (2008). Iodine-deficiency disorders. Lancet (London, England), 372(9645), 1251–1262. https://doi.org/10.1016/S0140-6736(08)61005-3

[2677] Zimmermann, M. B., Hess, S. Y., Adou, P., Toresanni, T., Wegmüller, R., & Hurrell, R. F. (2003). Thyroid size and goiter prevalence after introduction of iodized salt: a 5-y prospective study in schoolchildren in Côte d'Ivoire. The American journal of clinical nutrition, 77(3), 663–667. https://doi.org/10.1093/ajcn/77.3.663

[2678] Suzuki, H., Higuchi, T., Sawa, K., Ohtaki, S., & Horiuchi, Y. (1965). "Endemic coast goitre" in Hokkaido, Japan. Acta endocrinologica, 50(2), 161–176.

[2679] Zimmermann, M. B., Ito, Y., Hess, S. Y., Fujieda, K., & Molinari, L. (2005). High thyroid volume in children with excess dietary iodine intakes. The American Journal of Clinical Nutrition, 81(4), 840–844. doi:10.1093/ajcn/81.4.840

[2680] Medani, A. M., Elnour, A. A., & Saeed, A. M. (2013). Excessive iodine intake, water chemicals and endemic goitre in a Sudanese coastal area. Public health nutrition, 16(9), 1586–1592. https://doi.org/10.1017/S1368980012004685

[2681] Henjum, S., Barikmo, I., Gjerlaug, A. K., Mohamed-Lehabib, A., Oshaug, A., Strand, T. A., & Torheim, L. E. (2010). Endemic goitre and excessive iodine in urine and drinking water among Saharawi refugee children. Public health nutrition, 13(9), 1472–1477. https://doi.org/10.1017/S1368980010000650

[2682] Seal, A. J., Creeke, P. I., Gnat, D., Abdalla, F., & Mirghani, Z. (2006). Excess dietary iodine intake in long-term African refugees. Public Health Nutrition, 9(1), 35–39. doi:10.1079/phn2005830

[2683] Markou, K., Georgopoulos, N., Kyriazopoulou, V., & Vagenakis, A. G. (2001). Iodine-Induced hypothyroidism. Thyroid : official journal of the American Thyroid Association, 11(5), 501–510. https://doi.org/10.1089/105072501300176462

[2684] Laurberg, P., Pedersen, K. M., Vestergaard, H., & Sigurdsson, G. (1991). High incidence of multinodular toxic goitre in the elderly population in a low iodine intake area vs. high incidence of Graves' disease in the young in a high iodine intake area: comparative surveys of thyrotoxicosis epidemiology in East-Jutland Denmark and Iceland. Journal of internal medicine, 229(5), 415–420. https://doi.org/10.1111/j.1365-2796.1991.tb00368.x

[2685] Weng, W., Dong, M., Zhang, J., Yang, J., Zhang, B., & Zhao, X. (2017). A PRISMA-compliant systematic review and meta-analysis of the relationship between thyroid disease and different levels of iodine intake in mainland China. Medicine, 96(25), e7279. doi:10.1097/md.0000000000007279

[2686] Flores-Rebollar, A., Moreno-Castañeda, L., Vega-Servín, N. S., López-Carrasco, G., & Ruiz-Juvera, A. (2015). PREVALENCE OF AUTOIMMUNE THYROIDITIS AND THYROID DYSFUNCTION IN HEALTHY ADULT MEXICANS WITH A SLIGHTLY EXCESSIVE IODINE INTAKE. Nutricion hospitalaria, 32(2), 918–924. https://doi.org/10.3305/nh.2015.32.2.9246

[2687] Luo, Y., Kawashima, A., Ishido, Y., Yoshihara, A., Oda, K., Hiroi, N., Ito, T., Ishii, N., & Suzuki, K. (2014). Iodine excess as an environmental risk factor for autoimmune thyroid disease. International journal of molecular sciences, 15(7), 12895–12912. https://doi.org/10.3390/ijms150712895

[2688] Ferrari, S. M., Fallahi, P., Antonelli, A., & Benvenga, S. (2017). Environmental Issues in Thyroid Diseases. Frontiers in endocrinology, 8, 50. https://doi.org/10.3389/fendo.2017.00050

[2689] Pedersen, I. B., Knudsen, N., Jørgensen, T., Perrild, H., Ovesen, L., & Laurberg, P. (2003). Thyroid peroxidase and thyroglobulin autoantibodies in a large survey of populations with mild and moderate iodine deficiency. Clinical endocrinology, 58(1), 36–42. https://doi.org/10.1046/j.1365-2265.2003.01633.x

[2690] Leung, A. M., & Braverman, L. E. (2014). Consequences of excess iodine. Nature reviews. Endocrinology, 10(3), 136–142. https://doi.org/10.1038/nrendo.2013.251

[2691] Leung, A. M., & Braverman, L. E. (2014). Consequences of excess iodine. Nature reviews. Endocrinology, 10(3), 136–142. https://doi.org/10.1038/nrendo.2013.251

[2692] Laurberg, P., Cerqueira, C., Ovesen, L., Rasmussen, L. B., Perrild, H., Andersen, S., Pedersen, I. B., & Carlé, A. (2010). Iodine intake as a determinant of thyroid disorders in populations. Best practice &

research. Clinical endocrinology & metabolism, 24(1), 13–27. https://doi.org/10.1016/j.beem.2009.08.013

[2693] Teng, W., Shan, Z., Teng, X., Guan, H., Li, Y., Teng, D., … Li, C. (2006). Effect of Iodine Intake on Thyroid Diseases in China. New England Journal of Medicine, 354(26), 2783–2793. doi:10.1056/nejmoa054022

[2694] Farebrother, J., Zimmermann, M. B., & Andersson, M. (2019). Excess iodine intake: sources, assessment, and effects on thyroid function. Annals of the New York Academy of Sciences, 1446(1), 44–65. https://doi.org/10.1111/nyas.14041

[2695] Girgis, C. M., Champion, B. L., & Wall, J. R. (2011). Current concepts in Graves' disease. Therapeutic Advances in Endocrinology and Metabolism, 2(3), 135–144. doi:10.1177/2042018811408488

[2696] Nall (2018) 'Autoimmune arthritis: Types, symptoms, and treatment', Medical News Today, Accessed Online Dec 22 2020: https://www.medicalnewstoday.com/articles/322975

[2697] Fiducia, M., Lauretta, R., Lunghi, R., Kyanvash, S., & Pallotti, S. (2007). Tiroidite di Hashimoto e parametri di autoimmunità. Studio descrittivo [Hashimoto's thyroiditis and autoimmunity parameters: descriptive study]. Minerva medica, 98(2), 95–99.

[2698] Zhang, Y., Dai, J., Wu, T., Yang, N., & Yin, Z. (2014). The study of the coexistence of Hashimoto's thyroiditis with papillary thyroid carcinoma. Journal of cancer research and clinical oncology, 140(6), 1021–1026. https://doi.org/10.1007/s00432-014-1629-z

[2699] Wajner, S. M., Goemann, I. M., Bueno, A. L., Larsen, P. R., & Maia, A. L. (2011). IL-6 promotes nonthyroidal illness syndrome by blocking thyroxine activation while promoting thyroid hormone inactivation in human cells. Journal of Clinical Investigation, 121(5), 1834–1845. doi:10.1172/jci44678

[2700] Wirth, C. D., Blum, M. R., da Costa, B. R., Baumgartner, C., Collet, T. H., Medici, M., Peeters, R. P., Aujesky, D., Bauer, D. C., & Rodondi, N. (2014). Subclinical thyroid dysfunction and the risk for fractures: a systematic review and meta-analysis. Annals of internal medicine, 161(3), 189–199. https://doi.org/10.7326/M14-0125

[2701] Onigata K. (2014). '[Thyroid hormone and skeletal metabolism]', Clinical calcium, 24(6), 821–827.

[2702] Tamura, K., Takayama, S., Ishii, T., Mawaribuchi, S., Takamatsu, N., & Ito, M. (2015). Apoptosis and differentiation of Xenopus tail-derived myoblasts by thyroid hormone. Journal of molecular endocrinology, 54(3), 185–192. https://doi.org/10.1530/JME-14-0327

[2703] Robertson et al (1940) 'Mucinase: A Bacterial Enzyme Which Hydrolyzes Synoval Fluid Mucin and Other Mucins', J. Biol. Chem. 1940, 133:261-276.

[2704] Benton, D. (2010). The influence of dietary status on the cognitive performance of children. Molecular Nutrition & Food Research, 54(4), 457–470. doi:10.1002/mnfr.200900158

[2705] Garmendia Madariaga, A., Santos Palacios, S., Guillén-Grima, F., & Galofré, J. C. (2014). The Incidence and Prevalence of Thyroid Dysfunction in Europe: A Meta-Analysis. The Journal of Clinical Endocrinology & Metabolism, 99(3), 923–931. doi:10.1210/jc.2013-2409

[2706] Tunbridge, W. M., Evered, D. C., Hall, R., Appleton, D., Brewis, M., Clark, F., Evans, J. G., Young, E., Bird, T., & Smith, P. A. (1977). The spectrum of thyroid disease in a community: the Whickham survey. Clinical endocrinology, 7(6), 481–493. https://doi.org/10.1111/j.1365-2265.1977.tb01340.x

[2707] Hollowell, J. G., Staehling, N. W., Flanders, W. D., Hannon, W. H., Gunter, E. W., Spencer, C. A., & Braverman, L. E. (2002). Serum TSH, T(4), and thyroid antibodies in the United States population (1988 to 1994): National Health and Nutrition Examination Survey (NHANES III). The Journal of clinical endocrinology and metabolism, 87(2), 489–499. https://doi.org/10.1210/jcem.87.2.8182

[2708] Fade, J. V., Franklyn, J. A., Cross, K. W., Jones, S. C., & Sheppard, M. C. (1991). Prevalence and follow-up of abnormal thyrotrophin (TSH) concentrations in the elderly in the United Kingdom. Clinical Endocrinology, 34(1), 77–84. doi:10.1111/j.1365-2265.1991.tb01739.x

[2709] Åsvold, B. O., Vatten, L. J., & Bjøro, T. (2013). Changes in the prevalence of hypothyroidism: the HUNT Study in Norway. European Journal of Endocrinology, 169(5), 613–620. doi:10.1530/eje-13-0459

[2710] Canaris, G. J., Manowitz, N. R., Mayor, G., & Ridgway, E. C. (2000). The Colorado Thyroid Disease Prevalence Study. Archives of Internal Medicine, 160(4), 526. doi:10.1001/archinte.160.4.526

[2711] McGrogan, A., Seaman, H. E., Wright, J. W., & de Vries, C. S. (2008). The incidence of autoimmune thyroid disease: a systematic review of the literature. Clinical endocrinology, 69(5), 687–696. https://doi.org/10.1111/j.1365-2265.2008.03338.x

[2712] Vanderpump, M. P. J. (2011). The epidemiology of thyroid disease. British Medical Bulletin, 99(1), 39–51. doi:10.1093/bmb/ldr030

[2713] Taylor, P. N., Albrecht, D., Scholz, A., Gutierrez-Buey, G., Lazarus, J. H., Dayan, C. M., & Okosieme, O. E. (2018). Global epidemiology of hyperthyroidism and hypothyroidism. Nature reviews. Endocrinology, 14(5), 301–316. https://doi.org/10.1038/nrendo.2018.18

[2714] Garmendia Madariaga, A., Santos Palacios, S., Guillén-Grima, F., & Galofré, J. C. (2014). The Incidence and Prevalence of Thyroid Dysfunction in Europe: A Meta-Analysis. The Journal of Clinical Endocrinology & Metabolism, 99(3), 923–931. doi:10.1210/jc.2013-2409

[2715] Bülow Pedersen, I., Laurberg, P., Knudsen, N., Jørgensen, T., Perrild, H., Ovesen, L., & Rasmussen, L. B. (2007). An Increased Incidence of Overt Hypothyroidism after Iodine Fortification of Salt in

Denmark: A Prospective Population Study. The Journal of Clinical Endocrinology & Metabolism, 92(8), 3122–3127. doi:10.1210/jc.2007-0732

[2716] Boelaert, K., Newby, P. R., Simmonds, M. J., Holder, R. L., Carr-Smith, J. D., Heward, J. M., Manji, N., Allahabadia, A., Armitage, M., Chatterjee, K. V., Lazarus, J. H., Pearce, S. H., Vaidya, B., Gough, S. C., & Franklyn, J. A. (2010). Prevalence and relative risk of other autoimmune diseases in subjects with autoimmune thyroid disease. The American journal of medicine, 123(2), 183.e1–183.e1839. https://doi.org/10.1016/j.amjmed.2009.06.030

[2717] Schultheiss, U. T., Teumer, A., Medici, M., Li, Y., Daya, N., Chaker, L., Homuth, G., Uitterlinden, A. G., Nauck, M., Hofman, A., Selvin, E., Völzke, H., Peeters, R. P., & Köttgen, A. (2015). A genetic risk score for thyroid peroxidase antibodies associates with clinical thyroid disease in community-based populations. The Journal of clinical endocrinology and metabolism, 100(5), E799–E807. https://doi.org/10.1210/jc.2014-4352

[2718] Marinò, M., Latrofa, F., Menconi, F., Chiovato, L., & Vitti, P. (2015). Role of genetic and non-genetic factors in the etiology of Graves' disease. Journal of endocrinological investigation, 38(3), 283–294. https://doi.org/10.1007/s40618-014-0214-2

[2719] Bülow Pedersen, I., Knudsen, N., Carlé, A., Schomburg, L., Köhrle, J., Jørgensen, T., … Laurberg, P. (2013). Serum selenium is low in newly diagnosed Graves' disease: a population-based study. Clinical Endocrinology, 79(4), 584–590. doi:10.1111/cen.12185

[2720] Tomer, Y. & Davies, T. F. (1993) Infection, thyroid disease, and autoimmunity. Endocr. Rev. 14, 107–120.

[2721] Blomberg, M., Feldt-Rasmussen, U., Andersen, K. K., & Kjaer, S. K. (2012). Thyroid cancer in Denmark 1943-2008, before and after iodine supplementation. International journal of cancer, 131(10), 2360–2366. https://doi.org/10.1002/ijc.27497

[2722] Zimmermann, M. B., & Galetti, V. (2015). Iodine intake as a risk factor for thyroid cancer: a comprehensive review of animal and human studies. Thyroid research, 8, 8. https://doi.org/10.1186/s13044-015-0020-8

[2723] Lee, J. H., Hwang, Y., Song, R. Y., Yi, J. W., Yu, H. W., Kim, S. J., Chai, Y. J., Choi, J. Y., Lee, K. E., & Park, S. K. (2017). Relationship between iodine levels and papillary thyroid carcinoma: A systematic review and meta-analysis. Head & neck, 39(8), 1711–1718. https://doi.org/10.1002/hed.24797

[2724] Zimmerman, M. B., & Galetti, V. (2015). Iodine intake as a risk factor for thyroid cancer: a comprehensive review of animal and human studies. Thyroid research, 8, 8. https://doi.org/10.1186/s13044-015-0020-8

[2725] Cao, L.-Z., Peng, X.-D., Xie, J.-P., Yang, F.-H., Wen, H.-L., & Li, S. (2017). The relationship between iodine intake and the risk of thyroid cancer. Medicine, 96(20), e6734. doi:10.1097/md.0000000000006734

[2726] Aceves, C., Anguiano, B., & Delgado, G. (2013). The extrathyronine actions of iodine as antioxidant, apoptotic, and differentiation factor in various tissues. Thyroid : official journal of the American Thyroid Association, 23(8), 938–946. https://doi.org/10.1089/thy.2012.0579

[2727] Nauman, J., & Wolff, J. (1993). Iodide prophylaxis in Poland after the Chernobyl reactor accident: benefits and risks. The American journal of medicine, 94(5), 524–532. https://doi.org/10.1016/0002-9343(93)90089-8

[2728] Center for Drug Evaluation and Research, Food and Drug Administration. Guidance. Potassium iodide as a thyroid blocking agent in radiation emergencies. December 2001.

[2729] National Cancer Institute (2019) 'Get the Facts about Exposure to I-131 Radiation', National Institute of Health, Accessed Online Dec 23 2020: https://www.cancer.gov/about-cancer/causes-prevention/risk/radiation/i-131

[2730] CDC (2018) 'Potassium Iodide (KI)', Radiation Emergencies & Your Health, Accessed Online Dec 23 2020: https://www.cdc.gov/nceh/radiation/emergencies/

[2731] CDC (2018) 'Potassium Iodide (KI)', Radiation Emergencies & Your Health, Treatments, Accessed Online Dec 29 2020: https://www.cdc.gov/nceh/radiation/emergencies/ki.htm

[2732] Meikle, A. W. (2004). The Interrelationships Between Thyroid Dysfunction and Hypogonadism in Men and Boys. Thyroid, 14(supplement 1), 17–25. doi:10.1089/105072504323024552

[2733] Meikle A. W. (2004). The interrelationships between thyroid dysfunction and hypogonadism in men and boys. Thyroid : official journal of the American Thyroid Association, 14 Suppl 1, S17–S25. https://doi.org/10.1089/105072504323024552

[2734] Krysiak, R., Kowalcze, K., & Okopień, B. (2019). The effect of testosterone on thyroid autoimmunity in euthyroid men with Hashimoto's thyroiditis and low testosterone levels. Journal of clinical pharmacy and therapeutics, 44(5), 742–749. https://doi.org/10.1111/jcpt.12987

[2735] Chen, D., Yan, Y., Huang, H., Dong, Q., & Tian, H. (2018). The association between subclinical hypothyroidism and erectile dysfunction. Pakistan journal of medical sciences, 34(3), 621–625. https://doi.org/10.12669/pjms.343.14330

[2736] Knudsen, N., Laurberg, P., Rasmussen, L. B., Bülow, I., Perrild, H., Ovesen, L., & Jørgensen, T. (2005). Small Differences in Thyroid Function May Be Important for Body Mass Index and the

Occurrence of Obesity in the Population. The Journal of Clinical Endocrinology & Metabolism, 90(7), 4019–4024. doi:10.1210/jc.2004-2225

[2737] Fox, C. S., Pencina, M. J., D'Agostino, R. B., Murabito, J. M., Seely, E. W., Pearce, E. N., & Vasan, R. S. (2008). Relations of thyroid function to body weight: cross-sectional and longitudinal observations in a community-based sample. Archives of internal medicine, 168(6), 587–592. https://doi.org/10.1001/archinte.168.6.587

[2738] Stone N. J. (1994). Secondary causes of hyperlipidemia. The Medical clinics of North America, 78(1), 117–141. https://doi.org/10.1016/s0025-7125(16)30179-1

[2739] Al-Tonsi, A. A., Abdel-Gayoum, A. A., & Saad, M. (2004). The secondary dyslipidemia and deranged serum phosphate concentration in thyroid disorders. Experimental and molecular pathology, 76(2), 182–187. https://doi.org/10.1016/j.yexmp.2003.10.006

[2740] Cutting, W. C., Rytand, D. A., & Tainter, M. L. (1934). RELATIONSHIP BETWEEN BLOOD CHOLESTEROL AND INCREASED METABOLISM FROM DINITROPHENOL AND THYROID. The Journal of clinical investigation, 13(4), 547–552. https://doi.org/10.1172/JCI100604

[2741] Tzotzas, T., Krassas, G. E., Konstantinidis, T., & Bougoulia, M. (2000). Changes in lipoprotein(a) levels in overt and subclinical hypothyroidism before and during treatment. Thyroid : official journal of the American Thyroid Association, 10(9), 803–808. https://doi.org/10.1089/thy.2000.10.803

[2742] de Bruin, T. W., van Barlingen, H., van Linde-Sibenius Trip, M., van Vuurst de Vries, A. R., Akveld, M. J., & Erkelens, D. W. (1993). Lipoprotein(a) and apolipoprotein B plasma concentrations in hypothyroid, euthyroid, and hyperthyroid subjects. The Journal of clinical endocrinology and metabolism, 76(1), 121–126. https://doi.org/10.1210/jcem.76.1.8421075

[2743] Zalewski, A., & Macphee, C. (2005). Role of lipoprotein-associated phospholipase A2 in atherosclerosis: biology, epidemiology, and possible therapeutic target. Arteriosclerosis, thrombosis, and vascular biology, 25(5), 923–931. https://doi.org/10.1161/01.ATV.0000160551.21962.a7

[2744] Packard, C. J., O'Reilly, D. S., Caslake, M. J., McMahon, A. D., Ford, I., Cooney, J., Macphee, C. H., Suckling, K. E., Krishna, M., Wilkinson, F. E., Rumley, A., & Lowe, G. D. (2000). Lipoprotein-associated phospholipase A2 as an independent predictor of coronary heart disease. West of Scotland Coronary Prevention Study Group. The New England journal of medicine, 343(16), 1148–1155. https://doi.org/10.1056/NEJM200010193431603

[2745] Jublanc, C., Bruckert, E., Giral, P., Chapman, M. J., Leenhardt, L., Carreau, V., & Turpin, G. (2004). Relationship of circulating C-reactive protein levels to thyroid status and cardiovascular risk in hyperlipidemic euthyroid subjects: low free thyroxine is associated with elevated hsCRP. Atherosclerosis, 172(1), 7–11. https://doi.org/10.1016/j.atherosclerosis.2003.09.009

[2746] Gullberg, H., Rudling, M., Forrest, D., Angelin, B., & Vennström, B. (2000). Thyroid hormone receptor beta-deficient mice show complete loss of the normal cholesterol 7alpha-hydroxylase (CYP7A) response to thyroid hormone but display enhanced resistance to dietary cholesterol. Molecular endocrinology (Baltimore, Md.), 14(11), 1739–1749. https://doi.org/10.1210/mend.14.11.0548

[2747] Rizos, C. V., Elisaf, M. S., & Liberopoulos, E. N. (2011). Effects of thyroid dysfunction on lipid profile. The open cardiovascular medicine journal, 5, 76–84. https://doi.org/10.2174/1874192401105010076

[2748] Abrams, J. J., & Grundy, S. M. (1981). Cholesterol metabolism in hypothyroidism and hyperthyroidism in man. Journal of lipid research, 22(2), 323–338.

[2749] Brenta and Duntas (2016) 'Thyroid hormones: a potential ally', HORMONES 2016, 15(4):500-510.

[2750] Gavin, L. A., McMahon, F., & Moeller, M. (1985). Modulation of Adipose Lipoprotein Lipase by Thyroid Hormone and Diabetes: The Significance of the Low T3 State. Diabetes, 34(12), 1266–1271. doi:10.2337/diab.34.12.1266

[2751] Shin, D. J., & Osborne, T. F. (2003). Thyroid hormone regulation and cholesterol metabolism are connected through Sterol Regulatory Element-Binding Protein-2 (SREBP-2). The Journal of biological chemistry, 278(36), 34114–34118. https://doi.org/10.1074/jbc.M305417200

[2752] Bakker, O., Hudig, F., Meijssen, S., & Wiersinga, W. M. (1998). Effects of triiodothyronine and amiodarone on the promoter of the human LDL receptor gene. Biochemical and biophysical research communications, 249(2), 517–521. https://doi.org/10.1006/bbrc.1998.9174

[2753] Faure, P., Oziol, L., Artur, Y., & Chomard, P. (2004). Thyroid hormone (T3) and its acetic derivative (TA3) protect low-density lipoproteins from oxidation by different mechanisms. Biochimie, 86(6), 411–418. https://doi.org/10.1016/j.biochi.2004.04.009

[2754] Willard, D. L., Leung, A. M., & Pearce, E. N. (2014). Thyroid Function Testing in Patients With Newly Diagnosed Hyperlipidemia. JAMA Internal Medicine, 174(2), 287. doi:10.1001/jamainternmed.2013.12188

[2755] Elder, J., McLelland, A., O'Reilly, D. S., Packard, C. J., Series, J. J., & Shepherd, J. (1990). The relationship between serum cholesterol and serum thyrotropin, thyroxine and tri-iodothyronine concentrations in suspected hypothyroidism. Annals of clinical biochemistry, 27 (Pt 2), 110–113. https://doi.org/10.1177/000456329002700204

[2756] Danese, M. D., Ladenson, P. W., Meinert, C. L., & Powe, N. R. (2000). Clinical review 115: effect of thyroxine therapy on serum lipoproteins in patients with mild thyroid failure: a quantitative review of the literature. The Journal of clinical endocrinology and metabolism, 85(9), 2993–3001. https://doi.org/10.1210/jcem.85.9.6841

[2757] Costantini, F., Pierdomenico, S. D., De Cesare, D., De Remigis, P., Bucciarelli, T., Bittolo-Bon, G., Cazzolato, G., Nubile, G., Guagnano, M. T., Sensi, S., Cuccurullo, F., & Mezzetti, A. (1998). Effect of thyroid function on LDL oxidation. Arteriosclerosis, thrombosis, and vascular biology, 18(5), 732–737. https://doi.org/10.1161/01.atv.18.5.732

[2758] Wang, F., Tan, Y., Wang, C., Zhang, X., Zhao, Y., Song, X., ... Zhao, J. (2012). Thyroid-Stimulating Hormone Levels within the Reference Range Are Associated with Serum Lipid Profiles Independent of Thyroid Hormones. The Journal of Clinical Endocrinology & Metabolism, 97(8), 2724–2731. doi:10.1210/jc.2012-1133

[2759] Wang, F., Tan, Y., Wang, C., Zhang, X., Zhao, Y., Song, X., ... Zhao, J. (2012). Thyroid-Stimulating Hormone Levels within the Reference Range Are Associated with Serum Lipid Profiles Independent of Thyroid Hormones. The Journal of Clinical Endocrinology & Metabolism, 97(8), 2724–2731. doi:10.1210/jc.2012-1133

[2760] Aviram, M., Luboshitzky, R., & Brook, J. G. (1982). Lipid and lipoprotein pattern in thyroid dysfunction and the effect of therapy. Clinical biochemistry, 15(1), 62–66. https://doi.org/10.1016/s0009-9120(82)90529-x

[2761] Kung, A. W., Pang, R. W., Lauder, I., Lam, K. S., & Janus, E. D. (1995). Changes in serum lipoprotein(a) and lipids during treatment of hyperthyroidism. Clinical chemistry, 41(2), 226–231.

[2762] Rizos, C. V. (2011). Effects of Thyroid Dysfunction on Lipid Profile. The Open Cardiovascular Medicine Journal, 5(1), 76–84. doi:10.2174/1874192401105010076

[2763] Singh-Manoux, A., Gimeno, D., Kivimaki, M., Brunner, E., & Marmot, M. G. (2008). Low HDL cholesterol is a risk factor for deficit and decline in memory in midlife: the Whitehall II study. Arteriosclerosis, thrombosis, and vascular biology, 28(8), 1556–1562. https://doi.org/10.1161/ATVBAHA.108.163998

[2764] Suarez E. C. (1999). Relations of trait depression and anxiety to low lipid and lipoprotein concentrations in healthy young adult women. Psychosomatic medicine, 61(3), 273–279. https://doi.org/10.1097/00006842-199905000-00004

[2765] Onder, G., Landi, F., Volpato, S., Fellin, R., Carbonin, P., Gambassi, G., & Bernabei, R. (2003). Serum cholesterol levels and in-hospital mortality in the elderly. The American journal of medicine, 115(4), 265–271. https://doi.org/10.1016/s0002-9343(03)00354-1

[2766] Rodondi, N., den Elzen, W. P., Bauer, D. C., Cappola, A. R., Razvi, S., Walsh, J. P., Asvold, B. O., Iervasi, G., Imaizumi, M., Collet, T. H., Bremner, A., Maisonneuve, P., Sgarbi, J. A., Khaw, K. T., Vanderpump, M. P., Newman, A. B., Cornuz, J., Franklyn, J. A., Westendorp, R. G., Vittinghoff, E., ... Thyroid Studies Collaboration (2010). Subclinical hypothyroidism and the risk of coronary heart disease and mortality. JAMA, 304(12), 1365–1374. https://doi.org/10.1001/jama.2010.1361

[2767] Klein, I., & Ojamaa, K. (2001). Thyroid hormone and the cardiovascular system. The New England journal of medicine, 344(7), 501–509. https://doi.org/10.1056/NEJM200102153440707

[2768] Jabbar, A., Pingitore, A., Pearce, S. H., Zaman, A., Iervasi, G., & Razvi, S. (2017). Thyroid hormones and cardiovascular disease. Nature reviews. Cardiology, 14(1), 39–55. https://doi.org/10.1038/nrcardio.2016.174

[2769] Klein, I., & Danzi, S. (2007). Thyroid Disease and the Heart. Circulation, 116(15), 1725–1735. doi:10.1161/circulationaha.106.678326

[2770] Farrell A. P. (2002). Coronary arteriosclerosis in salmon: growing old or growing fast?. Comparative biochemistry and physiology. Part A, Molecular & integrative physiology, 132(4), 723–735. https://doi.org/10.1016/s1095-6433(02)00126-5

[2771] Walsh, C. J., Luer, C. A., Bodine, A. B., Smith, C. A., Cox, H. L., Noyes, D. R., & Maura, G. (2006). Elasmobranch immune cells as a source of novel tumor cell inhibitors: Implications for public health. Integrative and comparative biology, 46(6), 1072–1081. https://doi.org/10.1093/icb/icl041

[2772] Iwata, A., Morrison, M. L., & Roth, M. B. (2014). Iodide protects heart tissue from reperfusion injury. PloS one, 9(11), e112458. https://doi.org/10.1371/journal.pone.0112458

[2773] Prummel, M. F. (1993). Smoking and Risk of Graves' Disease. JAMA: The Journal of the American Medical Association, 269(4), 479. doi:10.1001/jama.1993.03500040045034

[2774] Thyroid-Stimulating Hormone–Receptor Antibody and Thyroid Hormone Concentrations in Smokers vs Nonsmokers With Graves Disease Treated With Carbimazole. (2009). JAMA, 301(2), 162. doi:10.1001/jama.2008.931

[2775] Brix, T. H., Hansen, P. S., Kyvik, K. O., & Hegedüs, L. (2000). Cigarette Smoking and Risk of Clinically Overt Thyroid Disease. Archives of Internal Medicine, 160(5). doi:10.1001/archinte.160.5.661

[2776] NIH (2020) 'Iodine: Fact Sheet for Health Professionals', Dietary Supplement Fact Sheets, Accessed Online Dec 20 2020: https://ods.od.nih.gov/factsheets/Iodine-HealthProfessional/

[2777] World Health Organization & Food and Agriculture Organization of the United Nations. (2004). 'Vitamin and mineral requirements in human nutrition'. Geneva, Switzerland: WHO. Accessed Online Dec 20 2020: https://www.who.int/nutrition/publications/micronutrients/9241546123/en/

[2778] Institute of Medicine (US) Panel on Micronutrients (2001) 'Dietary Reference Intakes for Vitamin A, Vitamin K, Arsenic, Boron, Chromium, Copper, Iodine, Iron, Manganese, Molybdenum, Nickel, Silicon, Vanadium, and Zinc', Washington (DC): National Academies Press (US); 2001.

[2779] Gardner, D. F., Centor, R. M., & Utiger, R. D. (1988). Effects of low dose oral iodide supplementation on thyroid function in normal men. Clinical endocrinology, 28(3), 283–288. https://doi.org/10.1111/j.1365-2265.1988.tb01214.x

[2780] El-Shafie K. T. (2003). Clinical presentation of hypothyroidism. Journal of family & community medicine, 10(1), 55–58.

[2781] Chow, C. C., Phillips, D. I., Lazarus, J. H., & Parkes, A. B. (1991). Effect of low dose iodide supplementation on thyroid function in potentially susceptible subjects: are dietary iodide levels in Britain acceptable?. Clinical endocrinology, 34(5), 413–416. https://doi.org/10.1111/j.1365-2265.1991.tb00314.x

[2782] Farebrother, J., Zimmermann, M. B., & Andersson, M. (2019). Excess iodine intake: sources, assessment, and effects on thyroid function. Annals of the New York Academy of Sciences. doi:10.1111/nyas.14041

[2783] World Health Organization. 1989. Toxological evaluation of certain food additives and contaminants. WHO Food Additives Series 24. Prepared by: The 33rd Meeting of the Joint FAO/WHO Expert Committee on Food Additives (JECFA). Geneva, Switzerland: World Health Organization.

[2784] Patrick L. (2008). Iodine: deficiency and therapeutic considerations. Alternative medicine review : a journal of clinical therapeutic, 13(2), 116–127.

[2785] de Benoist et al (2008) 'Iodine deficiency in 2007: Global progress since 2003', Food and Nutrition Bulletin, vol. 29, no. 3 © 2008, The United Nations University, Accessed Online Dec 21 2020: https://www.who.int/nutrition/publications/micronutrients/FNBvol29N3sep08.pdf

[2786] Vitti, P., Delange, F., Pinchera, A., Zimmermann, M., & Dunn, J. T. (2003). Europe is iodine deficient. Lancet (London, England), 361(9364), 1226. https://doi.org/10.1016/S0140-6736(03)12935-2

[2787] Vanderpump, M. P., Lazarus, J. H., Smyth, P. P., Laurberg, P., Holder, R. L., Boelaert, K., & Franklyn, J. A. (2011). Iodine status of UK schoolgirls: a cross-sectional survey. The Lancet, 377(9782), 2007–2012. doi:10.1016/s0140-6736(11)60693-4

[2788] Dissanayake, C. B., Chandrajith, R., & Tobschall, H. J. (1999). The iodine cycle in the tropical environment — implications on iodine deficiency disorders. International Journal of Environmental Studies, 56(3), 357–372. doi:10.1080/00207239908711210

[2789] Darnton-Hill and Delange (2007) 'Iodine deficiency in Europe: A continuing public health problem', World Health Organization, Accessed Online Dec 23 2020: https://www.who.int/nutrition/publications/micronutrients/iodine_deficiency/9789241593960/en/

[2790] Piccone (2011) 'The Silent Epidemic of Iodine Deficiency', Life Extension Magazine, Accessed Online Dec 30 2020: https://www.lifeextension.com/magazine/2011/10/the-silent-epidemic-of-iodine-deficiency

[2791] Hoption Cann S. A. (2006). Hypothesis: dietary iodine intake in the etiology of cardiovascular disease. Journal of the American College of Nutrition, 25(1), 1–11. https://doi.org/10.1080/07315724.2006.10719508

[2792] Pearce E. N. (2007). National trends in iodine nutrition: is everyone getting enough?. Thyroid : official journal of the American Thyroid Association, 17(9), 823–827. https://doi.org/10.1089/thy.2007.0102

[2793] Abt, E., Spungen, J., Pouillot, R., Gamalo-Siebers, M., & Wirtz, M. (2016). Update on dietary intake of perchlorate and iodine from U.S. food and drug administration's total diet study: 2008–2012. Journal of Exposure Science & Environmental Epidemiology, 28(1), 21–30. doi:10.1038/jes.2016.78

[2794] Aguayo et al (2003) 'Sierra Leone - Investing in nutrition to reduce poverty: A call for action', Public Health Nutrition 6(7):653-7, DOI: 10.1079/PHN2003484

[2795] Abuye, C., & Berhane, Y. (2007). The goitre rate, its association with reproductive failure, and the knowledge of iodine deficiency disorders (IDD) among women in Ethiopia: Cross-section community based study. BMC Public Health, 7(1). doi:10.1186/1471-2458-7-316

[2796] Egbuta, J., Onyezili, F., & Vanormelingen, K. (2003). Impact evaluation of efforts to eliminate iodine deficiency disorders in Nigeria. Public health nutrition, 6(2), 169–173. https://doi.org/10.1079/PHN2002413

[2797] Okosieme O. E. (2006). Impact of iodination on thyroid pathology in Africa. Journal of the Royal Society of Medicine, 99(8), 396–401. https://doi.org/10.1258/jrsm.99.8.396

[2798] The Iodine Global Network (2019) 'Global scorecard of iodine nutrition in 2019 in the general population based on school-age children (SAC)', IGN: Zurich, Switzerland, Accessed Online Dec 21 2020: https://www.ign.org/cm_data/Global_Scorecard_2019_SAC.pdf

[2799] Fuge, R., & Johnson, C. C. (2015). Iodine and human health, the role of environmental geochemistry and diet, a review. Applied Geochemistry, 63, 282–302. doi:10.1016/j.apgeochem.2015.09.013

[2800] Assey, V. D., Greiner, T., Mzee, R. K., Abuu, H., Mgoba, C., Kimboka, S., & Peterson, S. (2006). Iodine deficiency persists in the Zanzibar Islands of Tanzania. Food and nutrition bulletin, 27(4), 292–299. https://doi.org/10.1177/156482650602700402

[2801] Colin, C., Leblanc, C., Wagner, E., Delage, L., Leize-Wagner, E., Van Dorsselaer, A., Kloareg, B., & Potin, P. (2003). The brown algal kelp Laminaria digitata features distinct bromoperoxidase and iodoperoxidase activities. The Journal of biological chemistry, 278(26), 23545–23552. https://doi.org/10.1074/jbc.M300247200

[2802] Carpenter, L. J., Sturges, W. T., Penkett, S. A., Liss, P. S., Alicke, B., Hebestreit, K., & Platt, U. (1999). Short-lived alkyl iodides and bromides at Mace Head, Ireland: Links to biogenic sources and halogen oxide production. Journal of Geophysical Research: Atmospheres, 104(D1), 1679–1689. doi:10.1029/98jd02746

[2803] Pedersén, M., Collén, J., Abrahamson, J., & Ekdahl, A. (1996). Production of Halocarbons from Seaweeds: An Oxidative Stress Reaction? Sci. Mar., 60: 257-63

[2804] Kupper, F. C., Carpenter, L. J., McFiggans, G. B., Palmer, C. J., Waite, T. J., Boneberg, E.-M., … Feiters, M. C. (2008). Iodide accumulation provides kelp with an inorganic antioxidant impacting atmospheric chemistry. Proceedings of the National Academy of Sciences, 105(19), 6954–6958. doi:10.1073/pnas.0709959105

[2805] Fuse Y. (2017). Iodine and Thyroid Function: A Historical Review of Goiter and the Current Iodine Status in Japan. Pediatric endocrinology reviews : PER, 14 Suppl 1(Suppl 1), 260–270. https://doi.org/10.17458/per.vol14.2017.f.iodinethyroidfunction

[2806] Nagataki S. (2008). The average of dietary iodine intake due to the ingestion of seaweeds is 1.2 mg/day in Japan. Thyroid : official journal of the American Thyroid Association, 18(6), 667–668. https://doi.org/10.1089/thy.2007.0379

[2807] Zava, T. T., & Zava, D. T. (2011). Assessment of Japanese iodine intake based on seaweed consumption in Japan: A literature-based analysis. Thyroid research, 4, 14. https://doi.org/10.1186/1756-6614-4-14

[2808] Teas, J., Pino, S., Critchley, A., & Braverman, L. E. (2004). Variability of iodine content in common commercially available edible seaweeds. Thyroid : official journal of the American Thyroid Association, 14(10), 836–841. https://doi.org/10.1089/thy.2004.14.836

[2809] Pearce et al (2004) 'Sources of Dietary Iodine: Bread, Cows' Milk, and Infant Formula in the Boston Area', The Journal of Clinical Endocrinology & Metabolism, Volume 89, Issue 7, 1 July 2004, Pages 3421–3424, https://doi.org/10.1210/jc.2003-032002

[2810] Thomson, B. M., Vannoort, R. W., & Haslemore, R. M. (2008). Dietary exposure and trends of exposure to nutrient elements iodine, iron, selenium and sodium from the 2003-4 New Zealand Total Diet Survey. The British journal of nutrition, 99(3), 614–625. https://doi.org/10.1017/S0007114507812001

[2811] Haldimann, M., Alt, A., Blanc, A., & Blondeau, K. (2005). Iodine content of food groups. Journal of Food Composition and Analysis, 18(6), 461–471. doi:10.1016/j.jfca.2004.06.003

[2812] El-Ghawi, U. M., & Al-Sadeq, A. A. (2006). Determination of Iodine in Libyan Food Samples Using Epithermal Instrumental Neutron Activation Analysis. Biological Trace Element Research, 111(1-3), 31–40. doi:10.1385/bter:111:1:31

[2813] World Health Organization Department of Nutrition for Health and Development (2004) 'Iodine Status Worldwide', WHO Global Database on Iodine Deficiency, Geneva, Accessed Online Dec 29 2020: https://apps.who.int/iris/bitstream/handle/10665/43010/9241592001.pdf

[2814] Pennington JAT, Schoen SA, Salmon GD, Young B, Johnson RD, Marts RW. Composition of Core Foods of the U.S. Food Supply, 1982-1991. III. Copper, Manganese, Selenium, and Iodine. J Food Comp Anal. 1995;8(2):171-217.

[2815] Hedberg, C. W., Fishbein, D. B., Janssen, R. S., Meyers, B., McMillen, J. M., MacDonald, K. L., White, K. E., Huss, L. J., Hurwitz, E. S., & Farhie, J. R. (1987). An outbreak of thyrotoxicosis caused by the consumption of bovine thyroid gland in ground beef. The New England journal of medicine, 316(16), 993–998. https://doi.org/10.1056/NEJM198704163161605

[2816] Parmar, M. S., & Sturge, C. (2003). Recurrent hamburger thyrotoxicosis. CMAJ : Canadian Medical Association journal = journal de l'Association medicale canadienne, 169(5), 415–417.

[2817] Lucie Wartique, Lucie Pothen, Nathalie Pirson, Michel P. Hermans, Michel Lambert & Halil Yildiz (2017) An unusual cause of epidemic thyrotoxicosis, Acta Clinica Belgica, 72:6, 451-453, DOI: 10.1080/17843286.2017.1309336

[2818] Jeong, K. U., Lee, H. S., & Hwang, J. S. (2014). Effects of short-term potassium iodide treatment for thyrotoxicosis due to Graves disease in children and adolescents. Annals of pediatric endocrinology & metabolism, 19(4), 197–201. https://doi.org/10.6065/apem.2014.19.4.197

[2819] Barikmo, I., Henjum, S., Dahl, L., Oshaug, A., & Torheim, L. E. (2011). Environmental implication of iodine in water, milk and other foods used in Saharawi refugees camps in Tindouf, Algeria. Journal of Food Composition and Analysis, 24(4-5), 637–641. doi:10.1016/j.jfca.2010.10.003

[2820] Van der Reijden, O. L., Zimmermann, M. B., & Galetti, V. (2017). Iodine in dairy milk: Sources, concentrations and importance to human health. Best Practice & Research Clinical Endocrinology & Metabolism, 31(4), 385–395. doi:10.1016/j.beem.2017.10.004

[2821] Flachowsky, G., Franke, K., Meyer, U., Leiterer, M., & Schöne, F. (2014). Influencing factors on iodine content of cow milk. European journal of nutrition, 53(2), 351–365. https://doi.org/10.1007/s00394-013-0597-4

[2822] Phillips D. I. (1997). Iodine, milk, and the elimination of endemic goitre in Britain: the story of an accidental public health triumph. Journal of epidemiology and community health, 51(4), 391–393. https://doi.org/10.1136/jech.51.4.391

[2823] Phillips, D. I. (1997). Iodine, milk, and the elimination of endemic goitre in Britain: the story of an accidental public health triumph. Journal of Epidemiology & Community Health, 51(4), 391–393. doi:10.1136/jech.51.4.391

[2824] Ershow, A. G., Skeaff, S. A., Merkel, J. M., & Pehrsson, P. R. (2018). Development of Databases on Iodine in Foods and Dietary Supplements. Nutrients, 10(1), 100. https://doi.org/10.3390/nu10010100

[2825] Stinca, S., Andersson, M., Herter-Aeberli, I., Chabaa, L., Cherkaoui, M., El Ansari, N., Aboussad, A., Weibel, S., & Zimmermann, M. B. (2017). Moderate-to-Severe Iodine Deficiency in the "First 1000 Days" Causes More Thyroid Hypofunction in Infants Than in Pregnant or Lactating Women. The Journal of nutrition, 147(4), 589–595. https://doi.org/10.3945/jn.116.244665

[2826] Farebrother, J., Zimmermann, M. B., Assey, V., Castro, M. C., Cherkaoui, M., Fingerhut, R., ... Andersson, M. (2019). Thyroglobulin Is Markedly Elevated in 6- to 24-Month-Old Infants at Both Low and High Iodine Intakes and Suggests a Narrow Optimal Iodine Intake Range. Thyroid, 29(2), 268–277. doi:10.1089/thy.2018.0321

[2827] Morreale de Escobar, G, Obregon, MJ, & Escobar del Rey, F. (2004). Role of thyroid hormone during early brain development, European Journal of Endocrinology Eur J Endocrinol, 151(Suppl_3), U25-U37. Retrieved Dec 21, 2020, from https://eje.bioscientifica.com/view/journals/eje/151/Suppl_3/U25.xml

[2828] Zimmermann M. B. (2011). The role of iodine in human growth and development. Seminars in cell & developmental biology, 22(6), 645–652. https://doi.org/10.1016/j.semcdb.2011.07.009

[2829] Cao, X. Y., Jiang, X. M., Dou, Z. H., Rakeman, M. A., Zhang, M. L., O'Donnell, K., Ma, T., Amette, K., DeLong, N., & DeLong, G. R. (1994). Timing of vulnerability of the brain to iodine deficiency in endemic cretinism. The New England journal of medicine, 331(26), 1739–1744. https://doi.org/10.1056/NEJM199412293312603

[2830] Cobra, C., Muhilal, Rusmil, K., Rustama, D., Djatnika, Suwardi, S. S., ... Semba, R. D. (1997). Infant Survival Is Improved by Oral Iodine Supplementation. The Journal of Nutrition, 127(4), 574–578. doi:10.1093/jn/127.4.574

[2831] Pharoah, P. O., Buttfield, I. H., & Hetzel, B. S. (1971). Neurological damage to the fetus resulting from severe iodine deficiency during pregnancy. Lancet (London, England), 1(7694), 308–310. https://doi.org/10.1016/s0140-6736(71)91040-3

[2832] Wan Nazaimoon, W. M., Osman, A., Wu, L. L., & Khalid, B. A. (1996). Effects of iodine deficiency on insulin-like growth factor-I, insulin-like growth factor-binding protein-3 levels and height attainment in malnourished children. Clinical endocrinology, 45(1), 79–83.

[2833] Zimmermann, M. B., Jooste, P. L., Mabapa, N. S., Mbhenyane, X., Schoeman, S., Biebinger, R., Chaouki, N., Bozo, M., Grimci, L., & Bridson, J. (2007). Treatment of iodine deficiency in school-age children increases insulin-like growth factor (IGF)-I and IGF binding protein-3 concentrations and improves somatic growth. The Journal of clinical endocrinology and metabolism, 92(2), 437–442. https://doi.org/10.1210/jc.2006-1901

[2834] Hynes, K. L., Otahal, P., Burgess, J. R., Oddy, W. H., & Hay, I. (2017). Reduced Educational Outcomes Persist into Adolescence Following Mild Iodine Deficiency in Utero, Despite Adequacy in Childhood: 15-Year Follow-Up of the Gestational Iodine Cohort Investigating Auditory Processing Speed and Working Memory. Nutrients, 9(12), 1354. https://doi.org/10.3390/nu9121354

[2835] Bath, S. C., Steer, C. D., Golding, J., Emmett, P., & Rayman, M. P. (2013). Effect of inadequate iodine status in UK pregnant women on cognitive outcomes in their children: results from the Avon Longitudinal Study of Parents and Children (ALSPAC). Lancet (London, England), 382(9889), 331–337. https://doi.org/10.1016/S0140-6736(13)60436-5

[2836] Pearce, E. N., Bazrafshan, H. R., He, X., Pino, S., & Braverman, L. E. (2004). Dietary iodine in pregnant women from the Boston, Massachusetts area. Thyroid : official journal of the American Thyroid Association, 14(4), 327–328. https://doi.org/10.1089/105072504323031013

[2837] Toloza, F. J. K., Motahari, H., & Maraka, S. (2020). Consequences of Severe Iodine Deficiency in Pregnancy: Evidence in Humans. Frontiers in Endocrinology, 11. doi:10.3389/fendo.2020.00409

[2838] Bleichrodt et al (1987) 'Developmental disorders associated with severe iodine deficiency', In: Hetzel B, Dunn J, Stanbury J, eds. 'The prevention and control of iodine deficiency disorders.' Amsterdam: Elsevier, 1987: 65–84.

[2839] Qian et al (2005) 'The effects of iodine on intelligence in children: A meta-analysis of studies conducted in China', Asia Pacific Journal of Clinical Nutrition 14(1):32-42.

657

[2840] Boyages, S. C., Collins, J. K., Maberly, G. F., Jupp, J. J., Morris, J., & Eastman, C. J. (1989). Iodine deficiency impairs intellectual and neuromotor development in apparently-normal persons. A study of rural inhabitants of north-central China. Medical Journal of Australia, 150(12), 676-682.

[2841] Stanbury J B. 'The clinical pattern of cretinism as seen in Highland Equador', in Stanbury, J B and Kroc R L (eds) op. cit. pp3-17.

[2842] Zimmermann, M. B., Connolly, K., Bozo, M., Bridson, J., Rohner, F., & Grimci, L. (2006). Iodine supplementation improves cognition in iodine-deficient schoolchildren in Albania: a randomized, controlled, double-blind study. The American Journal of Clinical Nutrition, 83(1), 108–114. doi:10.1093/ajcn/83.1.108

[2843] Public Health Committee of the American Thyroid Association, Becker, D. V., Braverman, L. E., Delange, F., Dunn, J. T., Franklyn, J. A., Hollowell, J. G., Lamm, S. H., Mitchell, M. L., Pearce, E., Robbins, J., & Rovet, J. F. (2006). Iodine supplementation for pregnancy and lactation-United States and Canada: recommendations of the American Thyroid Association. Thyroid : official journal of the American Thyroid Association, 16(10), 949–951. https://doi.org/10.1089/thy.2006.16.949

[2844] Foster H. D. (1993). The iodine-selenium connection: its possible roles in intelligence, cretinism, sudden infant death syndrome, breast cancer and multiple sclerosis. Medical hypotheses, 40(1), 61–65. https://doi.org/10.1016/0306-9877(93)90198-y

[2845] NIH (2020) 'Iodine: Fact Sheet for Health Professionals', Dietary Supplement Fact Sheets, Accessed Online Dec 29 2020: https://ods.od.nih.gov/factsheets/Iodine-HealthProfessional/

[2846] Trumbo, P., Yates, A. A., Schlicker, S., & Poos, M. (2001). Dietary reference intakes: vitamin A, vitamin K, arsenic, boron, chromium, copper, iodine, iron, manganese, molybdenum, nickel, silicon, vanadium, and zinc. Journal of the American Dietetic Association, 101(3), 294–301. https://doi.org/10.1016/S0002-8223(01)00078-5

[2847] Zimmermann M. B. (2009). Iodine deficiency in pregnancy and the effects of maternal iodine supplementation on the offspring: a review. The American journal of clinical nutrition, 89(2), 668S–72S. https://doi.org/10.3945/ajcn.2008.26811C

[2848] Alexander, E. K., Pearce, E. N., Brent, G. A., Brown, R. S., Chen, H., Dosiou, C., Grobman, W. A., Laurberg, P., Lazarus, J. H., Mandel, S. J., Peeters, R. P., & Sullivan, S. (2017). 2017 Guidelines of the American Thyroid Association for the Diagnosis and Management of Thyroid Disease During Pregnancy and the Postpartum. Thyroid : official journal of the American Thyroid Association, 27(3), 315–389. https://doi.org/10.1089/thy.2016.0457

[2849] Council on Environmental Health, Rogan, W. J., Paulson, J. A., Baum, C., Brock-Utne, A. C., Brumberg, H. L., Campbell, C. C., Lanphear, B. P., Lowry, J. A., Osterhoudt, K. C., Sandel, M. T., Spanier, A., & Trasande, L. (2014). Iodine deficiency, pollutant chemicals, and the thyroid: new information on an old problem. Pediatrics, 133(6), 1163–1166. https://doi.org/10.1542/peds.2014-0900

[2850] Gupta, P. M., Gahche, J. J., Herrick, K. A., Ershow, A. G., Potischman, N., & Perrine, C. G. (2018). Use of Iodine-Containing Dietary Supplements Remains Low among Women of Reproductive Age in the United States: NHANES 2011-2014. Nutrients, 10(4), 422. https://doi.org/10.3390/nu10040422

[2851] Rebagliato, M., Murcia, M., Espada, M., Alvarez-Pedrerol, M., Bolúmar, F., Vioque, J., Basterrechea, M., Blarduni, E., Ramón, R., Guxens, M., Foradada, C. M., Ballester, F., Ibarluzea, J., & Sunyer, J. (2010). Iodine intake and maternal thyroid function during pregnancy. Epidemiology (Cambridge, Mass.), 21(1), 62–69. https://doi.org/10.1097/EDE.0b013e3181c1592b

[2852] Aakre, I., Bjøro, T., Norheim, I., Strand, T. A., Barikmo, I., & Henjum, S. (2015). Excessive iodine intake and thyroid dysfunction among lactating Saharawi women. Journal of Trace Elements in Medicine and Biology, 31, 279–284. doi:10.1016/j.jtemb.2014.09.009

[2853] Liu, L., Wang, D., Liu, P., Meng, F., Wen, D., Jia, Q., … Shen, H. (2015). The relationship between iodine nutrition and thyroid disease in lactating women with different iodine intakes. British Journal of Nutrition, 114(9), 1487–1495. doi:10.1017/s0007114515003128

[2854] Chung, H. R., Shin, C. H., Yang, S. W., Choi, C. W., & Kim, B. I. (2009). Subclinical hypothyroidism in Korean preterm infants associated with high levels of iodine in breast milk. The Journal of clinical endocrinology and metabolism, 94(11), 4444–4447. https://doi.org/10.1210/jc.2009-0632

[2855] Moon, S., & Kim, J. (1999). Iodine content of human milk and dietary iodine intake of Korean lactating mothers. International journal of food sciences and nutrition, 50(3), 165–171. https://doi.org/10.1080/096374899101201

[2856] Wang, J., Hallinger, D. R., Murr, A. S., Buckalew, A. R., Simmons, S. O., Laws, S. C., & Stoker, T. E. (2018). High-Throughput Screening and Quantitative Chemical Ranking for Sodium-Iodide Symporter Inhibitors in ToxCast Phase I Chemical Library. Environmental science & technology, 52(9), 5417–5426. https://doi.org/10.1021/acs.est.7b06145

[2857] Mervish et al (2016) 'Thyroid Antagonists (Perchlorate, Thiocyanate, and Nitrate) and Childhood Growth in a Longitudinal Study of U.S. Girls', Environmental Health Perspectives 124:4 CID: https://doi.org/10.1289/ehp.1409309

658

[2858] Llorente-Esteban, A., Manville, R. W., Reyna-Neyra, A., Abbott, G. W., Amzel, L. M., & Carrasco, N. (2020). Allosteric regulation of mammalian Na+/I− symporter activity by perchlorate. Nature Structural & Molecular Biology, 27(6), 533–539. doi:10.1038/s41594-020-0417-5

[2859] Blount, B. C., Valentin-Blasini, L., Osterloh, J. D., Mauldin, J. P., & Pirkle, J. L. (2006). Perchlorate Exposure of the US Population, 2001–2002. Journal of Exposure Science & Environmental Epidemiology, 17(4), 400–407. doi:10.1038/sj.jes.7500535

[2860] Waugh D. T. (2019). Fluoride Exposure Induces Inhibition of Sodium/Iodide Symporter (NIS) Contributing to Impaired Iodine Absorption and Iodine Deficiency: Molecular Mechanisms of Inhibition and Implications for Public Health. International journal of environmental research and public health, 16(6), 1086. https://doi.org/10.3390/ijerph16061086

[2861] European Union. (2015). 'Commission Delegated Regulation (EU) 2016/127 of 25 September 2015 supplementing Regulation (EU) No 609/2013 of the European Parliament and of the Council as regards the specific compositional and information requirements for infant formula and follow-on formula and as regards requirements on information relating to infant and young child feeding'. Brussels: European Union.

[2862] Dold, S., Zimmermann, M. B., Aboussad, A., Cherkaoui, M., Jia, Q., Jukic, T., ... Andersson, M. (2017). Breast Milk Iodine Concentration Is a More Accurate Biomarker of Iodine Status Than Urinary Iodine Concentration in Exclusively Breastfeeding Women. The Journal of Nutrition, 147(4), 528–537. doi:10.3945/jn.116.242560

[2863] Lee, S. Y., Stagnaro-Green, A., MacKay, D., Wong, A. W., & Pearce, E. N. (2017). Iodine Contents in Prenatal Vitamins in the United States. Thyroid, 27(8), 1101–1102. doi:10.1089/thy.2017.0097

[2864] Restani, P., Persico, A., Ballabio, C., Moro, E., Fuggetta, D., & Colombo, M. L. (2008). Analysis of food supplements containing iodine: a survey of Italian market. Clinical Toxicology, 46(4), 282–286. doi:10.1080/15563650701373788

[2865] NIH (2020) 'Iodine: Health Professional Fact Sheet', Dietary Supplement Fact Sheets, Accessed Online Dec 21 2020: https://ods.od.nih.gov/factsheets/Iodine-HealthProfessional/

[2866] USDA (2020) 'USDA, FDA and ODS-NIH Database for the Iodine Content of Common Foods Release 1.0 (2020)', Iodine, Accessed Online Dec 21 2020: https://www.ars.usda.gov/northeast-area/beltsville-md-bhnrc/beltsville-human-nutrition-research-center/methods-and-application-of-food-composition-laboratory/mafcl-site-pages/iodine/

[2867] Pehrsson, P. R., Patterson, K. Y., Spungen, J. H., Wirtz, M. S., Andrews, K. W., Dwyer, J. T., & Swanson, C. A. (2016). Iodine in food- and dietary supplement-composition databases. The American journal of clinical nutrition, 104 Suppl 3(Suppl 3), 868S–76S. https://doi.org/10.3945/ajcn.115.110064

[2868] College of Agriculture and Life Sciences (2019) 'Glucosinolates (Goitrogenic Glycosides)', Department of Animal Science - Plants Poisonous to Livestock, Accessed Online Dec 23 2020: http://poisonousplants.ansci.cornell.edu/toxicagents/glucosin.html

[2869] Petre (2017) 'Are Goitrogens in Foods Harmful?', Healthline, Accessed Online Dec 23 2020: https://www.healthline.com/nutrition/goitrogens-in-foods

[2870] Rungapamestry, V., Duncan, A. J., Fuller, Z., & Ratcliffe, B. (2007). Effect of cooking brassica vegetables on the subsequent hydrolysis and metabolic fate of glucosinolates. The Proceedings of the Nutrition Society, 66(1), 69–81. https://doi.org/10.1017/S0029665107005319

[2871] McMillan, M., Spinks, E. A., & Fenwick, G. R. (1986). Preliminary Observations on the Effect of Dietary Brussels Sprouts on Thyroid Function. Human Toxicology, 5(1), 15–19. https://doi.org/10.1177/096032718600500104

[2872] National Cancer Institute (2012) 'Cruciferous Vegetables and Cancer Prevention', Cancer Causes and Prevention, NIH, Accessed Online Dec 23 2020: https://www.cancer.gov/about-cancer/causes-prevention/risk/diet/cruciferous-vegetables-fact-sheet

[2873] Hecht S. S. (2000). Inhibition of carcinogenesis by isothiocyanates. Drug metabolism reviews, 32(3-4), 395–411. https://doi.org/10.1081/dmr-100102342

[2874] Murillo, G., & Mehta, R. G. (2001). Cruciferous vegetables and cancer prevention. Nutrition and cancer, 41(1-2), 17–28. https://doi.org/10.1080/01635581.2001.9680607

[2875] Zhou, Y., Samson, M., Francon, J., & Blondeau, J. P. (1992). Thyroid hormone concentrative uptake in rat erythrocytes. Involvement of the tryptophan transport system T in countertransport of tri-iodothyronine and aromatic amino acids. The Biochemical journal, 281 (Pt 1)(Pt 1), 81–86. https://doi.org/10.1042/bj2810081

[2876] Zhou, Y., Samson, M., Osty, J., Francon, J., & Blondeau, J. P. (1990). Evidence for a close link between the thyroid hormone transport system and the aromatic amino acid transport system T in erythrocytes. The Journal of biological chemistry, 265(28), 17000–17004.

[2877] Samson, M., Osty, J., Francon, J., & Blondeau, J. P. (1992). Triiodothyronine binding sites in the rat erythrocyte membrane: involvement in triiodothyronine transport and relation to the tryptophan transport System T. Biochimica et biophysica acta, 1108(1), 91–98. https://doi.org/10.1016/0005-2736(92)90118-6

[2878] Yan, Z., & Hinkle, P. M. (1993). Saturable, stereospecific transport of 3,5,3'-triiodo-L-thyronine and L-thyroxine into GH4C1 pituitary cells. The Journal of biological chemistry, 268(27), 20179–20184.

[2879] Lim, C. F., Loidl, N. M., Kennedy, J. A., Topliss, D. J., & Stockigt, J. R. (1996). Drug effects on triiodothyronine uptake by rat anterior pituitary cells in vitro. Experimental and clinical endocrinology & diabetes : official journal, German Society of Endocrinology [and] German Diabetes Association, 104(2), 151–157. https://doi.org/10.1055/s-0029-1211437

[2880] Kragie, L., Forrester, M. L., Cody, V., & McCourt, M. (1994). Computer-assisted molecular modeling of benzodiazepine and thyromimetic inhibitors of the HepG2 iodothyronine membrane transporter. Molecular endocrinology (Baltimore, Md.), 8(3), 382–391. https://doi.org/10.1210/mend.8.3.8015555

[2881] Topliss, D. J., Scholz, G. H., Kolliniatis, E., Barlow, J. W., & Stockigt, J. R. (1993). Influence of calmodulin antagonists and calcium channel blockers on triiodothyronine uptake by rat hepatoma and myoblast cell lines. Metabolism: clinical and experimental, 42(3), 376–380. https://doi.org/10.1016/0026-0495(93)90090-b

[2882] Kragie, L., & Doyle, D. (1992). Benzodiazepines inhibit temperature-dependent L-[125I]triiodothyronine accumulation into human liver, human neuroblast, and rat pituitary cell lines. Endocrinology, 130(3), 1211–1216. https://doi.org/10.1210/endo.130.3.1537286

[2883] Topliss, D. J., Kolliniatis, E., Barlow, J. W., Lim, C. F., & Stockigt, J. R. (1989). Uptake of 3,5,3'-triiodothyronine by cultured rat hepatoma cells is inhibitable by nonbile acid cholephils, diphenylhydantoin, and nonsteroidal antiinflammatory drugs. Endocrinology, 124(2), 980–986. https://doi.org/10.1210/endo-124-2-980

[2884] Scholz, G. H., Vieweg, S., Uhlig, M., Thormann, M., Klossek, P., Goldmann, S., & Hofmann, H. J. (1997). Inhibition of thyroid hormone uptake by calcium antagonists of the dihydropyridine class. Journal of medicinal chemistry, 40(10), 1530–1538. https://doi.org/10.1021/jm9604989

[2885] Topliss, D. J., Kolliniatis, E., Barlow, J. W., Lim, C. F., & Stockigt, J. R. (1989). Uptake of 3,5,3'-triiodothyronine by cultured rat hepatoma cells is inhibitable by nonbile acid cholephils, diphenylhydantoin, and nonsteroidal antiinflammatory drugs. Endocrinology, 124(2), 980–986. https://doi.org/10.1210/endo-124-2-980

[2886] Sarne, D. (2016). Effects of the Environment, Chemicals and Drugs on Thyroid Function. In K. R. Feingold (Eds.) et. al., Endotext. MDText.com, Inc.

[2887] Goldberg, A. S., Tirona, R. G., Asher, L. J., Kim, R. B., & Van Uum, S. H. M. (2013). Ciprofloxacin and Rifampin Have Opposite Effects on Levothyroxine Absorption. Thyroid, 23(11), 1374–1378. doi:10.1089/thy.2013.0014

[2888] Pollock, A. J., Seibert, T., & Allen, D. B. (2016). Severe and Persistent Thyroid Dysfunction Associated with Tetracycline-Antibiotic Treatment in Youth. The Journal of pediatrics, 173, 232–234. https://doi.org/10.1016/j.jpeds.2016.03.034

[2889] Munivenkatappa, S., Anil, S., Naik, B., Volkmann, T., Sagili, K. D., Akshatha, J. S., … Moonan, P. K. (2016). Drug-Induced Hypothyroidism during Anti-Tuberculosis Treatment of Multidrug-Resistant Tuberculosis: Notes from the Field. Journal of Tuberculosis Research, 04(03), 105–110. doi:10.4236/jtr.2016.43013

[2890] Bostancı, I., Sanoglu, A., Ergin, H., Akşit, A., Cinbiş, M., & Aklın, N. (2001). Neonatal Goiter Caused by Expectorant Usage. Journal of Pediatric Endocrinology and Metabolism, 14(8). doi:10.1515/jpem-2001-0815

[2891] Tokinaga et al (2006) 'HMG-coa reductase inhibitors (statins) might cause high elevations of creatine phosphokinase (CK) in patients with unnoticed hypothyroidism', Endocr J. Jun;53(3):401-5.

[2892] Răcătăianu, N., Bolboacă, S. D., Sitar-Tăut, A. V., Mârza, S., Moga, D., Valea, A., & Ghervan, C. (2018). The effect of Metformin treatment in obese insulin-resistant patients with euthyroid goiter. Acta clinica Belgica, 73(5), 317–323. https://doi.org/10.1080/17843286.2018.1439273

[2893] Ittermann, T., Markus, M. R., Schipf, S., Derwahl, M., Meisinger, C., & Völzke, H. (2013). Metformin inhibits goitrogenous effects of type 2 diabetes. European journal of endocrinology, 169(1), 9–15. https://doi.org/10.1530/EJE-13-0101

[2894] Knight, B. A., Shields, B. M., He, X., Pearce, E. N., Braverman, L. E., Sturley, R., & Vaidya, B. (2018). Effect of perchlorate and thiocyanate exposure on thyroid function of pregnant women from South-West England: a cohort study. Thyroid Research, 11(1). doi:10.1186/s13044-018-0053-x

[2895] Sanchez, C. A., Krieger, R. I., Khandaker, N., Moore, R. C., Holts, K. C., & Neidel, L. L. (2005). Accumulation and Perchlorate Exposure Potential of Lettuce Produced in the Lower Colorado River Region. Journal of Agricultural and Food Chemistry, 53(13), 5479–5486. doi:10.1021/jf050380d

[2896] Wadden, T. A., Mason, G., Foster, G. D., Stunkard, A. J., & Prange, A. J. (1990). Effects of a very low calorie diet on weight, thyroid hormones and mood. International journal of obesity, 14(3), 249–258.

[2897] Fliers, E., Kalsbeek, A., & Boelen, A. (2014). MECHANISMS IN ENDOCRINOLOGY: Beyond the fixed setpoint of the hypothalamus–pituitary–thyroid axis. European Journal of Endocrinology, 171(5), R197–R208. doi:10.1530/eje-14-0285

[2898] Fothergill, E., Guo, J., Howard, L., Kerns, J. C., Knuth, N. D., Brychta, R., ... Hall, K. D. (2016). Persistent metabolic adaptation 6 years after "The Biggest Loser" competition. Obesity, 24(8), 1612–1619. doi:10.1002/oby.21538

[2899] Byrne, N. M., Sainsbury, A., King, N. A., Hills, A. P., & Wood, R. E. (2017). Intermittent energy restriction improves weight loss efficiency in obese men: the MATADOR study. International Journal of Obesity, 42(2), 129–138. doi:10.1038/ijo.2017.206

[2900] Chan, J. L., Heist, K., DePaoli, A. M., Veldhuis, J. D., & Mantzoros, C. S. (2003). The role of falling leptin levels in the neuroendocrine and metabolic adaptation to short-term starvation in healthy men. Journal of Clinical Investigation, 111(9), 1409–1421. doi:10.1172/jci200317490

[2901] Azizi, F. (1978). Effect of dietary composition on fasting-induced changes in serum thyroid hormones and thyrotropin. Metabolism, 27(8), 935–942. doi:10.1016/0026-0495(78)90137-3

[2902] CARLSON, H. E., DRENICK, E. J., CHOPRA, I. J., & HERSHMAN, J. M. (1977). Alterations in Basal and TRH-Stimulated Serum Levels of Thyrotropin, Prolactin, and Thyroid Hormones in Starved Obese Men. The Journal of Clinical Endocrinology & Metabolism, 45(4), 707–713. doi:10.1210/jcem-45-4-707

[2903] Anita Boelen, Wilmar Maarten Wiersinga, and Eric Fliers.Thyroid.Feb 2008.123-129.http://doi.org/10.1089/thy.2007.0253

[2904] Ucci, Renzini, Russi, Mangialardo, Cammarata, Cavioli, ... Verga-Falzacappa. (2019). Thyroid Hormone Protects from Fasting-Induced Skeletal Muscle Atrophy by Promoting Metabolic Adaptation. International Journal of Molecular Sciences, 20(22), 5754. doi:10.3390/ijms20225754

[2905] Azizi F, Rasouli HA, Beheshti S. Evaluation of certain hormones and blood constituents during Islamic fasting month. Med Assoc Thailand. 1986;69:57A.

[2906] Raza, S., Unnikrishnan, A., Ahmad, J., Azad, K., Pathan, M. F., Ishtiaq, O., ... Baruah, M. (2012). Thyroid diseases and Ramadan. Indian Journal of Endocrinology and Metabolism, 16(4), 522. doi:10.4103/2230-8210.98001

[2907] Sulimani RA. The effects of Ramadan fasting on thyroid functions in healthy male subjects. Nutrition Research. 1988;8(5):549–52. doi: 10.1016/s0271-5317(88)80076-9

[2908] Ahmadinejad Z, Ziaee V, Rezaee M, Yarmohammadi Y, Shaikh H. The effect of ramadan fasting on thyroid hormone profile: A cohort study. Pak J Biol Sci. 2006;9 doi: 10.3923/pjbs.2006.1999.2002.

[2909] De Jong, M., Docter, R., Van Der Hoek, H. J., Vos, R. A., Krenning, E. P., & Hennemann, G. (1992). Transport of 3,5,3'-triiodothyronine into the perfused rat liver and subsequent metabolism are inhibited by fasting. Endocrinology, 131(1), 463–470. https://doi.org/10.1210/endo.131.1.1612027

[2910] Bodoky, G., Yang, Z. J., Meguid, M. M., Laviano, A., & Szeverenyi, N. (1995). Effects of fasting, intermittent feeding, or continuous parenteral nutrition on rat liver and brain energy metabolism as assessed by 31P-NMR. Physiology & behavior, 58(3), 521–527. https://doi.org/10.1016/0031-9384(95)00078-w

[2911] De Jong, M., Docter, R., Bernard, B. F., van der Heijden, J. T., van Toor, H., Krenning, E. P., & Hennemann, G. (1994). T4 uptake into the perfused rat liver and liver T4 uptake in humans are inhibited by fructose. The American journal of physiology, 266(5 Pt 1), E768–E775. https://doi.org/10.1152/ajpendo.1994.266.5.E768

[2912] De Jong, M., Docter, R., Bernard, B. F., van der Heijden, J. T., van Toor, H., Krenning, E. P., & Hennemann, G. (1994). T4 uptake into the perfused rat liver and liver T4 uptake in humans are inhibited by fructose. The American journal of physiology, 266(5 Pt 1), E768–E775. https://doi.org/10.1152/ajpendo.1994.266.5.E768

[2913] Greene, H. L., Wilson, F. A., Hefferan, P., Terry, A. B., Moran, J. R., Slonim, A. E., Claus, T. H., & Burr, I. M. (1978). ATP depletion, a possible role in the pathogenesis of hyperuricemia in glycogen storage disease type I. The Journal of clinical investigation, 62(2), 321–328. https://doi.org/10.1172/JCI109132

[2914] Birdsong, W. T., Fierro, L., Williams, F. G., Spelta, V., Naves, L. A., Knowles, M., ... McCleskey, E. W. (2010). Sensing Muscle Ischemia: Coincident Detection of Acid and ATP via Interplay of Two Ion Channels. Neuron, 68(4), 739–749. doi:10.1016/j.neuron.2010.09.029

[2915] Nadolnik, L. I. (2011). Stress and the thyroid gland. Biochemistry (Moscow) Supplement Series B: Biomedical Chemistry, 5(2), 103–112. doi:10.1134/s1990750811020119

[2916] Brown-Grant, K., Harris, G. W., & Reichlin, S. (1954). The effect of emotional and physical stress on thyroid activity in the rabbit. The Journal of Physiology, 126(1), 29–40. doi:10.1113/jphysiol.1954.sp005189

[2917] Jung, S. J., Kang, J. H., Roberts, A. L., Nishimi, K., Chen, Q., Sumner, J. A., Kubzansky, L., & Koenen, K. C. (2019). Posttraumatic stress disorder and incidence of thyroid dysfunction in women. Psychological medicine, 49(15), 2551–2560. https://doi.org/10.1017/S0033291718003495

[2918] Burman, K. D., Smallridge, R. C., Osburne, R., Dimond, R. C., Whorton, N. E., Kesler, P., & Wartofsky, L. (1980). Nature of suppressed TSH secretion during undernutrition: Effect of fasting and refeeding on TSH responses to prolonged TRH infusions. Metabolism, 29(1), 46–52. doi:10.1016/0026-0495(80)90097-9

[2919] Azizi, F. (1978). Effect of dietary composition on fasting-induced changes in serum thyroid hormones and thyrotropin. Metabolism, 27(8), 935–942. doi:10.1016/0026-0495(78)90137-3

[2920] Spaulding, S. W., Chopra, I. J., Sherwin, R. S., & Lyall, S. S. (1976). EFFECT OF CALORIC RESTRICTION AND DIETARY COMPOSITION ON SERUM T3AND REVERSE T3IN MAN. The Journal of Clinical Endocrinology & Metabolism, 42(1), 197–200. doi:10.1210/jcem-42-1-197

[2921] Paz-Filho, G., Wong, M.-L., Licinio, J., & Mastronardi, C. (2012). Leptin therapy, insulin sensitivity, and glucose homeostasis. Indian Journal of Endocrinology and Metabolism, 16(9), 549. doi:10.4103/2230-8210.105571

[2922] Berglund, E. D., Vianna, C. R., Donato, J., Kim, M. H., Chuang, J.-C., Lee, C. E., … Elmquist, J. K. (2012). Direct leptin action on POMC neurons regulates glucose homeostasis and hepatic insulin sensitivity in mice. Journal of Clinical Investigation, 122(3), 1000–1009. doi:10.1172/jci59816

[2923] Fery et al (1982) 'Hormonal and metabolic changes induced by an isocaloric isoproteinic ketogenic diet in healthy subjects', Diabete Metab. 1982 Dec;8(4):299-305.

[2924] Kinzig, K. P., Honors, M. A., & Hargrave, S. L. (2010). Insulin sensitivity and glucose tolerance are altered by maintenance on a ketogenic diet. Endocrinology, 151(7), 3105–3114. https://doi.org/10.1210/en.2010-0175

[2925] Boden et al (2005). Effect of a low-carbohydrate diet on appetite, blood glucose levels, and insulin resistance in obese patients with type 2 diabetes. Annals of internal medicine, 142(6), 403–411. https://doi.org/10.7326/0003-4819-142-6-200503150-00006

[2926] Kaptein EM 1986 Thyroid hormone metabolism in illness. In: Hennemann G, ed. Thyroid hormone metabolism. New York: Marcel Dekker; 297–333

[2927] Kaptein, E. M., Feinstein, E. I., Nicoloff, J. T., & Massry, S. G. (1983). Serum reverse triiodothyronine and thyroxine kinetics in patients with chronic renal failure. The Journal of clinical endocrinology and metabolism, 57(1), 181–189. https://doi.org/10.1210/jcem-57-1-181

[2928] Dold, S., Zimmermann, M. B., Jukic, T., Kusic, Z., Jia, Q., Sang, Z., Quirino, A., San Luis, T., Fingerhut, R., Kupka, R., Timmer, A., Garrett, G. S., & Andersson, M. (2018). Universal Salt Iodization Provides Sufficient Dietary Iodine to Achieve Adequate Iodine Nutrition during the First 1000 Days: A Cross-Sectional Multicenter Study. The Journal of nutrition, 148(4), 587–598. https://doi.org/10.1093/jn/nxy015

[2929] Cooper LF, Barber EM, Mitchell HS. Nutrition in Health and Disease, 9th ed. J.B. Lippincott Co, Philadelphia. 1943, pg 66.

[2930] McClure R. D. (1935). GOITER PROPHYLAXIS WITH IODIZED SALT. Science (New York, N.Y.), 82(2129), 370–371. https://doi.org/10.1126/science.82.2129.370

[2931] Delange, F., Bürgi, H., Chen, Z. P., & Dunn, J. T. (2002). World status of monitoring iodine deficiency disorders control programs. Thyroid : official journal of the American Thyroid Association, 12(10), 915–924. https://doi.org/10.1089/105072502761016557

[2932] World Health Organization. 2014. Guideline: fortification of food-grade salt with iodine for the prevention and control of iodine deficiency disorders. Geneva, Switzerland: World Health Organization.

[2933] Dasgupta, P. K., Liu, Y., & Dyke, J. V. (2008). Iodine nutrition: iodine content of iodized salt in the United States. Environmental science & technology, 42(4), 1315–1323. https://doi.org/10.1021/es0719071

[2934] Farebrother, J., Zimmermann, M. B., Abdallah, F., Assey, V., Fingerhut, R., Gichohi-Wainaina, W. N., Hussein, I., Makokha, A., Sagno, K., Untoro, J., Watts, M., & Andersson, M. (2018). Effect of Excess Iodine Intake from Iodized Salt and/or Groundwater Iodine on Thyroid Function in Nonpregnant and Pregnant Women, Infants, and Children: A Multicenter Study in East Africa. Thyroid : official journal of the American Thyroid Association, 28(9), 1198–1210. https://doi.org/10.1089/thy.2018.0234

[2935] Diosady, L. L., Alberti, J. 0., Mannar, M. G. V., & Stone, T. G. (1997). Stability of Iodine in Iodized Salt Used for Correction of Iodine-Deficiency Disorders. Food and Nutrition Bulletin, 18(4), 1–9. https://doi.org/10.1177/156482659701800409

[2936] Diosady, L. L., Alberti, J. O., Mannar, M. G. V., & FitzGerald, S. (1998). Stability of Iodine in Iodized Salt Used for Correction of Iodine-Deficiency Disorders. II. Food and Nutrition Bulletin, 19(3), 240–250. doi:10.1177/156482659801900306

[2937] Wang, G. Y., Zhou, R. H., Wang, Z., Shi, L., & Sun, M. (1999). Effects of storage and cooking on the iodine content in iodized salt and study on monitoring iodine content in iodized salt. Biomedical and environmental sciences : BES, 12(1), 1–9.

[2938] Horton (2006) 'The economics of food fortification'. J Nutr 2006; 136: 1068–71.

[2939] Caulfield et al (2006). 'Stunting, wasting, and micronutrient deficiency disorders 2006'. In: Dean T, Jamison DT, Breman JG, et al. Disease control priorities in developing countries, 2nd edn. New York: Oxford University Press, 2006: 551–68.

[2940] Engle PL, Black MM, Behrman JR, et al; International Child Development Steering Group. Strategies to avoid the loss of developmental potential in more than 200 million children in the developing world. Lancet 2007; 369: 229–42.

[2941] Katagiri, R., Yuan, X., Kobayashi, S., & Sasaki, S. (2017). Effect of excess iodine intake on thyroid diseases in different populations: A systematic review and meta-analyses including observational studies. PloS one, 12(3), e0173722. https://doi.org/10.1371/journal.pone.0173722

[2942] Bajuk, V., Zaletel, K., Pirnat, E., Hojker, S., & Gaberšček, S. (2017). Effects of Adequate Iodine Supply on the Incidence of Iodine-Induced Thyroid Disorders in Slovenia. Thyroid, 27(4), 558–566. doi:10.1089/thy.2016.0186

[2943] Zaletel, K., Gaberscek, S., & Pirnat, E. (2011). Ten-year follow-up of thyroid epidemiology in Slovenia after increase in salt iodization. Croatian medical journal, 52(5), 615–621. https://doi.org/10.3325/cmj.2011.52.615

[2944] Aghini Lombardi, F., Fiore, E., Tonacchera, M., Antonangeli, L., Rago, T., Frigeri, M., Provenzale, A. M., Montanelli, L., Grasso, L., Pinchera, A., & Vitti, P. (2013). The effect of voluntary iodine prophylaxis in a small rural community: the Pescopagano survey 15 years later. The Journal of clinical endocrinology and metabolism, 98(3), 1031–1039. https://doi.org/10.1210/jc.2012-2960

[2945] Gołkowski, F., Buziak-Bereza, M., Trofimiuk, M., Bałdys-Waligórska, A., Szybiński, Z., & Huszno, B. (2007). Increased prevalence of hyperthyroidism as an early and transient side-effect of implementing iodine prophylaxis. Public Health Nutrition, 10(8), 799–802. doi:10.1017/s1368980007585939

[2946] Premawardhana, L. D., Parkes, A. B., Smyth, P. P., Wijeyaratne, C. N., Jayasinghe, A., de Silva, D. G., & Lazarus, J. H. (2000). Increased prevalence of thyroglobulin antibodies in Sri Lankan schoolgirls-- is iodine the cause?. European journal of endocrinology, 143(2), 185–188. https://doi.org/10.1530/eje.0.1430185

[2947] Fountoulakis, S., Philippou, G., & Tsatsoulis, A. (2007). The role of iodine in the evolution of thyroid disease in Greece: from endemic goiter to thyroid autoimmunity. Hormones (Athens, Greece), 6(1), 25–35.

[2948] Miranda, D. M., Massom, J. N., Catarino, R. M., Santos, R. T., Toyoda, S. S., Marone, M. M., Tomimori, E. K., & Monte, O. (2015). Impact of nutritional iodine optimization on rates of thyroid hypoechogenicity and autoimmune thyroiditis: a cross-sectional, comparative study. Thyroid : official journal of the American Thyroid Association, 25(1), 118–124. https://doi.org/10.1089/thy.2014.0182

[2949] Pedersen, I. B., Knudsen, N., Carlé, A., Vejbjerg, P., Jørgensen, T., Perrild, H., Ovesen, L., Rasmussen, L. B., & Laurberg, P. (2011). A cautious iodization programme bringing iodine intake to a low recommended level is associated with an increase in the prevalence of thyroid autoantibodies in the population. Clinical endocrinology, 75(1), 120–126. https://doi.org/10.1111/j.1365-2265.2011.04008.x

[2950] Bourdoux, P. P., Ermans, A. M., Mukalay wa Mukalay, A., Filetti, S., & Vigneri, R. (1996). Iodine-induced thyrotoxicosis in Kivu, Zaire. Lancet (London, England), 347(9000), 552–553. https://doi.org/10.1016/s0140-6736(96)91188-5

[2951] Delange, F., de Benoist, B., & Alnwick, D. (1999). Risks of iodine-induced hyperthyroidism after correction of iodine deficiency by iodized salt. Thyroid : official journal of the American Thyroid Association, 9(6), 545–556. https://doi.org/10.1089/thy.1999.9.545

[2952] Iodine Global Network. (2017). 'Global Scorecard of Iodine Nutrition in 2017 in the general population and in pregnant women'. IGN: Zurich, Switzerland, Accessed Online Dec 20 2020: https://www.ign.org/cm_data/IGN_Global_Scorecard_AllPop_and_PW_May2017.pdf

[2953] Bülow Pedersen, I., Laurberg, P., Knudsen, N., Jørgensen, T., Perrild, H., Ovesen, L., & Rasmussen, L. B. (2006). Increase in incidence of hyperthyroidism predominantly occurs in young people after iodine fortification of salt in Denmark. The Journal of clinical endocrinology and metabolism, 91(10), 3830–3834. https://doi.org/10.1210/jc.2006-0652

[2954] Stanbury, J. B., Ermans, A. E., Bourdoux, P., Todd, C., Oken, E., Tonglet, R., Vidor, G., Braverman, L. E., & Medeiros-Neto, G. (1998). Iodine-induced hyperthyroidism: occurrence and epidemiology. Thyroid : official journal of the American Thyroid Association, 8(1), 83–100. https://doi.org/10.1089/thy.1998.8.83

[2955] Petersen, M., Knudsen, N., Carlé, A., Andersen, S., Jørgensen, T., Perrild, H., Ovesen, L., Rasmussen, L. B., Thuesen, B. H., & Pedersen, I. B. (2018). Thyrotoxicosis after iodine fortification. A 21-year Danish population-based study. Clinical endocrinology, 89(3), 360–366. https://doi.org/10.1111/cen.13751

[2956] Ursella, S., Testa, A., Mazzone, M., & Gentiloni Silveri, N. (2006). Amiodarone-induced thyroid dysfunction in clinical practice. European review for medical and pharmacological sciences, 10(5), 269–278.

[2957] U.S. Food and Drug Administration. Food Labeling: Revision of the Nutrition and Supplement Facts Labels.external link disclaimer 2016.

[2958] NIH (2020) 'Iodine: Health Professional Fact Sheet', Iodine, Accessed Online Dec 21 2020: https://ods.od.nih.gov/factsheets/Iodine-HealthProfessional/

[2959] Johnson, C.C.. 2003 The geochemistry of iodine and its application to environmental strategies for reducing the risk from iodine deficiency disorders (IDD). Nottingham, UK, British Geological Survey, 54pp. (CR/03/057N) (Unpublished)

[2960] Pichel, N., & Vivar, M. (2017). A critical review on iodine presence in drinking water access at the Saharawi refugee camps (Tindouf, Algeria). Journal of Trace Elements in Medicine and Biology, 42, 32–38. doi:10.1016/j.jtemb.2017.03.011

[2961] Watts, M. J., O'Reilly, J., Maricelli, A., Coleman, A., Ander, E. L., & Ward, N. I. (2010). A snapshot of environmental iodine and selenium in La Pampa and San Juan provinces of Argentina. Journal of Geochemical Exploration, 107(2), 87–93. doi:10.1016/j.gexplo.2009.11.002

[2962] Teng, W., Shan, Z., Teng, X., Guan, H., Li, Y., Teng, D., ... Li, C. (2006). Effect of Iodine Intake on Thyroid Diseases in China. New England Journal of Medicine, 354(26), 2783–2793. doi:10.1056/nejmoa054022

[2963] Voutchkova, D. D., Ernstsen, V., Hansen, B., Sørensen, B. L., Zhang, C., & Kristiansen, S. M. (2014). Assessment of spatial variation in drinking water iodine and its implications for dietary intake: A new conceptual model for Denmark. Science of The Total Environment, 493, 432–444. doi:10.1016/j.scitotenv.2014.06.008

[2964] Reimann, C., Bjorvatn, K., Frengstad, B., Melaku, Z., Tekle-Haimanot, R., & Siewers, U. (2003). Drinking water quality in the Ethiopian section of the East African Rift Valley I—data and health aspects. Science of The Total Environment, 311(1-3), 65–80. doi:10.1016/s0048-9697(03)00137-2

[2965] Watts, M.J., D.R.S. Middleton, O. Humphrey, et al. 2018. Measurements to apportion micronutrient status in Western Kenya, Poster presentation. In 34th International Conference 'Geochemistry for Sustainable Development', Livingstone, Zambia.

[2966] Kassim, I. A. R., Moloney, G., Busili, A., Nur, A. Y., Paron, P., Jooste, P., ... Seal, A. J. (2014). Iodine Intake in Somalia Is Excessive and Associated with the Source of Household Drinking Water. The Journal of Nutrition, 144(3), 375–381. doi:10.3945/jn.113.176693

[2967] Sang, Z., Chen, W., Shen, J., Tan, L., Zhao, N., Liu, H., ... Zhang, W. (2013). Long-Term Exposure to Excessive Iodine from Water Is Associated with Thyroid Dysfunction in Children. The Journal of Nutrition, 143(12), 2038–2043. doi:10.3945/jn.113.179135

[2968] Li, M., D. Liu, C. Qu, et al. 1987. Endemic goitre in central China caused by excessive iodine intake. Lancet 2: 257–259.

[2969] Shen, H., Liu, S., Sun, D., Zhang, S., Su, X., Shen, Y., & Han, H. (2011). Geographical distribution of drinking-water with high iodine level and association between high iodine level in drinking-water and goitre: a Chinese national investigation. British Journal of Nutrition, 106(2), 243–247. doi:10.1017/s0007114511000055

[2970] Endemic goiter associated with high iodine intake. (2000). American Journal of Public Health, 90(10), 1633–1635. doi:10.2105/ajph.90.10.1633

[2971] Pearce, E. N., Gerber, A. R., Gootnick, D. B., Khan, L. K., Li, R., Pino, S., & Braverman, L. E. (2002). Effects of chronic iodine excess in a cohort of long-term American workers in West Africa. The Journal of clinical endocrinology and metabolism, 87(12), 5499–5502. https://doi.org/10.1210/jc.2002-020692

[2972] McMonigal, K.A., L.E. Braverman, J.T. Dunn, et al. 2000. Thyroid function changes related to use of iodinated water in the U.S. Space Program. Aviat. Space Environ. Med. 71: 1120–1125.

[2973] Lowe, D. O., Knowles, S. R., Weber, E. A., Railton, C. J., & Shear, N. H. (2006). Povidone-iodine-induced burn: case report and review of the literature. Pharmacotherapy, 26(11), 1641–1645. https://doi.org/10.1592/phco.26.11.1641

[2974] Smyth P. P. (2003). Role of iodine in antioxidant defence in thyroid and breast disease. BioFactors (Oxford, England), 19(3-4), 121–130. https://doi.org/10.1002/biof.5520190304

[2975] Xu, J., Liu, X. L., Yang, X. F., Guo, H. L., Zhao, L. N., & Sun, X. F. (2011). Supplemental selenium alleviates the toxic effects of excessive iodine on thyroid. Biological trace element research, 141(1-3), 110–118. https://doi.org/10.1007/s12011-010-8728-8

[2976] Boehm I. (2008). Seafood allergy and radiocontrast media: are physicians propagating a myth?. The American journal of medicine, 121(8), e19. https://doi.org/10.1016/j.amjmed.2008.03.035

[2977] Lombardo, P., Nairz, K., & Boehm, I. (2019). Patients' safety and the "iodine allergy" - How should we manage patients with iodine allergy before they receive an iodinated contrast medium?. European journal of radiology, 116, 150–151. https://doi.org/10.1016/j.ejrad.2019.05.002

[2978] Rousset and Dunn (2004) 'Thyroid hormone synthesis and secretion'. In: DeGroot LE, Hannemann G, eds. The Thyroid and Its Diseases.

[2979] Zimmermann, M. B., & Andersson, M. (2012). Assessment of iodine nutrition in populations: past, present, and future. Nutrition reviews, 70(10), 553–570. https://doi.org/10.1111/j.1753-4887.2012.00528.x

[2980] Rohner, F., Zimmermann, M., Jooste, P., Pandav, C., Caldwell, K., Raghavan, R., & Raiten, D. J. (2014). Biomarkers of nutrition for development--iodine review. The Journal of nutrition, 144(8), 1322S–1342S. https://doi.org/10.3945/jn.113.181974

[2981] Vejbjerg, P., Knudsen, N., Perrild, H., Laurberg, P., Andersen, S., Rasmussen, L. B., Ovesen, L., & Jørgensen, T. (2009). Estimation of iodine intake from various urinary iodine measurements in population studies. Thyroid : official journal of the American Thyroid Association, 19(11), 1281–1286. https://doi.org/10.1089/thy.2009.0094

[2982] König, F., Andersson, M., Hotz, K., Aeberli, I., & Zimmermann, M. B. (2011). Ten repeat collections for urinary iodine from spot samples or 24-hour samples are needed to reliably estimate individual iodine status in women. The Journal of nutrition, 141(11), 2049–2054. https://doi.org/10.3945/jn.111.144071

[2983] Gordon, R. C., Rose, M. C., Skeaff, S. A., Gray, A. R., Morgan, K. M., & Ruffman, T. (2009). Iodine supplementation improves cognition in mildly iodine-deficient children. The American journal of clinical nutrition, 90(5), 1264–1271. https://doi.org/10.3945/ajcn.2009.28145

[2984] World Health Organization (2013) 'Urinary iodine concentrations for determining iodine status in populations', WHO/NMH/NHD/EPG/13.1, Accessed Online Dec 23 2020: https://www.who.int/vmnis/indicators/urinaryiodine/en/

[2985] Haddow, J. E., McClain, M. R., Palomaki, G. E., & Hollowell, J. G. (2007). Urine iodine measurements, creatinine adjustment, and thyroid deficiency in an adult United States population. The Journal of clinical endocrinology and metabolism, 92(3), 1019–1022. https://doi.org/10.1210/jc.2006-2156

[2986] Caldwell, K. L., Jones, R., & Hollowell, J. G. (2005). Urinary Iodine Concentration: United States National Health and Nutrition Examination Survey 2001–2002. Thyroid, 15(7), 692–699. doi:10.1089/thy.2005.15.692

[2987] Caldwell, K. L., Miller, G. A., Wang, R. Y., Jain, R. B., & Jones, R. L. (2008). Iodine status of the U.S. population, National Health and Nutrition Examination Survey 2003-2004. Thyroid : official journal of the American Thyroid Association, 18(11), 1207–1214. https://doi.org/10.1089/thy.2008.0161

[2988] Perrine, C. G., Herrick, K., Serdula, M. K., & Sullivan, K. M. (2010). Some subgroups of reproductive age women in the United States may be at risk for iodine deficiency. The Journal of nutrition, 140(8), 1489–1494. https://doi.org/10.3945/jn.109.120147

[2989] Perrine, C. G., Herrick, K. A., Gupta, P. M., & Caldwell, K. L. (2019). Iodine Status of Pregnant Women and Women of Reproductive Age in the United States. Thyroid : official journal of the American Thyroid Association, 29(1), 153–154. https://doi.org/10.1089/thy.2018.0345

[2990] Charlton, K. E., Gemming, L., Yeatman, H., & Ma, G. (2010). Suboptimal iodine status of Australian pregnant women reflects poor knowledge and practices related to iodine nutrition. Nutrition (Burbank, Los Angeles County, Calif.), 26(10), 963–968. https://doi.org/10.1016/j.nut.2009.08.016

[2991] Tayie, F. A., & Jourdan, K. (2010). Hypertension, dietary salt restriction, and iodine deficiency among adults. American journal of hypertension, 23(10), 1095–1102. https://doi.org/10.1038/ajh.2010.120

[2992] Li, M., & Eastman, C. J. (2010). Neonatal TSH screening: is it a sensitive and reliable tool for monitoring iodine status in populations?. Best practice & research. Clinical endocrinology & metabolism, 24(1), 63–75. https://doi.org/10.1016/j.beem.2009.08.007

[2993] Biondi (2013) 'The Normal TSH Reference Range: What Has Changed in the Last Decade?', The Journal of Clinical Endocrinology & Metabolism, Volume 98, Issue 9, 1 September 2013, Pages 3584–3587, https://doi.org/10.1210/jc.2013-2760

[2994] Hollowell, J. G., Staehling, N. W., Flanders, W. D., Hannon, W. H., Gunter, E. W., Spencer, C. A., & Braverman, L. E. (2002). Serum TSH, T(4), and thyroid antibodies in the United States population (1988 to 1994): National Health and Nutrition Examination Survey (NHANES III). The Journal of clinical endocrinology and metabolism, 87(2), 489–499. https://doi.org/10.1210/jcem.87.2.8182

[2995] Sullivan et al (1997) 'Use of Thyroid Stimulating Hormone Testing in Newborns to Identify Iodine Deficiency', The Journal of Nutrition, Volume 127, Issue 1, January 1997, Pages 55–58, https://doi.org/10.1093/jn/127.1.55

[2996] Vadiveloo, T., Donnan, P. T., Murphy, M. J., & Leese, G. P. (2013). Age- and Gender-Specific TSH Reference Intervals in People With No Obvious Thyroid Disease in Tayside, Scotland: The Thyroid Epidemiology, Audit, and Research Study (TEARS). The Journal of Clinical Endocrinology & Metabolism, 98(3), 1147–1153. doi:10.1210/jc.2012-3191

[2997] Sunde RA. Selenium. In: Ross AC, Caballero B, Cousins RJ, Tucker KL, Ziegler TR, eds. Modern Nutrition in Health and Disease. 11th ed. Philadelphia, PA: Lippincott Williams & Wilkins; 2012:225-37

[2998] Reeves, M. A., & Hoffmann, P. R. (2009). The human selenoproteome: recent insights into functions and regulation. Cellular and molecular life sciences : CMLS, 66(15), 2457–2478. https://doi.org/10.1007/s00018-009-0032-4

[2999] Sunde RA. Selenium. In: Bowman B, Russell R, eds. Present Knowledge in Nutrition. 9th ed. Washington, DC: International Life Sciences Institute; 2006:480-97

[3000] Schomburg L. (2011). Selenium, selenoproteins and the thyroid gland: interactions in health and disease. Nature reviews. Endocrinology, 8(3), 160–171. https://doi.org/10.1038/nrendo.2011.174

[3001] Schomburg, L. (2011). Selenium, selenoproteins and the thyroid gland: interactions in health and disease. Nature Reviews Endocrinology, 8(3), 160–171. doi:10.1038/nrendo.2011.174

[3002] Berry, M. J., Kieffer, J. D., Harney, J. W., & Larsen, P. R. (1991). Selenocysteine confers the biochemical properties characteristic of the type I iodothyronine deiodinase. The Journal of biological chemistry, 266(22), 14155–14158.

[3003] Dickson, R. C., & Tomlinson, R. H. (1967). Selenium in blood and human tissues. Clinica Chimica Acta, 16(2), 311–321. doi:10.1016/0009-8981(67)90197-0

665

[3004] Beckett, G. J., & Arthur, J. R. (2005). Selenium and endocrine systems. The Journal of endocrinology, 184(3), 455–465. https://doi.org/10.1677/joe.1.05971

[3005] Köhrle, J., & Gärtner, R. (2009). Selenium and thyroid. Best practice & research. Clinical endocrinology & metabolism, 23(6), 815–827. https://doi.org/10.1016/j.beem.2009.08.002

[3006] Flohe, L., Günzler, W. A., & Schock, H. H. (1973). Glutathione peroxidase: a selenoenzyme. FEBS letters, 32(1), 132–134. https://doi.org/10.1016/0014-5793(73)80755-0

[3007] Ekholm, R., & Björkman, U. (1997). Glutathione peroxidase degrades intracellular hydrogen peroxide and thereby inhibits intracellular protein iodination in thyroid epithelium. Endocrinology, 138(7), 2871–2878. https://doi.org/10.1210/endo.138.7.5222

[3008] Lehmann, P., Rank, P., Hallfeldt, K. L., Krebs, B., & Gärtner, R. (2006). Dose-related influence of sodium selenite on apoptosis in human thyroid follicles in vitro induced by iodine, EGF, TGF-beta, and H2O2. Biological trace element research, 112(2), 119–130. https://doi.org/10.1385/BTER:112:2:119

[3009] Sedighi, O., Makhlough, A., Shokrzadeh, M., & Hoorshad, S. (2014). Association between plasma selenium and glutathione peroxidase levels and severity of diabetic nephropathy in patients with type two diabetes mellitus. Nephro-urology monthly, 6(5), e21355. https://doi.org/10.5812/numonthly.21355

[3010] Olivieri, O., Girelli, D., Stanzial, A. M., Rossi, L., Bassi, A., & Corrocher, R. (1996). Selenium, zinc, and thyroid hormones in healthy subjects: low T3/T4 ratio in the elderly is related to impaired selenium status. Biological trace element research, 51(1), 31–41. https://doi.org/10.1007/BF02790145

[3011] Drutel, A., Archambeaud, F., & Caron, P. (2013). Selenium and the thyroid gland: more good news for clinicians. Clinical Endocrinology, 78(2), 155–164. doi:10.1111/cen.12066

[3012] Tamura, T., & Stadtman, T. C. (1996). A new selenoprotein from human lung adenocarcinoma cells: purification, properties, and thioredoxin reductase activity. Proceedings of the National Academy of Sciences of the United States of America, 93(3), 1006–1011. https://doi.org/10.1073/pnas.93.3.1006

[3013] Lee, S. R., Kim, J. R., Kwon, K. S., Yoon, H. W., Levine, R. L., Ginsburg, A., & Rhee, S. G. (1999). Molecular cloning and characterization of a mitochondrial selenocysteine-containing thioredoxin reductase from rat liver. The Journal of biological chemistry, 274(8), 4722–4734. https://doi.org/10.1074/jbc.274.8.4722

[3014] Sun, Q. A., Kirnarsky, L., Sherman, S., & Gladyshev, V. N. (2001). Selenoprotein oxidoreductase with specificity for thioredoxin and glutathione systems. Proceedings of the National Academy of Sciences of the United States of America, 98(7), 3673–3678. https://doi.org/10.1073/pnas.051454398

[3015] Green W. L. (1968). Inhibition of thyroidal iodotyrosine deiodination by tyrosine analogues. Endocrinology, 83(2), 336–347. https://doi.org/10.1210/endo-83-2-336

[3016] QUERIDO, A., STANBURY, J. B., KASSENAAR, A. A., & MEIJER, J. W. (1956). The metabolism of iodotyrosines. III. Di-iodotyrosine deshalogenating activity of human thyroid tissue. The Journal of clinical endocrinology and metabolism, 16(8), 1096–1101. https://doi.org/10.1210/jcem-16-8-1096

[3017] Callebaut, I., Curcio-Morelli, C., Mornon, J. P., Gereben, B., Buettner, C., Huang, S., Castro, B., Fonseca, T. L., Harney, J. W., Larsen, P. R., & Bianco, A. C. (2003). The iodothyronine selenodeiodinases are thioredoxin-fold family proteins containing a glycoside hydrolase clan GH-A-like structure. The Journal of biological chemistry, 278(38), 36887–36896. https://doi.org/10.1074/jbc.M305725200

[3018] Rokita, S. E., Adler, J. M., McTamney, P. M., & Watson, J. A., Jr (2010). Efficient use and recycling of the micronutrient iodide in mammals. Biochimie, 92(9), 1227–1235. https://doi.org/10.1016/j.biochi.2010.02.013

[3019] Knobel, M., & Medeiros-Neto, G. (2003). An outline of inherited disorders of the thyroid hormone generating system. Thyroid : official journal of the American Thyroid Association, 13(8), 771–801. https://doi.org/10.1089/105072503768499671

[3020] Thomas, S. R., McTamney, P. M., Adler, J. M., Laronde-Leblanc, N., & Rokita, S. E. (2009). Crystal structure of iodotyrosine deiodinase, a novel flavoprotein responsible for iodide salvage in thyroid glands. The Journal of biological chemistry, 284(29), 19659–19667. https://doi.org/10.1074/jbc.M109.013458

[3021] Lever, E. G., Medeiros-Neto, G. A., & DeGroot, L. J. (1983). Inherited disorders of thyroid metabolism. Endocrine reviews, 4(3), 213–239. https://doi.org/10.1210/edrv-4-3-213

[3022] Bates, J. M., Spate, V. L., Morris, J. S., St Germain, D. L., & Galton, V. A. (2000). Effects of selenium deficiency on tissue selenium content, deiodinase activity, and thyroid hormone economy in the rat during development. Endocrinology, 141(7), 2490–2500. https://doi.org/10.1210/endo.141.7.7571

[3023] Köhrle J. (1990). Thyrotropin (TSH) action on thyroid hormone deiodination and secretion: one aspect of thyrotropin regulation of thyroid cell biology. Hormone and metabolic research. Supplement series, 23, 18–28.

[3024] Contempre, B., Dumont, J. E., Ngo, B., Thilly, C. H., Diplock, A. T., & Vanderpas, J. (1991). Effect of selenium supplementation in hypothyroid subjects of an iodine and selenium deficient area: the possible danger of indiscriminate supplementation of iodine-deficient subjects with selenium. The Journal of clinical endocrinology and metabolism, 73(1), 213–215. https://doi.org/10.1210/jcem-73-1-213

[3025] Olivieri, O., Girelli, D., Azzini, M., Stanzial, A. M., Russo, C., Ferroni, M., & Corrocher, R. (1995). Low selenium status in the elderly influences thyroid hormones. Clinical science, 89(6), 637–642. https://doi.org/10.1042/cs0890637

666

[3026] Duffield, A. J., Thomson, C. D., Hill, K. E., & Williams, S. (1999). An estimation of selenium requirements for New Zealanders. The American journal of clinical nutrition, 70(5), 896–903. https://doi.org/10.1093/ajcn/70.5.896

[3027] Barcza Stockler-Pinto, M., Carrero, J. J., De Carvalho Cardoso Weide, L., Franciscato Cozzolino, S. M., & Mafra, D. (2015). EFFECT OF SELENIUM SUPPLEMENTATION VIA BRAZIL NUT (BERTHOLLETIA EXCELSA, HBK) ON THYROID HORMONES LEVELS IN HEMODIALYSIS PATIENTS: A PILOT STUDY. Nutricion hospitalaria, 32(4), 1808–1812. https://doi.org/10.3305/nh.2015.32.4.9384

[3028] Kauf, E., Dawczynski, H., Jahreis, G., Janitzky, E., & Winnefeld, K. (1994). Sodium selenite therapy and thyroid-hormone status in cystic fibrosis and congenital hypothyroidism. Biological trace element research, 40(3), 247–253. https://doi.org/10.1007/BF02950797

[3029] Calomme, M. R., Vanderpas, J. B., François, B., Van Caillie-Bertrand, M., Herchuelz, A., Vanovervelt, N., Van Hoorebeke, C., & Vanden Berghe, D. A. (1995). Thyroid function parameters during a selenium repletion/depletion study in phenylketonuric subjects. Experientia, 51(12), 1208–1215. https://doi.org/10.1007/BF01944738

[3030] Köhrle J. (2005). Selenium and the control of thyroid hormone metabolism. Thyroid : official journal of the American Thyroid Association, 15(8), 841–853. https://doi.org/10.1089/thy.2005.15.841

[3031] Lassen, K. O., & Hørder, M. (1994). Selenium status and the effect of organic and inorganic selenium supplementation in a group of elderly people in Denmark. Scandinavian journal of clinical and laboratory investigation, 54(8), 585–590. https://doi.org/10.3109/00365519409087535

[3032] Rayman, M. P., Thompson, A. J., Bekaert, B., Catterick, J., Galassini, R., Hall, E., Warren-Perry, M., & Beckett, G. J. (2008). Randomized controlled trial of the effect of selenium supplementation on thyroid function in the elderly in the United Kingdom. The American journal of clinical nutrition, 87(2), 370–378. https://doi.org/10.1093/ajcn/87.2.370

[3033] Thomson, C. D., McLachlan, S. K., Grant, A. M., Paterson, E., & Lillico, A. J. (2005). The effect of selenium on thyroid status in a population with marginal selenium and iodine status. The British journal of nutrition, 94(6), 962–968. https://doi.org/10.1079/bjn20051564

[3034] Hawkes, W. C., Keim, N. L., Diane Richter, B., Gustafson, M. B., Gale, B., Mackey, B. E., & Bonnel, E. L. (2008). High-selenium yeast supplementation in free-living North American men: no effect on thyroid hormone metabolism or body composition. Journal of trace elements in medicine and biology : organ of the Society for Minerals and Trace Elements (GMS), 22(2), 131–142. https://doi.org/10.1016/j.jtemb.2007.11.005

[3035] Rasmussen, L. B., Schomburg, L., Köhrle, J., Pedersen, I. B., Hollenbach, B., Hög, A., Ovesen, L., Perrild, H., & Laurberg, P. (2011). Selenium status, thyroid volume, and multiple nodule formation in an area with mild iodine deficiency. European journal of endocrinology, 164(4), 585–590. https://doi.org/10.1530/EJE-10-1026

[3036] SAMIR, M., & AWADY, M. Y. (1998). Serum selenium levels in multinodular goitre. Clinical Otolaryngology and Allied Sciences, 23(6), 512–514. doi:10.1046/j.1365-2273.1998.2360512.x

[3037] Derumeaux, H., Valeix, P., Castetbon, K., Bensimon, M., Boutron-Ruault, M. C., Arnaud, J., & Hercberg, S. (2003). Association of selenium with thyroid volume and echostructure in 35- to 60-year-old French adults. European journal of endocrinology, 148(3), 309–315. https://doi.org/10.1530/eje.0.1480309

[3038] Rasmussen, L. B., Schomburg, L., Köhrle, J., Pedersen, I. B., Hollenbach, B., Hög, A., Ovesen, L., Perrild, H., & Laurberg, P. (2011). Selenium status, thyroid volume, and multiple nodule formation in an area with mild iodine deficiency. European journal of endocrinology, 164(4), 585–590. https://doi.org/10.1530/EJE-10-1026

[3039] Derumeaux, H., Valeix, P., Castetbon, K., Bensimon, M., Boutron-Ruault, M. C., Arnaud, J., & Hercberg, S. (2003). Association of selenium with thyroid volume and echostructure in 35- to 60-year-old French adults. European journal of endocrinology, 148(3), 309–315. https://doi.org/10.1530/eje.0.1480309

[3040] Beeson (1941) 'The Mineral Composition of Crops with Particular Reference to the Soils in which They Were Grown', U.S. Department of Agriculture, Accessed Online Dec 25 2020: https://play.google.com/store/books/details?id=yDv_1zUAnigC&rdid=book-yDv_1zUAnigC&rdot=1

[3041] Zimmermann, M. B., Adou, P., Torresani, T., Zeder, C., & Hurrell, R. F. (2000). Effect of oral iodized oil on thyroid size and thyroid hormone metabolism in children with concurrent selenium and iodine deficiency. European journal of clinical nutrition, 54(3), 209–213. https://doi.org/10.1038/sj.ejcn.1600921

[3042] Jellum, E., Andersen, A., Lund-Larsen, P., Theodorsen, L., & Orjasaeter, H. (1993). The JANUS serum bank. The Science of the total environment, 139-140, 527–535. https://doi.org/10.1016/0048-9697(93)90049-c

[3043] Kucharzewski, M., Braziewicz, J., Majewska, U., & Góźdź, S. (2002). Concentration of selenium in the whole blood and the thyroid tissue of patients with various thyroid diseases. Biological trace element research, 88(1), 25–30. https://doi.org/10.1385/BTER:88:1:25

[3044] Sugawara, M., Sugawara, Y., Wen, K., & Giulivi, C. (2002). Generation of oxygen free radicals in thyroid cells and inhibition of thyroid peroxidase. Experimental biology and medicine (Maywood, N.J.), 227(2), 141–146. https://doi.org/10.1177/153537020222700209

[3045] Allen, N. E., Appleby, P. N., Roddam, A. W., Tjønneland, A., Johnsen, N. F., Overvad, K., Boeing, H., Weikert, S., Kaaks, R., Linseisen, J., Trichopoulou, A., Misirli, G., Trichopoulos, D., Sacerdote, C., Grioni, S., Palli, D., Tumino, R., Bueno-de-Mesquita, H. B., Kiemeney, L. A., Barricarte, A., ... European Prospective Investigation into Cancer and Nutrition (2008). Plasma selenium concentration and prostate cancer risk: results from the European Prospective Investigation into Cancer and Nutrition (EPIC). The American journal of clinical nutrition, 88(6), 1567–1575. https://doi.org/10.3945/ajcn.2008.26205

[3046] Dennert, G., Zwahlen, M., Brinkman, M., Vinceti, M., Zeegers, M. P., & Horneber, M. (2011). Selenium for preventing cancer. The Cochrane database of systematic reviews, (5), CD005195. https://doi.org/10.1002/14651858.CD005195.pub2

[3047] Brinkman, M., Reulen, R. C., Kellen, E., Buntinx, F., & Zeegers, M. P. (2006). Are men with low selenium levels at increased risk of prostate cancer?. European journal of cancer (Oxford, England : 1990), 42(15), 2463–2471. https://doi.org/10.1016/j.ejca.2006.02.027

[3048] Duffield-Lillico, A. J., Dalkin, B. L., Reid, M. E., Turnbull, B. W., Slate, E. H., Jacobs, E. T., Marshall, J. R., Clark, L. C., & Nutritional Prevention of Cancer Study Group (2003). Selenium supplementation, baseline plasma selenium status and incidence of prostate cancer: an analysis of the complete treatment period of the Nutritional Prevention of Cancer Trial. BJU international, 91(7), 608–612. https://doi.org/10.1046/j.1464-410x.2003.04167.x

[3049] Klein, E. A., Thompson, I. M., Jr, Tangen, C. M., Crowley, J. J., Lucia, M. S., Goodman, P. J., Minasian, L. M., Ford, L. G., Parnes, H. L., Gaziano, J. M., Karp, D. D., Lieber, M. M., Walther, P. J., Klotz, L., Parsons, J. K., Chin, J. L., Darke, A. K., Lippman, S. M., Goodman, G. E., Meyskens, F. L., Jr, ... Baker, L. H. (2011). Vitamin E and the risk of prostate cancer: the Selenium and Vitamin E Cancer Prevention Trial (SELECT). JAMA, 306(14), 1549–1556. https://doi.org/10.1001/jama.2011.1437

[3050] Lippman, S. M., Klein, E. A., Goodman, P. J., Lucia, M. S., Thompson, I. M., Ford, L. G., Parnes, H. L., Minasian, L. M., Gaziano, J. M., Hartline, J. A., Parsons, J. K., Bearden, J. D., 3rd, Crawford, E. D., Goodman, G. E., Claudio, J., Winquist, E., Cook, E. D., Karp, D. D., Walther, P., Lieber, M. M., ... Coltman, C. A., Jr (2009). Effect of selenium and vitamin E on risk of prostate cancer and other cancers: the Selenium and Vitamin E Cancer Prevention Trial (SELECT). JAMA, 301(1), 39–51. https://doi.org/10.1001/jama.2008.864

[3051] Toulis, K. A., Anastasilakis, A. D., Tzellos, T. G., Goulis, D. G., & Kouvelas, D. (2010). Selenium supplementation in the treatment of Hashimoto's thyroiditis: a systematic review and a meta-analysis. Thyroid : official journal of the American Thyroid Association, 20(10), 1163–1173. https://doi.org/10.1089/thy.2009.0351

[3052] Gärtner, R., Gasnier, B. C. H., Dietrich, J. W., Krebs, B., & Angstwurm, M. W. A. (2002). Selenium Supplementation in Patients with Autoimmune Thyroiditis Decreases Thyroid Peroxidase Antibodies Concentrations. The Journal of Clinical Endocrinology & Metabolism, 87(4), 1687–1691. doi:10.1210/jcem.87.4.8421

[3053] Duntas, L. H., Mantzou, E., & Koutras, D. A. (2003). Effects of a six month treatment with selenomethionine in patients with autoimmune thyroiditis. European journal of endocrinology, 148(4), 389–393. https://doi.org/10.1530/eje.0.1480389

[3054] Gärtner, R., & Gasnier, B. C. (2003). Selenium in the treatment of autoimmune thyroiditis. BioFactors (Oxford, England), 19(3-4), 165–170. https://doi.org/10.1002/biof.5520190309

[3055] Mazokopakis, E. E., Papadakis, J. A., Papadomanolaki, M. G., Batistakis, A. G., Giannakopoulos, T. G., Protopapadakis, E. E., & Ganotakis, E. S. (2007). Effects of 12 months treatment with L-selenomethionine on serum anti-TPO Levels in Patients with Hashimoto's thyroiditis. Thyroid : official journal of the American Thyroid Association, 17(7), 609–612. https://doi.org/10.1089/thy.2007.0040

[3056] Turker, O., Kumanlioglu, K., Karapolat, I., & Dogan, I. (2006). Selenium treatment in autoimmune thyroiditis: 9-month follow-up with variable doses. The Journal of endocrinology, 190(1), 151–156. https://doi.org/10.1677/joe.1.06661

[3057] Pearce, E. N., Farwell, A. P., & Braverman, L. E. (2003). Thyroiditis. The New England journal of medicine, 348(26), 2646–2655. https://doi.org/10.1056/NEJMra021194

[3058] Duntas L. H. (2008). Environmental factors and autoimmune thyroiditis. Nature clinical practice. Endocrinology & metabolism, 4(8), 454–460. https://doi.org/10.1038/ncpendmet0896

[3059] Negro, R., Greco, G., Mangieri, T., Pezzarossa, A., Dazzi, D., & Hassan, H. (2007). The influence of selenium supplementation on postpartum thyroid status in pregnant women with thyroid peroxidase autoantibodies. The Journal of clinical endocrinology and metabolism, 92(4), 1263–1268. https://doi.org/10.1210/jc.2006-1821

[3060] Reid, S. M., Middleton, P., Cossich, M. C., & Crowther, C. A. (2010). Interventions for clinical and subclinical hypothyroidism in pregnancy. The Cochrane database of systematic reviews, (7), CD007752. https://doi.org/10.1002/14651858.CD007752.pub2

[3061] Nacamulli, D., Mian, C., Petricca, D., Lazzarotto, F., Barollo, S., Pozza, D., Masiero, S., Faggian, D., Plebani, M., Girelli, M. E., Mantero, F., & Betterle, C. (2010). Influence of physiological dietary selenium supplementation on the natural course of autoimmune thyroiditis. Clinical endocrinology, 73(4), 535–539. https://doi.org/10.1111/j.1365-2265.2009.03758.x

[3062] Karanikas, G., Schuetz, M., Wahl, K., Paul, M., Kontur, S., Pietschmann, P., Kletter, K., Dudczak, R., & Willheim, M. (2005). Relation of anti-TPO autoantibody titre and T-lymphocyte cytokine production patterns in Hashimoto's thyroiditis. Clinical endocrinology, 63(2), 191–196. https://doi.org/10.1111/j.1365-2265.2005.02324.x

[3063] Komosinska-Vassev, K., Olczyk, K., Kucharz, E. J., Marcisz, C., Winsz-Szczotka, K., & Kotulska, A. (2000). Free radical activity and antioxidant defense mechanisms in patients with hyperthyroidism due to Graves' disease during therapy. Clinica chimica acta; international journal of clinical chemistry, 300(1-2), 107–117. https://doi.org/10.1016/s0009-8981(00)00306-5

[3064] Abalovich, M., Llesuy, S., Gutierrez, S., & Repetto, M. (2003). Peripheral parameters of oxidative stress in Graves' disease: the effects of methimazole and 131 iodine treatments. Clinical endocrinology, 59(3), 321–327. https://doi.org/10.1046/j.1365-2265.2003.01850.x

[3065] Bacić Vrca, V., Skreb, F., Cepelak, I., & Mayer, L. (2004). Supplementation with antioxidants in the treatment of Graves' disease: the effect on the extracellular antioxidative parameters. Acta pharmaceutica (Zagreb, Croatia), 54(2), 79–89.

[3066] Marcocci, C., Kahaly, G. J., Krassas, G. E., Bartalena, L., Prummel, M., Stahl, M., Altea, M. A., Nardi, M., Pitz, S., Boboridis, K., Sivelli, P., von Arx, G., Mourits, M. P., Baldeschi, L., Bencivelli, W., Wiersinga, W., & European Group on Graves' Orbitopathy (2011). Selenium and the course of mild Graves' orbitopathy. The New England journal of medicine, 364(20), 1920–1931. https://doi.org/10.1056/NEJMoa1012985

[3067] Chen J. (2012). An original discovery: selenium deficiency and Keshan disease (an endemic heart disease). Asia Pacific journal of clinical nutrition, 21(3), 320–326.

[3068] Twagirumukiza, M., Nkeramihigo, E., Seminega, B., Gasakure, E., Boccara, F., & Barbaro, G. (2007). Prevalence of dilated cardiomyopathy in HIV-infected African patients not receiving HAART: a multicenter, observational, prospective, cohort study in Rwanda. Current HIV research, 5(1), 129–137. https://doi.org/10.2174/157016207779316288

[3069] Baum, M. K., Shor-Posner, G., Lai, S., Zhang, G., Lai, H., Fletcher, M. A., Sauberlich, H., & Page, J. B. (1997). High risk of HIV-related mortality is associated with selenium deficiency. Journal of acquired immune deficiency syndromes and human retrovirology : official publication of the International Retrovirology Association, 15(5), 370–374. https://doi.org/10.1097/00042560-199708150-00007

[3070] Kupka, R., Msamanga, G. I., Spiegelman, D., Rifai, N., Hunter, D. J., & Fawzi, W. W. (2005). Selenium levels in relation to morbidity and mortality among children born to HIV-infected mothers. European journal of clinical nutrition, 59(11), 1250–1258. https://doi.org/10.1038/sj.ejcn.1602236

[3071] Campa, A., Shor-Posner, G., Indacochea, F., Zhang, G., Lai, H., Asthana, D., Scott, G. B., & Baum, M. K. (1999). Mortality risk in selenium-deficient HIV-positive children. Journal of acquired immune deficiency syndromes and human retrovirology : official publication of the International Retrovirology Association, 20(5), 508–513. https://doi.org/10.1097/00042560-199904150-00015

[3072] Burbano, X., Miguez-Burbano, M. J., McCollister, K., Zhang, G., Rodriguez, A., Ruiz, P., Lecusay, R., & Shor-Posner, G. (2002). Impact of a selenium chemoprevention clinical trial on hospital admissions of HIV-infected participants. HIV clinical trials, 3(6), 483–491. https://doi.org/10.1310/A7LC-7C9V-EWKF-2Y0H

[3073] Hurwitz, B. E., Klaus, J. R., Llabre, M. M., Gonzalez, A., Lawrence, P. J., Maher, K. J., Greeson, J. M., Baum, M. K., Shor-Posner, G., Skyler, J. S., & Schneiderman, N. (2007). Suppression of human immunodeficiency virus type 1 viral load with selenium supplementation: a randomized controlled trial. Archives of internal medicine, 167(2), 148–154. https://doi.org/10.1001/archinte.167.2.148

[3074] Flores-Mateo, G., Navas-Acien, A., Pastor-Barriuso, R., & Guallar, E. (2006). Selenium and coronary heart disease: a meta-analysis. The American journal of clinical nutrition, 84(4), 762–773. https://doi.org/10.1093/ajcn/84.4.762

[3075] Bleys, J., Navas-Acien, A., & Guallar, E. (2008). Serum selenium levels and all-cause, cancer, and cardiovascular mortality among US adults. Archives of internal medicine, 168(4), 404–410. https://doi.org/10.1001/archinternmed.2007.74

[3076] Xun, P., Liu, K., Morris, J. S., Daviglus, M. L., & He, K. (2010). Longitudinal association between toenail selenium levels and measures of subclinical atherosclerosis: the CARDIA trace element study. Atherosclerosis, 210(2), 662–667. https://doi.org/10.1016/j.atherosclerosis.2010.01.021

[3077] Bleys, J., Navas-Acien, A., Laclaustra, M., Pastor-Barriuso, R., Menke, A., Ordovas, J., Stranges, S., & Guallar, E. (2009). Serum selenium and peripheral arterial disease: results from the national health and nutrition examination survey, 2003-2004. American journal of epidemiology, 169(8), 996–1003. https://doi.org/10.1093/aje/kwn414

669

[3078] Rees, K., Hartley, L., Day, C., Flowers, N., Clarke, A., & Stranges, S. (2013). Selenium supplementation for the primary prevention of cardiovascular disease. The Cochrane database of systematic reviews, 2013(1), CD009671. https://doi.org/10.1002/14651858.CD009671.pub2

[3079] Alehagen, U., Aaseth, J., Alexander, J., & Johansson, P. (2018). Still reduced cardiovascular mortality 12 years after supplementation with selenium and coenzyme Q10 for four years: A validation of previous 10-year follow-up results of a prospective randomized double-blind placebo-controlled trial in elderly. PloS one, 13(4), e0193120. https://doi.org/10.1371/journal.pone.0193120

[3080] Alehagen, U., Johansson, P., Björnstedt, M., Rosén, A., & Dahlström, U. (2013). Cardiovascular mortality and N-terminal-proBNP reduced after combined selenium and coenzyme Q10 supplementation: a 5-year prospective randomized double-blind placebo-controlled trial among elderly Swedish citizens. International journal of cardiology, 167(5), 1860–1866. https://doi.org/10.1016/j.ijcard.2012.04.156

[3081] Zhang, X., Liu, C., Guo, J., & Song, Y. (2016). Selenium status and cardiovascular diseases: meta-analysis of prospective observational studies and randomized controlled trials. European journal of clinical nutrition, 70(2), 162–169. https://doi.org/10.1038/ejcn.2015.78

[3082] Kuria, A., Tian, H., Li, M., Wang, Y., Aaseth, J. O., Zang, J., & Cao, Y. (2020). Selenium status in the body and cardiovascular disease: a systematic review and meta-analysis. Critical Reviews in Food Science and Nutrition, 1–10. doi:10.1080/10408398.2020.1803200

[3083] Benstoem, C., Goetzenich, A., Kraemer, S., Borosch, S., Manzanares, W., Hardy, G., & Stoppe, C. (2015). Selenium and its supplementation in cardiovascular disease--what do we know?. Nutrients, 7(5), 3094–3118. https://doi.org/10.3390/nu7053094

[3084] Navas-Acien, A., Bleys, J., & Guallar, E. (2008). Selenium intake and cardiovascular risk: what is new?. Current opinion in lipidology, 19(1), 43–49. https://doi.org/10.1097/MOL.0b013e3282f2b261

[3085] Flores-Mateo, G., Navas-Acien, A., Pastor-Barriuso, R., & Guallar, E. (2006). Selenium and coronary heart disease: a meta-analysis. The American Journal of Clinical Nutrition, 84(4), 762–773. doi:10.1093/ajcn/84.4.762

[3086] Liu, H., Xu, H., & Huang, K. (2017). Selenium in the prevention of atherosclerosis and its underlying mechanisms. Metallomics : integrated biometal science, 9(1), 21–37. https://doi.org/10.1039/c6mt00195e

[3087] Arbogast, S., & Ferreiro, A. (2010). Selenoproteins and protection against oxidative stress: selenoprotein N as a novel player at the crossroads of redox signaling and calcium homeostasis. Antioxidants & redox signaling, 12(7), 893–904. https://doi.org/10.1089/ars.2009.2890

[3088] Moskovitz, J., Bar-Noy, S., Williams, W. M., Requena, J., Berlett, B. S., & Stadtman, E. R. (2001). Methionine sulfoxide reductase (MsrA) is a regulator of antioxidant defense and lifespan in mammals. Proceedings of the National Academy of Sciences of the United States of America, 98(23), 12920–12925. https://doi.org/10.1073/pnas.231472998

[3089] Rock, C., & Moos, P. J. (2010). Selenoprotein P protects cells from lipid hydroperoxides generated by 15-LOX-1. Prostaglandins, leukotrienes, and essential fatty acids, 83(4-6), 203–210. https://doi.org/10.1016/j.plefa.2010.08.006

[3090] Aviram, M., & Fuhrman, B. (1998). LDL oxidation by arterial wall macrophages depends on the oxidative status in the lipoprotein and in the cells: role of prooxidants vs. antioxidants. Molecular and cellular biochemistry, 188(1-2), 149–159.

[3091] Rayman, M. P., Stranges, S., Griffin, B. A., Pastor-Barriuso, R., & Guallar, E. (2011). Effect of supplementation with high-selenium yeast on plasma lipids: a randomized trial. Annals of internal medicine, 154(10), 656–665. https://doi.org/10.7326/0003-4819-154-10-201105170-00005

[3092] Schwenke, D. C., & Behr, S. R. (1998). Vitamin E combined with selenium inhibits atherosclerosis in hypercholesterolemic rabbits independently of effects on plasma cholesterol concentrations. Circulation research, 83(4), 366–377. https://doi.org/10.1161/01.res.83.4.366

[3093] Venardos, K., Harrison, G., Headrick, J., & Perkins, A. (2004). Effects of dietary selenium on glutathione peroxidase and thioredoxin reductase activity and recovery from cardiac ischemia-reperfusion. Journal of trace elements in medicine and biology : organ of the Society for Minerals and Trace Elements (GMS), 18(1), 81–88. https://doi.org/10.1016/j.jtemb.2004.01.001

[3094] Tanguy, S., Boucher, F., Besse, S., Ducros, V., Favier, A., & de Leiris, J. (1998). Trace elements and cardioprotection: increasing endogenous glutathione peroxidase activity by oral selenium supplementation in rats limits reperfusion-induced arrhythmias. Journal of trace elements in medicine and biology : organ of the Society for Minerals and Trace Elements (GMS), 12(1), 28–38. https://doi.org/10.1016/S0946-672X(98)80018-7

[3095] Jin, R. C., Mahoney, C. E., Coleman Anderson, L., Ottaviano, F., Croce, K., Leopold, J. A., Zhang, Y. Y., Tang, S. S., Handy, D. E., & Loscalzo, J. (2011). Glutathione peroxidase-3 deficiency promotes platelet-dependent thrombosis in vivo. Circulation, 123(18), 1963–1973. https://doi.org/10.1161/CIRCULATIONAHA.110.000034

[3096] Brigelius-Flohé, R., Banning, A., & Schnurr, K. (2003). Selenium-dependent enzymes in endothelial cell function. Antioxidants & redox signaling, 5(2), 205–215. https://doi.org/10.1089/152308603764816569

670

[3097] Wortmann, M., Schneider, M., Pircher, J., Hellfritsch, J., Aichler, M., Vegi, N., Kölle, P., Kuhlencordt, P., Walch, A., Pohl, U., Bornkamm, G. W., Conrad, M., & Beck, H. (2013). Combined deficiency in glutathione peroxidase 4 and vitamin E causes multiorgan thrombus formation and early death in mice. Circulation research, 113(4), 408–417. https://doi.org/10.1161/CIRCRESAHA.113.279984

[3098] Rotruck, J. T., Pope, A. L., Ganther, H. E., Swanson, A. B., Hafeman, D. G., & Hoekstra, W. G. (1973). Selenium: biochemical role as a component of glutathione peroxidase. Science (New York, N.Y.), 179(4073), 588–590. https://doi.org/10.1126/science.179.4073.588

[3099] Okuyama, H., Langsjoen, P. H., Hamazaki, T., Ogushi, Y., Hama, R., Kobayashi, T., & Uchino, H. (2015). Statins stimulate atherosclerosis and heart failure: pharmacological mechanisms. Expert review of clinical pharmacology, 8(2), 189–199. https://doi.org/10.1586/17512433.2015.1011125

[3100] Lubos, E., Sinning, C. R., Schnabel, R. B., Wild, P. S., Zeller, T., Rupprecht, H. J., Bickel, C., Lackner, K. J., Peetz, D., Loscalzo, J., Münzel, T., & Blankenberg, S. (2010). Serum selenium and prognosis in cardiovascular disease: results from the AtheroGene study. Atherosclerosis, 209(1), 271–277. https://doi.org/10.1016/j.atherosclerosis.2009.09.008

[3101] Bomer, N., Grote Beverborg, N., Hoes, M. F., Streng, K. W., Vermeer, M., Dokter, M. M., … Meer, P. (2019). Selenium and outcome in heart failure. European Journal of Heart Failure, 22(8), 1415–1423. doi:10.1002/ejhf.1644

[3102] Berndt, C., Lillig, C. H., & Holmgren, A. (2007). Thiol-based mechanisms of the thioredoxin and glutaredoxin systems: implications for diseases in the cardiovascular system. American journal of physiology. Heart and circulatory physiology, 292(3), H1227–H1236. https://doi.org/10.1152/ajpheart.01162.2006

[3103] Ago, T., & Sadoshima, J. (2006). Thioredoxin and ventricular remodeling. Journal of molecular and cellular cardiology, 41(5), 762–773. https://doi.org/10.1016/j.yjmcc.2006.08.006

[3104] Yamamoto, M., Yang, G., Hong, C., Liu, J., Holle, E., Yu, X., Wagner, T., Vatner, S. F., & Sadoshima, J. (2003). Inhibition of endogenous thioredoxin in the heart increases oxidative stress and cardiac hypertrophy. The Journal of clinical investigation, 112(9), 1395–1406. https://doi.org/10.1172/JCI17700

[3105] Jirong, Y., Huiyun, P., Zhongzhe, Y., Birong, D., Weimin, L., Ming, Y., & Yi, S. (2012). Sodium selenite for treatment of Kashin-Beck disease in children: a systematic review of randomised controlled trials. Osteoarthritis and cartilage, 20(7), 605–613. https://doi.org/10.1016/j.joca.2012.02.012

[3106] Moreno-Reyes, R., Suetens, C., Mathieu, F., Begaux, F., Zhu, D., Rivera, M. T., Boelaert, M., Nève, J., Perlmutter, N., & Vanderpas, J. (1998). Kashin-Beck osteoarthropathy in rural Tibet in relation to selenium and iodine status. The New England journal of medicine, 339(16), 1112–1120. https://doi.org/10.1056/NEJM199810153391604

[3107] Akbaraly, T. N., Hininger-Favier, I., Carrière, I., Arnaud, J., Gourlet, V., Roussel, A. M., & Berr, C. (2007). Plasma selenium over time and cognitive decline in the elderly. Epidemiology (Cambridge, Mass.), 18(1), 52–58. https://doi.org/10.1097/01.ede.0000248202.83695.4e

[3108] Shahar, A., Patel, K. V., Semba, R. D., Bandinelli, S., Shahar, D. R., Ferrucci, L., & Guralnik, J. M. (2010). Plasma selenium is positively related to performance in neurological tasks assessing coordination and motor speed. Movement disorders : official journal of the Movement Disorder Society, 25(12), 1909–1915. https://doi.org/10.1002/mds.23218

[3109] Loef, M., Schrauzer, G. N., & Walach, H. (2011). Selenium and Alzheimer's disease: a systematic review. Journal of Alzheimer's disease : JAD, 26(1), 81–104. https://doi.org/10.3233/JAD-2011-110414

[3110] Berr, C., Balansard, B., Arnaud, J., Roussel, A. M., & Alpérovitch, A. (2000). Cognitive decline is associated with systemic oxidative stress: the EVA study. Etude du Vieillissement Artériel. Journal of the American Geriatrics Society, 48(10), 1285–1291. https://doi.org/10.1111/j.1532-5415.2000.tb02603.x

[3111] Perkins, A. J., Hendrie, H. C., Callahan, C. M., Gao, S., Unverzagt, F. W., Xu, Y., Hall, K. S., & Hui, S. L. (1999). Association of antioxidants with memory in a multiethnic elderly sample using the Third National Health and Nutrition Examination Survey. American journal of epidemiology, 150(1), 37–44. https://doi.org/10.1093/oxfordjournals.aje.a009915

[3112] Kesse-Guyot, E., Fezeu, L., Jeandel, C., Ferry, M., Andreeva, V., Amieva, H., Hercberg, S., & Galan, P. (2011). French adults' cognitive performance after daily supplementation with antioxidant vitamins and minerals at nutritional doses: a post hoc analysis of the Supplementation in Vitamins and Mineral Antioxidants (SU.VI.MAX) trial. The American journal of clinical nutrition, 94(3), 892–899. https://doi.org/10.3945/ajcn.110.007815

[3113] Rastogi, S. C., Clausen, J., & Srivastava, K. C. (1976). Selenium and lead: Mutual detoxifying effects. Toxicology, 6(3), 377–388. doi:10.1016/0300-483x(76)90041-x

[3114] Stone, C. L., & Soares, J. H., Jr (1976). The effect of dietary selenium level on lead toxicity in the Japanese quail. Poultry science, 55(1), 341–349. https://doi.org/10.3382/ps.0550341

[3115] Chang, L. W. (1983). Protective effects of selenium against methylmercury neurotoxicity: a morphological and biochemical study. Experimental Pathology, 23(3), 143–156. doi:10.1016/s0232-1513(83)80052-8

[3116] Carvalho, C. M., Chew, E. H., Hashemy, S. I., Lu, J., & Holmgren, A. (2008). Inhibition of the human thioredoxin system. A molecular mechanism of mercury toxicity. The Journal of biological chemistry, 283(18), 11913–11923. https://doi.org/10.1074/jbc.M710133200

[3117] Yamashita, Y., Yabu, T., & Yamashita, M. (2010). Discovery of the strong antioxidant selenoneine in tuna and selenium redox metabolism. World journal of biological chemistry, 1(5), 144–150. https://doi.org/10.4331/wjbc.v1.i5.144

[3118] Gribble, M. O., Karimi, R., Feingold, B. J., Nyland, J. F., O'Hara, T. M., Gladyshev, M. I., & Chen, C. Y. (2016). Mercury, selenium and fish oils in marine food webs and implications for human health. Journal of the Marine Biological Association of the United Kingdom. Marine Biological Association of the United Kingdom, 96(1), 43–59. https://doi.org/10.1017/S0025315415001356

[3119] Feng, R., Wei, C., & Tu, S. (2013). The roles of selenium in protecting plants against abiotic stresses. Environmental and Experimental Botany, 87, 58–68. doi:10.1016/j.envexpbot.2012.09.002

[3120] Hamilton S. J. (2004). Review of selenium toxicity in the aquatic food chain. The Science of the total environment, 326(1-3), 1–31. https://doi.org/10.1016/j.scitotenv.2004.01.019

[3121] Severo, J. S., Morais, J., de Freitas, T., Andrade, A., Feitosa, M. M., Fontenelle, L. C., de Oliveira, A., Cruz, K., & do Nascimento Marreiro, D. (2019). The Role of Zinc in Thyroid Hormones Metabolism. International journal for vitamin and nutrition research. Internationale Zeitschrift fur Vitamin- und Ernahrungsforschung. Journal international de vitaminologie et de nutrition, 89(1-2), 80–88. https://doi.org/10.1024/0300-9831/a000262

[3122] Berzelius, J.J. (1818). "Lettre de M. Berzelius à M. Berthollet sur deux métaux nouveaux" [Letter from Mr. Berzelius to Mr. Berthollet on two new metals]. Annales de Chimie et de Physique. 2nd series (in French). 7: 199–206. From p. 203: "Cependant, pour rappeler les rapports de cette dernière avec le tellure, je l'ai nommée sélénium." (However, in order to recall the relationships of this latter [substance (viz, selenium)] to tellurium, I have named it "selenium".)

[3123] Duntas, L. H., & Benvenga, S. (2014). Selenium: an element for life. Endocrine, 48(3), 756–775. doi:10.1007/s12020-014-0477-6

[3124] Smith, Willoughby (1873). "The action of light on selenium". Journal of the Society of Telegraph Engineers. 2 (4): 31–33.

[3125] Bonnier Corporation (1876). "Action of light on selenium". Popular Science. 10 (1): 116.

[3126] Kabata-Pendias A. (1998). Geochemistry of selenium. Journal of environmental pathology, toxicology and oncology : official organ of the International Society for Environmental Toxicology and Cancer, 17(3-4), 173–177.

[3127] Terry EN, Diamond AM. Selenium. In: Erdman JW, Macdonald IA, Zeisel SH, eds. Present Knowledge in Nutrition. 10th ed. Washington, DC: Wiley-Blackwell; 2012:568-87

[3128] Amouroux, D., Liss, P. S., Tessier, E., Hamren-Larsson, M., & Donard, O. F. . (2001). Role of oceans as biogenic sources of selenium. Earth and Planetary Science Letters, 189(3-4), 277–283. doi:10.1016/s0012-821x(01)00370-3

[3129] Institute of Medicine, Food and Nutrition Board. Dietary Reference Intakes: Vitamin C, Vitamin E, Selenium, and Carotenoids. National Academy Press, Washington, DC, 2000.

[3130] Institute of Medicine (US) Panel on Dietary Antioxidants and Related Compounds, "Vitamin C, vitamin E, selenium, and β-carotene and other carotenoids: overview, antioxidant definition, and relationship to chronic disease," in Dietary Reference Intakes for Vitamin C, Vitamin E, Selenium, and Carotenoids, N. A. P. (US), Ed., Washington (DC), USA, 2000.

[3131] Panel on Dietary Antioxidants and Related Compounds, Subcommittees on Upper Reference Levels of Nutrients and Interpretation and Uses of DRIs, Standing Committee on the Scientific Evaluation of Dietary Reference Intakes, Food and Nutrition Board, Institute of Medicine (August 15, 2000). Dietary Reference Intakes for Vitamin C, Vitamin E, Selenium, and Carotenoids. Institute of Medicine. pp. 314–315.

[3132] Yang, G. Q., & Xia, Y. M. (1995). Studies on human dietary requirements and safe range of dietary intakes of selenium in China and their application in the prevention of related endemic diseases. Biomedical and environmental sciences : BES, 8(3), 187–201.

[3133] Agency for Toxic Substances and Disease Registry (ATSDR), in Toxicologic Profile for Selenium, US Department of Health and Human Services, Public Health Service, Atlanta, GA, USA, 2003.

[3134] MacFarquhar, J. K., Broussard, D. L., Melstrom, P., Hutchinson, R., Wolkin, A., Martin, C., Burk, R. F., Dunn, J. R., Green, A. L., Hammond, R., Schaffner, W., & Jones, T. F. (2010). Acute selenium toxicity associated with a dietary supplement. Archives of internal medicine, 170(3), 256–261. https://doi.org/10.1001/archinternmed.2009.495

[3135] Yang, G., & Zhou, R. (1994). Further observations on the human maximum safe dietary selenium intake in a seleniferous area of China. Journal of trace elements and electrolytes in health and disease, 8(3-4), 159–165.

[3136] Rocourt, C., & Cheng, W.-H. (2013). Selenium Supranutrition: Are the Potential Benefits of Chemoprevention Outweighed by the Promotion of Diabetes and Insulin Resistance? Nutrients, 5(4), 1349–1365. doi:10.3390/nu5041349

3137 Rayman M. P. (2008). Food-chain selenium and human health: emphasis on intake. The British journal of nutrition, 100(2), 254–268. https://doi.org/10.1017/S0007114508939830

3138 U.S. Department of Agriculture, Agricultural Research Service. What We Eat in Americaexternal link disclaimer, 2009-2010

3139 Kafai, M. R., & Ganji, V. (2003). Sex, age, geographical location, smoking, and alcohol consumption influence serum selenium concentrations in the USA: third National Health and Nutrition Examination Survey, 1988-1994. Journal of trace elements in medicine and biology : organ of the Society for Minerals and Trace Elements (GMS), 17(1), 13–18. https://doi.org/10.1016/S0946-672X(03)80040-8

3140 Rayman M. P. (2012). Selenium and human health. Lancet (London, England), 379(9822), 1256–1268. https://doi.org/10.1016/S0140-6736(11)61452-9

3141 Park, K., Rimm, E., Siscovick, D., Spiegelman, D., Morris, J. S., & Mozaffarian, D. (2011). Demographic and lifestyle factors and selenium levels in men and women in the U.S. Nutrition Research and Practice, 5(4), 357. doi:10.4162/nrp.2011.5.4.357

3142 NIH (2020) 'Selenium: Fact Sheet for Health Professionals', Accessed Online Dec 19 2020: https://ods.od.nih.gov/factsheets/Selenium-HealthProfessional/

3143 Barclay, M. N. I., MacPherson, A., & Dixon, J. (1995). Selenium Content of a Range of UK Foods. Journal of Food Composition and Analysis, 8(4), 307–318. doi:10.1006/jfca.1995.1025

3144 Tonelli, M., Wiebe, N., Hemmelgarn, B., Klarenbach, S., Field, C., Manns, B., Thadhani, R., Gill, J., & Alberta Kidney Disease Network (2009). Trace elements in hemodialysis patients: a systematic review and meta-analysis. BMC medicine, 7, 25. https://doi.org/10.1186/1741-7015-7-25

3145 Stone, C. A., Kawai, K., Kupka, R., & Fawzi, W. W. (2010). Role of selenium in HIV infection. Nutrition reviews, 68(11), 671–681. https://doi.org/10.1111/j.1753-4887.2010.00337.x

3146 Sieja, K., & Talerczyk, M. (2004). Selenium as an element in the treatment of ovarian cancer in women receiving chemotherapy. Gynecologic oncology, 93(2), 320–327. https://doi.org/10.1016/j.ygyno.2003.12.013

3147 Vernie, L. N., de Goeij, J. J., Zegers, C., de Vries, M., Baldew, G. S., & McVie, J. G. (1988). Cisplatin-induced changes of selenium levels and glutathione peroxidase activities in blood of testis tumor patients. Cancer letters, 40(1), 83–91. https://doi.org/10.1016/0304-3835(88)90265-0

3148 Burk, R. F. (2006). Effects of Chemical Form of Selenium on Plasma Biomarkers in a High-Dose Human Supplementation Trial. Cancer Epidemiology Biomarkers & Prevention, 15(4), 804–810. doi:10.1158/1055-9965.epi-05-0950

3149 Schrauzer G. N. (2000). Selenomethionine: a review of its nutritional significance, metabolism and toxicity. The Journal of nutrition, 130(7), 1653–1656. https://doi.org/10.1093/jn/130.7.1653

3150 Hardy, G., Hardy, I., & Manzanares, W. (2012). Selenium supplementation in the critically ill. Nutrition in clinical practice : official publication of the American Society for Parenteral and Enteral Nutrition, 27(1), 21–33. https://doi.org/10.1177/0884533611434116

3151 Sunde RA. Selenium. In: Coates PM, Betz JM, Blackman MR, et al., eds. Encyclopedia of Dietary Supplements. 2nd ed. London and New York: Informa Healthcare; 2010:711-8

3152 Laclaustra, M., Stranges, S., Navas-Acien, A., Ordovas, J. M., & Guallar, E. (2010). Serum selenium and serum lipids in US adults: National Health and Nutrition Examination Survey (NHANES) 2003-2004. Atherosclerosis, 210(2), 643–648. https://doi.org/10.1016/j.atherosclerosis.2010.01.005

3153 Xun, P., Bujnowski, D., Liu, K., Morris, J. S., Guo, Z., & He, K. (2011). Distribution of toenail selenium levels in young adult Caucasians and African Americans in the United States: the CARDIA Trace Element Study. Environmental research, 111(4), 514–519. https://doi.org/10.1016/j.envres.2011.01.016

3154 Niskar, A. S., Paschal, D. C., Kieszak, S. M., Flegal, K. M., Bowman, B., Gunter, E. W., Pirkle, J. L., Rubin, C., Sampson, E. J., & McGeehin, M. (2003). Serum selenium levels in the US population: Third National Health and Nutrition Examination Survey, 1988-1994. Biological trace element research, 91(1), 1–10. https://doi.org/10.1385/BTER:91:1:1

3155 Xia, Y., Hill, K. E., Byrne, D. W., Xu, J., & Burk, R. F. (2005). Effectiveness of selenium supplements in a low-selenium area of China. The American Journal of Clinical Nutrition, 81(4), 829–834. doi:10.1093/ajcn/81.4.829

3156 Maxwell, C., & Volpe, S. L. (2007). Effect of Zinc Supplementation on Thyroid Hormone Function. Annals of Nutrition and Metabolism, 51(2), 188–194. doi:10.1159/000103324

3157 Morley, J. E., Gordon, J., & Hershman, J. M. (1980). Zinc deficiency, chronic starvation, and hypothalamic-pituitary-thyroid function. The American Journal of Clinical Nutrition, 33(8), 1767–1770. doi:10.1093/ajcn/33.8.1767

3158 Fujimoto, S., Indo, Y., Higashi, A., Matsuda, I., Kashiwabara, N., & Nakashima, I. (1986). Conversion of thyroxine into tri-iodothyronine in zinc deficient rat liver. Journal of pediatric gastroenterology and nutrition, 5(5), 799–805. https://doi.org/10.1097/00005176-198609000-00023

3159 Pathak, R., Dhawan, D., & Pathak, A. (2010). Effect of Zinc Supplementation on the Status of Thyroid Hormones and Na, K, and Ca Levels in Blood Following Ethanol Feeding. Biological Trace Element Research, 140(2), 208–214. doi:10.1007/s12011-010-8691-4

[3160] Oliver, J. W., Sachan, D. S., Su, P., & Applehans, F. M. (1987). Effects of zinc deficiency on thyroid function. Drug-nutrient interactions, 5(2), 113–124.

[3161] Betsy, A., Binitha, M., & Sarita, S. (2013). Zinc deficiency associated with hypothyroidism: an overlooked cause of severe alopecia. International journal of trichology, 5(1), 40–42. https://doi.org/10.4103/0974-7753.114714

[3162] Eftekhari, M. H., Keshavarz, S. A., Jalali, M., Elguero, E., Eshraghian, M. R., & Simondon, K. B. (2006). The relationship between iron status and thyroid hormone concentration in iron-deficient adolescent Iranian girls. Asia Pacific journal of clinical nutrition, 15(1), 50–55.

[3163] Zimmermann, M. B., & Köhrle, J. (2002). The impact of iron and selenium deficiencies on iodine and thyroid metabolism: biochemistry and relevance to public health. Thyroid : official journal of the American Thyroid Association, 12(10), 867–878. https://doi.org/10.1089/105072502761016494

[3164] Eftekhari, M. H., Keshavarz, S. A., Jalali, M., Elguero, E., Eshraghian, M. R., & Simondon, K. B. (2006). The relationship between iron status and thyroid hormone concentration in iron-deficient adolescent Iranian girls. Asia Pacific journal of clinical nutrition, 15(1), 50–55.

[3165] Beard, J., Tobin, B., & Green, W. (1989). Evidence for thyroid hormone deficiency in iron-deficient anemic rats. The Journal of nutrition, 119(5), 772–778. https://doi.org/10.1093/jn/119.5.772

[3166] Tamagno, G., De Carlo, E., Murialdo, G., & Scandellari, C. (2007). A possible link between genetic hemochromatosis and autoimmune thyroiditis. Minerva medica, 98(6), 769–772.

[3167] Abdulzahra, M. S., Al-Hakeim, H. K., & Ridha, M. M. (2011). Study of the effect of iron overload on the function of endocrine glands in male thalassemia patients. Asian journal of transfusion science, 5(2), 127–131. https://doi.org/10.4103/0973-6247.83236

[3168] Fuchs, F. D., & Whelton, P. K. (2020). High Blood Pressure and Cardiovascular Disease. Hypertension, 75(2), 285–292. doi:10.1161/hypertensionaha.119.14240

[3169] Franklin, S. S., & Wong, N. D. (2013). Hypertension and Cardiovascular Disease: Contributions of the Framingham Heart Study. Global Heart, 8(1), 49. doi:10.1016/j.gheart.2012.12.004

[3170] Lopez, A. D., & Mathers, C. D. (2006). Measuring the global burden of disease and epidemiological transitions: 2002-2030. Annals of tropical medicine and parasitology, 100(5-6), 481–499. https://doi.org/10.1179/136485906X97417

[3171] World Health Organization (2019) 'Hypertension', Health Topics, Fact Sheets, Accessed Online Dec 28 2020: https://www.who.int/news-room/fact-sheets/detail/hypertension

[3172] Rigaud and Forette (2001) 'Hypertension in Older Adults', The Journals of Gerontology: Series A, Volume 56, Issue 4, 1 April 2001, Pages M217–M225, https://doi.org/10.1093/gerona/56.4.M217

[3173] Roger, V. L., Go, A. S., Lloyd-Jones, D. M., Benjamin, E. J., Berry, J. D., Borden, W. B., Bravata, D. M., Dai, S., Ford, E. S., Fox, C. S., Fullerton, H. J., Gillespie, C., Hailpern, S. M., Heit, J. A., Howard, V. J., Kissela, B. M., Kittner, S. J., Lackland, D. T., Lichtman, J. H., Lisabeth, L. D., … American Heart Association Statistics Committee and Stroke Statistics Subcommittee (2012). Executive summary: heart disease and stroke statistics--2012 update: a report from the American Heart Association. Circulation, 125(1), 188–197. https://doi.org/10.1161/CIR.0b013e3182456d46

[3174] Hall, J. E., do Carmo, J. M., da Silva, A. A., Wang, Z., & Hall, M. E. (2015). Obesity-Induced Hypertension. Circulation Research, 116(6), 991–1006. doi:10.1161/circresaha.116.305697

[3175] Dimeo, F., Pagonas, N., Seibert, F., Arndt, R., Zidek, W., & Westhoff, T. H. (2012). Aerobic Exercise Reduces Blood Pressure in Resistant Hypertension. Hypertension, 60(3), 653–658. doi:10.1161/hypertensionaha.112.197780

[3176] Beilin, L. J., & Puddey, I. B. (2006). Alcohol and Hypertension. Hypertension, 47(6), 1035–1038. doi:10.1161/01.hyp.0000218586.21932.3c

[3177] Primatesta, P., Falaschetti, E., Gupta, S., Marmot, M. G., & Poulter, N. R. (2001). Association Between Smoking and Blood Pressure. Hypertension, 37(2), 187–193. doi:10.1161/01.hyp.37.2.187

[3178] Babu, G. R., Murthy, G., Ana, Y., Patel, P., Deepa, R., Neelon, S., Kinra, S., & Reddy, K. S. (2018). Association of obesity with hypertension and type 2 diabetes mellitus in India: A meta-analysis of observational studies. World journal of diabetes, 9(1), 40–52. https://doi.org/10.4239/wjd.v9.i1.40

[3179] Saad, M. F., Rewers, M., Selby, J., Howard, G., Jinagouda, S., Fahmi, S., … Haffner, S. M. (2004). Insulin Resistance and Hypertension. Hypertension, 43(6), 1324–1331. doi:10.1161/01.hyp.0000128019.19363.f9

[3180] Rosário, R., Santos, R., Lopes, L., Agostinis-Sobrinho, C., Moreira, C., Mota, J., … Abreu, S. (2018). Fruit, vegetable consumption and blood pressure in healthy adolescents: A longitudinal analysis from the LabMed study. Nutrition, Metabolism and Cardiovascular Diseases, 28(10), 1075–1080. doi:10.1016/j.numecd.2018.05.014

[3181] Utsugi, M. T., Ohkubo, T., Kikuya, M., Kurimoto, A., Sato, R. I., Suzuki, K., Metoki, H., Hara, A., Tsubono, Y., & Imai, Y. (2008). Fruit and vegetable consumption and the risk of hypertension determined by self measurement of blood pressure at home: the Ohasama study. Hypertension research : official journal of the Japanese Society of Hypertension, 31(7), 1435–1443. https://doi.org/10.1291/hypres.31.1435

[3182] Borgi, L., Muraki, I., Satija, A., Willett, W. C., Rimm, E. B., & Forman, J. P. (2016). Fruit and Vegetable Consumption and the Incidence of Hypertension in Three Prospective Cohort Studies. Hypertension, 67(2), 288–293. doi:10.1161/hypertensionaha.115.06497

[3183] Wang, L., Manson, J. E., Gaziano, J. M., Buring, J. E., & Sesso, H. D. (2012). Fruit and Vegetable Intake and the Risk of Hypertension in Middle-Aged and Older Women. American Journal of Hypertension, 25(2), 180–189. doi:10.1038/ajh.2011.186

[3184] Zhang, Z., Cogswell, M. E., Gillespie, C., Fang, J., Loustalot, F., Dai, S., Carriquiry, A. L., Kuklina, E. V., Hong, Y., Merritt, R., & Yang, Q. (2013). Association between usual sodium and potassium intake and blood pressure and hypertension among U.S. adults: NHANES 2005-2010. PloS one, 8(10), e75289. https://doi.org/10.1371/journal.pone.0075289

[3185] Whelton, P. K., & He, J. (2014). Health effects of sodium and potassium in humans. Current opinion in lipidology, 25(1), 75–79. https://doi.org/10.1097/MOL.0000000000000033

[3186] Mente, A., O'Donnell, M. J., Rangarajan, S., McQueen, M. J., Poirier, P., Wielgosz, A., Morrison, H., Li, W., Wang, X., Di, C., Mony, P., Devanath, A., Rosengren, A., Oguz, A., Zatonska, K., Yusufali, A. H., Lopez-Jaramillo, P., Avezum, A., Ismail, N., Lanas, F., ... PURE Investigators (2014). Association of urinary sodium and potassium excretion with blood pressure. The New England journal of medicine, 371(7), 601–611. https://doi.org/10.1056/NEJMoa1311989

[3187] Jackson, S. L., Cogswell, M. E., Zhao, L., Terry, A. L., Wang, C. Y., Wright, J., Coleman King, S. M., Bowman, B., Chen, T. C., Merritt, R., & Loria, C. M. (2018). Association Between Urinary Sodium and Potassium Excretion and Blood Pressure Among Adults in the United States: National Health and Nutrition Examination Survey, 2014. Circulation, 137(3), 237–246. https://doi.org/10.1161/CIRCULATIONAHA.117.029193

[3188] D'Elia, L., Barba, G., Cappuccio, F. P., & Strazzullo, P. (2011). Potassium intake, stroke, and cardiovascular disease a meta-analysis of prospective studies. Journal of the American College of Cardiology, 57(10), 1210–1219. https://doi.org/10.1016/j.jacc.2010.09.070

[3189] Tobian, L. (1989). High Potassium Diets During Hypertension Reduce Arterial Endothelial Injury, Stroke Mortality Rate, Arterial Hypertrophy, and Renal Lesions Without Lowering Blood Pressure. Salt and Hypertension, 218–234. doi:10.1007/978-3-642-73917-0_20

[3190] Roger, V. L., Go, A. S., Lloyd-Jones, D. M., Benjamin, E. J., Berry, J. D., Borden, W. B., Bravata, D. M., Dai, S., Ford, E. S., Fox, C. S., Fullerton, H. J., Gillespie, C., Hailpern, S. M., Heit, J. A., Howard, V. J., Kissela, B. M., Kittner, S. J., Lackland, D. T., Lichtman, J. H., Lisabeth, L. D., ... American Heart Association Statistics Committee and Stroke Statistics Subcommittee (2012). Executive summary: heart disease and stroke statistics--2012 update: a report from the American Heart Association. Circulation, 125(1), 188–197. https://doi.org/10.1161/CIR.0b013e3182456d46

[3191] Preuss HG, Clouatre DL. Sodium, chloride, and potassium. In: Erdman JW, Macdonald IA, Zeisel SH, eds. Present Knowledge in Nutrition. 10th ed. Washington, DC: Wiley-Blackwell; 2012:475-92.

[3192] Youn J. H. (2013). Gut sensing of potassium intake and its role in potassium homeostasis. Seminars in nephrology, 33(3), 248–256. https://doi.org/10.1016/j.semnephrol.2013.04.005

[3193] Leggett, R. W., & Williams, L. R. (1986). A model for the kinetics of potassium in healthy humans. Physics in medicine and biology, 31(1), 23–42. https://doi.org/10.1088/0031-9155/31/1/003

[3194] Hinderling P. H. (2016). The Pharmacokinetics of Potassium in Humans Is Unusual. Journal of clinical pharmacology, 56(10), 1212–1220. https://doi.org/10.1002/jcph.713

[3195] Stone, M. S., Martyn, L., & Weaver, C. M. (2016). Potassium Intake, Bioavailability, Hypertension, and Glucose Control. Nutrients, 8(7), 444. https://doi.org/10.3390/nu8070444

[3196] Palmer B. F. (2015). Regulation of Potassium Homeostasis. Clinical journal of the American Society of Nephrology : CJASN, 10(6), 1050–1060. https://doi.org/10.2215/CJN.08580813

[3197] Ismail-Beigi, F. (1993). Thyroid hormone regulation of Na,K-ATPase expression. Trends in Endocrinology & Metabolism, 4(5), 152–155. doi:10.1016/1043-2760(93)90104-m

[3198] Shao, Y., Ojamaa, K., Klein, I., & Ismail-Beigi, F. (2000). Thyroid hormone stimulates Na, K-ATPase gene expression in the hemodynamically unloaded heterotopically transplanted rat heart. Thyroid : official journal of the American Thyroid Association, 10(9), 753–759. https://doi.org/10.1089/thy.2000.10.753

[3199] LeGrow, A. B., Fielding, D. C., & Pressley, T. A. (1999). Stimulation of Na,K-ATPase by hypothyroidism in the thyroid gland. The Journal of endocrinology, 160(3), 453–460. https://doi.org/10.1677/joe.0.1600453

[3200] Unwin, R. J., Luft, F. C., & Shirley, D. G. (2011). Pathophysiology and management of hypokalemia: a clinical perspective. Nature reviews. Nephrology, 7(2), 75–84. https://doi.org/10.1038/nrneph.2010.175

[3201] GINSBURG J. M. (1962). Equilibration of potassium in blood and tissues. The American journal of digestive diseases, 7, 34–42. https://doi.org/10.1007/BF02231928

[3202] Aronson, P. S., & Giebisch, G. (2011). Effects of pH on potassium: new explanations for old observations. Journal of the American Society of Nephrology : JASN, 22(11), 1981–1989. https://doi.org/10.1681/ASN.2011040414

675

[3203] Bushinsky, D. A., Riordon, D. R., Chan, J. S., & Krieger, N. S. (1997). Decreased potassium stimulates bone resorption. The American journal of physiology, 272(6 Pt 2), F774–F780. https://doi.org/10.1152/ajprenal.1997.272.6.F774

[3204] Lemann, J., Gray, R. W., & Pleuss, J. A. (1989). Potassium bicarbonate, but not sodium bicarbonate, reduces urinary calcium excretion and improves calcium balance in healthy men. Kidney International, 35(2), 688–695. doi:10.1038/ki.1989.40

[3205] Sebastian, A., & Morris, R. C., Jr (1994). Improved mineral balance and skeletal metabolism in postmenopausal women treated with potassium bicarbonate. The New England journal of medicine, 331(4), 279. https://doi.org/10.1056/NEJM199407283310421

[3206] Potassium may help fight osteoporosis. Potassium citrate increases bone-beneficial calcium retention. (2008). DukeMedicine healthnews, Suppl, 9.

[3207] Zhu, K., Devine, A., & Prince, R. L. (2009). The effects of high potassium consumption on bone mineral density in a prospective cohort study of elderly postmenopausal women. Osteoporosis international : a journal established as result of cooperation between the European Foundation for Osteoporosis and the National Osteoporosis Foundation of the USA, 20(2), 335–340. https://doi.org/10.1007/s00198-008-0666-3

[3208] Hanley, D. A., & Whiting, S. J. (2013). Does a high dietary acid content cause bone loss, and can bone loss be prevented with an alkaline diet?. Journal of clinical densitometry : the official journal of the International Society for Clinical Densitometry, 16(4), 420–425. https://doi.org/10.1016/j.jocd.2013.08.014

[3209] Tucker, K. L., Hannan, M. T., Chen, H., Cupples, L. A., Wilson, P. W., & Kiel, D. P. (1999). Potassium, magnesium, and fruit and vegetable intakes are associated with greater bone mineral density in elderly men and women. The American journal of clinical nutrition, 69(4), 727–736. https://doi.org/10.1093/ajcn/69.4.727

[3210] Frassetto, L., Morris, R. C., Jr, & Sebastian, A. (1997). Potassium bicarbonate reduces urinary nitrogen excretion in postmenopausal women. The Journal of clinical endocrinology and metabolism, 82(1), 254–259. https://doi.org/10.1210/jcem.82.1.3663

[3211] Parry, S. M., & Puthucheary, Z. A. (2015). The impact of extended bed rest on the musculoskeletal system in the critical care environment. Extreme Physiology & Medicine, 4(1). doi:10.1186/s13728-015-0036-7

[3212] Bosutti, A., Salanova, M., Blottner, D., Buehlmeier, J., Mulder, E., Rittweger, J., Yap, M. H., Ganse, B., & Degens, H. (2016). Whey protein with potassium bicarbonate supplement attenuates the reduction in muscle oxidative capacity during 19 days of bed rest. Journal of applied physiology (Bethesda, Md. : 1985), 121(4), 838–848. https://doi.org/10.1152/japplphysiol.00936.2015

[3213] LaMonte, M. J., Wactawski-Wende, J., Larson, J. C., Mai, X., Robbins, J. A., … LeBoff, M. S. (2019). Association of Physical Activity and Fracture Risk Among Postmenopausal Women. JAMA Network Open, 2(10), e1914084. doi:10.1001/jamanetworkopen.2019.14084

[3214] Stein, T. P., Schluter, M. D., Leskiw, M. J., & Boden, G. (1999). Attenuation of the protein wasting associated with bed rest by branched-chain amino acids. Nutrition, 15(9), 656–660. doi:10.1016/s0899-9007(99)00120-3

[3215] Vormann and Goedecke (2006) 'Acid-Base Homeostasis: Latent Acidosis as a Cause of Chronic Diseases', Schweiz. Zschr. GanzheitsMedizin 18, 255–266 (2006).

[3216] Marunaka Y. (2018). The Proposal of Molecular Mechanisms of Weak Organic Acids Intake-Induced Improvement of Insulin Resistance in Diabetes Mellitus via Elevation of Interstitial Fluid pH. International journal of molecular sciences, 19(10), 3244. https://doi.org/10.3390/ijms19103244

[3217] Bonjour J. P. (2013). Nutritional disturbance in acid-base balance and osteoporosis: a hypothesis that disregards the essential homeostatic role of the kidney. The British journal of nutrition, 110(7), 1168–1177. https://doi.org/10.1017/S0007114513000962

[3218] Goraya, N., Simoni, J., Jo, C. H., & Wesson, D. E. (2013). A comparison of treating metabolic acidosis in CKD stage 4 hypertensive kidney disease with fruits and vegetables or sodium bicarbonate. Clinical journal of the American Society of Nephrology : CJASN, 8(3), 371–381. https://doi.org/10.2215/CJN.02430312

[3219] Goraya, N., Simoni, J., Jo, C., & Wesson, D. E. (2012). Dietary acid reduction with fruits and vegetables or bicarbonate attenuates kidney injury in patients with a moderately reduced glomerular filtration rate due to hypertensive nephropathy. Kidney international, 81(1), 86–93. https://doi.org/10.1038/ki.2011.313

[3220] Goraya, N., Simoni, J., Jo, C. H., & Wesson, D. E. (2014). Treatment of metabolic acidosis in patients with stage 3 chronic kidney disease with fruits and vegetables or oral bicarbonate reduces urine angiotensinogen and preserves glomerular filtration rate. Kidney international, 86(5), 1031–1038. https://doi.org/10.1038/ki.2014.83

[3221] Sebastian, A., Harris, S. T., Ottaway, J. H., Todd, K. M., & Morris, R. C., Jr (1994). Improved mineral balance and skeletal metabolism in postmenopausal women treated with potassium bicarbonate. The New England journal of medicine, 330(25), 1776–1781. https://doi.org/10.1056/NEJM199406233302502

[3222] Frassetto, L., Morris, R. C., Jr, & Sebastian, A. (1997). Potassium bicarbonate reduces urinary nitrogen excretion in postmenopausal women. The Journal of clinical endocrinology and metabolism, 82(1), 254–259. https://doi.org/10.1210/jcem.82.1.3663

[3223] Ceglia, L., Harris, S. S., Abrams, S. A., Rasmussen, H. M., Dallal, G. E., & Dawson-Hughes, B. (2009). Potassium bicarbonate attenuates the urinary nitrogen excretion that accompanies an increase in dietary protein and may promote calcium absorption. The Journal of clinical endocrinology and metabolism, 94(2), 645–653. https://doi.org/10.1210/jc.2008-1796

[3224] Ceglia, L., & Dawson-Hughes, B. (2017). Increasing alkali supplementation decreases urinary nitrogen excretion when adjusted for same day nitrogen intake. Osteoporosis international : a journal established as result of cooperation between the European Foundation for Osteoporosis and the National Osteoporosis Foundation of the USA, 28(12), 3355–3359. https://doi.org/10.1007/s00198-017-4196-8

[3225] Dawson-Hughes, B., Harris, S. S., Palermo, N. J., Gilhooly, C. H., Shea, M. K., Fielding, R. A., & Ceglia, L. (2015). Potassium Bicarbonate Supplementation Lowers Bone Turnover and Calcium Excretion in Older Men and Women: A Randomized Dose-Finding Trial. Journal of bone and mineral research : the official journal of the American Society for Bone and Mineral Research, 30(11), 2103–2111. https://doi.org/10.1002/jbmr.2554

[3226] Halperin M. L. (1982). Metabolism and acid-base physiology. Artificial organs, 6(4), 357–362. https://doi.org/10.1111/j.1525-1594.1982.tb04126.x

[3227] Hu J-F, Zhao X-H, Parpia B, Campbell TC (1993) Dietary intakes and urinary excretion of calcium and acids: a crosssectional study of women in China. Am J Clin Nutr 58:398–406

[3228] BLATHERWICK, N. R. (1914). THE SPECIFIC ROLE OF FOODS IN RELATION TO THE COMPOSITION OF THE URINE. Archives of Internal Medicine, XIV(3), 409. doi:10.1001/archinte.1914.00070150122008

[3229] Mardon, J., Habauzit, V., Trzeciakiewicz, A., Davicco, M. J., Lebecque, P., Mercier, S., Tressol, J. C., Horcajada, M. N., Demigné, C., & Coxam, V. (2008). Long-term intake of a high-protein diet with or without potassium citrate modulates acid-base metabolism, but not bone status, in male rats. The Journal of nutrition, 138(4), 718–724. https://doi.org/10.1093/jn/138.4.718

[3230] Eaton, S. B. (2006). The ancestral human diet: what was it and should it be a paradigm for contemporary nutrition? Proceedings of the Nutrition Society, 65(1), 1–6. doi:10.1079/pns2005471

[3231] Frassetto, L., Morris, R. C., Jr, Sellmeyer, D. E., Todd, K., & Sebastian, A. (2001). Diet, evolution and aging--the pathophysiologic effects of the post-agricultural inversion of the potassium-to-sodium and base-to-chloride ratios in the human diet. European journal of nutrition, 40(5), 200–213. https://doi.org/10.1007/s394-001-8347-4

[3232] Sellmeyer DE, Stone KL, Sebastian A, Cummings SR (2001) A high ratio of dietary animal to vegetable protein increases the rate of bone loss and the risk of fracture in postmenopausal women. Am J Clin Nutr 73:118–122

[3233] New, S. A., & Millward, D. J. (2003). Calcium, protein, and fruit and vegetables as dietary determinants of bone health. The American Journal of Clinical Nutrition, 77(5), 1340–1341. doi:10.1093/ajcn/77.5.1340

[3234] König, D., Muser, K., Dickhuth, H. H., Berg, A., & Deibert, P. (2009). Effect of a supplement rich in alkaline minerals on acid-base balance in humans. Nutrition journal, 8, 23. https://doi.org/10.1186/1475-2891-8-23

[3235] Goraya, N., Simoni, J., Jo, C. H., & Wesson, D. E. (2013). A comparison of treating metabolic acidosis in CKD stage 4 hypertensive kidney disease with fruits and vegetables or sodium bicarbonate. Clinical journal of the American Society of Nephrology : CJASN, 8(3), 371–381. https://doi.org/10.2215/CJN.02430312

[3236] Lanham-New, S. A. (2008). The Balance of Bone Health: Tipping the Scales in Favor of Potassium-Rich, Bicarbonate-Rich Foods. The Journal of Nutrition, 138(1), 172S–177S. doi:10.1093/jn/138.1.172s

[3237] Addison W. L. (1928). The Use of Sodium Chloride, Potassium Chloride, Sodium Bromide, and Potassium Bromide in Cases of Arterial Hypertension which are Amenable to Potassium Chloride. Canadian Medical Association journal, 18(3), 281–285.

[3238] Dahl, L. K., Leitl, G., & Heine, M. (1972). Influence of dietary potassium and sodium/potassium molar ratios on the development of salt hypertension. The Journal of experimental medicine, 136(2), 318–330. https://doi.org/10.1084/jem.136.2.318

[3239] Morris RC, Jr., Sebastian A, Forman A, Tanaka M, Schmidlin O (1999) Normotensive salt sensitivity: effects of race and dietary potassium. Hypertension 33:18–23

[3240] Dahl, L. K. (1972). Salt and hypertension. The American Journal of Clinical Nutrition, 25(2), 231–244. doi:10.1093/ajcn/25.2.231

[3241] Myers, J. B., & Morgan, T. O. (1984). Effect of alteration in sodium chloride intake on blood pressure of normotensive subjects. Journal of cardiovascular pharmacology, 6 Suppl 1, S204–S209. https://doi.org/10.1097/00005344-198400061-00032

[3242] Gleibermann, L. (1973). Blood pressure and dietary salt in human populations. Ecology of Food and Nutrition, 2(2), 143–156. doi:10.1080/03670244.1973.9990329

677

[3243] Poulter, N., Khaw, K. T., Hopwood, B. E., Mugambi, M., Peart, W. S., & Sever, P. S. (1984). Salt and blood pressure in various populations. Journal of cardiovascular pharmacology, 6 Suppl 1, S197–S203. https://doi.org/10.1097/00005344-198400061-00031

[3244] Kawasaki, T., Delea, C. S., Bartter, F. C., & Smith, H. (1978). The effect of high-sodium and low-sodium intakes on blood pressure and other related variables in human subjects with idiopathic hypertension. The American journal of medicine, 64(2), 193–198. https://doi.org/10.1016/0002-9343(78)90045-1

[3245] Warren, S. E., & O'Connor, D. T. (1981). The antihypertensive mechanism of sodium restriction. Journal of cardiovascular pharmacology, 3(4), 781–790. https://doi.org/10.1097/00005344-198107000-00011

[3246] Bayer, R., Johns, D. M., & Galea, S. (2012). Salt And Public Health: Contested Science And The Challenge Of Evidence-Based Decision Making. Health Affairs, 31(12), 2738–2746. doi:10.1377/hlthaff.2012.0554

[3247] Overlack, A., Ruppert, M., Kolloch, R., Göbel, B., Kraft, K., Diehl, J., … Stumpe, K. O. (1993). Divergent hemodynamic and hormonal responses to varying salt intake in normotensive subjects. Hypertension, 22(3), 331–338. doi:10.1161/01.hyp.22.3.331

[3248] Kuehn, B. M. (2017). How Low Is Too Low With Salt in Heart Failure? Randomized Studies Needed to Resolve Concern. Circulation, 136(6), 597–598. doi:10.1161/circulationaha.117.030211

[3249] Tasdemir, V., Oguz, A. K., Sayın, I., & Ergun, I. (2015). Hyponatremia in the outpatient setting: clinical characteristics, risk factors, and outcome. International urology and nephrology, 47(12), 1977–1983. https://doi.org/10.1007/s11255-015-1134-6

[3250] Brands, M. W., & Manhiani, M. M. (2012). Sodium-retaining effect of insulin in diabetes. American journal of physiology. Regulatory, integrative and comparative physiology, 303(11), R1101–R1109. https://doi.org/10.1152/ajpregu.00390.2012

[3251] Yatabe, M. S., Yatabe, J., Yoneda, M., Watanabe, T., Otsuki, M., Felder, R. A., Jose, P. A., & Sanada, H. (2010). Salt sensitivity is associated with insulin resistance, sympathetic overactivity, and decreased suppression of circulating renin activity in lean patients with essential hypertension. The American journal of clinical nutrition, 92(1), 77–82. https://doi.org/10.3945/ajcn.2009.29028

[3252] Kurtz and Morris (1983) 'Dietary chloride as a determinant of "sodium-dependent" hypertension', Science, Vol. 222, Issue 4628, pp. 1139-1141, DOI: 10.1126/science.6648527

[3253] Luft, F. C., Zemel, M. B., Sowers, J. A., Fineberg, N. S., & Weinberger, M. H. (1990). Sodium bicarbonate and sodium chloride: effects on blood pressure and electrolyte homeostasis in normal and hypertensive man. Journal of hypertension, 8(7), 663–670. https://doi.org/10.1097/00004872-199007000-00010

[3254] Tanaka, M., Schmidlin, O., Olson, J. L., Yi, S. L., & Morris, R. C. (2001). Chloride-sensitive renal microangiopathy in the stroke-prone spontaneously hypertensive rat. Kidney international, 59(3), 1066–1076. https://doi.org/10.1046/j.1523-1755.2001.0590031066.x

[3255] He, F. J., & MacGregor, G. A. (2008). Beneficial effects of potassium on human health. Physiologia plantarum, 133(4), 725–735. https://doi.org/10.1111/j.1399-3054.2007.01033.x

[3256] Sullivan, J. M. (1991). Salt sensitivity. Definition, conception, methodology, and long-term issues. Hypertension, 17(1 Suppl), I61–I61. doi:10.1161/01.hyp.17.1_suppl.i61

[3257] Ascherio, A., Rimm, E. B., Hernán, M. A., Giovannucci, E. L., Kawachi, I., Stampfer, M. J., & Willett, W. C. (1998). Intake of Potassium, Magnesium, Calcium, and Fiber and Risk of Stroke Among US Men. Circulation, 98(12), 1198–1204. doi:10.1161/01.cir.98.12.1198

[3258] Bazzano, L. A., He, J., Ogden, L. G., Loria, C., Vupputuri, S., Myers, L., & Whelton, P. K. (2001). Dietary Potassium Intake and Risk of Stroke in US Men and Women. Stroke, 32(7), 1473–1480. doi:10.1161/01.str.32.7.1473

[3259] Whang, R. (1984). Predictors of Clinical Hypomagnesemia. Archives of Internal Medicine, 144(9), 1794. doi:10.1001/archinte.1984.00350210112019

[3260] Young, D. B., Lin, H., & McCabe, R. D. (1995). Potassium's cardiovascular protective mechanisms. The American journal of physiology, 268(4 Pt 2), R825–R837. https://doi.org/10.1152/ajpregu.1995.268.4.R825

[3261] Haddy, F. J., Vanhoutte, P. M., & Feletou, M. (2006). Role of potassium in regulating blood flow and blood pressure. American journal of physiology. Regulatory, integrative and comparative physiology, 290(3), R546–R552. https://doi.org/10.1152/ajpregu.00491.2005

[3262] Houston M. C. (2011). The importance of potassium in managing hypertension. Current hypertension reports, 13(4), 309–317. https://doi.org/10.1007/s11906-011-0197-8

[3263] Zillich, A. J., Garg, J., Basu, S., Bakris, G. L., & Carter, B. L. (2006). Thiazide diuretics, potassium, and the development of diabetes: a quantitative review. Hypertension (Dallas, Tex. : 1979), 48(2), 219–224. https://doi.org/10.1161/01.HYP.0000231552.10054.aa

[3264] Chatterjee, R., Yeh, H. C., Edelman, D., & Brancati, F. (2011). Potassium and risk of Type 2 diabetes. Expert review of endocrinology & metabolism, 6(5), 665–672. https://doi.org/10.1586/eem.11.60

[3265] Helderman, J. H., Elahi, D., Andersen, D. K., Raizes, G. S., Tobin, J. D., Shocken, D., & Andres, R. (1983). Prevention of the glucose intolerance of thiazide diuretics by maintenance of body potassium. Diabetes, 32(2), 106–111. https://doi.org/10.2337/diab.32.2.106

[3266] Sarafidis, P. A., Georgianos, P. I., & Lasaridis, A. N. (2010). Diuretics in clinical practice. Part II: electrolyte and acid-base disorders complicating diuretic therapy. Expert opinion on drug safety, 9(2), 259–273. https://doi.org/10.1517/14740330903499257

[3267] SAGILD, U., ANDERSEN, V., & ANDREASEN, P. B. (1961). Glucose tolerance and insulin responsiveness in experimental potassium depletion. Acta medica Scandinavica, 169, 243–251. https://doi.org/10.1111/j.0954-6820.1961.tb07829.x

[3268] Rowe, J. W., Tobin, J. D., Rosa, R. M., & Andres, R. (1980). Effect of experimental potassium deficiency on glucose and insulin metabolism. Metabolism, 29(6), 498–502. doi:10.1016/0026-0495(80)90074-8

[3269] Ekmekcioglu, C., Elmadfa, I., Meyer, A. L., & Moeslinger, T. (2016). The role of dietary potassium in hypertension and diabetes. Journal of physiology and biochemistry, 72(1), 93–106. https://doi.org/10.1007/s13105-015-0449-1

[3270] Oria-Hernández, J., Cabrera, N., Pérez-Montfort, R., & Ramírez-Silva, L. (2005). Pyruvate kinase revisited: the activating effect of K+. The Journal of biological chemistry, 280(45), 37924–37929. https://doi.org/10.1074/jbc.M508490200

[3271] Toney, M., Hohenester, E., Cowan, S., & Jansonius, J. (1993). Dialkylglycine decarboxylase structure: bifunctional active site and alkali metal sites. Science, 261(5122), 756–759. doi:10.1126/science.8342040

[3272] Colditz, G. A., Manson, J. E., Stampfer, M. J., Rosner, B., Willett, W. C., & Speizer, F. E. (1992). Diet and risk of clinical diabetes in women. The American journal of clinical nutrition, 55(5), 1018–1023. https://doi.org/10.1093/ajcn/55.5.1018

[3273] Chatterjee, R., Colangelo, L. A., Yeh, H. C., Anderson, C. A., Daviglus, M. L., Liu, K., & Brancati, F. L. (2012). Potassium intake and risk of incident type 2 diabetes mellitus: the Coronary Artery Risk Development in Young Adults (CARDIA) Study. Diabetologia, 55(5), 1295–1303. https://doi.org/10.1007/s00125-012-2487-3

[3274] Chatterjee, R., Yeh, H. C., Shafi, T., Selvin, E., Anderson, C., Pankow, J. S., Miller, E., & Brancati, F. (2010). Serum and dietary potassium and risk of incident type 2 diabetes mellitus: The Atherosclerosis Risk in Communities (ARIC) study. Archives of internal medicine, 170(19), 1745–1751. https://doi.org/10.1001/archinternmed.2010.362

[3275] DeFronzo, R. A., Felig, P., Ferrannini, E., & Wahren, J. (1980). Effect of graded doses of insulin on splanchnic and peripheral potassium metabolism in man. The American journal of physiology, 238(5), E421–E427. https://doi.org/10.1152/ajpendo.1980.238.5.E421

[3276] Sterns, R. H., Grieff, M., & Bernstein, P. L. (2016). Treatment of hyperkalemia: something old, something new. Kidney international, 89(3), 546–554. https://doi.org/10.1016/j.kint.2015.11.018

[3277] Chatterjee, R., Yeh, H. C., Shafi, T., Anderson, C., Pankow, J. S., Miller, E. R., Levine, D., Selvin, E., & Brancati, F. L. (2011). Serum potassium and the racial disparity in diabetes risk: the Atherosclerosis Risk in Communities (ARIC) Study. The American journal of clinical nutrition, 93(5), 1087–1091. https://doi.org/10.3945/ajcn.110.007286

[3278] Chatterjee, R., Davenport, C. A., Svetkey, L. P., Batch, B. C., Lin, P. H., Ramachandran, V. S., Fox, E. R., Harman, J., Yeh, H. C., Selvin, E., Correa, A., Butler, K., & Edelman, D. (2017). Serum potassium is a predictor of incident diabetes in African Americans with normal aldosterone: the Jackson Heart Study. The American journal of clinical nutrition, 105(2), 442–449. https://doi.org/10.3945/ajcn.116.143255

[3279] Lee, H., Lee, J., Hwang, S. S., Kim, S., Chin, H. J., Han, J. S., & Heo, N. J. (2013). Potassium intake and the prevalence of metabolic syndrome: the Korean National Health and Nutrition Examination Survey 2008-2010. PloS one, 8(1), e55106. https://doi.org/10.1371/journal.pone.0055106

[3280] Vašák, Milan; Schnabl, Joachim (2016). "Chapter 8. Sodium and Potassium Ions in Proteins and Enzyme Catalysis". In Astrid, Sigel; Helmut, Sigel; Roland K.O., Sigel (eds.). The Alkali Metal Ions: Their Role in Life. Metal Ions in Life Sciences. 16. Springer. pp. 259–290. doi:10.1007/978-4-319-21756-7_8

[3281] Boyer et al (1942) 'THE ROLE OF POTASSIUM IN MUSCLE Phosphorylations', J. Biol. Chem. 1942, 146:673-682.

[3282] Milne, J. L. S. (2013). Structure and Regulation of Pyruvate Dehydrogenases. Encyclopedia of Biological Chemistry, 321–328. doi:10.1016/b978-0-12-378630-2.00079-7

[3283] Andersson, C. E., & Mowbray, S. L. (2002). Activation of ribokinase by monovalent cations. Journal of Molecular Biology, 315(3), 409–419. doi:10.1006/jmbi.2001.5248

[3284] Machius, M., Chuang, J. L., Wynn, R. M., Tomchick, D. R., & Chuang, D. T. (2001). Structure of rat BCKD kinase: nucleotide-induced domain communication in a mitochondrial protein kinase. Proceedings of the National Academy of Sciences of the United States of America, 98(20), 11218–11223. https://doi.org/10.1073/pnas.201220098

[3285] Villeret, V., Huang, S., Fromm, H. J., & Lipscomb, W. N. (1995). Crystallographic evidence for the action of potassium, thallium, and lithium ions on fructose-1,6-bisphosphatase. Proceedings of the

National Academy of Sciences of the United States of America, 92(19), 8916–8920. https://doi.org/10.1073/pnas.92.19.8916

[3286] Shibata, N., Masuda, J., Tobimatsu, T., Toraya, T., Suto, K., Morimoto, Y., & Yasuoka, N. (1999). A new mode of B12 binding and the direct participation of a potassium ion in enzyme catalysis: X-ray structure of diol dehydratase. Structure, 7(8), 997–1008. doi:10.1016/s0969-2126(99)80126-9

[3287] O'Brien, M. C., & McKay, D. B. (1995). How Potassium Affects the Activity of the Molecular Chaperone Hsc70. Journal of Biological Chemistry, 270(5), 2247–2250. doi:10.1074/jbc.270.5.2247

[3288] Flaherty, K. M., DeLuca-Flaherty, C., & McKay, D. B. (1990). Three-dimensional structure of the ATPase fragment of a 70K heat-shock cognate protein. Nature, 346(6285), 623–628. https://doi.org/10.1038/346623a0

[3289] Ramos, R. J., Albersen, M., Vringer, E., Bosma, M., Zwakenberg, S., Zwartkruis, F., Jans, J., & Verhoeven-Duif, N. M. (2019). Discovery of pyridoxal reductase activity as part of human vitamin B6 metabolism. Biochimica et biophysica acta. General subjects, 1863(6), 1088–1097. https://doi.org/10.1016/j.bbagen.2019.03.019

[3290] Lin, C. R., Cheng, J. K., Wu, C. H., Chen, K. H., & Liu, C. K. (2017). Epigenetic suppression of potassium-chloride co-transporter 2 expression in inflammatory pain induced by complete Freund's adjuvant (CFA). European journal of pain (London, England), 21(2), 309–321. https://doi.org/10.1002/ejp.925

[3291] Riera, T. V., Zheng, L., Josephine, H. R., Min, D., Yang, W., & Hedstrom, L. (2011). Allosteric activation via kinetic control: potassium accelerates a conformational change in IMP dehydrogenase. Biochemistry, 50(39), 8508–8518. https://doi.org/10.1021/bi200785s

[3292] Isupov, M. N., Antson, A. A., Dodson, E. J., Dodson, G. G., Dementieva, I. S., Zakomirdina, L. N., Wilson, K. S., Dauter, Z., Lebedev, A. A., & Harutyunyan, E. H. (1998). Crystal structure of tryptophanase. Journal of molecular biology, 276(3), 603–623. https://doi.org/10.1006/jmbi.1997.1561

[3293] Milić, D., Matković-Čalogović, D., Demidkina, T. V., Kulikova, V. V., Sinitzina, N. I., & Antson, A. A. (2006). Structures of Apo- and Holo-Tyrosine Phenol-lyase Reveal a Catalytically Critical Closed Conformation and Suggest a Mechanism for Activation by K+Ions†,‡. Biochemistry, 45(24), 7544–7552. doi:10.1021/bi0601858

[3294] Curhan, G. C., Willett, W. C., Speizer, F. E., Spiegelman, D., & Stampfer, M. J. (1997). Comparison of dietary calcium with supplemental calcium and other nutrients as factors affecting the risk for kidney stones in women. Annals of internal medicine, 126(7), 497–504. https://doi.org/10.7326/0003-4819-126-7-199704010-00001

[3295] Curhan, G. C., Willett, W. C., Rimm, E. B., & Stampfer, M. J. (1993). A prospective study of dietary calcium and other nutrients and the risk of symptomatic kidney stones. The New England journal of medicine, 328(12), 833–838. https://doi.org/10.1056/NEJM199303253281203

[3296] Barcelo, P., Wuhl, O., Servitge, E., Rousaud, A., & Pak, C. Y. (1993). Randomized double-blind study of potassium citrate in idiopathic hypocitraturic calcium nephrolithiasis. The Journal of urology, 150(6), 1761–1764. https://doi.org/10.1016/s0022-5347(17)35888-3

[3297] Phillips, R., Hanchanale, V. S., Myatt, A., Somani, B., Nabi, G., & Biyani, C. S. (2015). Citrate salts for preventing and treating calcium containing kidney stones in adults. The Cochrane database of systematic reviews, (10), CD010057. https://doi.org/10.1002/14651858.CD010057.pub2

[3298] Maalouf, N. M., Moe, O. W., Adams-Huet, B., & Sakhaee, K. (2011). Hypercalciuria associated with high dietary protein intake is not due to acid load. The Journal of clinical endocrinology and metabolism, 96(12), 3733–3740. https://doi.org/10.1210/jc.2011-1531

[3299] Goraya, N., Simoni, J., Jo, C., & Wesson, D. E. (2012). Dietary acid reduction with fruits and vegetables or bicarbonate attenuates kidney injury in patients with a moderately reduced glomerular filtration rate due to hypertensive nephropathy. Kidney international, 81(1), 86–93. https://doi.org/10.1038/ki.2011.313

[3300] Goraya, N., Simoni, J., Jo, C.-H., & Wesson, D. E. (2013). A Comparison of Treating Metabolic Acidosis in CKD Stage 4 Hypertensive Kidney Disease with Fruits and Vegetables or Sodium Bicarbonate. Clinical Journal of the American Society of Nephrology, 8(3), 371–381. doi:10.2215/cjn.02430312

[3301] Demigné, C., Sabboh, H., Rémésy, C., & Meneton, P. (2004). Protective effects of high dietary potassium: nutritional and metabolic aspects. The Journal of nutrition, 134(11), 2903–2906. https://doi.org/10.1093/jn/134.11.2903

[3302] Musto, D., Rispo, A., Testa, A., Sasso, F., & Castiglione, F. (2013). Hypokalemic myopathy in inflammatory bowel diseases. Journal of Crohn's & colitis, 7(8), 680. https://doi.org/10.1016/j.crohns.2013.01.005

[3303] Welch, A. A., Fransen, H., Jenab, M., Boutron-Ruault, M. C., Tumino, R., Agnoli, C., Ericson, U., Johansson, I., Ferrari, P., Engeset, D., Lund, E., Lentjes, M., Key, T., Touvier, M., Niravong, M., Larrañaga, N., Rodríguez, L., Ocké, M. C., Peeters, P. H., Tjønneland, A., … Bingham, S. (2009). Variation in intakes of calcium, phosphorus, magnesium, iron and potassium in 10 countries in the

European Prospective Investigation into Cancer and Nutrition study. European journal of clinical nutrition, 63 Suppl 4, S101–S121. https://doi.org/10.1038/ejcn.2009.77

[3304] Public Health England; Food Standards Agency. National Diet and Nutrition Survey: Results from Years 1, 2, 3 and 4 (Combined) of the Rolling Programme (2008/2009–2011/2012); Public Health England: London, UK, 2014.

[3305] Keast, D. R., Fulgoni, V. L., 3rd, Nicklas, T. A., & O'Neil, C. E. (2013). Food sources of energy and nutrients among children in the United States: National Health and Nutrition Examination Survey 2003–2006. Nutrients, 5(1), 283–301. https://doi.org/10.3390/nu5010283

[3306] O'Neil, C. E., Keast, D. R., Fulgoni, V. L., & Nicklas, T. A. (2012). Food sources of energy and nutrients among adults in the US: NHANES 2003–2006. Nutrients, 4(12), 2097–2120. https://doi.org/10.3390/nu4122097

[3307] Chan, Q., Stamler, J., Brown, I. J., Daviglus, M. L., Van Horn, L., … Elliott, P. (2013). Relation of raw and cooked vegetable consumption to blood pressure: the INTERMAP Study. Journal of Human Hypertension, 28(6), 353–359. doi:10.1038/jhh.2013.115

[3308] Greenwood, Norman N.; Earnshaw, Alan (1997). Chemistry of the Elements (2nd ed.). Butterworth-Heinemann. pp 73. ISBN 978-0-08-037941-8.

[3309] Panel on Dietary Reference Intakes for Electrolytes and Water; Standing Committee on the Scientific Evaluation of Dietary Reference Intakes; Food and Nutrition Board; Institute of Medicine. Dietary Reference Intakes for Water, Potassium, Sodium, Chloride, and Sulfate; The National Academies Press: Washington, DC, USA, 2005.

[3310] World Health Organization (WHO). Guideline: Potassium Intake for Adults and Children; WHO: Geneva, Switzerland, 2012.

[3311] Chobanian, A. V., Bakris, G. L., Black, H. R., Cushman, W. C., Green, L. A., Izzo, J. L., Jr, Jones, D. W., Materson, B. J., Oparil, S., Wright, J. T., Jr, Roccella, E. J., Joint National Committee on Prevention, Detection, Evaluation, and Treatment of High Blood Pressure. National Heart, Lung, and Blood Institute, & National High Blood Pressure Education Program Coordinating Committee (2003). Seventh report of the Joint National Committee on Prevention, Detection, Evaluation, and Treatment of High Blood Pressure. Hypertension (Dallas, Tex. : 1979), 42(6), 1206–1252. https://doi.org/10.1161/01.HYP.0000107251.49515.c2

[3312] McCarron, D. A. (1991). A consensus approach to electrolytes and blood pressure. Could we all be right? Hypertension, 17(1_Suppl), I170–I170. doi:10.1161/01.hyp.17.1_suppl.i170

[3313] Fulgoni, V. L., 3rd, Keast, D. R., Bailey, R. L., & Dwyer, J. (2011). Foods, fortificants, and supplements: Where do Americans get their nutrients?. The Journal of nutrition, 141(10), 1847–1854. https://doi.org/10.3945/jn.111.142257

[3314] DeSalvo, K. B., Olson, R., & Casavale, K. O. (2016). Dietary Guidelines for Americans. JAMA, 315(5), 457–458. https://doi.org/10.1001/jama.2015.18396

[3315] Cogswell, M. E., Zhang, Z., Carriquiry, A. L., Gunn, J. P., Kuklina, E. V., Saydah, S. H., Yang, Q., & Moshfegh, A. J. (2012). Sodium and potassium intakes among US adults: NHANES 2003-2008. The American journal of clinical nutrition, 96(3), 647–657. https://doi.org/10.3945/ajcn.112.034413

[3316] National Centre for Chronic Disease Prevention and Health Promotion. Highlights: Sodium and potassium intakes among us infants and preschool children, 2003–2010. Am. J. Clin. Nutr. 2013, 98, 1113–1122.

[3317] O'Neil, C. E., Keast, D. R., Fulgoni, V. L., & Nicklas, T. A. (2012). Food sources of energy and nutrients among adults in the US: NHANES 2003–2006. Nutrients, 4(12), 2097–2120. https://doi.org/10.3390/nu4122097

[3318] Welch, A. A., Fransen, H., Jenab, M., Boutron-Ruault, M. C., Tumino, R., Agnoli, C., Ericson, U., Johansson, I., Ferrari, P., Engeset, D., Lund, E., Lentjes, M., Key, T., Touvier, M., Niravong, M., Larrañaga, N., Rodríguez, L., Ocké, M. C., Peeters, P. H., Tjønneland, A., … Bingham, S. (2009). Variation in intakes of calcium, phosphorus, magnesium, iron and potassium in 10 countries in the European Prospective Investigation into Cancer and Nutrition study. European journal of clinical nutrition, 63 Suppl 4, S101–S121. https://doi.org/10.1038/ejcn.2009.77

[3319] Du, S., Batis, C., Wang, H., Zhang, B., Zhang, J., & Popkin, B. M. (2014). Understanding the patterns and trends of sodium intake, potassium intake, and sodium to potassium ratio and their effect on hypertension in China. The American journal of clinical nutrition, 99(2), 334–343. https://doi.org/10.3945/ajcn.113.059121

[3320] Chinese Nutrition Society. Chinese Adults 18–49 Dietary Reference Intakes; Standards Press of China: Beijing, China, 2013.

[3321] Lee, H. S., Duffey, K. J., & Popkin, B. M. (2013). Sodium and potassium intake patterns and trends in South Korea. Journal of human hypertension, 27(5), 298–303. https://doi.org/10.1038/jhh.2012.43

[3322] Eaton, S. B., & Konner, M. (1985). Paleolithic nutrition. A consideration of its nature and current implications. The New England journal of medicine, 312(5), 283–289. https://doi.org/10.1056/NEJM198501313120505

681

[3323] Denton D (1982) Hunger for salt, an anthropological, physiological and medical analysis. Springer Berlin, Heidelberg, New York, pp 573–575

[3324] Khaw, K. T., & Barrett-Connor, E. (1984). Dietary potassium and blood pressure in a population. The American Journal of Clinical Nutrition, 39(6), 963–968. doi:10.1093/ajcn/39.6.963

[3325] Langford H. G. (1983). Dietary potassium and hypertension: epidemiologic data. Annals of internal medicine, 98(5 Pt 2), 770–772. https://doi.org/10.7326/0003-4819-98-5-770

[3326] FDA (2020) 'Sodium in Your Diet: Use the Nutrition Facts Label and Reduce Your Intake', Nutrition Education Resources & Materials, Accessed Online Dec 30 2020: https://www.fda.gov/food/nutrition-education-resources-materials/sodium-your-diet

[3327] Barlow, R. J., Connell, M. A., Levendig, B. J., Gear, J. S., & Milne, F. J. (1982). A comparative study of urinary sodium and potassium excretion in normotensive urban black and white South African males. South African medical journal = Suid-Afrikaanse tydskrif vir geneeskunde, 62(25), 939–941.

[3328] Grim, C. E., Luft, F. C., Miller, J. Z., Meneely, G. R., Battarbee, H. D., Hames, C. G., & Dahl, L. K. (1980). Racial differences in blood pressure in Evans County, Georgia: relationship to sodium and potassium intake and plasma renin activity. Journal of chronic diseases, 33(2), 87–94. https://doi.org/10.1016/0021-9681(80)90032-6

[3329] Eaton, S. B., & Konner, M. (1985). Paleolithic Nutrition. New England Journal of Medicine, 312(5), 283–289. doi:10.1056/nejm198501313120505

[3330] Konner, M., & Eaton, S. B. (2010). Paleolithic nutrition: twenty-five years later. Nutrition in clinical practice : official publication of the American Society for Parenteral and Enteral Nutrition, 25(6), 594–602. https://doi.org/10.1177/0884533610385702

[3331] Wrangham, R., & Conklin-Brittain, N. (2003). "Cooking as a biological trait." Comparative Biochemistry and Physiology Part A: Molecular & Integrative Physiology, 136(1), 35–46. doi:10.1016/s1095-6433(03)00020-5

[3332] KARKANAS, P., SHAHACKGROSS, R., AYALON, A., BARMATTHEWS, M., BARKAI, R., FRUMKIN, A., … STINER, M. (2007). Evidence for habitual use of fire at the end of the Lower Paleolithic: Site-formation processes at Qesem Cave, Israel. Journal of Human Evolution, 53(2), 197–212. doi:10.1016/j.jhevol.2007.04.002

[3333] Appel, L. J., Moore, T. J., Obarzanek, E., Vollmer, W. M., Svetkey, L. P., Sacks, F. M., … Harsha, D. W. (1997). A Clinical Trial of the Effects of Dietary Patterns on Blood Pressure. New England Journal of Medicine, 336(16), 1117–1124. doi:10.1056/nejm199704173361601

[3334] Khaw, K. T., & Rose, G. (1982). Population study of blood pressure and associated factors in St Lucia, West Indies. International journal of epidemiology, 11(4), 372–377. https://doi.org/10.1093/ije/11.4.372

[3335] Whelton, P. K., & He, J. (1999). Potassium in preventing and treating high blood pressure. Seminars in nephrology, 19(5), 494–499.

[3336] Graudal, N. A., Galløe, A. M., & Garred, P. (1998). Effects of Sodium Restriction on Blood Pressure, Renin, Aldosterone, Catecholamines, Cholesterols, and Triglyceride. JAMA, 279(17), 1383. doi:10.1001/jama.279.17.1383

[3337] Filippini, T., Violi, F., D'Amico, R., & Vinceti, M. (2017). The effect of potassium supplementation on blood pressure in hypertensive subjects: A systematic review and meta-analysis. International journal of cardiology, 230, 127–135. https://doi.org/10.1016/j.ijcard.2016.12.048

[3338] Binia, A., Jaeger, J., Hu, Y., Singh, A., & Zimmermann, D. (2015). Daily potassium intake and sodium-to-potassium ratio in the reduction of blood pressure: a meta-analysis of randomized controlled trials. Journal of hypertension, 33(8), 1509–1520. https://doi.org/10.1097/HJH.0000000000000611

[3339] Sacks, F. M., Willett, W. C., Smith, A., Brown, L. E., Rosner, B., & Moore, T. J. (1998). Effect on blood pressure of potassium, calcium, and magnesium in women with low habitual intake. Hypertension (Dallas, Tex. : 1979), 31(1), 131–138. https://doi.org/10.1161/01.hyp.31.1.131

[3340] Dickinson, H. O., Nicolson, D. J., Campbell, F., Beyer, F. R., & Mason, J. (2006). Potassium supplementation for the management of primary hypertension in adults. The Cochrane database of systematic reviews, (3), CD004641. https://doi.org/10.1002/14651858.CD004641.pub2

[3341] Khaw, K. T., & Barrett-Connor, E. (1987). Dietary potassium and stroke-associated mortality. A 12-year prospective population study. The New England journal of medicine, 316(5), 235–240. https://doi.org/10.1056/NEJM198701293160502

[3342] He, J., Tell, G. S., Tang, Y. C., Mo, P. S., & He, G. Q. (1991). Relation of electrolytes to blood pressure in men. The Yi people study. Hypertension, 17(3), 378–385. doi:10.1161/01.hyp.17.3.378

[3343] Reed, D., McGee, D., Yano, K., & Hankin, J. (1985). Diet, blood pressure, and multicollinearity. Hypertension (Dallas, Tex. : 1979), 7(3 Pt 1), 405–410.

[3344] D'Elia, L., Barba, G., Cappuccio, F. P., & Strazzullo, P. (2011). Potassium intake, stroke, and cardiovascular disease a meta-analysis of prospective studies. Journal of the American College of Cardiology, 57(10), 1210–1219. https://doi.org/10.1016/j.jacc.2010.09.070

[3345] Aburto, N. J., Hanson, S., Gutierrez, H., Hooper, L., Elliott, P., & Cappuccio, F. P. (2013). Effect of increased potassium intake on cardiovascular risk factors and disease: systematic review and meta-analyses. BMJ (Clinical research ed.), 346, f1378. https://doi.org/10.1136/bmj.f1378

682

[3346] Mannix, E. T., Farber, M. O., Aronoff, G. R., Brier, M. E., Weinberger, M. H., Palange, P., & Manfredi, F. (1996). Hemodynamic, renal, and hormonal responses to lower body positive pressure in human subjects. The Journal of laboratory and clinical medicine, 128(6), 585–593. https://doi.org/10.1016/s0022-2143(96)90131-6

[3347] Bauer, J. H., & Gauntner, W. C. (1979). Effect of potassium chloride on plasma renin activity and plasma aldosterone during sodium restriction in normal man. Kidney International, 15(3), 286–293. doi:10.1038/ki.1979.37

[3348] Palmer, B. F., & Clegg, D. J. (2016). Achieving the Benefits of a High-Potassium, Paleolithic Diet, Without the Toxicity. Mayo Clinic Proceedings, 91(4), 496–508. doi:10.1016/j.mayocp.2016.01.012

[3349] Krishna and Kapoor (1991) 'Potassium Depletion Exacerbates Essential Hypertension', Ann Intern Med.1991;115:77-83.

[3350] Ueshima, H., Tanigaki, M., Iida, M., Shimamoto, M., Konishi, M., & Komachi, Y. (1981). Hypertension, salt, and potassium. Lancet (London, England), 1(8218), 504. https://doi.org/10.1016/s0140-6736(81)91895-x

[3351] NIH (2020) 'Potassium: Fact Sheet for Health Professionals', Dietary Supplement Fact Sheets, Accessed Online Dec 26 2020: https://ods.od.nih.gov/factsheets/Potassium-HealthProfessional/

[3352] U.S. Department of Agriculture, Agricultural Research Service. FoodData Centralexternal link disclaimer, 2019.

[3353] USDA (2015) '2015-2020 Dietary Guidelines for Americans', December 2015. Available at http://health.gov/dietaryguidelines/2015/guidelines/.

[3354] SELF Nutrition Data (2018) 'Foods highest in Potassium', Accessed Online Dec 26 2020: https://nutritiondata.self.com/foods-000122000000000000000-w.html

[3355] McGill, C. R., Kurilich, A. C., & Davignon, J. (2013). The role of potatoes and potato components in cardiometabolic health: a review. Annals of medicine, 45(7), 467–473. https://doi.org/10.3109/07853890.2013.813633

[3356] Macdonald-Clarke, C. J., Martin, B. R., McCabe, L. D., McCabe, G. P., Lachcik, P. J., Wastney, M., & Weaver, C. M. (2016). Bioavailability of potassium from potatoes and potassium gluconate: a randomized dose response trial. The American journal of clinical nutrition, 104(2), 346–353. https://doi.org/10.3945/ajcn.115.127225

[3357] Beyer, F. R., Dickinson, H. O., Nicolson, D., Ford, G. A., & Mason, J. (2006). Combined calcium, magnesium and potassium supplementation for the management of primary hypertension in adults. Cochrane Database of Systematic Reviews. doi:10.1002/14651858.cd004805.pub2

[3358] Whelton, P. K., He, J., Cutler, J. A., Brancati, F. L., Appel, L. J., Follmann, D., & Klag, M. J. (1997). Effects of oral potassium on blood pressure. Meta-analysis of randomized controlled clinical trials. JAMA, 277(20), 1624–1632. https://doi.org/10.1001/jama.1997.03540440058033

[3359] Cappuccio, F. P., & MacGregor, G. A. (1991). Does potassium supplementation lower blood pressure? A meta-analysis of published trials. Journal of hypertension, 9(5), 465–473. https://doi.org/10.1097/00004872-199105000-00011

[3360] Geleijnse, J. M., Kok, F. J., & Grobbee, D. E. (2003). Blood pressure response to changes in sodium and potassium intake: a metaregression analysis of randomised trials. Journal of human hypertension, 17(7), 471–480. https://doi.org/10.1038/sj.jhh.1001575

[3361] Cappuccio, F. P., & MacGregor, G. A. (1991). Does potassium supplementation lower blood pressure? A meta-analysis of published trials. Journal of hypertension, 9(5), 465–473. https://doi.org/10.1097/00004872-199105000-00011

[3362] Houston M. C. (2011). The importance of potassium in managing hypertension. Current hypertension reports, 13(4), 309–317. https://doi.org/10.1007/s11906-011-0197-8

[3363] Whelton, P. K., He, J., Cutler, J. A., Brancati, F. L., Appel, L. J., Follmann, D., & Klag, M. J. (1997). Effects of oral potassium on blood pressure. Meta-analysis of randomized controlled clinical trials. JAMA, 277(20), 1624–1632. https://doi.org/10.1001/jama.1997.03540440058033

[3364] Dickinson, H. O., Nicolson, D., Campbell, F., Beyer, F. R., & Mason, J. (2006). Potassium supplementation for the management of primary hypertension in adults. Cochrane Database of Systematic Reviews. doi:10.1002/14651858.cd004641.pub2

[3365] U.S. Food and Drug Administration. List of Drug Products That Have Been Withdrawn or Removed from the Market for Reasons of Safety or Effectiveness. Federal Register 1998;63.

[3366] U.S. Food and Drug Administration. Code of Federal Regulations Title 21. 21CFR201.306. Potassium salt preparations intended for oral ingestion by man. 2017.

[3367] Levene D. L. (1973). The absorption of potassium chloride--liquid vs. tablet. Canadian Medical Association journal, 108(12), 1480–passim.

[3368] Riccardella, D., & Dwyer, J. (1985). Salt substitutes and medicinal potassium sources: risks and benefits. Journal of the American Dietetic Association, 85(4), 471–474.

[3369] Kunis, C. L., & Charney, A. N. (1981). Potassium and renal failure. Comprehensive therapy, 7(3), 29–33.

683

[3370] Institute of Medicine. Dietary Reference Intakes for Water, Potassium, Sodium, Chloride, and Sulfate. Washington, DC; 2005.

[3371] Shils, M.E.; Shike, M. Modern Nutrition in Health and Disease; Lippincott Williams & Wilkins: Baltimore, MD, USA, 2006.

[3372] SQUIRES, R. D., & HUTH, E. J. (1959). Experimental potassium depletion in normal human subjects. I. Relation of ionic intakes to the renal conservation of potassium. The Journal of clinical investigation, 38(7), 1134–1148. https://doi.org/10.1172/JCI103890

[3373] Levene D. L. (1973). Potassium chloride: absorption and excretion. Canadian Medical Association journal, 108(7), 853–855.

[3374] Bia, M. J., & DeFronzo, R. A. (1981). Extrarenal potassium homeostasis. The American journal of physiology, 240(4), F257–F268. https://doi.org/10.1152/ajprenal.1981.240.4.F257

[3375] Jasani, B. M., & Edmonds, C. J. (1971). Kinetics of potassium distribution in man using isotope dilution and whole-body counting. Metabolism, 20(12), 1099–1106. doi:10.1016/0026-0495(71)90034-5

[3376] Ludlow M. (1993). Renal handling of potassium. ANNA journal, 20(1), 52–58.

[3377] Penton, D., Czogalla, J., & Loffing, J. (2015). Dietary potassium and the renal control of salt balance and blood pressure. Pflugers Archiv: European journal of physiology, 467(3), 513–530. https://doi.org/10.1007/s00424-014-1673-1

[3378] Meneton, P., Loffing, J., & Warnock, D. G. (2004). Sodium and potassium handling by the aldosterone-sensitive distal nephron: the pivotal role of the distal and connecting tubule. American journal of physiology. Renal physiology, 287(4), F593–F601. https://doi.org/10.1152/ajprenal.00454.2003

[3379] Ohno, Y., Sone, M., Inagaki, N., Yamasaki, T., Ogawa, O., Takeda, Y., Kurihara, I., Itoh, H., Umakoshi, H., Tsuiki, M., Ichijo, T., Katabami, T., Tanaka, Y., Wada, N., Shibayama, Y., Yoshimoto, T., Ogawa, Y., Kawashima, J., Takahashi, K., Fujita, M., … JPAS Study Group (2018). Prevalence of Cardiovascular Disease and Its Risk Factors in Primary Aldosteronism: A Multicenter Study in Japan. Hypertension (Dallas, Tex. : 1979), 71(3), 530–537. https://doi.org/10.1161/HYPERTENSIONAHA.117.10263

[3380] Hurwitz, S., Cohen, R. J., & Williams, G. H. (2004). Diurnal variation of aldosterone and plasma renin activity: timing relation to melatonin and cortisol and consistency after prolonged bed rest. Journal of Applied Physiology, 96(4), 1406–1414. doi:10.1152/japplphysiol.00611.2003

[3381] Graudal, N. A., Galløe, A. M., & Garred, P. (1998). Effects of sodium restriction on blood pressure, renin, aldosterone, catecholamines, cholesterols, and triglyceride: a meta-analysis. JAMA, 279(17), 1383–1391. https://doi.org/10.1001/jama.279.17.1383

[3382] Miller, W. L., Borgeson, D. D., Grantham, J. A., Luchner, A., Redfield, M. M., & Burnett, J. C., Jr (2015). Dietary sodium modulation of aldosterone activation and renal function during the progression of experimental heart failure. European journal of heart failure, 17(2), 144–150. https://doi.org/10.1002/ejhf.212

[3383] Viera, A. J., & Wouk, N. (2015). Potassium Disorders: Hypokalemia and Hyperkalemia. American family physician, 92(6), 487–495.

[3384] Paice, B. J., Paterson, K. R., Onyanga-Omara, F., Donnelly, T., Gray, J. M., & Lawson, D. H. (1986). Record linkage study of hypokalaemia in hospitalized patients. Postgraduate medical journal, 62(725), 187–191. https://doi.org/10.1136/pgmj.62.725.187

[3385] Lippi, G., Favaloro, E. J., Montagnana, M., & Guidi, G. C. (2010). Prevalence of hypokalaemia: the experience of a large academic hospital. Internal medicine journal, 40(4), 315–316. https://doi.org/10.1111/j.1445-5994.2009.02146.x

[3386] Huang, C. L., & Kuo, E. (2007). Mechanism of hypokalemia in magnesium deficiency. Journal of the American Society of Nephrology : JASN, 18(10), 2649–2652. https://doi.org/10.1681/ASN.2007070792

[3387] Epstein M. (2009). Hyperkalemia as a constraint to therapy with combination Renin-Angiotensin system blockade: the elephant in the room. Journal of clinical hypertension (Greenwich, Conn.), 11(2), 55–60. https://doi.org/10.1111/j.1751-7176.2008.00071.x

[3388] Raebel M. A. (2012). Hyperkalemia associated with use of angiotensin-converting enzyme inhibitors and angiotensin receptor blockers. Cardiovascular therapeutics, 30(3), e156–e166. https://doi.org/10.1111/j.1755-5922.2010.00258.x

[3389] Lehnhardt, A., & Kemper, M. J. (2011). Pathogenesis, diagnosis and management of hyperkalemia. Pediatric nephrology (Berlin, Germany), 26(3), 377–384. https://doi.org/10.1007/s00467-010-1699-3

[3390] Patrick J. (1977). Assessment of body potassium stores. Kidney international, 11(6), 476–490. https://doi.org/10.1038/ki.1977.65

[3391] Nielsen FH. Manganese, molybdenum, boron, silicon and other trace elements. In: Marriott B, Birt D, Stallings G, Yates A, editors. Present knowledge in nutrition. 11th ed. Amsterdam: Elsevier. In press.

[3392] Nielsen, F. H., & Meacham, S. L. (2011). Growing Evidence for Human Health Benefits of Boron. Journal of Evidence-Based Complementary & Alternative Medicine, 16(3), 169–180. doi:10.1177/2156587211407638

[3393] Penland J. G. (1998). The importance of boron nutrition for brain and psychological function. Biological trace element research, 66(1-3), 299–317. https://doi.org/10.1007/BF02783144

[3394] Cui, Y., Winton, M. I., Zhang, Z. F., Rainey, C., Marshall, J., De Kernion, J. B., & Eckhert, C. D. (2004). Dietary boron intake and prostate cancer risk. Oncology reports, 11(4), 887–892.

[3395] Barranco, W. T., Hudak, P. F., & Eckhert, C. D. (2007). Evaluation of ecological and in vitro effects of boron on prostate cancer risk (United States). Cancer causes & control : CCC, 18(1), 71–77. https://doi.org/10.1007/s10552-006-0077-8

[3396] Mahabir, S., Spitz, M. R., Barrera, S. L., Dong, Y. Q., Eastham, C., & Forman, M. R. (2008). Dietary boron and hormone replacement therapy as risk factors for lung cancer in women. American journal of epidemiology, 167(9), 1070–1080. https://doi.org/10.1093/aje/kwn021

[3397] Hunt, C. D. (2003). Dietary boron: An overview of the evidence for its role in immune function. The Journal of Trace Elements in Experimental Medicine, 16(4), 291–306. doi:10.1002/jtra.10041

[3398] Meacham, S. L., Taper, L. J., & Volpe, S. L. (1994). Effects of boron supplementation on bone mineral density and dietary, blood, and urinary calcium, phosphorus, magnesium, and boron in female athletes. Environmental health perspectives, 102 Suppl 7(Suppl 7), 79–82. https://doi.org/10.1289/ehp.94102s779

[3399] Hall, I., Chen, S., Rajendran, K., Sood, A., Spielvogel, B., & Shih, J. (1994). Hypolipidemic, Anti-Obesity, Anti-Inflammatory, Anti-Osteoporotic, and Anti-Neoplastic Properties of Amine Carboxyboranes. Environmental Health Perspectives, 102, 21-30. doi:10.2307/3431958

[3400] Meacham, S. L., Taper, L. J., & Volpe, S. L. (1995). Effect of boron supplementation on blood and urinary calcium, magnesium, and phosphorus, and urinary boron in athletic and sedentary women. The American Journal of Clinical Nutrition, 61(2), 341–345. doi:10.1093/ajcn/61.2.341

[3401] WILSON, J. H., & RUSZLER, P. L. (1998). Long term effects of boron on layer bone strength and production parameters. British Poultry Science, 39(1), 11–15. doi:10.1080/00071669889312

[3402] Nielsen FH. Boron. In: Merian E, Anke M, Ihnat M, Stoeppler M, editors. Elements and their compounds in the environment. Occurrence, analysis and biological relevance. Vol. 3: Nonmetals, particular aspects. 2nd ed. Weinheim: Wiley-VCH Verlag; 2004. p. 1251-60.

[3403] Goldbach, H. E., & Wimmer, M. A. (2007). Boron in plants and animals: Is there a role beyond cell-wall structure? Journal of Plant Nutrition and Soil Science, 170(1), 39–48. doi:10.1002/jpln.200625161

[3404] Ploquin (1967) 'Le bore dans l'alimentation'. Bull. Soc. Sci. Hyg. Aliment. 55, 70-113.

[3405] Nielsen, F. H., & Eckhert, C. D. (2020). Boron. Advances in nutrition (Bethesda, Md.), 11(2), 461–462. https://doi.org/10.1093/advances/nmz110

[3406] Oiwa, Y., Kitayama, K., Kobayashi, M., & Matoh, T. (2013). Boron deprivation immediately causes cell death in growing roots ofArabidopsis thaliana(L.) Heynh. Soil Science and Plant Nutrition, 59(4), 621–627. doi:10.1080/00380768.2013.813382

[3407] Fort, D. J., Stover, E. L., Strong, P. L., Murray, F. J., & Keen, C. L. (1999). Chronic Feeding of a Low Boron Diet Adversely Affects Reproduction and Development in Xenopus laevis. The Journal of Nutrition, 129(11), 2055–2060. doi:10.1093/jn/129.11.2055

[3408] Fort et al (1999) 'Adverse effects from low dietary and environmental boron exposure on reproduction, development, and maturation in Xenopus laevis', The Journal of Trace Elements in Experimental Medicine 12(3):175 - 185

[3409] Lanoue et al (1999) 'Adverse effects of a low boron environment on the preimplantation development of mouse embryos in vitro', J Trace Elem Exp Med 1999;12:235.

[3410] Travis NJ, Cocks EJ. (1984) 'The Tincal Trail: A History of Borax.', London, UK: Harraps.

[3411] Weimer, Alan W. (1997). Carbide, Nitride and Boride Materials Synthesis and Processing. Chapman & Hall (London, New York).

[3412] Calvert (2009) 'Boron', University of Denver, Accessed Online Jan 05 2021: http://mysite.du.edu/~jcalvert/phys/boron.htm

[3413] Garrett, Donald E. (1998). Borates: handbook of deposits, processing, properties, and use. Academic Press. pp. 102, 385–386.

[3414] Davy H (1809). "An account of some new analytical researches on the nature of certain bodies, particularly the alkalies, phosphorus, sulphur, carbonaceous matter, and the acids hitherto undecomposed: with some general observations on chemical theory". Philosophical Transactions of the Royal Society of London. 99: 39–104. doi:10.1098/rstl.1809.0005

[3415] Moore, J. A., & Expert Scientific Committee. (1997). An assessment of boric acid and borax using the IEHR Evaluative process for assessing human developmental and reproductive toxicity of agents. Reproductive Toxicology, 11(1), 123–160. doi:10.1016/s0890-6238(96)00204-3

[3416] Jansen, J. A., Andersen, J., & Schou, J. S. (1984). Boric acid single dose pharmacokinetics after intravenous administration to man. Archives of toxicology, 55(1), 64–67. https://doi.org/10.1007/BF00316588

[3417] Kot, F. S. (2008). Boron sources, speciation and its potential impact on health. Reviews in Environmental Science and Bio/Technology, 8(1), 3–28. doi:10.1007/s11157-008-9140-0

[3418] Bolaños, L., Lukaszewski, K., Bonilla, I., & Blevins, D. (2004). Why boron? Plant Physiology and Biochemistry, 42(11), 907–912. doi:10.1016/j.plaphy.2004.11.002

[3419] Furukawa, Y., Horiuchi, M., & Kakegawa, T. (2013). Selective Stabilization of Ribose by Borate. Origins of Life and Evolution of Biospheres, 43(4-5), 353–361. doi:10.1007/s11084-013-9350-5

[3420] Teitelbaum, J. E., Johnson, C., & St Cyr, J. (2006). The use of D-ribose in chronic fatigue syndrome and fibromyalgia: a pilot study. Journal of alternative and complementary medicine (New York, N.Y.), 12(9), 857–862. https://doi.org/10.1089/acm.2006.12.857

[3421] Nielsen F. H. (2014). Update on human health effects of boron. Journal of trace elements in medicine and biology : organ of the Society for Minerals and Trace Elements (GMS), 28(4), 383–387. https://doi.org/10.1016/j.jtemb.2014.06.023

[3422] Kim, D. H., Marbois, B. N., Faull, K. F., & Eckhert, C. D. (2003). Esterification of borate with NAD+ and NADH as studied by electrospray ionization mass spectrometry and11B NMR spectroscopy. Journal of Mass Spectrometry, 38(6), 632–640. doi:10.1002/jms.476

[3423] Ralston, N. V. ., & Hunt, C. D. (2001). Diadenosine phosphates and S-adenosylmethionine: novel boron binding biomolecules detected by capillary electrophoresis. Biochimica et Biophysica Acta (BBA) - General Subjects, 1527(1-2), 20–30. doi:10.1016/s0304-4165(01)00130-1

[3424] Loenen W. A. (2006). S-adenosylmethionine: jack of all trades and master of everything?. Biochemical Society transactions, 34(Pt 2), 330–333. https://doi.org/10.1042/BST20060330

[3425] Kim, D. H., Hee, S. Q., Norris, A. J., Faull, K. F., & Eckhert, C. D. (2006). Boric acid inhibits adenosine diphosphate-ribosyl cyclase non-competitively. Journal of Chromatography A, 1115(1-2), 246–252. doi:10.1016/j.chroma.2006.02.066

[3426] Henderson, K., Stella, S. L., Kobylewski, S., & Eckhert, C. D. (2009). Receptor activated Ca(2+) release is inhibited by boric acid in prostate cancer cells. PloS one, 4(6), e6009. https://doi.org/10.1371/journal.pone.0006009

[3427] Korkmaz, M., Uzgören, E., Bakirdere, S., Aydin, F., & Ataman, O. Y. (2007). Effects of dietary boron on cervical cytopathology and on micronucleus frequency in exfoliated buccal cells. Environmental toxicology, 22(1), 17–25. https://doi.org/10.1002/tox.20229

[3428] Scorei I. R. (2011). Calcium fructoborate: plant-based dietary boron as potential medicine for cancer therapy. Frontiers in bioscience (Scholar edition), 3, 205–215. https://doi.org/10.2741/s145

[3429] Mahabir, S., Spitz, M. R., Barrera, S. L., Dong, Y. Q., Eastham, C., & Forman, M. R. (2008). Dietary boron and hormone replacement therapy as risk factors for lung cancer in women. American journal of epidemiology, 167(9), 1070–1080. https://doi.org/10.1093/aje/kwn021

[3430] Müezzinoğlu, T., Korkmaz, M., Neşe, N., Bakırdere, S., Arslan, Y., Ataman, O. Y., & Lekili, M. (2011). Prevalence of prostate cancer in high boron-exposed population: a community-based study. Biological trace element research, 144(1-3), 49–57. https://doi.org/10.1007/s12011-011-9023-z

[3431] Barranco, W. T., & Eckhert, C. D. (2006). Cellular changes in boric acid-treated DU-145 prostate cancer cells. British journal of cancer, 94(6), 884–890. https://doi.org/10.1038/sj.bjc.6603009

[3432] Barranco, W. T., & Eckhert, C. D. (2004). Boric acid inhibits human prostate cancer cell proliferation. Cancer letters, 216(1), 21–29. https://doi.org/10.1016/j.canlet.2004.06.001

[3433] Kobylewski, S. E., Henderson, K. A., Yamada, K. E., & Eckhert, C. D. (2017). Activation of the EIF2α/ATF4 and ATF6 Pathways in DU-145 Cells by Boric Acid at the Concentration Reported in Men at the US Mean Boron Intake. Biological trace element research, 176(2), 278–293. https://doi.org/10.1007/s12011-016-0824-y

[3434] Yamada, K. E., & Eckhert, C. D. (2019). Boric Acid Activation of eIF2α and Nrf2 Is PERK Dependent: a Mechanism that Explains How Boron Prevents DNA Damage and Enhances Antioxidant Status. Biological trace element research, 188(1), 2–10. https://doi.org/10.1007/s12011-018-1498-4

[3435] Türkez, H., Geyikoğlu, F., Tatar, A., Keleş, S., & Özkan, A. (2007). Effects of Some Boron Compounds on Peripheral Human Blood. Zeitschrift Für Naturforschung C, 62(11-12), 889–896. doi:10.1515/znc-2007-11-1218

[3436] Nielsen F. H. (1994). Biochemical and physiologic consequences of boron deprivation in humans. Environmental health perspectives, 102 Suppl 7(Suppl 7), 59–63. https://doi.org/10.1289/ehp.94102s759

[3437] Nielsen F. H. (1994). Biochemical and physiologic consequences of boron deprivation in humans. Environmental health perspectives, 102 Suppl 7(Suppl 7), 59–63. https://doi.org/10.1289/ehp.94102s759

[3438] Türkez, H., Geyikoğlu, F., Tatar, A., Keleş, S., & Özkan, A. (2007). Effects of Some Boron Compounds on Peripheral Human Blood. Zeitschrift Für Naturforschung C, 62(11-12), 889–896. doi:10.1515/znc-2007-11-1218

[3439] Turkez, H., Geyikoglu, F., Tatar, A., Keles, M. S., & Kaplan, I. (2012). The effects of some boron compounds against heavy metal toxicity in human blood. Experimental and toxicologic pathology : official journal of the Gesellschaft fur Toxikologische Pathologie, 64(1-2), 93–101. https://doi.org/10.1016/j.etp.2010.06.011

[3440] Travers, R. L., Rennie, G. C., & Newnham, R. E. (1990). Boron and Arthritis: The Results of a Double-blind Pilot Study. Journal of Nutritional Medicine, 1(2), 127–132. doi:10.3109/13590849009003147

[3441] Hunt, C.D. and Idso, J.P. (1999), Dietary boron as a physiological regulator of the normal inflammatory response: A review and current research progress. J. Trace Elem. Exp. Med., 12: 221-233. https://doi.org/10.1002/(SICI)1520-670X(1999)12:3<221::AID-JTRA6>3.0.CO;2-X

686

[3442] Belver, A., & Donaire, J. P. (1983). Partial Purification of Soluble Lipoxygenase of Sunflower Cotyledons: Action of Boron on the Enzyme and Lipid Constituents. Zeitschrift Für Pflanzenphysiologie, 109(4), 309–317. doi:10.1016/s0044-328x(83)80114-7

[3443] Rajendran, K., Chen, S., Sood, A., Spielvogel, B., & Hall, I. (1995). The anti-osteoporotic activity of amine-carboxyboranes in rodents. Biomedicine & Pharmacotherapy, 49(3), 131–140. doi:10.1016/0753-3322(96)82606-0

[3444] Rogoveanu, O. C., Mogoşanu, G. D., Bejenaru, C., Bejenaru, L. E., Croitoru, O., Neamţu, J., Pietrzkowski, Z., Reyes-Izquierdo, T., Biţă, A., Scorei, I. D., & Scorei, R. I. (2015). Effects of Calcium Fructoborate on Levels of C-Reactive Protein, Total Cholesterol, Low-Density Lipoprotein, Triglycerides, IL-1β, IL-6, and MCP-1: a Double-blind, Placebo-controlled Clinical Study. Biological trace element research, 163(1-2), 124–131. https://doi.org/10.1007/s12011-014-0155-9

[3445] Hakki, S. S., Bozkurt, B. S., & Hakki, E. E. (2010). Boron regulates mineralized tissue-associated proteins in osteoblasts (MC3T3-E1). Journal of Trace Elements in Medicine and Biology, 24(4), 243–250. doi:10.1016/j.jtemb.2010.03.003

[3446] Uluisik I, Kaya A, Fomenko DE, Karakaya HC, Carlson BA, Gladyshev VN, et al. (2011) Boron Stress Activates the General Amino Acid Control Mechanism and Inhibits Protein Synthesis. PLoS ONE 6(11): e27772. https://doi.org/10.1371/journal.pone.0027772

[3447] Newnham RE. How boron is being used in medical practice. In: Goldbach HE, Rerkasem B, Wimmer MA, Brown PH, Thellier M, Bell RW, eds. Boron in Plant and Animal Nutrition. New York, NY: Kluwer Academic/Plenum; 2002:59-62.

[3448] Peng, X., Lingxia, Z., Schrauzer, G. N., & Xiong, G. (2000). Selenium, Boron, and Germanium Deficiency in the Etiology of Kashin-Beck Disease. Biological Trace Element Research, 77(3), 193–198. doi:10.1385/bter:77:3:193

[3449] Newnham R. E. (1994). Essentiality of boron for healthy bones and joints. Environmental health perspectives, 102 Suppl 7(Suppl 7), 83–85. https://doi.org/10.1289/ehp.94102s783

[3450] Pietrzkowski, Z., Phelan, M. J., Keller, R., Shu, C., Argumedo, R., & Reyes-Izquierdo, T. (2014). Short-term efficacy of calcium fructoborate on subjects with knee discomfort: a comparative, double-blind, placebo-controlled clinical study. Clinical interventions in aging, 9, 895–899. https://doi.org/10.2147/CIA.S64590

[3451] Nielsen, F. H., & Stoecker, B. J. (2009). Boron and fish oil have different beneficial effects on strength and trabecular microarchitecture of bone. Journal of trace elements in medicine and biology : organ of the Society for Minerals and Trace Elements (GMS), 23(3), 195–203. https://doi.org/10.1016/j.jtemb.2009.03.003

[3452] Kim, M. H., Bae, Y. J., Lee, Y. S., & Choi, M. K. (2008). Estimation of boron intake and its relation with bone mineral density in free-living Korean female subjects. Biological trace element research, 125(3), 213–222. https://doi.org/10.1007/s12011-008-8176-x

[3453] Rondanelli, M., Faliva, M. A., Peroni, G., Infantino, V., Gasparri, C., Iannello, G., … Tartara, A. (2020). Pivotal role of boron supplementation on bone health: A narrative review. Journal of Trace Elements in Medicine and Biology, 62, 126577. doi:10.1016/j.jtemb.2020.126577

[3454] Nielsen F. H. (1990). Studies on the relationship between boron and magnesium which possibly affects the formation and maintenance of bones. Magnesium and trace elements, 9(2), 61–69.

[3455] Nielsen, F. H., Hunt, C. D., Mullen, L. M., & Hunt, J. R. (1987). Effect of dietary boron on mineral, estrogen, and testosterone metabolism in postmenopausal women. FASEB journal : official publication of the Federation of American Societies for Experimental Biology, 1(5), 394–397.

[3456] Beattie, J. H., & Peace, H. S. (1993). The influence of a low-boron diet and boron supplementation on bone, major mineral and sex steroid metabolism in postmenopausal women. The British journal of nutrition, 69(3), 871–884. https://doi.org/10.1079/bjn19930087

[3457] Meacham, S. L., Taper, L. J., & Volpe, S. L. (1994). Effects of boron supplementation on bone mineral density and dietary, blood, and urinary calcium, phosphorus, magnesium, and boron in female athletes. Environmental health perspectives, 102 Suppl 7(Suppl 7), 79–82. https://doi.org/10.1289/ehp.94102s779

[3458] Nielsen, F. H. (1998). The justification for providing dietary guidance for the nutritional intake of boron. Biological Trace Element Research, 66(1-3), 319–330. doi:10.1007/bf02783145

[3459] Hunt CD, Nielsen FH (1981) Interaction between boron and cholecalciferol in the chick. In: McC Howell J, Gawthorne JM, White CL (eds) Trace element metabolism in man and animals (TEMA-4). Australian Academy of Science, Canberra, pp 597–600

[3460] Hunt C. D. (1989). Dietary boron modified the effects of magnesium and molybdenum on mineral metabolism in the cholecalciferol-deficient chick. Biological trace element research, 22(2), 201–220. https://doi.org/10.1007/BF02916650

[3461] Hegsted, M., Keenan, M. J., Siver, F., & Wozniak, P. (1991). Effect of boron on vitamin D deficient rats. Biological trace element research, 28(3), 243–255. https://doi.org/10.1007/BF02990471

[3462] Naghii, M. R., & Samman, S. (1997). The effect of boron on plasma testosterone and plasma lipids in rats. Nutrition Research, 17(3), 523–531. doi:10.1016/s0271-5317(97)00017-1

687

[3463] Dupre, J. N., Keenan, M. J., Hegsted, M., & Brudevold, A. M. (1994). Effects of dietary boron in rats fed a vitamin D-deficient diet. Environmental health perspectives, 102 Suppl 7(Suppl 7), 55–58. https://doi.org/10.1289/ehp.94102s755

[3464] Nielsen, F. H, Mullen, L. M, & Gallagher, S. K. (1990). Effect of boron depletion and repletion on blood indicators of calcium status in humans fed a magnesium-low diet. Journal of trace elements in experimental medicine, 3, 45.

[3465] Nielsen, F.H. (1996), Evidence for the nutritional essentiality of boron. J. Trace Elem. Exp. Med., 9: 215-229. https://doi.org/10.1002/(SICI)1520-670X(1996)9:4<215::AID-JTRA7>3.0.CO;2-P

[3466] Miljkovic, D., Miljkovic, N., & McCarty, M. F. (2004). Up-regulatory impact of boron on vitamin D function -- does it reflect inhibition of 24-hydroxylase?. Medical hypotheses, 63(6), 1054–1056. https://doi.org/10.1016/j.mehy.2003.12.053

[3467] Nielsen, F. H., Hunt, C. D., Mullen, L. M., & Hunt, J. R. (1987). Effect of dietary boron on mineral, estrogen, and testosterone metabolism in postmenopausal women. FASEB journal : official publication of the Federation of American Societies for Experimental Biology, 1(5), 394–397.

[3468] Naghii, M. R., & Samman, S. (1997). The effect of boron supplementation on its urinary excretion and selected cardiovascular risk factors in healthy male subjects. Biological trace element research, 56(3), 273–286. https://doi.org/10.1007/BF02785299

[3469] Naghii, M. R., Mofid, M., Asgari, A. R., Hedayati, M., & Daneshpour, M. S. (2011). Comparative effects of daily and weekly boron supplementation on plasma steroid hormones and proinflammatory cytokines. Journal of trace elements in medicine and biology : organ of the Society for Minerals and Trace Elements (GMS), 25(1), 54–58. https://doi.org/10.1016/j.jtemb.2010.10.001

[3470] Naghii, M. R., & Samman, S. (1997). The effect of boron supplementation on its urinary excretion and selected cardiovascular risk factors in healthy male subjects. Biological trace element research, 56(3), 273–286. https://doi.org/10.1007/BF02785299

[3471] Pilz, S., Frisch, S., Koertke, H., Kuhn, J., Dreier, J., Obermayer-Pietsch, B., Wehr, E., & Zittermann, A. (2011). Effect of vitamin D supplementation on testosterone levels in men. Hormone and metabolic research = Hormon- und Stoffwechselforschung = Hormones et metabolisme, 43(3), 223–225. https://doi.org/10.1055/s-0030-1269854

[3472] Penland J. G. (1994). Dietary boron, brain function, and cognitive performance. Environmental health perspectives, 102 Suppl 7(Suppl 7), 65–72. https://doi.org/10.1289/ehp.94102s765

[3473] Penland (1995) 'Quantitative analysis of EEG effects following experimental marginal magnesium and boron deprivation.', Magnesium Research, 01 Dec 1995, 8(4):341-358

[3474] Penland, J. G. (1998). The importance of boron nutrition for brain and psychological function. Biological Trace Element Research, 66(1-3), 299–317. doi:10.1007/bf02783144

[3475] Penland J. G. (1994). Dietary boron, brain function, and cognitive performance. Environmental health perspectives, 102 Suppl 7(Suppl 7), 65–72. https://doi.org/10.1289/ehp.94102s765

[3476] Penland, J. G, & Eberhardt, M. J. (1993). Effects of dietary boron and magnesium on brain function of mature male and female Long-Evans rats. Journal of trace elements in experimental medicine, 6, 53.

[3477] Eckhert, C.D. and Rowe, R.I. (1999), Embryonic dysplasia and adult retinal dystrophy in boron-deficient zebrafish. J. Trace Elem. Exp. Med., 12: 213-219. https://doi.org/10.1002/(SICI)1520-670X(1999)12:3<213::AID-JTRA5>3.0.CO;2-0

[3478] Zhu, Z., Liao, H., Liu, S., Zhang, J., Chen, Y., & Wang, W. (2020). Cross-sectional study of the association between age-related macular degeneration and arthritis in the National Health and Nutrition Examination Survey 2005–2008. BMJ Open, 10(12), e035805. doi:10.1136/bmjopen-2019-035805

[3479] Huel G, Yazbeck C, Burnel D, Missy P, Kloppmann W (2004) Environmental boron exposure and activity of d-aminolevulinic acid dehydratase (ALA-D) in a newborn population. Toxicol Sci 80:304–309. doi:10.1093/toxsci/kfh165

[3480] World Health Organization. Boron. In: Trace elements in human nutrition and health. Geneva, 1996.

[3481] Nielsen F. H. (1998). The justification for providing dietary guidance for the nutritional intake of boron. Biological trace element research, 66(1-3), 319–330. https://doi.org/10.1007/BF02783145

[3482] Medline (2020) 'Boron', NIH, Herbs and Supplements, Accessed Online Jan 04 2021: https://medlineplus.gov/druginfo/natural/894.html

[3483] Panel on Micronutrients, Subcommittees on Upper Reference Levels of Nutrients and of Interpretation and Uses of Dietary Reference Intakes; Standing Committee on the Scientific Evaluation of Dietary Reference Intakes; Food and Nutrition Board; Institute of Medicine. Dietary Reference Intakes for Vitamin A, Vitamin K, Arsenic, Boron, Chromium, Copper, Iodine, Iron, Manganese, Molybdenum, Nickel, Silicon, Vanadium, and Zinc. Washington, DC: National Academy Press; 2002.

[3484] World Health Organization, International Programme on Chemical Safety. Environmental Health Criteria 204 Boron. Geneva, Switzerland: World Health Organization; 1998.

[3485] EFSA Panel on Dietetic Products, Nutrition and Allergies, 2004. Opinion of the Scientific Panel on Dietetic products, nutrition and allergies [NDA] related to the Tolerable Upper Intake Level of Boron (Sodium Borate and Boric Acid). EFSA Journal 2004; 2(8):80, 22 pp. doi:10.2903/j.efsa.2004.80

[3486] Institute of Medicine (US) Panel on Micronutrients. (2001). Dietary Reference Intakes for Vitamin A, Vitamin K, Arsenic, Boron, Chromium, Copper, Iodine, Iron, Manganese, Molybdenum, Nickel, Silicon, Vanadium, and Zinc. National Academies Press (US).

[3487] Kim, M. H., Bae, Y. J., Lee, Y. S., & Choi, M. K. (2008). Estimation of boron intake and its relation with bone mineral density in free-living Korean female subjects. Biological trace element research, 125(3), 213–222. https://doi.org/10.1007/s12011-008-8176-x

[3488] Rainey, C., & Nyquist, L. (1998). Multicountry estimation of dietary boron intake. Biological trace element research, 66(1-3), 79–86. https://doi.org/10.1007/BF02783128

[3489] Hunt, C. D., Shuler, T. R., & Mullen, L. M. (1991). Concentration of boron and other elements in human foods and personal-care products. Journal of the American Dietetic Association, 91(5), 558–568.

[3490] Hooshmand, S., & Arjmandi, B. H. (2009). Viewpoint: dried plum, an emerging functional food that may effectively improve bone health. Ageing research reviews, 8(2), 122–127. https://doi.org/10.1016/j.arr.2009.01.002

[3491] Hooshmand, S., Chai, S. C., Saadat, R. L., Payton, M. E., Brummel-Smith, K., & Arjmandi, B. H. (2011). Comparative effects of dried plum and dried apple on bone in postmenopausal women. The British journal of nutrition, 106(6), 923–930. https://doi.org/10.1017/S000711451100119X

[3492] Saiki, M.K., Jennings, M.R. & Brumbaugh, W.G. Boron, molybdenum, and selenium in aquatic food chains from the lower San Joaquin river and its tributaries, California. Arch. Environ. Contam. Toxicol. 24, 307–319 (1993). https://doi.org/10.1007/BF01128729

[3493] World Health Organization IPoCS. Boron. In: Environmental Health Criteria 204. Geneva. 1998.

[3494] Miwa, K., Takano, J., Omori, H., Seki, M., Shinozaki, K., & Fujiwara, T. (2007). Plants Tolerant of High Boron Levels. Science, 318(5855), 1417–1417. doi:10.1126/science.1146634

[3495] Matterson KJ. Borate ore discovery, mining and beneficiation. Sect. A3, vol 5, Suppl to Mellor's Comprehensive Treatise on Inorganic and Theoretical Chemistry (Thompson R, Welch AJE eds). New York:Longman,1980.

[3496] Garrett (1998) 'Borates: Handbook of Deposits, Processing, Properties, and Use', Academic Press, ISBN: 978-0-12-276060-0.

[3497] Rainey, C. J., Nyquist, L. A., Christensen, R. E., Strong, P. L., Culver, B. D., & Coughlin, J. R. (1999). Daily boron intake from the American diet. Journal of the American Dietetic Association, 99(3), 335–340. https://doi.org/10.1016/S0002-8223(99)00085-1

[3498] Rainey, C. J., Nyquist, L. A., Christensen, R. E., Strong, P. L., Culver, B. D., & Coughlin, J. R. (1999). Daily boron intake from the American diet. Journal of the American Dietetic Association, 99(3), 335–340. https://doi.org/10.1016/S0002-8223(99)00085-1

[3499] Anderson R. R. (1992). Comparison of trace elements in milk of four species. Journal of dairy science, 75(11), 3050–3055. https://doi.org/10.3168/jds.S0022-0302(92)78068-0

[3500] Murray F. J. (1995). A human health risk assessment of boron (boric acid and borax) in drinking water. Regulatory toxicology and pharmacology : RTP, 22(3), 221–230. https://doi.org/10.1006/rtph.1995.0004

[3501] Yazbeck, C., Kloppmann, W., Cottier, R., Sahuquillo, J., Debotte, G., & Huel, G. (2005). Health Impact Evaluation of Boron in Drinking Water: A Geographical Risk Assessment in Northern France. Environmental Geochemistry and Health, 27(5-6), 419–427. doi:10.1007/s10653-005-1796-6

[3502] World Health Organization. Guidelines for Drinking Water Quality. Geneva, Switzerland: World Health Organization; 1993.

[3503] Şayli, B. S. (1998). An assessment of fertility in boron-exposed turkish subpopulations. Biological Trace Element Research, 66(1-3), 409–422. doi:10.1007/bf02783152

[3504] Howe, P. D. (1998). A review of boron effects in the environment. Biological Trace Element Research, 66(1-3), 153–166. doi:10.1007/bf02783135

[3505] NIH (2020) 'Boron: Fact Sheet for Health Professionals', Dietary Supplement Fact Sheets, Accessed Online Jan 02 2021: https://ods.od.nih.gov/factsheets/Boron-HealthProfessional/

[3506] M R Naghii, P M Wall & S Samman (1996) The boron content of selected foods and the estimation of its daily intake among free-living subjects., Journal of the American College of Nutrition, 15:6, 614-619, DOI: 10.1080/07315724.1996.10718638

[3507] Pizzorno, Lara. "Nothing boring about boron." Integrative Medicine: A Clinician's Journal 14, no. 4 (2015): 35.

[3508] Richold M. (1998). Boron exposure from consumer products. Biological trace element research, 66(1-3), 121–129. https://doi.org/10.1007/BF02783132

[3509] Uluisik, I., Karakaya, H. C., & Koc, A. (2018). The importance of boron in biological systems. Journal of trace elements in medicine and biology : organ of the Society for Minerals and Trace Elements (GMS), 45, 156–162. https://doi.org/10.1016/j.jtemb.2017.10.008

[3510] Draize, J. H., & Kelley, E. A. (1959). The urinary excretion of boric acid preparations following oral administration and topical applications to intact and damaged skin of rabbits. Toxicology and Applied Pharmacology, 1(3), 267–276. doi:10.1016/0041-008x(59)90111-5

689

[3511] Sutherland, B., Woodhouse, L.R., Strong, P. and King, J.C. (1999), Boron balance in humans. J. Trace Elem. Exp. Med., 12: 271-284. https://doi.org/10.1002/(SICI)1520-670X(1999)12:3<271::AID-JTRA10>3.0.CO;2-B

[3512] Khaliq, H., Juming, Z., & Ke-Mei, P. (2018). The Physiological Role of Boron on Health. Biological trace element research, 186(1), 31–51. https://doi.org/10.1007/s12011-018-1284-3

[3513] Jansen, J. A., Andersen, J., & Schou, J. S. (1984). Boric acid single dose pharmacokinetics after intravenous administration to man. Archives of Toxicology, 55(1), 64–67. doi:10.1007/bf00316588

[3514] Sutherland, B., Strong, P., & King, J. C. (1998). Determining human dietary requirements for boron. Biological trace element research, 66(1-3), 193–204. https://doi.org/10.1007/BF02783138

[3515] Culver, B. D., Shen, P. T., Taylor, T. H., Lee-Feldstein, A., Anton-Culver, H., & Strong, P. L. (1994). The relationship of blood- and urine-boron to boron exposure in borax-workers and usefulness of urine-boron as an exposure marker. Environmental health perspectives, 102 Suppl 7(Suppl 7), 133–137. https://doi.org/10.1289/ehp.94102s7133

[3516] Duydu et al (2012) 'Exposure assessment of boron in Bandırma boric acid production plant', Journal of Trace Elements in Medicine and Biology, Volume 26, Issues 2–3, June 2012, Pages 161-164.

[3517] Litovitz, T. L., Klein-Schwartz, W., Oderda, G. M., & Schmitz, B. F. (1988). Clinical manifestations of toxicity in a series of 784 boric acid ingestions. The American journal of emergency medicine, 6(3), 209–213. https://doi.org/10.1016/0735-6757(88)90001-0

[3518] Litovitz, T. L., Klein-Schwartz, W., Oderda, G. M., & Schmitz, B. F. (1988). Clinical manifestations of toxicity in a series of 784 boric acid ingestions. The American Journal of Emergency Medicine, 6(3), 209–213. doi:10.1016/0735-6757(88)90001-0

[3519] Restuccio, A., Mortensen, M. E., & Kelley, M. T. (1992). Fatal ingestion of boric acid in an adult. The American Journal of Emergency Medicine, 10(6), 545–547. doi:10.1016/0735-6757(92)90180-6

[3520] Ishii, Y., Fujizuka, N., Takahashi, T., Shimizu, K., Tuchida, A., Yano, S., Naruse, T., & Chishiro, T. (1993). A fatal case of acute boric acid poisoning. Journal of toxicology. Clinical toxicology, 31(2), 345–352. https://doi.org/10.3109/15563659309000402

[3521] Schillinger, B. M., Berstein, M., Goldberg, L. A., & Shalita, A. R. (1982). Boric acid poisoning. Journal of the American Academy of Dermatology, 7(5), 667–673. doi:10.1016/s0190-9622(82)70149-5

[3522] Gordon V (Ed) 1987 The case of the toxic life-preserver. Borax Review No. 2, 10-12.

[3523] Wiley (1904) 'Influence of Food Preservation and Artificial Colors on Digestion and Health: I. Boric Acid and Borax'. Washington, DC: Government Printing Office; 1904. US Department of Agriculture Bulletin No 84, Pt 1

[3524] Pongsavee M. (2009). Effect of borax on immune cell proliferation and sister chromatid exchange in human chromosomes. Journal of occupational medicine and toxicology (London, England), 4, 27. https://doi.org/10.1186/1745-6673-4-27

[3525] Halliburton W. D. (1900). Remarks on the Use of Borax and Formaldehyde as Preservatives of Food. British medical journal, 2(2062), 1–2. https://doi.org/10.1136/bmj.2.2062.1

[3526] A Model for Estimation of the Nasal Dose of Sodium Borate for Use in an Epidemiological Study of Workers Experiencing Irritant Symptoms. (1994). The Annals of Occupational Hygiene. doi:10.1093/annhyg/38.inhaled_particles_vii.533

[3527] Locksley, H.B. , and Farr, L.E. (1955). Tolerance of large doses of sodium borate intravenously by patients receiving neutron capture therapy. J. Pharmacol. Exp. Ther. 114, 484–9.

[3528] Popova, E. V., Tinkov, A. A., Ajsuvakova, O. P., Skalnaya, M. G., & Skalny, A. V. (2017). Boron - A potential goiterogen?. Medical hypotheses, 104, 63–67. https://doi.org/10.1016/j.mehy.2017.05.024

[3529] Ali, S. E., Thoen, E., Evensen, Ø., Wiik-Nielsen, J., Gamil, A. A., & Skaar, I. (2014). Mitochondrial dysfunction is involved in the toxic activity of boric acid against Saprolegnia. PloS one, 9(10), e110343. https://doi.org/10.1371/journal.pone.0110343

[3530] Naghii, M. R., Mofid, M., Asgari, A. R., Hedayati, M., & Daneshpour, M. S. (2011). Comparative effects of daily and weekly boron supplementation on plasma steroid hormones and proinflammatory cytokines. Journal of trace elements in medicine and biology : organ of the Society for Minerals and Trace Elements (GMS), 25(1), 54–58. https://doi.org/10.1016/j.jtemb.2010.10.001

[3531] Ferrando, A. A., & Green, N. R. (1993). The Effect of Boron Supplementation on Lean Body Mass, Plasma Testosterone Levels, and Strength in Male Bodybuilders. International Journal of Sport Nutrition, 3(2), 140–149. doi:10.1123/ijsn.3.2.140

[3532] Scorei, R., Mitrut, P., Petrisor, I., & Scorei, I. (2011). A double-blind, placebo-controlled pilot study to evaluate the effect of calcium fructoborate on systemic inflammation and dyslipidemia markers for middle-aged people with primary osteoarthritis. Biological trace element research, 144(1-3), 253–263. https://doi.org/10.1007/s12011-011-9083-0

[3533] Mogoşanu, G. D., Biţă, A., Bejenaru, L. E., Bejenaru, C., Croitoru, O., Răü, G., Rogoveanu, O. C., Florescu, D. N., Neamţu, J., Scorei, I. D., & Scorei, R. I. (2016). Calcium Fructoborate for Bone and Cardiovascular Health. Biological trace element research, 172(2), 277–281. https://doi.org/10.1007/s12011-015-0590-2

[3534] Dessordi, R., Spirlandeli, A. L., Zamarioli, A., Volpon, J. B., & Navarro, A. M. (2017). Boron supplementation improves bone health of non-obese diabetic mice. Journal of trace elements in medicine and biology : organ of the Society for Minerals and Trace Elements (GMS), 39, 169–175. https://doi.org/10.1016/j.jtemb.2016.09.011

[3535] Chapin, R. E., Ku, W. W., Kenney, M. A., McCoy, H., Gladen, B., Wine, R. N., Wilson, R., & Elwell, M. R. (1997). The effects of dietary boron on bone strength in rats. Fundamental and applied toxicology : official journal of the Society of Toxicology, 35(2), 205–215. https://doi.org/10.1006/faat.1996.2275

[3536] Armstrong, T. A., Spears, J. W., Crenshaw, T. D., & Nielsen, F. H. (2000). Boron supplementation of a semipurified diet for weanling pigs improves feed efficiency and bone strength characteristics and alters plasma lipid metabolites. The Journal of nutrition, 130(10), 2575–2581. https://doi.org/10.1093/jn/130.10.2575

[3537] Pinto et al (1978) 'Increased urinary riboflavin excretion resulting from boric acid ingestion', Journal of Laboratory and Clinical Medicine 92(1):126-34.

[3538] Köse, D. A., Zumreoglu-Karan, B., Sahin, O., & Büyükgüngör, O. (2014). Boric acid complexes with thiamine (vitamin B1) and pyridoxine (vitamin B6). Inorganica Chimica Acta, 413, 77–83. doi:10.1016/j.ica.2013.12.045

[3539] Kim, D.H., Faull, K.F. and Eckhert, C.D. (2010), Investigating the Complex Formation between Boron and Riboflavin using Electrospray Ionization Mass Spectrometry and Fluorescence Spectroscopy. FASEB J, 24: 537.13-537.13. https://doi.org/10.1096/fasebj.24.1_supplement.537.13

[3540] Chassard-Bouchaud, C., Galle, P., Escaig, F., & Miyawaki, M. (1984). Bioaccumulation de lithium par les organismes marins des zones côtières européennes, américaines et asiatiques: étude microanalytique par émission ionique secondaire [Bioaccumulation of lithium by marine organisms in European, American, and Asian coastal zones: microanalytic study using secondary ion emission]. Comptes rendus de l'Academie des sciences. Serie III, Sciences de la vie, 299(18), 719–724.

[3541] Birch NJ. Lithium in medicine. In: Berthon G, ed. Handbook of Metal-Ligand Interactions in Biological Fluids. Bioinorganic Medicine, Vol 2. Marcel Dekker. New York, 1995,pp.1274-1281.

[3542] Lieb, J., & Zeff, A. (1978). Lithium treatment of chronic cluster headaches. The British journal of psychiatry : the journal of mental science, 133, 556–558. https://doi.org/10.1192/bjp.133.6.556

[3543] Vanyo L, Vu T, Ramos M, Amin J, Conners S, Bateman R, Tisman G: Lithium induced perturbations of vitamin B12, folic acid and DNA metabolism. In Schrauzer GN, Klippel, KF (eds): Lithium in Biology and Medicine. Weinheim: VCH Verlag, pp 17–30, 1991.

[3544] Schrauzer, G. N., & Shrestha, K. P. (1990). Lithium in drinking water and the incidences of crimes, suicides, and arrests related to drug addictions. Biological trace element research, 25(2), 105–113. https://doi.org/10.1007/BF02990271

[3545] Dawson EB (1991) The relationship of tap water and physiological levels of lithium to mental hospital admission and homicide in Texas. In: Schrauzer GN, Klippel KF (eds) Lithium in biology and medicine. VCH Verlag, Weinheim, pp 171–187

[3546] Dawson, E. B., Moore, T. D., & McGanity, W. J. (1972). Relationship of lithium metabolism to mental hospital admission and homicide. Diseases of the nervous system, 33(8), 546–556.

[3547] Schrauzer, G. N., & de Vroey, E. (1994). Effects of nutritional lithium supplementation on mood. Biological Trace Element Research, 40(1), 89–101. doi:10.1007/bf02916824

[3548] Anke M, Arnhold W, Groppel B, Krause U. The biological importance of lithium. In: Schrauzer GN, Klippel K-F, eds. Lithium in Biology and Medicine. VCH Publishers, Weinheim, 1990,pp.148-167.

[3549] Patt, E. L., Pickett, E. E., & O'Dell, B. L. (1978). Effect of dietary lithium levels on tissue lithium concentrations, growth rate, and reproduction in the rat. Bioinorganic Chemistry, 9(4), 299–310. doi:10.1016/s0006-3061(00)80024-1

[3550] Anke M, Grlin M, Groppel B, Kronemann H. The biological importance oflithium. In: Anke M, Schneider H-J, eds. Mengen-und Spurenelemente. Karl-Marx- Universitat, Leipzig, 1981,pp:217-239.

[3551] Yacobi, S., & Ornoy, A. (2008). Is lithium a real teratogen? What can we conclude from the prospective versus retrospective studies? A review. The Israel journal of psychiatry and related sciences, 45(2), 95–106.

[3552] Rossetti, L., Giaccari, A., Klein-Robbenhaar, E., & Vogel, L. R. (1990). Insulinomimetic properties of trace elements and characterization of their in vivo mode of action. Diabetes, 39(10), 1243–1250. https://doi.org/10.2337/diab.39.10.1243

[3553] Amdisen A. (1977). Serum level monitoring and clinical pharmacokinetics of lithium. Clinical pharmacokinetics, 2(2), 73–92. https://doi.org/10.2165/00003088-197702020-00001

[3554] Birch NJ. Lithium in medicine. In: Berthon G, ed. Handbook of Metal-Ligand Interactions in Biological Fluids. Bioinorganic Medicine, Vol 2. Marcel Dekker, New York, 1995,pp. 1274–1281.

[3555] Schrauzer G. N. (2002). Lithium: occurrence, dietary intakes, nutritional essentiality. Journal of the American College of Nutrition, 21(1), 14–21. https://doi.org/10.1080/07315724.2002.10719188

[3556] Drugs.com (2020) 'Lithium Orotate', Wolters Kluwer Health, Accessed Online Jan 08 2021: https://www.drugs.com/npp/lithium-orotate.html

[3557] Anke M, Arnhold B, Glei M, Mu¨ller M, Illing H, Scha¨fer U, Jaritz M. Essentiality and toxicity of lithium. In T. Kosla (ed): "Lithium in the Trophic Chain Soil-Plant-Animal-Man." Warsaw: Proceedings of International Symposium, 17–42.

[3558] SCHROEDER, H. A., BALASSA, J. J., & TIPTON, I. H. (1963). ABNORMAL TRACE METALS IN MAN--VANADIUM. Journal of chronic diseases, 16, 1047–1071. https://doi.org/10.1016/0021-9681(63)90041-9

[3559] Anke M, Groppel B, Gruhn K, Langer M, Arnhold W. The essentiality of vanadium for animals. In: Anke M, Baumann W, Bräunlich H, Bruckner C, Groppel B, Grün M, eds. 6th International Trace Element Symposium, Vol 1. Friedrich-Schiller-Universitat, Jena, 1989,pp. 17–27.

[3560] Orvig et al (1995) 'Vanadium compounds as insulin mimics.', Metal Ions in Biological Systems, 01 Jan 1995, 31:575-594.

[3561] Boyd, D. W., & Kustin, K. (1984). Vanadium: a versatile biochemical effector with an elusive biological function. Advances in inorganic biochemistry, 6, 311–365.

[3562] Stern, A., Yin, X., Tsang, S. S., Davison, A., & Moon, J. (1993). Vanadium as a modulator of cellular regulatory cascades and oncogene expression. Biochemistry and cell biology = Biochimie et biologie cellulaire, 71(3-4), 103–112. https://doi.org/10.1139/o93-018

[3563] Carmignani M, Boscolo P, Ripanti G, Porcelli G, Volpe AR. Mechanisms of the vanadate-induced arterial hypertension only in part depend on the levels of exposure. In: Anke M, Meissner D, Mills CF, eds. Trace Elements in Man and Animals–TEMA 8. Verlag Media Touristik, Gersdorf, 1993,pp. 971–975.

[3564] Cohen, N., Halberstam, M., Shlimovich, P., Chang, C. J., Shamoon, H., & Rossetti, L. (1995). Oral vanadyl sulfate improves hepatic and peripheral insulin sensitivity in patients with non-insulin-dependent diabetes mellitus. The Journal of clinical investigation, 95(6), 2501–2509. https://doi.org/10.1172/JCI117951

[3565] Halberstam, M., Cohen, N., Shlimovich, P., Rossetti, L., & Shamoon, H. (1996). Oral Vanadyl Sulfate Improves Insulin Sensitivity in NIDDM but Not in Obese Nondiabetic Subjects. Diabetes, 45(5), 659–666. doi:10.2337/diab.45.5.659

[3566] Goldfine, A. B., Simonson, D. C., Folli, F., Patti, M. E., & Kahn, C. R. (1995). Metabolic effects of sodium metavanadate in humans with insulin-dependent and noninsulin-dependent diabetes mellitus in vivo and in vitro studies. The Journal of clinical endocrinology and metabolism, 80(11), 3311–3320. https://doi.org/10.1210/jcem.80.11.7593444

[3567] Nielsen FH. Other Trace Elements. In: Ziegler EE, Filer LJ Jr, eds. Present Knowledge in Nutrition. ILSI Press, Washington, DC, 1996,pp. 353–376.

[3568] Jiang, P., Ni, Z., Wang, B., Ma, B., Duan, H., Li, X., Ma, X., Wei, Q., Ji, X., Liu, Q., Xing, S., & Li, M. (2017). Acute toxicity, twenty-eight days repeated dose toxicity and genotoxicity of vanadyl trehalose in kunming mice. Regulatory toxicology and pharmacology : RTP, 85, 86–97. https://doi.org/10.1016/j.yrtph.2017.02.001

[3569] Myron, D. R., Zimmerman, T. J., Shuler, T. R., Klevay, L. M., Lee, D. E., & Nielsen, F. H. (1978). Intake of nickel and vanadium by humans. A survey of selected diets. The American journal of clinical nutrition, 31(3), 527–531. https://doi.org/10.1093/ajcn/31.3.527

[3570] Byrne, A. R., & Kosta, L. (1978). Vanadium in foods and in human body fluids and tissues. The Science of the total environment, 10(1), 17–30. https://doi.org/10.1016/0048-9697(78)90046-3

[3571] Myron, D. R., Givand, S. H., & Nielsen, F. H. (1977). Vanadium content of selected foods as determined by flameless atomic absorption spectroscopy. Journal of Agricultural and Food Chemistry, 25(2), 297–300. doi:10.1021/jf60210a036

[3572] Spears J. W. (1984). Nickel as a "newer trace element" in the nutrition of domestic animals. Journal of animal science, 59(3), 823–835. https://doi.org/10.2527/jas1984.593823x

[3573] Nielsen, F. H., Shuler, T. R., McLeod, T. G., & Zimmerman, T. J. (1984). Nickel influences iron metabolism through physiologic, pharmacologic and toxicologic mechanisms in the rat. The Journal of nutrition, 114(7), 1280–1288. https://doi.org/10.1093/jn/114.7.1280

[3574] Nielsen, F. H., Uthus, E. O., Poellot, R. A., & Shuler, T. R. (1993). Dietary vitamin B12, sulfur amino acids, and odd-chain fatty acids affect the responses of rats to nickel deprivation. Biological trace element research, 37(1), 1–15. https://doi.org/10.1007/BF02789397

[3575] Nielsen FH, Zimmerman TJ, Shuler TR, Brossait B, Uthus EO. Evidence for a cooperative metabolic relationship between nickel and vitamin Bit in rats. J Trace Elem Exp Med 1989; 2: 21–29.

[3576] Malinow M. R. (1996). Plasma homocyst(e)ine: a risk factor for arterial occlusive diseases. The Journal of nutrition, 126(4 Suppl), 1238S–43S. https://doi.org/10.1093/jn/126.suppl_4.1238S

[3577] Anke M, Angelow L, Müller M, Glei M. Dietary trace element intake and excretion of man. In: Anke M, Meissner D, Mills CF, eds. Trace Elements in Man and Animals-TEMA 8. Verlag Media Touristik, Gersdorf 1993,pp:180–188..

[3578] Cronin E, DiMichiel AD, Brown SS. Oral challenge in nickel-sensitive women with hand eczema. In: Brown SS, Sunderman FW Jr, eds. Nickel Toxicology. Academic Press, New York,1980,pp:149–152..

3579 Pennington, J. A., & Jones, J. W. (1987). Molybdenum, nickel, cobalt, vanadium, and strontium in total diets. Journal of the American Dietetic Association, 87(12), 1644–1650.

3580 Carlisle, E. M. (1981). Silicon in Bone Formation. Silicon and Siliceous Structures in Biological Systems, 69–94. doi:10.1007/978-1-4612-5944-2_4

3581 Seaborn CD, Nielsen FH. Silicon: A nutritional beneficence for bones, brains, and blood vessels? Nutr Today 1993; 28: 13–18.

3582 Carlisle E. M. (1974). Proceedings: Silicon as an essential element. Federation proceedings, 33(6), 1758–1766.

3583 Gouget MA. Athérome expérimental et silicate de soude. La Presse Medicale 1911; 97: 1005–1006.

3584 Nasolodin, V. V., Rusin, V., & Vorob'ev, V. A. (1987). Obmen tsinka i kremniia u sportsmenov vysokoĭ kvalifikatsii pri bol'shikh sportivnykh nagruzkakh [Zinc and silicon metabolism in highly trained athletes during heavy exercise]. Voprosy pitaniia, (4), 37–39.

3585 Kelsay, J. L., Behall, K. M., & Prather, E. S. (1979). Effect of fiber from fruits and vegetables on metabolic responses of human subjects, II. Calcium, magnesium, iron, and silicon balances. The American journal of clinical nutrition, 32(9), 1876–1880. https://doi.org/10.1093/ajcn/32.9.1876

3586 Pennington, J. A. T. (1991). Silicon in foods and diets. Food Additives and Contaminants, 8(1), 97–118. doi:10.1080/02652039109373959

3587 Boyera, N., Galey, I., & Bernard, B. A. (1998). Effect of vitamin C and its derivatives on collagen synthesis and cross-linking by normal human fibroblasts. International journal of cosmetic science, 20(3), 151–158. https://doi.org/10.1046/j.1467-2494.1998.171747.x

3588 Yamada K. (2013). Cobalt: its role in health and disease. Metal ions in life sciences, 13, 295–320. https://doi.org/10.1007/978-94-007-7500-8_9

3589 Christen, W. G., Ajani, U. A., Glynn, R. J., & Hennekens, C. H. (2000). Blood Levels of Homocysteine and Increased Risks of Cardiovascular Disease. Archives of Internal Medicine, 160(4), 422. doi:10.1001/archinte.160.4.422

3590 Daly, C., Fitzgerald, A. P., O'Callaghan, P., Collins, P., Cooney, M. T., Graham, I. M., & COMAC Group (2009). Homocysteine increases the risk associated with hyperlipidaemia. European journal of cardiovascular prevention and rehabilitation : official journal of the European Society of Cardiology, Working Groups on Epidemiology & Prevention and Cardiac Rehabilitation and Exercise Physiology, 16(2), 150–155. https://doi.org/10.1097/HJR.0b013e32831e1185

3591 Clarke, R., Smith, A. D., Jobst, K. A., Refsum, H., Sutton, L., & Ueland, P. M. (1998). Folate, vitamin B12, and serum total homocysteine levels in confirmed Alzheimer disease. Archives of neurology, 55(11), 1449–1455. https://doi.org/10.1001/archneur.55.11.1449

3592 McDowell, Lee Russell (2008). Vitamins in Animal and Human Nutrition (2nd ed.). Hoboken: John Wiley & Sons. p. 525.

3593 Snook, Laurence C. (1962). "Cobalt : its use to control wasting disease". Journal of the Department of Agriculture, Western Australia. 4. 3 (11): 844–852.

3594 Vieira-Makings, E., Metz, J., Van der Westhuyzen, J., Bottiglieri, T., & Chanarin, I. (1990). Cobalamin neuropathy. Is S-adenosylhomocysteine toxicity a factor?. The Biochemical journal, 266(3), 707–711. https://doi.org/10.1042/bj2660707

3595 Watanabe, T., Kaji, R., Oka, N., Bara, W., & Kimura, J. (1994). Ultra-high dose methylcobalamin promotes nerve regeneration in experimental acrylamide neuropathy. Journal of the neurological sciences, 122(2), 140–143. https://doi.org/10.1016/0022-510x(94)90290-9

3596 NIH (2021) 'Pernicious Anemia', Accessed Online Feb 16 2021: https://www.nhlbi.nih.gov/health-topics/pernicious-anemia

3597 Chan, C. Q., Low, L. L., & Lee, K. H. (2016). Oral Vitamin B12 Replacement for the Treatment of Pernicious Anemia. Frontiers in medicine, 3, 38. https://doi.org/10.3389/fmed.2016.00038

3598 Roth (2016) 'DRI / RDA for Nickel and Cobalt + Vit C - E - B12 - B15', Dr. Ronald Roth's Research Library on Cellular Nutrition and Health Disorders, Cellular Nutrition, Accessed Online Feb 16 2021: https://acu-cell.com/nico2.html

3599 NIH (2020) 'Vitamin B12: Fact Sheet for Health Professionals', Accessed Online Feb 16 2021: https://ods.od.nih.gov/factsheets/VitaminB12-HealthProfessional/

3600 Donaldson, J.D. and Beyersmann, D. (2005). Cobalt and Cobalt Compounds. In Ullmann's Encyclopedia of Industrial Chemistry, (Ed.). https://doi.org/10.1002/14356007.a07_281.pub2

3601 Morin, Y., Têtu, A., & Mercier, G. (1969). Québec beer-drinkers' cardiomyopathy: clinical and hemodynamic aspects. Annals of the New York Academy of Sciences, 156(1), 566–576. https://doi.org/10.1111/j.1749-6632.1969.tb16751.x

3602 Bendell L. I. (2009). Survey of levels of cadmium in oysters, mussels, clams and scallops from the Pacific Northwest coast of Canada. Food additives & contaminants. Part B, Surveillance, 2(2), 131–139. https://doi.org/10.1080/19440040903367765

3603 Copes, R., Clark, N. A., Rideout, K., Palaty, J., & Teschke, K. (2008). Uptake of cadmium from Pacific oysters (Crassostrea gigas) in British Columbia oyster growers. Environmental research, 107(2), 160–169. https://doi.org/10.1016/j.envres.2008.01.014

[3604] Kruzynski G. M. (2004). Cadmium in oysters and scallops: the BC experience. Toxicology letters, 148(3), 159–169. https://doi.org/10.1016/j.toxlet.2003.10.030

[3605] Bach, L., Sonne, C., Rigét, F. F., Dietz, R., & Asmund, G. (2014). A simple method to reduce the risk of cadmium exposure from consumption of Iceland scallops (Chlamys islandica) fished in Greenland. Environment international, 69, 100–103. https://doi.org/10.1016/j.envint.2014.04.008

[3606] Bendell L. I. (2010). Cadmium in shellfish: the British Columbia, Canada experience--a mini-review. Toxicology letters, 198(1), 7–12. https://doi.org/10.1016/j.toxlet.2010.04.012

[3607] Ziegler (1996) 'Present Knowledge in Nutrition, 7th ed.', Washington, DC: International Life Sciences Institute.

[3608] Baker (2007) 'The dehydration of sucrose', Education in Chemistry, Royal Society of Chemistry, Accessed Online Jan 19 2021: https://edu.rsc.org/exhibition-chemistry/the-dehydration-of-sucrose/2020073.article

[3609] Madhu (2013) 'Difference Between Sulfur, Sulfate and Sulfite', Chemistry, Difference.com, Accessed Online Jan 15 2021: https://www.differencebetween.com/difference-between-sulfur-and-vs-sulfate-and-vs-sulfite/

[3610] Gupta, A. K., & Nicol, K. (2004). The use of sulfur in dermatology. Journal of drugs in dermatology : JDD, 3(4), 427–431.

[3611] Yunming, Z. (1986). Ancient Chinese Sulfur Manufacturing Processes. Isis, 77(3), 487–497. doi:10.1086/354207

[3612] Lin, A. N., Reimer, R. J., & Carter, D. M. (1988). Sulfur revisited. Journal of the American Academy of Dermatology, 18(3), 553–558. doi:10.1016/s0190-9622(88)70079-1

[3613] Tarimci, N., Sener, S., & Kilinç, T. (1997). Topical sodium sulfacetamide/sulfur lotion. Journal of clinical pharmacy and therapeutics, 22(4), 301. https://doi.org/10.1046/j.1365-2710.1997.9975099.x

[3614] Berardesca, E., Cameli, N., Cavallotti, C., Levy, J. L., Piérard, G. E., & de Paoli Ambrosi, G. (2008). Combined effects of silymarin and methylsulfonylmethane in the management of rosacea: clinical and instrumental evaluation. Journal of cosmetic dermatology, 7(1), 8–14. https://doi.org/10.1111/j.1473-2165.2008.00355.x

[3615] Verhagen, A. P., Bierma-Zeinstra, S. M., Boers, M., Cardoso, J. R., Lambeck, J., de Bie, R., & de Vet, H. C. (2007). Balneotherapy for osteoarthritis. Cochrane Database of Systematic Reviews. doi:10.1002/14651858.cd006864

[3616] Costantino, M., Filippelli, A., Quenau, P., Nicolas, J.-P., & Coiro, V. (2012). Rôle de l'eau minérale sulfurée dans la SPA thérapie de l'arthrose. Therapies, 67(1), 43–48. doi:10.2515/therapie/2012002

[3617] Salami, A. (2010). Sulphurous thermal water inhalations in the treatment of chronic rhinosinusitis. Rhinology Journal, 48(1). doi:10.4193/rhin09.065

[3618] Yamagishi, S., & Matsui, T. (2016). Protective role of sulphoraphane against vascular complications in diabetes. Pharmaceutical biology, 54(10), 2329–2339. https://doi.org/10.3109/13880209.2016.1138314

[3619] Zhang, X., Shu, X. O., Xiang, Y. B., Yang, G., Li, H., Gao, J., Cai, H., Gao, Y. T., & Zheng, W. (2011). Cruciferous vegetable consumption is associated with a reduced risk of total and cardiovascular disease mortality. The American journal of clinical nutrition, 94(1), 240–246. https://doi.org/10.3945/ajcn.110.009340

[3620] Olson K. R. (2012). Mitochondrial adaptations to utilize hydrogen sulfide for energy and signaling. Journal of comparative physiology. B, Biochemical, systemic, and environmental physiology, 182(7), 881–897. https://doi.org/10.1007/s00360-012-0654-y

[3621] Overmann, J., & van Gemerden, H. (2000). Microbial interactions involving sulfur bacteria: implications for the ecology and evolution of bacterial communities. FEMS microbiology reviews, 24(5), 591–599. https://doi.org/10.1111/j.1574-6976.2000.tb00560.x

[3622] Kletzin, A., Urich, T., Müller, F., Bandeiras, T. M., & Gomes, C. M. (2004). Dissimilatory Oxidation and Reduction of Elemental Sulfur in Thermophilic Archaea. Journal of Bioenergetics and Biomembranes, 36(1), 77–91. doi:10.1023/b:jobb.0000019600.36757.8c

[3623] Barton, L. L., & Fauque, G. D. (2009). Biochemistry, physiology and biotechnology of sulfate-reducing bacteria. Advances in applied microbiology, 68, 41–98. https://doi.org/10.1016/S0065-2164(09)01202-7

[3624] Muyzer G, Stams AJ. 2008. The ecology and biotechnology of sulphate-reducing bacteria. Nat. Rev. Microbiol. 6:441–54

[3625] Ghosh, W., & Dam, B. (2009). Biochemistry and molecular biology of lithotrophic sulfur oxidation by taxonomically and ecologically diverse bacteria and archaea. FEMS microbiology reviews, 33(6), 999–1043. https://doi.org/10.1111/j.1574-6976.2009.00187.x

[3626] Kabil, O., Vitvitsky, V., & Banerjee, R. (2014). Sulfur as a signaling nutrient through hydrogen sulfide. Annual review of nutrition, 34, 171–205. https://doi.org/10.1146/annurev-nutr-071813-105654

[3627] DiNicolantonio, J. J., OKeefe, J. H., & McCarty, M. F. (2017). Boosting endogenous production of vasoprotective hydrogen sulfide via supplementation with taurine and N-acetylcysteine: a novel way to promote cardiovascular health. Open Heart, 4(1), e000600. doi:10.1136/openhrt-2017-000600

[3628] McCarty, M. F., O'Keefe, J. H., & DiNicolantonio, J. J. (2019). A diet rich in taurine, cysteine, folate, B12 and betaine may lessen risk for Alzheimer's disease by boosting brain synthesis of hydrogen sulfide. Medical hypotheses, 132, 109356. https://doi.org/10.1016/j.mehy.2019.109356

[3629] Bos, E. M., van Goor, H., Joles, J. A., Whiteman, M., & Leuvenink, H. G. (2015). Hydrogen sulfide: physiological properties and therapeutic potential in ischaemia. British journal of pharmacology, 172(6), 1479–1493. https://doi.org/10.1111/bph.12869

[3630] DUPERRON, S., GUEZI, H., GAUDRON, S. M., POP RISTOVA, P., WENZHÖFER, F., & BOETIUS, A. (2011). Relative abundances of methane- and sulphur-oxidising symbionts in the gills of a cold seep mussel and link to their potential energy sources. Geobiology, 9(6), 481–491. doi:10.1111/j.1472-4669.2011.00300.x

[3631] Arndt, C., Gaill, F., & Felbeck, H. (2001). Anaerobic sulfur metabolism in thiotrophic symbioses. The Journal of experimental biology, 204(Pt 4), 741–750.

[3632] Szabo, C., Ransy, C., Módis, K., Andriamihaja, M., Murghes, B., Coletta, C., Olah, G., Yanagi, K., & Bouillaud, F. (2014). Regulation of mitochondrial bioenergetic function by hydrogen sulfide. Part I. Biochemical and physiological mechanisms. British journal of pharmacology, 171(8), 2099–2122. https://doi.org/10.1111/bph.12369

[3633] Grimble R. F. (2006). The effects of sulfur amino acid intake on immune function in humans. The Journal of nutrition, 136(6 Suppl), 1660S–1665S. https://doi.org/10.1093/jn/136.6.1660S

[3634] Courtney-Martin and Pencharz (2016) 'Chapter 19 - Sulfur Amino Acids Metabolism From Protein Synthesis to Glutathione', The Molecular Nutrition of Amino Acids and Proteins, 2016, Pages 265-286.

[3635] Speiser, A., Silbermann, M., Dong, Y., Haberland, S., Uslu, V. V., Wang, S., Bangash, S., Reichelt, M., Meyer, A. J., Wirtz, M., & Hell, R. (2018). Sulfur Partitioning between Glutathione and Protein Synthesis Determines Plant Growth. Plant physiology, 177(3), 927–937. https://doi.org/10.1104/pp.18.00421

[3636] Bahadoran, Z., Mirmiran, P., Hosseinpanah, F., Hedayati, M., Hosseinpour-Niazi, S., & Azizi, F. (2011). Broccoli sprouts reduce oxidative stress in type 2 diabetes: a randomized double-blind clinical trial. European journal of clinical nutrition, 65(8), 972–977. https://doi.org/10.1038/ejcn.2011.59

[3637] Bogaards, J. J., Verhagen, H., Willems, M. I., van Poppel, G., & van Bladeren, P. J. (1994). Consumption of Brussels sprouts results in elevated alpha-class glutathione S-transferase levels in human blood plasma. Carcinogenesis, 15(5), 1073–1075. https://doi.org/10.1093/carcin/15.5.1073

[3638] Moore, L. E., Brennan, P., Karami, S., Hung, R. J., Hsu, C., Boffetta, P., Toro, J., Zaridze, D., Janout, V., Bencko, V., Navratilova, M., Szeszenia-Dabrowska, N., Mates, D., Mukeria, A., Holcatova, I., Welch, R., Chanock, S., Rothman, N., & Chow, W. H. (2007). Glutathione S-transferase polymorphisms, cruciferous vegetable intake and cancer risk in the Central and Eastern European Kidney Cancer Study. Carcinogenesis, 28(9), 1960–1964. https://doi.org/10.1093/carcin/bgm151

[3639] Margalit, A., Hauser, S. D., Zweifel, B. S., Anderson, M. A., & Isakson, P. C. (1998). Regulation of prostaglandin biosynthesis in vivo by glutathione. The American journal of physiology, 274(2), R294–R302. https://doi.org/10.1152/ajpregu.1998.274.2.R294

[3640] Honda, Y., Kessoku, T., Sumida, Y., Kobayashi, T., Kato, T., Ogawa, Y., … Nakajima, A. (2017). Efficacy of glutathione for the treatment of nonalcoholic fatty liver disease: an open-label, single-arm, multicenter, pilot study. BMC Gastroenterology, 17(1). doi:10.1186/s12876-017-0652-3

[3641] Scheidleder, B., Holzer, F., & Marktl, W. (2000). Einfluss von Schwefeltrinkkuren auf Parameter des Lipidstoffwechsels, den antioxidativen Status und die Konzentration von Peroxiden bei Kurpatienten [Effect of sulfur administration on lipid levels, antioxidant status and peroxide concentration in health resort patients]. Forschende Komplementarmedizin und klassische Naturheilkunde = Research in complementary and natural classical medicine, 7(2), 75–78. https://doi.org/10.1159/000021313

[3642] Ekmekcioglu, C., Strauss-Blasche, G., Holzer, F., & Marktl, W. (2002). Effect of Sulfur Baths on Antioxidative Defense Systems, Peroxide Concentrations and Lipid Levels in Patients with Degenerative Osteoarthritis. Complementary Medicine Research, 9(4), 216–220. doi:10.1159/000066031

[3643] Hoshi, T., & Heinemann, S. (2001). Regulation of cell function by methionine oxidation and reduction. The Journal of physiology, 531(Pt 1), 1–11. https://doi.org/10.1111/j.1469-7793.2001.0001j.x

[3644] Dröge, W., Kinscherf, R., Hildebrandt, W., & Schmitt, T. (2006). The deficit in low molecular weight thiols as a target for antiageing therapy. Current drug targets, 7(11), 1505–1512. https://doi.org/10.2174/138945010607011505

[3645] Dröge W. (2005). Oxidative stress and ageing: is ageing a cysteine deficiency syndrome?. Philosophical transactions of the Royal Society of London. Series B, Biological sciences, 360(1464), 2355–2372. https://doi.org/10.1098/rstb.2005.1770

[3646] Brzóska, K., Meczyńska, S., & Kruszewski, M. (2006). Iron-sulfur cluster proteins: electron transfer and beyond. Acta biochimica Polonica, 53(4), 685–691.

[3647] Rouault T. A. (2012). Biogenesis of iron-sulfur clusters in mammalian cells: new insights and relevance to human disease. Disease models & mechanisms, 5(2), 155–164. https://doi.org/10.1242/dmm.009019

695

[3648] Guan, P., & Wang, N. (2014). Mammalian target of rapamycin coordinates iron metabolism with iron-sulfur cluster assembly enzyme and tristetraprolin. Nutrition (Burbank, Los Angeles County, Calif.), 30(9), 968–974. https://doi.org/10.1016/j.nut.2013.12.016

[3649] Sancak, Y. et al (2008) 'The Rag GTPases bind raptor and mediate amino acid signaling to mTORC1', Science, Vol 320(5882), p 1496-501.

[3650] Wolfson, RL. et al (2016) 'Sestrin2 is a leucine sensor for the mTORC1 pathway', Science, Vol 351(6268), p 43-8.

[3651] Nimni, M. E., Han, B., & Cordoba, F. (2007). Are we getting enough sulfur in our diet? Nutrition & Metabolism, 4(1), 24. doi:10.1186/1743-7075-4-24

[3652] Dröge, W., & Holm, E. (1997). Role of cysteine and glutathione in HIV infection and other diseases associated with muscle wasting and immunological dysfunction. FASEB journal : official publication of the Federation of American Societies for Experimental Biology, 11(13), 1077–1089. https://doi.org/10.1096/fasebj.11.13.9367343

[3653] Martensson and Meister (1989) 'Mitochondrial damage in muscle occurs after marked depletion of glutathione and is prevented by giving glutathione monoester', PNAS January 1, 1989 86 (2) 471-475; https://doi.org/10.1073/pnas.86.2.471

[3654] Roth (2016) 'Low Sulfur Levels in Alzheimer's Disease', Acu-Cell, Disorders, Accessed Online Jan 19 2021: https://acu-cell.com/dis-alz.html

[3655] Christen, Y. (2000). Oxidative stress and Alzheimer disease. The American Journal of Clinical Nutrition, 71(2), 621S–629S. doi:10.1093/ajcn/71.2.621s

[3656] Bonda, D. J., Wang, X., Perry, G., Nunomura, A., Tabaton, M., Zhu, X., & Smith, M. A. (2010). Oxidative stress in Alzheimer disease: a possibility for prevention. Neuropharmacology, 59(4-5), 290–294. https://doi.org/10.1016/j.neuropharm.2010.04.005

[3657] Tomljenovic L. (2011). Aluminum and Alzheimer's disease: after a century of controversy, is there a plausible link?. Journal of Alzheimer's disease : JAD, 23(4), 567–598. https://doi.org/10.3233/JAD-2010-101494

[3658] Mirza, A., King, A., Troakes, C., & Exley, C. (2017). Aluminium in brain tissue in familial Alzheimer's disease. Journal of Trace Elements in Medicine and Biology, 40, 30–36. doi:10.1016/j.jtemb.2016.12.001

[3659] The Sulphur Institute 'Sulphur and the Human Body', www.sulphurinstitute.org, Accessed Online Jan 28 2021: https://www.sulphurinstitute.org/pub/?id=8c64bf34-bc30-5bd9-0719-f6de83f7e841

[3660] Axelson M. (1985). 25-Hydroxyvitamin D3 3-sulphate is a major circulating form of vitamin D in man. FEBS letters, 191(2), 171–175. https://doi.org/10.1016/0014-5793(85)80002-8

[3661] Nagubandi, S., Londowski, J. M., Bollman, S., Tietz, P., & Kumar, R. (1981). Synthesis and biological activity of vitamin D3 3 beta-sulfate. Role of vitamin D3 sulfates in calcium homeostasis. The Journal of biological chemistry, 256(11), 5536–5539.

[3662] Reeve, L. E., DeLuca, H. F., & Schnoes, H. K. (1981). Synthesis and biological activity of vitamin D3-sulfate. The Journal of biological chemistry, 256(2), 823–826.

[3663] Lakdawala, D., & Widdowson, E. (1977). VITAMIN-D IN HUMAN MILK. The Lancet, 309(8004), 167–168. doi:10.1016/s0140-6736(77)91764-0

[3664] Roberts, K.D. and Lieberman, S. (1970) in: Chemical and Biological Aspects of Steroid Conjugation (Bernstein, S. and Solomon, S. eds) pp.219-290, Springer, Berlin.

[3665] Kawabe, S., Ikuta, T., Ohba, M., Chida, K., Ueda, E., Yamanishi, K., & Kuroki, T. (1998). Cholesterol sulfate activates transcription of transglutaminase 1 gene in normal human keratinocytes. The Journal of investigative dermatology, 111(6), 1098–1102. https://doi.org/10.1046/j.1523-1747.1998.00441.x

[3666] Jetten, A. M., George, M. A., Nervi, C., Boone, L. R., & Rearick, J. I. (1989). Increased cholesterol sulfate and cholesterol sulfotransferase activity in relation to the multi-step process of differentiation in human epidermal keratinocytes. The Journal of investigative dermatology, 92(2), 203–209. https://doi.org/10.1111/1523-1747.ep12276731

[3667] Merten, M., Dong, J. F., Lopez, J. A., & Thiagarajan, P. (2001). Cholesterol Sulfate. Circulation, 103(16), 2032–2034. doi:10.1161/01.cir.103.16.2032

[3668] Hanyu, O., Nakae, H., Miida, T., Higashi, Y., Fuda, H., Endo, M., Kohjitani, A., Sone, H., & Strott, C. A. (2012). Cholesterol sulfate induces expression of the skin barrier protein filaggrin in normal human epidermal keratinocytes through induction of RORα. Biochemical and biophysical research communications, 428(1), 99–104. https://doi.org/10.1016/j.bbrc.2012.10.013

[3669] McGrath, J. A., & Uitto, J. (2008). The filaggrin story: novel insights into skin-barrier function and disease. Trends in molecular medicine, 14(1), 20–27. https://doi.org/10.1016/j.molmed.2007.10.006

[3670] Sandilands, A., Sutherland, C., Irvine, A. D., & McLean, W. H. I. (2009). Filaggrin in the frontline: role in skin barrier function and disease. Journal of Cell Science, 122(9), 1285–1294. doi:10.1242/jcs.033969

[3671] Kitson, N., Monck, M., Wong, K., Thewalt, J., & Cullis, P. (1992). The influence of cholesterol 3-sulphate on phase behaviour and hydrocarbon order in model membrane systems. Biochimica et biophysica acta, 1111(1), 127–133. https://doi.org/10.1016/0005-2736(92)90282-q

[3672] Cheetham, J. J., R. M. Epand, M. Andrews, and T. D. Flanagan. 1990. Cholesterol sulfate inhibits the fusion of Sendai virus to biological and model membranes. J. Biol. Chem. 265: 12404–12409.

[3673] Roberts, K. D. (1987). Sterol sulfates in the epididymis; synthesis and possible function in the reproductive process. Journal of Steroid Biochemistry, 27(1-3), 337–341. doi:10.1016/0022-4731(87)90325-6

[3674] Williams, M. L., Hughes-Fulford, M., & Elias, P. M. (1985). Inhibition of 3-hydroxy-3-methylglutaryl coenzyme A reductase activity and sterol synthesis by cholesterol sulfate in cultured fibroblasts. Biochimica et biophysica acta, 845(3), 349–357. https://doi.org/10.1016/0167-4889(85)90198-3

[3675] Seneff, S., Davidson, R. M., Lauritzen, A., Samsel, A., & Wainwright, G. (2015). A novel hypothesis for atherosclerosis as a cholesterol sulfate deficiency syndrome. Theoretical biology & medical modelling, 12, 9. https://doi.org/10.1186/s12976-015-0006-1

[3676] Hochberg, R. B., S. Ladany, M. Welch, and S. Lieberman. 1974. Cholesterol and cholesterol sulfate as substrates for the adrenal side-chain cleavage enzyme. Biochemistry. 13: 1938–1945.

[3677] Roberts, K. D., Bandy, L., & Lieberman, S. (1967). The conversion of cholesterol-3H-sulfate-35S into pregnenolone-3H-sulfate-35S by sonicated bovine adrenal mitochondria. Biochemical and Biophysical Research Communications, 29(5), 741–746. doi:10.1016/0006-291x(67)90280-x

[3678] ROBERTS, K. D., BANDI, L., CALVIN, H. I., DRUCKER, W. D., & LIEBERMAN, S. (1964). EVIDENCE THAT STEROID SULFATES SERVE AS BIOSYNTHETIC INTERMEDIATES. IV. CONVERSION OF CHOLESTEROL SULFATE IN VIVO TO URINARY C-19 AND C-21 STEROIDAL SULFATES. Biochemistry, 3, 1983–1988. https://doi.org/10.1021/bi00900a034

[3679] Seo, Y. K., Mirkheshti, N., Song, C. S., Kim, S., Dodds, S., Ahn, S. C., Christy, B., Mendez-Meza, R., Ittmann, M. M., Abboud-Werner, S., & Chatterjee, B. (2013). SULT2B1b sulfotransferase: induction by vitamin D receptor and reduced expression in prostate cancer. Molecular endocrinology (Baltimore, Md.), 27(6), 925–939. https://doi.org/10.1210/me.2012-1369

[3680] de Agostini et al (2008) 'Human Follicular Fluid Heparan Sulfate Contains Abundant 3-O-Sulfated Chains with Anticoagulant Activity*', GLYCOBIOLOGY AND EXTRACELLULAR MATRICES, VOLUME 283, ISSUE 42, P28115-28124, OCTOBER 17, 2008

[3681] Cooper ID, Crofts CAP, DiNicolantonio JJ, et alRelationships between hyperinsulinaemia, magnesium, vitamin D, thrombosis and COVID-19: rationale for clinical managementOpen Heart 2020;7:e001356. doi: 10.1136/openhrt-2020-001356

[3682] Merten, M., Dong, J. F., Lopez, J. A., & Thiagarajan, P. (2001). Cholesterol sulfate: a new adhesive molecule for platelets. Circulation, 103(16), 2032–2034. https://doi.org/10.1161/01.cir.103.16.2032

[3683] Iwamori, M., Y. Iwamori, and N. Ito. 1999. Regulation of the activities of thrombin and plasmin by cholesterol sulfate as a physiological inhibitor in human plasma. J. Biol. Chem. 125: 594–601.

[3684] Goldberg I. J. (1996). Lipoprotein lipase and lipolysis: central roles in lipoprotein metabolism and atherogenesis. Journal of lipid research, 37(4), 693–707.

[3685] Hartman and Kilianska (2012) 'Lipoprotein lipase; a new prognostic factor in chronic lymphocytic leukemia', Wspolczesna Onkol 2012; 16 (5): 474–479. DOI: https://doi.org/10.5114/wo.2012.32476

[3686] Myocardial Infarction Genetics and CARDIoGRAM Exome Consortia Investigators, Stitziel, N. O., Stirrups, K. E., Masca, N. G., Erdmann, J., Ferrario, P. G., König, I. R., Weeke, P. E., Webb, T. R., Auer, P. L., Schick, U. M., Lu, Y., Zhang, H., Dube, M. P., Goel, A., Farrall, M., Peloso, G. M., Won, H. H., Do, R., van Iperen, E., … Schunkert, H. (2016). Coding Variation in ANGPTL4, LPL, and SVEP1 and the Risk of Coronary Disease. The New England journal of medicine, 374(12), 1134–1144. https://doi.org/10.1056/NEJMoa1507652

[3687] Xie, C., Wang, Z., Liu, X. et al. The common biological basis for common complex diseases: evidence from lipoprotein lipase gene. Eur J Hum Genet 18, 3–7 (2010). https://doi.org/10.1038/ejhg.2009.134

[3688] Kersten, S. (2014). Physiological regulation of lipoprotein lipase. Biochimica et biophysica acta, 1841 7, 919-33 .

[3689] Saari, T. J., Raiko, J., U-Din, M., Niemi, T., Taittonen, M., Laine, J., … Virtanen, K. A. (2020). Basal and cold-induced fatty acid uptake of human brown adipose tissue is impaired in obesity. Scientific Reports, 10(1). doi:10.1038/s41598-020-71197-2

[3690] Inoue et al (2006) 'Compartmentalization of the exocyst complex in lipid rafts controls Glut4 vesicle tethering.', Molecular Biology of the Cell, 08 Mar 2006, 17(5):2303-2311, DOI: 10.1091/mbc.e06-01-0030.

[3691] Yamagishi, S., Matsui, T., Ueda, S., Nakamura, K., & Imaizumi, T. (2007). Advanced glycation end products (AGEs) and cardiovascular disease (CVD) in diabetes. Cardiovascular & hematological agents in medicinal chemistry, 5(3), 236–240. https://doi.org/10.2174/187152507781058681

[3692] Brownlee, M., Cerami, A., & Vlassara, H. (1988). Advanced glycosylation end products in tissue and the biochemical basis of diabetic complications. The New England journal of medicine, 318(20), 1315–1321. https://doi.org/10.1056/NEJM198805193182007

[3693] Bodiga, V. L., Eda, S. R., & Bodiga, S. (2014). Advanced glycation end products: role in pathology of diabetic cardiomyopathy. Heart failure reviews, 19(1), 49–63. https://doi.org/10.1007/s10741-013-9374-y

697

[3694] Brownlee M. (2001). Biochemistry and molecular cell biology of diabetic complications. Nature, 414(6865), 813–820. https://doi.org/10.1038/414813a

[3695] Li, Y. M., & Dickson, D. W. (1997). Enhanced binding of advanced glycation endproducts (AGE) by the ApoE4 isoform links the mechanism of plaque deposition in Alzheimer's disease. Neuroscience letters, 226(3), 155–158. https://doi.org/10.1016/s0304-3940(97)00266-8

[3696] Seneff, S., Wainwright, G., & Mascitelli, L. (2011). Is the metabolic syndrome caused by a high fructose, and relatively low fat, low cholesterol diet?. Archives of medical science : AMS, 7(1), 8–20. https://doi.org/10.5114/aoms.2011.20598

[3697] Ma, Y., Xu, L., Rodriguez-Agudo, D., Li, X., Heuman, D. M., Hylemon, P. B., Pandak, W. M., & Ren, S. (2008). 25-Hydroxycholesterol-3-sulfate regulates macrophage lipid metabolism via the LXR/SREBP-1 signaling pathway. American journal of physiology. Endocrinology and metabolism, 295(6), E1369–E1379. https://doi.org/10.1152/ajpendo.90555.2008

[3698] Sharma, A. K., Sharma, V. R., Gupta, G. K., Ashraf, G. M., & Kamal, M. A. (2019). Advanced Glycation End Products (AGEs), Glutathione and Breast Cancer: Factors, Mechanism and Therapeutic Interventions. Current drug metabolism, 20(1), 65–71. https://doi.org/10.2174/1389200219666180912104342

[3699] Loo, M. (2009). Lifestyle Approaches. Integrative Medicine for Children, 37–57. doi:10.1016/b978-141602299-2.10004-0

[3700] Baker D. H. (1986). Utilization of isomers and analogs of amino acids and other sulfur-containing compounds. Progress in food & nutrition science, 10(1-2), 133–178.

[3701] Parcell S. (2002). Sulfur in human nutrition and applications in medicine. Alternative medicine review : a journal of clinical therapeutic, 7(1), 22–44.

[3702] van der Kraan, P. M., Vitters, E. L., de Vries, B. J., & van den Berg, W. B. (1990). High susceptibility of human articular cartilage glycosaminoglycan synthesis to changes in inorganic sulfate availability. Journal of orthopaedic research : official publication of the Orthopaedic Research Society, 8(4), 565–571. https://doi.org/10.1002/jor.1100080413

[3703] McAlindon, T. E., LaValley, M. P., Gulin, J. P., & Felson, D. T. (2000). Glucosamine and chondroitin for treatment of osteoarthritis: a systematic quality assessment and meta-analysis. JAMA, 283(11), 1469–1475. https://doi.org/10.1001/jama.283.11.1469

[3704] King, D. E., & Xiang, J. (2020). Glucosamine/Chondroitin and Mortality in a US NHANES Cohort. The Journal of the American Board of Family Medicine, 33(6), 842–847. doi:10.3122/jabfm.2020.06.200110

[3705] Ma, H., Li, X., Sun, D., Zhou, T., Ley, S. H., Gustat, J., … Qi, L. (2019). Association of habitual glucosamine use with risk of cardiovascular disease: prospective study in UK Biobank. BMJ, l1628. doi:10.1136/bmj.l1628

[3706] Nimni, M., Cordoba, F., Strates, B., & Han, B. (2006). Chondroitin Sulfate and Sulfur Containing Chondroprotective Agents: Is there a Basis for their Pharmacological Action? Current Rheumatology Reviews, 2(2), 137–149. doi:10.2174/157339706776876017

[3707] Kleinman, W. A., & Richie, J. P., Jr (2000). Status of glutathione and other thiols and disulfides in human plasma. Biochemical pharmacology, 60(1), 19–29. https://doi.org/10.1016/s0006-2952(00)00293-8

[3708] Jones, D. P., Kagan, V. E., Aust, S. D., Reed, D. J., & Omaye, S. T. (1995). Impact of nutrients on cellular lipid peroxidation and antioxidant defense system. Fundamental and applied toxicology : official journal of the Society of Toxicology, 26(1), 1–7. https://doi.org/10.1006/faat.1995.1069

[3709] Nguyen, D., Hsu, J. W., Jahoor, F., & Sekhar, R. V. (2014). Effect of increasing glutathione with cysteine and glycine supplementation on mitochondrial fuel oxidation, insulin sensitivity, and body composition in older HIV-infected patients. The Journal of clinical endocrinology and metabolism, 99(1), 169–177. https://doi.org/10.1210/jc.2013-2376

[3710] Dröge and Breitkreutz (1999) 'N-acetyl-cysteine in the therapy of HIV-positive patients', Current Opinion in Clinical Nutrition and Metabolic Care: November 1999 - Volume 2 - Issue 6 - p 493-498.

[3711] Viscomi, C., Burlina, A. B., Dweikat, I., Savoiardo, M., Lamperti, C., Hildebrandt, T., Tiranti, V., & Zeviani, M. (2010). Combined treatment with oral metronidazole and N-acetylcysteine is effective in ethylmalonic encephalopathy. Nature medicine, 16(8), 869–871. https://doi.org/10.1038/nm.2188

[3712] Yarema, M., Chopra, P., Sivilotti, M., Johnson, D., Nettel-Aguirre, A., Bailey, B., Victorino, C., Gosselin, S., Purssell, R., Thompson, M., Spyker, D., & Rumack, B. (2018). Anaphylactoid Reactions to Intravenous N-Acetylcysteine during Treatment for Acetaminophen Poisoning. Journal of medical toxicology : official journal of the American College of Medical Toxicology, 14(2), 120–127. https://doi.org/10.1007/s13181-018-0653-9

[3713] Coulson, J., & Thompson, J. P. (2010). Paracetamol (acetaminophen) attenuates in vitro mast cell and peripheral blood mononucleocyte cell histamine release induced by N-acetylcysteine. Clinical toxicology (Philadelphia, Pa.), 48(2), 111–114. https://doi.org/10.3109/15563650903520959

[3714] Sandilands, E. A., & Bateman, D. N. (2009). Adverse reactions associated with acetylcysteine. Clinical toxicology (Philadelphia, Pa.), 47(2), 81–88. https://doi.org/10.1080/15563650802665587

[3715] Tsikas et al (2014) 'N-Acetylcysteine (NAC) inhibits renal nitrite and nitrate reabsorption in healthy subjects and in patients undergoing cardiac surgery: Risk of nitric oxide (NO) bioavailability loss by NAC?', International Journal of Cardiology 177 (2014) 30–33.

[3716] Chesney (1985) 'Taurine: its biological role and clinical implications.', Advances in Pediatrics, 01 Jan 1985, 32:1-42.

[3717] Kagan et al (1992) 'Dihydrolipoic acid—a universal antioxidant both in the membrane and in the aqueous phase: Reduction of peroxyl, ascorbyl and chromanoxyl radicals, Biochemical Pharmacology, Volume 44, Issue 8, 20 October 1992, Pages 1637-1649.

[3718] Kagan et al (1990) 'Antioxidant effects of ubiquinones in microsomes and mitochondria are mediated by tocopherol recycling', Biochemical and Biophysical Research Communications, Volume 169, Issue 3, 29 June 1990, Pages 851-857.

[3719] Hultberg, B., Andersson, A., & Isaksson, A. (2002). Lipoic acid increases glutathione production and enhances the effect of mercury in human cell lines. Toxicology, 175(1-3), 103–110. https://doi.org/10.1016/s0300-483x(02)00060-4

[3720] Kolb, K.H., Jaenicke, G., Kramer, M. and Schulze, P.E. (1967), ABSORPTION, DISTRIBUTION AND ELIMINATION OF LABELED DIMETHYL SULFOXIDE IN MAN AND ANIMALS. Annals of the New York Academy of Sciences, 141: 85-95. https://doi.org/10.1111/j.1749-6632.1967.tb34869.x

[3721] Jacob, S. W., & Herschler, R. (1983). Dimethyl sulfoxide after twenty years. Annals of the New York Academy of Sciences, 411, xiii–xvii. https://doi.org/10.1111/j.1749-6632.1983.tb4 /276.x

[3722] Fox, R.B. and Fox, W.K. (1983), DIMETHYL SULFOXIDE PREVENTS HYDROXYL RADICAL-MEDIATED DEPOLYMERIZATION OF HYALURONIC ACID*. Annals of the New York Academy of Sciences, 411: 14-18. https://doi.org/10.1111/j.1749-6632.1983.tb47280.x

[3723] Barrager, E., Veltmann, J. R., Schauss, A. G., & Schiller, R. N. (2002). A Multicentered, Open-Label Trial on the Safety and Efficacy of Methylsulfonylmethane in the Treatment of Seasonal Allergic Rhinitis. The Journal of Alternative and Complementary Medicine, 8(2), 167–173. doi:10.1089/107555302317371451

[3724] Brien, S., Prescott, P., Bashir, N., Lewith, H., & Lewith, G. (2008). Systematic review of the nutritional supplements dimethyl sulfoxide (DMSO) and methylsulfonylmethane (MSM) in the treatment of osteoarthritis. Osteoarthritis and Cartilage, 16(11), 1277–1288. doi:10.1016/j.joca.2008.03.002

[3725] Nakhostin-Roohi, B., Niknam, Z., Vaezi, N., Mohammadi, S., & Bohlooli, S. (2013). Effect of single dose administration of methylsulfonylmethane on oxidative stress following acute exhaustive exercise. Iranian journal of pharmaceutical research : IJPR, 12(4), 845–853.

[3726] Withee, E. D., Tippens, K. M., Dehen, R., Tibbitts, D., Hanes, D., & Zwickey, H. (2017). Effects of Methylsulfonylmethane (MSM) on exercise-induced oxidative stress, muscle damage, and pain following a half-marathon: a double-blind, randomized, placebo-controlled trial. Journal of the International Society of Sports Nutrition, 14, 24. https://doi.org/10.1186/s12970-017-0181-z

[3727] Brien, S., Prescott, P., & Lewith, G. (2011). Meta-analysis of the related nutritional supplements dimethyl sulfoxide and methylsulfonylmethane in the treatment of osteoarthritis of the knee. Evidence-based complementary and alternative medicine : eCAM, 2011, 528403. https://doi.org/10.1093/ecam/nep045

[3728] Ahn, H., Kim, J., Lee, M. J., Kim, Y. J., Cho, Y. W., & Lee, G. S. (2015). Methylsulfonylmethane inhibits NLRP3 inflammasome activation. Cytokine, 71(2), 223–231. https://doi.org/10.1016/j.cyto.2014.11.001

[3729] Joksimovic, N., Spasovski, G., Joksimovic, V., Andreevski, V., Zuccari, C., & Omini, C. F. (2012). Efficacy and tolerability of hyaluronic acid, tea tree oil and methyl-sulfonyl-methane in a new gel medical device for treatment of haemorrhoids in a double-blind, placebo-controlled clinical trial. Updates in surgery, 64(3), 195–201. https://doi.org/10.1007/s13304-012-0153-4

[3730] Sousa-Lima, I., Park, S. Y., Chung, M., Jung, H. J., Kang, M. C., Gaspar, J. M., Seo, J. A., Macedo, M. P., Park, K. S., Mantzoros, C., Lee, S. H., & Kim, Y. B. (2016). Methylsulfonylmethane (MSM), an organosulfur compound, is effective against obesity-induced metabolic disorders in mice. Metabolism: clinical and experimental, 65(10), 1508–1521. https://doi.org/10.1016/j.metabol.2016.07.007

[3731] Chiang, P. K., Gordon, R. K., Tal, J., Zeng, G. C., Doctor, B. P., Pardhasaradhi, K., & McCann, P. P. (1996). S-Adenosylmethionine and methylation. FASEB journal : official publication of the Federation of American Societies for Experimental Biology, 10(4), 471–480.

[3732] Richmond, V. L. (1986). Incorporation of methylsulfonylmethane sulfur into guinea pig serum proteins. Life Sciences, 39(3), 263–268. doi:10.1016/0024-3205(86)90540-0

[3733] Uden, S., Bilton, D., Nathan, L., Hunt, L. P., Main, C., & Braganza, J. M. (1990). Antioxidant therapy for recurrent pancreatitis: placebo-controlled trial. Alimentary pharmacology & therapeutics, 4(4), 357–371. https://doi.org/10.1111/j.1365-2036.1990.tb00482.x

[3734] Müller et al (1996) 'Elevated plasma concentration of reduced homocysteine in patients with human immunodeficiency virus infection', The American Journal of Clinical Nutrition, Volume 63, Issue 2, February 1996, Pages 242–248, https://doi.org/10.1093/ajcn/63.2.242

[3735] Prescott L. F. (1981). Treatment of severe acetaminophen poisoning with intravenous acetylcysteine. Archives of internal medicine, 141(3 Spec No), 386–389. https://doi.org/10.1001/archinte.141.3.386

[3736] Flanagan, R. J., & Meredith, T. J. (1991). Use of N-acetylcysteine in clinical toxicology. The American Journal of Medicine, 91(3), S131–S139. doi:10.1016/0002-9343(91)90296-a

[3737] Grandjean, E. M., Berthet, P. H., Ruffmann, R., & Leuenberger, P. (2000). Cost-effectiveness analysis of oral N-acetylcysteine as a preventive treatment in chronic bronchitis. Pharmacological research, 42(1), 39–50. https://doi.org/10.1006/phrs.1999.0647

[3738] Stey, C., Steurer, J., Bachmann, S., Medici, T. C., & Tramèr, M. R. (2000). The effect of oral N-acetylcysteine in chronic bronchitis: a quantitative systematic review. The European respiratory journal, 16(2), 253–262. https://doi.org/10.1034/j.1399-3003.2000.16b12.x

[3739] De Rosa, S. C., Zaretsky, M. D., Dubs, J. G., Roederer, M., Anderson, M., Green, A., Mitra, D., Watanabe, N., Nakamura, H., Tjioe, I., Deresinski, S. C., Moore, W. A., Ela, S. W., Parks, D., Herzenberg, L. A., & Herzenberg, L. A. (2000). N-acetylcysteine replenishes glutathione in HIV infection. European journal of clinical investigation, 30(10), 915–929. https://doi.org/10.1046/j.1365-2362.2000.00736.x

[3740] Akerlund, B., Jarstrand, C., Lindeke, B., Sönnerborg, A., Akerblad, A. C., & Rasool, O. (1996). Effect of N-acetylcysteine(NAC) treatment on HIV-1 infection: a double-blind placebo-controlled trial. European journal of clinical pharmacology, 50(6), 457–461. https://doi.org/10.1007/s002280050140

[3741] de Quay, B., Malinverni, R., & Lauterburg, B. H. (1992). Glutathione depletion in HIV-infected patients: role of cysteine deficiency and effect of oral N-acetylcysteine. AIDS (London, England), 6(8), 815–819.

[3742] ROEDERER, M., ELA, S. W., STAAL, F. J. T., HERZENBERG, L. A., & HERZENBERG, L. A. (1992). N-Acetylcysteine: A New Approach to Anti-HIV Therapy. AIDS Research and Human Retroviruses, 8(2), 209–217. doi:10.1089/aid.1992.8.209

[3743] Baker, D. H., & Czarnecki-Maulden, G. L. (1987). Pharmacologic role of cysteine in ameliorating or exacerbating mineral toxicities. The Journal of nutrition, 117(6), 1003–1010. https://doi.org/10.1093/jn/117.6.1003

[3744] Stephney Whillier, Julia E. Raftos, Bogdan Chapman & Philip W. Kuchel (2009) Role of N-acetylcysteine and cystine in glutathione synthesis in human erythrocytes, Redox Report, 14:3, 115-124, DOI: 10.1179/135100009X392539

[3745] Crome, P., Vale, J. A., Volans, G. N., Widdop, B., & Goulding, R. (1976). Oral methionine in the treatment of severe paracetamol (Acetaminophen) overdose. Lancet (London, England), 2(7990), 829–830. https://doi.org/10.1016/s0140-6736(76)91211-3

[3746] Meininger, V., Flamier, A., Phan, T., Ferris, O., Uzan, A., & Lefur, G. (1982). Traitement de la maladie de Parkinson par la L. méthionine. Premiers résultats [L-Methionine treatment of Parkinson's disease: preliminary results]. Revue neurologique, 138(4), 297–303.

[3747] Tabakoff, B., Eriksson, C.J.P. and von Wartburg, J.-P. (1989), Methionine Lowers Circulating Levels of Acetaldehyde after Ethanol Ingestion. Alcoholism: Clinical and Experimental Research, 13: 164-171. https://doi.org/10.1111/j.1530-0277.1989.tb00304.x

[3748] Azuma, J., Sawamura, A., & Awata, N. (1992). Usefulness of taurine in chronic congestive heart failure and its prospective application. Japanese circulation journal, 56(1), 95–99. https://doi.org/10.1253/jcj.56.95

[3749] Azuma et al (1985), Therapeutic effect of taurine in congestive heart failure: A double-blind crossover trial. Clin Cardiol, 8: 276-282. https://doi.org/10.1002/clc.4960080507

[3750] Franconi, F., Loizzo, A., Ghirlanda, G., & Seghieri, G. (2006). Taurine supplementation and diabetes mellitus. Current opinion in clinical nutrition and metabolic care, 9(1), 32–36. https://doi.org/10.1097/01.mco.0000196141.65362.46

[3751] Militante et al (2000) 'The role of taurine in the pathogenesis of the cardiomyopathy of insulin-dependent diabetes mellitus', Cardiovascular Research, Volume 46, Issue 3, June 2000, Pages 393–402, https://doi.org/10.1016/S0008-6363(00)00025-0

[3752] Devamanoharan, P. S., Ali, A. H., & Varma, S. D. (1997). Prevention of lens protein glycation by taurine. Molecular and cellular biochemistry, 177(1-2), 245–250. https://doi.org/10.1023/a:1006863322454

[3753] Heinämäki, A. A., Muhonen, A. S., & Piha, R. S. (1986). Taurine and other free amino acids in the retina, vitreous, lens, iris-ciliary body, and cornea of the rat eye. Neurochemical research, 11(4), 535–542. https://doi.org/10.1007/BF00965323

[3754] Baskin, S. I., Cohn, E. M., & Kocsis, J. J. (1977). The effect of age on taurine levels in eye tissues. Experimental Eye Research, 24(3), 315–319. doi:10.1016/0014-4835(77)90170-1

[3755] Franconi, F., Bennardini, F., Mattana, A., Miceli, M., Ciuti, M., Milan, M., … Seghieri, G. (1994). Taurine Levels in Plasma and Platelets in Insulin-Dependent and Non-Insulin-Dependent Diabetes Mellitus: Correlation with Platelet Aggregation. Taurine in Health and Disease, 419–424. doi:10.1007/978-1-4899-1471-2_45

[3756] Franconi, F., Bennardini, F., Mattana, A., Miceli, M., Ciuti, M., Mian, M., Gironi, A., Anichini, R., & Seghieri, G. (1995). Plasma and platelet taurine are reduced in subjects with insulin-dependent diabetes mellitus: effects of taurine supplementation. The American journal of clinical nutrition, 61(5), 1115–1119. https://doi.org/10.1093/ajcn/61.4.1115

[3757] Murakami, S., Kondo-Ohta, Y., & Tomisawa, K. (1999). Improvement in cholesterol metabolism in mice given chronic treatment of taurine and fed a high-fat diet. Life sciences, 64(1), 83–91. https://doi.org/10.1016/s0024-3205(98)00536-0

[3758] Chen, W., Guo, J. X., & Chang, P. (2012). The effect of taurine on cholesterol metabolism. Molecular nutrition & food research, 56(5), 681–690. https://doi.org/10.1002/mnfr.201100799

[3759] Anyanwu, E., & Harding, G. F. (1993). The involvement of taurine in the action mechanism of sodium valproate (VPA) in the treatment of epilepsy. Acta physiologica, pharmacologica et therapeutica latinoamericana : organo de la Asociacion Latinoamericana de Ciencias Fisiologicas y [de] la Asociacion Latinoamericana de Farmacologia, 43(1-2), 20–27.

[3760] Marchesi, G. F., Quattrini, A., Scarpino, O., & Dellantonio, R. (1975). Effetti terapeutici della taurina nella epilessia. Indagine clinica e polifisiografica [Therapeutic effects of taurine in epilepsy: a clinical and polyphysiographic study (author's transl)]. Rivista di patologia nervosa e mentale, 96(3), 166–184.

[3761] Oh, S. J., Lee, H. J., Jeong, Y. J., Nam, K. R., Kang, K. J., Han, S. J., Lee, K. C., Lee, Y. J., & Choi, J. Y. (2020). Evaluation of the neuroprotective effect of taurine in Alzheimer's disease using functional molecular imaging. Scientific reports, 10(1), 15551. https://doi.org/10.1038/s41598-020-72755-4

[3762] Jakaria, M., Azam, S., Haque, M. E., Jo, S.-H., Uddin, M. S., Kim, I.-S., & Choi, D.-K. (2019). Taurine and its analogs in neurological disorders: Focus on therapeutic potential and molecular mechanisms. Redox Biology, 24, 101223. doi:10.1016/j.redox.2019.101223

[3763] Carrasco, S., Codoceo, R., Prieto, G., Lama, R., & Polanco, I. (1990). Effect of taurine supplements on growth, fat absorption and bile acid on cystic fibrosis. Acta Universitatis Carolinae. Medica, 36(1-4), 152–156.

[3764] Merli, M., Bertasi, S., Servi, R., Diamanti, S., Martino, F., De Santis, A., Goffredo, F., Quattrucci, S., Antonelli, M., & Angelico, M. (1994). Effect of a medium dose of ursodeoxycholic acid with or without taurine supplementation on the nutritional status of patients with cystic fibrosis: a randomized, placebo-controlled, crossover trial. Journal of pediatric gastroenterology and nutrition, 19(2), 198–203. https://doi.org/10.1097/00005176-199408000-00010

[3765] Smith et al (1991) 'Taurine Decreases Fecal Fatty Acid and Sterol Excretion in Cystic Fibrosis: A Randomized Double-blind Trial', Am J Dis Child. 1991;145(12):1401-1404. doi:10.1001/archpedi.1991.02160120069022

[3766] Tedeschi, M. (1991). The role of glutathione in combination with cisplatin in the treatment of ovarian cancer. Cancer Treatment Reviews, 18(4), 253–259. doi:10.1016/0305-7372(91)90016-s

[3767] Bohm et al (1990) 'Efficacy and safety of high-dose cisplatin and cyclophosphamide with glutathione protection in the treatment of bulky advanced epithelial ovarian cancer', Cancer Chemother. Pharmacol. 25, 355–360 (1990). https://doi.org/10.1007/BF00686237

[3768] Cascinu, S., Cordella, L., Del Ferro, E., Fronzoni, M., & Catalano, G. (1995). Neuroprotective effect of reduced glutathione on cisplatin-based chemotherapy in advanced gastric cancer: a randomized double-blind placebo-controlled trial. Journal of clinical oncology : official journal of the American Society of Clinical Oncology, 13(1), 26–32. https://doi.org/10.1200/JCO.1995.13.1.26

[3769] Julius, M., Lang, C. A., Gleiberman, L., Harburg, E., DiFranceisco, W., & Schork, A. (1994). Glutathione and morbidity in a community-based sample of elderly. Journal of clinical epidemiology, 47(9), 1021–1026. https://doi.org/10.1016/0895-4356(94)90117-1

[3770] Lenzi, A., Culasso, F., Gandini, L., Lombardo, F., & Dondero, F. (1993). Placebo-controlled, double-blind, cross-over trial of glutathione therapy in male infertility. Human reproduction (Oxford, England), 8(10), 1657–1662. https://doi.org/10.1093/oxfordjournals.humrep.a137909

[3771] Ziegler, D., Hanefeld, M., Ruhnau, K. J., Hasche, H., Lobisch, M., Schütte, K., Kerum, G., & Malessa, R. (1999). Treatment of symptomatic diabetic polyneuropathy with the antioxidant alpha-lipoic acid: a 7-month multicenter randomized controlled trial (ALADIN III Study). ALADIN III Study Group. Alpha-Lipoic Acid in Diabetic Neuropathy. Diabetes care, 22(8), 1296–1301. https://doi.org/10.2337/diacare.22.8.1296

[3772] Ziegler, D., Reljanovic, M., Mehnert, H., & Gries, F. A. (1999). Alpha-lipoic acid in the treatment of diabetic polyneuropathy in Germany: current evidence from clinical trials. Experimental and clinical endocrinology & diabetes : official journal, German Society of Endocrinology [and] German Diabetes Association, 107(7), 421–430. https://doi.org/10.1055/s-0029-1212132

[3773] Ziegler, D., Hanefeld, M., Ruhnau, K. J., Meissner, H. P., Lobisch, M., Schütte, K., & Gries, F. A. (1995). Treatment of symptomatic diabetic peripheral neuropathy with the anti-oxidant alpha-lipoic acid. A 3-week multicentre randomized controlled trial (ALADIN Study). Diabetologia, 38(12), 1425–1433. https://doi.org/10.1007/BF00400603

[3774] Ruhnau, K. J., Meissner, H. P., Finn, J. R., Reljanovic, M., Lobisch, M., Schütte, K., Nehrdich, D., Tritschler, H. J., Mehnert, H., & Ziegler, D. (1999). Effects of 3-week oral treatment with the antioxidant thioctic acid (alpha-lipoic acid) in symptomatic diabetic polyneuropathy. Diabetic medicine : a journal of the British Diabetic Association, 16(12), 1040–1043. https://doi.org/10.1046/j.1464-5491.1999.00190.x

701

[3775] Suzuki, Y. J., Tsuchiya, M., & Packer, L. (1992). Lipoate Prevents Glucose-Induced Protein Modifications. Free Radical Research Communications, 17(3), 211–217. doi:10.3109/10715769209068167

[3776] Akbari, M., Ostadmohammadi, V., Tabrizi, R., Mobini, M., Lankarani, K. B., Moosazadeh, M., … Asemi, Z. (2018). The effects of alpha-lipoic acid supplementation on inflammatory markers among patients with metabolic syndrome and related disorders: a systematic review and meta-analysis of randomized controlled trials. Nutrition & Metabolism, 15(1). doi:10.1186/s12986-018-0274-y

[3777] Debbi, E. M., Agar, G., Fichman, G., Ziv, Y. B., Kardosh, R., Halperin, N., Elbaz, A., Beer, Y., & Debi, R. (2011). Efficacy of methylsulfonylmethane supplementation on osteoarthritis of the knee: a randomized controlled study. BMC complementary and alternative medicine, 11, 50. https://doi.org/10.1186/1472-6882-11-50

[3778] Kim, L. S., Axelrod, L. J., Howard, P., Buratovich, N., & Waters, R. F. (2006). Efficacy of methylsulfonylmethane (MSM) in osteoarthritis pain of the knee: a pilot clinical trial. Osteoarthritis and cartilage, 14(3), 286–294. https://doi.org/10.1016/j.joca.2005.10.003

[3779] Childs S. J. (1994). Dimethyl sulfone (DMSO2) in the treatment of interstitial cystitis. The Urologic clinics of North America, 21(1), 85–88.

[3780] Xu, G., Zhou, T., Gu, Y., Wang, Q., Shariff, M., Gu, P., Nguyen, T., Shi, R., & Rao, J. (2015). Evaluation of the Effect of Mega MSM on Improving Joint Function in Populations Experiencing Joint Degeneration. International journal of biomedical science : IJBS, 11(2), 54–60.

[3781] Withee, E.D., Tippens, K.M., Dehen, R. et al. Effects of Methylsulfonylmethane (MSM) on exercise-induced oxidative stress, muscle damage, and pain following a half-marathon: a double-blind, randomized, placebo-controlled trial. J Int Soc Sports Nutr 14, 24 (2017). https://doi.org/10.1186/s12970-017-0181-z

[3782] Withee, E. D., Tippens, K. M., Dehen, R., & Hanes, D. (2015). Effects of MSM on exercise-induced muscle and joint pain: a pilot study. Journal of the International Society of Sports Nutrition, 12(Suppl 1), P8. https://doi.org/10.1186/1550-2783-12-S1-P8

[3783] Kagan, B. L., Sultzer, D. L., Rosenlicht, N., & Gerner, R. H. (1990). Oral S-adenosylmethionine in depression: a randomized, double-blind, placebo-controlled trial. The American journal of psychiatry, 147(5), 591–595. https://doi.org/10.1176/ajp.147.5.591

[3784] Bell, K. M., Plon, L., Bunney, W. E., Jr, & Potkin, S. G. (1988). S-adenosylmethionine treatment of depression: a controlled clinical trial. The American journal of psychiatry, 145(9), 1110–1114. https://doi.org/10.1176/ajp.145.9.1110

[3785] Galizia et al (2016) 'S-adenosyl methionine (SAMe) for depression in adults. Cochrane Database of Systematic Reviews 2016, Issue 10. Art. No.: CD011286. DOI: 10.1002/14651858.CD011286.pub2

[3786] Tavoni, A., Vitali, C., Bombardieri, S., & Pasero, G. (1987). Evaluation of S-adenosylmethionine in primary fibromyalgia. A double-blind crossover study. The American journal of medicine, 83(5A), 107–110. https://doi.org/10.1016/0002-9343(87)90862-x

[3787] Jacobsen, S., Danneskiold-Samsøe, B., & Andersen, R. B. (1991). Oral S-adenosylmethionine in primary fibromyalgia. Double-blind clinical evaluation. Scandinavian journal of rheumatology, 20(4), 294–302. https://doi.org/10.3109/03009749109096803

[3788] di Padova C. (1987). S-adenosylmethionine in the treatment of osteoarthritis. Review of the clinical studies. The American journal of medicine, 83(5A), 60–65. https://doi.org/10.1016/0002-9343(87)90853-9

[3789] Maccagno, A., Di Giorgio, E. E., Caston, O. L., & Sagasta, C. L. (1987). Double-blind controlled clinical trial of oral S-adenosylmethionine versus piroxicam in knee osteoarthritis. The American journal of medicine, 83(5A), 72–77. https://doi.org/10.1016/0002-9343(87)90855-2

[3790] König B. (1987). A long-term (two years) clinical trial with S-adenosylmethionine for the treatment of osteoarthritis. The American journal of medicine, 83(5A), 89–94. https://doi.org/10.1016/0002-9343(87)90859-x

[3791] Visioli, F., Colombo, C., Monti, S., Giulidori, P., & Galli, C. (1998). S-adenosyl-L-methionine: role in phosphatidylcholine synthesis and in vitro effects on the ethanol-induced alterations of lipid metabolism. Pharmacological research, 37(3), 203–206. https://doi.org/10.1006/phrs.1997.0282

[3792] Mato, J. M., Cámara, J., Fernández de Paz, J., Caballería, L., Coll, S., Caballero, A., García-Buey, L., Beltrán, J., Benita, V., Caballería, J., Solà, R., Moreno-Otero, R., Barrao, F., Martín-Duce, A., Correa, J. A., Parés, A., Barrao, E., García-Magaz, I., Puerta, J. L., Moreno, J., … Rodés, J. (1999). S-adenosylmethionine in alcoholic liver cirrhosis: a randomized, placebo-controlled, double-blind, multicenter clinical trial. Journal of hepatology, 30(6), 1081–1089. https://doi.org/10.1016/s0168-8278(99)80263-3

[3793] Le Bon, A. M., & Siess, M. H. (2000). Organosulfur compounds from Allium and the chemoprevention of cancer. Drug metabolism and drug interactions, 17(1-4), 51–79. https://doi.org/10.1515/dmdi.2000.17.1-4.51

[3794] Fenwick, G. R., & Hanley, A. B. (1985). The genus Allium--Part 1. Critical reviews in food science and nutrition, 22(3), 199–271. https://doi.org/10.1080/10408398509527415

3795 Joung, Y. H., Na, Y. M., Yoo, Y. B., Darvin, P., Sp, N., Kang, D. Y., Kim, S. Y., Kim, H. S., Choi, Y. H., Lee, H. K., Park, K. D., Cho, B. W., Kim, H. S., Park, J. H., & Yang, Y. M. (2014). Combination of AG490, a Jak2 inhibitor, and methylsulfonylmethane synergistically suppresses bladder tumor growth via the Jak2/STAT3 pathway. International journal of oncology, 44(3), 883–895. https://doi.org/10.3892/ijo.2014.2250

3796 Kim, J. H., Shin, H. J., Ha, H. L., Park, Y. H., Kwon, T. H., Jung, M. R., Moon, H. B., Cho, E. S., Son, H. Y., & Yu, D. Y. (2014). Methylsulfonylmethane suppresses hepatic tumor development through activation of apoptosis. World journal of hepatology, 6(2), 98–106. https://doi.org/10.4254/wjh.v6.i2.98

3797 Lim, E. J., Hong, D. Y., Park, J. H., Joung, Y. H., Darvin, P., Kim, S. Y., Na, Y. M., Hwang, T. S., Ye, S. K., Moon, E. S., Cho, B. W., Do Park, K., Lee, H. K., Park, T., & Yang, Y. M. (2012). Methylsulfonylmethane suppresses breast cancer growth by down-regulating STAT3 and STAT5b pathways. PloS one, 7(4), e33361. https://doi.org/10.1371/journal.pone.0033361

3798 Foye W. O. (1992). Sulfur compounds in therapy: radiation-protective agents, amphetamines, and mucopolysaccharide sulfation. The Annals of pharmacotherapy, 26(9), 1144–1147. https://doi.org/10.1177/106002809202600918

3799 Zhou, Y., Zhuang, W., Hu, W., Liu, G., Wu, T., & Wu, X. (2011). Consumption of Large Amounts of Allium Vegetables Reduces Risk for Gastric Cancer in a Meta-analysis. Gastroenterology, 141(1), 80–89. doi:10.1053/j.gastro.2011.03.057

3800 Wu, X., Shi, J., Fang, W., Guo, X., Zhang, L., Liu, Y., & Li, Z. (2019). Allium vegetables are associated with reduced risk of colorectal cancer: A hospital-based matched case-control study in China. Asia-Pacific Journal of Clinical Oncology, 15(5). doi:10.1111/ajco.13133

3801 Turati, F., Pelucchi, C., Guercio, V., La Vecchia, C., & Galeone, C. (2015). Allium vegetable intake and gastric cancer: a case-control study and meta-analysis. Molecular nutrition & food research, 59(1), 171–179. https://doi.org/10.1002/mnfr.201400496

3802 Wu, X., Shi, J., Fang, W. X., Guo, X. Y., Zhang, L. Y., Liu, Y. P., & Li, Z. (2019). Allium vegetables are associated with reduced risk of colorectal cancer: A hospital-based matched case-control study in China. Asia-Pacific journal of clinical oncology, 15(5), e132–e141. https://doi.org/10.1111/ajco.13133

3803 Dorant, E., van den Brandt, P., Goldbohm, R., & Sturmans, F. (1996). Consumption of onions and a reduced risk of stomach carcinoma. Gastroenterology, 110(1), 12–20. doi:10.1053/gast.1996.v110.pm8536847

3804 Hu, J., La Vecchia, C., Negri, E., Chatenoud, L., Bosetti, C., Jia, X., Liu, R., Huang, G., Bi, D., & Wang, C. (1999). Diet and brain cancer in adults: a case-control study in northeast China. International journal of cancer, 81(1), 20–23. https://doi.org/10.1002/(sici)1097-0215(19990331)81:1<20::aid-ijc4>3.0.co;2-2

3805 Steinmetz, K. A., Kushi, L. H., Bostick, R. M., Folsom, A. R., & Potter, J. D. (1994). Vegetables, fruit, and colon cancer in the Iowa Women's Health Study. American journal of epidemiology, 139(1), 1–15. https://doi.org/10.1093/oxfordjournals.aje.a116921

3806 Augusti (1996) 'Therapeutic values of onion (Allium cepa L.) and garlic (Allium sativum L.)', Indian Journal of Experimental Biology, 01 Jul 1996, 34(7):634-640.

3807 Wan, Q., Li, N., Du, L., Zhao, R., Yi, M., Xu, Q., & Zhou, Y. (2019). Allium vegetable consumption and health: An umbrella review of meta-analyses of multiple health outcomes. Food Science & Nutrition, 7(8), 2451–2470. doi:10.1002/fsn3.1117

3808 Schwingshackl, L., Missbach, B., & Hoffmann, G. (2016). An umbrella review of garlic intake and risk of cardiovascular disease. Phytomedicine : international journal of phytotherapy and phytopharmacology, 23(11), 1127–1133. https://doi.org/10.1016/j.phymed.2015.10.015

3809 Jung, E. S., Park, S. H., Choi, E. K., Ryu, B. H., Park, B. H., Kim, D. S., Kim, Y. G., & Chae, S. W. (2014). Reduction of blood lipid parameters by a 12-wk supplementation of aged black garlic: a randomized controlled trial. Nutrition (Burbank, Los Angeles County, Calif.), 30(9), 1034–1039. https://doi.org/10.1016/j.nut.2014.02.014

3810 Alali, F. Q., El-Elimat, T., Khalid, L., Hudaib, R., Al-Shehabi, T. S., & Eid, A. H. (2017). Garlic for Cardiovascular Disease: Prevention or Treatment?. Current pharmaceutical design, 23(7), 1028–1041. https://doi.org/10.2174/1381612822666161010124530

3811 Zhao, Y., & Zhao, B. (2013). Oxidative Stress and the Pathogenesis of Alzheimer's Disease. Oxidative Medicine and Cellular Longevity, 2013, 1–10. doi:10.1155/2013/316523

3812 Bianchini, F., & Vainio, H. (2001). Allium vegetables and organosulfur compounds: do they help prevent cancer?. Environmental health perspectives, 109(9), 893–902. https://doi.org/10.1289/ehp.01109893

3813 Sparnins, V. L., Barany, G., & Wattenberg, L. W. (1988). Effects of organosulfur compounds from garlic and onions on benzo[a]pyrene-induced neoplasia and glutathione S-transferase activity in the mouse. Carcinogenesis, 9(1), 131–134. https://doi.org/10.1093/carcin/9.1.131

3814 Song, K., & Milner, J. A. (2001). The influence of heating on the anticancer properties of garlic. The Journal of nutrition, 131(3s), 1054S–7S. https://doi.org/10.1093/jn/131.3.1054S

703

[3815] Cavagnaro, P. F., Camargo, A., Galmarini, C. R., & Simon, P. W. (2007). Effect of cooking on garlic (Allium sativum L.) antiplatelet activity and thiosulfinates content. Journal of agricultural and food chemistry, 55(4), 1280–1288. https://doi.org/10.1021/jf062587s

[3816] Song, K., & Milner, J. A. (1999). Heating garlic inhibits its ability to suppress 7, 12-dimethylbenz(a)anthracene-induced DNA adduct formation in rat mammary tissue. The Journal of nutrition, 129(3), 657–661. https://doi.org/10.1093/jn/129.3.657

[3817] de Figueiredo et al (2015). The antioxidant properties of organosulfur compounds (sulforaphane). Recent patents on endocrine, metabolic & immune drug discovery, 9(1), 24–39. https://doi.org/10.2174/1872214809666150505164138

[3818] Bahadoran, Z., Mirmiran, P., & Azizi, F. (2013). Potential efficacy of broccoli sprouts as a unique supplement for management of type 2 diabetes and its complications. Journal of medicinal food, 16(5), 375–382. https://doi.org/10.1089/jmf.2012.2559

[3819] Senanayake et al (2012). The dietary phase 2 protein inducer sulforaphane can normalize the kidney epigenome and improve blood pressure in hypertensive rats. American journal of hypertension, 25(2), 229–235. https://doi.org/10.1038/ajh.2011.200

[3820] Kim et al (2016) 'Sulforaphane epigenetically enhances neuronal BDNF expression and TrkB signaling pathways', Mol. Nutr. Food Res. 2017, 1600194.

[3821] Riedl, M. A., Saxon, A., & Diaz-Sanchez, D. (2009). Oral sulforaphane increases Phase II antioxidant enzymes in the human upper airway. Clinical immunology (Orlando, Fla.), 130(3), 244–251. https://doi.org/10.1016/j.clim.2008.10.007

[3822] Armah et al (2015). Diet rich in high glucoraphanin broccoli reduces plasma LDL cholesterol: Evidence from randomised controlled trials. Molecular nutrition & food research, 59(5), 918–926. https://doi.org/10.1002/mnfr.201400863

[3823] Kim, H. J., Barajas, B., Wang, M., & Nel, A. E. (2008). Nrf2 activation by sulforaphane restores the age-related decrease of T(H)1 immunity: role of dendritic cells. The Journal of allergy and clinical immunology, 121(5), 1255–1261.e7. https://doi.org/10.1016/j.jaci.2008.01.016

[3824] Johansson, N. L., Pavia, C. S., & Chiao, J. W. (2008). Growth inhibition of a spectrum of bacterial and fungal pathogens by sulforaphane, an isothiocyanate product found in broccoli and other cruciferous vegetables. Planta medica, 74(7), 747–750. https://doi.org/10.1055/s-2008-1074520

[3825] Bahadoran, Z., Mirmiran, P., & Azizi, F. (2013). Potential efficacy of broccoli sprouts as a unique supplement for management of type 2 diabetes and its complications. Journal of medicinal food, 16(5), 375–382. https://doi.org/10.1089/jmf.2012.2559

[3826] Kikuchi et al (2015). Sulforaphane-rich broccoli sprout extract improves hepatic abnormalities in male subjects. World journal of gastroenterology, 21(43), 12457–12467. https://doi.org/10.3748/wjg.v21.i43.12457

[3827] Kim et al (2017). Sulforaphane epigenetically enhances neuronal BDNF expression and TrkB signaling pathways. Molecular nutrition & food research, 61(2), 10.1002/mnfr.201600194. https://doi.org/10.1002/mnfr.201600194

[3828] Bauman et al (2016) 'Prevention of Carcinogen-Induced Oral Cancer by Sulforaphane', Cancer Prev Res July 1 2016 (9) (7) 547-557; DOI: 10.1158/1940-6207.CAPR-15-0290

[3829] Leone et al (2017) 'Sulforaphane for the chemoprevention of bladder cancer: molecular mechanism targeted approach', Oncotarget. 2017; 8: 35412-35424. Retrieved from https://www.oncotarget.com/article/16015/

[3830] Tortorella et al (2015). Dietary Sulforaphane in Cancer Chemoprevention: The Role of Epigenetic Regulation and HDAC Inhibition. Antioxidants & redox signaling, 22(16), 1382–1424. https://doi.org/10.1089/ars.2014.6097

[3831] Sedlak, T. W., Nucifora, L. G., Koga, M., Shaffer, L. S., Higgs, C., Tanaka, T., Wang, A. M., Coughlin, J. M., Barker, P. B., Fahey, J. W., & Sawa, A. (2018). Sulforaphane Augments Glutathione and Influences Brain Metabolites in Human Subjects: A Clinical Pilot Study. Molecular neuropsychiatry, 3(4), 214–222. https://doi.org/10.1159/000487639

[3832] Kim, J. K., & Park, S. U. (2016). Current potential health benefits of sulforaphane. EXCLI journal, 15, 571–577. https://doi.org/10.17179/excli2016-485

[3833] Bogaards, J. J. P., Verhagen, H., Willems, M. I., Poppel, G. van, & Bladeren, P. J. va. (1994). Consumption of Brussels sprouts results in elevated α-class glutathione S-transferase levels in human blood plasma. Carcinogenesis, 15(5), 1073–1075. doi:10.1093/carcin/15.5.1073

[3834] Doleman, J. et al. (2017). The contribution of alliaceous and cruciferous vegetables to dietary sulphur intake. Food chemistry 234: 38–45.

[3835] https://www.ncbi.nlm.nih.gov/pubmed/22752583
[3836] https://www.sciencedirect.com/science/article/abs/pii/S0024320518306593
[3837] https://www.ncbi.nlm.nih.gov/pmc/articles/PMC5403866/

[3838] Juge, N., Mithen, R. F., & Traka, M. (2007). Molecular basis for chemoprevention by sulforaphane: a comprehensive review. Cellular and Molecular Life Sciences, 64(9), 1105–1127. doi:10.1007/s00018-007-6484-5

[3839] Sharma et al (2010). Role of Lipid Peroxidation in Cellular Responses tod,l-Sulforaphane, a Promising Cancer Chemopreventive Agent. Biochemistry, 49(14), 3191–3202. doi:10.1021/bi100104e

[3840] Baier et al (2014). Off-target effects of sulforaphane include the derepression of long terminal repeats through histone acetylation events. The Journal of Nutritional Biochemistry, 25(6), 665–668. doi:10.1016/j.jnutbio.2014.02.007

[3841] Socala et al (2017) 'Increased seizure susceptibility and other toxicity symptoms following acute sulforaphane treatment in mice', April 2017Toxicology and Applied Pharmacology 326.

[3842] Houghton, C. A., Fassett, R. G., & Coombes, J. S. (2016). Sulforaphane and Other Nutrigenomic Nrf2 Activators: Can the Clinician's Expectation Be Matched by the Reality?. Oxidative medicine and cellular longevity, 2016, 7857186. https://doi.org/10.1155/2016/7857186

[3843] Yuan, G., Sun, B., Yuan, J., & Wang, Q. (2009). Effects of different cooking methods on health-promoting compounds of broccoli. Journal of Zhejiang University SCIENCE B, 10(8), 580–588. doi:10.1631/jzus.b0920051

[3844] https://www.ncbi.nlm.nih.gov/pubmed/29806738

[3845] https://www.ncbi.nlm.nih.gov/pmc/articles/PMC2668525/

[3846] Smith, T. K. (2003). Effects of Brassica vegetable juice on the induction of apoptosis and aberrant crypt foci in rat colonic mucosal crypts in vivo. Carcinogenesis, 24(3), 491–495. doi:10.1093/carcin/24.3.491

[3847] Marcus, J. B. (2013). Vitamin and Mineral Basics: The ABCs of Healthy Foods and Beverages, Including Phytonutrients and Functional Foods. Culinary Nutrition, 279–331. doi:10.1016/b978-0-12-391882-6.00007-8

[3848] Nimni, M. E., Han, B., & Cordoba, F. (2007). Are we getting enough sulfur in our diet?. Nutrition & metabolism, 4, 24. https://doi.org/10.1186/1743-7075-4-24

[3849] McNally, M. E., Atkinson, S. A., & Cole, D. E. C. (1991). Contribution of Sulfate and Sulfoesters to Total Sulfur Intake in Infants Fed Human Milk. The Journal of Nutrition, 121(8), 1250–1254. doi:10.1093/jn/121.8.1250

[3850] S. CJC. Sulfur Deficiency. Purdue University Department of Agronomy: Soil Fertility Update. 2017.

[3851] Jez, J. (Ed.). (2008). Sulfur: A Missing Link between Soils, Crops, and Nutrition. Agronomy Monographs. doi:10.2134/agronmonogr50

[3852] Asia Pacific Journal of Clinical Nutrition (1998) 'SULPHUR', Elements, Accessed Online Jan 27 2021: http://apjcn.nhri.org.tw/server/info/books-phds/books/foodfacts/html/data/data5g.html

[3853] Lee, H. R., Cho, S. D., Lee, W. K., Kim, G. H., & Shim, S. M. (2014). Digestive recovery of sulfur-methyl-L-methionine and its bioaccessibility in Kimchi cabbages using a simulated in vitro digestion model system. Journal of the science of food and agriculture, 94(1), 109–112. https://doi.org/10.1002/jsfa.6205

[3854] Szabo C. (2018). A timeline of hydrogen sulfide (H2S) research: From environmental toxin to biological mediator. Biochemical pharmacology, 149, 5–19. https://doi.org/10.1016/j.bcp.2017.09.010

[3855] Paul, B. D., & Snyder, S. H. (2012). H2S signalling through protein sulfhydration and beyond. Nature reviews. Molecular cell biology, 13(8), 499–507. https://doi.org/10.1038/nrm3391

[3856] Wang R. (2012). Physiological implications of hydrogen sulfide: a whiff exploration that blossomed. Physiological reviews, 92(2), 791–896. https://doi.org/10.1152/physrev.00017.2011

[3857] Olson, K. R. (2013). Hydrogen sulfide: both feet on the gas and none on the brake? Frontiers in Physiology, 4. doi:10.3389/fphys.2013.00002

[3858] Szabo, C., & Papapetropoulos, A. (2017). International Union of Basic and Clinical Pharmacology. CII: Pharmacological Modulation of H2S Levels: H2S Donors and H2S Biosynthesis Inhibitors. Pharmacological reviews, 69(4), 497–564. https://doi.org/10.1124/pr.117.014050

[3859] T., Hancock, John (2017). Cell signalling (Fourth ed.). Oxford, United Kingdom.

[3860] Meng, G., Zhao, S., Xie, L., Han, Y., & Ji, Y. (2018). Protein S-sulfhydration by hydrogen sulfide in cardiovascular system. British journal of pharmacology, 175(8), 1146–1156. https://doi.org/10.1111/bph.13825

[3861] Kanagy, N. L., Szabo, C., & Papapetropoulos, A. (2017). Vascular biology of hydrogen sulfide. American journal of physiology. Cell physiology, 312(5), C537–C549. https://doi.org/10.1152/ajpcell.00329.2016

[3862] van Goor, H., van den Born, J. C., Hillebrands, J. L., & Joles, J. A. (2016). Hydrogen sulfide in hypertension. Current opinion in nephrology and hypertension, 25(2), 107–113. https://doi.org/10.1097/MNH.0000000000000206

[3863] Polhemus, D. J., & Lefer, D. J. (2014). Emergence of hydrogen sulfide as an endogenous gaseous signaling molecule in cardiovascular disease. Circulation research, 114(4), 730–737. https://doi.org/10.1161/CIRCRESAHA.114.300505

[3864] Zhao, W., Zhang, J., Lu, Y., & Wang, R. (2001). The vasorelaxant effect of H(2)S as a novel endogenous gaseous K(ATP) channel opener. The EMBO journal, 20(21), 6008–6016. https://doi.org/10.1093/emboj/20.21.6008

[3865] Zhao, W., & Wang, R. (2002). H(2)S-induced vasorelaxation and underlying cellular and molecular mechanisms. American journal of physiology. Heart and circulatory physiology, 283(2), H474–H480. https://doi.org/10.1152/ajpheart.00013.2002

[3866] Zhao, W., & Wang, R. (2002). H2S-induced vasorelaxation and underlying cellular and molecular mechanisms. American Journal of Physiology-Heart and Circulatory Physiology, 283(2), H474–H480. doi:10.1152/ajpheart.00013.2002

[3867] Wang, R., Szabo, C., Ichinose, F., Ahmed, A., Whiteman, M., & Papapetropoulos, A. (2015). The role of H2S bioavailability in endothelial dysfunction. Trends in pharmacological sciences, 36(9), 568–578. https://doi.org/10.1016/j.tips.2015.05.007

[3868] Szabo C. (2017). Hydrogen sulfide, an enhancer of vascular nitric oxide signaling: mechanisms and implications. American journal of physiology. Cell physiology, 312(1), C3–C15. https://doi.org/10.1152/ajpcell.00282.2016

[3869] Eberhardt, M., Dux, M., Namer, B., Miljkovic, J., Cordasic, N., Will, C., Kichko, T. I., de la Roche, J., Fischer, M., Suárez, S. A., Bikiel, D., Dorsch, K., Leffler, A., Babes, A., Lampert, A., Lennerz, J. K., Jacobi, J., Martí, M. A., Doctorovich, F., Högestätt, E. D., … Filipovic, M. R. (2014). H2S and NO cooperatively regulate vascular tone by activating a neuroendocrine HNO-TRPA1-CGRP signalling pathway. Nature communications, 5, 4381. https://doi.org/10.1038/ncomms5381

[3870] Coletta, C., Papapetropoulos, A., Erdelyi, K., Olah, G., Módis, K., Panopoulos, P., Asimakopoulou, A., Gerö, D., Sharina, I., Martin, E., & Szabo, C. (2012). Hydrogen sulfide and nitric oxide are mutually dependent in the regulation of angiogenesis and endothelium-dependent vasorelaxation. Proceedings of the National Academy of Sciences of the United States of America, 109(23), 9161–9166. https://doi.org/10.1073/pnas.1202916109

[3871] Zhang, Y., & Hogg, N. (2005). S-Nitrosothiols: cellular formation and transport. Free radical biology & medicine, 38(7), 831–838. https://doi.org/10.1016/j.freeradbiomed.2004.12.016

[3872] Whiteman, M., Li, L., Kostetski, I., Chu, S. H., Siau, J. L., Bhatia, M., & Moore, P. K. (2006). Evidence for the formation of a novel nitrosothiol from the gaseous mediators nitric oxide and hydrogen sulphide. Biochemical and biophysical research communications, 343(1), 303–310. https://doi.org/10.1016/j.bbrc.2006.02.154

[3873] King, A. L., Polhemus, D. J., Bhushan, S., Otsuka, H., Kondo, K., Nicholson, C. K., Bradley, J. M., Islam, K. N., Calvert, J. W., Tao, Y. X., Dugas, T. R., Kelley, E. E., Elrod, J. W., Huang, P. L., Wang, R., & Lefer, D. J. (2014). Hydrogen sulfide cytoprotective signaling is endothelial nitric oxide synthase-nitric oxide dependent. Proceedings of the National Academy of Sciences of the United States of America, 111(8), 3182–3187. https://doi.org/10.1073/pnas.1321871111

[3874] Wang R. (2003). The gasotransmitter role of hydrogen sulfide. Antioxidants & redox signaling, 5(4), 493–501. https://doi.org/10.1089/152308603768295249

[3875] Wang R. (2002). Two's company, three's a crowd: can H2S be the third endogenous gaseous transmitter?. FASEB journal : official publication of the Federation of American Societies for Experimental Biology, 16(13), 1792–1798. https://doi.org/10.1096/fj.02-0211hyp

[3876] Benavides, G. A., Squadrito, G. L., Mills, R. W., Patel, H. D., Isbell, T. S., Patel, R. P., Darley-Usmar, V. M., Doeller, J. E., & Kraus, D. W. (2007). Hydrogen sulfide mediates the vasoactivity of garlic. Proceedings of the National Academy of Sciences of the United States of America, 104(46), 17977–17982. https://doi.org/10.1073/pnas.0705710104

[3877] Katsouda, A., Bibli, S. I., Pyriochou, A., Szabo, C., & Papapetropoulos, A. (2016). Regulation and role of endogenously produced hydrogen sulfide in angiogenesis. Pharmacological research, 113(Pt A), 175–185. https://doi.org/10.1016/j.phrs.2016.08.026

[3878] Papapetropoulos, A., Pyriochou, A., Altaany, Z., Yang, G., Marazioti, A., Zhou, Z., Jeschke, M. G., Branski, L. K., Herndon, D. N., Wang, R., & Szabó, C. (2009). Hydrogen sulfide is an endogenous stimulator of angiogenesis. Proceedings of the National Academy of Sciences of the United States of America, 106(51), 21972–21977. https://doi.org/10.1073/pnas.0908047106

[3879] Jiang HL, Wu HC, Li ZL, Geng B, Tang CS. 2005. [Changes of the new gaseous transmitter H2S in

[3880] Wang, Y., Zhao, X., Jin, H., Wei, H., Li, W., Bu, D., Tang, X., Ren, Y., Tang, C., & Du, J. (2009). Role of hydrogen sulfide in the development of atherosclerotic lesions in apolipoprotein E knockout mice. Arteriosclerosis, thrombosis, and vascular biology, 29(2), 173–179. https://doi.org/10.1161/ATVBAHA.108.179333

[3881] Krishnan, N., Fu, C., Pappin, D. J., & Tonks, N. K. (2011). H2S-Induced Sulfhydration of the Phosphatase PTP1B and Its Role in the Endoplasmic Reticulum Stress Response. Science Signaling, 4(203), ra86–ra86. doi:10.1126/scisignal.2002329

[3882] Calvert, J. W., Jha, S., Gundewar, S., Elrod, J. W., Ramachandran, A., Pattillo, C. B., Kevil, C. G., & Lefer, D. J. (2009). Hydrogen sulfide mediates cardioprotection through Nrf2 signaling. Circulation research, 105(4), 365–374. https://doi.org/10.1161/CIRCRESAHA.109.199919

[3883] Elrod, J. W., Calvert, J. W., Morrison, J., Doeller, J. E., Kraus, D. W., Tao, L., Jiao, X., Scalia, R., Kiss, L., Szabo, C., Kimura, H., Chow, C. W., & Lefer, D. J. (2007). Hydrogen sulfide attenuates myocardial ischemia-reperfusion injury by preservation of mitochondrial function. Proceedings of the National Academy of Sciences of the United States of America, 104(39), 15560–15565. https://doi.org/10.1073/pnas.0705891104

[3884] Cao, X., & Bian, J. S. (2016). The Role of Hydrogen Sulfide in Renal System. Frontiers in pharmacology, 7, 385. https://doi.org/10.3389/fphar.2016.00385

[3885] Koning, A. M., Frenay, A. R., Leuvenink, H. G., & van Goor, H. (2015). Hydrogen sulfide in renal physiology, disease and transplantation--the smell of renal protection. Nitric oxide : biology and chemistry, 46, 37–49. https://doi.org/10.1016/j.niox.2015.01.005

[3886] Feliers, D., Lee, H. J., & Kasinath, B. S. (2016). Hydrogen Sulfide in Renal Physiology and Disease. Antioxidants & redox signaling, 25(13), 720–731. https://doi.org/10.1089/ars.2015.6596

[3887] Lu, M., Liu, Y.-H., Goh, H. S., Wang, J. J. X., Yong, Q.-C., Wang, R., & Bian, J.-S. (2010). Hydrogen Sulfide Inhibits Plasma Renin Activity. Journal of the American Society of Nephrology, 21(6), 993–1002. doi:10.1681/asn.2009090949

[3888] Bełtowski J. (2010). Hypoxia in the renal medulla: implications for hydrogen sulfide signaling. The Journal of pharmacology and experimental therapeutics, 334(2), 358–363. https://doi.org/10.1124/jpet.110.166637

[3889] Mimura, I., & Nangaku, M. (2010). The suffocating kidney: tubulointerstitial hypoxia in end-stage renal disease. Nature reviews. Nephrology, 6(11), 667–678. https://doi.org/10.1038/nrneph.2010.124

[3890] Jiang, D., Zhang, Y., Yang, M., Wang, S., Jiang, Z., & Li, Z. (2013). Exogenous hydrogen sulfide prevents kidney damage following unilateral ureteral obstruction. Neurourology and Urodynamics, 33(5), 538–543. doi:10.1002/nau.22450

[3891] Song, K., Wang, F., Li, Q., Shi, Y.-B., Zheng, H.-F., Peng, H., … Hu, L.-F. (2014). Hydrogen sulfide inhibits the renal fibrosis of obstructive nephropathy. Kidney International, 85(6), 1318–1329. doi:10.1038/ki.2013.449

[3892] Jung, K.-J., Jang, H.-S., Kim, J. I., Han, S. J., Park, J.-W., & Park, K. M. (2013). Involvement of hydrogen sulfide and homocysteine transsulfuration pathway in the progression of kidney fibrosis after ureteral obstruction. Biochimica et Biophysica Acta (BBA) - Molecular Basis of Disease, 1832(12), 1989–1997. doi:10.1016/j.bbadis.2013.06.015

[3893] Kimura, Y., & Kimura, H. (2004). Hydrogen sulfide protects neurons from oxidative stress. FASEB journal : official publication of the Federation of American Societies for Experimental Biology, 18(10), 1165–1167. https://doi.org/10.1096/fj.04-1815fje

[3894] Kimura, Y., Goto, Y., & Kimura, H. (2010). Hydrogen sulfide increases glutathione production and suppresses oxidative stress in mitochondria. Antioxidants & redox signaling, 12(1), 1–13. https://doi.org/10.1089/ars.2008.2282

[3895] Snyder S. The rotten smell of memory: it's a gas. Science News. 1996;149:116.

[3896] Abe, K., & Kimura, H. (1996). The possible role of hydrogen sulfide as an endogenous neuromodulator. The Journal of neuroscience : the official journal of the Society for Neuroscience, 16(3), 1066–1071. https://doi.org/10.1523/JNEUROSCI.16-03-01066.1996

[3897] Whiteman, M., Armstrong, J. S., Chu, S. H., Jia-Ling, S., Wong, B. S., Cheung, N. S., Halliwell, B., & Moore, P. K. (2004). The novel neuromodulator hydrogen sulfide: an endogenous peroxynitrite 'scavenger'?. Journal of neurochemistry, 90(3), 765–768. https://doi.org/10.1111/j.1471-4159.2004.02617.x

[3898] Ishigami, M., Hiraki, K., Umemura, K., Ogasawara, Y., Ishii, K., & Kimura, H. (2009). A source of hydrogen sulfide and a mechanism of its release in the brain. Antioxidants & redox signaling, 11(2), 205–214. https://doi.org/10.1089/ars.2008.2132

[3899] Eto, K., Asada, T., Arima, K., Makifuchi, T., & Kimura, H. (2002). Brain hydrogen sulfide is severely decreased in Alzheimer's disease. Biochemical and biophysical research communications, 293(5), 1485–1488. https://doi.org/10.1016/S0006-291X(02)00422-9

[3900] Sen, N., Paul, B. D., Gadalla, M. M., Mustafa, A. K., Sen, T., Xu, R., Kim, S., & Snyder, S. H. (2012). Hydrogen sulfide-linked sulfhydration of NF-κB mediates its antiapoptotic actions. Molecular cell, 45(1), 13–24. https://doi.org/10.1016/j.molcel.2011.10.021

[3901] Zanardo, R. C., Brancaleone, V., Distrutti, E., Fiorucci, S., Cirino, G., & Wallace, J. L. (2006). Hydrogen sulfide is an endogenous modulator of leukocyte-mediated inflammation. FASEB journal : official publication of the Federation of American Societies for Experimental Biology, 20(12), 2118–2120. https://doi.org/10.1096/fj.06-6270fje

[3902] Oh, G. S., Pae, H. O., Lee, B. S., Kim, B. N., Kim, J. M., Kim, H. R., Jeon, S. B., Jeon, W. K., Chae, H. J., & Chung, H. T. (2006). Hydrogen sulfide inhibits nitric oxide production and nuclear factor-kappaB via heme oxygenase-1 expression in RAW264.7 macrophages stimulated with lipopolysaccharide. Free radical biology & medicine, 41(1), 106–119. https://doi.org/10.1016/j.freeradbiomed.2006.03.021

[3903] Li, L., Bhatia, M., Zhu, Y. Z., Zhu, Y. C., Ramnath, R. D., Wang, Z. J., Anuar, F. B., Whiteman, M., Salto-Tellez, M., & Moore, P. K. (2005). Hydrogen sulfide is a novel mediator of lipopolysaccharide-induced inflammation in the mouse. FASEB journal : official publication of the Federation of American Societies for Experimental Biology, 19(9), 1196–1198. https://doi.org/10.1096/fj.04-3583fje

[3904] Goslar, T., Marš, T., & Podbregar, M. (2011). Total plasma sulfide as a marker of shock severity in nonsurgical adult patients. Shock (Augusta, Ga.), 36(4), 350–355. https://doi.org/10.1097/SHK.0b013e31822bcfd0

[3905] Fiorucci, S., Antonelli, E., Distrutti, E., Rizzo, G., Mencarelli, A., Orlandi, S., Zanardo, R., Renga, B., Di Sante, M., Morelli, A., Cirino, G., & Wallace, J. L. (2005). Inhibition of hydrogen sulfide generation contributes to gastric injury caused by anti-inflammatory nonsteroidal drugs. Gastroenterology, 129(4), 1210–1224. https://doi.org/10.1053/j.gastro.2005.07.060

[3906] Suliman, H. B., & Piantadosi, C. A. (2014). Mitochondrial biogenesis: regulation by endogenous gases during inflammation and organ stress. Current pharmaceutical design, 20(35), 5653–5662. https://doi.org/10.2174/1381612820666140306095717

[3907] Predmore, B. L., Lefer, D. J., & Gojon, G. (2012). Hydrogen Sulfide in Biochemistry and Medicine. Antioxidants & Redox Signaling, 17(1), 119–140. doi:10.1089/ars.2012.4612

[3908] Sun, W.-H., Liu, F., Chen, Y., & Zhu, Y.-C. (2012). Hydrogen sulfide decreases the levels of ROS by inhibiting mitochondrial complex IV and increasing SOD activities in cardiomyocytes under ischemia/reperfusion. Biochemical and Biophysical Research Communications, 421(2), 164–169. doi:10.1016/j.bbrc.2012.03.121

[3909] Magierowski, M., Magierowska, K., Kwiecien, S., & Brzozowski, T. (2015). Gaseous mediators nitric oxide and hydrogen sulfide in the mechanism of gastrointestinal integrity, protection and ulcer healing. Molecules (Basel, Switzerland), 20(5), 9099–9123. https://doi.org/10.3390/molecules20059099

[3910] Singh, S. B., & Lin, H. C. (2015). Hydrogen Sulfide in Physiology and Diseases of the Digestive Tract. Microorganisms, 3(4), 866–889. https://doi.org/10.3390/microorganisms3040866

[3911] Miller, D. L., & Roth, M. B. (2007). Hydrogen sulfide increases thermotolerance and lifespan in Caenorhabditis elegans. Proceedings of the National Academy of Sciences, 104(51), 20618–20622. doi:10.1073/pnas.0710191104

[3912] Qabazard, B., Li, L., Gruber, J., Peh, M. T., Ng, L. F., Kumar, S. D., Rose, P., Tan, C. H., Dymock, B. W., Wei, F., Swain, S. C., Halliwell, B., Stürzenbaum, S. R., & Moore, P. K. (2014). Hydrogen sulfide is an endogenous regulator of aging in Caenorhabditis elegans. Antioxidants & redox signaling, 20(16), 2621–2630. https://doi.org/10.1089/ars.2013.5448

[3913] Shatalin, K., Shatalina, E., Mironov, A., & Nudler, E. (2011). H2S: a universal defense against antibiotics in bacteria. Science (New York, N.Y.), 334(6058), 986–990. https://doi.org/10.1126/science.1209855

[3914] Blackstone, E. (2005). H2S Induces a Suspended Animation-Like State in Mice. Science, 308(5721), 518–518. doi:10.1126/science.1108581

[3915] National Institute of Aging (2018) 'Calorie Restriction and Fasting Diets: What Do We Know?', Health Information, Accessed Online Jan 16 2021: https://www.nia.nih.gov/health/calorie-restriction-and-fasting-diets-what-do-we-know

[3916] Hine, C., Harputlugil, E., Zhang, Y., Ruckenstuhl, C., Lee, B. C., Brace, L., Longchamp, A., Treviño-Villarreal, J. H., Mejia, P., Ozaki, C. K., Wang, R., Gladyshev, V. N., Madeo, F., Mair, W. B., & Mitchell, J. R. (2015). Endogenous hydrogen sulfide production is essential for dietary restriction benefits. Cell, 160(1-2), 132–144. https://doi.org/10.1016/j.cell.2014.11.048

[3917] Abdrashitova, A. T., Panova, T. N., & Belolapenko, I. A. (2011). Meditsina truda i promyshlennaia ekologiia, (7), 10–16.

[3918] Huang, C. W., & Moore, P. K. (2015). H2S Synthesizing Enzymes: Biochemistry and Molecular Aspects. Handbook of experimental pharmacology, 230, 3–25. https://doi.org/10.1007/978-3-319-18144-8_1

[3919] Kabil, O., & Banerjee, R. (2014). Enzymology of H2S biogenesis, decay and signaling. Antioxidants & redox signaling, 20(5), 770–782. https://doi.org/10.1089/ars.2013.5339

[3920] Kabil, O., Vitvitsky, V., Xie, P., & Banerjee, R. (2011). The quantitative significance of the transsulfuration enzymes for H2S production in murine tissues. Antioxidants & redox signaling, 15(2), 363–372. https://doi.org/10.1089/ars.2010.3781

[3921] Lu SC. 2013. Glutathione synthesis. Biochim. Biophys. Acta 1830:3143–53

[3922] Huxtable RJ. 1992. Physiological actions of taurine. Physiol. Rev. 72:101–63

[3923] Korendyaseva, T. K., Kuvatov, D. N., Volkov, V. A., Martinov, M. V., Vitvitsky, V. M., Banerjee, R., & Ataullakhanov, F. I. (2008). An allosteric mechanism for switching between parallel tracks in mammalian sulfur metabolism. PLoS computational biology, 4(5), e1000076. https://doi.org/10.1371/journal.pcbi.1000076

[3924] du Vigneaud V, Loring HS, Craft H. The oxidation of the sulfur of homocystine, methionine, and S-methylcysteine in the animal body. J Biol Chem. 1934;105:481.

[3925] du Vigneaud V, Brown GB, Chandler JP. The synthesis of ll-S-(β-amino- βcarboxyethyl) homocysteine and the replacement by it of cystine in the diet. J Biol Chem. 1942;143:59.

[3926] Binkley F, du Vigneaud V. The formation of cysteine from homocysteine and serine by liver tissue of rats. J Biol Chem. 1942;144:507.

[3927] Ingenbleek, Y., & Kimura, H. (2013). Nutritional essentiality of sulfur in health and disease. Nutrition reviews, 71(7), 413–432. https://doi.org/10.1111/nure.12050

[3928] Finkelstein JD. 2000. Pathways and regulation of homocysteine metabolism in mammals. Semin. Thromb. Hemost. 26:219–25

[3929] ISHII, I., AKAHOSHI, N., YU, X.-N., KOBAYASHI, Y., NAMEKATA, K., KOMAKI, G., & KIMURA, H. (2004). Murine cystathionine γ-lyase: complete cDNA and genomic sequences, promoter activity, tissue distribution and developmental expression. Biochemical Journal, 381(1), 113–123. doi:10.1042/bj20040243

[3930] Vitvitsky, V., Thomas, M., Ghorpade, A., Gendelman, H. E., & Banerjee, R. (2006). A functional transsulfuration pathway in the brain links to glutathione homeostasis. The Journal of biological chemistry, 281(47), 35785–35793. https://doi.org/10.1074/jbc.M602799200

[3931] Mosharov, E., Cranford, M. R., & Banerjee, R. (2000). The quantitatively important relationship between homocysteine metabolism and glutathione synthesis by the transsulfuration pathway and its regulation by redox changes. Biochemistry, 39(42), 13005–13011. https://doi.org/10.1021/bi001088w

[3932] Cho, E. S., Hovanec-Brown, J., Tomanek, R. J., & Stegink, L. D. (1991). Propargylglycine infusion effects on tissue glutathione levels, plasma amino acid concentrations and tissue morphology in parenterally-fed growing rats. The Journal of nutrition, 121(6), 785–794. https://doi.org/10.1093/jn/121.6.785

[3933] Triguero, A., Barber, T., García, C., Puertes, I. R., Sastre, J., & Viña, J. R. (1997). Liver intracellular L-cysteine concentration is maintained after inhibition of the trans-sulfuration pathway by propargylglycine in rats. British Journal of Nutrition, 78(5), 823–831. doi:10.1079/bjn19970198

[3934] Beatty, P. W., & Reed, D. J. (1980). Involvement of the cystathionine pathway in the biosynthesis of glutathione by isolated rat hepatocytes. Archives of biochemistry and biophysics, 204(1), 80–87. https://doi.org/10.1016/0003-9861(80)90009-0

[3935] Garg, S. K., Yan, Z., Vitvitsky, V., & Banerjee, R. (2011). Differential dependence on cysteine from transsulfuration versus transport during T cell activation. Antioxidants & redox signaling, 15(1), 39–47. https://doi.org/10.1089/ars.2010.3496

[3936] Vitvitsky, V., Mosharov, E., Tritt, M., Ataullakhanov, F., & Banerjee, R. (2003). Redox regulation of homocysteine-dependent glutathione synthesis. Redox report : communications in free radical research, 8(1), 57–63. https://doi.org/10.1179/135100003125001260

[3937] SNOKE, J. E., & BLOCH, K. (1954). The Biosynthesis of Glutathione. Glutathione, 129–137. doi:10.1016/b978-1-4832-2900-3.50014-6

[3938] Grotheer, P., Marshall, M., & Simonne, A. (2019). Sulfites: Separating Fact from Fiction. EDIS, 2005(5). Retrieved from https://journals.flvc.org/edis/article/view/114835

[3939] Challen R. G. (1990). Sulphite content of Australian pharmaceutical products. The Medical journal of Australia, 152(4), 196–198. https://doi.org/10.5694/j.1326-5377.1990.tb125149.x

[3940] Ijssennagger, N., van der Meer, R., & van Mil, S. (2016). Sulfide as a Mucus Barrier-Breaker in Inflammatory Bowel Disease?. Trends in molecular medicine, 22(3), 190–199. https://doi.org/10.1016/j.molmed.2016.01.002

[3941] Vally, H., & Misso, N. L. (2012). Adverse reactions to the sulphite additives. Gastroenterology and hepatology from bed to bench, 5(1), 16–23.

[3942] Bold J. (2012). Considerations for the diagnosis and management of sulphite sensitivity. Gastroenterology and hepatology from bed to bench, 5(1), 3–6.

[3943] Stohs, S. J., & Miller, M. J. S. (2014). A case study involving allergic reactions to sulfur-containing compounds including, sulfite, taurine, acesulfame potassium and sulfonamides. Food and Chemical Toxicology, 63, 240–243. doi:10.1016/j.fct.2013.11.008

[3944] Silva, M., Gama, J., Pinto, N., Pivi, G., Brancal, H., Carvalho, L., Loureiro, V., & Patto, M. V. (2019). Sulfite concentration and the occurrence of headache in young adults: a prospective study. European journal of clinical nutrition, 73(9), 1316–1322. https://doi.org/10.1038/s41430-019-0420-2

[3945] Panconesi A. (2008). Alcohol and migraine: trigger factor, consumption, mechanisms. A review. The journal of headache and pain, 9(1), 19–27. https://doi.org/10.1007/s10194-008-0006-1

[3946] Pitcher, M. C., & Cummings, J. H. (1996). Hydrogen sulphide: a bacterial toxin in ulcerative colitis? Gut, 39(1), 1–4. doi:10.1136/gut.39.1.1

[3947] Pitcher MCL, Beatty ER, Gibson GR, et al. (1995) Incidence and activities of sulphate-reducing bacteria in patients with ulcerative colitis. Gut 36:A63.

[3948] Pitcher et al (1995) Salicylates inhibit bacterial sulphide production within the colonic lumen in ulcerative colitis. Gut 37:A15.

[3949] Christl, S. U., Gibson, G. R., & Cummings, J. H. (1992). Role of dietary sulphate in the regulation of methanogenesis in the human large intestine. Gut, 33(9), 1234–1238. https://doi.org/10.1136/gut.33.9.1234

[3950] Backer, L. C. (2000). Assessing the Acute Gastrointestinal Effects of Ingesting Naturally Occurring, High Levels of Sulfate in Drinking Water. Critical Reviews in Clinical Laboratory Sciences, 37(4), 389–400. doi:10.1080/10408360091174259

[3951] EPA (2012) 'Sulfate in Drinking Water', Drinking Water, Accessed Online Jan 21 2021: https://archive.epa.gov/water/archive/web/html/sulfate.html

[3952] Ikem et al (2002) 'Chemical quality of bottled waters from three cities in eastern Alabama', Science of The Total Environment, Volume 285, Issues 1–3, 21 February 2002, Pages 165-175.

[3953] Allen, H. E., Halley-Henderson, M. A., & Hass, C. N. (1989). Chemical composition of bottled mineral water. Archives of environmental health, 44(2), 102–116. https://doi.org/10.1080/00039896.1989.9934383

[3954] EPA (1999) 'Health Effects from Exposure to High Levels of Sulfate in Drinking Water Study'. EPA 815/R/99/001. Washington, DC: Office of Water, EPA.

[3955] Heizer, W. D., Sandler, R. S., Seal, E., Jr, Murray, S. C., Busby, M. G., Schliebe, B. G., & Pusek, S. N. (1997). Intestinal effects of sulfate in drinking water on normal human subjects. Digestive diseases and sciences, 42(5), 1055–1061. https://doi.org/10.1023/a:1018801522760

[3956] Cocchetto, D.M. and Levy, G. (1981), Absorption of orally administered sodium sulfate in humans. J. Pharm. Sci., 70: 331-333. https://doi.org/10.1002/jps.2600700330

[3957] Florin, T. H. J., Neale, G., Goretski, S., & Cummings, J. H. (1993). The Sulfate Content of Foods and Beverages. Journal of Food Composition and Analysis, 6(2), 140–151. doi:10.1006/jfca.1993.1016

[3958] Cole, D. E. C., & Evrovski, J. (2000). The Clinical Chemistry of Inorganic Sulfate. Critical Reviews in Clinical Laboratory Sciences, 37(4), 299–344. doi:10.1080/10408360091174231

[3959] Cardin, C. J., & Mason, J. (1975). Sulphate transport by rat ileum. Effect of molybdate and other anions. Biochimica et biophysica acta, 394(1), 46–54. https://doi.org/10.1016/0005-2736(75)90203-5

[3960] Batt E. R. (1969). Sulfate accumulation by mouse intestine: influence of age and other factors. The American journal of physiology, 217(4), 1101–1104. https://doi.org/10.1152/ajplegacy.1969.217.4.1101

[3961] ANAST, C., KENNEDY, R., VOLK, G., & ADAMSON, L. (1965). IN VITRO STUDIES OF SULFATE TRANSPORT BY THE SMALL INTESTINE OF THE RAT, RABBIT, AND HAMSTER. The Journal of laboratory and clinical medicine, 65, 903–911.

[3962] Florin, T., Neale, G., Gibson, G. R., Christl, S. U., & Cummings, J. H. (1991). Metabolism of dietary sulphate: absorption and excretion in humans. Gut, 32(7), 766–773. https://doi.org/10.1136/gut.32.7.766

[3963] Ahearn, G. A., & Murer, H. (1984). Functional roles of Na+ and H+ in SO 4 2− transport by rabbit ileal brush border membrane vesicles. The Journal of Membrane Biology, 78(3), 177–186. doi:10.1007/bf01925966

[3964] Miller et al (2001). Heat-damaged protein has reduced ileal true digestibility of cysteine and aspartic acid in chicks. J. Anim. Sci, 79(suppl 1), 65.

[3965] Bauer J. H. (1976). Oral administration of radioactive sulfate to measure extracellular fluid space in man. Journal of applied physiology, 40(4), 648–650. https://doi.org/10.1152/jappl.1976.40.4.648

[3966] Ramani, S. K., & Ismael, A. H. (1990). Barium Sulfate Absorption and Sensitivity. Radiology, 174(3), 895–896. doi:10.1148/radiology.174.3.895d

[3967] Roediger, W. E. W., Moore, J., & Babidge, W. (1997). Digestive Diseases and Sciences, 42(8), 1571–1579. doi:10.1023/a:1018851723920

[3968] Kurpad, A. V., Regan, M. M., Varalakshmi, S., Vasudevan, J., Gnanou, J., Raj, T., & Young, V. R. (2003). Daily methionine requirements of healthy Indian men, measured by a 24-h indicator amino acid oxidation and balance technique. The American Journal of Clinical Nutrition, 77(5), 1198–1205. doi:10.1093/ajcn/77.5.1198

[3969] Irwin, M. I., & Hegsted, D. M. (1971). A conspectus of research on amino acid requirements of man. The Journal of nutrition, 101(4), 539–566. https://doi.org/10.1093/jn/101.4.539

[3970] Fukagawa, N. K., & Galbraith, R. A. (2004). Advancing Age and Other Factors Influencing the Balance between Amino Acid Requirements and Toxicity. The Journal of Nutrition, 134(6), 1569S–1574S. doi:10.1093/jn/134.6.1569s

[3971] Young, V. R., Wagner, D. A., Burini, R., & Storch, K. J. (1991). Methionine kinetics and balance at the 1985 FAO/WHO/UNU intake requirement in adult men studied with L-[2H3-methyl-1-13C]methionine as a tracer. The American Journal of Clinical Nutrition, 54(2), 377–385. doi:10.1093/ajcn/54.2.377

[3972] Storch, K. J., Wagner, D. A., Burke, J. F., & Young, V. R. (1988). Quantitative study in vivo of methionine cycle in humans using [methyl-2H3]- and [1-13C]methionine. The American journal of physiology, 255(3 Pt 1), E322–E331. https://doi.org/10.1152/ajpendo.1988.255.3.E322

[3973] Tuttle, S. G., Bassett, S. H., Griffith, W. H., Mulcare, D. B., & Swendseid, M. E. (1965). FURTHER OBSERVATIONS ON THE AMINO ACID REQUIREMENTS OF OLDER MEN. II. METHIONINE AND LYSINE. The American journal of clinical nutrition, 16, 229–231. https://doi.org/10.1093/ajcn/16.2.229

[3974] van de Poll, M. C., Dejong, C. H., & Soeters, P. B. (2006). Adequate range for sulfur-containing amino acids and biomarkers for their excess: lessons from enteral and parenteral nutrition. The Journal of nutrition, 136(6 Suppl), 1694S–1700S. https://doi.org/10.1093/jn/136.6.1694S

[3975] Kurpad AV, Regan MM, Varalakshmi S, Gnanou J, Lingappa A, Young VR. 2004. Effect of cystine on the methionine requirement of healthy Indian men determined by using the 24-h indicator amino acid balance approach. Am. J. Clin. Nutr. 80:1526–35

[3976] ROSE, W. C., & WIXOM, R. L. (1955). The amino acid requirements of man. XIII. The sparing effect of cystine on the methionine requirement. The Journal of biological chemistry, 216(2), 753–773.

[3977] Humayun, M. A., Turner, J. M., Elango, R., Rafii, M., Langos, V., Ball, R. O., & Pencharz, P. B. (2006). Minimum methionine requirement and cysteine sparing of methionine in healthy school-age children. The American Journal of Clinical Nutrition, 84(5), 1080–1085. doi:10.1093/ajcn/84.5.1080

[3978] Laidlaw, S. A., Shultz, T. D., Cecchino, J. T., & Kopple, J. D. (1988). Plasma and urine taurine levels in vegans. The American journal of clinical nutrition, 47(4), 660–663. https://doi.org/10.1093/ajcn/47.4.660

[3979] Dickey LE, Cutrufelli R, et al. Nutrition Monitoring Division. Composition of Foods Raw, Processed, Prepared, 1992; Supplement, 1993. U.S. Dept. of Agriculture Human Nutrition Information Service.

[3980] Nimni, M. E., Han, B., & Cordoba, F. (2007). Are we getting enough sulfur in our diet?. Nutrition & metabolism, 4, 24. https://doi.org/10.1186/1743-7075-4-24

[3981] Zlotkin, S. H., & Anderson, G. H. (1982). Sulfur balances in intravenously fed infants: effects of cysteine supplementation. The American journal of clinical nutrition, 36(5), 862–867. https://doi.org/10.1093/ajcn/36.5.862

[3982] Sabry, Z. I., Shadarevian, S. B., Cowan, J. W., & Campbell, J. A. (1965). Relationship of dietary intake of sulphur amino-acids to urinary excretion of inorganic sulphate in man. Nature, 206(987), 931–933. https://doi.org/10.1038/206931b0

[3983] Houterman (1965) 'Is urinary sulfate a biomarker for the intake of animal protein and meat?', Cancer Letters, 01 Mar 1997, 114(1-2):295-296, DOI: 10.1016/s0304-3835(97)04684-3

[3984] Greer, F. R., McCormick, A., & Loker, J. (1986). Increased urinary excretion of inorganic sulfate in premature infants fed bovine milk protein. The Journal of pediatrics, 109(4), 692–697. https://doi.org/10.1016/s0022-3476(86)80244-x

[3985] van den Born, J. C., Frenay, A. S., Koning, A. M., Bachtler, M., Riphagen, I. J., Minović, I., Feelisch, M., Dekker, M. M., Bulthuis, M., Gansevoort, R. T., Hillebrands, J. L., Pasch, A., Bakker, S., & van Goor, H. (2019). Urinary Excretion of Sulfur Metabolites and Risk of Cardiovascular Events and All-Cause Mortality in the General Population. Antioxidants & redox signaling, 30(17), 1999–2010. https://doi.org/10.1089/ars.2017.7040

[3986] Said, M. Y., Post, A., Minović, I., van Londen, M., van Goor, H., Postmus, D., Heiner-Fokkema, M. R., van den Berg, E., Pasch, A., Navis, G., & Bakker, S. (2020). Urinary sulfate excretion and risk of late graft failure in renal transplant recipients - a prospective cohort study. Transplant international : official journal of the European Society for Organ Transplantation, 33(7), 752–761. https://doi.org/10.1111/tri.13600

[3987] Florin, T., Neale, G., Gibson, G. R., Christl, S. U., & Cummings, J. H. (1991). Metabolism of dietary sulphate: absorption and excretion in humans. Gut, 32(7), 766–773. https://doi.org/10.1136/gut.32.7.766

[3988] Lin, J. H., & Levy, G. (1983). Renal clearance of inorganic sulfate in rats: effect of acetaminophen-induced depletion of endogenous sulfate. Journal of pharmaceutical sciences, 72(3), 213–217. https://doi.org/10.1002/jps.2600720303

[3989] Tschöpe, W., & Ritz, E. (1985). Sulfur-containing amino acids are a major determinant of urinary calcium. Mineral and electrolyte metabolism, 11(3), 137–139.

[3990] Gregus, Z., Kim, H. J., Madhu, C., Liu, Y., Rozman, P., & Klaassen, C. D. (1994). Sulfation of acetaminophen and acetaminophen-induced alterations in sulfate and 3'-phosphoadenosine 5'-phosphosulfate homeostasis in rats with deficient dietary intake of sulfur. Drug metabolism and disposition: the biological fate of chemicals, 22(5), 725–730.

[3991] Lin, J. H., & Levy, G. (1983). Renal clearance of inorganic sulfate in rats: effect of acetaminophen-induced depletion of endogenous sulfate. Journal of pharmaceutical sciences, 72(3), 213–217. https://doi.org/10.1002/jps.2600720303

[3992] McLean, A. E., Armstrong, G. R., & Beales, D. (1989). Effect of D- or L-methionine and cysteine on the growth inhibitory effects of feeding 1% paracetamol to rats. Biochemical pharmacology, 38(2), 347–352. https://doi.org/10.1016/0006-2952(89)90048-8

[3993] https://www.ncbi.nlm.nih.gov/pubmed/25926513

[3994] Loren Cordain, Janette Brand Miller, S Boyd Eaton, Neil Mann, Susanne HA Holt, John D Speth; Plant-animal subsistence ratios and macronutrient energy estimations in worldwide hunter-gatherer diets, The American Journal of Clinical Nutrition, Volume 71, Issue 3, 1 March 2000, Pages 682–692

[3995] Rodriguez, N. R. (2015). Introduction to Protein Summit 2.0: continued exploration of the impact of high-quality protein on optimal health. The American Journal of Clinical Nutrition, 101(6), 1317S–1319S. doi:10.3945/ajcn.114.083980

[3996] Campbell, W. W., Crim, M. C., Dallal, G. E., Young, V. R., & Evans, W. J. (1994). Increased protein requirements in elderly people: new data and retrospective reassessments. The American journal of clinical nutrition, 60(4), 501–509. https://doi.org/10.1093/ajcn/60.4.501

[3997] Chernoff R. (2004). Protein and older adults. Journal of the American College of Nutrition, 23(6 Suppl), 627S–630S. https://doi.org/10.1080/07315724.2004.10719434

[3998] Kurpad, A. V., & Vaz, M. (2000). Protein and amino acid requirements in the elderly. European journal of clinical nutrition, 54 Suppl 3, S131–S142. https://doi.org/10.1038/sj.ejcn.1601035

[3999] Young V. R. (1990). Protein and amino acid metabolism with reference to aging and the elderly. Progress in clinical and biological research, 326, 279–300.

[4000] Morley J. E. (1997). Anorexia of aging: physiologic and pathologic. The American journal of clinical nutrition, 66(4), 760–773. https://doi.org/10.1093/ajcn/66.4.760

[4001] Wolfe R. R. (2012). The role of dietary protein in optimizing muscle mass, function and health outcomes in older individuals. The British journal of nutrition, 108 Suppl 2, S88–S93. https://doi.org/10.1017/S0007114512002590

[4002] Kerstetter, J. E., Kenny, A. M., & Insogna, K. L. (2011). Dietary protein and skeletal health: a review of recent human research. Current opinion in lipidology, 22(1), 16–20. https://doi.org/10.1097/MOL.0b013e3283419441

[4003] Bonjour J. P. (2005). Dietary protein: an essential nutrient for bone health. Journal of the American College of Nutrition, 24(6 Suppl), 526S–36S. https://doi.org/10.1080/07315724.2005.10719501

[4004] Campbell, W. W., Trappe, T. A., Wolfe, R. R., & Evans, W. J. (2001). The recommended dietary allowance for protein may not be adequate for older people to maintain skeletal muscle. The journals of gerontology. Series A, Biological sciences and medical sciences, 56(6), M373–M380. https://doi.org/10.1093/gerona/56.6.m373

[4005] Wycherley, T. P., Moran, L. J., Clifton, P. M., Noakes, M., & Brinkworth, G. D. (2012). Effects of energy-restricted high-protein, low-fat compared with standard-protein, low-fat diets: a meta-analysis of randomized controlled trials. The American journal of clinical nutrition, 96(6), 1281–1298. https://doi.org/10.3945/ajcn.112.044321

[4006] Wycherley, T. P., Moran, L. J., Clifton, P. M., Noakes, M., & Brinkworth, G. D. (2012). Effects of energy-restricted high-protein, low-fat compared with standard-protein, low-fat diets: a meta-analysis of randomized controlled trials. The American journal of clinical nutrition, 96(6), 1281–1298. https://doi.org/10.3945/ajcn.112.044321

[4007] Weigle, D. S., Breen, P. A., Matthys, C. C., Callahan, H. S., Meeuws, K. E., Burden, V. R., & Purnell, J. Q. (2005). A high-protein diet induces sustained reductions in appetite, ad libitum caloric intake, and body weight despite compensatory changes in diurnal plasma leptin and ghrelin concentrations. The American journal of clinical nutrition, 82(1), 41–48. https://doi.org/10.1093/ajcn.82.1.41

[4008] Bosse, J. D., & Dixon, B. M. (2012). Dietary protein to maximize resistance training: a review and examination of protein spread and change theories. Journal of the International Society of Sports Nutrition, 9(1), 42. https://doi.org/10.1186/1550-2783-9-42

[4009] Dietary protein for athletes: From requirements to optimum adaptation. Phillips SM, Van Loon LJ. J Sports Sci. 2011;29 Suppl 1:S29-38.

[4010] Breitkreutz, R., Babylon, A., Hack, V., Schuster, K., Tokus, M., Böhles, H., Hagmüller, E., Edler, L., Holm, E., & Dröge, W. (2000). Effect of carnitine on muscular glutamate uptake and intramuscular glutathione in malignant diseases. British journal of cancer, 82(2), 399–403. https://doi.org/10.1054/bjoc.1999.0933

[4011] Lyons, J., Rauh-Pfeiffer, A., Yu, Y. M., Lu, X. M., Zurakowski, D., Tompkins, R. G., Ajami, A. M., Young, V. R., & Castillo, L. (2000). Blood glutathione synthesis rates in healthy adults receiving a sulfur amino acid-free diet. Proceedings of the National Academy of Sciences of the United States of America, 97(10), 5071–5076. https://doi.org/10.1073/pnas.090083297

[4012] Flagg et al (1994) Dietary glutathione intake in humans and the relationship between intake and plasma total glutathione level, Nutrition and Cancer, 21:1, 33-46, DOI: 10.1080/01635589409514302

[4013] Jones, D. P., Coates, R. J., Flagg, E. W., Eley, J. W., Block, G., Greenberg, R. S., Gunter, E. W., & Jackson, B. (1992). Glutathione in foods listed in the National Cancer Institute's Health Habits and History Food Frequency Questionnaire. Nutrition and cancer, 17(1), 57–75. https://doi.org/10.1080/01635589209514173

[4014] Zavorsky, G. S., Kubow, S., Grey, V., Riverin, V., & Lands, L. C. (2007). An open-label dose-response study of lymphocyte glutathione levels in healthy men and women receiving pressurized whey protein isolate supplements. International journal of food sciences and nutrition, 58(6), 429–436. https://doi.org/10.1080/09637480701253581

[4015] Flaim, C., Kob, M., Di Pierro, A. M., Herrmann, M., & Lucchin, L. (2017). Effects of a whey protein supplementation on oxidative stress, body composition and glucose metabolism among overweight people affected by diabetes mellitus or impaired fasting glucose: A pilot study. The Journal of nutritional biochemistry, 50, 95–102. https://doi.org/10.1016/j.jnutbio.2017.05.003

[4016] Abenavoli, L., Capasso, R., Milic, N., & Capasso, F. (2010). Milk thistle in liver diseases: past, present, future. Phytotherapy research : PTR, 24(10), 1423–1432. https://doi.org/10.1002/ptr.3207

[4017] Kiruthiga, P. V., Pandian, S. K., & Devi, K. P. (2010). Silymarin protects PBMC against B(a)P induced toxicity by replenishing redox status and modulating glutathione metabolizing enzymes--an in vitro study. Toxicology and applied pharmacology, 247(2), 116–128. https://doi.org/10.1016/j.taap.2010.06.004

[4018] Muriel, P., Garciapiña, T., Perez-Alvarez, V., & Mourelle, M. (1992). Silymarin protects against paracetamol-induced lipid peroxidation and liver damage. Journal of applied toxicology : JAT, 12(6), 439–442. https://doi.org/10.1002/jat.2550120613

[4019] Biswas, S. K., McClure, D., Jimenez, L. A., Megson, I. L., & Rahman, I. (2005). Curcumin induces glutathione biosynthesis and inhibits NF-kappaB activation and interleukin-8 release in alveolar epithelial cells: mechanism of free radical scavenging activity. Antioxidants & redox signaling, 7(1-2), 32–41. https://doi.org/10.1089/ars.2005.7.32

[4020] Ward, M., McNulty, H., McPartlin, J., Strain, J. J., Weir, D. G., & Scott, J. M. (2001). Effect of supplemental methionine on plasma homocysteine concentrations in healthy men: a preliminary study. International journal for vitamin and nutrition research. Internationale Zeitschrift fur Vitamin- und Ernahrungsforschung. Journal international de vitaminologie et de nutrition, 71(1), 82–86. https://doi.org/10.1024/0300-9831.71.1.82

[4021] Verhoef, P., van Vliet, T., Olthof, M. R., & Katan, M. B. (2005). A high-protein diet increases postprandial but not fasting plasma total homocysteine concentrations: a dietary controlled, crossover trial in healthy volunteers. The American journal of clinical nutrition, 82(3), 553–558. https://doi.org/10.1093/ajcn.82.3.553

[4022] Ditscheid, B., Fünfstück, R., Busch, M., Schubert, R., Gerth, J., & Jahreis, G. (2005). Effect of L-methionine supplementation on plasma homocysteine and other free amino acids: a placebo-controlled double-blind cross-over study. European journal of clinical nutrition, 59(6), 768–775. https://doi.org/10.1038/sj.ejcn.1602138

[4023] Barter, P. J., & Rye, K.-A. (2006). Homocysteine and Cardiovascular Disease. Circulation Research, 99(6), 565–566. doi:10.1161/01.res.0000243583.39694.1f

[4024] Kraus, J. P., Janosík, M., Kozich, V., Mandell, R., Shih, V., Sperandeo, M. P., Sebastio, G., de Franchis, R., Andria, G., Kluijtmans, L. A., Blom, H., Boers, G. H., Gordon, R. B., Kamoun, P., Tsai, M. Y., Kruger, W. D., Koch, H. G., Ohura, T., & Gaustadnes, M. (1999). Cystathionine beta-synthase mutations in homocystinuria. Human mutation, 13(5), 362–375. https://doi.org/10.1002/(SICI)1098-1004(1999)13:5<362::AID-HUMU4>3.0.CO;2-K

[4025] Beard and Bearden (2001) 'Vascular complications of cystathionine -synthase deficiency:', Am J Physiol Heart Circ Physiol 300: H13–H26, 2011.

[4026] Finkelstein, J. D. (2006). Inborn Errors of Sulfur-Containing Amino Acid Metabolism. The Journal of Nutrition, 136(6), 1750S–1754S. doi:10.1093/jn/136.6.1750s

[4027] Mudd, S. H., Skovby, F., Levy, H. L., Pettigrew, K. D., Wilcken, B., Pyeritz, R. E., Andria, G., Boers, G. H., Bromberg, I. L., & Cerone, R. (1985). The natural history of homocystinuria due to cystathionine beta-synthase deficiency. American journal of human genetics, 37(1), 1–31.

[4028] Wang, J., & Hegele, R. A. (2003). Genomic basis of cystathioninuria (MIM 219500) revealed by multiple mutations in cystathionine gamma-lyase (CTH). Human genetics, 112(4), 404–408. https://doi.org/10.1007/s00439-003-0906-8

[4029] https://www.ncbi.nlm.nih.gov/pmc/articles/PMC5008916/

[4030] Ruckenstuhl et al (2014) 'Lifespan extension by methionine restriction requires autophagy-dependent vacuolar acidification', PLoS Genet. 2014 May 1;10(5):e1004347. doi: 10.1371/journal.pgen.1004347. eCollection 2014 May.

[4031] Speakman JR, Mitchell SE, Mazidi M. Calories or protein? The effect of dietary restriction on lifespan in rodents is explained by calories alone. Exp Gerontol.2016 Dec 15;86:28-38. doi: 10.1016/j.exger.2016.03.011. Epub 2016 Mar 19. Review.PubMed PMID: 27006163.

[4032] Pugh TD, Oberley TD, Weindruch R. Dietary intervention at middle age: caloric restriction but not dehydroepiandrosterone sulfate increases lifespan and lifetime cancer incidence in mice. Cancer Res. 1999 Apr 1;59(7):1642-8. PubMed PMID: 10197641.

[4033] Davis TA, Bales CW, Beauchene RE. Differential effects of dietary caloric and protein restriction in the aging rat. Exp Gerontol. 1983;18(6):427-35. PubMed PMID: 6673988.

[4034] Richardson B. (2003). DNA methylation and autoimmune disease. Clinical immunology (Orlando, Fla.), 109(1), 72–79. https://doi.org/10.1016/s1521-6616(03)00206-7

[4035] Cellarier, E., Durando, X., Vasson, M. P., Farges, M. C., Demiden, A., Maurizis, J. C., Madelmont, J. C., & Chollet, P. (2003). Methionine dependency and cancer treatment. Cancer treatment reviews, 29(6), 489–499. https://doi.org/10.1016/s0305-7372(03)00118-x

[4036] Wood, J. M., Decker, H., Hartmann, H., Chavan, B., Rokos, H., Spencer, J. D., Hasse, S., Thornton, M. J., Shalbaf, M., Paus, R., & Schallreuter, K. U. (2009). Senile hair graying: H2O2-mediated oxidative stress affects human hair color by blunting methionine sulfoxide repair. FASEB journal : official

713

publication of the Federation of American Societies for Experimental Biology, 23(7), 2065–2075. https://doi.org/10.1096/fj.08-125435

[4037] Bin, P., Huang, R., & Zhou, X. (2017). Oxidation Resistance of the Sulfur Amino Acids: Methionine and Cysteine. BioMed research international, 2017, 9584932. https://doi.org/10.1155/2017/9584932

[4038] Hunter, E. A., & Grimble, R. F. (1997). Dietary sulphur amino acid adequacy influences glutathione synthesis and glutathione-dependent enzymes during the inflammatory response to endotoxin and tumour necrosis factor-alpha in rats. Clinical science (London, England : 1979), 92(3), 297–305. https://doi.org/10.1042/cs0920297

[4039] https://www.fasebj.org/doi/abs/10.1096/fasebj.25.1_supplement.528.2

[4040] American College Of Chest Physicians. (2000, October 19). New Study Supports Chicken Soup As A Cold Remedy. ScienceDaily. Retrieved January 24, 2021 from www.sciencedaily.com/releases/2000/10/001018075252.htm

[4041] Rennard, B. O., Ertl, R. F., Gossman, G. L., Robbins, R. A., & Rennard, S. I. (2000). Chicken soup inhibits neutrophil chemotaxis in vitro. Chest, 118(4), 1150–1157. https://doi.org/10.1378/chest.118.4.1150

[4042] Zajac J, Shrestha A, Patel P, Poretsky L (2009). "The Main Events in the History of Diabetes Mellitus". In Poretsky L (ed.). Principles of diabetes mellitus (2nd ed.). New York: Springer. pp. 3–16. ISBN 978-0-387-09840-1. OCLC 663097550

[4043] Papaspyros NS. The history of diabetes. In: Verlag GT, ed. The History of Diabetes Mellitus. Stuttgart: Thieme; 1964:4–5.

[4044] Mandal (2019) 'History of Diabetes', News Medical Life Sciences, Accessed Online Jan 17 2021: https://www.news-medical.net/health/History-of-Diabetes.aspx

[4045] Papaspyros NS. The history of diabetes. In: Verlag GT, ed. The History of Diabetes Mellitus. Stuttgart: Thieme; 1964:4.

[4046] Sanders LJ. From Thebes to Toronto and the 21st century: an incredible journey. Diabetes Spect. 2002;15:56–60.

[4047] Medvei VC. The Greco – Roman period. In: Medvei VC, ed. The History of Clinical Endocrinology: A Comprehensive Account of Endocrinology from Earliest Times to the Present Day. New York: Parthenon Publishing; 1993:34, 37.

[4048] Medvei VC. The 16th century and the Renaissance. In: Medvei VC, ed. The History of Clinical Endocrinology: A Comprehensive Account of Endocrinology from Earliest Times to the Present Day. New York: Parthenon Publishing; 1993:55–56.

[4049] Medvei VC. The 18th century and the beginning of the 19th century. In: Medvei VC, ed. The History of Clinical Endocrinology: A Comprehensive Account of Endocrinology from Earliest Times to the Present Day. New York: Parthenon Publishing; 1993:97.

[4050] GBD 2015 Disease and Injury Incidence and Prevalence Collaborators (2016). Global, regional, and national incidence, prevalence, and years lived with disability for 310 diseases and injuries, 1990-2015: a systematic analysis for the Global Burden of Disease Study 2015. Lancet (London, England), 388(10053), 1545–1602. https://doi.org/10.1016/S0140-6736(16)31678-6

[4051] Danaei, G., Finucane, M. M., Lu, Y., Singh, G. M., Cowan, M. J., Paciorek, C. J., Lin, J. K., Farzadfar, F., Khang, Y. H., Stevens, G. A., Rao, M., Ali, M. K., Riley, L. M., Robinson, C. A., Ezzati, M., & Global Burden of Metabolic Risk Factors of Chronic Diseases Collaborating Group (Blood Glucose) (2011). National, regional, and global trends in fasting plasma glucose and diabetes prevalence since 1980: systematic analysis of health examination surveys and epidemiological studies with 370 country-years and 2·7 million participants. Lancet (London, England), 378(9785), 31–40. https://doi.org/10.1016/S0140-6736(11)60679-X

[4052] Menke et al (2015) 'Prevalence of and Trends in Diabetes Among Adults in the United States, 1988-2012', JAMA. 2015;314(10):1021-1029. doi:10.1001/jama.2015.10029

[4053] Gardner, David G.; Shoback, Dolores, eds. (2011). "Chapter 17: Pancreatic hormones & diabetes mellitus". Greenspan's basic & clinical endocrinology (9th ed.). New York: McGraw-Hill Medical. ISBN 978-0-07-162243-1. OCLC 613429053

[4054] Chiang, J. L., Kirkman, M. S., Laffel, L. M., Peters, A. L., & Type 1 Diabetes Sourcebook Authors (2014). Type 1 diabetes through the life span: a position statement of the American Diabetes Association. Diabetes care, 37(7), 2034–2054. https://doi.org/10.2337/dc14-1140

[4055] World Health Organization (2009) 'GLOBAL HEALTH RISKS: Mortality and burden of disease attributable to selected major risks', WHO Library Cataloguing-in-Publication Data, Accessed Online Jan 13 2021: https://www.who.int/healthinfo/global_burden_disease/GlobalHealthRisks_report_full.pdf

[4056] Mathers, C. D., & Loncar, D. (2006). Projections of Global Mortality and Burden of Disease from 2002 to 2030. PLoS Medicine, 3(11), e442. doi:10.1371/journal.pmed.0030442

[4057] World Health Organization (2011) 'Global status report on noncommunicable diseases 2010: Description of the global burden of NCDs, their risk factors and determinants', Noncommunicable diseases and mental health, Accessed Online Jan 13 2021: https://www.who.int/nmh/publications/ncd_report2010/en/

714

[4058] Bitzur R. (2011). Diabetes and cardiovascular disease: when it comes to lipids, statins are all you need. Diabetes care, 34 Suppl 2(Suppl 2), S380–S382. https://doi.org/10.2337/dc11-s256

[4059] Shah, A. D., Langenberg, C., Rapsomaniki, E., Denaxas, S., Pujades-Rodriguez, M., Gale, C. P., … Hemingway, H. (2015). Type 2 diabetes and incidence of cardiovascular diseases: a cohort study in 1·9 million people. The Lancet Diabetes & Endocrinology, 3(2), 105–113. doi:10.1016/s2213-8587(14)70219-0

[4060] Ho, J. E., Paultre, F., & Mosca, L. (2003). Is Diabetes Mellitus a Cardiovascular Disease Risk Equivalent for Fatal Stroke in Women? Stroke, 34(12), 2812–2816. doi:10.1161/01.str.0000102901.41780.5c

[4061] Morrish, N. J., Wang, S.-L., Stevens, L. K., Fuller, J. H., & Keen, H. (2001). Mortality and causes of death in the WHO multinational study of vascular disease in diabetes. Diabetologia, 44(S2), S14–S21. doi:10.1007/pl00002934

[4062] NIDDK (2017) 'Diabetic Kidney Disease', Preventing Diabetes Problems, Accessed Online Jan 13 2021: https://www.niddk.nih.gov/health-information/diabetes/overview/preventing-problems/diabetic-kidney-disease

[4063] Roglic, G., Unwin, N., Bennett, P. H., Mathers, C., Tuomilehto, J., Nag, S., … King, H. (2005). The Burden of Mortality Attributable to Diabetes: Realistic estimates for the year 2000. Diabetes Care, 28(9), 2130–2135. doi:10.2337/diacare.28.9.2130

[4064] Boulton A. J. (1998). Lowering the risk of neuropathy, foot ulcers and amputations. Diabetic medicine : a journal of the British Diabetic Association, 15 Suppl 4, S57–S59. https://doi.org/10.1002/(sici)1096-9136(1998120)15:4+3.3.co;2-4

[4065] Dwyer, M. S., Melton, L. J., 3rd, Ballard, D. J., Palumbo, P. J., Trautmann, J. C., & Chu, C. P. (1985). Incidence of diabetic retinopathy and blindness: a population-based study in Rochester, Minnesota. Diabetes care, 8(4), 316–322. https://doi.org/10.2337/diacare.8.4.316

[4066] Pasquier F. (2010). Diabetes and cognitive impairment: how to evaluate the cognitive status?. Diabetes & metabolism, 36 Suppl 3, S100–S105. https://doi.org/10.1016/S1262-3636(10)70475-4

[4067] CDC (2019) 'Insulin Resistance and Diabetes', Type 2 Diabetes, Accessed Online Jan 13 2021: https://www.cdc.gov/diabetes/basics/insulin-resistance.html

[4068] Smyth, S., & Heron, A. (2006). Diabetes and obesity: the twin epidemics. Nature medicine, 12(1), 75–80. https://doi.org/10.1038/nm0106-75

[4069] World Health Organization. (1999). Definition, diagnosis and classification of diabetes mellitus and its complications : report of a WHO consultation. Part 1, Diagnosis and classification of diabetes mellitus. World Health Organization. https://apps.who.int/iris/handle/10665/66040

[4070] Daneman D. (2006). Type 1 diabetes. Lancet (London, England), 367(9513), 847–858. https://doi.org/10.1016/S0140-6736(06)68341-4

[4071] Streeten, D. H. P., Gerstein, M. M., Marmor, B. M., & Doisy, R. J. (1965). Reduced Glucose Tolerance in Elderly Human Subjects. Diabetes, 14(9), 579–583. doi:10.2337/diab.14.9.579

[4072] Tfayli, H., & Arslanian, S. (2009). Pathophysiology of type 2 diabetes mellitus in youth: the evolving chameleon. Arquivos brasileiros de endocrinologia e metabologia, 53(2), 165–174. https://doi.org/10.1590/s0004-27302009000200008

[4073] Kraft (2020) 'Detection of Diabetes Mellitus In Situ (Occult Diabetes)', Meridian Valley Labs, Accessed Online Jan 18 2021: http://meridianvalleylab.com/wp-content/uploads/2012/08/GITT-Article-Re-type1.pdf

[4074] DiNicolantonio, J. J., Bhutani, J., OKeefe, J. H., & Crofts, C. (2017). Postprandial insulin assay as the earliest biomarker for diagnosing pre-diabetes, type 2 diabetes and increased cardiovascular risk. Open heart, 4(2), e000656. https://doi.org/10.1136/openhrt-2017-000656

[4075] World Health Organization (2013) 'Diabetes', Fact Sheets, Accessed Online Jan 13 2021 https://web.archive.org/web/20130826174444/http://www.who.int/mediacentre/factsheets/fs312/en/

[4076] American Diabetes Association (2010). Diagnosis and classification of diabetes mellitus. Diabetes care, 33 Suppl 1(Suppl 1), S62–S69. https://doi.org/10.2337/dc10-S062

[4077] Vijan S. (2010). In the clinic. Type 2 diabetes. Annals of internal medicine, 152(5), ITC31–ITC316. https://doi.org/10.7326/0003-4819-152-5-201003020-01003

[4078] International Expert Committee (2009). International Expert Committee report on the role of the A1C assay in the diagnosis of diabetes. Diabetes care, 32(7), 1327–1334. https://doi.org/10.2337/dc09-9033

[4079] Raina Elley, C., & Kenealy, T. (2008). Lifestyle interventions reduced the long-term risk of diabetes in adults with impaired glucose tolerance. Evidence-based medicine, 13(6), 173. https://doi.org/10.1136/ebm.13.6.173

[4080] Schellenberg et al (2013) 'Lifestyle Interventions for Patients With and at Risk for Type 2 Diabetes', Ann Intern Med.2013;159:543-551. [Epub ahead of print 15 October 2013]. doi:10.7326/0003-4819-159-8-201310150-00007

[4081] NIDDK (2020) 'Diabetes Prevention Program (DPP)', Diabetes, Accessed Online Jan 13 2021: https://www.niddk.nih.gov/about-niddk/research-areas/diabetes/diabetes-prevention-program-dpp

[4082] Zanuso, S., Jimenez, A., Pugliese, G., Corigliano, G., & Balducci, S. (2010). Exercise for the management of type 2 diabetes: a review of the evidence. Acta diabetologica, 47(1), 15–22. https://doi.org/10.1007/s00592-009-0126-3

[4083] O'Gorman, D. J., & Krook, A. (2011). Exercise and the treatment of diabetes and obesity. The Medical clinics of North America, 95(5), 953–969. https://doi.org/10.1016/j.mcna.2011.06.007

[4084] Kyu, H. H., Bachman, V. F., Alexander, L. T., Mumford, J. E., Afshin, A., Estep, K., Veerman, J. L., Delwiche, K., Iannarone, M. L., Moyer, M. L., Cercy, K., Vos, T., Murray, C. J., & Forouzanfar, M. H. (2016). Physical activity and risk of breast cancer, colon cancer, diabetes, ischemic heart disease, and ischemic stroke events: systematic review and dose-response meta-analysis for the Global Burden of Disease Study 2013. BMJ (Clinical research ed.), 354, i3857. https://doi.org/10.1136/bmj.i3857

[4085] Koutroumpakis, E., Jozwik, B., Aguilar, D., & Taegtmeyer, H. (2020). Strategies of Unloading the Failing Heart from Metabolic Stress. The American journal of medicine, 133(3), 290–296. https://doi.org/10.1016/j.amjmed.2019.08.035

[4086] Schwingshackl, L., Hoffmann, G., Lampousi, A. M., Knüppel, S., Iqbal, K., Schwedhelm, C., Bechthold, A., Schlesinger, S., & Boeing, H. (2017). Food groups and risk of type 2 diabetes mellitus: a systematic review and meta-analysis of prospective studies. European journal of epidemiology, 32(5), 363–375. https://doi.org/10.1007/s10654-017-0246-y

[4087] Carter, P., Gray, L. J., Troughton, J., Khunti, K., & Davies, M. J. (2010). Fruit and vegetable intake and incidence of type 2 diabetes mellitus: systematic review and meta-analysis. BMJ (Clinical research ed.), 341, c4229. https://doi.org/10.1136/bmj.c4229

[4088] Xi, B., Li, S., Liu, Z., Tian, H., Yin, X., Huai, P., Tang, W., Zhou, D., & Steffen, L. M. (2014). Intake of fruit juice and incidence of type 2 diabetes: a systematic review and meta-analysis. PloS one, 9(3), e93471. https://doi.org/10.1371/journal.pone.0093471

[4089] Reynolds, A., Mann, J., Cummings, J., Winter, N., Mete, E., & Te Morenga, L. (2019). Carbohydrate quality and human health: a series of systematic reviews and meta-analyses. The Lancet, 393(10170), 434–445. doi:10.1016/s0140-6736(18)31809-9

[4090] Maruthur, N.M., Tseng, E., Hutfless, S., Wilson, L., Suarez-Cuervo, C., Berger, Z., Chu, Y., Iyoha, E., Segal, J., & Bolen, S. (2016). Diabetes Medications as Monotherapy or Metformin-Based Combination Therapy for Type 2 Diabetes. Annals of Internal Medicine, 164, 740-751.

[4091] Thukral, A., Selvan, C., Chakraborty, P. P., Roy, A., Goswami, S., Bhattacharjee, R., … Chowdhury, S. (2013). Case Studies in Insulin Therapy: The Last Arrow in the Treatment Quiver. Clinical Diabetes, 31(4), 175–178. doi:10.2337/diaclin.31.4.175

[4092] Haw, J. S., Galaviz, K. I., Straus, A. N., Kowalski, A. J., Magee, M. J., Weber, M. B., Wei, J., Narayan, K., & Ali, M. K. (2017). Long-term Sustainability of Diabetes Prevention Approaches: A Systematic Review and Meta-analysis of Randomized Clinical Trials. JAMA internal medicine, 177(12), 1808–1817. https://doi.org/10.1001/jamainternmed.2017.6040

[4093] Takaya, J., Higashino, H., & Kobayashi, Y. (2004). Intracellular magnesium and insulin resistance. Magnesium research, 17(2), 126–136.

[4094] Rosique-Esteban, N., Guasch-Ferré, M., Hernández-Alonso, P., & Salas-Salvadó, J. (2018). Dietary Magnesium and Cardiovascular Disease: A Review with Emphasis in Epidemiological Studies. Nutrients, 10(2), 168. doi:10.3390/nu10020168

[4095] De Baaij, J. H. F., Hoenderop, J. G. J., & Bindels, R. J. M. (2015). Magnesium in Man: Implications for Health and Disease. Physiological Reviews, 95(1), 1–46. doi:10.1152/physrev.00012.2014

[4096] Kleefstra, N., Houweling, S. T., Groenier, K. H., & Bilo, H. J. (2010). Characterization of the metabolic and physiologic response to chromium supplementation in subjects with type 2 diabetes mellitus. Metabolism: clinical and experimental, 59(11), e17. https://doi.org/10.1016/j.metabol.2010.07.016

[4097] Mertz, W. (1993). Chromium in Human Nutrition: A Review. The Journal of Nutrition, 123(4), 626–633. doi:10.1093/jn/123.4.626

[4098] DiNicolantonio, J. J., & OKeefe, J. H. (2017). Added sugars drive coronary heart disease via insulin resistance and hyperinsulinaemia: a new paradigm. Open heart, 4(2), e000729. https://doi.org/10.1136/openhrt-2017-000729

[4099] DiNicolantonio, J. J., O'Keefe, J. H., & Lucan, S. C. (2015). Added fructose: a principal driver of type 2 diabetes mellitus and its consequences. Mayo Clinic proceedings, 90(3), 372–381. https://doi.org/10.1016/j.mayocp.2014.12.019

[4100] Malik, V. S., Popkin, B. M., Bray, G. A., Després, J. P., & Hu, F. B. (2010). Sugar-sweetened beverages, obesity, type 2 diabetes mellitus, and cardiovascular disease risk. Circulation, 121(11), 1356–1364. https://doi.org/10.1161/CIRCULATIONAHA.109.876185

[4101] Malik, V. S., Popkin, B. M., Bray, G. A., Després, J. P., Willett, W. C., & Hu, F. B. (2010). Sugar-sweetened beverages and risk of metabolic syndrome and type 2 diabetes: a meta-analysis. Diabetes care, 33(11), 2477–2483. https://doi.org/10.2337/dc10-1079

[4102] Garaulet, M., Pérez-Llamas, F., Pérez-Ayala, M., Martínez, P., de Medina, F. S., Tebar, F. J., & Zamora, S. (2001). Site-specific differences in the fatty acid composition of abdominal adipose tissue in an obese population from a Mediterranean area: relation with dietary fatty acids, plasma lipid profile, serum insulin, and central obesity. The American journal of clinical nutrition, 74(5), 585–591. https://doi.org/10.1093/ajcn/74.5.585

[4103] Deol, P., Fahrmann, J., Yang, J., Evans, J. R., Rizo, A., Grapov, D., ... Sladek, F. M. (2017). Omega-6 and omega-3 oxylipins are implicated in soybean oil-induced obesity in mice. Scientific Reports, 7(1). doi:10.1038/s41598-017-12624-9

[4104] Risérus, U., Willett, W. C., & Hu, F. B. (2009). Dietary fats and prevention of type 2 diabetes. Progress in lipid research, 48(1), 44–51. https://doi.org/10.1016/j.plipres.2008.10.002

[4105] Hu, E. A., Pan, A., Malik, V., & Sun, Q. (2012). White rice consumption and risk of type 2 diabetes: meta-analysis and systematic review. BMJ (Clinical research ed.), 344, e1454. https://doi.org/10.1136/bmj.e1454

[4106] Lee, I. M., Shiroma, E. J., Lobelo, F., Puska, P., Blair, S. N., Katzmarzyk, P. T., & Lancet Physical Activity Series Working Group (2012). Effect of physical inactivity on major non-communicable diseases worldwide: an analysis of burden of disease and life expectancy. Lancet (London, England), 380(9838), 219–229. https://doi.org/10.1016/S0140-6736(12)61031-9

[4107] Abdullah, A., Peeters, A., de Courten, M., & Stoelwinder, J. (2010). The magnitude of association between overweight and obesity and the risk of diabetes: a meta-analysis of prospective cohort studies. Diabetes research and clinical practice, 89(3), 309–319. https://doi.org/10.1016/j.diabres.2010.04.012

[4108] Gastaldelli, A., Miyazaki, Y., Pettiti, M., Matsuda, M., Mahankali, S., Santini, E., ... Ferrannini, E. (2002). Metabolic Effects of Visceral Fat Accumulation in Type 2 Diabetes. The Journal of Clinical Endocrinology & Metabolism, 87(11), 5098–5103. doi:10.1210/jc.2002-020696

[4109] Nielsen, F. H., Milne, D. B., Klevay, L. M., Gallagher, S., & Johnson, L. (2007). Dietary magnesium deficiency induces heart rhythm changes, impairs glucose tolerance, and decreases serum cholesterol in post menopausal women. Journal of the American College of Nutrition, 26(2), 121–132. https://doi.org/10.1080/07315724.2007.10719593

[4110] Resnick, L. M., Altura, B. T., Gupta, R. K., Laragh, J. H., Alderman, M. H., & Altura, B. M. (1993). Intracellular and extracellular magnesium depletion in type 2 (non-insulin-dependent) diabetes mellitus. Diabetologia, 36(8), 767–770. https://doi.org/10.1007/BF00401149

[4111] Nadler, J. L., Buchanan, T., Natarajan, R., Antonipillai, I., Bergman, R., & Rude, R. (1993). Magnesium deficiency produces insulin resistance and increased thromboxane synthesis. Hypertension, 21(6_pt_2), 1024–1029. doi:10.1161/01.hyp.21.6.1024

[4112] Wälti, M. K., Zimmermann, M. B., Spinas, G. A., & Hurrell, R. F. (2003). Low plasma magnesium in type 2 diabetes. Swiss medical weekly, 133(19-20), 289–292.

[4113] de Lourdes Lima et al (2006) '[Magnesium deficiency and insulin resistance in patients with type 2 diabetes mellitus]', Arquivos Brasileiros de Endocrinologia & Metabologia 49(6):959-63

[4114] Solati et al (2014) 'Oral magnesium supplementation in type II diabetic patients.', Medical Journal of the Islamic Republic of Iran, 15 Jul 2014, 28:67

[4115] Anderson R. A. (1981). Nutritional role of chromium. The Science of the total environment, 17(1), 13–29. https://doi.org/10.1016/0048-9697(81)90104-2

[4116] Brownley, K. A., Boettiger, C. A., Young, L., & Cefalu, W. T. (2015). Dietary chromium supplementation for targeted treatment of diabetes patients with comorbid depression and binge eating. Medical hypotheses, 85(1), 45–48. https://doi.org/10.1016/j.mehy.2015.03.020

[4117] Pan, A., Wang, Y., Talaei, M., Hu, F. B., & Wu, T. (2015). Relation of active, passive, and quitting smoking with incident type 2 diabetes: a systematic review and meta-analysis. The lancet. Diabetes & endocrinology, 3(12), 958–967. https://doi.org/10.1016/S2213-8587(15)00316-2

[4118] Lind, L., & Lind, P. M. (2012). Can persistent organic pollutants and plastic-associated chemicals cause cardiovascular disease?. Journal of internal medicine, 271(6), 537–553. https://doi.org/10.1111/j.1365-2796.2012.02536.x

[4119] Touma, C., & Pannain, S. (2011). Does lack of sleep cause diabetes?. Cleveland Clinic journal of medicine, 78(8), 549–558. https://doi.org/10.3949/ccjm.78a.10165

[4120] Saad, F., & Gooren, L. (2009). The role of testosterone in the metabolic syndrome: a review. The Journal of steroid biochemistry and molecular biology, 114(1-2), 40–43. https://doi.org/10.1016/j.jsbmb.2008.12.022

[4121] Farrell, J. B., Deshmukh, A., & Baghaie, A. A. (2008). Low testosterone and the association with type 2 diabetes. The Diabetes educator, 34(5), 799–806. https://doi.org/10.1177/0145721708323100

[4122] Seida, J. C., Mitri, J., Colmers, I. N., Majumdar, S. R., Davidson, M. B., Edwards, A. L., Hanley, D. A., Pittas, A. G., Tjosvold, L., & Johnson, J. A. (2014). Clinical review: Effect of vitamin D3 supplementation on improving glucose homeostasis and preventing diabetes: a systematic review and meta-analysis. The Journal of clinical endocrinology and metabolism, 99(10), 3551–3560. https://doi.org/10.1210/jc.2014-2136

[4123] Mertz et al (1988) 'IS CHROMIUM ESSENTIAL FOR HUMANS? Nutrition Reviews, Volume 46, Issue 1, January 1988, Pages 17–20, https://doi.org/10.1111/j.1753-4887.1988.tb05348.x

717

[4124] Liu, L., Cui, W. M., Zhang, S. W., Kong, F. H., Pedersen, M. A., Wen, Y., & Lv, J. P. (2015). Effect of glucose tolerance factor (GTF) from high chromium yeast on glucose metabolism in insulin-resistant 3T3-L1 adipocytes. RSC Advances, 5(5), 3482–3490. doi:10.1039/c4ra10343b

[4125] Barrett, J., Brien, P. O., & De Jesus, J. P. (1985). Chromium(III) and the glucose tolerance factor. Polyhedron, 4(1), 1–14. doi:10.1016/s0277-5387(00)84214-x

[4126] Bahijiri, S. M., Mira, S. A., Mufti, A. M., & Ajabnoor, M. A. (2000). The effects of inorganic chromium and brewer's yeast supplementation on glucose tolerance, serum lipids and drug dosage in individuals with type 2 diabetes. Saudi medical journal, 21(9), 831–837.

[4127] Racek, J., Trefil, L., Rajdl, D., Mudrová, V., Hunter, D., & Senft, V. (2006). Influence of chromium-enriched yeast on blood glucose and insulin variables, blood lipids, and markers of oxidative stress in subjects with type 2 diabetes mellitus. Biological trace element research, 109(3), 215–230. https://doi.org/10.1385/BTER:109:3:215

[4128] Li, Y.-C. (1994). Effects of brewer's yeast on glucose tolerance and serum lipids in Chinese adults. Biological Trace Element Research, 41(3), 341–347. doi:10.1007/bf02917434

[4129] Doisy et al (1976) 'Chromium Metabolism in Man and Biochemical Effects', in Trace Elements in Human Health and Disease, Volume II: Essential and Toxic Elements, Academic Press, New York, pp 79-80.

[4130] Urberg, M., & Zemel, M. B. (1987). Evidence for synergism between chromium and nicotinic acid in the control of glucose tolerance in elderly humans. Metabolism: clinical and experimental, 36(9), 896–899. https://doi.org/10.1016/0026-0495(87)90100-4

[4131] Schroeder H. A. (1966). Chromium deficiency in rats: a syndrome simulating diabetes mellitus with retarded growth. The Journal of nutrition, 88(4), 439–445. https://doi.org/10.1093/jn/88.4.439

[4132] Schroeder, H. A. (1965). Diabetic-like serum glucose levels in chromium deficient rats. Life Sciences, 4(21), 2057–2062. doi:10.1016/0024-3205(65)90322-x

[4133] Padmavathi, I. J., Rao, K. R., Venu, L., Ganeshan, M., Kumar, K. A., Rao, C., Harishankar, N., Ismail, A., & Raghunath, M. (2010). Chronic maternal dietary chromium restriction modulates visceral adiposity: probable underlying mechanisms. Diabetes, 59(1), 98–104. https://doi.org/10.2337/db09-0779

[4134] Esen Gursel, F., & Tekeli, S. K. (2009). The effects of feeding with different levels of zinc and chromium on plasma thiobarbituric acid reactive substances and antioxidant enzymes in rats. Polish journal of veterinary sciences, 12(1), 35–39.

[4135] Balk, E. M., Tatsioni, A., Lichtenstein, A. H., Lau, J., & Pittas, A. G. (2007). Effect of Chromium Supplementation on Glucose Metabolism and Lipids: A systematic review of randomized controlled trials. Diabetes Care, 30(8), 2154–2163. doi:10.2337/dc06-0996

[4136] Jeejeebhoy, K. N., Chu, R. C., Marliss, E. B., Greenberg, G. R., & Bruce-Robertson, A. (1977). Chromium deficiency, glucose intolerance, and neuropathy reversed by chromium supplementation, in a patient receiving long-term total parenteral nutrition. The American journal of clinical nutrition, 30(4), 531–538. https://doi.org/10.1093/ajcn/30.4.531

[4137] Anderson R. A. (1993). Recent advances in the clinical and biochemical effects of chromium deficiency. Progress in clinical and biological research, 380, 221–234.

[4138] Stehle, P., Stoffel-Wagner, B., & Kuhn, K. S. (2016). Parenteral trace element provision: recent clinical research and practical conclusions. European journal of clinical nutrition, 70(8), 886–893. https://doi.org/10.1038/ejcn.2016.53

[4139] Freund, H., Atamian, S., & Fischer, J. E. (1979). Chromium deficiency during total parenteral nutrition. JAMA, 241(5), 496–498.

[4140] Brown, R. O., Forloines-Lynn, S., Cross, R. E., & Heizer, W. D. (1986). Chromium deficiency after long-term total parenteral nutrition. Digestive diseases and sciences, 31(6), 661–664. https://doi.org/10.1007/BF01318699

[4141] Fessler T. A. (2013). Trace elements in parenteral nutrition: a practical guide for dosage and monitoring for adult patients. Nutrition in clinical practice : official publication of the American Society for Parenteral and Enteral Nutrition, 28(6), 722–729. https://doi.org/10.1177/0884533613506596

[4142] National Toxicology Program (2018) 'Hexavalent Chromium Factsheet', U.S. Department of Health and Human Services, NIH, Accessed Online Jan 11 2021: https://www.niehs.nih.gov/health/materials/hexavalent_chromium_508.pdf

[4143] Wise, S. S., & Wise, J. P., Sr (2012). Chromium and genomic stability. Mutation research, 733(1-2), 78–82. https://doi.org/10.1016/j.mrfmmm.2011.12.002

[4144] Agency for Toxic Substances and Disease Registry (2012) 'ToxFAQs™ for Chromium', Toxic Substances Portal, Accessed Online Jan 12 2021: https://web.archive.org/web/20140708162618/http://www.atsdr.cdc.gov/toxfaqs/TF.asp?id=61&tid=17

[4145] Basketter, D., Horev, L., Slodovnik, D., Merimes, S., Trattner, A., & Ingber, A. (2001). Investigation of the threshold for allergic reactivity to chromium. Contact dermatitis, 44(2), 70–74. https://doi.org/10.1034/j.1600-0536.2001.440202.x

[4146] Vincent J. B. (2013). Chromium: is it essential, pharmacologically relevant, or toxic?. Metal ions in life sciences, 13, 171–198. https://doi.org/10.1007/978-94-007-7500-8_6

[4147] Indian Council of Medical Research (2009) 'NUTRIENT REQUIREMENTS AND RECOMMENDED DIETARY ALLOWANCES FOR INDIANS', A Report of the Expert Group of the Indian Council of Medical Research, NATIONAL INSTITUTE OF NUTRITION, Accessed Online Jan 12 2021: https://web.archive.org/web/20160615094048/http://icmr.nic.in/final/RDA-2010.pdf#

[4148] EFSA NDA Panel (EFSA Panel on Dietetic Products, Nutrition and Allergies), 2014. Scientific Opinion on Dietary Reference Values for chromium. EFSA Journal 2014; 12(10):3845, 25 pp. doi:10.2903/j.efsa.2014.3845

[4149] Institute of Medicine (US) Panel on Micronutrients. (2001). Dietary Reference Intakes for Vitamin A, Vitamin K, Arsenic, Boron, Chromium, Copper, Iodine, Iron, Manganese, Molybdenum, Nickel, Silicon, Vanadium, and Zinc. National Academies Press (US).

[4150] Mertz W. (1969). Chromium occurrence and function in biological systems. Physiological reviews, 49(2), 163–239. https://doi.org/10.1152/physrev.1969.49.2.163

[4151] NIH (2020) 'Chromium: Fact Sheet for Health Professionals', Dietary Supplement Fact Sheets, Accessed Online Jan 18 2021: https://ods.od.nih.gov/factsheets/Chromium-HealthProfessional/

[4152] Food and Nutrition Board. Recommended Dietary Allowances. 9th ed National Academy of Sciences; Washington, DC, USA: 1980.

[4153] WHO (1996) 'Chromium' In: Trace elements in human nutrition and health, Geneva, 155-60. Accessed Online Jan 11 2021: https://www.who.int/nutrition/publications/micronutrients/9241561734/en/

[4154] Sasaki, S. (2017). Dietary Reference Intakes for Japanese (2015): an Outline and Its Academic and Practical Significance. Nippon Eiyo Shokuryo Gakkaishi, 70(2), 53–59. doi:10.4327/jsnfs.70.53

[4155] U. S. Food and Drug Administration (2016) 'Food Labeling: Revision of the Nutrition and Supplement Facts Labels', Docket No. FDA-2012-N-1210, Accessed Online Jan 11 2021: https://www.federalregister.gov/documents/2016/05/27/2016-11867/food-labeling-revision-of-the-nutrition-and-supplement-facts-labels

[4156] Trumbo, P. R., & Ellwood, K. C. (2006). Chromium picolinate intake and risk of type 2 diabetes: an evidence-based review by the United States Food and Drug Administration. Nutrition reviews, 64(8), 357–363. https://doi.org/10.1111/j.1753-4887.2006.tb00220.x

[4157] Emord (2005) 'Qualified Health Claims: Letter of Enforcement Discretion - Chromium Picolinate and Insulin Resistance(Docket No. 2004Q-0144)', U.S. Food and Drug Administration, Labeling & Nutrition, Accessed Online Jan 12 2021: https://wayback.archive-it.org/7993/20171114183739/https://www.fda.gov/Food/IngredientsPackagingLabeling/LabelingNutrition/ucm073017.htm

[4158] American Diabetes Association (2015). (4) Foundations of care: education, nutrition, physical activity, smoking cessation, psychosocial care, and immunization. Diabetes care, 38 Suppl, S20–S30. https://doi.org/10.2337/dc15-S007

[4159] American Diabetes Association (2010). Standards of medical care in diabetes--2010. Diabetes care, 33 Suppl 1(Suppl 1), S11–S61. https://doi.org/10.2337/dc10-S011

[4160] European Food Safety Authority (EFSA) (2010) 'Scientific Opinion on the substantiation of health claims related to chromium and contribution to normal macronutrient metabolism (ID 260, 401, 4665, 4666, 4667), maintenance of normal blood glucose concentrations (ID 262, 4667), contribution to the maintenance or achievement of a normal body weight (ID 339, 4665, 4666), and reduction of tiredness and fatigue (ID 261) pursuant to Article 13(1) of Regulation (EC) No 1924/2006', EFSA Panel on Dietetic Products, Nutrition and Allergies (NDA), Accessed Online Jan 12 2021: https://efsa.onlinelibrary.wiley.com/doi/epdf/10.2903/j.efsa.2010.1732

[4161] Moradi, F., Kooshki, F., Nokhostin, F., Khoshbaten, M., Bazyar, H., & Pourghassem Gargari, B. (2021). A pilot study of the effects of chromium picolinate supplementation on serum fetuin-A, metabolic and inflammatory factors in patients with nonalcoholic fatty liver disease: A double-blind, placebo-controlled trial. Journal of Trace Elements in Medicine and Biology, 63, 126659. doi:10.1016/j.jtemb.2020.126659

[4162] Paiva, A. N., Lima, J. G. de, Medeiros, A. C. Q. de, Figueiredo, H. A. O., Andrade, R. L. de, Ururahy, M. A. G., ... Almeida, M. das G. (2015). Beneficial effects of oral chromium picolinate supplementation on glycemic control in patients with type 2 diabetes: A randomized clinical study. Journal of Trace Elements in Medicine and Biology, 32, 66–72. doi:10.1016/j.jtemb.2015.05.006

[4163] Stearns, D. M., Belbruno, J. J., & Wetterhahn, K. E. (1995). A prediction of chromium(III) accumulation in humans from chromium dietary supplements. FASEB journal : official publication of the Federation of American Societies for Experimental Biology, 9(15), 1650–1657. https://doi.org/10.1096/fasebj.9.15.8529846

[4164] Hopkins, L. L., Jr, Ransome-Kuti, O., & Majaj, A. S. (1968). Improvement of impaired carbohydrate metabolism by chromium 3 in manourished infants. The American journal of clinical nutrition, 21(3), 203–211. https://doi.org/10.1093/ajcn/21.3.203

[4165] Gürson, C. T., & Saner, G. (1973). Effects of chromium supplementation on growth in marasmic protein--calorie malnutrition. The American journal of clinical nutrition, 26(9), 988–991. https://doi.org/10.1093/ajcn/26.9.988

[4166] Gürson, C. T., & Saner, G. (1971). Effect of chromium on glucose utilization in marasmic protein-calorie malnutrition. The American journal of clinical nutrition, 24(11), 1313–1319. https://doi.org/10.1093/ajcn/24.11.1313

[4167] Kantor, E. D., Rehm, C. D., Du, M., White, E., & Giovannucci, E. L. (2016). Trends in Dietary Supplement Use Among US Adults From 1999-2012. JAMA, 316(14), 1464–1474. https://doi.org/10.1001/jama.2016.14403

[4168] Costello, R. B., Dwyer, J. T., & Bailey, R. L. (2016). Chromium supplements for glycemic control in type 2 diabetes: limited evidence of effectiveness. Nutrition reviews, 74(7), 455–468. https://doi.org/10.1093/nutrit/nuw011

[4169] Amato, P., Morales, A. J., & Yen, S. S. C. (2000). Effects of Chromium Picolinate Supplementation on Insulin Sensitivity, Serum Lipids, and Body Composition in Healthy, Nonobese, Older Men and Women. The Journals of Gerontology Series A: Biological Sciences and Medical Sciences, 55(5), M260–M263. doi:10.1093/gerona/55.5.m260

[4170] Wilson, B. E., & Gondy, A. (1995). Effects of chromium supplementation on fasting insulin levels and lipid parameters in healthy, non-obese young subjects. Diabetes research and clinical practice, 28(3), 179–184. https://doi.org/10.1016/0168-8227(95)01097-w

[4171] Di Bona, K. R., Love, S., Rhodes, N. R., McAdory, D., Sinha, S. H., Kern, N., Kent, J., Strickland, J., Wilson, A., Beaird, J., Ramage, J., Rasco, J. F., & Vincent, J. B. (2011). Chromium is not an essential trace element for mammals: effects of a "low-chromium" diet. Journal of biological inorganic chemistry : JBIC : a publication of the Society of Biological Inorganic Chemistry, 16(3), 381–390. https://doi.org/10.1007/s00775-010-0734-y

[4172] Anderson, R. A., Cheng, N., Bryden, N. A., Polansky, M. M., Cheng, N., Chi, J., & Feng, J. (1997). Elevated intakes of supplemental chromium improve glucose and insulin variables in individuals with type 2 diabetes. Diabetes, 46(11), 1786–1791. https://doi.org/10.2337/diab.46.11.1786

[4173] Science Direct (2020) 'Low-Molecular-Weight Chromium-Binding Substance', Biochemistry, Genetics and Molecular Biology, Accessed Online Jan 10 2021: https://www.sciencedirect.com/topics/biochemistry-genetics-and-molecular-biology/low-molecular-weight-chromium-binding-substance

[4174] Davis, C. M., & Vincent, J. B. (1997). Chromium oligopeptide activates insulin receptor tyrosine kinase activity. Biochemistry, 36(15), 4382–4385. https://doi.org/10.1021/bi963154t

[4175] Vincent J. B. (1999). Mechanisms of chromium action: low-molecular-weight chromium-binding substance. Journal of the American College of Nutrition, 18(1), 6–12. https://doi.org/10.1080/07315724.1999.10718821

[4176] Vincent J. B. (2015). Is the Pharmacological Mode of Action of Chromium(III) as a Second Messenger?. Biological trace element research, 166(1), 7–12. https://doi.org/10.1007/s12011-015-0231-9

[4177] Salloum, Z, Lehoux, EA, Harper, M-E, Catelas, I. Effects of cobalt and chromium ions on glycolytic flux and the stabilization of hypoxia-inducible factor-1α in macrophages in vitro. J Orthop Res. 2021; 39: 112– 120. https://doi.org/10.1002/jor.24758

[4178] Mertz, W. (1981). THE INTERACTION BETWEEN CHROMIUM AND INSULIN. Nutrition, Digestion, Metabolism, 101–105. doi:10.1016/b978-0-08-026825-5.50019-x

[4179] Phung et al (2010) 'Improved Glucose Control Associated with i.v. Chromium Administration in Two Patients Receiving Enteral Nutrition', Am J Health Syst Pharm. 2010;67(7):535-541

[4180] Piotrowska, A., Pilch, W., Czerwińska-Ledwig, O., Zuziak, R., Siwek, A., Wolak, M., & Nowak, G. (2019). The Possibilities of Using Chromium Salts as an Agent Supporting Treatment of Polycystic Ovary Syndrome. Biological trace element research, 192(2), 91–97. https://doi.org/10.1007/s12011-019-1654-5

[4181] Tang, X. L., Sun, Z., & Gong, L. (2018). Chromium supplementation in women with polycystic ovary syndrome: Systematic review and meta-analysis. The journal of obstetrics and gynaecology research, 44(1), 134–143. https://doi.org/10.1111/jog.13462

[4182] Maleki, V., Izadi, A., Farsad-Naeimi, A., & Alizadeh, M. (2018). Chromium supplementation does not improve weight loss or metabolic and hormonal variables in patients with polycystic ovary syndrome: A systematic review. Nutrition research (New York, N.Y.), 56, 1–10. https://doi.org/10.1016/j.nutres.2018.04.003

[4183] Fazelian, S., Rouhani, M. H., Bank, S. S., & Amani, R. (2017). Chromium supplementation and polycystic ovary syndrome: A systematic review and meta-analysis. Journal of trace elements in medicine and biology : organ of the Society for Minerals and Trace Elements (GMS), 42, 92–96. https://doi.org/10.1016/j.jtemb.2017.04.008

[4184] Heshmati, J., Omani-Samani, R., Vesali, S., Maroufizadeh, S., Rezaeinejad, M., Razavi, M., & Sepidarkish, M. (2018). The Effects of Supplementation with Chromium on Insulin Resistance Indices in Women with Polycystic Ovarian Syndrome: A Systematic Review and Meta-Analysis of Randomized Clinical Trials. Hormone and metabolic research = Hormon- und Stoffwechselforschung = Hormones et metabolisme, 50(3), 193–200. https://doi.org/10.1055/s-0044-101835

[4185] Gibson, R.S., Scythes, C.A. Chromium, selenium, and other trace element intakes of a selected sample of Canadian premenopausal women. Biol Trace Elem Res 6, 105–116 (1984). https://doi.org/10.1007/BF02916928

[4186] Pittler, M. H., Stevinson, C., & Ernst, E. (2003). Chromium picolinate for reducing body weight: meta-analysis of randomized trials. International journal of obesity and related metabolic disorders : journal of the International Association for the Study of Obesity, 27(4), 522–529. https://doi.org/10.1038/sj.ijo.0802262

[4187] Onakpoya, I., Posadzki, P., & Ernst, E. (2013). Chromium supplementation in overweight and obesity: a systematic review and meta-analysis of randomized clinical trials. Obesity reviews : an official journal of the International Association for the Study of Obesity, 14(6), 496–507. https://doi.org/10.1111/obr.12026

[4188] Willoughby, D., Hewlings, S., & Kalman, D. (2018). Body Composition Changes in Weight Loss: Strategies and Supplementation for Maintaining Lean Body Mass, a Brief Review. Nutrients, 10(12), 1876. https://doi.org/10.3390/nu10121876

[4189] Tian, H., Guo, X., Wang, X., He, Z., Sun, R., Ge, S., & Zhang, Z. (2013). Chromium picolinate supplementation for overweight or obese adults. The Cochrane database of systematic reviews, 2013(11), CD010063. https://doi.org/10.1002/14651858.CD010063.pub2

[4190] Tsang, C., Taghizadeh, M., Aghabagheri, E., Asemi, Z., & Jafarnejad, S. (2019). A meta-analysis of the effect of chromium supplementation on anthropometric indices of subjects with overweight or obesity. Clinical obesity, 9(4), e12313. https://doi.org/10.1111/cob.12313

[4191] Manore M. M. (2012). Dietary supplements for improving body composition and reducing body weight: where is the evidence?. International journal of sport nutrition and exercise metabolism, 22(2), 139–154. https://doi.org/10.1123/ijsnem.22.2.139

[4192] Anton, S. D., Morrison, C. D., Cefalu, W. T., Martin, C. K., Coulon, S., Geiselman, P., Han, H., White, C. L., & Williamson, D. A. (2008). Effects of chromium picolinate on food intake and satiety. Diabetes technology & therapeutics, 10(5), 405–412. https://doi.org/10.1089/dia.2007.0292

[4193] Vincent J. B. (2003). The potential value and toxicity of chromium picolinate as a nutritional supplement, weight loss agent and muscle development agent. Sports medicine (Auckland, N.Z.), 33(3), 213–230. https://doi.org/10.2165/00007256-200333030-00004

[4194] Lefavi, R. G., Anderson, R. A., Keith, R. E., Wilson, G. D., McMillan, J. L., & Stone, M. H. (1992). Efficacy of chromium supplementation in athletes: emphasis on anabolism. International journal of sport nutrition, 2(2), 111–122. https://doi.org/10.1123/ijsn.2.2.111

[4195] Evans GW. The effect of chromium picolinate on insulin controlled parameters in humans. Int J Biosocial Med Res 1989; 11: 163–80.

[4196] Kaats, G. R., Blum, K., Fisher, J. A., & Adelman, J. A. (1996). Effects of chromium picolinate supplementation on body composition: a randomized, double-masked, placebo-controlled study. Current Therapeutic Research, 57(10), 747–756. doi:10.1016/s0011-393x(96)80080-4

[4197] Hallmark et al (1996) 'Effects of chromium and resistive training on muscle strength and body composition', Medicine & Science in Sports & Exercise: January 1996 - Volume 28 - Issue 1 - p 139-144.

[4198] Clancy, S. P., Clarkson, P. M., DeCheke, M. E., Nosaka, K., Freedson, P. S., Cunningham, J. J., & Valentine, B. (1994). Effects of chromium picolinate supplementation on body composition, strength, and urinary chromium loss in football players. International journal of sport nutrition, 4(2), 142–153. https://doi.org/10.1123/ijsn.4.2.142

[4199] Maughan, R. J., Burke, L. M., Dvorak, J., Larson-Meyer, D. E., Peeling, P., Phillips, S. M., Rawson, E. S., Walsh, N. P., Garthe, I., Geyer, H., Meeusen, R., van Loon, L., Shirreffs, S. M., Spriet, L. L., Stuart, M., Vernec, A., Currell, K., Ali, V. M., Budgett, R., Ljungqvist, A., … Engebretsen, L. (2018). IOC Consensus Statement: Dietary Supplements and the High-Performance Athlete. International journal of sport nutrition and exercise metabolism, 28(2), 104–125. https://doi.org/10.1123/ijsnem.2018-0020

[4200] DiNicolantonio, J. J., O'Keefe, J. H., & Wilson, W. (2018). Subclinical magnesium deficiency: a principal driver of cardiovascular disease and a public health crisis. Open Heart, 5(1), e000668. doi:10.1136/openhrt-2017-000668

[4201] Anderson, R. A., Polansky, M. M., Bryden, N. A., Roginski, E. E., Patterson, K. Y., & Reamer, D. C. (1982). Effect of Exercise (Running) on Serum Glucose, Insulin, Glucagon, and Chromium Excretion. Diabetes, 31(3), 212–216. doi:10.2337/diab.31.3.212

[4202] Anderson, R. A., Polansky, M. M., & Bryden, N. A. (1984). Acute effects on chromium, copper, zinc, and selected clinical variables in urine and serum of male runners. Biological Trace Element Research, 6(4), 327–336. doi:10.1007/bf02989240

[4203] Lukaski, H. C., Bolonchuk, W. W., Siders, W. A., & Milne, D. B. (1996). Chromium supplementation and resistance training: effects on body composition, strength, and trace element status of men. The American Journal of Clinical Nutrition, 63(6), 954–965. doi:10.1093/ajcn/63.6.954

[4204] Anderson, R. A. (n.d.). New Insights on the Trace Elements, Chromium, Copper and Zinc, and Exercise. Medicine and Sport Science, 38–58. doi:10.1159/000420239

721

[4205] Anderson, R. A., Bryden, N. A., Polansky, M. M., & Deuster, P. A. (1988). Exercise effects on chromium excretion of trained and untrained men consuming a constant diet. Journal of Applied Physiology, 64(1), 249–252. doi:10.1152/jappl.1988.64.1.249

[4206] Bunker, V. W., Lawson, M. S., Delves, H. T., & Clayton, B. E. (1984). The uptake and excretion of chromium by the elderly. The American Journal of Clinical Nutrition, 39(5), 797–802. doi:10.1093/ajcn/39.5.797

[4207] CONSOLAZIO, C. F., NELSON, R. A., MATOUSH, L. O., HUGHES, R. C., & URONE, P. (1964). THE TRACE MINERAL LOSSES IN SWEAT. REP NO. 284. Report. U.S. Army Medical Research and Nutrition Laboratory, 1–14.

[4208] Saraymen et al (2004) 'Sweat Copper, Zinc, Iron, Magnesium and Chromium Levels in National Wrestler', İnönü Üniversitesi Tıp Fakültesi Dergisi 11(1) 7-10.

[4209] European Food Safety Authority NDA Panel. Scientific Opinion on Dietary Reference Values for chromium. EFSA Journal 2014;12(10):3845.

[4210] Bunker, V. W., Lawson, M. S., Delves, H. T., & Clayton, B. E. (1984). The uptake and excretion of chromium by the elderly. The American Journal of Clinical Nutrition, 39(5), 797–802. doi:10.1093/ajcn/39.5.797

[4211] Jamilian, M., Zadeh Modarres, S., Amiri Siavashani, M., Karimi, M., Mafi, A., Ostadmohammadi, V., & Asemi, Z. (2018). The Influences of Chromium Supplementation on Glycemic Control, Markers of Cardio-Metabolic Risk, and Oxidative Stress in Infertile Polycystic ovary Syndrome Women Candidate for In vitro Fertilization: a Randomized, Double-Blind, Placebo-Controlled Trial. Biological trace element research, 185(1), 48–55. https://doi.org/10.1007/s12011-017-1236-3

[4212] Press RI, Geller J, Evans GW. The effect of chromium picolinate on serum cholesterol and apolipoprotein fractions in human subjects. The Western Journal of Medicine. 1990 Jan;152(1):41-45.

[4213] Gunton, J. E., Cheung, N. W., Hitchman, R., Hams, G., O'Sullivan, C., Foster-Powell, K., & McElduff, A. (2005). Chromium supplementation does not improve glucose tolerance, insulin sensitivity, or lipid profile: a randomized, placebo-controlled, double-blind trial of supplementation in subjects with impaired glucose tolerance. Diabetes care, 28(3), 712–713. https://doi.org/10.2337/diacare.28.3.712

[4214] Abdollahi, M., Farshchi, A., Nikfar, S., & Seyedifar, M. (2013). Effect of chromium on glucose and lipid profiles in patients with type 2 diabetes; a meta-analysis review of randomized trials. Journal of pharmacy & pharmaceutical sciences : a publication of the Canadian Society for Pharmaceutical Sciences, Societe canadienne des sciences pharmaceutiques, 16(1), 99–114. https://doi.org/10.18433/j3g022

[4215] Balk, E. M., Tatsioni, A., Lichtenstein, A. H., Lau, J., & Pittas, A. G. (2007). Effect of chromium supplementation on glucose metabolism and lipids: a systematic review of randomized controlled trials. Diabetes care, 30(8), 2154–2163. https://doi.org/10.2337/dc06-0996

[4216] Huang, H., Chen, G., Dong, Y., Zhu, Y., & Chen, H. (2018). Chromium supplementation for adjuvant treatment of type 2 diabetes mellitus: Results from a pooled analysis. Molecular nutrition & food research, 62(1), 10.1002/mnfr.201700438. https://doi.org/10.1002/mnfr.201700438

[4217] Suksomboon, N., Poolsup, N., & Yuwanakorn, A. (2014). Systematic review and meta-analysis of the efficacy and safety of chromium supplementation in diabetes. Journal of clinical pharmacy and therapeutics, 39(3), 292–306. https://doi.org/10.1111/jcpt.12147

[4218] Riales, R., & Albrink, M. J. (1981). Effect of chromium chloride supplementation on glucose tolerance and serum lipids including high-density lipoprotein of adult men. The American journal of clinical nutrition, 34(12), 2670–2678. https://doi.org/10.1093/ajcn/34.12.2670

[4219] Lima, K. V. G., Lima, R. P. A., Gonçalves, M. C. R., Faintuch, J., Morais, L. C. S. L., Asciutti, L. S. R., & Costa, M. J. C. (2013). High Frequency of Serum Chromium Deficiency and Association of Chromium with Triglyceride and Cholesterol Concentrations in Patients Awaiting Bariatric Surgery. Obesity Surgery, 24(5), 771–776. doi:10.1007/s11695-013-1132-7

[4220] Bai, J., Xun, P., Morris, S., Jacobs, D. R., Jr, Liu, K., & He, K. (2015). Chromium exposure and incidence of metabolic syndrome among American young adults over a 23-year follow-up: the CARDIA Trace Element Study. Scientific reports, 5, 15606. https://doi.org/10.1038/srep15606

[4221] Guallar, E., Jiménez, F. J., van 't Veer, P., Bode, P., Riemersma, R. A., Gómez-Aracena, J., Kark, J. D., Arab, L., Kok, F. J., Martín-Moreno, J. M., & EURAMIC-Heavy Metals and Myocardial Infraction Study Group (2005). Low toenail chromium concentration and increased risk of nonfatal myocardial infarction. American journal of epidemiology, 162(2), 157–164. https://doi.org/10.1093/aje/kwi180

[4222] Chung, J. H., & Yum, K. S. (2012). Correlation of hair mineral concentrations with insulin resistance in Korean males. Biological trace element research, 150(1-3), 26–30. https://doi.org/10.1007/s12011-012-9474-x

[4223] Forte, G., Bocca, B., Peruzzu, A., Tolu, F., Asara, Y., Farace, C., Oggiano, R., & Madeddu, R. (2013). Blood metals concentration in type 1 and type 2 diabetics. Biological trace element research, 156(1-3), 79–90. https://doi.org/10.1007/s12011-013-9858-6

[4224] Zhou, W., Vazin, M., Yu, T., Ding, J., & Liu, J. (2016). In Vitro Selection of Chromium-Dependent DNAzymes for Sensing Chromium(III) and Chromium(VI). Chemistry - A European Journal, 22(28), 9835–9840. doi:10.1002/chem.201601426

[4225] Thor, M. Y., Harnack, L., King, D., Jasthi, B., & Pettit, J. (2011). Evaluation of the comprehensiveness and reliability of the chromium composition of foods in the literature (). Journal of food composition and analysis : an official publication of the United Nations University, International Network of Food Data Systems, 24(8), 1147–1152. https://doi.org/10.1016/j.jfca.2011.04.006

[4226] Lovkova, M., Buzuk, G. N., Sokolova, S. M., Kliment'eva, N. I., Ponomareva, S. M., Shelepova, O. V., & Vorotnitskaia, I. E. (1996). Lekarstvennue rasteniia--kontsentratory khroma. Rol' khroma v metabolizme alkaloidov [Medicinal plants--concentrators of chromium. The role of chromium in alkaloid metabolism]. Izvestiia Akademii nauk. Seriia biologicheskaia, (5), 552–564.

[4227] Toepfer, E. W., Mertz, W., Roginski, E. E., & Polansky, M. M. (1973). Chromium in foods in relation to biological activity. Journal of agricultural and food chemistry, 21(1), 69–71. https://doi.org/10.1021/jf60185a008

[4228] Offenbacher, E. G., & Pi-Sunyer, F. X. (1980). Beneficial effect of chromium-rich yeast on glucose tolerance and blood lipids in elderly subjects. Diabetes, 29(11), 919–925. https://doi.org/10.2337/diab.29.11.919

[4229] Anderson R. A. (2008). Chromium and polyphenols from cinnamon improve insulin sensitivity. The Proceedings of the Nutrition Society, 67(1), 48–53. https://doi.org/10.1017/S0029665108006010

[4230] Bakshi, A., & Panigrahi, A. K. (2018). A comprehensive review on chromium induced alterations in fresh water fishes. Toxicology reports, 5, 440–447. https://doi.org/10.1016/j.toxrep.2018.03.007

[4231] WASHINGTON (AFP) (2010) 'US water has large amounts of likely carcinogen: study', Yahoo News, Accessed Online Jan 12 2021: https://web.archive.org/web/20101224075935if_/http://news.yahoo.com/s/afp/healthusenvironmentpollutionwater/print

[4232] Mossop R. T. (1986). The geography of diabetes and vascular occlusive disease in relation to chromium. The Central African journal of medicine, 32(6), 137–140.

[4233] Kumpulainen J, Tahvonen R (1989) Report on the activities of the sub-network on trace elements status in food. In: Report on the Consultation of the European Cooperation Research Network on Trace Elements. Lausanne, Switzerland, 5.–8.9. 1989, FAO, Rome

[4234] Vincent JB. Chromium: Properties and Determination In: Caballero B, Finglas PM, Toldra F, eds. Encyclopedia of Food and Health: Academic Press; 2016:114-8.

[4235] Czerniejewski CP, et al. The minerals of wheat flour and bread. Cereal chem. 1964

[4236] Casey, C. E., Hambidge, K. M., & Neville, M. C. (1985). Studies in human lactation: zinc, copper, manganese and chromium in human milk in the first month of lactation. The American journal of clinical nutrition, 41(6), 1193–1200. https://doi.org/10.1093/ajcn/41.6.1193

[4237] Carter, J. P., Kattab, A., Abd-el-Hadi, K., Davis, J. T., el Gholmy, A., & Patwardhan, V. N. (1968). Chromium (3) in hypoglycemia and in impaired glucose utilization in kwashiorkor. The American journal of clinical nutrition, 21(3), 195–202. https://doi.org/10.1093/ajcn/21.3.195

[4238] Versieck J. (1985). Trace elements in human body fluids and tissues. Critical reviews in clinical laboratory sciences, 22(2), 97–184. https://doi.org/10.3109/10408368509165788

[4239] Kumpulainen, J., & Vuori, E. (1980). Longitudinal study of chromium in human milk. The American journal of clinical nutrition, 33(11), 2299–2302. https://doi.org/10.1093/ajcn/33.11.2299

[4240] Xia, W., Hu, J., Zhang, B., Li, Y., Wise, J. P., Sr, Bassig, B. A., Zhou, A., Savitz, D. A., Xiong, C., Zhao, J., du, X., Zhou, Y., Pan, X., Yang, J., Wu, C., Jiang, M., Peng, Y., Qian, Z., Zheng, T., & Xu, S. (2016). A case-control study of maternal exposure to chromium and infant low birth weight in China. Chemosphere, 144, 1484–1489. https://doi.org/10.1016/j.chemosphere.2015.10.006

[4241] Schroeder (1967) 'Cadmium, Chromium, and Cardiovascular Disease', Circulation, Volume XXXV, March 1967.

[4242] Gibson, R. S., & Scythes, C. A. (1984). Chromium, selenium, and other trace element intakes of a selected sample of Canadian premenopausal women. Biological Trace Element Research, 6(2), 105–116. doi:10.1007/bf02916928

[4243] Grijalva Haro, M. I., Ballesteros Vázquez, M. N., & Cabrera Pacheco, R. M. (2001). Contenido de cromo en alimentos y estimación de su ingestión dietaria en el noroeste de México [Chromium content in foods and dietary intake estimation in the Northwest of Mexico]. Archivos latinoamericanos de nutricion, 51(1), 105–110.

[4244] Anon. Food Monitoring in Denmark--Nutrients and Contaminants 1983-1987, The National Food Agency of Denmark, ed., 1990, p. 176.

[4245] S. Wyttenbach, S. Bajo, and L. Tobler (1987) in Trace Element--Analytical Chemistry in Medicine and Biology, vol. 4, P. Bratter and P. Schramel, eds., Walter de Gruyter & Co., Berlin, 1987, p. 169.

[4246] Roussel, A.-M., Andriollo-Sanchez, M., Ferry, M., Bryden, N. A., & Anderson, R. A. (2007). Food chromium content, dietary chromium intake and related biological variables in French free-living elderly. British Journal of Nutrition, 98(2), 326–331. doi:10.1017/s000711450770168x

[4247] Lendinez, E., Lorenzo, M. ., Cabrera, C., & López, M. . (2001). Chromium in basic foods of the Spanish diet: seafood, cereals, vegetables, olive oils and dairy products. Science of The Total Environment, 278(1-3), 183–189. doi:10.1016/s0048-9697(01)00647-7

[4248] Kumpulainen J. T. (1992). Chromium content of foods and diets. Biological trace element research, 32, 9–18. https://doi.org/10.1007/BF02784582

[4249] Trace Elements in Man and Animals 7Monography, Proceedings, Round Tables, and Discussions of the Seventh International Symposium on Trace Elements in Man and Animals (TEMA 7), held May 20–25, 1990 at Hotel Libertas, Dubrovnik, Croatia Berislav Momčilović, ed. (1992). Biological Trace Element Research, 35(2), 201–201. doi:10.1007/bf02783730

[4250] TIPTON, I. H., SCHROEDER, H. A., PERRY, H. M., Jr, & COOK, M. J. (1965). TRACE ELEMENTS IN HUMAN TISSUE. 3. SUBJECTS FROM AFRICA, THE NEAR AND FAR EAST AND EUROPE. Health physics, 11, 403–451. https://doi.org/10.1097/00004032-196505000-00006

[4251] Levine, R. A., Streeten, D. H. P., & Doisy, R. J. (1968). Effects of oral chromium supplementation on the glucose tolerance of elderly human subjects. Metabolism, 17(2), 114–125. doi:10.1016/0026-0495(68)90137-6

[4252] Bunker, V. W., Lawson, M. S., Delves, H. T., & Clayton, B. E. (1984). The uptake and excretion of chromium by the elderly. The American journal of clinical nutrition, 39(5), 797–802. https://doi.org/10.1093/ajcn/39.5.797

[4253] Anderson, R. A., Polansky, M. M., Bryden, N. A., & Canary, J. J. (1991). Supplemental-chromium effects on glucose, insulin, glucagon, and urinary chromium losses in subjects consuming controlled low-chromium diets. The American journal of clinical nutrition, 54(5), 909–916. https://doi.org/10.1093/ajcn/54.5.909

[4254] NIH (2020) 'Chromium: Fact Sheet for Health Professionals', Accessed Online Jan 10 2021: https://ods.od.nih.gov/factsheets/chromium-HealthProfessional/

[4255] Anderson, R. A., Bryden, N. A., & Polansky, M. M. (1992). Dietary chromium intake. Freely chosen diets, institutional diet, and individual foods. Biological trace element research, 32, 117–121. https://doi.org/10.1007/BF02784595

[4256] Rêczajska et al (2005) 'Determination of chromium content of food and beverages of plant origin', Polish journal of food and nutrition sciences 14, no. 55 (2005): 2.

[4257] WebMD (2020) 'Top Foods High in Chromium', Diet & Weight Management, Accessed Online Jan 10 2021: https://www.webmd.com/diet/foods-high-in-chromium#2

[4258] Kuligowski, J., & Halperin, K. M. (1992). Stainless steel cookware as a significant source of nickel, chromium, and iron. Archives of environmental contamination and toxicology, 23(2), 211–215. https://doi.org/10.1007/BF00212277

[4259] Kamerud, K. L., Hobbie, K. A., & Anderson, K. A. (2013). Stainless steel leaches nickel and chromium into foods during cooking. Journal of agricultural and food chemistry, 61(39), 9495–9501. https://doi.org/10.1021/jf402400v

[4260] Kumpulainen, J., Vuori, E., Mäkinen, S., & Kara, R. (1980). Dietary chromium intake of lactating Finnish mothers: effect on the Cr content of their breast milk. The British journal of nutrition, 44(3), 257–263. https://doi.org/10.1079/bjn19800039

[4261] Kumpulainen J. T. (1992). Chromium content of foods and diets. Biological trace element research, 32, 9–18. https://doi.org/10.1007/BF02784582

[4262] Wolf, W., Mertz, W., & Masironi, R. (1974). Determination of chromium in refined and unrefined sugars by oxygen plasma ashing flameless atomic absorption. Journal of agricultural and food chemistry, 22(6), 1037–1042. https://doi.org/10.1021/jf60196a014

[4263] Levin ME and Recant L. Diabetes and the environment. Arch Environ Health (Chicago) 12:621. 1966

[4264] Schroeder H. A. (1967). Cadmium, chromium, and cardiovascular disease. Circulation, 35(3), 570–582. https://doi.org/10.1161/01.cir.35.3.570

[4265] Anderson, R. A., & Kozlovsky, A. S. (1985). Chromium intake, absorption and excretion of subjects consuming self-selected diets. The American journal of clinical nutrition, 41(6), 1177–1183. https://doi.org/10.1093/ajcn/41.6.1177

[4266] Glinsmann et al (1966) 'Plasma Chromium after Glucose Administration', Science 27 May 1966: Vol. 152, Issue 3726, pp. 1243-1245, DOI: 10.1126/science.152.3726.1243

[4267] Bahijri, S. M., & Alissa, E. M. (2011). Increased insulin resistance is associated with increased urinary excretion of chromium in non-diabetic, normotensive Saudi adults. Journal of clinical biochemistry and nutrition, 49(3), 164–168. https://doi.org/10.3164/jcbn.10-148

[4268] Stoecker B. Chromium. In: Shils M, Shike M, Ross A, Caballero B, Cousins R, eds. Modern Nutrition in Health and Disease. Philadelphia: Lippincott, Williams & Wilkins; 2006:332-337.

[4269] Seaborn, C. D., & Stoecker, B. J. (1990). Effects of antacid or ascorbic acid on tissue accumulation and urinary excretion of 51chromium. Nutrition Research, 10(12), 1401–1407. doi:10.1016/s0271-5317(05)80132-0

[4270] Food and Nutrition Board, Institute of Medicine. Chromium. Dietary reference intakes for vitamin A, vitamin K, boron, chromium, copper, iodine, iron, manganese, molybdenum, nickel, silicon, vanadium, and zinc. Washington, D.C.: National Academy Press; 2001:197-223.

[4271] Kozlovsky, A. S., Moser, P. B., Reiser, S., & Anderson, R. A. (1986). Effects of diets high in simple sugars on urinary chromium losses. Metabolism: clinical and experimental, 35(6), 515–518. https://doi.org/10.1016/0026-0495(86)90007-7

[4272] Anderson et al (1990) 'Urinary chromium excretion and insulinogenic properties of carbohydrates', The American Journal of Clinical Nutrition, Volume 51, Issue 5, May 1990, Pages 864–868, https://doi.org/10.1093/ajcn/51.5.864

[4273] Morris et al (1985) 'Plasma chromium and chromium excretion in diabetes', Clinical Chemistry 31(2):334-5, DOI: 10.1093/clinchem/31.2.334

[4274] Anderson, R. A., Bryden, N. A., Polansky, M. M., & Thorp, J. W. (1991). Effects of carbohydrate loading and underwater exercise on circulating cortisol, insulin and urinary losses of chromium and zinc. European Journal of Applied Physiology and Occupational Physiology, 63(2), 146–150. doi:10.1007/bf00235185

[4275] Afridi, H. I., Kazi, T. G., Talpur, F. N., Arain, S., Arain, S. S., Kazi, N., Panhwar, A. H., & Brahman, K. D. (2014). Evaluation of chromium and manganese in biological samples (scalp hair, blood and urine) of tuberculosis and diarrhea male human immunodeficiency virus patients. Clinical laboratory, 60(8), 1333–1341. https://doi.org/10.7754/clin.lab.2013.130736

[4276] Harris (1977) 'Different metal-binding properties of the two sites of human transferrin', Biochemistry 1977, 16, 3, 560–564

[4277] Stearns D. M. (2000). Is chromium a trace essential metal?. BioFactors (Oxford, England), 11(3), 149–162. https://doi.org/10.1002/biof.5520110301

[4278] Clodfelder, B.J., Emamaullee, J., Hepburn, D.D. et al. The trail of chromium(III) in vivo from the blood to the urine: the roles of transferrin and chromodulin. JBIC 6, 608–617 (2001). https://doi.org/10.1007/s007750100238

[4279] Geir Bjorklund*, Vera Stejskal, Mauricio A. Urbina, Maryam Dadar, Salvatore Chirumbolo and Joachim Mutter, "Metals and Parkinson's Disease: Mechanisms and Biochemical Processes", Current Medicinal Chemistry (2018) 25: 2198. https://doi.org/10.2174/0929867325666171129124616

[4280] Mold, Matthew; Cottle, Jason; Exley, Christopher. 2019. "Aluminium in Brain Tissue in Epilepsy: A Case Report from Camelford" Int. J. Environ. Res. Public Health 16, no. 12: 2129.

[4281] Mold, M., Umar, D., King, A., & Exley, C. (2018). Aluminium in brain tissue in autism. Journal of Trace Elements in Medicine and Biology, 46, 76–82. doi:10.1016/j.jtemb.2017.11.012

[4282] McFarland et al (2020) 'Acute exposure and chronic retention of aluminum in three vaccine schedules and effects of genetic and environmental variation', Journal of Trace Elements in Medicine and Biology, Volume 58, March 2020, 126444

[4283] Martin, J., Wang, Z. Q., Zhang, X. H., Wachtel, D., Volaufova, J., Matthews, D. E., & Cefalu, W. T. (2006). Chromium picolinate supplementation attenuates body weight gain and increases insulin sensitivity in subjects with type 2 diabetes. Diabetes care, 29(8), 1826–1832. https://doi.org/10.2337/dc06-0254

[4284] John-Kalarickal, J., Pearlman, G., & Carlson, H. E. (2007). New medications which decrease levothyroxine absorption. Thyroid : official journal of the American Thyroid Association, 17(8), 763–765. https://doi.org/10.1089/thy.2007.0060

[4285] Ravina, A., Slezak, L., Mirsky, N. and Anderson, R.A. (1999), Control of steroid-induced diabetes with supplemental chromium. J. Trace Elem. Exp. Med., 12: 375-378. https://doi.org/10.1002/(SICI)1520-670X(1999)12:4<375::AID-JTRA11>3.0.CO;2-R

[4286] Ravina, A., Slezak, L., Mirsky, N., Bryden, N. A., & Anderson, R. A. (1999). Reversal of corticosteroid-induced diabetes mellitus with supplemental chromium. Diabetic medicine : a journal of the British Diabetic Association, 16(2), 164–167. https://doi.org/10.1046/j.1464-5491.1999.00004.x

[4287] Fowler J. F., Jr (2000). Systemic contact dermatitis caused by oral chromium picolinate. Cutis, 65(2), 116.

[4288] Vincent J. B. (2003). The potential value and toxicity of chromium picolinate as a nutritional supplement, weight loss agent and muscle development agent. Sports medicine (Auckland, N.Z.), 33(3), 213–230. https://doi.org/10.2165/00007256-200333030-00004

[4289] UCSF Benioff Children's Hospital (2019) 'Serum Chromium', Medical Tests, Accessed Online Jan 13 2021: https://www.ucsfbenioffchildrens.org/tests/003359.html

[4290] UCSF Health (2019) 'Chromium - blood test', Medical Tests, Accessed Online Jan 13 2021: https://www.ucsfhealth.org/medical-tests/chromium---blood-test

[4291] Mayo Clinic Laboratories (2021) 'Chromium, Serum', Test ID: CRS, Accessed Online Jan 13 2021: https://www.mayocliniclabs.com/test-catalog/Clinical+and+Interpretive/8638

[4292] Jantzen, C., Jørgensen, H. L., Duus, B. R., Sporring, S. L., & Lauritzen, J. B. (2013). Chromium and cobalt ion concentrations in blood and serum following various types of metal-on-metal hip arthroplasties: a literature overview. Acta orthopaedica, 84(3), 229–236. https://doi.org/10.3109/17453674.2013.792034

[4293] Agency for Toxic Substances and Disease Registry (2008) 'Chromium Toxicity', Clinical Assessment - Laboratory Tests, Accessed Online Jan 13 2021: https://www.atsdr.cdc.gov/csem/csem.asp?csem=10&po=12

[4294] Price JW. Elevated Chromium Levels and Prosthetic Joint Implants. J Am Osteopath Assoc 2011;111(9):548–550.

[4295] Carter (2019) 'What are the benefits and effects of manganese?', Medical News Today, Accessed Online Feb 07 2021: https://www.medicalnewstoday.com/articles/325636#health-benefits

[4296] Freeland-Graves, J., Llanes, C., 1994. Models to study manganese deficiency. In: Klimis-Tavantzis, D.J. (Ed.), Manganese in Health and Disease. CRC Press, Boca Raton, FL, pp. 115–120.

[4297] Keen, C. L., Ensunsa, J. L., Watson, M. H., Baly, D. K., Donovan, S. M., Monaco, M. H., & Clegg, M. S. (1999). Nutritional aspects of manganese from experimental studies. NeuroToxicology, 20(2-3), 213-224.

[4298] Xu, Y., Miriyala, S., Fang, F., Bakthavatchalu, V., Noel, T., Schell, D. M., … St Clair, D. K. (2014). Manganese superoxide dismutase deficiency triggers mitochondrial uncoupling and the Warburg effect. Oncogene, 34(32), 4229–4237. doi:10.1038/onc.2014.355

[4299] Alessio, L., Campagna, M., & Lucchini, R. (2007). From lead to manganese through mercury: mythology, science, and lessons for prevention. American journal of industrial medicine, 50(11), 779–787. https://doi.org/10.1002/ajim.20524

[4300] Sayre, E. V., & Smith, R. W. (1961). Compositional Categories of Ancient Glass. Science (New York, N.Y.), 133(3467), 1824–1826. https://doi.org/10.1126/science.133.3467.1824

[4301] Chalmin, E.; Vignaud, C.; Salomon, H.; Farges, F.; Susini, J.; Menu, M. (2006). "Minerals discovered in paleolithic black pigments by transmission electron microscopy and micro-X-ray absorption near-edge structure". Applied Physics A. 83 (12): 213–218.

[4302] American Chemistry (2005) 'Chlorine Compound of the Month: Silver Chloride: Helping Us Get the Picture', Chlorine Chemistry, Accessed Online Feb 10 2021: https://chlorine.americanchemistry.com/Science-Center/Chlorine-Compound-of-the-Month-Library/Silver-Chloride-Helping-Us-Get-the-Picture/

[4303] Olsen, Sverre E.; Tangstad, Merete; Lindstad, Tor (2007). "History of omanganese". Production of Manganese Ferroalloys. Tapir Academic Press. pp. 11–12.

[4304] Bae, Y. J., & Kim, M. H. (2008). Manganese supplementation improves mineral density of the spine and femur and serum osteocalcin in rats. Biological trace element research, 124(1), 28–34. https://doi.org/10.1007/s12011-008-8119-6

[4305] Reginster JY, Strause LG, Saltman P, Franchimont P. Trace elements and postmenopausal osteoporosis: a preliminary study of decreased serum manganese. Med Sci Res 1988; 16: 337–338.

[4306] Němčíková et al (2009) 'Relationship of serum manganese and copper levels to bone density and quality in postmenopausal women. A pilot study', Osteologicky Bulletin 14(3):97-100.

[4307] Zofková, I., Nemcikova, P., & Matucha, P. (2013). Trace elements and bone health. Clinical chemistry and laboratory medicine, 51(8), 1555–1561. https://doi.org/10.1515/cclm-2012-0868

[4308] Odabasi, E., Turan, M., Aydin, A., Akay, C., & Kutlu, M. (2008). Magnesium, zinc, copper, manganese, and selenium levels in postmenopausal women with osteoporosis. Can magnesium play a key role in osteoporosis?. Annals of the Academy of Medicine, Singapore, 37(7), 564–567.

[4309] Wang, L., Yu, H., Yang, G., Zhang, Y., Wang, W., Su, T., Ma, W., Yang, F., Chen, L., He, L., Ma, Y., & Zhang, Y. (2015). Correlation between bone mineral density and serum trace element contents of elderly males in Beijing urban area. International journal of clinical and experimental medicine, 8(10), 19250–19257.

[4310] Strause, L., Saltman, P., & Glowacki, J. (1987). The effect of deficiencies of manganese and copper on osteoinduction and on resorption of bone particles in rats. Calcified tissue international, 41(3), 145–150. https://doi.org/10.1007/BF02563794

[4311] FROST, G., ASLING, C. W., & NELSON, M. M. (1959). Skeletal deformities in manganese-deficient rats. The Anatomical record, 134, 37–53. https://doi.org/10.1002/ar.1091340105

[4312] Zhou, Q., Einert, M., Schmitt, H., Wang, Z., Pankratz, F., Olivier, C. B., Bode, C., Liao, J. K., & Moser, M. (2016). MnTBAP increases BMPR-II expression in endothelial cells and attenuates vascular inflammation. Vascular pharmacology, 84, 67–73. https://doi.org/10.1016/j.vph.2016.07.001

[4313] Martin-Montañez, E., Pavia, J., Santin, L. J., Boraldi, F., Estivill-Torrus, G., Aguirre, J. A., & Garcia-Fernandez, M. (2014). Involvement of IGF-II receptors in the antioxidant and neuroprotective effects of IGF-II on adult cortical neuronal cultures. Biochimica et biophysica acta, 1842(7), 1041–1051. https://doi.org/10.1016/j.bbadis.2014.03.010

[4314] Zhou, B., Su, X., Su, D., Zeng, F., Wang, M. H., Huang, L., Huang, E., Zhu, Y., Zhao, D., He, D., Zhu, X., Yeoh, E., Zhang, R., & Ding, G. (2016). Dietary intake of manganese and the risk of the metabolic syndrome in a Chinese population. The British journal of nutrition, 116(5), 853–863. https://doi.org/10.1017/S0007114516002580

[4315] Choi, M.-K., & Bae, Y.-J. (2013). Relationship between Dietary Magnesium, Manganese, and Copper and Metabolic Syndrome Risk in Korean Adults: The Korea National Health and Nutrition Examination Survey (2007–2008). Biological Trace Element Research, 156(1-3), 56–66. doi:10.1007/s12011-013-9852-z

[4316] Li, Y., Guo, H., Wu, M., & Liu, M. (2013). Serum and dietary antioxidant status is associated with lower prevalence of the metabolic syndrome in a study in Shanghai, China. Asia Pacific journal of clinical nutrition, 22(1), 60–68. https://doi.org/10.6133/apjcn.2013.22.1.06

[4317] Rhee, S. Y., Hwang, Y. C., Woo, J. T., Sinn, D. H., Chin, S. O., Chon, S., & Kim, Y. S. (2013). Blood lead is significantly associated with metabolic syndrome in Korean adults: an analysis based on the Korea National Health and Nutrition Examination Survey (KNHANES), 2008. Cardiovascular diabetology, 12, 9. https://doi.org/10.1186/1475-2840-12-9

[4318] Ballinger, S. W., Patterson, C., Knight-Lozano, C. A., Burow, D. L., Conklin, C. A., Hu, Z., Reuf, J., Horaist, C., Lebovitz, R., Hunter, G. C., McIntyre, K., & Runge, M. S. (2002). Mitochondrial integrity and function in atherogenesis. Circulation, 106(5), 544–549. https://doi.org/10.1161/01.cir.0000023921.93743.89

[4319] Ross R. (1999). Atherosclerosis--an inflammatory disease. The New England journal of medicine, 340(2), 115–126. https://doi.org/10.1056/NEJM199901143400207

[4320] Heinecke, J. W. (1998). Oxidants and antioxidants in the pathogenesis of atherosclerosis: implications for the oxidized low density lipoprotein hypothesis. Atherosclerosis, 141(1), 1–15. doi:10.1016/s0021-9150(98)00173-7

[4321] Fang, X., Weintraub, N. L., Rios, C. D., Chappell, D. A., Zwacka, R. M., Engelhardt, J. F., Oberley, L. W., Yan, T., Heistad, D. D., & Spector, A. A. (1998). Overexpression of human superoxide dismutase inhibits oxidation of low-density lipoprotein by endothelial cells. Circulation research, 82(12), 1289–1297. https://doi.org/10.1161/01.res.82.12.1289

[4322] Malecki, E. A., & Greger, J. L. (1996). Manganese Protects against Heart Mitochondrial Lipid Peroxidation in Rats Fed High Levels of Polyunsaturated Fatty Acids. The Journal of Nutrition, 126(1), 27–33. doi:10.1093/jn/126.1.27

[4323] Kinscherf, R., Claus, R., Wagner, M., Gehrke, C., Kamencic, H., Hou, D., Nauen, O., Schmiedt, W., Kovacs, G., Pill, J., Metz, J., & Deigner, H. P. (1998). Apoptosis caused by oxidized LDL is manganese superoxide dismutase and p53 dependent. FASEB journal : official publication of the Federation of American Societies for Experimental Biology, 12(6), 461–467. https://doi.org/10.1096/fasebj.12.6.461

[4324] Jiang, F., Guo, Y., Salvemini, D., & Dusting, G. J. (2003). Superoxide dismutase mimetic M40403 improves endothelial function in apolipoprotein(E)-deficient mice. British Journal of Pharmacology, 139(6), 1127–1134. doi:10.1038/sj.bjp.0705354

[4325] Lozhkin, A. P., Biktagirov, T. B., Abdul'ianov, V. A., Gorshkov, O. V., Timonina, E. V., Mamin, G. V., Orlinskiĭ, S. B., Silkin, N. I., Chernov, V. M., Khaĭrullin, R. N., Salakhov, M., & Il'inskaia, O. N. (2012). Biomeditsinskaia khimiia, 58(3), 291–299. https://doi.org/10.18097/pbmc20125803291

[4326] Zhou, Q., Einert, M., Schmitt, H., Wang, Z., Pankratz, F., Olivier, C. B., Bode, C., Liao, J. K., & Moser, M. (2016). MnTBAP increases BMPR-II expression in endothelial cells and attenuates vascular inflammation. Vascular pharmacology, 84, 67–73. https://doi.org/10.1016/j.vph.2016.07.001

[4327] Ilyas, A., & Shah, M. H. (2016). Multivariate statistical evaluation of trace metal levels in the blood of atherosclerosis patients in comparison with healthy subjects. Heliyon, 2(1), e00054. doi:10.1016/j.heliyon.2015.e00054

[4328] Pires, K. M., Ilkun, O., Valente, M., & Boudina, S. (2014). Treatment with a SOD mimetic reduces visceral adiposity, adipocyte death, and adipose tissue inflammation in high fat-fed mice. Obesity (Silver Spring, Md.), 22(1), 178–187. https://doi.org/10.1002/oby.20465

[4329] Kobayashi, H., Matsuda, M., Fukuhara, A., Komuro, R., & Shimomura, I. (2009). Dysregulated glutathione metabolism links to impaired insulin action in adipocytes. American journal of physiology. Endocrinology and metabolism, 296(6), E1326–E1334. https://doi.org/10.1152/ajpendo.90921.2008

[4330] Ko, S. H., Park, J. H., Kim, S. Y., Lee, S. W., Chun, S. S., & Park, E. (2014). Antioxidant Effects of Spinach (Spinacia oleracea L.) Supplementation in Hyperlipidemic Rats. Preventive nutrition and food science, 19(1), 19–26. https://doi.org/10.3746/pnf.2014.19.1.019

[4331] Rezazadeh, A., & Yazdanparast, R. (2014). Prevention of nonalcoholic steatohepatitis in rats by two manganese-salen complexes. Iranian biomedical journal, 18(1), 41–48. https://doi.org/10.6091/ibj.1201.2013

[4332] Laurent, A., Nicco, C., Tran Van Nhieu, J., Borderie, D., Chéreau, C., Conti, F., … Batteux, F. (2004). Pivotal role of superoxide anion and beneficial effect of antioxidant molecules in murine steatohepatitis. Hepatology, 39(5), 1277–1285. doi:10.1002/hep.20177

[4333] Rotter, I., Kosik-Bogacka, D., Dołęgowska, B., Safranow, K., Lubkowska, A., & Laszczyńska, M. (2015). Relationship between the concentrations of heavy metals and bioelements in aging men with metabolic syndrome. International journal of environmental research and public health, 12(4), 3944–3961. https://doi.org/10.3390/ijerph120403944

[4334] Zhou, B., Su, X., Su, D., Zeng, F., Wang, M. H., Huang, L., Huang, E., Zhu, Y., Zhao, D., He, D., Zhu, X., Yeoh, E., Zhang, R., & Ding, G. (2016). Dietary intake of manganese and the risk of the metabolic syndrome in a Chinese population. The British journal of nutrition, 116(5), 853–863. https://doi.org/10.1017/S0007114516002580

[4335] Fan, Y., Zhang, C., & Bu, J. (2017). Relationship between Selected Serum Metallic Elements and Obesity in Children and Adolescent in the U.S. Nutrients, 9(2), 104. https://doi.org/10.3390/nu9020104

[4336] Hoehn, K. L., Salmon, A. B., Hohnen-Behrens, C., Turner, N., Hoy, A. J., Maghzal, G. J., … James, D. E. (2009). Insulin resistance is a cellular antioxidant defense mechanism. Proceedings of the National Academy of Sciences, 106(42), 17787–17792. doi:10.1073/pnas.0902380106

[4337] Goto, H., Nishikawa, T., Sonoda, K., Kondo, T., Kukidome, D., Fujisawa, K., … Araki, E. (2008). Endothelial MnSOD overexpression prevents retinal VEGF expression in diabetic mice. Biochemical and Biophysical Research Communications, 366(3), 814–820. doi:10.1016/j.bbrc.2007.12.041

[4338] Kowluru, R. A., Kowluru, V., Xiong, Y., & Ho, Y.-S. (2006). Overexpression of mitochondrial superoxide dismutase in mice protects the retina from diabetes-induced oxidative stress. Free Radical Biology and Medicine, 41(8), 1191–1196. doi:10.1016/j.freeradbiomed.2006.01.012

[4339] Vincent, A. M., Russell, J. W., Sullivan, K. A., Backus, C., Hayes, J. M., McLean, L. L., & Feldman, E. L. (2007). SOD2 protects neurons from injury in cell culture and animal models of diabetic neuropathy. Experimental neurology, 208(2), 216–227. https://doi.org/10.1016/j.expneurol.2007.07.017

[4340] Shen, X., Zheng, S., Metreveli, N. S., & Epstein, P. N. (2006). Protection of Cardiac Mitochondria by Overexpression of MnSOD Reduces Diabetic Cardiomyopathy. Diabetes, 55(3), 798–805. doi:10.2337/diabetes.55.03.06.db05-1039

[4341] Burlet, E., & Jain, S. K. (2017). Manganese supplementation increases adiponectin and lowers ICAM-1 and creatinine blood levels in Zucker type 2 diabetic rats, and downregulates ICAM-1 by upregulating adiponectin multimerization protein (DsbA-L) in endothelial cells. Molecular and cellular biochemistry, 429(1-2), 1–10. https://doi.org/10.1007/s11010-016-2931-7

[4342] Burlet, E., & Jain, S. K. (2013). Manganese supplementation reduces high glucose-induced monocyte adhesion to endothelial cells and endothelial dysfunction in Zucker diabetic fatty rats. The Journal of biological chemistry, 288(9), 6409–6416. https://doi.org/10.1074/jbc.M112.447805

[4343] Lee, S. H., Jouihan, H. A., Cooksey, R. C., Jones, D., Kim, H. J., Winge, D. R., & McClain, D. A. (2013). Manganese supplementation protects against diet-induced diabetes in wild type mice by enhancing insulin secretion. Endocrinology, 154(3), 1029–1038. https://doi.org/10.1210/en.2012-1445

[4344] Hurley, L. S., Keen, C. L., & Baly, D. L. (1984). Manganese deficiency and toxicity: Effects on carbohydrate metabolism in the rat. NeuroToxicology, 5(1), 97-104.

[4345] BALY, D., LONNERDAL, B., & KEEN, C. (1985). Effects of high doses of manganese on carbohydrate homeostasis☆. Toxicology Letters, 25(1), 95–102. doi:10.1016/0378-4274(85)90106-7

[4346] Burch, R. E., Williams, R. V., Hahn, H. K., Jetton, M. M., & Sullivan, J. F. (1975). Tissue trace element and enzyme content in pigs fed a low manganese diet. I. Arelationship between manganese and selenium. The Journal of laboratory and clinical medicine, 86(1), 132–139.

[4347] Shan, Z., Chen, S., Sun, T., Luo, C., Guo, Y., Yu, X., … Liu, L. (2016). U-Shaped Association between Plasma Manganese Levels and Type 2 Diabetes. Environmental Health Perspectives, 124(12), 1876–1881. doi:10.1289/ehp176

[4348] Kazi, T. G., Afridi, H. I., Kazi, N., Jamali, M. K., Arain, M. B., Jalbani, N., & Kandhro, G. A. (2008). Copper, chromium, manganese, iron, nickel, and zinc levels in biological samples of diabetes mellitus patients. Biological trace element research, 122(1), 1–18. https://doi.org/10.1007/s12011-007-8062-y

[4349] Li, X. T., Yu, P. F., Gao, Y., Guo, W. H., Wang, J., Liu, X., Gu, A. H., Ji, G. X., Dong, Q., Wang, B. S., Cao, Y., Zhu, B. L., & Xiao, H. (2017). Association between Plasma Metal Levels and Diabetes Risk: a Case-control Study in China. Biomedical and environmental sciences : BES, 30(7), 482–491. https://doi.org/10.3967/bes2017.064

[4350] Jitrapakdee, S., St Maurice, M., Rayment, I., Cleland, W. W., Wallace, J. C., & Attwood, P. V. (2008). Structure, mechanism and regulation of pyruvate carboxylase. The Biochemical journal, 413(3), 369–387. https://doi.org/10.1042/BJ20080709

[4351] Jitrapakdee, S., Nezic, M. G., Cassady, A. I., Khew-Goodall, Y., & Wallace, J. C. (2002). Molecular cloning and domain structure of chicken pyruvate carboxylase. Biochemical and biophysical research communications, 295(2), 387–393. https://doi.org/10.1016/s0006-291x(02)00651-4

[4352] Rothman, D. L., Magnusson, I., Katz, L. D., Shulman, R. G., & Shulman, G. I. (1991). Quantitation of hepatic glycogenolysis and gluconeogenesis in fasting humans with 13C NMR. Science (New York, N.Y.), 254(5031), 573–576. https://doi.org/10.1126/science.1948033

[4353] Stark, R., Pasquel, F., Turcu, A., Pongratz, R. L., Roden, M., Cline, G. W., Shulman, G. I., & Kibbey, R. G. (2009). Phosphoenolpyruvate cycling via mitochondrial phosphoenolpyruvate carboxykinase links anaplerosis and mitochondrial GTP with insulin secretion. The Journal of biological chemistry, 284(39), 26578–26590. https://doi.org/10.1074/jbc.M109.011775

[4354] Jitrapakdee, S., Walker, M. E., & Wallace, J. C. (1996). Identification of novel alternatively spliced pyruvate carboxylase mRNAs with divergent 5'-untranslated regions which are expressed in a tissue-specific manner. Biochemical and biophysical research communications, 223(3), 695–700. https://doi.org/10.1006/bbrc.1996.0958

[4355] Wu, G., & Morris, S. M., Jr (1998). Arginine metabolism: nitric oxide and beyond. The Biochemical journal, 336 (Pt 1)(Pt 1), 1–17. https://doi.org/10.1042/bj3360001

[4356] Di Costanzo, L., Moulin, M., Haertlein, M., Meilleur, F., & Christianson, D. W. (2007). Expression, purification, assay, and crystal structure of perdeuterated human arginase I. Archives of biochemistry and biophysics, 465(1), 82–89. https://doi.org/10.1016/j.abb.2007.04.036

[4357] Iyer, R. K., Yoo, P. K., Kern, R. M., Rozengurt, N., Tsoa, R., O'Brien, W. E., Yu, H., Grody, W. W., & Cederbaum, S. D. (2002). Mouse model for human arginase deficiency. Molecular and cellular biology, 22(13), 4491–4498. https://doi.org/10.1128/mcb.22.13.4491-4498.2002

[4358] Berg, JM; Tymoczko, JL; Stryer, L (2002). "23.4: Ammonium Ion is Converted into Urea in Most Terrestrial Vertebrates". Biochemistry (5th ed.). Accessed Online Feb 06 2021: https://www.ncbi.nlm.nih.gov/books/NBK22450/

[4359] Qiu, J., Thapaliya, S., Runkana, A., Yang, Y., Tsien, C., Mohan, M. L., Narayanan, A., Eghtesad, B., Mozdziak, P. E., McDonald, C., Stark, G. R., Welle, S., Naga Prasad, S. V., & Dasarathy, S. (2013). Hyperammonemia in cirrhosis induces transcriptional regulation of myostatin by an NF-κB-mediated mechanism. Proceedings of the National Academy of Sciences of the United States of America, 110(45), 18162–18167. https://doi.org/10.1073/pnas.1317049110

[4360] Olde Damink, S. W., Jalan, R., Deutz, N. E., Redhead, D. N., Dejong, C. H., Hynd, P., Jalan, R. A., Hayes, P. C., & Soeters, P. B. (2003). The kidney plays a major role in the hyperammonemia seen after simulated or actual GI bleeding in patients with cirrhosis. Hepatology (Baltimore, Md.), 37(6), 1277–1285. https://doi.org/10.1053/jhep.2003.50221

[4361] Judd, Sandra (2010). Genetic Disorders Sourcebook. Omnigraphics. p. 225. ISBN 978 0 7808 1076 1.

[4362] Liaw, S. H., Kuo, I., & Eisenberg, D. (1995). Discovery of the ammonium substrate site on glutamine synthetase, a third cation binding site. Protein science : a publication of the Protein Society, 4(11), 2358–2365. https://doi.org/10.1002/pro.5560041114

[4363] Eisenberg, D., Gill, H. S., Pfluegl, G. M., & Rotstein, S. H. (2000). Structure-function relationships of glutamine synthetases. Biochimica et biophysica acta, 1477(1-2), 122–145. https://doi.org/10.1016/s0167-4838(99)00270-8

[4364] Newsholme, P. (2001). Why Is L-Glutamine Metabolism Important to Cells of the Immune System in Health, Postinjury, Surgery or Infection?2. The Journal of Nutrition, 131(9), 2515S–2522S. doi:10.1093/jn/131.9.2515s

[4365] Calder, P. & Yaqoob, P. (1999). Glutamine and the immune system. Amino Acids 17 (3): 227–241. Review.

[4366] Chang, W-K. & Yang, K. & Shaio, M.-F. (1999). Effect of Glutamine on Th1 and Th2 Cytokine Responses of Human Peripheral Blood Mononuclear Cells. Clinical Immunology 93 (3): 294–301.

[4367] Zhou, Q. et al. (2019). Randomised placebo-controlled trial of dietary glutamine supplements for postinfectious irritable bowel syndrome. Gut 68 (6): 996–1002.

[4368] Rao, R., & Samak, G. (2012). Role of Glutamine in Protection of Intestinal Epithelial Tight Junctions. Journal of Epithelial Biology & Pharmacology 5 (Suppl 1-M7): 47–54.

[4369] Krajewski, W. W., Collins, R., Holmberg-Schiavone, L., Jones, T. A., Karlberg, T., & Mowbray, S. L. (2008). Crystal structures of mammalian glutamine synthetases illustrate substrate-induced conformational changes and provide opportunities for drug and herbicide design. Journal of molecular biology, 375(1), 217–228. https://doi.org/10.1016/j.jmb.2007.10.029

[4370] Suárez, I., Bodega, G., & Fernández, B. (2002). Glutamine synthetase in brain: effect of ammonia. Neurochemistry international, 41(2-3), 123–142. https://doi.org/10.1016/s0197-0186(02)00033-5

[4371] Yokel, R. A. (2009). Manganese Flux Across the Blood–Brain Barrier. NeuroMolecular Medicine, 11(4), 297–310. doi:10.1007/s12017-009-8101-2

[4372] Avila, D. S., Puntel, R. L., & Aschner, M. (2013). Manganese in health and disease. Metal ions in life sciences, 13, 199–227. https://doi.org/10.1007/978-94-007-7500-8_7

[4373] Jiang, Y., & Zheng, W. (2005). Cardiovascular toxicities upon manganese exposure. Cardiovascular toxicology, 5(4), 345–354. https://doi.org/10.1385/ct:5:4:345

[4374] Roth J. A. (2006). Homeostatic and toxic mechanisms regulating manganese uptake, retention, and elimination. Biological research, 39(1), 45–57. https://doi.org/10.4067/s0716-97602006000100006

[4375] Lu, C. S., Huang, C. C., Chu, N. S., & Calne, D. B. (1994). Levodopa failure in chronic manganism. Neurology, 44(9), 1600–1602. https://doi.org/10.1212/wnl.44.9.1600

[4376] Li, G. J., Zhang, L. L., Lu, L., Wu, P., & Zheng, W. (2004). Occupational exposure to welding fume among welders: alterations of manganese, iron, zinc, copper, and lead in body fluids and the oxidative stress status. Journal of occupational and environmental medicine, 46(3), 241–248. https://doi.org/10.1097/01.jom.0000116900.49159.03

[4377] Zheng, W., Ren, S., & Graziano, J. H. (1998). Manganese inhibits mitochondrial aconitase: a mechanism of manganese neurotoxicity. Brain research, 799(2), 334–342. https://doi.org/10.1016/s0006-8993(98)00481-8

729

[4378] Zheng, W., Zhao, Q., Slavkovich, V., Aschner, M., & Graziano, J. H. (1999). Alteration of iron homeostasis following chronic exposure to manganese in rats. Brain research, 833(1), 125–132. https://doi.org/10.1016/s0006-8993(99)01558-9

[4379] Verity M. A. (1999). Manganese neurotoxicity: a mechanistic hypothesis. Neurotoxicology, 20(2-3), 489–497.

[4380] Zheng, W., & Zhao, Q. (2001). Iron overload following manganese exposure in cultured neuronal, but not neuroglial cells. Brain research, 897(1-2), 175–179. https://doi.org/10.1016/s0006-8993(01)02049-2

[4381] Aschner, M., 1997. Manganese neurotoxicity and oxidative damage. In: Connor, J.R. (Ed.), Metals and Oxidative Damage in Neurological Disorders. Plenum Press, New York, pp. 77–93.

[4382] DiNicolantonio, J. J., Mangan, D., & O'Keefe, J. H. (2018). Copper deficiency may be a leading cause of ischaemic heart disease. Open heart, 5(2), e000784. https://doi.org/10.1136/openhrt-2018-000784

[4383] Vayenas, D. V., Repanti, M., Vassilopoulos, A., & Papanastasiou, D. A. (1998). Influence of iron overload on manganese, zinc, and copper concentration in rat tissues in vivo: study of liver, spleen, and brain. International Journal of Clinical & Laboratory Research, 28(3), 183–186. doi:10.1007/s005990050041

[4384] Rao, K. V. R., & Norenberg, M. D. (2004). Manganese Induces the Mitochondrial Permeability Transition in Cultured Astrocytes. Journal of Biological Chemistry, 279(31), 32333–32338. doi:10.1074/jbc.m402096200

[4385] Sriram, K., Lin, G. X., Jefferson, A. M., Roberts, J. R., Wirth, O., Hayashi, Y., Krajnak, K. M., Soukup, J. M., Ghio, A. J., Reynolds, S. H., Castranova, V., Munson, A. E., & Antonini, J. M. (2010). Mitochondrial dysfunction and loss of Parkinson's disease-linked proteins contribute to neurotoxicity of manganese-containing welding fumes. FASEB journal : official publication of the Federation of American Societies for Experimental Biology, 24(12), 4989–5002. https://doi.org/10.1096/fj.10-163964

[4386] Malecki E. A. (2001). Manganese toxicity is associated with mitochondrial dysfunction and DNA fragmentation in rat primary striatal neurons. Brain research bulletin, 55(2), 225–228. https://doi.org/10.1016/s0361-9230(01)00456-7

[4387] Morello, M., Canini, A., Mattioli, P., Sorge, R. P., Alimonti, A., Bocca, B., Forte, G., Martorana, A., Bernardi, G., & Sancesario, G. (2008). Sub-cellular localization of manganese in the basal ganglia of normal and manganese-treated rats An electron spectroscopy imaging and electron energy-loss spectroscopy study. Neurotoxicology, 29(1), 60–72. https://doi.org/10.1016/j.neuro.2007.09.001

[4388] Gunter, R. E., Puskin, J. S., & Russell, P. R. (1975). Quantitative magnetic resonance studies of manganese uptake by mitochondria. Biophysical journal, 15(4), 319–333. https://doi.org/10.1016/S0006-3495(75)85822-X

[4389] Gavin et al (1990) 'Manganese and calcium efflux kinetics in brain mitochondria. Relevance to manganese toxicity', Biochemical Journal 266(2):329-34. DOI: 10.1042/bj2660329.

[4390] Gunter, T. E., & Puskin, J. S. (1972). Manganous ion as a spin label in studies of mitochondrial uptake of manganese. Biophysical journal, 12(6), 625–635. https://doi.org/10.1016/S0006-3495(72)86108-3

[4391] Gavin, C. E., Gunter, K. K., & Gunter, T. E. (1999). Manganese and calcium transport in mitochondria: implications for manganese toxicity. Neurotoxicology, 20(2-3), 445–453.

[4392] Hudnell H. K. (1999). Effects from environmental Mn exposures: a review of the evidence from non-occupational exposure studies. Neurotoxicology, 20(2-3), 379–397.

[4393] Ferraz, H. B., Bertolucci, P. H., Pereira, J. S., Lima, J. G., & Andrade, L. A. (1988). Chronic exposure to the fungicide maneb may produce symptoms and signs of CNS manganese intoxication. Neurology, 38(4), 550–553. https://doi.org/10.1212/wnl.38.4.550

[4394] Lynam, D. R., Roos, J. W., Pfeifer, G. D., Fort, B. F., & Pullin, T. G. (1999). Environmental effects and exposures to manganese from use of methylcyclopentadienyl manganese tricarbonyl (MMT) in gasoline. Neurotoxicology, 20(2-3), 145–150.

[4395] Kondakis, X. G., Makris, N., Leotsinidis, M., Prinou, M., & Papapetropoulos, T. (1989). Possible health effects of high manganese concentration in drinking water. Archives of environmental health, 44(3), 175–178. https://doi.org/10.1080/00039896.1989.9935883

[4396] Young, R. J., Critchley, J. A., Young, K. K., Freebairn, R. C., Reynolds, A. P., & Lolin, Y. I. (1996). Fatal acute hepatorenal failure following potassium permanganate ingestion. Human & experimental toxicology, 15(3), 259–261. https://doi.org/10.1177/096032719601500313

[4397] Ong, K. L., Tan, T. H., & Cheung, W. L. (1997). Potassium permanganate poisoning--a rare cause of fatal self poisoning. Emergency Medicine Journal, 14(1), 43–45. doi:10.1136/emj.14.1.43

[4398] Lauwerys, R., Roels, H., Genet, P., Toussaint, G., Bouckaert, A., & De Cooman, S. (1985). Fertility of male workers exposed to mercury vapor or to manganese dust: a questionnaire study. American journal of industrial medicine, 7(2), 171–176. https://doi.org/10.1002/ajim.4700070208

[4399] Huang, C. C., Chu, N. S., Lu, C. S., Wang, J. D., Tsai, J. L., Tzeng, J. L., Wolters, E. C., & Calne, D. B. (1989). Chronic manganese intoxication. Archives of neurology, 46(10), 1104–1106. https://doi.org/10.1001/archneur.1989.00520460090018

[4400] Bowler et al (2011) 'Prospective study on neurotoxic effects in manganese-exposed bridge construction welders', NeuroToxicology, Volume 32, Issue 5, October 2011, Pages 596-605.

[4401] Checkoway, H. (2010). Documenting neurotoxicity from occupational manganese exposure. Occupational and Environmental Medicine, 67(6), 362–363. doi:10.1136/oem.2009.047803

[4402] Occupational Safety and Health Administration (2021) 'OSHA Occupational Chemical Database', Directorate of Technical Support and Emergency Management (DTSEM), Accessed Online Feb 10 2021: https://www.osha.gov/chemicaldata/

[4403] CDC (2019) 'Manganese compounds and fume (as Mn)', NIOSH Pocket Guide to Chemical Hazards, Accessed Online Feb 10 2021: https://www.cdc.gov/niosh/npg/npgd0379.html

[4404] Talhout, R., Schulz, T., Florek, E., van Benthem, J., Wester, P., & Opperhuizen, A. (2011). Hazardous compounds in tobacco smoke. International journal of environmental research and public health, 8(2), 613–628. https://doi.org/10.3390/ijerph8020613

[4405] Bernhard, D., Rossmann, A., & Wick, G. (2005). Metals in cigarette smoke. IUBMB life, 57(12), 805–809. https://doi.org/10.1080/15216540500459667

[4406] Henriksson, J. (2000). Manganese Taken Up into the CNS via the Olfactory Pathway in Rats Affects Astrocytes. Toxicological Sciences, 55(2), 392–398. doi:10.1093/toxsci/55.2.392

[4407] Chen, P., Chakraborty, S., Mukhopadhyay, S., Lee, E., Paoliello, M. M., Bowman, A. B., & Aschner, M. (2015). Manganese homeostasis in the nervous system. Journal of neurochemistry, 134(4), 601–610. https://doi.org/10.1111/jnc.13170

[4408] Rubin, L. L., & Staddon, J. M. (1999). The cell biology of the blood-brain barrier. Annual review of neuroscience, 22, 11–28. https://doi.org/10.1146/annurev.neuro.22.1.11

[4409] Uchino, A., Noguchi, T., Nomiyama, K., Takase, Y., Nakazono, T., Nojiri, J., & Kudo, S. (2007). Manganese accumulation in the brain: MR imaging. Neuroradiology, 49(9), 715–720. https://doi.org/10.1007/s00234-007-0243-z

[4410] Sloot, W. N., Korf, J., Koster, J. F., de Wit, L. E. A., & Gramsbergen, J. B. P. (1996). Manganese-Induced Hydroxyl Radical Formation in Rat Striatum Is Not Attenuated by Dopamine Depletion or Iron Chelationin Vivo. Experimental Neurology, 138(2), 236–245. doi:10.1006/exnr.1996.0062

[4411] Bagga, P., & Patel, A. B. (2012). Regional cerebral metabolism in mouse under chronic manganese exposure: implications for manganism. Neurochemistry international, 60(2), 177–185. https://doi.org/10.1016/j.neuint.2011.10.016

[4412] Greger, J. L. (1998). Dietary Standards for Manganese: Overlap between Nutritional and Toxicological Studies. The Journal of Nutrition, 128(2), 368S–371S. doi:10.1093/jn/128.2.368s

[4413] Friedman, B. J., Freeland-Graves, J. H., Bales, C. W., Behmardi, F., Shorey-Kutschke, R. L., Willis, R. A., Crosby, J. B., Trickett, P. C., & Houston, S. D. (1987). Manganese balance and clinical observations in young men fed a manganese-deficient diet. The Journal of nutrition, 117(1), 133–143. https://doi.org/10.1093/jn/117.1.133

[4414] Penland, J. G., & Johnson, P. E. (1993). Dietary calcium and manganese effects on menstrual cycle symptoms. American journal of obstetrics and gynecology, 168(5), 1417–1423. https://doi.org/10.1016/s0002-9378(11)90775-3

[4415] NIH (2020) 'Manganese: Fact Sheet for Health Professionals', Accessed Online Feb 10 2021: https://ods.od.nih.gov/factsheets/Manganese-HealthProfessional/

[4416] Institute of Medicine. Food and Nutrition Board. Dietary Reference Intakes for Vitamin A, Vitamin K, Arsenic, Boron, Chromium, Copper, Iodine, Iron, Manganese, Molybdenum, Nickel, Silicon, Vanadium, and Zinc Washington, DC: National Academy Press; 2001.

[4417] Institute of Medicine (US) Panel on Micronutrients. Dietary Reference Intakes for Vitamin A, Vitamin K, Arsenic, Boron, Chromium, Copper, Iodine, Iron, Manganese, Molybdenum, Nickel, Silicon, Vanadium, and Zinc. Washington (DC): National Academies Press (US); 2001. 10, Manganese.

[4418] O'Neal, S. L., & Zheng, W. (2015). Manganese Toxicity Upon Overexposure: a Decade in Review. Current environmental health reports, 2(3), 315–328. https://doi.org/10.1007/s40572-015-0056-x

[4419] Pennington, J. A., & Young, B. E. (1991). Total diet study nutritional elements, 1982-1989. Journal of the American Dietetic Association, 91(2), 179–183.

[4420] Filippini, T., Cilloni, S., Malavolti, M., Violi, F., Malagoli, C., Tesauro, M., Bottecchi, I., Ferrari, A., Vescovi, L., & Vinceti, M. (2018). Dietary intake of cadmium, chromium, copper, manganese, selenium and zinc in a Northern Italy community. Journal of trace elements in medicine and biology : organ of the Society for Minerals and Trace Elements (GMS), 50, 508–517. https://doi.org/10.1016/j.jtemb.2018.03.001

[4421] Agency for Toxic Substances and Disease Registry (ATSDR), 2000. Toxicological profile for manganese. US Department of Health and Human Services, Public Health Service, Atlanta, GA.

[4422] National Academy of Sciences (NAS), 2001. Dietary Reference Intakes for Vitamin A, Vitamin K, Arsenic, Boron, Chromium, Copper, Iodine, Iron, Manganese, Molybdenum, Nickel, Silicon, Vanadium, and Zinc. Panel on Micronutrients, Subcommittees on Upper Reference Levels of Nutrients and of Interpretation and Use of Dietary Reference Intakes, and the Standing Committee on the Scientific Evaluation of Dietary Reference Intakes. Available from: <www.nap.edu/books/ 0309072794/html/>

[4423] Lönnerdal B. (1994). Nutritional aspects of soy formula. Acta paediatrica (Oslo, Norway : 1992). Supplement, 402, 105–108. https://doi.org/10.1111/j.1651-2227.1994.tb13371.x

[4424] Davidsson, L., Cederblad, A., Lönnerdal, B., & Sandström, B. (1989). Manganese absorption from human milk, cow's milk, and infant formulas in humans. American journal of diseases of children (1960), 143(7), 823–827. https://doi.org/10.1001/archpedi.1989.02150190073024

[4425] Zlotkin, S. H., Atkinson, S., & Lockitch, G. (1995). Trace Elements in Nutrition for Premature Infants. Clinics in Perinatology, 22(1), 223–240. doi:10.1016/s0095-5108(18)30310-5

[4426] Dörner, K., Dziadzka, S., Höhn, A., Sievers, E., Oldigs, H. D., Schulz-Lell, G., & Schaub, J. (1989). Longitudinal manganese and copper balances in young infants and preterm infants fed on breast-milk and adapted cow's milk formulas. The British journal of nutrition, 61(3), 559–572. https://doi.org/10.1079/bjn19890143

[4427] Schroeder, H. A., Balassa, J. J., & Tipton, I. H. (1966). Essential trace metals in man: Manganese. Journal of Chronic Diseases, 19(5), 545–571. doi:10.1016/0021-9681(66)90094-4

[4428] Collipp, P. J., Chen, S. Y., & Maitinsky, S. (1983). Manganese in infant formulas and learning disability. Annals of nutrition & metabolism, 27(6), 488–494. https://doi.org/10.1159/000176724

[4429] Tran, T. T., Chowanadisai, W., Crinella, F. M., Chicz-DeMet, A., & Lönnerdal, B. (2002). Effect of High Dietary Manganese Intake of Neonatal Rats on Tissue Mineral Accumulation, Striatal Dopamine Levels, and Neurodevelopmental Status. NeuroToxicology, 23(4-5), 635–643. doi:10.1016/s0161-813x(02)00091-8

[4430] Chen, L., Ding, G., Gao, Y., Wang, P., Shi, R., Huang, H., & Tian, Y. (2014). Manganese concentrations in maternal–infant blood and birth weight. Environmental Science and Pollution Research, 21(9), 6170–6175. doi:10.1007/s11356-013-2465-4

[4431] Zota, A. R., Ettinger, A. S., Bouchard, M., Amarasiriwardena, C. J., Schwartz, J., Hu, H., & Wright, R. O. (2009). Maternal blood manganese levels and infant birth weight. Epidemiology (Cambridge, Mass.), 20(3), 367–373. https://doi.org/10.1097/EDE.0b013e31819b93c0

[4432] Yu, X., Cao, L., & Yu, X. (2013). Elevated cord serum manganese level is associated with a neonatal high ponderal index. Environmental Research, 121, 79–83. doi:10.1016/j.envres.2012.11.002

[4433] Guan, H., Wang, M., Li, X., Piao, F., Li, Q., Xu, L., ... Yokoyama, K. (2013). Manganese concentrations in maternal and umbilical cord blood: related to birth size and environmental factors. European Journal of Public Health, 24(1), 150–157. doi:10.1093/eurpub/ckt033

[4434] Committee on Nutrition, American Academy of Pediatrics, 1985. Nutritional needs of low birth weight infants. Pediatrics 75, 976–986.

[4435] A.S.P.E.N. Report, 2004. Task Force for the Revision of Safe Practices for Parenteral Nutrition: Mirtallo, J., Canada, T., Johnson, D., Kumpf, V., Petersen, C., Sacks, G., Seres, D., Guenter, P. Special Report: Safe Practices for Parenteral. J. Parenter. Enteral. Nutr. 28, S39–S70.

[4436] Committee on Nutrition, American Academy of Pediatrics, 2003. In: Kleinman, R.E. (Ed.), Pediatric Nutrition Handbook, fifth ed.

[4437] Greger, J. L. (1998). Dietary Standards for Manganese: Overlap between Nutritional and Toxicological Studies. The Journal of Nutrition, 128(2), 368S–371S. doi:10.1093/jn/128.2.368s

[4438] Khan, K., Wasserman, G. A., Liu, X., Ahmed, E., Parvez, F., Slavkovich, V., ... Factor-Litvak, P. (2012). Manganese exposure from drinking water and children's academic achievement. NeuroToxicology, 33(1), 91–97. doi:10.1016/j.neuro.2011.12.002

[4439] DeSimone, L.A., 2009, Quality of water from domestic wells in principal aquifers of the United States, 1991–2004: U.S. Geological Survey Scientific Investigations Report 2008–5227, 139 p., available online at http://pubs.usgs.gov/sir/2008/5227.

[4440] Frisbie et al (2002) 'The concentrations of arsenic and other toxic elements in Bangladesh's drinking water.', Environmental Health Perspectives 110:11 CID: https://doi.org/10.1289/ehp.021101147

[4441] Khan, K., Factor-Litvak, P., Wasserman, G. A., Liu, X., Ahmed, E., Parvez, F., Slavkovich, V., Levy, D., Mey, J., van Geen, A., & Graziano, J. H. (2011). Manganese exposure from drinking water and children's classroom behavior in Bangladesh. Environmental health perspectives, 119(10), 1501–1506. https://doi.org/10.1289/ehp.1003397

[4442] Bouchard, M. F., Sauvé, S., Barbeau, B., Legrand, M., Brodeur, M. È., Bouffard, T., Limoges, E., Bellinger, D. C., & Mergler, D. (2011). Intellectual impairment in school-age children exposed to manganese from drinking water. Environmental health perspectives, 119(1), 138–143. https://doi.org/10.1289/ehp.1002321

[4443] Kondakis, X. G., Makris, N., Leotsinidis, M., Prinou, M., & Papapetropoulos, T. (1989). Possible health effects of high manganese concentration in drinking water. Archives of environmental health, 44(3), 175–178. https://doi.org/10.1080/00039896.1989.9935883

[4444] Ansari et al (2004). Essential Trace Metal (Zinc, Manganese, Copper and Iron) Levels in Plants of Medicinal Importance. Journal of Biological Sciences, 4(2), 95–99. doi:10.3923/jbs.2004.95.99

[4445] NIH (2020) 'Manganese', Fact Sheet for Consumers, Accessed Online Feb 06 2021: https://ods.od.nih.gov/factsheets/manganese-healthprofessional/

[4446] Jiang et al (2007) 'Brain magnetic resonance imaging and manganese concentrations in red blood cells of smelting workers: Search for biomarkers of manganese exposure', NeuroToxicology, Volume 28, Issue 1, January 2007, Pages 126-135.

[4447] Leblondel, G., & Allain, P. (1999). Manganese transport by caco-2 cells. Biological Trace Element Research, 67(1), 13–28. doi:10.1007/bf02784271

[4448] Mena, I., Horiuchi, K., Burke, K., & Cotzias, G. C. (1969). Chronic manganese poisoning. Individual susceptibility and absorption of iron. Neurology, 19(10), 1000–1006. https://doi.org/10.1212/wnl.19.10.1000

[4449] Hansen, S. L., Trakooljul, N., Liu, H. C., Moeser, A. J., & Spears, J. W. (2009). Iron transporters are differentially regulated by dietary iron, and modifications are associated with changes in manganese metabolism in young pigs. The Journal of nutrition, 139(8), 1474–1479. https://doi.org/10.3945/jn.109.105866

[4450] Garcia, S. J., Gellein, K., Syversen, T., & Aschner, M. (2006). Iron Deficient and Manganese Supplemented Diets Alter Metals and Transporters in the Developing Rat Brain. Toxicological Sciences, 95(1), 205–214. doi:10.1093/toxsci/kfl139

[4451] Lönnerdal, B., Keen, C. L., & Hurley, L. S. (1985). Manganese binding proteins in human and cow's milk. The American journal of clinical nutrition, 41(3), 550–559. https://doi.org/10.1093/ajcn/41.3.550

[4452] Davidson, L. A., & Lönnerdal, B. (1989). Fe-saturation and proteolysis of human lactoferrin: effect on brush-border receptor-mediated uptake of Fe and Mn. The American journal of physiology, 257(6 Pt 1), G930–G934. https://doi.org/10.1152/ajpgi.1989.257.6.G930

[4453] Davidsson, L., Cederblad, A., Lönnerdal, B., & Sandström, B. (1991). The effect of individual dietary components on manganese absorption in humans. The American Journal of Clinical Nutrition, 54(6), 1065–1070. doi:10.1093/ajcn/54.6.1065

[4454] Britton, A., & Cotzias, G. (1966). Dependence of manganese turnover on intake. American Journal of Physiology-Legacy Content, 211(1), 203–206. doi:10.1152/ajplegacy.1966.211.1.203

[4455] Davis, C. D., Zech, L., & Greger, J. L. (1993). Manganese Metabolism in Rats: An Improved Methodology for Assessing Gut Endogenous Losses. Experimental Biology and Medicine, 202(1), 103–108. doi:10.3181/00379727-202-43518

[4456] Finley, J. W. (1999). Manganese absorption and retention by young women is associated with serum ferritin concentration. The American Journal of Clinical Nutrition, 70(1), 37–43. doi:10.1093/ajcn/70.1.37

[4457] Finley, J. W., Johnson, P. E., & Johnson, L. K. (1994). Sex affects manganese absorption and retention by humans from a diet adequate in manganese. The American journal of clinical nutrition, 60(6), 949–955. https://doi.org/10.1093/ajcn/60.6.949

[4458] Raghib., M. H., Wai-Yee, C., & Rennert, M. O. (1986). Comparative biological availability of manganese from extrinsically labelled milk diets using sucking rats as a model. British Journal of Nutrition, 55(1), 49–58. doi:10.1079/bjn19860009

[4459] Keen, C. L., Bell, J. G., & Lönnerdal, B. (1986). The effect of age on manganese uptake and retention from milk and infant formulas in rats. The Journal of nutrition, 116(3), 395–402. https://doi.org/10.1093/jn/116.3.395

[4460] Ahmad, T. R., Higuchi, S., Bertaggia, E., Hung, A., Shanmugarajah, N., Guilz, N. C., Gamarra, J. R., & Haeusler, R. A. (2020). Bile acid composition regulates the manganese transporter Slc30a10 in intestine. The Journal of biological chemistry, 295(35), 12545–12558. https://doi.org/10.1074/jbc.RA120.012792

[4461] Malecki, E. A., Radzanowski, G. M., Radzanowski, T. J., Gallaher, D. D., & Greger, J. L. (1996). Biliary manganese excretion in conscious rats is affected by acute and chronic manganese intake but not by dietary fat. The Journal of nutrition, 126(2), 489–498. https://doi.org/10.1093/jn/126.2.489

[4462] Cotzias, G. C., Miller, S. T., Papavasiliou, P. S., & Tang, L. C. (1976). Interactions between manganese and brain dopamine. The Medical clinics of North America, 60(4), 729–738. https://doi.org/10.1016/s0025-7125(16)31856-9

[4463] Klaassen C. D. (1976). Biliary excretion of metals. Drug metabolism reviews, 5(2), 165–196. https://doi.org/10.3109/03602537609029977

[4464] Stastny, D., Vogel, R. S., & Picciano, M. F. (1984). Manganese intake and serum manganese concentration of human milk-fed and formula-fed infants. The American journal of clinical nutrition, 39(6), 872–878. https://doi.org/10.1093/ajcn/39.6.872

[4465] Papavasiliou, P. S., Miller, S. T., & Cotzias, G. C. (1966). Role of liver in regulating distribution and excretion of manganese. The American journal of physiology, 211(1), 211–216. https://doi.org/10.1152/ajplegacy.1966.211.1.211

[4466] Cotzias, G. C., Horiuchi, K., Fuenzalida, S., & Mena, I. (1968). Chronic manganese poisoning. Clearance of tissue manganese concentrations with persistance of the neurological picture. Neurology, 18(4), 376–382. https://doi.org/10.1212/wnl.18.4.376

[4467] Mahoney, J. P., & Small, W. J. (1968). Studies on manganese. Journal of Clinical Investigation, 47(3), 643–653. doi:10.1172/jci105760

[4468] Davidsson, L., Cederblad, A., Hagebø, E., Lönnerdal, B., & Sandström, B. (1988). Intrinsic and extrinsic labeling for studies of manganese absorption in humans. The Journal of nutrition, 118(12), 1517–1521. https://doi.org/10.1093/jn/118.12.1517

[4469] Aisen, P., Leibman, A., & Zweier, J. (1978). Stoichiometric and site characteristics of the binding of iron to human transferrin. Journal of Biological Chemistry, 253(6), 1930–1937. doi:10.1016/s0021-9258(19)62337-9

[4470] Inoue et al (2002) 'Structure, Function, and Expression Pattern of a Novel Sodium-coupled Citrate Transporter (NaCT) Cloned from Mammalian Brain', Journal of Biological Chemistry 277(42):39469-76, DOI: 10.1074/jbc.M207072200

[4471] Jenkitkasemwong, S., Wang, C. Y., Mackenzie, B., & Knutson, M. D. (2012). Physiologic implications of metal-ion transport by ZIP14 and ZIP8. Biometals : an international journal on the role of metal ions in biology, biochemistry, and medicine, 25(4), 643–655. https://doi.org/10.1007/s10534-012-9526-x

[4472] Moos, T., & Morgan, E. H. (2000). Transferrin and transferrin receptor function in brain barrier systems. Cellular and molecular neurobiology, 20(1), 77–95. https://doi.org/10.1023/a:1006948027674

[4473] Nam, H., Wang, C.-Y., Zhang, L., Zhang, W., Hojyo, S., Fukada, T., & Knutson, M. D. (2013). ZIP14 and DMT1 in the liver, pancreas, and heart are differentially regulated by iron deficiency and overload: implications for tissue iron uptake in iron-related disorders. Haematologica, 98(7), 1049–1057. doi:10.3324/haematol.2012.072314

[4474] Montes, S., Alcaraz-Zubeldia, M., Muriel, P., & Ríos, C. (2001). Striatal manganese accumulation induces changes in dopamine metabolism in the cirrhotic rat. Brain Research, 891(1-2), 123–129. doi:10.1016/s0006-8993(00)03208-x

[4475] Erikson, K. M., & Aschner, M. (2003). Manganese neurotoxicity and glutamate-GABA interaction. Neurochemistry international, 43(4-5), 475–480. https://doi.org/10.1016/s0197-0186(03)00037-8

[4476] Krieger, D., Krieger, S., Jansen, O., Gass, P., Theilmann, L., & Lichtnecker, H. (1995). Manganese and chronic hepatic encephalopathy. Lancet (London, England), 346(8970), 270–274. https://doi.org/10.1016/s0140-6736(95)92164-8

[4477] Ballatori, N., Miles, E., & Clarkson, T. W. (1987). Homeostatic control of manganese excretion in the neonatal rat. The American journal of physiology, 252(5 Pt 2), R842–R847. https://doi.org/10.1152/ajpregu.1987.252.5.R842

[4478] Ballatori, N. (2000). "12. Molecular mechanisms of hepatic metal transport". In Zalups, R.K.; Koropatnick, J. (eds.). Molecular Biology and Toxicology of Metals. Taylor & Francis. pp. 346–381.

[4479] REIMUND, J.-M., DIETEMANN, J.-L., WARTER, J.-M., BAUMANN, R., & DUCLOS, B. (2000). Factors associated to hypermanganesemia in patients receiving home parenteral nutrition. Clinical Nutrition, 19(5), 343–348. doi:10.1054/clnu.2000.0120

[4480] Ikeda, S., Yamaguchi, Y., Sera, Y., Ohshiro, H., Uchino, S., Yamashita, Y., & Ogawa, M. (2000). Manganese deposition in the globus pallidus in patients with biliary atresia. Transplantation, 69(11), 2339–2343. https://doi.org/10.1097/00007890-200006150-00021

[4481] Rose, C., Butterworth, R. F., Zayed, J., Normandin, L., Todd, K., Michalak, A., Spahr, L., Huet, P. M., & Pomier-Layrargues, G. (1999). Manganese deposition in basal ganglia structures results from both portal-systemic shunting and liver dysfunction. Gastroenterology, 117(3), 640–644. https://doi.org/10.1016/s0016-5085(99)70457-9

[4482] Rao, V. L., Giguère, J. F., Layrargues, G. P., & Butterworth, R. F. (1993). Increased activities of MAOA and MAOB in autopsied brain tissue from cirrhotic patients with hepatic encephalopathy. Brain research, 621(2), 349–352. https://doi.org/10.1016/0006-8993(93)90126-8

[4483] Fell, J. M., Reynolds, A. P., Meadows, N., Khan, K., Long, S. G., Quaghebeur, G., Taylor, W. J., & Milla, P. J. (1996). Manganese toxicity in children receiving long-term parenteral nutrition. Lancet (London, England), 347(9010), 1218–1221. https://doi.org/10.1016/s0140-6736(96)90735-7

[4484] Hambidge, K. M., Sokol, R. J., Fidanza, S. J., & Goodall, M. A. (1989). Plasma Manganese Concentrations in Infants and Children Receiving Parenteral Nutrition. Journal of Parenteral and Enteral Nutrition, 13(2), 168–171. doi:10.1177/0148607189013002168

[4485] ATSDR (2012) 'Toxicological profile for manganese (Draft for Public Comment)'. U.S. Department of Health and Human Services, Public Service.

[4486] Davis, C. D., & Greger, J. L. (1992). Longitudinal changes of manganese-dependent superoxide dismutase and other indexes of manganese and iron status in women. The American journal of clinical nutrition, 55(3), 747–752. https://doi.org/10.1093/ajcn/55.3.747

[4487] Greger, J. L., Davis, C. D., Suttie, J. W., & Lyle, B. J. (1990). Intake, serum concentrations, and urinary excretion of manganese by adult males. The American journal of clinical nutrition, 51(3), 457–461. https://doi.org/10.1093/ajcn/51.3.457

[4488] Zhang, L. L., Lu, L., Pan, Y. J., Ding, C. G., Xu, D. Y., Huang, C. F., Pan, X. F., & Zheng, W. (2015). Baseline blood levels of manganese, lead, cadmium, copper, and zinc in residents of Beijing suburb. Environmental research, 140, 10–17. https://doi.org/10.1016/j.envres.2015.03.008

[4489] Matsuda, A., Kimura, M., Kataoka, M., Ohkuma, S., Sato, M., & Itokawa, Y. (1989). Quantifying manganese in lymphocytes to assess manganese nutritional status. Clinical chemistry, 35(9), 1939–1941.

[4490] Leggett R. W. (2011). A biokinetic model for manganese. The Science of the total environment, 409(20), 4179–4186. https://doi.org/10.1016/j.scitotenv.2011.07.003

734

[4491] Aisen, P., Aasa, R., & Redfield, A. G. (1969). The chromium, manganese, and cobalt complexes of transferrin. The Journal of biological chemistry, 244(17), 4628–4633.

[4492] Harris and Chen (1994) 'Electron paramagnetic resonance and difference ultraviolet studies of Mn2+ binding to serum transferrin', Journal of Inorganic Biochemistry, Volume 54, Issue 1, April 1994, Pages 1-19.

[4493] Reaney et al (2002) 'Manganese Oxidation State and Its Implications for Toxicity', Chemical Research in Toxicology 2002 15 (9), 1119-1126.

[4494] Jursa, T., & Smith, D. R. (2009). Ceruloplasmin alters the tissue disposition and neurotoxicity of manganese, but not its loading onto transferrin. Toxicological sciences : an official journal of the Society of Toxicology, 107(1), 182–193. https://doi.org/10.1093/toxsci/kfn231

[4495] Archibald, F. S., & Tyree, C. (1987). Manganese poisoning and the attack of trivalent manganese upon catecholamines. Archives of biochemistry and biophysics, 256(2), 638–650. https://doi.org/10.1016/0003-9861(87)90621-7

[4496] Gunter, T. E., Gerstner, B., Gunter, K. K., Malecki, J., Gelein, R., Valentine, W. M., Aschner, M., & Yule, D. I. (2013). Manganese transport via the transferrin mechanism. Neurotoxicology, 34, 118–127. https://doi.org/10.1016/j.neuro.2012.10.018

[4497] Tuschl, K., Mills, P. B., & Clayton, P. T. (2013). Manganese and the brain. International review of neurobiology, 110, 277–312. https://doi.org/10.1016/B978-0-12-410502-7.00013-2

[4498] Keen, C.L., Zidenberg-Cherr, S., 1994. Manganese toxicity in humans and experimental animals, In: Klimis-Tavantzis, D.J. (Ed.), Manganese in Health and Disease. CRC Press, Boca Raton, FL, pp. 193–205.

[4499] Rehnberg, G. L., Hein, J. F., Carter, S. D., & Laskey, J. W. (1980). Chronic manganese oxide administration to preweanling rats: manganese accumulation and distribution. Journal of toxicology and environmental health, 6(1), 217–226. https://doi.org/10.1080/15287398009529844

[4500] Keen, C. L., Clegg, M. S., Lönnerdal, B., & Hurley, L. S. (1983). Whole-blood manganese as an indicator of body manganese. The New England journal of medicine, 308(20), 1230.

[4501] Rahil-Khazen, R., Bolann, B. J., Myking, A., & Ulvik, R. J. (2002). Multi-element analysis of trace element levels in human autopsy tissues by using inductively coupled atomic emission spectrometry technique (ICP-AES). Journal of trace elements in medicine and biology : organ of the Society for Minerals and Trace Elements (GMS), 16(1), 15–25. https://doi.org/10.1016/S0946-672X(02)80004-9

[4502] Schroeder, H. A., Balassa, J. J., & Tipton, I. H. (1966). Essential trace metals in man: Manganese. Journal of Chronic Diseases, 19(5), 545–571. doi:10.1016/0021-9681(66)90094-4

[4503] Pejović-Milić, A., Aslam, Chettle, D. R., Oudyk, J., Pysklywec, M. W., & Haines, T. (2009). Bone manganese as a biomarker of manganese exposure: a feasibility study. American journal of industrial medicine, 52(10), 742–750. https://doi.org/10.1002/ajim.20737

[4504] O'Neal, S. L., Hong, L., Fu, S., Jiang, W., Jones, A., Nie, L. H., & Zheng, W. (2014). Manganese accumulation in bone following chronic exposure in rats: Steady-state concentration and half-life in bone. Toxicology Letters, 229(1), 93–100. doi:10.1016/j.toxlet.2014.06.019

[4505] Saner, G., Dağoğlu, T., & Ozden, T. (1985). Hair manganese concentrations in newborns and their mothers. The American journal of clinical nutrition, 41(5), 1042–1044. https://doi.org/10.1093/ajcn/41.5.1042

[4506] Lide, David R., ed. (1994). "Molybdenum". CRC Handbook of Chemistry and Physics. 4. Chemical Rubber Publishing Company. p. 18.

[4507] Lansdown, A. R. (1999). Molybdenum disulphide lubrication. Tribology and Interface Engineering. 35. Elsevier.

[4508] Scheele (1779). "Versuche mit Wasserbley;Molybdaena". Svenska Vetensk. Academ. Handlingar. 40: 238.

[4509] Hjelm, P. J. (1788). "Versuche mit Molybdäna, und Reduction der selben Erde". Svenska Vetensk. Academ. Handlingar. 49: 268.

[4510] Millholland, Ray (August 1941). "Battle of the Billions: American industry mobilizes machines, materials, and men for a job as big as digging 40 Panama Canals in one year". Popular Science: 61.

[4511] Mendel, R. R., & Leimkühler, S. (2015). The biosynthesis of the molybdenum cofactors. Journal of biological inorganic chemistry : JBIC : a publication of the Society of Biological Inorganic Chemistry, 20(2), 337–347. https://doi.org/10.1007/s00775-014-1173-y

[4512] Wahl, B., Reichmann, D., Niks, D., Krompholz, N., Havemeyer, A., Clement, B., Messerschmidt, T., Rothkegel, M., Biester, H., Hille, R., Mendel, R. R., & Bittner, F. (2010). Biochemical and spectroscopic characterization of the human mitochondrial amidoxime reducing components hmARC-1 and hmARC-2 suggests the existence of a new molybdenum enzyme family in eukaryotes. The Journal of biological chemistry, 285(48), 37847–37859. https://doi.org/10.1074/jbc.M110.169532

[4513] Terao, M., Romão, M. J., Leimkühler, S., Bolis, M., Fratelli, M., Coelho, C., Santos-Silva, T., & Garattini, E. (2016). Structure and function of mammalian aldehyde oxidases. Archives of toxicology, 90(4), 753–780. https://doi.org/10.1007/s00204-016-1683-1

735

[4514] Ott, G., Havemeyer, A., & Clement, B. (2015). The mammalian molybdenum enzymes of mARC. Journal of biological inorganic chemistry : JBIC : a publication of the Society of Biological Inorganic Chemistry, 20(2), 265–275. https://doi.org/10.1007/s00775-014-1216-4

[4515] Beedham C. (1985). Molybdenum hydroxylases as drug-metabolizing enzymes. Drug metabolism reviews, 16(1-2), 119–156. https://doi.org/10.3109/03602538508991432

[4516] Burgess, B. K., & Lowe, D. J. (1996). Mechanism of Molybdenum Nitrogenase. Chemical reviews, 96(7), 2983–3012. https://doi.org/10.1021/cr950055x

[4517] Kim, J., & Rees, D. C. (1992). Structural models for the metal centers in the nitrogenase molybdenum-iron protein. Science (New York, N.Y.), 257(5077), 1677–1682. https://doi.org/10.1126/science.1529354

[4518] Reiss, J., & Johnson, J. L. (2003). Mutations in the molybdenum cofactor biosynthetic genes MOCS1, MOCS2, and GEPH. Human mutation, 21(6), 569–576. https://doi.org/10.1002/humu.10223

[4519] Cohen, H. J., Drew, R. T., Johnson, J. L., & Rajagopalan, K. V. (1973). Molecular basis of the biological function of molybdenum: the relationship between sulfite oxidase and the acute toxicity of bisulfite and SO2. Proceedings of the National Academy of Sciences of the United States of America, 70(12), 3655–3659. https://doi.org/10.1073/pnas.70.12.3655

[4520] Ichida, K., Aydin, H. I., Hosoyamada, M., Kalkanoglu, H. S., Dursun, A., Ohno, I., Coskun, T., Tokatli, A., Shibasaki, T., & Hosoya, T. (2006). A Turkish case with molybdenum cofactor deficiency. Nucleosides, nucleotides & nucleic acids, 25(9-11), 1087–1091. https://doi.org/10.1080/15257770600894022

[4521] Johnson, J. L., Wuebbens, M. M., Mandell, R., & Shih, V. E. (1989). Molybdenum cofactor biosynthesis in humans. Identification of two complementation groups of cofactor-deficient patients and preliminary characterization of a diffusible molybdopterin precursor. The Journal of clinical investigation, 83(3), 897–903. https://doi.org/10.1172/JCI113974

[4522] Bowhay, S. (2013). Two years experience of the treatment of molybdenum cofactor deficiency. Archives of Disease in Childhood, 98(6), e1–e1. doi:10.1136/archdischild-2013-303935a.26

[4523] Veldman, A., Santamaria-Araujo, J. A., Sollazzo, S., Pitt, J., Gianello, R., Yaplito-Lee, J., Wong, F., Ramsden, C. A., Reiss, J., Cook, I., Fairweather, J., & Schwarz, G. (2010). Successful treatment of molybdenum cofactor deficiency type A with cPMP. Pediatrics, 125(5), e1249–e1254. https://doi.org/10.1542/peds.2009-2192

[4524] Abumrad, N. N., Schneider, A. J., Steel, D., & Rogers, L. S. (1981). Amino acid intolerance during prolonged total parenteral nutrition reversed by molybdate therapy. The American journal of clinical nutrition, 34(11), 2551–2559. https://doi.org/10.1093/ajcn/34.11.2551

[4525] Schwarz, G., & Mendel, R. R. (2006). Molybdenum cofactor biosynthesis and molybdenum enzymes. Annual review of plant biology, 57, 623–647. https://doi.org/10.1146/annurev.arplant.57.032905.105437

[4526] Hover, B. M., Loksztejn, A., Ribeiro, A. A., & Yokoyama, K. (2013). Identification of a cyclic nucleotide as a cryptic intermediate in molybdenum cofactor biosynthesis. Journal of the American Chemical Society, 135(18), 7019–7032. https://doi.org/10.1021/ja401781t

[4527] Hover, B. M., Tonthat, N. K., Schumacher, M. A., & Yokoyama, K. (2015). Mechanism of pyranopterin ring formation in molybdenum cofactor biosynthesis. Proceedings of the National Academy of Sciences of the United States of America, 112(20), 6347–6352. https://doi.org/10.1073/pnas.1500697112

[4528] Broderick, J. B., Duffus, B. R., Duschene, K. S., & Shepard, E. M. (2014). Radical S-adenosylmethionine enzymes. Chemical reviews, 114(8), 4229–4317. https://doi.org/10.1021/cr4004709

[4529] Holliday, G. L., Akiva, E., Meng, E. C., Brown, S. D., Calhoun, S., Pieper, U., Sali, A., Booker, S. J., & Babbitt, P. C. (2018). Atlas of the Radical SAM Superfamily: Divergent Evolution of Function Using a "Plug and Play" Domain. Methods in enzymology, 606, 1–71. https://doi.org/10.1016/bs.mie.2018.06.004

[4530] Stiefel, E. I. (1998). "Transition metal sulfur chemistry and its relevance to molybdenum and tungsten enzymes". Pure Appl. Chem. 70 (4): 889–896.

[4531] Hille, R., Hall, J., & Basu, P. (2014). The mononuclear molybdenum enzymes. Chemical reviews, 114(7), 3963–4038. https://doi.org/10.1021/cr400443z

[4532] Kisker, C., Schindelin, H., Baas, D., Rétey, J., Meckenstock, R. U., & Kroneck, P. M. (1998). A structural comparison of molybdenum cofactor-containing enzymes. FEMS microbiology reviews, 22(5), 503–521. https://doi.org/10.1111/j.1574-6976.1998.tb00384.x

[4533] Cohen, H. J., Betcher-Lange, S., Kessler, D. L., & Rajagopalan, K. V. (1972). Hepatic sulfite oxidase. Congruency in mitochondria of prosthetic groups and activity. The Journal of biological chemistry, 247(23), 7759–7766.

[4534] NIH (2020) 'Manganese: Fact Sheet for Health Professionals', Accessed Online Feb 10 2021: https://ods.od.nih.gov/factsheets/Manganese-HealthProfessional/

[4535] Institute of Medicine (US) Panel on Micronutrients. Dietary Reference Intakes for Vitamin A, Vitamin K, Arsenic, Boron, Chromium, Copper, Iodine, Iron, Manganese, Molybdenum, Nickel, Silicon, Vanadium, and Zinc. Washington (DC): National Academies Press (US); 2001. 11, Molybdenum. Available from: https://www.ncbi.nlm.nih.gov/books/NBK222301/

[4536] Otten JJ, Hellwig JP, Meyers LD, eds. Institute of Medicine. Molybdenum. In: Dietary Reference Intakes: The essential guide to nutrient requirements. Washington DC: National Academies Press; 2006:357-61.

[4537] Anke M, Groppel B, Kronemann H, Grun M. 1985. Molybdenum supply and status in animals and human beings. Nutr Res 1:S180–S186.

[4538] Ngel, R. W., Price, N. O., & Miller, R. F. (1967). Copper, manganese, cobalt, and molybdenum balance in pre-adolescent girls. The Journal of nutrition, 92(2), 197–204. https://doi.org/10.1093/jn/92.2.197

[4539] Bremner I. (1979). The toxicity of cadmium, zinc and molybdenum and their effects on copper metabolism. The Proceedings of the Nutrition Society, 38(2), 235–242. https://doi.org/10.1079/pns19790037

[4540] Valli, V. E., McCarter, A., McSherry, B. J., & Robinson, G. A. (1969). Hematopoiesis and epiphyseal growth zones in rabbits with molybdenosis. American journal of veterinary research, 30(3), 435–445.

[4541] Ostrom CA, Van Reen R, Miller CW. 1961. Changes in the connective tissue of rats fed toxic diets containing molybdenum salts. J Dent Res 40:520–528.

[4542] McCarter A, Riddell PE, Robinson GA. 1962. Molybdenosis induced in laboratory rabbits. Can J Biochem Physiol 40:1415–1425.

[4543] ARRINGTON, L. R., & DAVIS, G. K. (1953). Molybdenum toxicity in the rabbit. The Journal of nutrition, 51(2), 295–304. https://doi.org/10.1093/jn/51.2.295

[4544] Deosthale, Y. G., & Gopalan, C. (1974). The effect of molybdenum levels in sorghum (Sorghum vulgare Pers.) on uric acid and copper excretion in man. The British journal of nutrition, 31(3), 351–355. https://doi.org/10.1079/bjn19740043

[4545] Turnlund JR, Keyes WR. 2000. Dietary molybdenum: Effect on copper absorption, excretion, and status in young men. In: Roussel AM, editor; Anderson RA, editor; , Favier A, editor. , eds. Trace Elements in Man and Animals 10. New York: Kluwer Academic.

[4546] Nouri, M., Chalian, H., Bahman, A., Mollahajian, H., Ahmadi-Faghih, M., Fakheri, H., & Soroush, A. (2008). Nail molybdenum and zinc contents in populations with low and moderate incidence of esophageal cancer. Archives of Iranian medicine, 11(4), 392–396.

[4547] Zheng, Liu; et al. (1982). "Geographical distribution of trace elements-deficient soils in China". Acta Ped. Sin. 19: 209–223.

[4548] Yang C. S. (1980). Research on esophageal cancer in China: a review. Cancer research, 40(8 Pt 1), 2633–2644.

[4549] Vyskocil, A., & Viau, C. (1999). Assessment of molybdenum toxicity in humans. Journal of applied toxicology : JAT, 19(3), 185–192. https://doi.org/10.1002/(sici)1099-1263(199905/06)19:3<185::aid-jat555>3.0.co;2-z

[4550] Wennig, R.; Kirsch, N. 1988. Molybdenum. In: Handbook on Toxicity of Inorganic Compounds. H.G. Seiler and H. Sigel, eds. Marcel Deker, Inc., New York. pp. 437-447.

[4551] KOVAL'SKII, V. V., IAROVAIA, G. A., & SHMAVONIAN, D. M. (1961). Zhurnal obshchei biologii, 22, 179–191.

[4552] Mertz, W. 1976. Defining trace element deficiencies and toxicities in man. In: Molybdenum in the Environment, vol. 1. W. Chappell and K.K. Peterson, eds. Marcel Dekker, Inc, New York. pp. 267-286.

[4553] Chappell WR, Meglen RR, Moure-Eraso R, Solomons CC, Tsongas TA, Walravens PA, Winston PW. 1979. Human Health Effects of Molybdenum in Drinking Water. EPA-600/1-79-006. Cincinnati, OH: U.S. Environmental Protection Agency, Health Effects Research Laboratory.

[4554] Lener J, Bibr B [1984]. Effects of molybdenum on the organism: a review. J Hyg Epidemiol Microbiol Immunol 29:405-419.

[4555] Avakajan, M.A. 1966b. The functional condition of the liver in workers in the copper and molybdenum industry: In: Information on the 2nd Scientific Conference of the Institute of Labor Hygiene and Occupational Pathology. Aiastan: Erevan. (Ref. Zh. Otd. Vyp. Farm. Khim. Sredstva Toksikol. No. 154789).

[4556] CDC (1994) 'Molybdenum (insoluble compounds, as Mo', Immediately Dangerous to Life or Health Concentrations (IDLH), Accessed Online Deb 10 2021: https://www.cdc.gov/niosh/idlh/7439987.html

[4557] Pennington, J. A., & Jones, J. W. (1987). Molybdenum, nickel, cobalt, vanadium, and strontium in total diets. Journal of the American Dietetic Association, 87(12), 1644–1650.

[4558] Hunt, C. D., & Meacham, S. L. (2001). Aluminum, boron, calcium, copper, iron, magnesium, manganese, molybdenum, phosphorus, potassium, sodium, and zinc: concentrations in common western foods and estimated daily intakes by infants; toddlers; and male and female adolescents, adults, and seniors in the United States. Journal of the American Dietetic Association, 101(9), 1058–1060. https://doi.org/10.1016/S0002-8223(01)00260-7

[4559] Novotny, J. A. (2011). Molybdenum Nutriture in Humans. Journal of Evidence-Based Complementary & Alternative Medicine, 16(3), 164–168. doi:10.1177/2156587211406732

[4560] Pennington, J. A., & Jones, J. W. (1987). Molybdenum, nickel, cobalt, vanadium, and strontium in total diets. Journal of the American Dietetic Association, 87(12), 1644–1650.

737

[4561] Tsongas, T. A., Meglen, R. R., Walravens, P. A., & Chappell, W. R. (1980). Molybdenum in the diet: an estimate of average daily intake in the United States. The American journal of clinical nutrition, 33(5), 1103–1107. https://doi.org/10.1093/ajcn/33.5.1103

[4562] Centers for Disease Control and Prevention. National Health and Nutrition Examination Survey (NHANES) III (1988-1994). Bethesda, Md: National Center for Health Statistics; 1996.

[4563] Friel, J. K., MacDonald, A. C., Mercer, C. N., Belkhode, S. L., Downton, G., Kwa, P. G., Aziz, K., & Andrews, W. L. (1999). Molybdenum requirements in low-birth-weight infants receiving parenteral and enteral nutrition. JPEN. Journal of parenteral and enteral nutrition, 23(3), 155–159. https://doi.org/10.1177/0148607199023003155

[4564] Sievers, E., Oldigs, H. D., Dörner, K., Kollmann, M., & Schaub, J. (2001). Molybdenum balance studies in premature male infants. European journal of pediatrics, 160(2), 109–113. https://doi.org/10.1007/s004310000649

[4565] Sievers, E., Dörner, K., Garbe-Schönberg, D., & Schaub, J. (2001). Molybdenum metabolism: stable isotope studies in infancy. Journal of trace elements in medicine and biology : organ of the Society for Minerals and Trace Elements (GMS), 15(2-3), 185–191. https://doi.org/10.1016/S0946-672X(01)80065-1

[4566] Biego, G. H., Joyeux, M., Hartemann, P., & Debry, G. (1998). Determination of mineral contents in different kinds of milk and estimation of dietary intake in infants. Food additives and contaminants, 15(7), 775–781. https://doi.org/10.1080/02652039809374709

[4567] Bougle, D., Bureau, F., Foucault, P., Duhamel, J. F., Muller, G., & Drosdowsky, M. (1988). Molybdenum content of term and preterm human milk during the first 2 months of lactation. The American journal of clinical nutrition, 48(3), 652–654. https://doi.org/10.1093/ajcn/48.3.652

[4568] Rossipal E, Krachler M. 1998. Pattern of trace elements in human milk during the course of lactation. Nutr Res 18:11–24.

[4569] Durfor CN, Becker E. Public water supplies of the 100 largest cities in the United States. U.S. Geological Survey water supply paper 1812. 1964. Washington DC. U.S. Government Printing Office.

[4570] U.S. Food and Drug Administration (2017) 'The Third Unregulated Contaminant Monitoring Rule (UCMR 3): Data Summary, January 2017', Accessed Online Feb 10 2021: https://www.epa.gov/sites/production/files/2017-02/documents/ucmr3-data-summary-january-2017.pdf

[4571] ASMANGULIAN T. A. (1965). PREDEL'NO DOPUSTIMAIA KONTSENTRATSIIA MOLIBDENA V VODE OTKRYTYKH VODOEMOV [MAXIMUM PERMISSIBLE CONCENTRATION OF MOLYBDENUM IN THE WATER OF OPEN RESERVOIRS]. Gigiena i sanitariia, 30, 6–11.

[4572] NIH (2020) 'Molybdenum: Fact Sheet for Health Professionals', Accessed Online Feb 10 2021: https://ods.od.nih.gov/factsheets/Molybdenum-HealthProfessional/

[4573] Novotny, J. A., & Turnlund, J. R. (2007). Molybdenum intake influences molybdenum kinetics in men. The Journal of nutrition, 137(1), 37–42. https://doi.org/10.1093/jn/137.1.37

[4574] Werner, E., Giussani, A., Heinrichs, U., Roth, P., & Greim, H. (1998). Biokinetic studies in humans with stable isotopes as tracers. Part 2: Uptake of molybdenum from aqueous solutions and labelled foodstuffs. Isotopes in environmental and health studies, 34(3), 297–301. https://doi.org/10.1080/10256019808234063

[4575] Turnlund, J. R., Keyes, W. R., & Peiffer, G. L. (1995). Molybdenum absorption, excretion, and retention studied with stable isotopes in young men at five intakes of dietary molybdenum. The American journal of clinical nutrition, 62(4), 790–796. https://doi.org/10.1093/ajcn/62.4.790

[4576] Novotny, J. A., & Turnlund, J. R. (2006). Molybdenum kinetics in men differ during molybdenum depletion and repletion. The Journal of nutrition, 136(4), 953–957. https://doi.org/10.1093/jn/136.4.953

[4577] Turnlund, J. R., Weaver, C. M., Kim, S. K., Keyes, W. R., Gizaw, Y., Thompson, K. H., & Peiffer, G. L. (1999). Molybdenum absorption and utilization in humans from soy and kale intrinsically labeled with stable isotopes of molybdenum. The American journal of clinical nutrition, 69(6), 1217–1223. https://doi.org/10.1093/ajcn/69.6.1217

[4578] Considine, Glenn D., ed. (2005). "Molybdenum". Van Nostrand's Encyclopedia of Chemistry. New York: Wiley-Interscience. pp. 1038–1040.

[4579] ATSDR (2014) 'Public Health Statement for Tungsten', CDC, Accessed Online Feb 10 2021: https://wwwn.cdc.gov/TSP/PHS/PHS.aspx?phsid=804&toxid=157

[4580] Holleman, Arnold F.; Wiberg, Egon (2001). Inorganic chemistry. Academic Press. p. 1384.

[4581] Turnlund, J. R., Keyes, W. R., Peiffer, G. L., & Chiang, G. (1995). Molybdenum absorption, excretion, and retention studied with stable isotopes in young men during depletion and repletion. The American journal of clinical nutrition, 61(5), 1102–1109. https://doi.org/10.1093/ajcn/61.4.1102

[4582] Curzon, M. E. J., Kubota, J., & Bibby, B. G. (1971). Environmental Effects of Molybdenum on Caries. Journal of Dental Research, 50(1), 74–77. doi:10.1177/00220345710500013401

[4583] Johnson, J. L., Waud, W. R., Rajagopalan, K. V., Duran, M., Beemer, F. A., & Wadman, S. K. (1980). Inborn errors of molybdenum metabolism: combined deficiencies of sulfite oxidase and xanthine

738

dehydrogenase in a patient lacking the molybdenum cofactor. Proceedings of the National Academy of Sciences of the United States of America, 77(6), 3715–3719. https://doi.org/10.1073/pnas.77.6.3715

[4584] Verseick, J., Hoste, J., Barbier, F., Vanballenberghe, L., DeRudder, J., & Cornelis, R. (1978). Determination of molybdenum in human serum by neutron activation analysis. Clinica chimica acta; international journal of clinical chemistry, 87(1), 135–140. https://doi.org/10.1016/0009-8981(78)90067-0

[4585] Verseick, J., Hoste, J., Barbier, F., Vanballenberghe, L., DeRudder, J., & Cornelis, R. (1978). Determination of molybdenum in human serum by neutron activation analysis. Clinica chimica acta; international journal of clinical chemistry, 87(1), 135–140. https://doi.org/10.1016/0009-8981(78)90067-0

[4586] Cantone, M. C., de Bartolo, D., Gambarini, G., Giussani, A., Ottolenghi, A., Pirola, L., Hansen, C., Roth, P., & Werner, E. (1995). Proton activation analysis of stable isotopes for a molybdenum biokinetics study in humans. Medical physics, 22(8), 1293–1298. https://doi.org/10.1118/1.597514

[4587] ROSOFF, B., & SPENCER, H. (1964). FATE OF MOLYBDENUM-99 IN MAN. Nature, 202, 410–411. https://doi.org/10.1038/202410a0

[4588] Turnlund, J. R., Keyes, W. R., Peiffer, G. L., & Chiang, G. (1995). Molybdenum absorption, excretion, and retention studied with stable isotopes in young men during depletion and repletion. The American journal of clinical nutrition, 61(5), 1102–1109. https://doi.org/10.1093/ajcn/61.4.1102

[4589] Turnlund, J. R., Keyes, W. R., & Peiffer, G. L. (1995). Molybdenum absorption, excretion, and retention studied with stable isotopes in young men at five intakes of dietary molybdenum. The American journal of clinical nutrition, 62(4), 790–796. https://doi.org/10.1093/ajcn/62.4.790

[4590] Paschal, D. C., Ting, B. G., Morrow, J. C., Pirkle, J. L., Jackson, R. J., Sampson, E. J., Miller, D. T., & Caldwell, K. L. (1998). Trace metals in urine of United States residents: reference range concentrations. Environmental research, 76(1), 53–59. https://doi.org/10.1006/enrs.1997.3793

[4591] Johnson JL, Rajagopalan KV, Wadman SK. 1993. Human molybdenum cofactor deficiency. In: Ayling JE, editor; Nair GM, editor; Baugh CM, editor. , eds. Chemistry and Biology of Pteridines and Folates . New York: Plenum Press. Pp.373–378.

[4592] Harris WS. Omega-3 fatty acids. In: Coates PM, Betz JM, Blackman MR, et al., eds. Encyclopedia of Dietary Supplements. 2nd ed. London and New York: Informa Healthcare; 2010:577-86.

[4593] Swanson, D., Block, R., & Mousa, S. A. (2012). Omega-3 Fatty Acids EPA and DHA: Health Benefits Throughout Life. Advances in Nutrition, 3(1), 1–7. doi:10.3945/an.111.000893

[4594] Ernster, L., & Dallner, G. (1995). Biochemical, physiological and medical aspects of ubiquinone function. Biochimica et biophysica acta, 1271(1), 195–204. https://doi.org/10.1016/0925-4439(95)00028-3

[4595] Lei, L., & Liu, Y. (2017). Efficacy of coenzyme Q10 in patients with cardiac failure: a meta-analysis of clinical trials. BMC cardiovascular disorders, 17(1), 196. https://doi.org/10.1186/s12872-017-0628-9

[4596] Martelli, A., Testai, L., Colletti, A., & Cicero, A. (2020). Coenzyme Q10: Clinical Applications in Cardiovascular Diseases. Antioxidants (Basel, Switzerland), 9(4), 341. https://doi.org/10.3390/antiox9040341

[4597] Ferguson L. R. (2010). Meat and cancer. Meat science, 84(2), 308–313. https://doi.org/10.1016/j.meatsci.2009.06.032

[4598] Zheng, W., & Lee, S. A. (2009). Well-done meat intake, heterocyclic amine exposure, and cancer risk. Nutrition and cancer, 61(4), 437–446. https://doi.org/10.1080/01635580802710741

[4599] Larsson, S. C., & Wolk, A. (2007). Coffee Consumption and Risk of Liver Cancer: A Meta-Analysis. Gastroenterology, 132(5), 1740–1745. doi:10.1053/j.gastro.2007.03.044

[4600] Tagliazucchi, D. (2015). Melanoidins from Coffee and Lipid Peroxidation. Coffee in Health and Disease Prevention, 859–867. doi:10.1016/b978-0-12-409517-5.00095-4

[4601] Devasagayam, T. P., Kamat, J. P., Mohan, H., & Kesavan, P. C. (1996). Caffeine as an antioxidant: inhibition of lipid peroxidation induced by reactive oxygen species. Biochimica et biophysica acta, 1282(1), 63–70. https://doi.org/10.1016/0005-2736(96)00040-5

[4602] Kromhout et al (1985). The inverse relation between fish consumption and 20-year mortality from coronary heart disease. The New England journal of medicine, 312(19), 1205–1209. https://doi.org/10.1056/NEJM198505093121901

[4603] Oomen et al (2000). Fish consumption and coronary heart disease mortality in Finland, Italy, and The Netherlands. American journal of epidemiology, 151(10), 999–1006. https://doi.org/10.1093/oxfordjournals.aje.a010144

[4604] Keli, S. O., Feskens, E. J., & Kromhout, D. (1994). Fish consumption and risk of stroke. The Zutphen Study. Stroke, 25(2), 328–332. https://doi.org/10.1161/01.str.25.2.328

[4605] Li et al (2019) 'Habitual tea drinking modulates brain efficiency: evidence from brain connectivity evaluation', Aging (Albany NY). 2019; 11:3876-3890. https://doi.org/10.18632/aging.102023

[4606] van Dam, R. M., & Hu, F. B. (2005). Coffee consumption and risk of type 2 diabetes: a systematic review. JAMA, 294(1), 97–104. https://doi.org/10.1001/jama.294.1.97

[4607] Maia, L., & de Mendonca, A. (2002). Does caffeine intake protect from Alzheimer's disease? European Journal of Neurology, 9(4), 377–382. doi:10.1046/j.1468-1331.2002.00421.x

[4608] Santos, C., Costa, J., Santos, J., Vaz-Carneiro, A., & Lunet, N. (2010). Caffeine intake and dementia: systematic review and meta-analysis. Journal of Alzheimer's disease : JAD, 20 Suppl 1, S187–S204. https://doi.org/10.3233/JAD-2010-091387

[4609] Larsson, S. C., & Wolk, A. (2007). Coffee Consumption and Risk of Liver Cancer: A Meta-Analysis. Gastroenterology, 132(5), 1740–1745. doi:10.1053/j.gastro.2007.03.044

[4610] Dmitrašinović et al (2016). ACTH, Cortisol and IL-6 Levels in Athletes Following Magnesium Supplementation. Journal of Medical Biochemistry, 35(4), 375–384. doi:10.1515/jomb-2016-0021

[4611] Basciano H et al (2005) 'Fructose, insulin resistance, and metabolic dyslipidemia', Nutrition & Metabolism20052:5.

[4612] Agarwal, S. P., Khanna, R., Karmarkar, R., Anwer, M. K., & Khar, R. K. (2007). Shilajit: a review. Phytotherapy research : PTR, 21(5), 401–405. https://doi.org/10.1002/ptr.2100

[4613] Visser S. A. (1987). Effect of humic substances on mitochondrial respiration and oxidative phosphorylation. The Science of the total environment, 62, 347–354. https://doi.org/10.1016/0048-9697(87)90521-3

[4614] Pandit, S., Biswas, S., Jana, U., De, R. K., Mukhopadhyay, S. C., & Biswas, T. K. (2016). Clinical evaluation of purified Shilajit on testosterone levels in healthy volunteers. Andrologia, 48(5), 570–575. https://doi.org/10.1111/and.12482

[4615] Stohs S. J. (2014). Safety and efficacy of shilajit (mumie, moomiyo). Phytotherapy research : PTR, 28(4), 475–479. https://doi.org/10.1002/ptr.5018

[4616] Carrasco-Gallardo, C., Guzmán, L., & Maccioni, R. B. (2012). Shilajit: a natural phytocomplex with potential procognitive activity. International journal of Alzheimer's disease, 2012, 674142. https://doi.org/10.1155/2012/674142

[4617] Carrasco-Gallardo, C., Farías, G. A., Fuentes, P., Crespo, F., & Maccioni, R. B. (2012). Can nutraceuticals prevent Alzheimer's disease? Potential therapeutic role of a formulation containing shilajit and complex B vitamins. Archives of medical research, 43(8), 699–704. https://doi.org/10.1016/j.arcmed.2012.10.010

[4618] Sharma, P., Jha, J., Shrinivas, V., Dwivedi, L. K., Suresh, P., & Sinha, M. (2003). Shilajit: evalution of its effects on blood chemistry of normal human subjects. Ancient science of life, 23(2), 114–119.

[4619] Goel, R. K., Banerjee, R. S., & Acharya, S. B. (1990). Antiulcerogenic and antiinflammatory studies with shilajit. Journal of ethnopharmacology, 29(1), 95–103. https://doi.org/10.1016/0378-8741(90)90102-y

[4620] Das, A., Datta, S., Rhea, B., Sinha, M., Veeraragavan, M., Gordillo, G., & Roy, S. (2016). The Human Skeletal Muscle Transcriptome in Response to Oral Shilajit Supplementation. Journal of medicinal food, 19(7), 701–709. https://doi.org/10.1089/jmf.2016.0010

[4621] Doosti, F., Dashti, S., Tabatabai, S. M., & Hosseinzadeh, H. (2013). Traditional Chinese and Indian medicine in the treatment of opioid-dependence: a review. Avicenna journal of phytomedicine, 3(3), 205–215.

[4622] Malekzadeh, G., Dashti-Rahmatabadi, M. H., Zanbagh, S., & Akhavi Mirab-bashii, A. (2015). Mumijo attenuates chemically induced inflammatory pain in mice. Alternative therapies in health and medicine, 21(2), 42–47.

[4623] Yin, H., Yang, E. J., Park, S. J., & Han, S. K. (2011). Glycine- and GABA-mimetic Actions of Shilajit on the Substantia Gelatinosa Neurons of the Trigeminal Subnucleus Caudalis in Mice. The Korean journal of physiology & pharmacology : official journal of the Korean Physiological Society and the Korean Society of Pharmacology, 15(5), 285–289. https://doi.org/10.4196/kjpp.2011.15.5.285

[4624] Bansal, P., & Banerjee, S. (2016). Effect of Withinia Somnifera and Shilajit on Alcohol Addiction in Mice. Pharmacognosy magazine, 12(Suppl 2), S121–S128. https://doi.org/10.4103/0973-1296.182170

[4625] Klučáková, M., & Pavlíková, M. (2017). Lignitic Humic Acids as Environmentally-Friendly Adsorbent for Heavy Metals. Journal of Chemistry, 2017, 1–5. doi:10.1155/2017/7169019

[4626] Rungapamestry V et al (2007) 'Effect of meal composition and cooking duration on the fate of sulforaphane following consumption of broccoli by healthy human subjects', Br J Nutr. 2007 Apr;97(4):644-52.

[4627] Yuan, G., Sun, B., Yuan, J., & Wang, Q. (2009). Effects of different cooking methods on health-promoting compounds of broccoli. Journal of Zhejiang University SCIENCE B, 10(8), 580–588. doi:10.1631/jzus.b0920051

[4628] Uribarri J et al (2010) 'Advanced Glycation End Products in Foods and a Practical Guide to Their Reduction in the Diet', Journal of the American Dietetic Association, Volume 110, Issue 6, June 2010, Pages 911-916.e12.

[4629] Nugent, A. P. (2005). Health properties of resistant starch. Nutrition Bulletin, 30(1), 27–54. doi:10.1111/j.1467-3010.2005.00481.x

[4630] Ferguson, L. R., Tasman-Jones, C., Englyst, H., & Harris, P. J. (2000). Comparative Effects of Three Resistant Starch Preparations on Transit Time and Short-Chain Fatty Acid Production in Rats. Nutrition and Cancer, 36(2), 230–237. doi:10.1207/s15327914nc3602_13

[4631] Donohoe, D. R., Garge, N., Zhang, X., Sun, W., O'Connell, T. M., Bunger, M. K., & Bultman, S. J. (2011). The microbiome and butyrate regulate energy metabolism and autophagy in the mammalian colon. Cell metabolism, 13(5), 517–526. https://doi.org/10.1016/j.cmet.2011.02.018

[4632] Maki, K. C., Pelkman, C. L., Finocchiaro, E. T., Kelley, K. M., Lawless, A. L., Schild, A. L., & Rains, T. M. (2012). Resistant Starch from High-Amylose Maize Increases Insulin Sensitivity in Overweight and Obese Men. The Journal of Nutrition, 142(4), 717–723. doi:10.3945/jn.111.152975

[4633] Robertson, M. D., Bickerton, A. S., Dennis, A. L., Vidal, H., & Frayn, K. N. (2005). Insulin-sensitizing effects of dietary resistant starch and effects on skeletal muscle and adipose tissue metabolism. The American Journal of Clinical Nutrition, 82(3), 559–567. doi:10.1093/ajcn/82.3.559

[4634] Murphy, M. M., Douglass, J. S., & Birkett, A. (2008). Resistant Starch Intakes in the United States. Journal of the American Dietetic Association, 108(1), 67–78. doi:10.1016/j.jada.2007.10.012

[4635] Moongngarm. (2013). CHEMICAL COMPOSITIONS AND RESISTANT STARCH CONTENT IN STARCHY FOODS. American Journal of Agricultural and Biological Sciences, 8(2), 107–113. doi:10.3844/ajabssp.2013.107.113

[4636] Wallace, T. C., McBurney, M., & Fulgoni, V. L., 3rd (2014). Multivitamin/mineral supplement contribution to micronutrient intakes in the United States, 2007-2010. Journal of the American College of Nutrition, 33(2), 94–102. https://doi.org/10.1080/07315724.2013.846806

[4637] Berardi (2020) 'How to fix a broken diet: 3 ways to get your eating on track.', Precision Nutrition, Accessed Online Nov 11 2020: https://www.precisionnutrition.com/fix-a-broken-diet

[4638] National Academies of Sciences, Engineering, and Medicine; Health and Medicine Division; Food and Nutrition Board; Committee to Review the Dietary Reference Intakes for Sodium and Potassium; Oria M, Harrison M, Stallings VA, editors. Dietary Reference Intakes for Sodium and Potassium. Washington (DC): National Academies Press (US); 2019 Mar 5. Potassium: Dietary Reference Intakes for Adequacy. Available from: https://www.ncbi.nlm.nih.gov/books/NBK545428/

[4639] DiNicolantonio, J. J., & OKeefe, J. H. (2017). Added sugars drive coronary heart disease via insulin resistance and hyperinsulinaemia: a new paradigm. Open Heart, 4(2), e000729. doi:10.1136/openhrt-2017-000729

[4640] DiNicolantonio, J. J., O'Keefe, J. H., & Lucan, S. C. (2015). Added Fructose. Mayo Clinic Proceedings, 90(3), 372–381. doi:10.1016/j.mayocp.2014.12.019

[4641] Basciano H et al (2005) 'Fructose, insulin resistance, and metabolic dyslipidemia', Nutrition & Metabolism20052:5.

[4642] Reiser, S., Michaelis, O. E., Cataland, S., & O'Dorisio, T. M. (1980). Effect of isocaloric exchange of dietary starch and sucrose in humans on the gastric inhibitory polypeptide response to a sucrose load. The American Journal of Clinical Nutrition, 33(9), 1907–1911. doi:10.1093/ajcn/33.9.1907

[4643] Reiser, S., Handler, H. B., Gardner, L. B., Hallfrisch, J. G., Michaelis, O. E., & Prather, E. S. (1979). Isocaloric exchange of dietary starch and sucrose in humans II. Effect on fasting blood insulin, glucose, and glucagon and on insulin and glucose response to a sucrose load. The American Journal of Clinical Nutrition, 32(11), 2206–2216. doi:10.1093/ajcn/32.11.2206

[4644] Gutman, R. A., Basilico, M. Z., Bernal, C. A., Chicco, A., & Lombardo, Y. B. (1987). Long-term hypertriglyceridemia and glucose intolerance in rats fed chronically an isocaloric sucrose-rich diet. Metabolism, 36(11), 1013–1020. doi:10.1016/0026-0495(87)90019-9

[4645] Beck-Nielsen, H., Pedersen, O., & Lindskov, H. O. (1980). Impaired cellular insulin binding and insulin sensitivity induced by high-fructose feeding in normal subjects. The American Journal of Clinical Nutrition, 33(2), 273–278. doi:10.1093/ajcn/33.2.273

[4646] Dunnigan, M. G., Fyfe, T., McKiddie, M. T., & Crosbie, S. M. (1970). The Effects of Isocaloric Exchange of Dietary Starch and Sucrose on Glucose Tolerance, Plasma Insulin and Serum Lipids in Man. Clinical Science, 38(1), 1–9. doi:10.1042/cs0380001

[4647] Yang, Q., Zhang, Z., Gregg, E. W., Flanders, W. D., Merritt, R., & Hu, F. B. (2014). Added Sugar Intake and Cardiovascular Diseases Mortality Among US Adults. JAMA Internal Medicine, 174(4), 516. doi:10.1001/jamainternmed.2013.13563

[4648] DiNicolantonio, J. J., Mangan, D., & O'Keefe, J. H. (2018). The fructose–copper connection: Added sugars induce fatty liver and insulin resistance via copper deficiency. Journal of Insulin Resistance, 3(1). doi:10.4102/jir.v3i1.43

[4649] Michael H et al (2008) 'Insulin Resistance and Hyperinsulinemia', Diabetes Care Feb 2008, 31 (Supplement 2) S262-S268.

[4650] Bergman et al (2006), Why Visceral Fat is Bad: Mechanisms of the Metabolic Syndrome. Obesity, 14: 16S-19S.

[4651] Balkau et al (2008). Physical activity and insulin sensitivity: the RISC study. Diabetes, 57(10), 2613–2618. https://doi.org/10.2337/db07-1605

[4652] Srikanthan, P. and Karlamangla, AS. (2011) 'Relative Muscle Mass Is Inversely Associated with Insulin Resistance and Prediabetes. Findings from The Third National Health and Nutrition Examination Survey', The Journal of Clinical Endocrinology & Metabolism, Volume 96, Issue 9, 1 September 2011, Pages 2898–2903.

[4653] Donga et al (2010). A Single Night of Partial Sleep Deprivation Induces Insulin Resistance in Multiple Metabolic Pathways in Healthy Subjects. The Journal of Clinical Endocrinology & Metabolism, 95(6), 2963–2968. doi:10.1210/jc.2009-2430

[4654] Clément L et al (2002) 'Dietary trans-10,cis-12 conjugated linoleic acid induces hyperinsulinemia and fatty liver in the mouse', J Lipid Res. 2002 Sep;43(9):1400-9.

[4655] Weintraub, M. S., Zechner, R., Brown, A., Eisenberg, S., & Breslow, J. L. (1988). Dietary polyunsaturated fats of the W-6 and W-3 series reduce postprandial lipoprotein levels. Chronic and acute effects of fat saturation on postprandial lipoprotein metabolism. Journal of Clinical Investigation, 82(6), 1884–1893. doi:10.1172/jci113806

[4656] Simopoulos, A. P., & DiNicolantonio, J. J. (2016). The importance of a balanced ω-6 to ω-3 ratio in the prevention and management of obesity. Open Heart, 3(2), e000385. doi:10.1136/openhrt-2015-000385

[4657] Garaulet, M., Pérez-Llamas, F., Pérez-Ayala, M., Martínez, P., de Medina, F. S., Tebar, F. J., & Zamora, S. (2001). Site-specific differences in the fatty acid composition of abdominal adipose tissue in an obese population from a Mediterranean area: relation with dietary fatty acids, plasma lipid profile, serum insulin, and central obesity. The American Journal of Clinical Nutrition, 74(5), 585–591. doi:10.1093/ajcn/74.5.585

[4658] Shoelson, S. E., Lee, J., & Goldfine, A. B. (2006). Inflammation and insulin resistance. The Journal of clinical investigation, 116(7), 1793-801.

[4659] G C Sturniolo, M C Montino, L Rossetto, A Martin, R D'Inca, A D'Odorico & R Naccarato (1991) Inhibition of gastric acid secretion reduces zinc absorption in man., Journal of the American College of Nutrition, 10:4, 372-375, DOI: 10.1080/07315724.1991.10718165

[4660] Sturniolo, G. C., Di Leo, V., Ferronato, A., D'Odorico, A., & D'Incà, R. (2001). Zinc Supplementation Tightens "Leaky Gut" in Crohn's Disease. Inflammatory Bowel Diseases, 7(2), 94–98. doi:10.1097/00054725-200105000-00003

[4661] Lee, H. S., Cui, L., Li, Y., Choi, J. S., Choi, J.-H., Li, Z., ... Yoon, K. C. (2016). Influence of Light Emitting Diode-Derived Blue Light Overexposure on Mouse Ocular Surface. PLOS ONE, 11(8), e0161041. doi:10.1371/journal.pone.0161041

[4662] Doll, S., & Conrad, M. (2017). Iron and ferroptosis: A still ill-defined liaison. IUBMB Life, 69(6), 423–434. doi:10.1002/iub.1616

[4663] Höhn, A., Jung, T., Grimm, S., & Grune, T. (2010). Lipofuscin-bound iron is a major intracellular source of oxidants: role in senescent cells. Free radical biology & medicine, 48(8), 1100–1108. https://doi.org/10.1016/j.freeradbiomed.2010.01.030

[4664] Corrao, G., Lepore, A. R., Torchio, P., Valenti, M., Galatola, G., D'Amicis, A., Aricó, S., & di Orio, F. (1994). The effect of drinking coffee and smoking cigarettes on the risk of cirrhosis associated with alcohol consumption. A case-control study. Provincial Group for the Study of Chronic Liver Disease. European journal of epidemiology, 10(6), 657–664. https://doi.org/10.1007/BF01719277

[4665] Bravi, F., Tavani, A., Bosetti, C., Boffetta, P., & La Vecchia, C. (2017). Coffee and the risk of hepatocellular carcinoma and chronic liver disease: a systematic review and meta-analysis of prospective studies. European journal of cancer prevention : the official journal of the European Cancer Prevention Organisation (ECP), 26(5), 368–377. https://doi.org/10.1097/CEJ.0000000000000252

[4666] Grant, D. M. (1991). Detoxification pathways in the liver. Journal of Inherited Metabolic Disease, 14(4), 421–430. doi:10.1007/bf01797915

[4667] Goyer R. A. (1997). Toxic and essential metal interactions. Annual review of nutrition, 17, 37–50. https://doi.org/10.1146/annurev.nutr.17.1.37

[4668] Fox, M. R., Tao, S. H., Stone, C. L., & Fry, B. E., Jr (1984). Effects of zinc, iron and copper deficiencies on cadmium in tissues of Japanese quail. Environmental health perspectives, 54, 57–65. https://doi.org/10.1289/ehp.845457

[4669] Sorkun, H. C., Bir, F., Akbulut, M., Divrikli, U., Erken, G., Demirhan, H., Duzcan, E., Elci, L., Celik, I., & Yozgatli, U. (2007). The effects of air pollution and smoking on placental cadmium, zinc concentration and metallothionein expression. Toxicology, 238(1), 15–22. https://doi.org/10.1016/j.tox.2007.05.020

[4670] Chmielnicka, J., Halatek, T., & Jedlińska, U. (1989). Correlation of cadmium-induced nephropathy and the metabolism of endogenous copper and zinc in rats. Ecotoxicology and Environmental Safety, 18(3), 268–276. doi:10.1016/0147-6513(89)90020-1

[4671] Ashby, S. L., King, L. J., & Parke, D. V. W. (1980). Effect of acute administration of cadmium on the disposition of copper, zinc, and iron in the rat. Environmental Research, 21(1), 177–185. doi:10.1016/0013-9351(80)90019-5

[4672] Bremner, I., & Campbell, J. K. (1978). Effect of copper and zinc status on susceptibility to cadmium intoxication. Environmental health perspectives, 25, 125–128. https://doi.org/10.1289/ehp.7825125

[4673] Sears, M. E., Kerr, K. J., & Bray, R. I. (2012). Arsenic, Cadmium, Lead, and Mercury in Sweat: A Systematic Review. Journal of Environmental and Public Health, 2012, 1–10. doi:10.1155/2012/184745

[4674] Genuis SJ, Birkholz D, Rodushkin I, et al. Blood, urine, and sweat (BUS) study: monitoring and elimination of bioaccumulated toxic elements. *Arch Environ Contam Toxicol* 2011;61:344-57.

[4675] Genuis SJ, Lane K, Birkholz D. Human Elimination of Organochlorine Pesticides: Blood, Urine, and Sweat Study. *BioMed research international* 2016;2016:1624643.

[4676] Ye, T., Tu, W., & Xu, G. (2013). Hot bath for the treatment of chronic renal failure. Renal Failure, 36(1), 126–130. doi:10.3109/0886022x.2013.832318

[4677] Turner, M. J., & Avolio, A. P. (2016). Does Replacing Sodium Excreted in Sweat Attenuate the Health Benefits of Physical Activity?. International journal of sport nutrition and exercise metabolism, 26(4), 377–389. https://doi.org/10.1123/ijsnem.2015-0233

[4678] Lara, B., Gallo-Salazar, C., Puente, C., Areces, F., Salinero, J. J., & Del Coso, J. (2016). Interindividual variability in sweat electrolyte concentration in marathoners. Journal of the International Society of Sports Nutrition, 13, 31. https://doi.org/10.1186/s12970-016-0141-z

[4679] Shirreffs, S. M., & Sawka, M. N. (2011). Fluid and electrolyte needs for training, competition, and recovery. Journal of sports sciences, 29 Suppl 1, S39–S46. https://doi.org/10.1080/02640414.2011.614269

[4680] Shirreffs et al (2007) 'Rehydration After Exercise in the Heat: A Comparison of 4 Commonly Used Drinks', International Journal of Sport Nutrition and Exercise Metabolism, 2007, 17, 244-258.

[4681] Kuberski, T., Roberts, A., Linehan, B., Bryden, R. N., & Teburae, M. (1979). Coconut water as a rehydration fluid. The New Zealand medical journal, 90(641), 98–100.

Made in United States
North Haven, CT
22 March 2024

50305414R00404